OCCUPATIONAL THERAPY

Enabling Function and Well-Being

SECOND EDITION

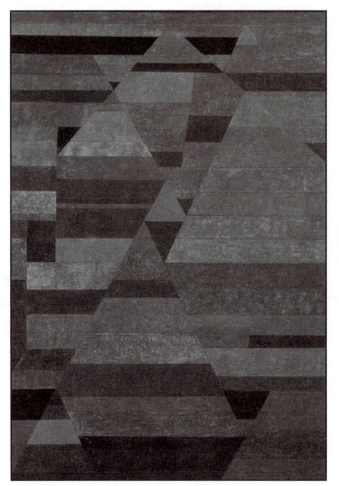

Nekropolis by Paul Klee

A NOTE ABOUT THE COVER ART

Paul Klee (1879-1940) was one of the most original masters of modern art. His well-known images evidence his clever and imaginative nature. Klee studied art in Munich, which in the early 20th century was an important center for abstract art. He later taught at the famous Bauhaus School, which was Germany's most advanced art school. Because his work was declared unsuitable by the Nazis, he moved to Switzerland in 1933, and was soon thereafter diagnosed with the progressive and disabling collagen disease, scleroderma. The effects of his condition, as well as the historical developments in Europe, influenced both the subject matter and the style of his later work. Thus, his work has special significance for occupational therapists because it so readily (and beautifully) illustrates the interconnectedness between daily occupations, health status, and one's environment.

OCCUPATIONAL THERAPY

Enabling Function and Well-Being

SECOND EDITION

Edited by

Charles H. Christiansen, EdD, OTR, OT(C), FAOTA
Dean, School of Allied Health Sciences
The University of Texas Medical Branch
Galveston, Texas

Carolyn M. Baum, PhD, OTR/C, FAOTA
Elias Michael, Director in Occupational Therapy
Washington University School of Medicine
St. Louis, Missouri

Publisher: John H. Bond
Editorial Director: Amy E. Drummond
Managing Editor: Debra Christy
Creative Director: Linda Baker

Cover artwork : Reproduction of *Nekropolis* by Paul Kleé; courtesy Christie's Images/SuperStock.

Disclaimers

"This publication is designed to provide accurate and authoritative information in regard to the subject matter covered. It is sold or distributed with the understanding that the publisher is not engaged in rendering legal, accounting, or other professional service. If legal advice or other expert assistance is required, the services of a competent professional person should be sought."

From the Declaration of Principles jointly adopted by the American Bar Association and a Committee of Publishers and Associations.

The procedures and practices described in this book should be used only by qualified practitioners in accordance with professional standards and in compliance with applicable statutes. Every effort has been made to ensure that the information presented is accurate and consistent with generally accepted practices. However, the editors, authors and publisher cannot accept responsibility for errors or omissions, or for the consequences of incorrect application of information. No warranty, express or implied, is made regarding the contents of this text.

Printed in the United States of America

Occupational therapy: enabling function and well-being/edited by Charles H. Christiansen, Carolyn M. Baum -- 2nd ed.
p. cm.
Includes bibliographical references and index.
ISBN 1-55642-248-2 (alk. paper)
1. Occupational therapy. I. Christiansen, Charles. II. Baum, Carolyn Manville.
[DNLM: 1. Occupational Therapy. WB 555 01427 1997]
RM735.036 1997
615.8'515--dc21
DNLM/DLC for Library of Congress   97-9050
                                                                   CIP

Published by: SLACK Incorporated
                   6900 Grove Road
                   Thorofare, NJ 08086 USA
                   Telephone: 609-848-1000
                   Fax: 609-853-5991

Contact SLACK Incorporated for more information about other books in this field or about the availability of our books from distributors outside the United States.

Authorization to photocopy items for internal or personal use, or the internal or personal use of specific clients, is granted by SLACK Incorporated, provided that the appropriate fee is paid directly to Copyright Clearance Center, 222 Rosewood Drive, Danvers, MA 01923 USA, 508-750-8400. Prior to photocopying items for educational classroom use, please contact the CCC at the address above. Please reference Account Number 9106324 for SLACK Incorporated's Professional Book Division.

For further information on CCC, check CCC Online at the following address: http://www.copyright.com.

Last digit is print number: 10 9 8 7 6 5 4 3 2 1

Dedication

No serious scholar in occupational therapy can deny the influence of three giants in the field, whose work will continue to inspire and challenge us: Adolph Meyer, Mary Reilly, and Wilma West. It is to their vision, energy, commitment and spirit that we dedicate this book.

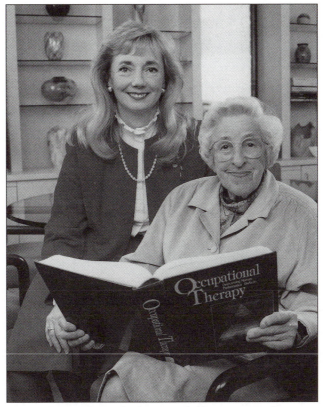

Wilma West with Mary Evert. Photo courtesy of
Gary Iglarsh.

Dedication to the First Edition

This book is dedicated to

Pamela, Erik, Kalle and Carrie Christiansen;

to Kirstin Baum;

and to our friends, colleagues

and students throughout the world.

Contents

SECTION ONE - CONTEXT AND DECISIONS FOR PRACTICE

SECTION FOUR - INTERVENTIONS: ACHIEVING FUNCTION AND WELL-BEING THROUGH OCCUPATION

APPENDICES:

Expanded Contents

SECTION ONE - CONTEXT AND DECISIONS FOR PRACTICE

Section Three - Extrinsic Social and Cultural Factors

First Edition Acknowledgments

We would like to acknowledge the efforts of the following contributing authors to the first edition of *Occupational Therapy*, without whom this book would not be possible.

Karin J. Barnes

James Berger

Barbara Borg

Carolyn Brayley

Mary Ann Bruce

Harriet Davidson

Elizabeth DePoy

Elizabeth Devereaux

Janet Duchek

Winnie Dunn

Shereen D. Farber

Ellen Kolodner

Douglas V. Krefting

Laura H. Krefting

Ruth E. Levine

Lela Llorens

Marion Minor

Karin Opacich

Barbara Boyt Schell

Richard K. Schwartz

Roger O. Smith

Jean Cole Spencer

Mary Sladky Struthers

Mary Warren

Contributing Authors

Beatriz C. Abreu, PhD, is Director of Occupational Therapy at the Transitional Learning Community at Galveston and Clinical Associate Professor at the University of Texas Medical Branch at Galveston. She earned her undergraduate degree in occupational therapy at the University of Puerto Rico and her M.A. in Psychology from The New School for Social Research at New York, and holds a Doctor of Philosophy in Occupational Therapy from New York University. Dr. Abreu has held various positions as a clinician, administrator, and faculty member, including services at State University of New York Downstate, Brooklyn, NY, New York University, and University of Southern California. She has received several honors and awards for her professional services, including one named after her from the New York Metropolitan Chapter. She is a Fellow of the American Occupational Therapy Association. Dr. Abreu has contributed to the occupational therapy literature and has delivered numerous invited presentations in cognitive rehabilitation throughout North America, South America, Japan, and China.

Carolyn Baum, PhD, OTR/C, FAOTA, is the Elias Michael Director and Assistant Professor of Occupational Therapy and Neurology at Washington University School of Medicine, St. Louis, MO. She has served as President of the American Occupational Therapy Association, President of the National Board for Certification of Occupational Therapy (formerly AOTCB), and has held numerous positions in the profession. She has served in a number of policy positions, most recently on the National Center for MEdical Rehabilitation Research at the National Institutes of Health, and a committee to make recommendations to Congress on future needs of rehabilitation and engineering at the Institute of Medicine. She has grants through the National Institute on Aging and the James S. McDonnell Foundation studying the impact of cognitive impairment on daily life.

Paula Bohr, PhD, OTR, is an occupational therapist with a background in industrial engineering. Her practice and research interests focus on evaluation of workers, analysis of work tasks, and assessment of work environments. She is Director of the Occupational Health and Ergonomics Laboratory at Washington University School of Medicine, Program in Occupational Therapy, St. Louis, Missouri, where she serves as a faculty member.

Bette R. Bonder, PhD, OTR/L, FAOTA, is a Professor in the Department of Health Sciences at Cleveland State University. Dr. Bonder received her baccalaureate degree in occupational therapy from Washington University, and her PhD in Counseling from Northwestern University. She is the author of *Psychopathology and Function, Second Edition* and editor of *Functional Performance in Older Adults*, as well as author of a number of papers focusing on mental health and gerontology. She is also the Editor of the *Occupational Therapy Journal of Research*.

Catherine E. Bridge, BA, MS, is a lecturer at the School of Occupational Therapy, Faculty of Health Sciences, University of Sydney. She earned her undergraduate degree in occupational therapy at Cumberland College of Health Sciences and holds a Masters degree in cognitive science from The University of New South Wales. Ms. Bridge is currently completing her PhD at the Faculty of Architecture, the University of Sydney, where she is an acknowledged expert in the area of environmental assessment and redesign. She has been the recipient of several major grants and has co-authored a number of publications including "Hoptions," a program designed to assist elder adults to make healthy choices. Ms. Bridge is a member of the Australian Association of Occupational Therapists (AAOT) and represents the NSW branch of AAOT on the access and mobility subcommittee of ACROD. She is also a referee for a number of professional journals.

Charles Christiansen, EdD, OTR, OT(C), FAOTA, is Dean of the School of Allied Health Sciences and Professor in the Department of Occupational Therapy at the University of Texas Medical Branch in Galveston, Texas. Dr. Christiansen earned his Bachelor's degree in occupational therapy in the School of Medicine at the University of North Dakota. He holds graduate degrees in Counseling Psychology and Education (respectively) from Ball State University and the University of Houston. Dr. Christiansen is a member of several scientific and professional societies, including the American Occupational Therapy Association, the Canadian Association of Occupational Therapists, and Sigma Xi. He is the founding editor of *The Occupational Therapy Journal of Research*, and author of over 70 scholarly papers, chapters, books and monographs, including *Ways of Living: Self Care Strategies for Special Needs*.

Barbara Acheson Cooper is Associate Professor, School of Rehabilitation Science, McMaster University, Hamilton, Canada, where she held the position of Associate Dean (Rehabilitation) from 1990-1996. She is a graduate of the combined program in Occupational Therapy and Physiotherapy from the University of Toronto, holds bachelors degrees in Art History and Fine Arts, a masters of Health Science, and a doctorate in Architecture (Aging and Environment). Dr. Cooper's research interests have focused on the development of non-handicapping environments for elderly people and the application of color in this context.

Mary Corcoran, PhD, OTR/L, FAOTA is an Associate Professor and Acting Chairman in the Department of Occupational Therapy, Thomas Jefferson University, Philadelphia, Pennsylvania. Dr. Corcoran received her bachelors degree in Occupational Therapy from Indiana University and her masters degree in Social Gerontology from the University of Pennsylvania in Philadelphia. She returned to the University of Pennsylvania for a doctorate in health planning, graduating in 1992. Dr. Corcoran has extensive clinical experience in home care of the elderly, particularly in environmental modifications to prevent and reduce functional problems. Dr. Corcoran conducts research, publishes and presents in the areas of Alzheimer's disease, care giving, environmental influences on behavior, and collaboration.

Janet Duchek, PhD, is Assistant Professor in the Program in Occupational Therapy and the Department of Neurology at Washington University School of Medicine in St. Louis. She holds a bachelor of arts in Psychology from the University of Missouri at St. Louis, and both a master of arts and a doctorate in Experimental Psychology from the University of South Carolina. Dr. Duchek's past professional experiences include faculty positions at the University of Kentucky and Iowa State University, and she served as Project Coordinator of the Memory and Aging Project at Washington University. Dr. Duchek has presented papers at professional meetings within and outside the United States and has published numerous book chapters and articles in professional journals on cognition. She has served on the editorial board of the *American Journal of Occupational Therapy* and serves as reviewer for various journals. Her research interests include cognitive mechanisms in healthy aging, Alzheimer's disease, head injury, and the relationships among attention, memory processing and everyday performance.

Winnie Dunn, PhD, OTR, FAOTA, is Professor and Chairperson of the Occupational Therapy Program at Kansas University Medical Center. Dr. Dunn earned a bachelor of science in Occupational Therapy and a master of science in Education/Learning Disabilities from the University of

Missouri, and holds a doctor of Philosophy degree in Neuroscience from the University of Kansas. She has held various positions in community based programs for children and families, such as early intervention and public school programs. She has served in the University Affiliated Programs at the University of Missouri and the University of Kansas, and has consulted in local, state and regional programs across the country. Dr. Dunn has received several honors and awards for her professional service. She is a Fellow of the American Occupational Therapy Association, received the Award of Merit, is a member of the Academy of Research for AOTF, and is faculty emeritus of Sensory Integration International. Dr. Dunn has published widely in professional journals, has served on the editorial boards for various publications, and is the editor of a book on pediatric occupational therapy practice, entitled *Pediatric Occupational Therapy: Facilitating Effective Service Provision.*

Dorothy Edwards, PhD, OTR, is an Assistant Professor in the Program in Occupational Therapy and the Department of Neurology at Washington University School of Medicine in St. Louis, MO. She holds a bachelor of science degree in Psychology from Loyola University of New Orleans and a doctorate in Experimental Psychology from Washington University in St. Louis. Dr. Edwards' previous experience includes many research projects which focused on the impact of services on frail elders in the community. She and Dr. Carolyn Baum were co-investigators in a project entitled "Functional Performance and Caregiver Stress," funded by the National Institute on Aging. She is currently the Principal Investigator of the Memory and Aging Project Satellite, the African American Outreach Program of the Washington University Alzheimer's Disease Research funded by the National Institute on Aging. Dr. Edwards has published widely in professional journals. Her research interests include functional outcomes and quality of life after acute brain injury, development of reliable and sensitive measures of occupational performance, and the impact of Alzheimer's Disease on African American elders and their families.

Patrick Fougeyrollas, PhD, was born in Paris, France in 1951. He is a social anthropologist, specializing in studies related to social integration of people with disabilities. From 1980 to 1986, he directed action research for the development of "On Equal Terms," the Quebec governmental social policy for people with disabilities. He was a founding member of the Quebec Committee and Canadian Society for ICIDH and principal researcher for the Quebec Classification on the Handicap Creation Process. He has been the president of the Canadian Society for ICIDH since 1990. From 1986 to 1996 he was Director of Professional Services in Centre Francois-Charon, a rehabilitation center in Quebec City, Canada. He is now

Scientific Director of the University Institute of Rehabilitation of Quebec City and Associate Professor, Department of Occupational Therapy, Laval University, Quebec City, Canada.

Nancy Gerein, PhD, has a background in nursing, health policy, and epidemiology. She has experience in health programs in Africa, Eastern Europe, and Canada. She spent several years as a health advisor in the Canadian International Development Agency, followed by two years at Queen's University, Kingston, Ontario, Canada, working on disability policy and community-based rehabilitation. Currently she is in Dhaka, Bangladesh working on a population health project funded by the World Bank and nine donor countries.

Laura Gitlin, PhD, is Professor in the Department of Occupational Therapy and Director of Research in the Center for Collaborative Research in the College of Allied Health Sciences at Thomas Jefferson University, Philadelphia, Pennsylvania. As part of her responsibilities, she will also be directing a new division on applied research that will focus on community and home-based interventions involving assistive devices and home modifications to improve the quality of life of older adults. Dr. Gitlin is a funded researcher, having received research and training grants from both federal agencies and private foundations, including the National Institute on Disability and Rehabilitation Research and the National Institute on Aging. She has presented numerous papers at scientific meetings, particularly in areas such as assistive technologies and home modifications for the elderly and their caregivers, clinical and collaborative research, and dementia management. She has published extensively in peer reviewed journals and has co-authored two books; one on research methodology published by Mosby Year Book, and one on grant writing for Health and Human Service professionals published by Springer.

David Gray, PhD is the Associate Director of Research and Professor of Occupational Therapy at the Washington University School of Medicine, St. Louis, MO. He is a member of the North American Collaborating Center (NACC) for the revision of the International Classification of Diseases, Disabilities and Handicaps (ICIDH). Dr. Gray was the Deputy Director of the National Center for Medical Rehabilitation Research (NCMRR) from 1990 through 1995. Dr. Gray was the health science administer at the NIH who developed a national research program in the area of learning disabilities. From 1986 to 1987, he directed the National Institute on Disability and Rehabilitation Research at the U.S. Department of Education in Washington DC.

Harlan Hahn, PhD is Professor of Political Science at the University of Southern California. He holds a doctorate in Political Science from Harvard University and an MS in Rehabilitation from California State University in Los Angeles. He has taught courses for 20 years on disability in society and written extensively on disability issues.

Betty Risteen Hasselkus, PhD, OTR, FAOTA, is Associate Professor in the Occupational Therapy Program, Department of Kinesiology at the University of Wisconsin-Madison; she served as Director of the Occupational Therapy Program from 1990 to 1996. Dr. Hasselkus earned her undergraduate degree in Occupational Therapy, her master of science degree in Physical Education, and her doctorate in Adult Education at the University of Wisconsin-Madison. She was elected to the AOTA Roster of Fellows in 1986 and served as Associate Editor of the *Occupational Therapy Journal of Research* from 1987 to 1991. From 1986 to 1989, she served as Chair, AOTA Gerontology Special Interest Section. Dr. Hasselkus' research focus is care giving for older people as it is provided by both family members and health care professionals. Research populations have included family caregivers in the community, family caregivers in the medical visit with an older patient, occupational therapists in geriatric practice, and care giving for the dying. Most recently, phenomenological interviews were carried out with the Alzheimer day care staff and family caregivers, focusing on satisfying and dissatisfying experiences and the everyday ethical dilemmas of dementia care. Dr. Hasselkus teaches undergraduate and graduate courses on aging and the independent living environment. Dr. Hasselkus is widely published in gerontology and occupational therapy journals; she currently serves on the editorial review boards for the *Journal of Applied Gerontology, The Occupational Therapy Journal of Research*, and *Physical and Occupational Therapy in Geriatrics*.

Douglas Hobson, PhD, is an Associate Professor in the Department of Rehabilitation Science and Technology and is Director of the Rehabilitation Technology Program at the University of Pittsburgh. Dr. Hobson began and directed the Rehabilitation Engineering Program at the University of Tennessee, Memphis, TN from 1974 to 1990. During the years from 1976-1981, the program was awarded a NIHR-REC grant for research and development of seating technology. Many of the seating principles now being taught to clinicians and suppliers were developed and communicated by the UT staff. The UT program co-hosted the International Seating Symposium, which is the single largest annual event in the seating field. Dr. Hobson currently serves as chairman of the SAE, ISO and the ANSI/RESNA-SOWHAT standards committees related to wheelchair securement and transport wheelchairs. Dr. Hobson served as the President of RESNA from

1991 to 1992, and is currently Chairman of the Education Committee.

Margo B. Holm, PhD, OTR/L, FAOTA, is Professor of Occupational Therapy at College Misericordia, Dallas, Pennsylvania; Professor Emeritus of Occupational Therapy, University of Puget Sound, Tacoma, Washington, and Adjunct Assistant Professor of Psychiatry, University of Pittsburgh, Pittsburgh, Pennsylvania. She received her bachelor of science degree in Occupational Therapy from the University of Minnesota, Minneapolis, Minnesota; her master of arts degree in Counseling from Pacific Lutheran University, Tacoma, Washington, and her doctor of Philosophy degree in Higher Education Administration from the University of Nebraska, Lincoln, Nebraska. She completed a post-doctoral fellowship in rehabilitation research in the Department of Psychiatry, School of Medicine, University of Pittsburgh, and was a Woodrow Wilson post-doctoral fellow at Hampton Institute, Hampton, Virginia. She has extensive clinical experience in psychiatry, work programming, geriatric medicine, and geriatric psychiatry. A Fellow of the American Occupational Therapy Association, she has served the profession on the Accreditation Council for Occupational Therapy Education, the Educational Essentials Review Committee, and the editorial boards of the *American Journal of Occupational Therapy* and *The Occupational Therapy Journal of Research*, among other contributions. She has over 50 publications on topics such as clinical reasoning, home health care, assistive technology, and work programming. She has lectured widely nationally and in Sweden, Germany and Taiwan. Her NIH-funded research focuses on functional assessment of older adults, functional outcomes of treatment for depression, and functional intervention for nursing home residents with dementia. While at the University of Puget Sound, she was named a John Lantz Senior Scholar and a Distinguished Professor.

Kathy Kniepmann, EdM, MPH, CHES, OTR/C, is Instructor and Coordinator of Student Activities at Washington University School of Medicine, Program in Occupational Therapy, St. Louis, Missouri. She earned undergraduate degrees in English Literature and Occupational Therapy at Washington University, then EdM and MPH degrees from Harvard University. She is also a certified health education specialist (CHES). Her clinical experience includes rehabilitation, mental health, and home health. She developed the Office of Health Education at Harvard University for students, faculty, staff and retirees in the University community. Ms. Kniepmann also helped students at Harvard to start one of the first college-based peer AIDS education programs in the United States. She is involved in education and program development for health promotion, prevention and multicultural awareness. Ms. Kniepmann was a founder of the Missouri Rural Health Association and is an honorary member of Pi Theta Epsilon.

Mary Law, PhD, OT(C), is Associate Professor, School of Rehabilitation Science, McMaster University, Hamilton, Canada, and Director of the Neurodevelopmental Clinical Research Unit at McMaster University. She holds an undergraduate degree in Occupational Therapy and graduate degrees in Clinical Epidemiology and Biostatistics and Urban and Regional Planning. Dr. Law's research interests center on environmental factors which support daily life participation of children with disabilities, evaluation of occupational therapy interventions with children, and methods to facilitate a client-centred occupational therapy practice.

Lori Letts, MA, OT(C), is Assistant Professor, School of Rehabilitation Science, McMaster University, Hamilton, Canada. She has a bachelors degree in Occupational Therapy, a masters in Urban and Regional Planning, and is currently enrolled in a doctoral program in Environmental Studies. Ms. Letts' research interests focus on the development of supportive environments for seniors and the development and validation of safety and mobility assessments for occupational therapists.

Leonard Matheson, PhD, is a pioneer in the field of Occupational Rehabilitation. He originated Work Hardening and set up the first program at Rancho Los Amigos Hospital in 1977. He is a consultant to employers, hospitals, rehabilitation centers, and governmental agencies throughout the United States and Canada and is the author of numerous peer-reviewed journal articles, professional papers, and textbook chapters. Dr. Matheson is Director of the Work Performance Laboratory and Assistant Professor at the Washington University School of Medicine Occupational Therapy Program in St. Louis.

Mary Ann McColl, PhD, OT(C), is Head of the Occupational Therapy Division, School of Rehabilitation Therapy and Associate Professor of Community Health and Epidemiology at Queen's University in Kingston, Ontario, Canada. Dr. McColl was previously Assistant Professor in the Department of Occupational Therapy at the University of Toronto, and Director of Research at Lyndhurst Spinal Cord Rehabilitation Centre in Toronto, Canada. Her research is on integration and participation of people with disabilities in support systems, communities, and society.

Marian A. Minor, PhD, PT, has an undergraduate degree in Physical Therapy from the University of Kansas, a masters of science in Public Health (MSPH) and a doctorate in Human Performance and Aging from the University of Missouri, Columbia, Missouri. Dr. Minor has been a clinician and community health educator; she is currently a researcher in the area of exercise and rheumatic diseases and an associate professor in the School of Health Related Professions at the University of Missouri.

Kenneth Ottenbacher, PhD, OTR, received baccalaureate degrees from the University of Montana and the University of Central Arkansas, and a masters degree in Special Education and Rehabilitation from the University of Tennessee at Knoxville. After completing his doctorate in Special Education at the University of Missouri-Columbia, Dr. Ottenbacher began his academic career at the University of Wisconsin-Madison, where he was a faculty member from 1982 to 1990. He joined the faculty at the State University of New York in Buffalo in 1990, where he served as Associate Dean for Academic Affairs and Research in the School of Health Related Professions. In 1994, he was appointed Associate Director of the Center for Functional Assessment Research in the Department of Rehabilitation Medicine at the State University of New York at Buffalo. In September 1995, Dr. Ottenbacher assumed the position of Vice Dean in the School of Allied Health Sciences at the University of Texas Medical Branch in Galveston. Dr. Ottenbacher is an occupational therapist with research interests in the development and application of design and measurement strategies appropriate for use in clinical environments. He has published more than 100 scientific/technical articles in refereed journals and is the author, coauthor or editor of four texts. Dr. Ottenbacher is past editor of the Occupational Therapy Journal of Research and a member of several editorial boards. He currently serves as the Statistical Consulting Editor for the *American Journal of Physical Medicine and Rehabilitation.*

Janet L. Poole, PhD, OTR, is Assistant Professor in the Departments of Orthopedics and Family and Community Medicine, School of Medicine, University of New Mexico. She earned her undergraduate degree in Occupational Therapy at Colorado State University, her master of arts degree in Education Psychology at the University of North Carolina, and her doctorate in Motor Learning/Motor Control from the University of Pittsburgh. Her clinical experiences and research interests are in assessment and treatment to improve function in individuals post stroke, and in hand impairments and functional ability in individuals with scleroderma. Dr. Poole has given numerous professional presentations and has several publications that apply theories of motor learning and motor control to occupational therapy and the treatment of individuals with physical disabilities. She is a Fellow of the American Occupational Therapy Association and continues to be an active member of that association as well as the Association of Rheumatology Health Professionals.

Patricia Rigby, MHSc, OT(C), is Assistant Professor, Department of Occupational Therapy, University of Toronto, and Research Occupational Therapist, Bloorview MacMillan Centre, Toronto. She holds an undergraduate degree in Occupational Therapy and a graduate degree in Health Sciences. Ms. Rigby's research focus includes play and playfulness, the written productivity of children, assistive technology in seating for children, and person-environment theory.

Joan C. Rogers, PhD, OTR/L, FAOTA, is Professor of Occupational Therapy, School of Health and Rehabilitation Sciences, and Assistant Professor of Psychiatry, School of Medicine at the University of Pittsburgh. She received her bachelors degree in Biology from Canisius College, Buffalo, New York; her masters degree in Occupational Therapy from the University of Southern California, Los Angeles, California; and her doctoral degree in Educational Psychology/Lifespan Human Development from the University of Illinois, Urbana, Illinois. She has published and lectured widely on topics related to clinical reasoning, gerontic practice, functional assessment, and assistive technology. Her research focuses on the validity of assessment methodologies and the relationship between impairment, disability, and handicap in various populations of older adults. Dr. Rogers has been honored by the American Occupational Therapy Association as a Fellow, an Eleanor Clarke Slagle Lecturer, and an Award of Merit recipient. She is a charter member of the Academy of Research of the American Occupational Therapy Foundation.

Susan Ayres Rosa, MS, OTR, received a bachelor of arts degree in 1967, a bachelor of science in Occupational Therapy in 1978, and a masters of science in Therapeutic Science in 1994 from the University of Wisconsin-Madison, where she is currently a doctoral candidate in the Department of Kinesiology. Ms. Rosa works as a teaching assistant in the Occupational Therapy program at the University of Wisconsin-Madison, assisting with courses in therapeutic use of activities, lifespan occupational performance, and adaptations in independent living. She has also given lectures to both undergraduates and graduate students on qualitative research approaches. Ms. Rosa's clinical experiences have been in the areas of acute care for adults in general medicine and surgery and geriatric rehabilitation. Her research background includes data collection for an epidemiological study of functional losses among the elderly during hospitalization and a qualitative study of work related satisfactions and dissatisfactions of occupational therapists. Her own research focuses on using qualitative approaches to understand the nature and meaning of occupational therapists' experiences of engagement in therapeutic relationships with their clients. Ms. Rosa was the recipient of the Marie L. Carns Fellowship in 1994.

Janette K. Schkade, PhD, OTR, received her AA in Liberal Arts from Lon Morris College and a BS in Business

Administration form Lamar University. She holds an MA and PhD in Psychology from the Univeristy of Texas at Arlington and an MOT from Texas Woman's University. She has served as a psychologist with the Texas Department of Mental Health and Mental Retardation and as an adjunct assistant professor in Psychology at the University of Texas at Arlington. She has been the Assistant Director and Director of Occupational Therapy at Texas Scottish Rite Hospital for Children, Dallas, Texas. Dr. Schkade is currently Professor and Dean, School of Occupational Therapy, Texas Woman's University. She has presented at numerous regional and national conferences and published in occupational therapy journals as well as those in related health care fields.

Sally Schultz, PhD, OTR, is an Associate Professor and Coordinator of Graduate Programs in Occupational Therapy at Texas Woman's University. She teaches in the entry-level, advanced master's, and doctoral programs. Her education includes a bachelor's degree in Business, and a master's degree in Counseling from Texas Tech University. In 1980, she completed a master of Occupational Therapy at Texas Woman's University. At that time, she was appointed Director of Acute Psychiatric Occupational Therapy at Presbyterian Hospital in Dallas, Texas. She began full-time teaching in 1985. Her doctorate in Behavioral Disorders of Children was completed at the University of North Texas in 1991. In addition to teaching, Dr. Schultz provides an ongoing program consultation and staff training to a Texas forensic psychiatric hospital. Her current research focuses on developing and testing a practice model for treating public school students with behavioral disorders.

Debra Stewart, BSc, OT(C), is a lecturer, School of Rehabilitation Science, McMaster University, Hamilton, Canada and a researcher in the Neurodevelopmental Clincial Research Unit at McMaster. She is currently working toward a master's in Clinical Epidemiology, where her research focuses on transition issues for adolescents and young adults with disabilities.

Susan Strong, MSc, OT(C), is an Occupational Therapist Researcher, Rehabilitation Services, Hamilton Psychiatric Hospital, and Clinical Professor, School of Rehabilitation Science, McMaster University, Hamilton, Ontario, Canada. She also holds a part-time research position at the Hamilton Psychiatric Hospital. In addition to person-environment-occupation relations, Ms. Stewart's research interests include the recovery process and meaningful occupations for persons with disabilities, vocational rehabilitation practices and functional capacity evaluations and measurement of effort.

Elaine Trefler, MEd, OTR, FAOTA, was trained as a physical and occupational therapist at the University of Toronto and earned a master's degree in Education with a focus on special education and rehabilitation at Memphis State University. She worked at the University of Tennessee at Memphis from 1974-1990 directing the continuing education program and working in service and applied research. From 1990 until moving to Pittsburgh in 1992, she operated a private practise in Canada with a focus on assistive technology provision. Her area of special interest is seating and wheeled mobility. She has published widely and is the principal author of a new book, *Seating and Wheeled Mobility for Persons with Physical Disabilities.* Ms. Trefler is responsible for many continuing education seminars and symposia in the broad scope of assistive technology. Ms. Trefler was awarded the honor of Fellow in the American Occupational Therapy Association in 1988 and became a Fellow of RESNA in June 1996. Currently, she is Assistant Professor in the Department of Rehabilitation Science and Technology, School of Health and Rehabilitation Science at the University of Pittsburgh.

Robyn L. Twible, Dip OT, MA, is a Lecturer in the School of Occupational Therapy, Faculty of Health Sciences, University of Sydney. Before joining the University in 1987, Ms. Twible gained extensive clinical and management experience in Australia, Britain, Southern Africa and the Middle East. Ms. Twible's professional research interests are in occupational therapy theory, clinical reasoning, health promotion, culture, community development and community based rehabilitation (CBR). Since 1988 she has been involved in a variety of CBR projects in areas including Fiji, Solomon Islands and India. Ms. Twible has numerous publications in the areas of health promotion and CBR. She is a member of the Australian Association of Occupational Therapists and has served on the executive board of the NSW branch. She is referee for the AAOT Journal and was invited to give the keynote address at the AAOT National Conference in 1995. Ms. Twible is also on the editorial board of the newly formed Asia-Pacific disability rehabilitation journal and is a curriculum consultant to the Sri Lanka Occupational Therapy School.

Fraser Valentine, MA, is a doctoral student in the Department of Political Science at the University of Toronto. He completed his masters of art degree in Canadian Studies at Carleton University and has worked as a research/policy analyst for the Canadian Association of Independent Living Centres (CAILC), a pan-Canadian disability organization, since 1993.

Foreword

The title of this volume's second edition signals a notable growth in both knowledge and perspective. From the title of "Overcoming Performance Deficits" to the current "Enabling Function and Well-Being" reflects an orientation that has moved from a principal concern with deficit and dysfunction to an all-inclusive concern for human performance. This development produces a broadened and more abstract interpretation of concepts and principles, client-centered theory constructs and a scholarly and timely exploration of the education and practice implications inherent in conceptualizing occupational therapy as a health science, distinguishable from a medical science.

Webster defines performance as "effectively carrying out"; as "taking action in accordance with requirements." Such a definition implies the existence of some criteria, some established expectations. Judgment then about the effectiveness of "the carrying out," of the "doing" combines the perceptions, the criteria and expectations of the performer as well as those of significant others. Performance from this point of view can thus be understood as a self-other dynamic with its many complex and diverse dimensions. Addressing this theme, and its increasing significance in the health care system of today, represents a marked contribution of this test. The relevance of occupational therapy to ways of living and to achieving a sense of well-being is a concept reflected throughout this volume, offering opportunities to question and explore the potential of occupational therapy.

In the Preface, the editors affirm that "a discipline's body of knowledge should always be evolving and its professionals always learning." The efficacy and stature of a profession defined by society in terms of the relevance and effectiveness of a profession to address what society views as its critical needs and interests. One significant characteristic of a full-fledged profession, therefore, is that its principles, concepts and body of knowledge be discernibly applicable to a broad spectrum of society's needs and interests. If occupational therapy is to continue to develop as a profession, it is essential that the discipline extend its exploration and study of its potential for responding to a wider range of societal needs.

The changing locus of treatment and rehabilitation from the hospital to community-based settings is bringing about alterations in what has traditionally been understood as encompassing treatment and rehabilitation regimens. With a significant portion of health care no longer occurring in the controlled environment of the hospital, the many variables impacting recovery and affecting health become far more evident. Society expects the professional to be able to address these as critical elements in attaining and sustaining health and well-being. These expectations provide occupational therapy with the opportunity, if not a mandate, to articulate and demonstrate the unique contributions that the profession can make to the needs and welfare of society.

The material presented in this volume does indeed add to the profession's knowledge base. It opens a number of doors for broadening that knowledge and for the exploration and study of the unique and differentiating constructs and principles of the discipline and the translation of these into practice. The pursuit of learning, the evolution of knowledge and theoretical constructs evident in this work represent a leap forward in the process of coming to understand and beginning to qualitatively affirm the rich potential inherent in the tenets of occupational therapy.

Gail S. Fidler, OTR, FAOTA
Pompano Beach, Florida

Preface

As we completed the second edition of this book, we were reminded of how important it was to do our work, share our ideas, and let people help us do it. When we wrote the first edition, there was no question with either of us who we wanted to write the foreword. There had been one occupational therapist who not only helped shape both our professional careers, but kept us both focused on our work and the mission of building a science to support occupational therapy practice. That person, Wilma West, passed away December 17, 1996, leaving hundreds of people that she inspired to carry on her vision. We number ourselves among her fortunate associates with pride. She not only gave us ideas, she stood by us and challenged us to keep going. We both feel Willie's presence in our daily lives and take comfort in the words of Brian Andreas (1994) who reminds us "that there are angels whose only job is to make sure you don't get too comfortable and fall asleep and miss your life" (p. 55). Willie will always be that angel for us and for others who insist that people who need occupational therapy services get them from knowledgeable, compassionate occupational therapists who understand that an individual's roles, tasks and occupations have meaning to them and can influence their health.

You don't take on a project like this book without listening to your colleagues and students. Yes, this book is lighter! It's more focused. And we are thrilled with the evolution of the science in our field since the first edition. We hope you are pleased with the book's evolution. The new title, *Occupational Therapy: Enabling Function and Well-Being*, evolved from a title we came to see as a deficit model (Overcoming Human Performance Deficits). Occupational therapists have always placed their emphasis on quality of life and well-being, and we thought it high time to state that more strongly. We have included some new contributors and some new chapters that provide a consumer perspective and address the social and societal issues more directly. We also welcome our colleagues from Canada and Australia who have strengthened our second edition. We hope the future brings much more international communication among occupational therapists.

When we wrote the first edition, we hoped it would be a useful portrait of the profession. We wanted students (whether new or life-long learners) to see an evolving body of knowledge organized with the intent of helping individuals overcome performance deficits. With this edition we have the same goal. A discipline's body of knowledge should always be evolving and its professionals should always be learning. We hope this second edition brings to each of you what it has brought to us. Occupational therapy has an amazing and rich knowledge base from which to draw, and fascinating questions yet to answer.

Editing a textbook offers a special opportunity for two busy people to take time for an important task and their own growth. With such an opportunity comes friendships and introductions to many talented people. We would like to thank all of our contributors. Their focus on occupation and occupational performance makes a very unique contribution to the discipline and to its practitioners. Special thanks also goes to the wonderful, talented people at SLACK Incorporated. Peter Slack has made a very strong commitment to produce quality professional publications for occupational therapists. He has implemented a vision, and we are happy to be a part of it. John Bond, the consummate organizer and a lovely man, has made working on this project a great experience. Everyone should have the opportunity to work with Amy Drummond, our Editorial Director. Her talent, humor, persistence and friendship has made this project fun and purposeful. We also thank all our other friends at SLACK, including Debra Christy, Managing Editor, for making this second edition a reality.

Only because we are loved and given emotional support by family and friends is it possible to commit the time for our own development to a task like this. "Thank you" seems too simple; we are truly grateful for the privilege.

cb and cc
St. Louis, MO.
January 20, 1997

REFERENCE

Andreas, B. (1994). *Still Mostly True.* Decorah, IA: Story People.

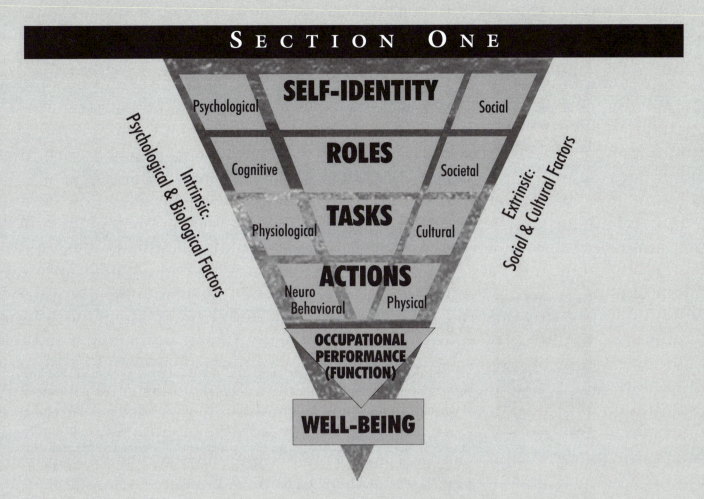

SELF-IDENTITY

Psychological

Social

ROLES

Cognitive

Societal

TASKS

Physiological

Cultural

ACTIONS

Neuro Behavioral

Physical

Intrinsic: Psychological & Biological Factors

Extrinsic: Social & Cultural Factors

OCCUPATIONAL PERFORMANCE (FUNCTION)

WELL-BEING

Context and Decisions for Practice

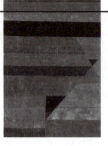

CHAPTER CONTENT OUTLINE

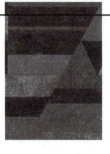

ABSTRACT

An understanding of occupation is essential as a foundation for occupational therapy practice. In this chapter, definitions of occupation are presented, and the many dimensions of occupations are described. It is emphasized that occupations are complex phenomena. Because complex phenomena are best understood through analysis and classification, approaches to classifying occupation are discussed. Definitions of related terms, such as purposeful activity and function, are reviewed and contrasted. Major categories of existing taxonomies are identified, including work, play, leisure and self-maintenance. Since occupation is also understood as a way of explaining how humans use time, typical patterns of occupation are discussed. Habits, routines and lifestyles are identified as types of recurring occupational patterns. The chapter continues with a consideration of the importance of narrative in providing an understanding of lives, and concludes with an overview of current issues in the study of occupation.

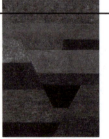

KEY TERMS

Occupation

Function

Purposeful activity

Taxonomy

Work

Play

Leisure

Narrative

Self-maintenance

Instrumental activities of daily living
(IADL)

Reductionism

REM

Lifestyle

Primatology

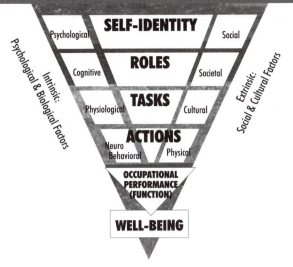

CHAPTER 1

Understanding Occupation

Definitions and Concepts

Charles Christiansen, EdD, OTR, OT(C), FAOTA, Carolyn Baum, PhD, OTR/C, FAOTA

OBJECTIVES

The information in this chapter is intended to help the reader:

1. define occupation and identify its several dimensions

2. appreciate that occupations are complex phenomena

3. distinguish among the terms occupation, function and purposeful activity

4. identify approaches for classifying occupation according to type and levels of complexity

5. compare work, play and leisure according to their defining characteristics

6. describe the allocation of time to various occupational categories in a typical day by able-bodied adults

7. understand social, psychological and physiological influences on time use

8. appreciate important issues in the study of occupation.

> *"The capacity to do something useful for yourself or others is key to personhood, whether it involves the ability to earn a living, cook a meal, put on shoes in the morning, or whatever other skill needs to be mastered at the moment."*
>
> —Mary Catherine Bateson, 1996 (p. 11)

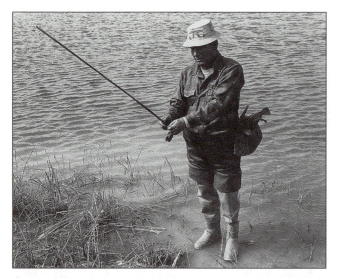

Figure 1-1. *Midstream.* Life-sized bronze sculpture by J. Seward Johnson, Jr. Image used courtesy of Sculpture Placement, Ltd. of Washington, D.C.

INTRODUCTION

As the introductory quotation from anthropologist Mary Catherine Bateson suggests, our daily occupations provide the basis for our feelings about ourselves. They enable us to declare our existence in the world and express our relationships with others. Yet, when illness or disability interfere with our ability to do things that are important to us, our overall health and well-being can be diminished. Clearly, there are important relationships among occupation, health and well-being. Although these relationships are not yet well understood, they inspired the development of innovative practices in medicine and nursing nearly a century ago. Put simply, the idea behind these practices was that occupations influence health. This powerful and important idea led to the development of the worldwide health profession known today as occupational therapy.

A full appreciation for the goals, practices and benefits of occupational therapy must begin with an exploration of occupation. In this chapter, our initial purposes are to define the concept and identify its many dimensions. Because occupation encompasses the many facets of life itself, it is by nature elaborate and difficult to understand. Much like a puzzle, its various pieces must be identified and arranged before a recognizable picture is apparent. But while the many dimensions of occupation contribute to its complexity, they also explain its rich, therapeutic potential.

Bibliographic citation of this chapter: Christiansen, C. & Baum, C. (1997). Understanding occupation: Definitions and concepts. In C. Christiansen & C. Baum (Eds.), *Occupational therapy: Enabling function and well-being* (2nd Ed.). Thorofare, NJ: SLACK Incorporated.

APPRECIATING THE COMPLEXITY OF OCCUPATIONS

We begin with a passage from the popular book and movie, *A River Runs Through It*, which describes the pursuit of fly fishing, one of many passions that can occupy the time and attention of people who enjoy outdoor activities. Fly fishing is one of life's occupations, and as such it serves as a particularly good example for beginning this section.

"..in a typical week of our childhood Paul and I probably received as many hours of instruction in fly fishing as we did in all other spiritual matters.

After my brother and I became good fishermen, we realized that our father was not a great fly caster, but he was accurate and stylish and wore a glove on his casting hand. As he buttoned his glove in preparation to giving us a lesson, he would say "It is an art that is performed on a four-count rhythm between ten and two o'clock." Norman Maclean (1976, p. 2)

To truly understand fly fishing, one must appreciate that it has many dimensions. First, it requires a capacity to plan, to organize, to sequence, and to move according to a particular technique which requires much practice. But it also has subtle creative and expressive qualities, so that casting a rod properly can be viewed as an art form as well as a skill.

The purpose of fly fishing is to provide enjoyment through doing it, and doing it well, rather than simply "catching a fish." In fact, in fly fishing, people "get hooked" in the sense that what they do, how they do it, and where they do it seem to come together to create a special experience, described by Maclean as almost spiritual in nature. Finally, in Maclean's passage, fly fishing is remembered as a boyhood activity that calls forth memories with special meaning. In *A River Runs Through It*, fly fishing symbolized special relationships, growing up, and meeting and mastering challenge.

The many facets of fly fishing illustrate the complexity of occupations. Occupations have dimensions related to performing them, involving abilities, skills and tools. Occupations have dimensions related to where they are done and under what circumstances, and they have dimensions related to their personal importance and meaning. And like fly fishing, occupations have a social dimension in that how we describe them, how we value them, and how they provide us with meaning can often depend on our relationships and experiences with other people (Figure 1-1).

OCCUPATION AND OCCUPATIONAL THERAPY

We have begun this book by describing occupations because an understanding of occupational therapy begins with a basic understanding of human occupation. As the excerpt on fly fishing illustrated, occupations are complex phenomena because they have many dimensions.

In the remaining parts of this chapter, occupation as a concept will be defined and reviewed. We will then describe the many dimensions of occupation. Because classification schemes (known as taxonomies) are vital to understanding any phenomenon, various ways for classifying occupation will be reviewed, including those which address types of occupation and their levels of complexity. Since engagement in occupations constitutes the purposeful use of time, studies of time use will be summarized. Finally, issues relevant to the study of occupation will be discussed.

DEFINING OCCUPATION

Occupation has been defined as the "ordinary and familiar things that people do every day" (Christiansen, Clark, Kielhofner, & Rogers, 1995; p. 1015). This simple definition appears in the first and only consensus paper on occupation published by the American Occupational Therapy Association (AOTA). Other published definitions of occupation from the occupational therapy literature are similar. For example, Clark, Parham, Carlson, Frank, Jackson, Pierce, Wolfe & Zemke (1991) define occupations as "chunks of daily activity that can be named in the lexicon of [the] culture" (p. 301). This definition suggests that occupations are the things people do everyday that can be named and described to others. The Canadian Association of Occupational Therapists (CAOT) defines occupations as "activities or tasks which engage a person's resources of time and energy; specifically self-care, productivity and leisure" (Canadian Association of Occupational Therapists, 1995, p. 140). This definition corresponds to one provided by Reed and Sanderson (1980). Finally, Kielhofner (1995) consolidates these definitions by describing human occupation as "doing culturally meaningful work, play or daily living tasks in the stream of time and in the contexts of one's physical and social world (p. 3)."

OCCUPATION, PURPOSEFUL ACTIVITY AND FUNCTION

Other authors in occupational therapy have described occupation differently, choosing to equate it with "purpose-

ful activity" or "function" (Henderson, Cermak & Coster et al. 1991; Wilcock, 1994). Evans proposed that occupation is the active or doing "process of a person engaged in goal-directed, intrinsically gratifying and culturally appropriate activity" (1987, p. 627). But there is something beyond the active or doing process that defines occupation. For example, meditation is purposeful and appropriate in all cultures, as well as gratifying. But typically it is not active.

The Uniform Terminology for Occupational Therapy (Third Edition), published by the AOTA in 1994, is a document written to "create common terminology for the profession and to capture the essence of occupational therapy succinctly for others" (p. 1047). Although the Uniform Terminology document does not define occupation, it does describe major performance areas of concern to occupational therapy practice. As we will discover later in this chapter, performance areas correspond to categories of occupation (such as self-maintenance, work, and play and rest). The Uniform Terminology document uses the term "purposeful activities" (rather than occupations) to describe these performance areas.

We prefer to make a distinction between occupation and purposeful activity by suggesting that while all occupation is purposeful activity, not all purposeful activity is occupation (Darnell & Heater, 1994). This is because many simple acts may be purposeful, but seem to become identifiable and meaningful to the person doing them only when they are done in combination with other acts. For example, replacing the lid on a trash can is a purposeful act, but would not itself constitute an occupation. In contrast, cleaning the house (of which trash removal is frequently a part) has group as well as individual meaning, and would qualify as an occupation in most definitions accepted by scholars of occupational therapy.

The late Wilma West, a significant figure in U.S. occupational therapy, was a frequent critic of those who used the terms activity and occupation interchangeably. She wrote: "the term occupation is infinitely more expressive and encompassing than purposeful activity" (p. 22). David Nelson (1997) has also emphasized the importance of using the term occupation rather than activity.

FUNCTION AND OCCUPATIONAL PERFORMANCE

The terms function or functional performance are often used in the medical literature to describe the ability of an individual to accomplish tasks of daily living. In an AOTA position paper, Baum & Edwards (1995) have observed that when occupational therapists in the United States use the term function, they refer to an individual's performance of activities, tasks and roles during daily occupations (occupational performance).

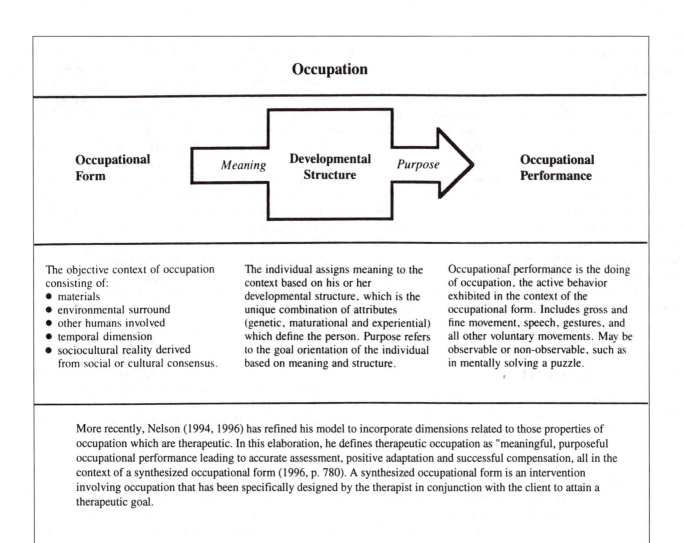

Occupation

Occupational Form	Meaning → Developmental Structure → Purpose	Occupational Performance
The objective context of occupation consisting of: • materials • environmental surround • other humans involved • temporal dimension • sociocultural reality derived from social or cultural consensus.	The individual assigns meaning to the context based on his or her developmental structure, which is the unique combination of attributes (genetic, maturational and experiential) which define the person. Purpose refers to the goal orientation of the individual based on meaning and structure.	Occupational performance is the doing of occupation, the active behavior exhibited in the context of the occupational form. Includes gross and fine movement, speech, gestures, and all other voluntary movements. May be observable or non-observable, such as in mentally solving a puzzle.

More recently, Nelson (1994, 1996) has refined his model to incorporate dimensions related to those properties of occupation which are therapeutic. In this elaboration, he defines therapeutic occupation as "meaningful, purposeful occupational performance leading to accurate assessment, positive adaptation and successful compensation, all in the context of a synthesized occupational form (1996, p. 780). A synthesized occupational form is an intervention involving occupation that has been specifically designed by the therapist in conjunction with the client to attain a therapeutic goal.

Figure 1-2. Occupation as the relationship between form and performance. Adapted from Nelson, D. L. (1988). Occupation: Form and performance. *American Journal of Occupational Therapy, 42*(10), 633-641. Reprinted with permission.

U.S. occupational therapist David Nelson (1988, 1996) has made important contributions to our thinking about occupation. Recognizing that people use the term *occupation* to mean active doing as well as that which is done, Nelson proposed a means of viewing occupation which reduces ambiguity by including both interpretations. In his schema, occupation is defined as the relationship between an occupational form and occupational performance. Occupational performance consists of the "doing" of occupation; whereas occupational form concerns the context of the doing, or the other elements of a "doing situation" which provide it with purpose and meaning. Consider, for example, the occupation of baking a cake for a special occasion using your grandmother's recipe. Using Nelson's concept, occupational performance would consist of the steps and actions involved in following the recipe as the cake is prepared. The "occupational form" in this instance imbues the act with meaning. It brings forth the

special memories of previous occasions, recollections of family traditions and relationships, and anticipation of good experiences to come.

For nearly a decade, Nelson and others have pursued studies designed to assess the impact of various aspects of occupational form on performance. These studies have shown generally that when the occupational form is enriched with characteristics that add dimension, such as meaning, materials or added purpose, performance or movement is enhanced.

In the illustration used above, it is easy to imagine that baking a cake for a festive occasion using a traditional family recipe would bring about considerably different performance than simply baking a cake to contribute to a bake sale. This is because there is different meaning associated with the two situations, even though the recipes and acts required to complete the task are exactly the same. A graphic depiction of Nelson's schema is presented in Figure 1-2.

As suggested earlier, we maintain that the component that distinguishes occupation from other "doing-related" terms is meaning. Occupations have purposes, they have process or doing components, and they have situations in which they are done. But most importantly, they have meaning for the person engaged in them. However, there is not yet agreement on the distinction between occupation and other terms related to doing among scholars in the field. With the profound growth of electronic communication and the development of professional journals having an international readership, agreement on a common definition of occupation for the field of occupational therapy will probably occur during the years ahead.

Achieving this agreement is important because definitions guide the research and scholarly work necessary for advancing theory and practice. For now, we must be content with accepting that occupations are human pursuits that: 1) are goal-directed or purposeful, 2) are performed in situations or contexts that influence them, 3) can be identified (named) by the doer and others, and 4) are meaningful. Chapters in this book are based on a particular point of view about occupations and their dimensions or structure.

TAXONOMIES

A taxonomy is a method for organizing phenomena, or objects or events in nature. In their everyday use of language, people describe and classify objects and events based on the differences they observe in them. These primitive classification systems have been called "folk taxonomies" (Cormack, 1971) and their purpose is to facilitate communication.

One example of a folk taxonomy is the common classification for produce, the edible products of plants. People classify produce as either fruits or vegetables, mostly unaware of the logic that creates this classification. But scientists recognize a much broader array of edible plants, with various important distinctions less important to the market shopper, but very important to science. Folk classifications used in everyday language are often not useful for science because they lack the precision and logic necessary in scientific classification. This will become evident later as we consider how everyday occupations are classified.

Just as folk taxonomies facilitate communication in everyday language, scientific taxonomies assist scientists and scholars in their communication by providing a means for identifying, labeling, grouping and comparing the characteristics of phenomena under study. Science is often concerned with understanding and explaining differences, and taxonomies permit such differences to be categorized according to rules.

The 18th century Swedish biologist Linneaus created one of the best known taxonomies for classifying plants and ani-

Why Classify? An Example

As a student entering a field where the ultimate goal of intervention is prevention, recovery or adaptation, it might not be obvious why it is important to classify the occupations of people. Unless they carefully understand what people do and why they do it, it will not be possible for occupational therapists to use occupations effectively in their everyday practice. Just as pharmacists know about the properties of drugs and how they can be used effectively in different situations, so too must occupational therapists become experts in understanding occupations if they are to effectively deal with the challenges of everyday living.

Consider this example: If a man has a stroke and through rehabilitation he is able to dress, bathe, feed and wash himself, it is natural to consider the challenges he faces in other aspects of his life. How should the occupational therapist approach these issues if the person is 35 years old, a father, a husband, a soccer coach and holds a position of instructor in computer science at the university? How will the therapist identify the relationships between his capacities and his occupations in order to affect the outcome of his care? What role will intrinsic factors (such as his personality, motivation, sensory abilities, and intellect) play? How will extrinsic factors (his background, family, culture, home situation, neighborhood, and community) influence his ability to live a satisfying lifestyle?

These are questions occupational therapists must address in order to gain the comprehensive understanding necessary to enable function and well-being. Each person needing services is unique. Occupations differ in the ability and skill necessary to perform them, in their capacity to meet psychological needs, and in their meaning to patients. The challenge to the occupational therapist is how to match an understanding of the patient with an understanding of daily occupations and environments in order to enable satisfactory daily living. Classification is a basic step toward understanding occupations.

mals (Figure 1-3). In this hierarchical system, each descending level becomes more precise as the plants or animals grouped and named share more characteristics in common.

In a similar way, the classification of everyday occupations requires that they be identified and grouped according to their properties or characteristics. If researchers hope to study, compare and understand daily occupations in a logical manner, methods for classifying them will need to be developed. This will lead to an improved understanding of those

Kingdom	Animal
Phylum	Chordate
Subphylum	Vertebrate
Class	Mammals
Order	Primates
Family	Hominids
Genus	Homo
Species	Sapiens

Figure 1-3. Example of classification developed by Swedish biologist Carl Linneaus.

aspects of occupations that are therapeutic in different situations (Nelson, 1994, 1996).

In the next section, we review some of the characteristics or dimensions used to classify occupations in current taxonomies. We also learn that classifying living things may be easier than classifying occupations.

CLASSIFYING OCCUPATION: LEVELS OF COMPLEXITY AND TYPES

Two major approaches toward classification are of particular interest to those studying occupation. The first type can be viewed as vertical or hierarchical in nature, where levels of complexity are distinguished, ranging from simple acts, such as turning the pages of a book, to more complex groups of goal-oriented tasks, such as completing a term paper or finishing a university degree.

In the second approach, types of occupation are grouped according to their similar properties. For example, hopscotch and kickball are types of play. Washing windows, sweeping floors and doing the laundry are typical household maintenance chores, while toileting, showering, and getting dressed each pertain to everyday self-care. Historically, occupational therapists have classified these occupations into the categories of play, work and self-care.

Despite the manner in which occupational therapists have classified occupations traditionally, studies have shown that people don't always agree on how to classify the same activ-

ity (Marino-Shorn, 1986; Yerxa and Locker, 1990). The classification of occupations is influenced by the situations in which they are performed (Bateson, 1979). Moreover, it is likely that the meaning of an occupation to the doer is ultimately a much more important factor than its classification.

Levels of Complexity

The concept of human occupation as a hierarchy of nested behaviors has been described by many writers, and has roots in occupational therapy and psychology (AOTA, 1995; Christiansen, 1991; Harré, Clarke & DeCarlo, 1985; Little, 1989; Nelson, 1988; Trombly, 1995). The term "nested" means that behavior can be viewed in recognizable segments which form a part of larger segments. A fishing outing can be viewed as a whole event, but this event can be explained or identified by the many tasks comprising the excursion. These range from packing the gear, to driving to the location, to actually doing the fishing, and so on. In turn, each of these tasks can be further subdivided into necessary actions, such as collecting the items in preparation for packing. Each act may have several steps that can be further analyzed and described. Here we use the term "nested"; other writers have described this phenomenon as enfolded or embedded occupations (Bateson, 1996).

A fishing outing can be viewed as part of a summer vacation, part of an eventful year with a loved one, or part of a lifetime of such outings. As we move up the hierarchy, the behavior described is more complex, accounts for greater periods of time, and it can be argued, is potentially more meaningful to the individual. Unfortunately, in occupational science, there are as yet no conventions for precisely naming or defining the levels of this hierarchy.

Harré, Clarke and DeCarlo (1985) have described this phenomenon in a slightly different way. In their view, this hierarchy has three levels: Behaviors, actions and acts. behaviors are movements, actions are intentional movements, and acts are movements with meaning in the culture. They note that the same movement can be used for different actions and acts, and that acts with the same meaning can be done with different actions and behaviors. For example, raising one finger in primary school can signal the need to go to the rest room; the same action by a football player at the end of the game can signal victory (and a lack of humility). Conversely, an act of affection can be exhibited through various actions, including a simple touch, a kiss, or through a thoughtful word. Actions become acts of meaning by noting their context, (i.e., where, when and by whom they are performed). Harré and colleagues (1985) argue that there is no simple one-to-one relationship between action and meaning.

It is clear that there are terms in the English language that suggest behaviors of various complexity. In the first edition of this book, we attempted to provide an hierarchical taxonomy of occupation, suggesting that activities were a part of tasks which, in turn, were parts of roles. In this edition, we have modified this hierarchy to promote consistency with other disciplines and to reflect current thinking. The reader should note that currently, no conventions exist for describing and measuring human occupation in a manner that proves useful for consistently and accurately capturing the differences between these levels of complexity.

Types of Occupation

While scholars in occupational therapy are just now beginning to agree on some of the categories that can be used to group occupations in a useful manner, some labels have already been widely used in everyday language. A popular folk taxonomy divides occupations into work and play (often viewed as work and non-work). Other approaches have classified occupations according to the extent to which they are chosen (obligatory versus voluntary), the degree of skill or practice required to engage in them (amateur versus professional), and whether they are typically done alone or with others (individual versus group).

Historically, most scholarly work on the classification of occupations has not been done by occupational therapists, but rather by sociologists, psychologists, economists, and experts in human factors. One important exception is the work of occupational therapist Kathlyn Reed (1984), who carefully reviewed models of practice and proposed a comprehensive "description of occupations" taxonomy. Although Reed identified major areas of occupation, she did not attempt to categorize these domains according to specific subtypes of activity or daily pursuit. Instead, she classified each subtype according to controlling elements, performance areas and roles (Table 1-1).

By including her list of performance areas under each occupational domain, Reed reflected the prevalent interest of occupational therapists in the performance analysis of specific occupations. Performance analysis focuses on questions such as: How is a specific occupation typically done?" and "What types of movement, thinking, sensing, feeling and interacting are necessary to engage successfully in that occupation?"

Despite the historical interest of occupational therapists in the "doing" of occupations and the underlying abilities and skills that enable their performance, it is necessary to look outside the field to find extensive research in this area. One notable research program was undertaken by Fleishman, a human factors engineer (Fleishman & Quaintance, 1984), who identified fifty-two abilities which can be used to classify the requirements of thousands of tasks. In theory, every purposeful act can be classified according to the extent to which abilities in these areas are necessary for its satisfacto-

---

TABLE 1-1

Occupational Therapy Taxonomy Developed by Reed

1.00 Philosophy and Assumptions
   1.10 Of humans
   1.20 Of health and adaptation
   1.30 Of occupations
   1.40 Of occupational therapy

2.00 Process
   2.10 Results or outcomes
     2.11 Objectives
     2.12 Goals
   2.20 Assessment
     2.21 Observation
     2.22 Interview
     2.23 Testing
   2.30 Planning
     2.31 Therapist control
     2.32 Testing
   2.40 Intervention
     2.41 Media and modalities
       2.411
       2.412
     2.42 Methods, techniques, approaches
       2.421
       2.422
     2.43 Equipment
       2.431
       2.432
     2.44 Prerequisite skills
       2.441
       2.442

3.00 Types of programs
   3.10 Prevent
   3.20 Develop
   3.30 Remediate
   3.40 Adjust
   3.50 Maintenance

From Reed, K. L. (1984). *Models of practice in occupational therapy* (pp. 96). Baltimore, MD: Williams and Wilkins. Reprinted with permission.

---

ry performance (Figure 1-4). Additional detail on the abilities identified by Fleishman is found in Chapter 3.

Occupations can also be classified according to the nature of the task. An early approach was developed by Fine (1974), who established that jobs can be classified according to what workers do in relation to data, people and things. His

Examples of Abilities Necessary to Perform Selected Tasks

ability: oral comprehension

<u>task</u>: Understand a lecture on occupational therapy.

<u>task</u>: Understand a commercial selling athletic footwear.

ability: inductive reasoning

<u>task</u>: Determine occupational performance dysfunction using observations and assessments.

<u>task</u>: Order a new menu item to determine if you like it.

ability: depth perception

<u>task</u>: Thread a needle.

<u>task</u>: Determine which of two warning signs is closest.

Figure 1-4. Examples of abilities necessary to perform selected tasks. Adapted with permission from Fleishman, E. A. (1975). *Development of ability requirements scales for analysis of Bell system jobs*. Bethesda, MD: Management Research Institute.

taxonomy led to the development of the job analysis system used by the United States Employment Service. The relation of specific jobs to data/persons/things has been a basis for rating occupations in the *Dictionary of Occupational Titles* and will be continued as part of the development of new job analysis systems for the United States Department of Labor.

In distinguishing among general categories of occupation, the most common classification used by occupational therapists uses the domains of work, play or leisure, self-maintenance (also referred to as self-care), and sleep. These categories have been convenient as general labels for communicating about and studying human occupation, largely because they account for the cycle of activities that constitutes the typical day, regardless of the culture being studied (Moore, 1995). Each of these general classifications will be discussed in the following sections.

Work

Work is defined traditionally as activity required for subsistence. Primeau (1995) has provided a useful review of the domain of work, noting that definitions of this category of occupation vary from that of paid employment to that which is the opposite of rest (or non-work). She illustrates one of

the difficulties in classifying occupation by noting that household work that is unpaid has discretionary characteristics (i.e., the worker typically has great choice in determining what is done), and such discretionary choice is usually typical of play, rest or leisure activities. Moreover, she points out that some people may derive relaxation and enjoyment out of performing household chores, thus exhibiting another characteristic typical of non-work activities. Another example is the sports "played" by professional athletes. These individuals often are paid generous salaries to perform their skills in tennis, baseball, soccer, hockey and other sports for admiring audiences. These same occupations are pursued by amateurs as freely chosen recreational and leisure pastimes.

The CAOT has used the term "productivity" as a more useful alternative to "work" (CAOT, 1991). Productivity is defined as: "Those activities and tasks which are done to enable the person to provide support to the self, family and society through the production of goods and services" (p. 141). Under the category of productivity, the Canadian taxonomy includes children's play. While it is widely accepted that much play in middle and later childhood involves imitation and rehearsal of adult work roles, it is also freely chosen, and therefore may not be appropriately classified as a productive occupation.

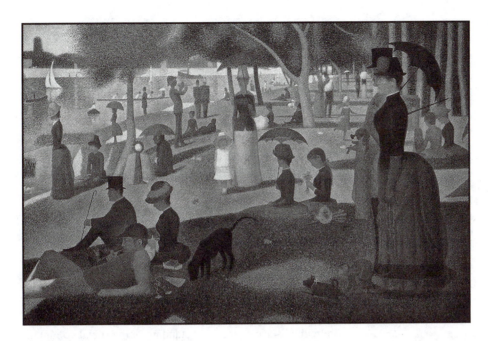

Figure 1-5. This work, painted by French artist Georges Pierre Seurat (1859-1891), now hangs in the Art Institute of Chicago. The subject in this large painting, done in the pointillist style Seurat introduced, is an island (La Grande Jatte) adopted by the Parisian middle class as a place of collective recreation. *A Sunday on La Grande Jatte - 1884,* oil on canvas, 1884-86, 207.5 x 308 cm, Helen Birch Bartlett Memorial Collection, 1926.224. Photograph © 1997, The Art Institute of Chicago. All rights reserved.

Play

The characteristics of choice, expression and development are also attributed to activities described as play, which constitutes the primary occupation of childhood. Play is also a term often used interchangeably with leisure to describe the non-work activities of adults.

In the recent history of the field, occupational therapists have adopted a functional view of childhood play. In this view, play is considered an important means for developing the motor and cognitive skills necessary for the competent performance of adult roles (Reilly, 1974; Robinson, 1977). Reilly suggested a progression from play in childhood to recreation in adulthood and leisure in retirement (1974, p. 60).

There is, however, another dimension of play described by Parham (1996). While recognizing that play is not easy to define as a category of occupation, Parham notes that play is motivated from within (intrinsic motivation) and that it is pleasurable. She agrees with an observation made by Takata (1974) that play is not defined by specific behaviors or activities but rather by attitudes and behavioral styles. Because of these characteristics, playfulness (or moments of play) can be experienced during (or enfolded within) work.

Whether or not play constitutes a classification similar to or different from leisure during adulthood has not been determined. We observe that some activities pursued as leisure activities, such as reading or gardening, are not considered play or playful in nature. Given these and other similar examples, it may be appropriate to classify play as a special type of leisure activity pursued as part of discretionary time.

Leisure

Leisure has been defined as a particular class of activity, as discretionary time, and as a state of mind (Gunter & Stanley, 1985). Freedom of choice in participation without a particular goal other than enjoyment seem to be the defining characteristics of leisure activity (Iso-Ahola, 1979). This "state of mind" philosophy dates back to the Greek philosophers Aristotle and Plato, who viewed leisure in terms of its opportunity for expression and self-development (Rybczynski, 1991) (Figure 1-5).

According to theories, leisure participation fulfills important psychological needs. Attempts to classify specific leisure occupations have been reported (Overs & Taylor, 1977; Holmberg, Rosen & Holland, 1990), but the validity of these classification systems has not been studied. More recently, Tinsley and Eldredge (1995) have proposed a taxonomy of leisure based on need gratification. Their classification identifies eleven clusters of leisure pursuits which fulfill identified needs, and was based on analysis of 82 leisure occupations.

Self-Care: Maintaining Oneself in a Social World

Those activities that are necessary for maintenance of the self within the environment constitute another major classification. Often included in this category are activities related to personal care (eating, grooming and hygiene), getting around (mobility), communicating, and performing basic tasks seen as fundamental to living in society. These include activities such as housecleaning, child care, banking, and shopping. Other terms used for this broad category include self-maintenance (Reed, 1984), activities of daily living (ADL) (AOTA, 1994) and instrumental activities of daily living (IADL)

Why Do People Participate in Leisure Pursuits?

Leisure pursuits meet different needs. Sometimes people want to do something different, or exciting, or creative, or competitive. Other times, they just want to relax. A study of 3771 subjects was done to determine the needs met by participation in various leisure activities. Subjects were presented a list of 82 common leisure activities and asked to select one with which they had the most experience. They then provided information on the extent to which that leisure activity met various psychological needs. The same leisure pursuit often met different needs for different participants. Analysis of the subjects' responses indicated psychological needs met by leisure participation fell into 11 major categories, as follows:

Agency	meeting a need for being active
Novelty	meeting a need for doing something different or unusual
Belongingness	meeting a need to be part of a group
Service	meeting a need to do something for others
Sensual Enjoyment	meeting a need to stimulate the senses
Cognitive Stimulation	meeting a need to exercise mental skill
Self-Expression	meeting a need to express individuality and identity
Creativity	meeting a need to be creative
Competition	meeting a need to compete directly with self or others
Vicarious Competition	meeting a need to compete indirectly with others
Relaxation	meeting a need to relax

From Tinsley, H. E. & Eldredge, B. D. (1995). Psychological benefits of leisure participation. A taxonomy of leisure activities based on their need gratifying properties. *Journal of Counseling Psychology, 42*(2) 123-132.

maintenance is *self-care,* the activities basic to caring for self (Christiansen, 1994; Christiansen & Ottenbacher, 1997).

M. Powell Lawton, a U.S. gerontologist, recognized that in order for a person to be self-reliant in any community, a level of competence is required that enables the accomplishment of tasks beyond those of basic self-care (which he referred to as physical self-maintenance). For this reason, Lawton identified use of the telephone, food preparation, housekeeping, laundry, shopping, money management, use of transportation, and medication management as important basic daily activities and proposed the term *instrumental activities of daily living* to describe them (Lawton, 1971).

Self-care tasks are viewed as necessary from a societal point of view (Christiansen, 1994). While eating and hygiene tasks are essential for survival and health, dressing and grooming are important to social interaction. This is because societies and cultures have many expectations for how people will behave in interacting with other members of their social group. These cultural role expectations influence an individual's acceptance and standing in the social community. If expectations are not met, people are at risk of losing their social standing, which in turn influences the degree of support and cooperation they receive from others.

Maintaining the support and cooperation of others in one's social sphere is important, because all group living animals (humans included) depend on others in their communities for meeting many of their needs. Social acceptance has much to do with involvement in organizations, success in employment, and self-identity. Not feeling part of the group (social isolation) can lead to alienation, problems with identity, and depression (Hogan, 1983).

The term *stigma* has been used to refer to the social devaluing that often accompanies differences in belief, behavior or appearance (Goffman, 1963). People whose abilities to perform self-care tasks are diminished or affected by physical or mental disability (or even economic circumstances) are at risk for stigma. Although social acceptance is influenced by both appearance and behavior, first impressions are typically dependent on appearance alone (Goffman, 1959). Disability can present special challenges for meeting the standards of dress and grooming considered acceptable by contemporary society. Limited access of homeless persons to everyday amenities such as toilets, showers, and clean clothes can produce the same stigma. A study of homeless men by Steiner, Looney, Hall & Wright (1995) found that poor social role functioning, rather than physical and cognitive abilities, was a major contributor to their poor quality of life.

While self-care tasks comprise a necessary, perhaps even obligatory category of occupations from the standpoint of survival, they also serve as foundations for existing in a social world. Social acceptance is essential to a healthy self-concept and to success in many facets of daily life, ranging

(Lawton, 1971). A review of how these terms have been used seems appropriate here.

When occupational therapists and others in rehabilitation use the term *activities of daily living,* they traditionally refer to personal care tasks including toileting, bathing, dressing, eating, and grooming (including oral hygiene). Another term which includes these tasks and those listed above as self-

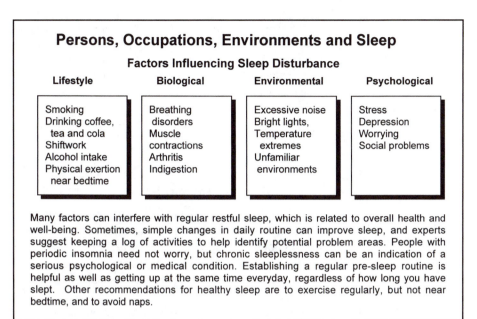

Figure 1-6. Persons, occupations, environments, and sleep.

from mate selection to career advancement (Hogan, 1983; Hogan & Sloan, 1991).

Sleep

Although it is seldom classified as a self-care occupation, sleep is clearly obligatory and necessary for self-maintenance. Humans spend approximately one-third of their lives in sleep. Because it occupies so much time, sleep has been studied extensively by psychologists, but very little by occupational therapists. Despite decades of study, however, little is known with certainty about the function of sleep.

Sleep is defined by behavioral and electrophysiological conditions. While they are asleep, organisms are quiet and devoid of movement. Brain waves indicate five distinct stages as evidenced by electroencephalographic (EEG) monitoring. In the final stage, characterized by the presence of rapid eye movement (REM), the EEG pattern is similar to wakefulness, yet the body has low muscle tone and is unresponsive to stimuli.

From an evolutionary perspective, scientists are puzzled at how sleep has survived as a behavior. During sleep, animals cannot do any of the adaptive behaviors necessary for survival of the species, such as procreation, self-protection, or getting nourishment. Current theories suggest that sleep provides important restorative functions by repairing tissue, allowing for the consolidation of memory traces and information, and conserving energy (Horne, 1983; Meddis, 1983; Webb, 1983).

Sleep needs in humans diminish with age. However, prolonged sleep deprivation can result in irritability, distortions in perception and orientation, and even hallucinations. These effects are not permanent. In fact, one study has shown that REM deprivation can have beneficial effects for people with depression (Smith & Wong, 1991). Because sleep forms part of the rest-activity cycle that influences human activity patterns and time use, it must be included in taxonomies of occupation and its influence must be considered in theories of occupation and well-being (Figure 1-6).

OCCUPATIONS AND TIME USE

Regardless of how they are named or classified, occupations constitute the use of time. During a person's life, the entire chronology from birth to death can be recorded as a series of occupations that differ according to various influences. These influences can be internal, such as a person's degree of arousal or internal motivation; or external, such as the location and social demands for performing them. As we will learn, the temporal nature of occupations (i.e., when, how often, and how long they are done) can be influenced by both internal and external factors. When we discuss time use, we are also describing the structure of lives. That is, we are attempting to describe the manner in which daily occupations can be viewed in a pattern which characterizes a person's lifestyle and life story.

In this section we begin with a review of literature that describes how time is used when activities are grouped into some of the main categories we have previously defined. This will lead logically to a discussion of other patterns of time use, including patterns of occupation over time, which are called lifestyles.

Much of the current information on time use comes from consumer research, although governmental agencies and scientists studying gerontology and leisure have also made use-

Sex Differences, Time Use, and Health

Two recent studies examined gender roles and health. The first compared time spent by men and women in various role-related activities, such as paid work, housework, child care, helping others, sleep, and active and passive leisure. Relationships between the amount of time men and women spent in these activities and their self-rated health were examined. Men reported better health than women. The researchers found that men and women do not differ in the amount of sleep they get nor in the time they allocate to passive leisure activities. However, the study showed that men spent twice as much time as women in paid employment, whereas women spent three and a half times as many hours per week in household labor than men.

The second study also showed that men reported better health than women. It found that men were more likely to walk and to exercise strenuously than women, but that their lifestyle advantage diminished with age because they were more likely to smoke and be overweight. The study also found that women were more likely to experience economic hardship and to do more unpaid domestic labor, both of which are associated with poorer health.

The studies also found evidence that household work is experienced differently by men and women. Women (in general) tend to spend a greater portion of their days performing household duties (whether or not they also perform paid work outside the home) and receive less recognition for these efforts. There is speculation that because household work is valued less than work outside the home (in many cultures), this may help explain why it is perceived as less gratifying by many women.

Overall, the studies suggest that many role-related tasks influence lifestyles and also contribute to health. They also indicate that the reason women experience more illness but live longer than men is related to their lifestyle rather than biological or physiological differences between the sexes.

From: Ross, C. E., & Bird, C. E. (1994). Sex stratification and health lifestyle: Consequences for men's and women's perceived health. *Journal of Health and Social Behavior, 35*(2), 161-178.

Bird, C. E., & Fremont, A. M. (1991). Gender, time use and health. *Journal of Health and Social Behavior, 32*(2), 114-129.

ful contributions to our general understanding of how people "spend" their time. The expression "spending time" is interesting, because it conveys a view of time that equates it with other commodities or resources. Modern society and its emphasis on consuming goods and services has influenced time use to the point that individuals may not realize the extent to which they fail to pursue activities that are meaningful to them (Peloquin, 1990).

MEASURING TIME USE

Time use studies depend on individuals to complete logs of their activities in sequence over a defined period, usually 24 or 48 hours. The accuracy of these logs or diaries is then typically checked by random observations or interviews of family members (proxy reporting) to establish their validity (Robinson, 1977).

Often, individuals are doing more than one activity at a time. A multinational time use study by Szalai (1972) identified that concurrent occupations may be described as primary and secondary. For example, a person may be listening to music and talking on the cellular phone while driving to work. In this example, driving to work would be the primary activity, while listening to music and talking on the phone would be secondary, since they are nested or enfolded within the primary act of driving to work. This further complicates the use of time as a measure of occupation.

In occupational therapy, a variety of instruments have been used to identify the time use of persons and their perceptions of that time. Watanabe (1968) developed a procedure known as the activity configuration, which is an interview designed to record the perceptions of the quality of activities in which a person engages during a typical week. A similar approach was developed by Mosey (1973). Cynkin (1979) and Neville (1980) proposed the use of a segmented circle (viewed as a clock or a pie graph) to record a day's activities. Baum (1993) developed a card sort to determine the percent of activities retained as a measure of time use in persons with Alzheimer disease. Other therapists have developed inventories to determine the frequency and time available for selected occupations, such as work or play (Moorhead, 1969; Takata, 1969). Although the approaches developed and used by occupational therapists vary in form, they have been consistent in their attention to recording the activity patterns and perceptions of individuals.

In contrast, the studies of time use by researchers outside occupational therapy have been interested in the activity patterns of groups. Unfortunately, the lack of consistent approaches to classifying activities has made detailed comparisons among these various studies difficult. However, since we know that each day has 24 hours, we can make reasonable

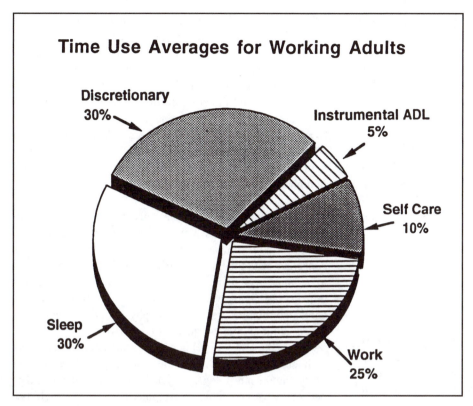

Figure 1-7. Time use averages for working adults.

assumptions about the amounts of time allocated for some categories of activity by knowing how much is given to others. For example, knowing that a person spends more time sleeping allows us to conclude that there is less time available for other activities.

GENERAL PATTERNS OF TIME USE

Time use studies indicate that for adults in the United States, on average, approximately 30% of a typical 24 hour day is spent sleeping, 10% is allocated to self-care activities (including eating), and another 10% is allocated to IADL, such as cooking, laundry, housecleaning, and marketing. For those who are employed, approximately 25% of one's day is spent on work (excluding breaks). Thus, nearly 60% of the waking day is devoted to obligatory or required activities, including employment, for a typically employed adult. This proportion of obligatory activity has also been found for adolescents (Kleiber, Larson & Csikszentmihalyi, 1986) (Figure 1-7).

There is international consistency in time allocation. Percentages reported for the United States are similar to data collected in other countries. Information on people in Sweden (Sjoberg & Magneberg, 1990), as well as analyses of time use by Germans (Baltes, Wahl & Schmid-Furstoss, 1990), Australians (Castles, 1994; Mercer, 1985) and Canadians (McKinnon, 1992), show remarkably consistent patterns, both for obligatory and discretionary categories of occupation, as well as in more specific areas of occupation, such as self-care and household maintenance.

THE FREQUENCY AND DURATION OF OCCUPATIONS

Studies have shown that the number of activities people perform during any given time segment may differ significantly. Also, the length of time spent in occupations seems to vary by category, and can reveal gender and role differences.

A study of adults in Germany (Baltes, Wahl & Schmid-Furstoss, 1990) found that, on average, people spent about twice as much time engaging in each leisure occupation as they did for each obligatory occupation. They also found that people who reported engaging in more obligatory activities also engaged in a greater number of discretionary activities. Thus, active people tend to be busy in all aspects of their lives, not just in one category or another. Researchers have theorized that some people have natural tendencies to be active, and this theory seems to be supported by studies of activity frequency (Stones & Kozma, 1986).

Patterns of Daily Occupation

Part of the predictability of life from day to day reflects the consistency of occupations. Obligatory occupations, such as self-care and sleep, are typically repeated as part of daily routines.

Some occupations become so engaging that they are pursued continuously to the exclusion of even obligatory occupations, sometimes with negative health consequences. For example, the popularity of computer games and the Internet have each created obsessive engagement in these pursuits by some people, perhaps because of their novelty.

Other occupations seem to have a self-perpetuating quality which encourages the individual to continue pursuing them. A preliminary study involving university students suggested that one important element of this phenomenon, which Carlson (1996) terms "occupational perseverance" (p. 145), was the individual's perceived progress toward meeting an important or valued goal. This tendency to continue pursuing an activity seems to be distinct from habits.

Habits

Some tasks are repeated so often that they become habitual, (i.e., performed on an automatic, preconscious level). In the extreme, recurring behavior may meet a strong physiological and psychological need, which is described as an addiction. Abuse of some substances with chemical agents, such as tobacco, alcohol, or mind-altering drugs, leads to addictive behaviors.

Interest in habitual influences on behavior dates back to the early years of occupational therapy, during a period when its founders pursued the strategy of "habit training" (Slagle, 1922; Kidner, 1924). At that time it was believed that habits reflected the organization of behavior.

Drawing from the work of Dewey (1922), Camic (1986) and Young (1988), a Model of Human Occupation proposed by Kielhofner (1995) describes habits as including these characteristics:
- they influence behavior in a semiautomatic way without need for conscious, deliberate action
- they are established through prior repetition of a series of acts and thus serve to organize smaller units of behavior
- they are more likely to occur in familiar environments.

Kielhofner describes habits as providing an internal map which helps us "locate ourselves in the midst of an external world" (1995, p. 66). Habits serve the purposes of conserving energy needed for attention and decision-making, while enabling us to do things we must do regularly without requiring high levels of motivation or energy.

Routines

Similarly, routines are occupations with established sequences, such as the morning ritual surrounding showering and dressing for the day. Routines provide an orderly structure for daily living as suggested in this description by Bond and Feather (1988), who wrote that "a routine has a stability about it that extends over time and pertains to a particular set of activities within a defined situation" (p. 328).

Studies have supported the idea that certain activities naturally take place at certain times of the day. For example, a study of the daily lives of older adults in Germany (Baltes, Wall and Schmid-Furstoss, 1990) observed that work and self-maintenance activities tended to predominate in the morning and early afternoon, whereas leisure and restful activities were associated with late afternoon and evening periods. Similar activity rhythms have been found in studies of higher order group living animals, such as mountain gorillas (Harcourt, 1977).

Studies have shown that our daily routines are influenced by biological factors, which has resulted in the specialized field of study known as *chronobiology*. Chronobiology is concerned with the internal physiological clocks which seem to regulate rest and activity cycles in animals, including humans (Halberg, Halberg, Barnum & Bittner, 1959). Circadian rhythms are among the physiological cycles influenced by these internal clocks (Figure 1-8).

Internal clocks depend on environmental timekeepers (zeitgebers), such as daily routines, to keep the body attuned to its natural physiological cycles. Thus, a vital link exists between what people do on a regular basis during each day, and their internal clocks. Both influence each other. Thus, shift workers or people who travel across time zones can be affected by the mismatch between their daily patterns of occupation and their internal clocks (Folkard, Minors & Waterhouse, 1985). The scientific term for this mismatch or lack of synchrony is "disentrainment." Psychiatrists have proposed that some types of depression may be the result of disentrainment (Ehlers, Frank & Kupfer, 1988; Hofer, 1984).

Aside from the influences of biological clocks, routines are also given structure by societal expectations and customs. For example, working for an employer imposes the routine of a workday, while business hours at a favorite store may dictate shopping routines, just as religious services influence the times when spiritual occupations occur on days of worship.

Viewed over extended periods, habits and routines comprise important dimensions of lifestyles, components of which have been shown to influence health and well-being. For example, regular exercise, rest and appropriate dietary habits are known lifestyle behaviors which can be influenced by daily routines. Additionally, adherence to therapeutic regimens, such as eating or taking medications at prescribed times, can also be influenced by habits and routines. Unfortunately, the extent to which habits and regular routines contribute to healthful consequences (independent of specific practices) has not been studied sufficiently. Similarly, studies are needed which examine the impact of emotional and physical illness on daily routines.

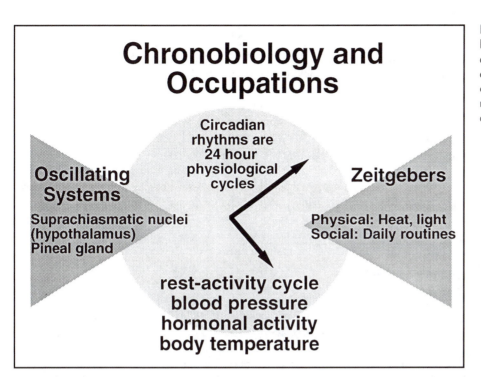

Chronobiology and Occupations

Circadian rhythms are 24 hour physiological cycles

Oscillating Systems

Suprachiasmatic nuclei (hypothalamus) Pineal gland

Zeitgebers

Physical: Heat, light Social: Daily routines

rest-activity cycle blood pressure hormonal activity body temperature

Figure 1-8. Daily activity is influenced by internal physiological clocks, which are themselves "set" by events in the environment, including daily occupations, particularly those of a regular nature. These timekeepers are called *zeitgebers*.

Lifestyles

Habits, routines, and occupational preferences help define lifestyles. Extending the ideas of Sobel (1981) and Elliott (1993), a lifestyle can be defined as a distinctive, selected mode of living with continuity over time that is both observable and recognizable, and through which an individual expresses his or her self-identity. Elliott (1993) notes that a routine or established way of dealing with personal needs and the demands of the environment, as well as an established and consistent pattern of involvement in a particular type of behavior, are also important characteristics of lifestyles. Thus, a lifestyle is not the totality of a person's behaviors, but a selected group of behaviors that is stable, patterned and predictable.

Some studies of lifestyle have attempted to identify types. Mitchell (1983) developed a typology of nine lifestyles based on analysis of people living in the United States. His study considered behaviors, values, and needs. Horley, Carroll & Little (1988) found evidence of the existence of three distinct lifestyle types through analysis of the organized goals or personal projects of two samples of people in Canada.

Most attention to measuring the impact of lifestyles on health and well-being has been directed toward behaviors that are health compromising or health enhancing. Behaviors in both areas often occur in clusters. That is, people who wear seat belts also tend to get adequate amounts of sleep, eat regular meals, exercise, and get regular medical and dental check-ups (Kulbock, Earls & Montgomery, 1988). Conversely, people who abuse substances are often involved in delinquent behavior (Osgood, 1991).

While studies of lifestyle have concentrated on problem behaviors related to prevention, there have been no comprehensive studies of lifestyles involving everyday behaviors and health or well-being. Current theories of lifestyle intervention emphasize the importance of environments, including communities, social networks, values, norms, social

How Does Emotional Illness Influence Daily Occupations?

A study of the daily lives of people with depression was reported in 1990 in the *American Journal of Occupational Therapy*. In this study, the author, occupational therapist Karen Larson, was interested in determining if significant life events before hospitalization may have contributed to depression. She also was interested in how the daily patterns of occupation changed over time.

Larson also found that the source of stress seemed to influence the patterns of occupation at home. Overall, as the number of stressors in a person's life increased, the amount of time spent on personal care decreased and the amount of time spent in passive recreation increased. As home and family stresses increased, personal care decreased. Interestingly, financial stress seemed to be associated with an increase in personal care.

From Larson, K. B. (1990). Activity patterns and life changes in people with depression. *American Journal of Occupational Therapy*, 44(10), 902-906.

sanctions, and opportunities for alternate behaviors, as factors important to influencing lifestyles.

Fidler (1996) suggests that each individual has a unique lifestyle profile which should be understood in terms of the extent to which it permits attention to four essential domains of living, which she identifies as self-maintenance, intrinsic gratification, social contribution, and interpersonal relatedness. According to Fidler, the extent to which an individual's lifestyle allows needs to be met in these four domains offers one method by which a person's need for occupational therapy services can be identified.

While lifestyles are useful ways of viewing an individual's occupations over time, they do not provide insight into the significance and meaning of those occupations. Occupations are given meaning over time as part of life stories. This subject constitutes an important concluding section in our survey of the complexities of occupation.

LIFE STORIES

Viewing the past, present and future as part of an unfolding story is an important mechanism in the meaning of everyday occupation, and is known as *narrative*. Narrative refers to the autobiographical stories through which lives are described and interpreted to the self and others. These stories provide a sense of unity and purpose by drawing together seemingly unrelated life actions (Polkinghorne, 1996; McAdams 1990, 1992). Jerome Bruner (1990) is convinced that the ability to make meaning of life events is so dependent on stories that he theorizes an innate or biological disposition to interpret events in the world through language.

It is believed that our sense of self, or social identity, is very much influenced by our ongoing interpretation of events through our life stories (Gergen and Gergen, 1988). Because our life stories are constantly being written and revised to incorporate new experiences, narrative can also serve as a motivational influence. That is, as we develop our life stories, we are guided by many possible scripts depending on the opportunities and options available to us (Markus & Nurius, 1986).

Occupational therapists must understand that their patients' or clients' lives are experienced not as categories of occupation but as meaningful events that are connected in an ongoing stream and are interpreted as stories (Clark, 1993). Viewing occupations as parts of life stories is a necessary part of identifying relevant goals and intervention processes. Mattingly and Fleming (1994), have studied this aspect of practice in great detail, using the term "narrative understanding" to describe it. They maintain that acquiring narrative understanding of patients and clients is an important part of the clinical reasoning of occupational therapists.

ISSUES IN THE STUDY OF OCCUPATION

Because occupation constitutes the process of living, it should not be surprising that many of the studies reported in the previous sections of this chapter demonstrate a relationship between what people do and their well-being. We know that our daily occupations influence health, since this was the very idea that motivated the founders of the field to begin a new profession early in the 20th century.

Most of the reported studies of occupation have been conducted by investigators outside occupational therapy. Their primary intent has been to answer questions for the primary benefit of other health, social and behavioral sciences disciplines. Understanding occupation from the point of view of occupational therapy requires a research program planned and conducted by researchers familiar with the field, its traditions, beliefs and practices. It was this realization that led many scholars in the field during the 1980s to call for more studies of occupation (Christiansen, 1981; Mosey, 1985; Yerxa, 1988).

In the late 1980s, the University of Southern California began a program of study in occupational science leading to the Ph.D. degree. Occupational science was described as a basic science (also known as an academic discipline) to study "universal issues about occupation without concern for their immediate application in occupational therapy" (Yerxa, Clark, Frank, Jackson, Parham, Pierce, Stein, & Zemke, 1989, p. 4). The basic mission of this new academic discipline has been described as understanding the forms, functions, and meanings of occupation as well as its relationship to human adaptation (Clark et al., 1991).

The perceived need to divide occupational science and occupational therapy has changed over time, but the debate continues on whether an academic discipline such as occupational science can flourish if scientists are distracted by the needs and concerns of a practice profession (Clark, Zemke, Frank et al., 1993; Mosey, 1993). Some scholars believe that deciding what to study should be based on an objective process that develops and tests theories which permit an understanding of occupation without concern for how the information gained from research will be applied. Others believe that one of the purposes of science is to develop theories which can be used for the advancement and greater good of humankind.

Wood (1996) proposes that the study of occupation should be conducted without constraints. She defines constraint-free study as "interdisciplinary scholarly inquiry that seeks to generate a deep understanding of how important occupations influence adaptation and health" (p. 327), and argues that the study of occupation should extend beyond service delivery, but not exclude it from its domain of concern. Wood has illustrated how primatology, particularly studies of the occupations of Chimpanzees and Bonobos, can

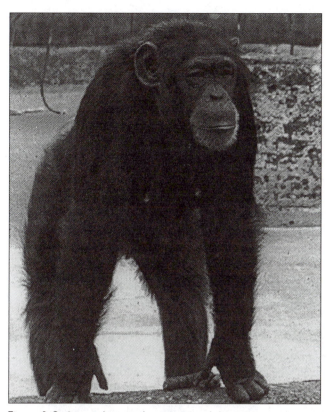

Figure 1-9. Primatology and occupational therapy.

provide important information to guide and inform occupational scientists, and that knowledge from occupational therapy can be used to improve the humane care and handling of primates in captivity (Wood, 1993) (Figure 1-9).

Another issue in the study of occupation concerns the appropriate methods for conducting research. Of particular concern are where data are gathered, on whom, and how these data are analyzed. Traditional basic sciences achieve control over the factors that influence research findings by relying on laboratory settings and comparisons. Using statistical procedures applied to large samples, they are able to determine the probability that observed changes are due to the factor being studied or the result of chance. Because they depend on statistics, these traditional quantitative approaches rely on the comparisons of groups of subjects and observations of change recorded through numerical measurement.

In contrast, some scholars have argued that the appropriate study of occupation requires approaches which observe behaviors in natural settings and capture the unique stories, meanings and complexities of particular individuals (Kielhofner, 1982; Hasselkus, 1991; Yerxa, 1991). Such approaches are described as naturalistic and qualitative. Ottenbacher (1992) has argued that the methods of science should depend on the questions being asked, rather than on a

---

Primatology and Occupational Therapy

The development of occupational science has created an interest in primatology, the study of non-human primates, as a means for better understanding how occupations contribute to health and well-being. Chimpanzees (pan trogolodytes) and humans (homosapiens) have less than 3% difference in their genetic composition (DNA), and share remarkable similarities in the anatomical structures of their brains.

Studies of primates have shown that they have language capability, can solve problems, and can use abstract symbols. They can also use objects as tools, as in the use of sticks to catch and eat termites. As community dwelling social animals, their patterns of daily behavior reflect their unique personalities.

Through research in the wild as well as in controlled conditions in regional primate laboratories, studies of primates may provide valuable insights into how environments influence daily occupations. They may also provide important information about how occupational patterns are socially influenced, and the conditions under which occupations, such as play, can influence adaptation and health.

From Wood, W. (1993). Occupation and the relevance of primatology to occupational therapy. *American Journal of Occupational Therapy, 47*(6), 515-522.

Goodall, J. (1995). Occupations of chimpanzee infants and mothers. In R. Zemke & F. Clark (Eds.), *Occupational science: The evolving discipline*. Philadelphia: F.A. Davis (pp. 31-42).

---

blanket endorsement of a particular approach. Carlson and Clark (1991) recommend the use and development of approaches which capture the unique qualities of individuals while permitting appropriate comparisons and generalizations to larger groups.

While nearly everyone concerned with the study of occupation agrees with the importance of theory-building, there is disagreement on what characteristics those theories should exhibit. Some argue that a single, unified theory would be best (Christiansen, 1981, 1991), while others have proposed that because of the diversity of practice, many theories and frames of reference are more appropriate (Mosey 1988; 1992). Much of this debate is complicated by the lack of consensus in defining concepts and terms.

Research is a way of coming to know and understand. In an important paper on knowledge in occupational therapy,

Wood (1996) argues that much of the field's knowledge falls within the domain of methods—knowing how—and far too little exists in the domain of understanding—knowing why. Certainly, there is much to be learned about human occupation that can be applied to the field of occupational therapy and lead to better theories. This will lead to improved strategies of intervention that will help our clients gain the skills necessary for accomplishing the goals or projects they wish to pursue.

The complexities described in the opening sections of this chapter provide a rich and important area for future research. We believe that an improved understanding of human occupation will come about more quickly if the importance of research is better valued, recognized and supported by professional societies and better integrated within the educational curricula of occupational therapy.

SUMMARY

This chapter began with a review of definitions and a description of the complexity of human occupation. We identified that occupations have dimensions relating to performance, meaning, social participation, and self-identity. We observed that occupations can be classified as variations in the use of time.

Traditional classifications of occupation were reviewed. In the traditional grouping by type, the categories of work, play, self-maintenance, leisure and sleep were defined. The complexity of performance and meaning of occupation over time was also described, suggesting the need for a hierarchy of terms ranging from actions to lifestyles, each encompassing greater segments of occupational behavior.

Since occupations constitute the use of time, general patterns of time use were described. Physiological factors, such as circadian rhythms, were also identified as influences on time use. Habits, routines, and lifestyles were identified as patterns of time use. The importance of narratives, or the life stories used by individuals to link events over time, was discussed.

The chapter concluded with a description of the evolution of occupational science and current issues in the study of occupation. We noted that the field has been burdened by the lack of consensus among its scholars and researchers, and has been hampered by a professional culture which undervalues the importance of theory and research.

The information in this chapter provides an important backdrop for viewing occupational therapy and for formulating a particular model of practice. Occupations are performed by persons in environments. Thus, three elements: persons, environments, and occupational performance, serve as convenient headings for organizing the main areas of focus for the model of occupational therapy described in this book. The Person-Environment Occupational Performance Model is described in greater detail in Chapter 3.

By studying these three areas of focus, we are able to better understand how occupations and the environments in which they are undertaken can influence individual health and well-being. By understanding these influences as concepts *before* they are applied as part of a practice model, we are able to better appreciate the many possibilities of occupation and less likely to view occupation in a narrow, restricted way, thus stripping it of its most important dimension—its meaning in the life of the individual.

STUDY QUESTIONS

1. Consider the leisure pursuit you most enjoy during your spare time. Can you describe it in terms of its performance requirements, meaning, social significance, and self-identity dimensions?

2. Identify the common elements in the definitions of occupation provided in this chapter. Compare and contrast the terms occupational performance, function, purposeful activity, and occupation.

3. Define the term "taxonomy" and describe its purposes.

4. Compare the occupational categories of play and leisure. Determine whether you believe they should be members of the same or different categories.

5. Identify influences on time use.

6. Define the term lifestyle. How does it differ from a life story?

7. Describe significant issues in the study of occupation.

RECOMMENDED READINGS

Baum, C. M. & Edwards, D. (1994). Position paper: Occupational Performance: Occupational therapy's definition of function. *American Journal of Occupational Therapy, 49*(10), 1019-1020.

Bruner, J. (1990). *Acts of Meaning*. Cambridge: Harvard University Press.

Christiansen, C. (1997). Acknowledging a spiritual dimension in occupational therapy. *American Journal of Occupational Therapy, 51*(3), 169-172.

Christiansen, C. (1994). A social framework for self-care intervention. In C. Christiansen (Ed.), *Ways of Living: Self Care Strategies for Special Needs*. Rockville, MD: American Occupational Therapy Association (pp. 1-26).

Christiansen, C. (1990). The perils of plurality. (Editorial). *Occupational Therapy Journal of Research, 10*(5), 259-265.

Christiansen, C. Clark, F., Kielhofner, G., & Rogers, J. (1995). Occupation: A Position paper. *American Journal of Occupational Therapy, 49*(10), 1015-1018.

Clark, F. A. (1993). Occupation embedded in real life: Interweaving occupational science and occupational therapy. *American Journal of Occupational Therapy, 47*(12), 1067-1078.

Engelhardt, H. T. (1977). Defining occupational therapy: The meaning of therapy and the virtues of occupation. *American Journal of Occupational Therapy, 31*(10), 666-672.

Fidler, G. S., & Fidler, J. W. (1978). Doing and becoming: Purposeful action and self-actualization. *American Journal of Occupational Therapy, 32*, 305-310.

Frank, G. (1994). The personal meaning of self-care. In C. Christiansen (Ed.), Ways of Living: Self Care Strategies for Special Needs. Rockville, MD: American Occupational Therapy Association (pp. 27-49).

Nelson, D. L. (1988). Occupation: Form and performance. *American Journal of Occupational Therapy, 42*, 633-641.

Polkinghorne, D. (1988). Narrative Knowing and the Human Sciences. Albany: State University of New York Press.

Szalai, A. (Ed.) (1972). *The Use of Time: Daily Activities of Urban and Suburban Populations in Twelve Countries.* The Hague: Mouton.

Wilcock, A. A. (1993). A theory of human need for occupation. *Journal of Occupational Science: Australia,* 1(1), 17-24.

Yerxa, E., Clark, F. A., Frank, G., Jackson, J., Parham, D., Pierce, D., Stein, C., and Zemke, R. (1989). An introduction to occupational science. A foundation for occupational therapy in the 21st century. In J. Johnson & E. J. Yerxa) (Eds.), *Occupational Science: The Foundation for New Models of Practice* (pp. 1-180). New York, Haworth.

REFERENCES

American Occupational Therapy Association. (1994). Uniform terminology for occupational therapy (third edition). *American Journal of Occupational Therapy, 48*(11), 1047-1054.

Baltes, M. M., Wahl, H. W., & Schmid-Furstoss, U. (1990). The daily life of elderly Germans: Activity patterns, personal control, and functional health. *Journal of Gerontology, 45*(4), 173-179.

Bateson, G. (1979). *Mind and nature: A necessary unity.* New York: Bantam.

Bateson, M. C. (1996). Enfolded activity and the concept of occupation. In R. Zemke, & F. Clark (Eds.), *Occupational science: The evolving discipline* (pp 5-12). Philadelphia: F. A. Davis.

Baum, C. M. (1995). The contribution of occupation to function in persons with Alzheimer Disease. *Journal of Occupational Science: Australia, 2*(2), 59-67.

Baum, C. M., & Edwards, D. (1993). Cognitive performance in senile dementia of the Alzheimer's Type: The Kitchen Task Assessment. *American Journal of Occupational Therapy, 47*(5), 431-436.

Baum, C. M., & Edwards, D. (1995). Position Paper: Occupational Performance: Occupational therapy's definition of function. *American Journal of Occupational Therapy, 49(10),* 1019-1020.

Baum, C. M., & Law, M. (1997). Occupational therapy practice:

Focusing on occupational performance. *American Journal of Occupational Therapy, 51*(4), 277-288.

Berger, P. L., & Luckmann, T. (1967). *The social construction of reality.* Garden City, New York: Doubleday & Company.

Bird, C. E., & Freemont, A. M. (1991). Gender, time use, and health. *Journal of Health and Social Behavior, 32,* 114-

Bond, M. J., & Feather, N. T. (1988). Some correlates of structure and purpose in the use of time. *Journal of Personality and Social Psychology, 55*(2), 321-329.

Brief, A. P., & Hollenbeck, J. R. (1985). Work and the quality of life. *International Journal of Psychology, 20,* 199-206.

Brief, A. P., & Nord, W. R. (1990). Work and non-work connections. In A. Brief & W. Nord (Eds.), *Meanings of occupational work* (pp. 171-199). Lexington, MA: Lexington Books.

Bruner, J. (1990). *Acts of meaning.* Cambridge: Harvard University Press.

Buss, D. & Block, J. (1980). Preschool activity level: Personality correlates and developmental implications. *Child Development, 51,* 401-408.

Camic, C. (1986). The matter of habit. *American Journal of Sociology, 91,* 1039-1087.

Canadian Association of Occupational Therapists. (1995). *Guidelines for the client-centred practice of occupational therapy.* Toronto, Canada: Author.

Carlson, M. (1995). The self perpetuation of occupations. In R. Zemke & F. Clark (Eds.), *Occupational Science: The emerging discipline* (pp. 143-158). Philadelphia: F. A. Davis.

Carlson, M. & Clark, F. (1991). The search for useful methodologies in occupational science. *American Journal of Occupational Therapy, 45,* 235-241.

Carlson, M., & Dunlea, A. (1995). The Issue Is—Further thoughts on the pitfalls of partition: A response to Mosey. *American Journal of Occupational Therapy, 49,* 73-81.

Castles, I. (1994). *How Australians use their time.* Canberra: Australian Bureau of Statistics.

Christiansen, C. (1990). The perils of plurality. *Occupational Therapy Journal of Research, 10,* 259-265.

Christiansen, C. (1996). Three perspectives on balance in occupation. In R. Zemke & F. Clark (Eds.), *Occupational science: The evolving discipline* (pp. 181-191). Philadelphia: F. A. Davis.

Christiansen, C. H. (1981). (Editorial) Toward resolution of crisis: Research requisites in occupational therapy. *Occupational Therapy Journal of Research, 1*(2), 115-125.

Christiansen, C. H. (1994a). A social-psychological approach to understanding self-care. In C. Christiansen (Ed.), *Ways of living: Self care strategies for special needs* (pp.1-26). Bethesda, MD: American Occupational Therapy Association.

Christiansen, C. H. (1994b). Classification and study in occupation: A review and discussion of taxonomies. *Journal of Occupational Science, Australia, 1*(3), 3-21.

Christiansen, C. H., Clark, F., Kielhofner, G., & Rogers, J. (1995). Position Paper: Occupation. *American Journal of Occupational Therapy, 49*(10), 1015-1018.

Christiansen, C. H., & Ottenbacher, K. (1997). Self care: Evaluation and management. In J. Delisa, B. Gans, & D. Currie et al (Eds.), *Rehabilitation medicine: Principles and practice.* Philadelphia:

J. B. Lippincott.

Clark, F. A. (1993). Occupation embedded in real life: Interweaving occupational science and occupational therapy. *American Journal of Occupational Therapy, 47*, 1067-1078.

Clark, F. A., Parham, D., Carlson, M. E., Frank, G., Jackson, J., Pierce, D., Wolfe, R., & Zemke, R. (1991). Occupational science: Academic innovation in the service of occupational therapy's future. *American Journal of Occupational Therapy, 45*, 300-310.

Clark, F. A., Zemke, R., Frank, G., Parkam, D., Neville-Jan, A., Hedricks, C., Carlson, M., Fazio, L., & Abreu, B. (1993). The issue is: Dangers inherent in the partition of occupational therapy and occupational science. *American Journal of Occupational Therapy, 47*, 184-186.

Cormack, R. M. (1971). A review of classification. *Journal of the Royal Statistical Society, 34*(3), 321-367.

Cskiszentmihalyi, M. (1993). Activity and happiness: Towards a science of occupation. *Journal of Occupational Science, Australia, 1*(1), 38-42.

Cynkin, S. (1979). *Occupational therapy: Toward health through activities*. Boston: Little, Brown.

Cynkin, S. & Robinson, A. M. (1990). *Occupational therapy and activities health: Toward health through activities*. Boston: Little Brown.

Darnell, J. L., & Heater, S. L. (1994). Occupational therapist or Activity Therapist—Which do you choose to be? *American Journal of Occupational Therapy, 48*, 467-468.

Dewey, J. (1922). *Human nature and conduct*. New York: Henry Holt & Company.

Egan M., & DeLaat, M. D. (1994). Considering spirituality in occupational therapy practice. *Canadian Journal of Occupational Therapy, 61*, 95-101.

Ehlers, C. L., Frank, E., & Kupfer, D. J. (1988). Social zeitgebers and biological rhythms: A unified approach to understanding the etiology of depression. *Archives of General Psychiatry, 45*, 948-952.

Elliott, D. S. (1993). Health enhancing and health compromising lifestyles. In S. G. Millstein, A. C. Petersen, & E. O. Nightingale (Eds.), *Promoting the health of adolescents*. (pp 119-145). New York: Oxford University Press.

Engelhardt, H. T. (1977). Defining occupational therapy: The meaning of therapy and the virtues of occupation. *American Journal of Occupational Therapy, 31*(10), 666-672.

Evans, A. K. (1987). Nationally speaking: Definition of occupation as the core concept of occupational therapy. *American Journal of Occupational Therapy, 41*, 627-628.

Fidler, G. S. (1996). Life-Style Performance: From profile to conceptual model. *American Journal of Occupational Therapy, 48*(11), 1006-1103.

Fleishman, E. (1975). Toward a taxonomy of human performance. *American Psychologist, 30*(12), 1127-1149.

Fleishman, E. A., & Quaintance, M. (1984). *Taxonomies of performance. The description of human tasks*. Orlando: Academic Press.

Folkard, S., Minors, D. S., & Waterhouse, J. M. (1985). Chronobiology and shift work: Current issues and trends. *Chronobiologia, 12*, 31-54.

Gärling, T., & Gärville, J. (1993). Psychological explanations of participation in everyday activities. In T. Gärling & R. G. Golledge (Eds.), *Behavior and environment: Psychological and geographical approaches*. New York: Elsevier.

Gergen, K. J., & Gergen, M. M. (1988). Narrative and the self as relationship. In L. Berkowitz (Ed.), *Advances in Experimental Social Psychology, 21*, 17-57.

Goffman, E. (1959). *The presentation of self in everyday life*. New York: Doubleday.

Goffman, E. (1963). *Stigma: Notes on the management of a spoiled identity*. Englewood Cliffs, NJ: Prentice-Hall.

Gramm, W. S. (1987). Labor, work and leisure: Human well-being and the optimal allocation of time. *Journal of Economic Issues, 21*, 167-188.

Gunter, B. G., & Stanley, J. (1985). Theoretical issues in leisure study. In B. G. Gunter, J. Stanley, & R. St. Clair (Eds.), *Transitions to leisure: Conceptual and human issues* (pp. 35-51). Lanham, MD: University Press of America.

Halberg, F., Halberg, E., Barnum, C. P., & Bittner, J. J. (1959). Physiologic 24 hour periodicity in human beings and mice, the lighting regimen and daily routine. In R. D. Withrow (Ed.), *Photoperiodicity and related phenomena in plants and animals* (pp. 803-878). Washington, D C: American Association for the Advancement of Science.

Harcourt, A. H. (1977). Activity periods and patterns of social interaction: A neglected problem. *Behaviour, 66*, 122-135.

Harré, R., Clarke, D., & DeCarlo, N. (1985). *Motives and mechanisms: An introduction to the psychology of action*. London: Methuen.

Hasselkus, B. R. (1991). Qualitative research: Not another orthodoxy. *Occupational Therapy Journal of Research, 11*(1), 1-7.

Henderson, A., Cermak, S., Coster, W., Murray, E., Trombly, C., & Tickle-Degnon, L. (1991). The issue is: Occupational science is multidimensional. *American Journal of Occupational Therapy, 45*, 370-372.

Hofer, M. A. (1984). Relationships as regulators: A psychobiologic perspective. *Psychosomatic Medicine, 46*(3), 183-198.

Hogan, R. (1983). A socioanalytic theory of personality. *Nebraska Symposium on Motivation, 30*, 55-89.

Hogan, R., & Sloan, T. (1991). Socioanalytic foundations for personality psychology. *Perspectives in Personality, 3*(Part B), 1-15.

Holbrook, M. B., & Lehmann, D. R. (1981). Allocating discretionary time: Complementarity among activities. *Journal of Consumer Research, 7*, 395-406.

Holmberg, K., Rosen, D., & Holland, J. L. (1990). *The leisure activities finder*. Odessa, FL: Psychological Assessment Resources.

Horley, J., Carroll, B., & Little, B. R. (1988). A typology of lifestyles. *Social Indicators Research, 20*, 383-398.

Horne, J. A. (1983). Mammalian sleep functions with particular reference to man. In A. Mayes (Ed.), *Sleep mechanisms and functions in humans and animals—an evolutionary perspective* (pp. 262-312). Wokingham, England: Van Nostrand-Reinhold.

Iso-Ahola, S. E. (1979). Basic dimensions of definitions of leisure. *Journal of Leisure Research, vol II*, 28-39.

Jacobs, K. (1994). Flow and the occupational therapy practitioner. *American Journal of Occupational Therapy, 48,* 989-995.

Kelly, J. R. (1972). Work and leisure: A simplified paradigm. *Journal of Leisure Research, 4,* 50-62.

Kerby, A. P. (1991). *Narrative and the self.* Bloomington: Indiana University Press.

Kidner, T. B. (1924). Work for the tuberculosis patient during and after cure: Part II. *Archives of Occupational Therapy, 3,* 169-193.

Kielhofner, G. (1977). Temporal adaptation: A conceptual framework for occupational therapy. *American Journal of Occupational Therapy, 31,* 235-242.

Kielhofner, G. (1982). Qualitative research: Part two. Methodological approaches and relevance to occupational therapy. *Occupational Therapy Journal of Research, 2,* 150-170.

Kielhofner, G. (1995). *A model of human occupation: Theory and application* (2nd ed.). Baltimore: Williams & Wilkins.

Kielhofner, G., & Burke, J. P. (1985). Components and determinants of human occupation. In Kielhofner, G. (Ed.), *A model of human occupation: Theory and application* (pp. 12-36). Baltimore: Williams & Wilkins.

Kleiber, D., Larson, R., & Csikszentmihalyi, M. (1986). The experience of leisure in adolescence. *Journal of Leisure Research, 18*(3), 169-173.

Kulbock, P., Earls, F., & Montgomery, A. (1988). Lifestyle and patterns of health and social behavior in high risk adolescents. *Advances in Nursing Science, 11,* 22-35.

Lawton, M. P. (1971). The functional assessment of elderly people. *Journal of the American Geriatrics Society, 19*(6), 465-481.

Lawton, M. P. (1990). Age and the performance of home tasks. *Human Factors, 32,* 527-536.

Little, B. R. (1989). Personal projects analysis: Trivial pursuits, magnificent obsessions and the search for coherence. In D. Buss & N. Cantor (Eds.), *Personality psychology: Recent trends and emerging directions* (pp. 15-31). New York: Springer-Verlag.

Loizos, C. (1966). Play in mammals. In P. Jewell & C. Loizos (Eds.), *Play, exploration and territory in mammals* (pp. 6-8). London: The Zoological Society.

Maclean, N. (1976). *A river runs through it.* Chicago: University of Chicago Press.

Mancuso, J. C., & Sarbin, T. R. (1983). The self-narrative in the enactment of roles. In T. R. Sarbin & K. E. Scheibe (Eds.), *Studies in social identity.* New York: Praeger.

Marino-Schorn, J. A. (1986). Morale, work and leisure in retirement. *Physical and Occupational Therapy in Geriatrics, 4*(2), 49-59.

Markus, H., & Nurius, P. (1986). Possible selves. *American Psychologist, 41,* 954-969.

Markus, H., & Ruvolo, A. (1980). *Possible selves: Personalized representations of goals.* In L. Pervin (Ed.), *Goal concepts in personality and social psychology* (pp. 211-241). Hilldale, NJ: Lawrence Erlbaum Associates.

Mattingly, C. (1991). The narrative nature of clinical reasoning. *American Journal of Occupational Therapy, 45,* 998-1005.

Mattingly, C., & Fleming (1994). *Clinical reasoning: Forms of inquiry in a therapeutic practice.* Philadelphia: F. A. Davis.

McAdams, D. (1990). Unity and purpose in human lives: The emergence of identity as a life story. In A. L. Rabin, R. A. Zuker, R. A. Emmons, & S. Frank (Eds.), *Studying persons and lives* (pp. 148-200). New York: Springer.

McAdams, D. (1992). Unity and purpose in human lives: The emergence of identity as a life story. In R. A. Zuker, et al (Eds.), *Personality structure in the life course* (pp. 323-376). New York: Springer.

McKinnon, A. L. (1992). Time use for self care, productivity and leisure among elderly Canadians. *Canadian Journal of Occupational Therapy, 59*(2), 102-110.

Meddis, R. (1983). The evolution of sleep. Theories in modern sleep research. In A. Mayes (Ed.), *Sleep mechanisms and functions in humans and animals—an evolutionary perspective* (pp. 57-106). Wokingham, England: Van Nostrand-Reinhold.

Meguro, K., Ueda, M., Yamaguchi, T., Sekita, Y., Yamazaki, H., Oikawa, Y., Kikuchi, Y., & Matsuzawa, T. (1990). Disturbance in daily sleep/wake patterns in patients with cognitive impairment and decreased daily activity. *Journal of the American Geriatric Society, 38,* 1176-1182.

Melges, F. T. (1982). *Time and the inner future: A temporal approach to psychiatric disorders.* New York: Wiley.

Mendelson, W. B. (1987). *Human sleep: Research and clinical care.* New York: Plenum.

Mercer, D. (1985). Australians' time use in work, homework and leisure: Changing profiles. *Australian and New Zealand Journal of Sociology, 21,* 371-384.

Meyer, A. (1922). The philosophy of occupation therapy. *Archives of Occupational Therapy, 1,* 10.

Mitchell, A. (1983). *The nine American lifestyles.* New York: Macmillan.

Moore, A. (1995). The band community: Synchronizing human activity cycles for group cooperation (pp 95-106). In R. Zemke & F. Clark (Eds.), *Occupational science: The evolving discipline.* Philadelphia: F. A. Davis.

Mosey, A. C. (1973). *Activities therapy.* New York: Raven Press.

Mosey, A. C. (1985). A monistic or pluralistic approach to professional identity. *American Journal of Occupational Therapy, 39*(8), 508-509.

Mosey, A. C. (1992). The issue is: Partition of occupational science and occupational therapy. *American Journal of Occupational Therapy, 46,* 851-855.

Mosey, A. C. (1993). The issue is: Partition of occupational science and occupational therapy: Sorting out some issues. *American Journal of Occupational Therapy, 47,* 751-754.

Moss, M. S., & Lawton, M. P. (1982). The time budgets of older people: A window on four lifestyles. *Journal of Gerontology, 37*(1) 115-123.

Nelson, D. (1988). Occupation: Form and performance. *American Journal of Occupational Therapy, 42,* 633-641.

Nelson, D. (1994). Occupational form, occupational performance and therapeutic occupation. In C. B. Royeen (Ed.), *AOTA self study series: The practice of the future: Putting occupation back into therapy* (pp. 9-48). Rockville, MD: American Occupational Therapy Association.

Nelson, D. (1996). Therapeutic occupation: a definition. *American Journal of Occupational Therapy, 50*(10), 775-782.

Neulinger, J. (1974). *The psychology of leisure: Research approaches to the study of leisure.* Springfield: Charles C. Thomas

Neville, A. (1980). Temporal adaptation: Application with short term psychiatric patients. *American Journal of Occupational Therapy, 34,* 328-331.

Osgood, D. W. (1991). *Covariation among adolescent health problems.* Background paper for U.S. Congress Office of Technology Assessment's Adolescent Health Project. Washington, DC: U.S. Government Printing Office.

Overs R. P., & Taylor, S. (1977). Avocational counseling instrumentation. In D. M. Compton & J. E. Goldstein (Eds.), *Perspectives of leisure counseling* (pp. 89-105). Alexandria, VA: National Recreation and Park Association.

Parham, L. D. (1996). Perspectives on play. In R. Zemke & F. Clark (Eds.), *Occupational science: The evolving discipline* (pp. 71-88). Philadelphia: F. A. Davis.

Peloquin, S. (1990). Time as a commodity. *American Journal of Occupational Therapy, 43,* 775-782.

Philipp, S. F. (1991). Spatial arrangement of personal constructs and frequency and duration of participation in leisure activities. *Perceptual and Motor Skills,* 963-969.

Polkinghorne, D. E. (1996). Transformative narratives: From victimic to agentic life plots. *American Journal of Occupational Therapy, 50*(4), 299-305.

Primeau, L. A. (1996a). Work and leisure: Transcending the dichotomy. *American Journal of Occupational Therapy, 50*(7), 569-577.

Primeau, L. A. (1996b). Work versus non-work: The case of household work. In R. Zemke & F. Clark (Eds.), *Occupational science: The evolving discipline* (pp. 57-70). Philadelphia: F. A. Davis.

Primeau, L. A. (1996c). Running as an occupation: Multiple meanings and purposes. In R. Zemke & F. Clark (Eds.), *Occupational science: The evolving discipline* (pp. 275-286). Philadelphia: F. A. Davis.

Reed, K. (1984). *Models of practice in occupational therapy.* Baltimore: Williams & Wilkins.

Reed, K., & Sanderson, S. R. (1980). *Concepts of occupational therapy.* Baltimore: Williams & Wilkins.

Reilly, M. (1969). The educational process. *American Journal of Occupational Therapy, 23,* 299-307.

Reilly, M. (1974). Defining a cobweb. In M. Reilly (Ed.), *Play as exploratory learning* (pp. 60). Beverly Hills, CA: Sage.

Robinson, J. P. (1977). *How Americans use time: A social-psychological analysis of everyday behavior.* New York: Praeger.

Rybczynski, W. (1991). *Waiting for the weekend.* Harmondsworth, England: Penguin Books.

Sarbin, T. R. (1989). Emotions as narrative emplotments. In J. M. Packer & R. B. Addison (Eds.), *Entering the circle: Hermeneutic investigation in psychology* (pp. 180-201). New York: State University of New York Press.

Schor, J. B. (1991). *The overworked American: The unexpected decline of leisure.* New York: Basic Books.

Scott, D., & Willits, F. K. (1989). Adolescent and adult leisure patterns: A 37 year follow-up study. *Leisure sciences, 11*(4), 323-336.

Seleen, D. (1982). The congruence between actual and desired use of time by older adults: A predictor of life satisfaction. *The Gerontologist, 22*(6), 95-99.

Shannon, P. D. (1970). The work-play model: A basis for occupational therapy programming in psychiatry. *The American Journal of Occupational Therapy, 24*(3), 215-218.

Sjoberg, L., & Magneberg, R. (1990). Action and emotion in everyday life. *Scandinavian Journal of Psychology, 31,* 9-27.

Slagle, E. C. (1922). Training aids for mental patients. *Archives of occupational therapy, 1,* 11-17,

Smith, C., & Wong, P. T. P. (1991). Paradoxical sleep increases predict successful learning in a complex operant task. *Behavioral Neuroscience, 105,* 282-288.

Sobel, M. E. (1981). *Lifestyle and social structure: Concepts, definitions, analysis.* New York: Academic Press.

Steiner, L. P., Looney, S. W., Hall, L. R., & Wright, K. M. (1995). Quality of life and functional status among homeless men attending a day shelter in Louisville, Kentucky. *Journal of the Kentucky Medical Association, 93*(5), 188-95.

Stones, M. J., & Kozma, A. (1986). Happiness and activities as propensities. *Journal of Gerontology, 41*(1), 85-90.

Szalai, A. (Ed.). (1972). *The use of time.* The Hague: Mouton.

Takata, N. (1969). The play history. *American Journal of Occupational Therapy, 23,* 314-318.

Takata, N. (1971). The play milieu—a preliminary proposal. *American Journal of Occupational Therapy, 25,* 281-292.

Tinsley, H. E., & Eldredge, B. D. (1995). Psychological benefits of leisure participation: A taxonomy of leisure activities based on their need gratifying properties. *Journal of Counseling Psychology, 42*(2), 123-132.

Tinsley, H. E., & Tinsley, D. J. (1982). A holistic model of leisure counseling. *Journal of Leisure Research, 14,* 100-116.

Trombly, C. A. (1995). Occupation: Purposefulness and meaningfulness as therapeutic mechanisms. The 1995 Eleanor Clarke Slagle Lecture. *American Journal of Occupational Therapy, 49,* 960-72.

Watanabe, S. (1968). Four concepts basic to the occupational therapy process. *American Journal of Occupational Therapy, 22,* 23-29.

Webb, W. B. (1983). Theories in modern sleep research. In A. Mayes (Ed.), *Sleep mechanisms and functions in humans and animals—an evolutionary perspective* (pp. 1-17). Wokingham, England: Van Nostrand-Reinhold.

Wesman, A. E. (1973). Personality and the subjective experience of time. *Journal of Personality Assessment, 37,* 103-114.

West, W. L. (1984). A reaffirmed philosophy and practice of occupational therapy for the 1980's. *American Journal of Occupational Therapy, 38,* 15-23.

Wilcock, A. (1993). A theory of the human need for occupation. *Occupational Science: Australia, 1*(1), 17-24.

Wood, W. (1993). Occupation and the relevance of primatology. *American Journal of Occupational Therapy, 47*(5), 515-528.

Wood, W. (1996). The value of studying occupation: An example with primate play. *American Journal of Occupational Therapy, 50*(5), 327-336.

Yerxa, E. J. (1988). Oversimplification: The hobgoblin of theory and practice in occupational therapy. *Canadian Journal of Occupational Therapy, 55,* 5-6.

Yerxa, E. J. (1991). Seeking a relevant, ethical and realistic way of knowing for occupational therapy. *American Journal of Occupational Therapy, 45,* 199-204.

Yerxa, E. J. (1995). Nationally speaking—Who is the keeper of occupational therapy's practice and knowledge? *American Journal of Occupational Therapy, 49,* 295-299.

Yerxa, E. J., Clark, F., Frank, G., Jackson, J., Parham, D., Pierce D., Stein, C., & Zemke, R. (1989). An introduction to occupational science: A foundation for occupational therapy in the 21st century. *Occupational Therapy in Health Care, 6*(1), 4.

Yerxa, E. J., & Locker, S. B. (1990). Quality of time use by adults with spinal cord injury. *American Journal of Occupational Therapy, 44*(4), 318-327.

Young, M. (1988). *The metronomic society*. Cambridge: Harvard University Press.

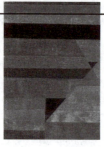

Chapter Content Outline

Abstract

Professional behaviors are built on a solid understanding of the key values and ethics of a field. This chapter introduces the developing practitioner to historical events, key relationships, values, ethics, and terminology that can be used by the clinician to shape interactions with clients and colleagues. It provides the core elements to help the clinician adopt an identity that will make a contribution, not only to the clients the clinician will serve but to the institutions who will employ him or her to provide services that will improve the health and well-being of a community.

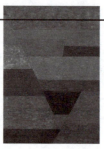

Key Terms

Client-centered

Disability

Disorder

Environmental (extrinsic) factors

Frames of reference

Function

Functional limitations

Handicapping situation

Health

Impairments

Occupational performance

Occupation

Pathophysiology

Person (intrinsic) factors

Social disadvantage

Societal limitations

Transaction

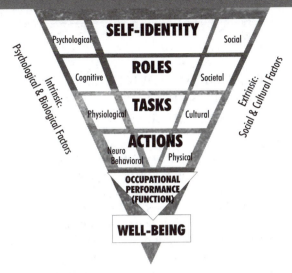

The Occupational Therapy Context

Philosophy- Principles- Practice

Carolyn Baum, PhD, OTR/C, FAOTA, Charles Christiansen, EdD, OTR, OT(C), FAOTA

OBJECTIVES

The information in this chapter is intended to help the reader:

1. understand that occupation is a key determinant of function and well-being

2. contrast the primary purposes of medicine and occupational therapy

3. articulate the profession's key values and ethics

4. understand key occupational therapy terms and how they relate to rehabilitation

5. have a general understanding of systems theory as a framework for evolving occupational therapy models

6. understand the interplay of person, environment and occupation that results in a transaction that is the unique contribution of occupational therapy to clients whose independence in threatened with disabling conditions.

"Our conception of man is that of an organism that maintains and balances itself in the world of reality and actuality by being in active life and active use."

Adolph Meyer, 1922

Early Occupational Therapy Leader
Eleanor Clarke Slagle
1876-1942

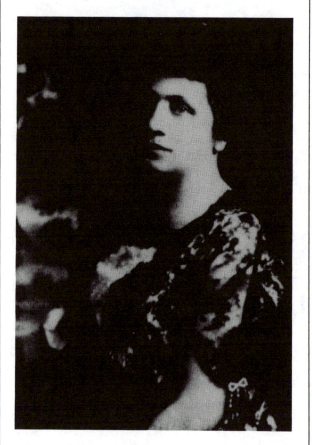

Eleanor Clarke Slagle: 1876-1942, the daughter of a prominent architect, was a founder of the Society for the Promotion of Occupation Therapy, now known as the American Occupational Therapy Association (AOTA). As an associate of Adolph Meyer and William Rush Dunton, she developed an appreciation for the importance of occupation to health and well-being, and served as the founding director for the Henry P. Favill School of Occupations in Chicago, the first organized school for occupational therapists in the United States. Later, she became the Director of Occupational Therapy for the New York State Department of Mental Hygiene, a position she held from 1921 until 1942. A strong leader and organizing influence of the AOTA, Mrs. Slagle was named honorary president in 1937 at a ceremony attended by Eleanor Roosevelt. Today, her legacy of strong leadership and devotion to challenge lives on in the Eleanor Clarke Slagle lectureship, one of the most prestigious honors awarded by the American Occupational Therapy Association. *From Bing, RK, Eleanor Clarke Slagle lectureship— 1981—Occupational Therapy revisited: a paraphrastic journey. American Journal of Occupational Therapy, 35(8), 511. Copyright 1981 by the American Occupational Therapy Association. Reprinted with permission.*

EVOLUTION OF AN IDENTITY: FRAMING THE NEED FOR OCCUPATIONAL THERAPY

Just as good health is often taken for granted, so too are everyday life experiences. The satisfaction of dining with friends and family, enjoying a walk in the park, or gaining a sense of accomplishment from seeing a garden blossom can be diminished by impaired senses, or diminished strength or movement resulting from injury or disease. But they need not be. The remarkable adaptability of the human body and the power of meaning and self-will provide many ways for people to derive satisfaction from life despite temporary or permanent limitations in function. When these resources are coupled with the skillful intervention of the occupational therapist, health-related functional performance limitations can often be overcome.

Whether the reason for a disruption in one's ability to perform daily activities is temporary, such as with the inconvenience of a broken arm, or permanent, such as that resulting from a traumatic injury that caused brain or structural injuries, the occupational therapist has the knowledge to help the person address the problems that limit functional performance. Through strategies of adaptation or compensation, occupational therapy makes it possible for the tasks and roles that are necessary to maintain daily life to continue.

Viewing health in the context of daily living has been a distinguishing characteristic of occupational therapy since its inception early in the 20th century. And while history has influenced its settings and modalities, occupational therapy has remained committed to its original purpose: that of helping people cope with the challenges of everyday living imposed by congenital anomalies, physical and emotional illnesses, accidents, the aging process, or environmental restriction.

The science supporting occupational therapy practice is evolving rapidly. It is important for the student and practitioner to be aware of recent developments so that intervention can be designed to take advantage of available knowledge. History is the best teacher. This is evident in the resurgence of many concepts that were first proposed when the field was founded, but lay dormant for many years. Occupational therapy will be better prepared to accommodate and influence the changes affecting health care tomorrow if we understand where we are today and how we got here. This requires a basic understanding of the history of Western medicine and a

Bibliographic citation of this chapter: Baum, C. & Christiansen, C. (1997). The occupational therapy context: Philosophy-principles-practice. In C. Christiansen & C. Baum (Eds.), *Occupational therapy: Enabling function and well-being* (2nd Ed.). Thorofare, NJ: SLACK Incorporated.

familiarity with early occupational therapy leaders and the ideas that influenced them (Bing, 1981).

AN HISTORICAL PERSPECTIVE

Occupational therapy is described as a health discipline rather than a medical discipline, because to be interested in the effects of disease or injury on everyday living is a uniquely non-medical phenomenon, at least as far as Western medicine has been concerned. This is because, traditionally, allopathic or traditional medicine has been organized around a mechanistic cause and effect model of scientific thought.

This mechanistic view had its roots in the 17th century work of the French philosopher and scientist, René Descartes, who believed that the mind and body should be viewed as separate. He emphasized a scientific approach based on reducing structures to their component parts and subjecting the parts to careful analysis. This approach led to the development of the germ theory of disease, advanced by the work of Koch and Pasteur, which further solidified a view of medical practice based on diagnosis and treatment. Today, the idea persists that the human being, like a machine, can be taken apart and reassembled if its structure and function are sufficiently well understood. It is commonly believed that simple cause and effect relationships can be used to explain most disease processes.

It is true that this tendency to explain by reducing the body to parts, such as bones, organs and cells, has been useful in helping medical science to explain the cause and identify the cure of many diseases and physical disorders. However, English bioscientist Thomas McKeown (1978) has argued convincingly that many other factors unrelated to medical intervention can also be used to explain the dramatic improvement in life expectancy over the past 150 years. Specifically, improved sanitation, nutrition, and birth control have each been identified as having played an important role in improving health status and life expectancy. Perhaps these factors are appreciated less than "miracle drugs" or vaccines because they are behavioral rather than mechanistic in nature and thus have not "fit well" within the orientation of contemporary medicine.

As described in Chapter 1, this preoccupation with component parts is frequently referred to as *reductionism*, and is reflected in the everyday use of medical terminology. Consider the word "function." Used by an occupational therapist, the term describes a behavior related to the performance of an activity, a task, or a role. In medicine, however, the term "function" is most often interpreted in its reductionistic sense, with biomedical scientists referring to the "function" of human organs; as reflected in such expressions as "pulmonary function" or "liver function."

Paradoxically, the successes of reductionistic practices in

The Roots of Occupational Therapy as Viewed by a Prominent Historian

In 1981, Dr. Robert K. Bing, professor of occupational therapy at the University of Texas Medical Branch in Galveston, identified several recurring patterns and themes in the history of occupational therapy (and before) as part of his Eleanor Clarke Slagle lecture. These themes and patterns are enduring philosophies:

1. There is an inextricable union of the mind and body; the employment of activity or occupation must be based on this precept, which is unique to occupational therapy.

2. Activity, inherently, contains modes the [individual] may employ to gain understanding of and ascendancy over one's feelings, actions and thoughts; these modes include the habits of attention and interest, the perceived usefulness of occupation as creative expression, the processes of learning, the acquisition of skill, and evidence of accomplishment.

3. Activity provides a balance between the practical and intellectual components of experience; therefore, a wide variety of activities must be accessible to meet human objectives for work, leisure and rest.

4. [The occupational therapist's] approach to the [person] is as significant to treatment and rehabilitation as is the selection and utilization of an activity.

5. Essential elements of occupational therapy practice are continuous observation, experimentation, empiricism, and analysis.

6. An appreciation of the pain that accompanies any illness or disability; a strong desire to reduce or remove it; a gentle firmness; and a knowledge of the patient's needs [and goals] are fundamental characteristics of the provider of therapeutic occupations.

7. Therapeutic processes and modes of treatment are synonymous with the processes of learning and methods of education.

8. The [person] is the product of his or her own efforts, not the article made nor the activity accomplished.

From Bing, R. K. (1981). Occupational therapy revisited: A paraphrastic journey. *American Journal of Occupational Therapy, 35*(8), 499-518.

---

medicine have helped emphasize their shortcomings. For example, it has been noted that developments in medicine and surgery during the past 50 years have prevented the deaths of thousands of persons who were critically ill, including many casualties from the World Wars. However, although a large number of these individuals have survived, they have been left

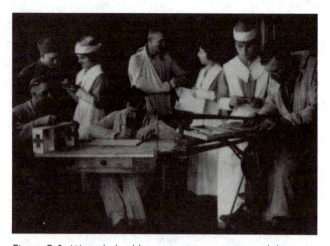

Figure 2-1. Wounded soldiers receiving occupational therapy at Camp Grant, Illinois, 1919. From Stattel, F. (1977). Occupational therapy: A sense of the past—focus on the present. *American Journal of Occupational Therapy, 31*(10), 649. Reprinted with permission.

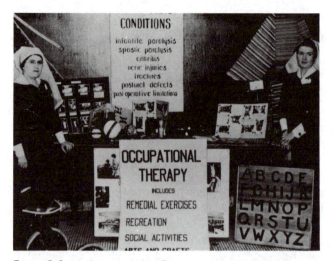

Figure 2-2. Medicine's early influence on occupational therapy is evident in this photo of an occupational therapy display at the Canadian National Exhibition, Toronto, Ontario, in the early 1930s. Photo courtesy the Canadian Association of Occupational Therapists.

with disabilities such as paralysis and amputations, for which medicine has no "cure." The specialty of physical medicine and rehabilitation was created in response to the needs of persons with disabling conditions, whose numbers have grown with developments in emergency medicine and trauma care. Advances in neonatal medicine have also led to the survival of greater numbers of infants with congenital problems who also require rehabilitation for their disabilities (Delisa, Martin & Currie, 1997) to overcome or avoid disabilities that can limit their potential to live independent lives (Figure 2-1).

HISTORICAL INFLUENCES OF MEDICINE

Medicine's successes with the reductionistic approach have also influenced the history of occupational therapy practice. For several decades beginning in the 1930s, practice became progressively less influenced by a view of function which was holistic and occupation-centered, in favor of practice techniques that emphasized components of function such as muscle strength, range of motion or disturbed thought processes. In fact, from the mid 1960s to the mid 1980s in the United States, occupational therapy's reimbursement was directly related to documentation of components of function. In this orientation, little consideration was given to how these components affected performance in day-to-day living. Fortunately, in the late 1970s, several prominent writers in the field expressed concern for this state of affairs and encouraged a return to the occupation-centered philosophy upon which the profession was first established (Figure 2-2).

Prominent among these was an article entitled "The

Derailment of Occupational Therapy," by Philip Shannon (1977). Shannon wrote:

> *"A new hypothesis has emerged that views man not as a creative being, capable of making choices and directing his own future, but as a mechanistic creature susceptible to manipulation and control via the application of techniques. The technique hypothesis, inspired by the principles of reductionism, subverts the occupational therapy hypothesis of man using his hands to influence the state of his own health"* (p. 233).

Later in the same year, Kielhofner and Burke (1977) provided a detailed account of various bases for practice during the first 60 years of occupational therapy in the United States. They traced the evolution of guiding principles in the field from its humanistic roots to the competing ideas of the 80s, noting that the paradigm of reductionism was reflected in three dominant treatment models that continued to influence practice. These were the kinesiological model, the psychoanalytic or interpersonal model, and the sensory integrative or neurological model. The authors concluded that advancement of the field would require a theoretical approach that went "beyond reductionism" and allowed an understanding of human adaptation, or "social man within a holistic theoretical framework."

In further emphasizing the distinction between occupational therapy and medicine, Rogers (1982) examined medicine and occupational therapy according to their views of the concepts of order, disorder and control. In her analysis, the concept of order refers to a desired state of affairs, which as

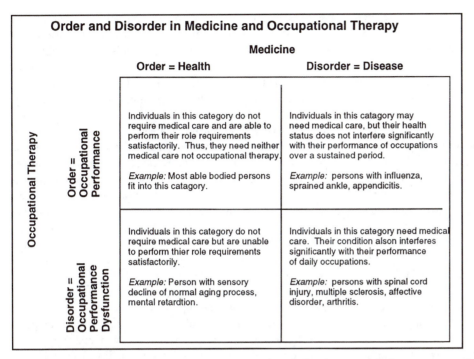

Figure 2-3. Order and disorder in medicine and occupational therapy. Adapted from Rogers, J. (1982). Order and disorder in medicine and occupational therapy. *American Journal of Occupational Therapy, 31*(1), 29-35.

defined by medicine is an absence of disease, and as defined by occupational therapy is competence in the performance of work, play or self-care "occupations." In contrast, disorder is defined as disease in medicine, and performance dysfunction in occupational therapy. Since access to occupational therapy services is greatly influenced by medical decisions, individuals who experience occupational performance problems that are not accompanied by disease have difficulty gaining access to occupational therapy services. On the other hand, there exists a category of individuals who require medical care but for whom no occupational therapy is required—because their conditions do not result in occupational performance dysfunction. Finally, many categories of illness and disease can result in impairment which influences occupational performance. According to Rogers, persons in this category constitute that group for whom occupational therapy services are most likely to be provided. In her comparative analysis, Rogers argued convincingly that through their emphasis on disease and functional deficit rather than occupational performance and competence, the biomedical influences on traditional health care have been a limiting factor in the development of occupational therapy (Figure 2-3).

A SHIFTING PARADIGM IN MEDICINE AND HEALTH CARE

As we approach the turn of the century, many health care systems are making a dramatic shift from a biomedical, acute-centered, and provider-driven approach to one that shares with the consumer the responsibility of employing healthy behaviors. This shift puts a much greater focus on occupational performance and the perceived well-being of the client, bringing occupational therapy and its body of knowledge to an advantageous position in the delivery of health care services. This approach requires the occupational therapist to focus on the long-term health needs of people and help them develop healthy behaviors which not only improve their health, but also minimize health-related costs associated with dysfunction (Baum & Law, 1997). The health professional of the future will be one who collaborates with patients and clients to plan and implement care, is able to communicate effectively, and works in teams to meet the primary health needs of the public (O'Neill, 1991). In the case of the occupational therapist, the successful clinician will assist clients to become actively engaged in their life activities.

This client-centered approach requires the occupational therapist to work collaboratively with individuals in the client's environment (family, teachers, independent living specialists, employers, neighbors, friends) to assist the client to obtain the skills and make the modifications to remove barriers that would create a social disadvantage (Baum & Law, 1997). This expanded role extends beyond the traditional biomedical approach to incorporate a broader socio-medical purpose, such as taking an active role in building healthy communities. In North America, the term "healthy communities" reflects an active recognition that the social, political and economic conditions of a region also influence health, and must be included in planning effective health delivery systems (Stern, 1990).

With the shifting paradigm in medicine, occupational therapy practice patterns are rapidly shifting. Occupational therapy practice has evolved to address the needs of persons in a number of environments which include health institutions, schools, work sites, and community (Baum & Law, 1997). As disability has become recognized as a public health problem, affecting not only individuals with disabling conditions and their immediate families, but also society (Pope & Tarlov, 1991) new approaches to care have emerged which are calling on occupational therapy skills.

About 35 million Americans (Pope & Tarlov, 1991), and 4 million Canadians (Statistics Canada, 1992), have a physical or mental impairment that interferes with their daily activities. This represents about 15% of the populations of each country. Yet only one in four persons with disability are so severe that they cannot work or participate in their communities (Baum & Law, 1997). Statistics are similar in other countries.

The definition of health has shifted from the absence of disease to address the physical, mental, and social well-being of the person and includes a focus on the individual's ability to function optimally in his or her environment. With this shift, a greater emphasis has been placed on health promotion and disease prevention and building healthy, supportive communities to reduce illness, disability and death. This approach addresses the importance of improving the physical environment and ensuring accessible and affordable health services for all (Premier's Council on Health, Well-being and Social Justice, 1993). Finally, the opportunities for occupational therapy to influence the health and function of persons with chronic disease or disabilities are moving into the mainstream.

As systems of health care change, society is also changing from a manufacturing to an information society (Drucker, 1989). These changes are having a profound impact on how business is conducted and how health care is delivered. To be effective in an information-oriented society, the effectiveness of services must be known. Occupational therapists must make their services understood by providers and clients who do not have an in-depth knowledge of health issues.

Another effect of the change to an information society has come to be known as the knowledge explosion. So much knowledge is available (and is changing so rapidly) that many occupational therapists have opted to become specialists as a way of limiting the knowledge required for them to know to be competent in practice. The need to access, interpret, and manage information efficiently requires changes in how therapists organize work.

To effectively meet the needs of their clients, therapists must work collaboratively, not so much across disciplines, but in project teams. For example, rather than working as a specialist with the sensory integrative needs of children, occupational therapists are now working on teams (clinical service lines) addressing the rehabilitation or habilitation needs of children as the experts in occupational performance. This expertise goes far beyond the child's sensory integrative needs to include all factors that affect the child's performance, including the school and family environment.

The payment structures supporting health care are changing in many countries. The business community and government, as well as the consumer, are asking questions about the value of services, demanding that satisfactory outcomes be obtained at reasonable costs. Because information technology now enables the linking of demographics, service provision, and outcome data, changes are occurring in the nature of practice. Many therapists (and other providers) are required to document treatment effectiveness by entering standard data into large data sets. There are many possible outcomes which can be used to determine service efficiency and value. Occupational therapists must be consistent in recognizing that their outcome is the client's reported improvement in occupational performance.

Outcomes are the results of care. After surgical amputation following trauma, the patient recovers and is typically discharged, often to a rehabilitation facility. This may take more or less time depending upon the health of the patient, his or her age, and whether complications (such as a post-surgical infection) occurred. The outcomes which could be examined in such an instance might include (among others) how long the patient was hospitalized, how satisfied the patient was with the hospitalization, and how much the episode of care cost.

The selection of outcomes is highly value-laden and depends on what is important to the person selecting the outcome. The total length of stay is important to the accountant and economist because these influence the overall cost of care. The occurrence of infections following surgery is important to the surgeon, nurse and epidemiologist, because these may reflect the competence of care. The amount of pain and discomfort, and the disruption of life caused by hospitalization, are important to all patients, because these influence the experience of care.

With patients who are discharged with altered life circumstances, (such as impaired cognitive function or paralysis) there is also the need to measure how well a person adapts to new life challenges, an altered self-identity, and social barriers. These outcomes may not be known for some time following discharge, and even then the extent to which the health care system and its rehabilitation providers contributed to that outcome will be difficult to determine. The point to be made is that quality and value are highly subjective dimensions, and that outcomes of interest to rehabilitation providers may be different than those of economists, surgeons, and others. They should, however, measure whether or not the patient or client is able to participate in those aspects of living necessary for meaning and satisfaction. In this respect, they will be closely aligned to the outcomes of importance to the client and relate to the client's perceived well-being.

If the client's goals are to be chief breadwinner in the family, rough-house with his dogs, and provide stability or be a good example for his son, how motivated will he be for interventions that are not a visible link for him to those goals? It is a challenge to the occupational therapist to use his or her knowledge to remove barriers to those goals through occupation and environmental modification. Perhaps the intervention can include vocational related tasks, a fitness program that involves his son, and maybe even his dogs. Not all occupational therapy needs to be delivered one to one by the clinician. In fact, it is more important to transfer the responsibility of recovery to the client early on who then organizes his or her own resources to maintain progress. In this way, the occupational therapist has become a coach and engages with the client in problem resolution. The outcome will result in a greater sense of well-being because the client is able to do that which he or she wants to do.

Another client states her goals to be the ability to organize her kitchen and her house, to plan ahead when she shops and the ability to do multiple tasks. These are realistic goals, but not goals that can be accomplished in a rehabilitation clinic. People with brain injury require strategies that involve new learning, and new learning in context. These goals, if met, will lead to improved satisfaction and well-being. Achieving these outcomes is facilitated when a patient or client and his or her family have the knowledge and skill to participate in recovery and to learn the behaviors that will sustain health and function over time. Being effective in this era of health care requires highly educated individuals who know how to work with and achieve the goals for the client and at the same time contribute to the goals of the organization as a whole.

PHILOSOPHICAL INFLUENCES ON PRACTICE

The values, beliefs and principles of a discipline have a major influence on its identity and development, and are known collectively as its *philosophy*. Shannon (1986) points out that philosophical issues fall into three dimensions: addressing the nature of humankind (metaphysics), how we come to know (epistemology) and values (axiology), which include beliefs about what is desirable and how we should conduct ourselves (p. 27).

Bockhoven (1971) and others have argued that the philosophical roots of occupational therapy practice can be traced to the moral treatment movement reflected in practices of some early 19th century mental hospitals. These approaches were designed to promote adaptation through involving patients in various activities which would promote the establishment of cultural values and moral principles.

Adolph Meyer, a noted psychiatrist and neurobiologist who taught at Johns Hopkins University and was a proponent of occupational therapy during its early years, is widely credited with making an important contribution to the development of philosophy in the field. In an address given at the fifth annual meeting of the National Society for the Promotion of Occupational Therapy at Baltimore, Maryland in 1921, Meyer suggested that occupational therapy represented an important manifestation of human philosophy, namely, "the valuation of time and work" (1922, p. 6) and the role of performance and completion in bringing meaning to life.

Meyer wrote that "man learns to organize time and he does it in terms of doing things" (p. 6), thus emphasizing his view of the importance of doing to achieving self-fulfillment. Meyer suggested that the view of mental illness as a problem of living rather than a structural, toxic or constitutional disorder, was an important characteristic of the field, and that occupational therapists could provide opportunities for the individual to work, to plan, to create, and to learn to use tools and materials. These opportunities, thought Meyer, would assist patients in gaining pleasure and pride in achievement. If we were to apply these concepts in today's practice, we would provide patients with an opportunity to use their minds in planning, organizing, sequencing, and carrying out a task (executive skills).

In summarizing Meyer's address, we can observe that he viewed the individual and health in a holistic rather than structural sense, and believed that engagement in occupations, or doing, provided a sense of reality, achievement and temporal organization. Meyer perceived occupational therapy as providing opportunities for engagement which would contribute to learning and improving one's sense of fulfillment and self-esteem. In doing so, he was proclaiming occupational therapy's concern for quality of life, and suggesting a clear relationship between the ability to perform daily occupations and one's life satisfaction (Figure 2-4).

Meyer's themes have been repeated in more recent contributions by scholars reflecting on the unique characteristics of the field. For example, Yerxa (1967) in her Eleanor Clarke Slagle address, emphasized the role of occupational therapy in providing opportunities for fulfillment in doing when she wrote:

"In occupational therapy, the patient experiences the reality of his physical environment and his capacity to function within it. Our clinics may be chambers of horror for some individuals as they confront their physical disability for the first time by trying to do

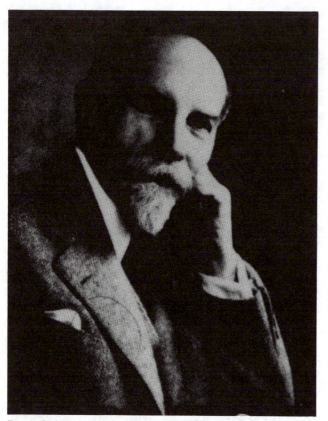

Figure 2-4. Dr. Adolph Meyer, early occupational therapy proponent and philosopher. (Fabian Bachrach photo.) Courtesy of the Archives of the American Psychiatric Association.

something, perhaps as simple as self-feeding. Yet, if the individual is to function with self actualization, he must discover both his limitations and his possibilities. We meet our responsibilities to the client when we provide opportunities to readjust his or her value system through the development of both new capacities and the ability to substitute for some lost capacities. We are like mirrors which can reflect, without the distortion of wish-fulfillment or self-deprecation, a true image of the client's potential" (p. 5).

Similarly, Fidler and Fidler (1978) emphasized the role of occupation, or doing, in gaining self-actualization when they wrote:

"The ability to adapt, to cope with the problems of everyday living, and to fulfill age-specific life roles requires a rich reservoir of experiences gathered from direct engagement with both human and non-human objects in one's environment. Doing is a process of investigating, trying out, and gaining evidence of one's capacities for experiencing, responding, managing, creating, and controlling. It is

through such action with feedback from both non-human and human objects that an individual comes to know the potential and limitations of self and the environment and achieves a sense of competence and intrinsic worth" (p. 306).

Both Elizabeth Yerxa and the Fidlers reaffirmed Adolph Meyer's beliefs and values in the opportunities occupational therapy affords for self-actualization. They also emphasized the role of the therapist in assisting the individual to cope with problems of everyday living and to adapt to limitations that interfere with competent role performance.

These philosophical foundations of practice must also be viewed in the wider context of cultural values. Western societies often value activity and self-reliance as contrasted with passivity and dependence. Bockhoven (1971) points out that moral treatment was influenced by cultural attitudes of communities in the Northeastern United States in the early nineteenth century. An important characteristic of this culture, derived from political and religious beliefs, was a respect for human individuality and rights of independent self-expression. To be sure, the widespread belief in the virtues of independence and self-reliance continue in some cultures. Perhaps because of this, there has been public support for the goals of rehabilitation when expressed in terms of increasing the patient's independence. As a rehabilitation discipline, occupational therapy has also inculcated this value, as reflected in some definitions of the field (Figure 2-5).

Rogers (1982) declared that functional independence is not only the core concept of occupational therapy theory, but also the goal of the occupational therapy process. Noting that the requirements for independence are competence and autonomy, she suggested that autonomy is reflected in the ability to make choices and have control over the environment. The opportunities afforded within occupational therapy practice for developing competence and teaching strategies for exerting autonomy make it unique among the rehabilitation disciplines.

This uniqueness led Engelhardt, a physician and philosopher, to describe occupational therapy as reflecting a "praxial," rather than a somatic, psychological, or even social work model of practice. Derived from the Greek word "praxis," or use of knowledge and skills, the term "praxial" captures the adaptive nature of engagement in occupations.

"In viewing humans as engaged in activities, realizing themselves through their occupation, occupational therapy supports a view of the whole person in function and adaptation often absent in somatic medicine, the psychological health care professions, and social work as well. The virtue of occupational therapy is engagement in the world" (Engelhardt, 1977, p. 672).

Year	Definition	Source
1922	Any activity, mental or physical, definitely prescribed and guided for the distinct purpose of contributing to, and hastening recovery from disease or injury.	Pattison, H.A. The trend of occupational therapy for the tuberculosis. Archives of Occupational Therapy,1: 19-24.
1947	Any activity, mental or physical, medically prescribed and professionally guided to aid a patient in recovery from disease or injury.	McNary, H. (1947) The scope of occupational therapy. In Willard, HS and Spackman, CS (Eds) Occupational Therapy. Philadelphia, JB Lippincott, p. 10
1962	Occupational therapy is the art and science of directing man's response to selected activity to promote and maintain health, to prevent disability, to evaluate behavior and to treat or train patients with physical or psychosocial dysfunction.	Official Definition Adopted by the Executive Board of the American Occupational Therapy Association, January, 1969
1972	The art and science of directing man's participation in selected tasks to restore, reinforce and enhance performance, facilitate learning of the skills and functions essential for adaptation and productivity, diminish or correct pathology, and to promote and maintain health.	Council on Standards, AOTA. Occupational Therapy: Its definition and functions.American Journal of Occupational Therapy, 26, 204-5, 1972.
1977	Occupational therapy is the application of occupation, any activity in which one engages for evaluation, diagnosis, and treatment of problems interfering with functional performance in persons impaired by physical illness or injury, emotional disorder, congenital or developmental disability or the aging process in order to achieve optimum functioning and for prevention and health maintenance.	AOTA Representative Assembly: Minutes. American Journal of Occupational Therapy, 31:599, 1977.
1981	Occupational therapy is use of purposeful activity with individuals who are limited by physical injury or illness, psychosocial dysfunction, developmental or learning disabilities, poverty and cultural differences, or the aging process in order to maximize independence, prevent disability and maintain health. The practice encompasses evaluation, treatment and consultation. Specific occupational therapy services include: teaching daily living skills, developing perceptual motor skills and sensory integrative functioning, developing play skills and prevocational and leisure capacities; designing and fabricating or applying selected orthotic and prosthetic devices and equipment; using specifically designed crafts and exercises to enhance functional performance; administering and interpreting tests such as manual muscle and range of motion; and adapting environments for the handicapped. These services are provided individually, in groups, or through social systems.	Official Definition for Licensure. Adopted by the AOTA Representative Assembly. Published in Minutes. Representative Assembly. American Journal of Occupational Therapy, 35, 798, 1981.
1986	Therapeutic use of self care-work and play activities to increase independent function, enhance development and prevent disability. May include adaptation of task or environment to achieve maximum independence and to enhance the quality of life.	AOTA Representative assembly, Minutes. American Journal of Occupational Therapy, 40, 852, 1986.

Figure 2-5. Views of occupational therapy as reflected in definitions of practice.

INDEPENDENCE AND INTERDEPENDENCE

The more recent rehabilitation literature has questioned the wisdom of declaring independence as an absolute goal in rehabilitation (Christiansen, 1994; Grady, 1995; Meier & Purtilo, 1994). The term "interdependence" communicates that those in societies depend on collaboration and cooperation, and that no community dwelling individual is truly independent. It also suggests that we can achieve something greater working with others than we can achieve working on our own. The concept of interdependence is embodied within the idea of occupational therapy as a helping profession. That is, by working with our clients and their families, we can achieve goals that we could not achieve working independently (Clark, Corcoran & Gitlin, 1995).

It is useful to conclude this section on the philosophical roots of occupational therapy by highlighting key beliefs and values which influence practice.

• "[A human] is an organism that maintains and balances itself in the world of reality and actuality by being in active life and active use...It is the use that we make of ourselves that gives the ultimate stamp to our every organ" (Meyer, 1922, p.1).

- Reilly (1962) suggests that human beings need to produce, create, master and improve their environment in order to achieve health and well-being.

- Fidler & Fidler (1963) conceptualized activity as a valuable vehicle to acquire, maintain or redevelop skills necessary to fulfill occupational roles and provide satisfaction.

- Individuals who perceive that they have control over their environments and can address obstacles derive satisfaction from their occupational roles (Burke, 1977; Sharrott and Cooper-Fraps, 1986).

- Function results from a series of complex relationships among cognitive, psychological, sensory, neuromotor, and physiological capabilities as the individual interacts with his or her environment (Christiansen, 1991).

- Occupational dysfunction can be viewed as a "breakdown in habits that leads to physiological deterioration with the concomitant loss of ability to perform competently in daily life" (Kielhofner, 1992, p. 30).

- When occupational therapists present the opportunity for individuals to engage in activity, not only does the individual's functional status improve (Baum, 1995), but occupational therapy makes explicit its unique contribution to the enhancement of human function.

- "...purposeful and fulfilling occupations can provide individuals with sufficient exercise to maintain homeostasis, to keep body parts and neuronal physiology and mental capacities functioning at peak efficiency, and enable maintenance and development of satisfying and stimulating social relationships.... if they are able, or encouraged to pursue this need, they will, apart from supplying sustenance for survival and safety, enhance their health" (Wilcock, 1993, p. 23).

These points can be summarized into the following enduring values which can serve as hypotheses for guiding treatment and should challenge students and faculty into action to empirically test these core principles.

1. Engagement in occupation is of value because it provides opportunities for individuals to influence their well-being by gaining fulfillment in living.

2. Through the experience of occupation (or doing), the individual is able to achieve mastery and competence by learning skills and strategies necessary for coping with problems and adapting to limitations.

3. As competence is gained and autonomy can be expressed, independence is achieved.

4. Autonomy implies choice and control over environmental circumstances. Thus, opportunities for exerting self-determination should be reflected in intervention strategies.

5. Choice and control extend to decisions about intervention, thus identifying occupational therapy as a collaborative process between the therapist and recipient of care. In this collaboration, the patient's values are respected.

6. Because of its focus on life performance, occupational therapy is neither somatic nor psychological, but concerned with the unity of body and mind in doing.

REFLECTING PHILOSOPHICAL VALUES IN PRACTICE: OCCUPATIONAL THERAPY ETHICS

The ethics of a profession are influenced by its founding beliefs and values, and no general text can be considered complete without addressing this aspect of practice. Ethics are philosophical stands on the rightness or appropriateness of various voluntary actions. The adoption of ethical principles is one characteristic often used to distinguish professions from other occupations (Vollmer & Mills, 1966).

Ethical principles form the basis for judgments and actions in practice. In acknowledging this, Rogers (1983) writes: "The ultimate question we, as clinicians, are challenged to answer is: What, among the many things that could be done for this patient, ought to be done? This is an ethical question" (p. 602).

This view has been substantiated by Hansen (1984, 1988), who studied the ethical dilemmas faced by occupational therapists in their daily practice. She found that deciding which type of treatment would be most effective was the most common. Other common ethical dilemmas faced by therapists included deciding whether to receive and act on referrals that are inappropriate, being unable to provide adequate therapy because of constraints in the work setting, and resolving disagreements between the therapist and patient or patient and family regarding treatment goals.

The most recent ethical document approved by the American Occupational Therapy Association (1994) identifies six principles of ethical responsibility ranging from concern for the welfare and dignity of the recipient of service to avoiding conflicts of interest. Future versions will incorporate the important ethics related to research. These include principles of informed consent, freedom of subjects to participate without coercion or prejudice, and integrity in data analysis and reporting. Ethical principles have meaning only inasmuch as they are reflected in the day-to-day practices of those who subscribe to them. Thus, it is incumbent on all practitioners in occupational therapy to be familiar with the principles and use them as guides to professional behavior (Figure 2-6).

Occupational Therapy Code of Ethics

Adopted by the Representative Assembly
American Occupational Therapy Association
July, 1994

PRINCIPLE 1: BENEFICENCE

Occupational therapy personnel shall demonstrate a concern for the well-being of the recipients of their services.

PRINCIPLE 2: AUTONOMY, PRIVACY, CONFIDENTIALITY

Occupational therapy personnel shall respect the rights of the recipients of the services.

PRINCIPLE 3: DUTIES

Occupational therapy personnel shall achieve and continually maintain high standards of competence.

PRINCIPLE 4: JUSTICE

Occupational therapy personnel shall comply with laws and Association policies guiding the profession of occupational therapy.

PRINCIPLE 5: VERACITY

Occupational therapy personnel shall provide accurate information about occupational therapy services.

PRINCIPLE 6: FIDELITY, VERACITY

Occupational therapy personnel shall treat colleagues and other professions with fairness, discretion and integrity.

Figure 2-6. Occupational Therapy Code of Ethics. Reprinted with permission from the American Occupational Therapy Association.

DESCRIBING DISABILITY: KEY TERMS AND DEFINITIONS

An understanding of several key concepts is necessary to appreciate fully how occupational therapy fits into the larger context of medicine and rehabilitation. Concepts from the World Health Organization (WHO) as well as the National Center for Medical Rehabilitation Research (NCMRR) in the United States are useful here. We acknowledge the pioneering work of Nagi (1976), who was among the first to examine the various causes and consequences of disability.

The traditional approach to medical care has focused on *impairments,* or the loss and/or abnormality of mental, emotional, physiological, or anatomical structure or function.

This term includes all losses or abnormalities, not just those attributable to the initial pathophysiology, and also includes pain as a limiting experience (NCMRR, 1993). When there is an interruption or interference of normal physiological and developmental processes or structures, a term that is used is *pathophysiology* (NCMRR, 1993).

Institutional based rehabilitation usually focuses on *functional limitations,* which have been defined as restrictions or lack of ability to perform an action or activity in the manner or within the range considered normal that results from impairment or failure of an individual to return to the preexisting level or function (NCMRR, 1993). The term *functional limitation* is synonymous with the term *performance components* used by many occupational therapists. In contrast,

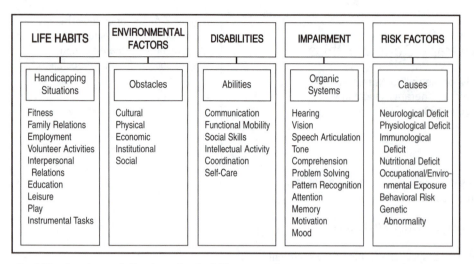

Figure 2-7. ICIDH Terminology.

disability has been defined as the inability to perform or a limitation in performing socially defined activities and roles expected of individuals within a social and physical environment as a result of internal or external factors and their interplay (NCMRR, 1993).

A *social disadvantage or handicap* for a given individual results when he or she is not able to fulfill a role that he or she expects or is required to fill. If the environment presents a barrier to the performance of an activity (a non-accessible building, an attitude of discrimination, or a policy that denies access) the barrier is defined as a *handicapping situation* (Fougeyrollas, 1994). When societal policy, attitudes, and actions, or lack of actions, create a physical, social, or financial barrier to access health care, housing or vocational/avocational opportunities, a term that is used is *societal limitation* (NCMRR, 1993).

When an occupational therapist approaches problem-solving with clients, three sets of information are basic to the plan. *Intrinsic factors* that must be considered are the neurobehavioral, cognitive, physical, and psychosocial strengths and deficits presented by the person. *Extrinsic or environmental* factors to be considered include the cultural, economic, institutional, political, and social context from the perspective of the person. *Occupational factors* include the self-maintenance, work, home, leisure, and family tasks and roles of the person. The unique term used by occupational therapy to express function is *occupational performance*. It reflects the individual's dynamic experience of engaging in daily occupations within the environment (Law & Baum, 1994).

MODELS FOR REHABILITATION SERVICES

Comprehensive rehabilitation models are now being developed that offer definitions and structures for facilitating

communication among health professionals and policy makers. Most health care services have focused on the impairment and functional limitation aspects of the human condition, however recent efforts to revise the International Classification of Impairment, Disabilities, and Handicap (ICIDH) of the WHO has led to debate that will result in improved definitions and systems of classification. This, in turn, will influence data collection that will be used by policy makers to build systems of care that facilitate independence in persons with disabilities. This is a worldwide effort.

The ICIDH is discussed throughout this book and is introduced here to familiarize the reader with key terms, concepts, and the factors that must be considered at each level. Figure 2-7 highlights the key terminology and concepts of the ICIDH model.

In 1993, the NCMRR developed an alternative classification system (Figure 2-8) to recognize the role that society plays in disability. Two categories differ from the ICIDH model: 1) The NCMRR classification puts special emphasis on a category called Functional Limitations. This category describes a limitation in the action or activity experienced by the individual who has sustained an impairment that continues to need attention if the individual is to avoid a disabling condition. This attention can include specific treatments to avoid or overcome disability, or it can include assistive technology that can serve to compensate for the loss of function incurred by the client; 2) The NCMRR model also explains a level identified as Societal Limitation. This level recognizes the environment and its role in supporting (or inhibiting) a person's social participation in work and in communities.

Whether the ICIDH or the NCMRR model is used in organizing assessments, interventions, and services, one issue is critical. Occupational therapists must place their primary focus at the level of the person-environment interaction so that occupational performance issues can be assessed and addressed in the occupational therapy plan. Person-environment issues are

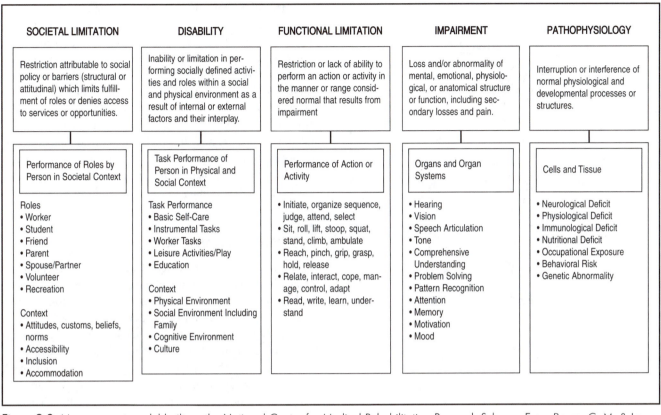

Figure 2-8. Measurement model built on the National Center for Medical Rehabilitation Research Scheme. From Baum, C. M. & Law, M. (1997). Occupational therapy practice: Focusing on occupational performance. *American Journal of Occupational Therapy, 51*(4), 277-288. Used with permission from the American Occupational Therapy Association.

addressed in the ICIDH model at the disability, environmental factors, and life habit levels and in the NCMRR model at the level of disabilities and societal limitations. When occupational performance issues are not addressed, the contributions of occupational therapy are not made explicit and the client is left to fend for him or herself with problems that will compromise his or her function and health.

INFLUENCING OUTCOMES

The health system is focusing on outcomes because of the need to be accountable, not only to the clients in need of services, but also to the third party who is paying the bill. With a shift in focus toward primary and secondary prevention, it is also important to know if interventions are successful in reducing the impact of secondary problems. Medical outcomes are being defined as well-being and quality of life; improved occupational performance is a critical construct in measuring quality of life regardless of the measure that is used. There is increasing evidence from research that client-centred practice improves not only the process but also the outcomes of care (Dunst, Trivette, Davis & Cornwall, 1988;

Dunst, Trivette, Boyd & Brookfield, 1994; Greenfield, Kaplan & Ware, 1985; Moxley-Haegert & Serbin, 1983; Stein & Jessop, 1991).

THE UNIQUE CONTRIBUTION OF OCCUPATIONAL THERAPY

As individuals engage in occupation, they use their motor and memory skills to enhance their performance and maintain both cognitive and physiological fitness (Baum & Law, 1997). Reilly (1962) proclaimed that "there is a reservoir of sensitivity and skill in the hands of man which can be tapped for his health [and a] rich adaptability and durability of the central nervous system which can be influenced by experience" (p. 89).

Being able "to do" requires the integration of factors within the individual (intrinsic) with those external to the individual, i.e., culture, economics, resources, and the physical and social environment (extrinsic). Of particular interest is how these environmental factors interact with the occupational structure of the individual (Baum & Law, 1997). Individuals who perceive that they have control over their

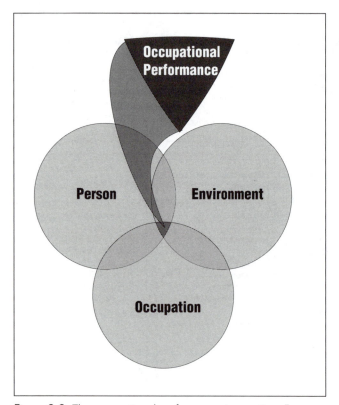

Figure 2-9. The occupational performance transaction. From Law, et al (1996).

environments and can address obstacles derive satisfaction from their occupational roles (Burke, 1977; Sharott and Cooper-Fraps, 1986). Thus, the unique contribution of occupational therapy is to maximize the fit between what it is the individual wants and needs to do and his or her capability to do it (Figure 2-9).

CONCEPTUAL SYSTEMS FOR GUIDING PRACTICE

While philosophical values and beliefs have an important and enduring influence on a profession's activities, they are not a sufficient basis for practice. There must also be systems for generating, organizing and applying knowledge that is useful to practice.

Typically, knowledge about the nature of things is derived from scientific disciplines in the form of theories. These abstract "truths" about nature may or may not be useful to scientific professions, which are concerned with the application of knowledge as it affects conditions in the real world. In the past, occupational therapy has been a scientific profession that draws much of its knowledge from other scientific disciplines and applies it in day-to-day practice.

In the future, this may change. The genesis and development of occupation science will contribute greatly to our understanding of how occupation influences health and well-being. Much credit should be extended to the pioneering efforts of Mary Reilly, Elizabeth Yerxa and Florence Clark and their colleagues at the University of Southern California for bringing focus to this initiative. Recently, scholars throughout the world have been contributing to our understanding of the relationship of occupation to function and well-being. The study of human occupation will provide more scientific guidance to the occupational therapy practitioners of the 21st century.

SYSTEMS THINKING

Because of the complexity of occupation, occupational therapy has benefited from the knowledge of systems which is developing in the worldwide scientific community. Systems are structures for understanding things which interact. It is thought that there are principles governing systems that influence their behavior. Systems thinking seeks a basic understanding of these principles in order to appreciate how a system changes or behaves over time. For our purposes here, systems thinking can be divided into general systems theory and complex systems theory.

GENERAL SYSTEMS THEORY

General systems theory (GST) is a label given to interdisciplinary efforts to identify the structural, behavioral and developmental features of living organisms (von Bertalanffy, 1969). General systems theory has evolved from attempts to identify general phenomena common to living organisms and to formulate theories from observations of those phenomena. One approach has been to view components of systems (or subsystems) as part of a hierarchy of complexity, with lower levels being governed or influenced by higher levels (Boulding, 1956).

An open system, such as a human being, is influenced by information (input), which is processed in some way and results in behavioral change (output). In open systems, behavioral change occurs in response to information or events in the environment. In humans, such change is called learning or adaptation.

Through GST, the relationships between the elements of a complex system, such as the human being, are more easily organized and understood. The principles can also be applied to groups in organizations to better understand the dynamics of organizational behavior (Senge, 1990).

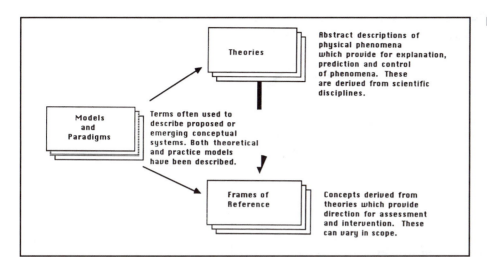

Figure 2-10. Types of conceptual tools.

COMPLEX SYSTEMS THEORY

A rapidly evolving approach to systems understanding is called complex systems theory or complexity theory. Other synonyms for this emerging area of science are chaos theory and dynamical systems theory. Complex systems theory represents the study of non-linear systems. Approaches in this area have roots in mathematics, physics and biology.

To best understand complex systems theory, it is useful to appreciate that much of science has evolved using models of nature with linear mathematics. Similarly, the study of systems has traditionally been approached using models of nature with linear mathematics. Similarly, the study of systems has traditionally been approached using mathematical models based on assumptions of linear (or highly predictable) relationships between the entities in the system. Often, however, these linear models have not been highly accurate predictors of what actually happens in nature.

Complex systems theory evolved in recognition of this disparity. By studying the disparity (or chaos) between linear predictions and actual behaviors of systems, scientists have determined that outcomes cannot be accurately predicted with models. Instead, the processes of systems can be studied to create the models. The unpredictability of complex systems is often attributed to a concept called "the butterfly effect." This idea (Llorenz, 1993) is that small changes in the starting conditions of a system can result in dramatically different outputs.

Non-linear approaches to modeling systems have broad application in many fields, and have already resulted in improved understanding of problems as diverse as heart arrhythmias, the origin of the universe, and the compression and encryption algorithms so vital to information science. In rehabilitation, complex systems theory is now being applied to our understanding of the processes involved in motor learning and nervous system function.

THEORIES, MODELS AND FRAMES OF REFERENCE

A review of the scholarly literature in occupational therapy quickly reveals that there is little agreement among writers about how to describe organized knowledge in the field. The terms theory, model, frame of reference, and paradigm have been variously used to describe subsets of the profession's knowledge. A theory can be viewed as a "tool for thinking" (Parham, 1987). This description applies equally well to model, frame of reference, and paradigm.

However, while each of the terms describes a conceptual tool, they should not be viewed as interchangeable. Theories are generally thought of as the products of the scientific disciplines, whose task it is to explain natural phenomena. Mosey (1985, 1989) argues that conceptual systems which organize applied knowledge in occupational therapy (mechanisms for linking theory to practice) are appropriately referred to as frames of reference. The term model is often used to describe a developing conceptual system (Figure 2-10).

Over the years, several writers have proposed that occupational therapy should adopt a single conceptual framework which is sufficiently broad so as to provide a means for applying to all areas of practice (Christiansen, 1981; Howe and Briggs, 1982; Kielhofner, 1982; King, 1978; Llorens, 1976; Reilly, 1966). Mosey (1985) contends that the profession has a tradition of multiple frames of reference, and therefore the selection of one unifying framework could be unnecessarily restrictive. The terms used by Mosey to describe multiple perspective versus single perspective approaches to practice are "pluralism" and "monism." In response, Christiansen (1991) argued that there are disadvantages to pluralism, and that occupational therapy theory can benefit from a unified theory, as well as greater consensus among scholars on key concepts and terms.

Yerxa has described this tendency to oversimplify in occu-

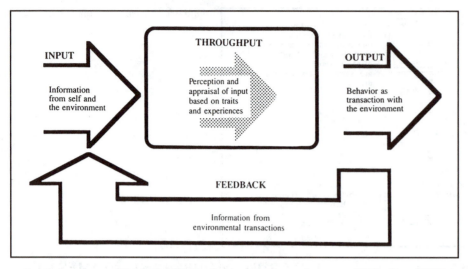

Figure 2-11. The human as an open system.

pational therapy as "the hobgoblin" of theory and practice. Writes Yerxa: "An essential quality of occupational therapy needs to be made more visible to the eye. That quality is the complexity of occupational therapy practice and the knowledge upon which it is based" (1988, p. 2). Yerxa suggests that viewing the person as a hierarchically arranged, complex open system which has interrelated levels of function can assist the therapist in understanding the complexities of occupational therapy practice. This view of the person requires an understanding of the complex factors which support the performance of a person in the tasks, occupations and roles of life. The Person-Environment Occupational Performance Model serves as a framework to simplify this task.

While there are many frames of reference in occupational therapy, varying widely in their scope and utility, we will be using the term "model" to describe the emerging work surrounding the issues of person, environment and occupation. Chapter 4 will discuss six developing models in occupational therapy.

PERSON ENVIRONMENT OCCUPATION TRANSACTIONS

The interplay between the human and its environment can be described as a transaction. Transactions between individuals and their surroundings occur at multiple levels as information (or energy) is fed into the system (input), processed (throughput) and output. At the level of the individual, output takes the form of behavior, the results of which influence the cycle through a feedback loop. This feedback portion of the cycle consists of information about one's performance which has been derived from the self and others (Figure 2-11).

It is within the context of performance transactions that individuals encounter the objects, people, conditions and events which stimulate development or maturation. As

Kielhofner (1985, p. 41) has suggested, although change is not always grossly apparent, experiences accumulate which reinforce or modify individual characteristics. Over time, changes become more evident, although the overall trend may be characterized by periods of varying organization or advancement. As the life cycle progresses, the desired course is one of greater satisfaction within one's environmental circumstances and an increasing sense of fulfillment through life's activities.

Performance is described as a transaction because individuals and their environments influence each other in a reciprocal manner. Transaction is the term suggested by Dewey and Bentley (1949) for processes involving object relationships within a system, and is a term that has been in use by social scientists for several decades. In addition to the suggestion of mutual influence, use of the term "transaction" implies a dynamic situation in which individuals alter their performance based on their perceptions of changing conditions in the environment.

An example may help to illustrate this point. While the morning routine of dressing is almost habitual for most of us, there is no doubt that it is influenced by our expectations of environmental encounter each day. Most of us select our most attractive clothes knowing we will be having lunch with an important person in our work setting. Similarly, our dressing habits at home may be influenced by the presence of house guests, as we elect to give up the comfortable but tattered housecoat in favor of apparel that we perceive will leave a more favorable impression. In either case, our behavior has been changed as the result of changes in our environment and our perception of the meaning of those changes as they affect our well-being.

As suggested by this example, people spend most of their waking hours engaged in occupations, which in addition to dressing and related self-maintenance activities include other productive and leisure pursuits. Thus, to speak of performance in occupational therapy is to refer to occupational performance. Viewing occupational performance as a transaction between the individual and the environment, which is influenced by that person's wants or needs and occupational requirements, provides a useful framework for viewing occupational therapy practice. This approach toward organizing information useful to practice can be referred to as the Person-Environment Occupational Performance Model.

Using this framework, factors that support the performance of individuals in their everyday lives are presented, including how such factors can be assessed, and strategies for overcoming performance deficits. This provides a way of organizing the complexity of occupations discussed in Chapter 1. The remainder of the text has been organized around this model, which is summarized in Chapter 3.

STUDY QUESTIONS

1. Occupational therapists are members of a team. What is the unique contribution occupational therapists bring to the team?

2. Discuss why and how occupational therapy has moved away from a reductionistic paradigm.

3. What are the core elements of client-centeredness?

4. What enduring principles did Adolph Meyer leave for future generations of occupational therapists?

5. Discuss doing versus telling and doing versus doing to.

6. Discuss how occupational therapies concerns fit into the ICIDH and NCMRR models which are guiding rehabilitation.

RECOMMENDED READINGS

Baum, C. M. (1980). Occupational therapists put care in the health system. *American Journal of Occupational Therapy, 24*(4), 505-516.

Bing, R. K. (1981). Occupational therapy revisited: a paraphrastic journey. *American Journal of Occupational Therapy, 35*(8), 499-518.

Engelhardt, H. T. (1977). Defining occupational therapy: The meaning of therapy and the virtues of occupation. *American Journal of Occupational Therapy, 31*(10), 666-672.

Kielhofner, G. & Burke, J. P. (1977). Occupational therapy after 60 years: An account of changing identity and knowledge. *American Journal of Occupational Therapy, 31*, 675-689.

Meyer, A. (1922). The philosophy of occupation therapy. *Archives of Occupational Therapy, 1*, 1-10.

Nagi, S. Z. (1976). An epidemiology of disability among adults in the United States. In *Health and Society*. Milbank Memorial Fund Quarterly, 54, 439-467.

Parsons, T. (1975). The sick role and the role of the physician reconsidered. *Health and Society*, 257-278.

Reilly, M. (1962). Occupational can be one of the great ideas of 20th century medicine. *American Journal of Occupational Therapy, 16*, 1-9.

Shannon, P. D. (1977). The derailment of occupational therapy. *American Journal of Occupational Therapy, 31*(4), 229-234.

Smith, M. B. (1974). Competence and adaptation: A perspective on therapeutic ends and means. *American Journal of Occupational Therapy, 28*(1), 11-15.

Wood, P. H. N. (1980). Appreciating the consequences of disease: The classification of impairments, disabilities and handicaps. *The WHO Chronicle, 34*, 376-380.

World Health Organization. (1980-1993). *International Classification of Impairments, Disabilities and Handicaps. A Manual Relating to the Consequences of Diseases.* Geneva: Author.

Yerxa, E. J. (1967). Authentic occupational therapy. *American Journal of Occupational Therapy, 21*, 1-9.

REFERENCES

American Occupational Therapy Association (1994). *Reference guide: American Occupational Therapy Code of Ethics.* Bethesda, MD: American Occupational Therapy Association.

Baum C. M. (1995). The contribution of occupation to function in persons with Alzheimer's disease. *Journal of Occupation Science: Australia, 2*(2), 59-67.

Baum, C. M., & Law, M. (1997), Occupational therapy practice: Focusing on occupational performance. *American Journal of Occupational Therapy, 51*(4) 277-288.

Bing, R. K. (1981). Occupational therapy revisited: A paraphrase journey. *American Journal of Occupational Therapy, 35*(8), 499-518.

Bockhoven, J. S. (1971). Legacy of moral treatment-1800's to 1910. *American Journal of Occupational Therapy, 25*, 223-225.

Boulding, K. E. (1956). General systems theory: The skeleton of science. *Management Science, 2*(3), 197-208, B. E. pp 81-97, CPIV 3-46RI.

Burke, J. P. (1977). A clinical perspective on motivation: pawn versus origin. *The American Journal of Occupational Therapy, 31*, 254-258.

Christiansen, C. (1991). Occupational therapy: Intervention for life performance. In C. Christiansen, & C. Baum (Eds.), *Occupational therapy: Overcoming human performance deficits* (pp 4-43). Thorofare, NJ: SLACK Incorporated.

Christiansen, C. (1994). A social framework for viewing self-care intervention. In C. Christiansen (Ed.), *Ways of living: Self care strategies for special needs* (pp. 1-27). Bethesda, MD: American Occupational Therapy Association.

Christiansen, C. H. (1981). Toward resolution of crisis: Research requisites in occupational therapy. *Occupational Therapy Journal of Research, 1*(2), 115-124.

Clark, C. A., Corcoran, M, & Gitlin, L. N. (1995). An exploratory study of how occupational therapists develop therapeutic relationships with family caregivers. *American Journal of Occupational Therapy, 49*(7), 587-594.

Delisa, J., Gans, B., & Currie, D. (1997). Rehabilitation medicine: Principles and practices (3rd Ed). Philadelphia: J. B. Lippincott.

Dewey, J. &. Bentley, A. F. (1949). *Knowing and the known.* Boston, MA: Beacon.

Drucker, P. F. (1989). *The new realities.* New York: Harper and Row.

Dunst D. J., Trivette C. M., Davis, M., & Cornwall, J. (1988). Enabling and empowering families of children with health impairments. *Children's Health Care, 17,* 71-81.

Dunst, D. J., Trivette, C. M., Boyd, K., & Brookfield, J. (1994). Help-giving practices and the self-efficacy appraisals of parents. In C. J. Dunst, C. M. Trivette, & A. G. Deal (Eds.), *Supporting and strengthening families (Vol. 1): Methods, strategies and practices.* Cambridge, MA: Brookline Books.

Engelhardt, H. T. (1977). Defining occupational therapy: The meaning of therapy and the virtues of occupation. *American Journal of Occupational Therapy, 31*(10), 666-672.

Fidler, G. S., & Fidler, J. W. (1978). Doing and becoming: Purposeful action and self-actualization. *American Journal of Occupational Therapy, 32,* 305-310.

Fidler, G. & Fidler J. (1963). *Occupational therapy: A communication process in psychiatry.* New York: Macmillan.

Gleick, J. (1987). *Chaos: The making of a new science.* New York: Viking-Penguin.

Grady, A. P. (1995). Building inclusive community: A challenge for occupational therapy. *American Journal of Occupational Therapy, 49*(4), 300-310.

Greenfield, S., Kaplan, S., & Ware, J. E. (1985). Expanding patient involvement in care: Effects on patient outcomes. *Annals of Internal Medicine, 102,* 520-528.

Hansen, R. A. (1984). *Moral reasoning of occupational therapists: Implications for education and practice.* Unpublished Doctoral Dissertation, Wayne State University,

Hansen, R. A. (1988). Ethics is the issue. *American Journal of Occupational Therapy, 42*(5), 279-281.

Howe, M. C., & Briggs, A. K. (1982). Ecological systems model for occupational therapy. *American Journal of Occupational Therapy, 36,* 322-327.

Kielhofner, G. (1982). A heritage of activity: Development of theory. *American Journal of Occupational Therapy, 36*(11), 723-730.

Kielhofner, G. (1985). *A model of human occupation: Theory and application.* Baltimore: Williams & Wilkins.

Kielhofner, G. (1992). *Conceptual foundations of occupational therapy.* Philadelphia: F. A Davis.

Kielhofner, G., & Burke, J. P. (1977). Occupational therapy after 60 years: An account of changing identity and knowledge. *American Journal of Occupational Therapy, 31,* 675-689.

King, L. J. (1978). Toward a science of adaptive responses. *American Journal of Occupational Therapy, 32,* 429-437.

Law, M., & Baum, C. M. (1994). A brief OT history: The importance of occupation in promoting and maintaining health. *Creating the future: A joint effort.* Can-Am Conference, Boston, Mass. July.

Llorens, L. A. (1976). *Application of developmental theory for health and rehabilitation.* Rockville, MD: American Occupational Therapy Association.

Lorenz, E. N. (1983). *The essence of chaos.* Seattle, WA: University of Washington Press.

McKeown, T. (1978). Determinants of health. *Human Nature, 1*(4), 60-67.

Meier, R. H. & Purtilo, R. B. Ethical issues and the patient-provider relationship. *American Journal of Physical Medicine and Rehabilitation, 73*(5), 365-366.

Meyer, A. (1922). The philosophy of occupation therapy. *Archives of Occupational Therapy, 1*(1), 1-10.

Mosey, A. C. (1985). A monistic or pluralistic approach to professional identity. *American Journal of Occupational Therapy, 39*(8), 504-509.

Mosey, A. C. (1989). The proper focus of scientific inquiry in occupational therapy: Frames of reference (Editorial). *Occupational Therapy Journal of Research, 9*(4), 195-201.

Moxley-Haegert, L., & Servin L. A. (1983). Developmental education for parents of delayed infants: Effects on parental motivation and children's development. *Child Development, 54,* 1324-1331.

Nagi, S. Z. (1976). An epidemiology of disability in the United States. *Milbank Memorial Fund Quarterly-Health and Society, 54*(4),439-467.

NCMRR (1993). *Research Plan for the National Center for Medical Rehabilitation Research. (*NIH Publication No. 93-3509). National Institutes of Health, Washington DC: U.S. Government Printing Office.

O'Neill, E. H. (1991). *Healthy America: Practitioners for 2005. An Agenda for Action.* A Report of the Pew Health Profession. San Francisco: The Pew Health Professions Commission.

Parham, L. D. (1987). Toward professionalism: The reflective therapist. *American Journal of Occupational Therapy, 41,* 555-561.

Pope, A. M., & Tarlov, A. R. (1991). *Disability in America: Toward a national agenda for prevention.* Washington, DC: National Academy Press.

Premier's Council on Health, Well-being and Social Justice (1993). *Our environment, our health.* Toronto: Author.

Reilly, M. (1962). Occupational therapy can be one of the great ideas of 20th century medicine. *The American Journal of Occupational Therapy, 16,* 87-105.

Reilly, M. (1966). A psychiatric occupational therapy program as a teaching model. *American Journal of Occupational Therapy, 20,* 61-67.

Rogers, J. C. (1982). Order and disorder in medicine and occupational therapy. *American Journal of Occupational Therapy, 36,* 29-35.

Rogers, J. C. (1983). Clinical reasoning: The ethics, science and art. *American Journal of Occupational Therapy, 37,* 601-616.

Senge, P. (1990). *The fifth discipline. The art and practice of the learning organization.* New York: Doubleday.

Shannon, P. D. (1977). The derailment of occupational therapy. *American Journal of Occupational Therapy, 31*(4), 229-234.

Shannon, P. D. (1986). Philosophical considerations for the practice of occupational therapy. In S. E. Ryan (Ed.), *The Certified Occupational Therapy Assistant: Roles and Responsibilities* (pp. 38-44). Thorofare, NJ: SLACK Incorporated.

Sharrot, G. W., & Cooper-Fraps, C. (1986). Theories of motivation in occupational therapy. *American Journal of Occupational Therapy, 40*(4), 249-257.

Statistics Canada (1992). *Canadian Health and Activity Limitation Survey.* Ottawa: Statistic Canada.

Stein, R. E. K. & Jessop, D. J. (1991). Long-term mental health effects of a pediatric home care program. *Pediatrics, 88,* 490-496.

Stern, R. (1990). Healthy communities: Reflections on building alliances in Canada. A view from the middle. *Health Promotion International, 5*(3), 225-231.

Vollmer, H. M., & Mills, D. L. (1966). *Professionalization.* Englewood Cliffs, NJ: Prentice-Hall.

von Bertalanffy, L. (1968). General systems theory: A critical review. In W. Buckley (Ed.), *Modern system's research for the behavioral scientist* (pp. 11-30). Chicago: Aldine.

Wilcock, A. (1993). A theory of the human need for occupation. *Occupational Science: Australia, 1*(1), 17-24.

Yerxa, E. (1967). Authentic occupational therapy. *American Journal of Occupational Therapy, 21,* 1-9.

Yerxa, E. (1988). Oversimplification: The hobgoblin of theory and practice in occupational therapy. *Canadian Journal of Occupational Therapy, 55* (1), 5-6.

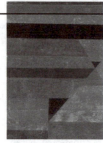

CHAPTER CONTENT OUTLINE

ABSTRACT

Because they constitute the essence of daily life, occupations are complex phenomena requiring conceptual frameworks of broad scope to explain them. Similarly, models for organizing occupational therapy intervention require similar breadth and depth. In this chapter, the Person-Environment Occupational Performance Model is presented. The origins of the model are traced, and its benefits are explained. Individuals are described as beings whose occupational behaviors are explained by psychological factors such as motivation, personality, values, and meaning. The chapter introduces other intrinsic performance enablers, which influence occupational choice and performance, including physiological factors related to general fitness, neuromotor structures, cognition, and emotion. A section on the environment describes how occupational performance is supported by extrinsic factors such as social expectations, cultural influences, and physical characteristics of the built environment. Collectively, these elements provide a structure for viewing occupations and for organizing approaches to occupational therapy intervention. A description of the intervention process, emphasizing a client-centered approach, concludes the chapter.

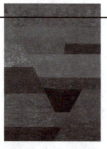

KEY TERMS

Internality

Motivation

Self-efficacy

Personality

Locus of control

Semantic differential

Values

Self-identity

Spiritual meaning

Occupational performance

Roles

Abilities

Skill

Intrinsic enablers of performance

Helplessness

Arousal

Client-centered

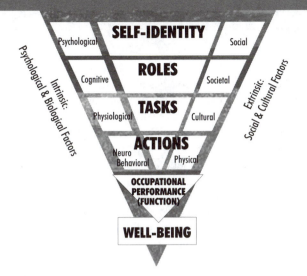

CHAPTER 3

Person-Environment Occupational Performance

A Conceptual Model for Practice

Charles Christiansen, EdD, OTR, OT(C), FAOTA, Carolyn Baum, PhD, OTR/C, FAOTA

OBJECTIVES

The information in this chapter is intended to help the reader:

1. understand the origins, elements and benefits of the Person-Environment Occupational Performance model as a conceptual framework for practice

2. appreciate various intrinsic and cognitive motivational influences on occupational choice and everyday behaviors

3. recognize the influence of personality traits on occupational preference

4. appreciate how values influence activity and meaning

5. describe structural relationships among actions, tasks, occupations and roles

6. list various performance enablers which influence abilities and skills

7. identify environmental characteristics that influence occupational performance

8. list steps in the occupational therapy intervention process

9. identify major intervention categories.

> *"In occupational therapy, the patient experiences the reality of his [or her] physical environment and his [or her] capacity to function within it."*
>
> Elizabeth J. Yerxa, 1967, p. 2

PURPOSE OF THIS CHAPTER

The purpose of this chapter is to present a framework for thinking about occupational therapy practice. In Chapter 1, we learned that classification systems are useful for naming and describing events and objects. In Chapter 2, the importance of using a model to organize intervention was stressed. A conceptual model, or framework for thinking, provides a means for organizing this information in a way that makes it useful for practice.

OVERVIEW OF THE MODEL

As its title suggests, the Person-Environment Occupational Performance Model has three major components. These three elements describe what people do in their daily lives, what motivates them, and how their personal characteristics combine with the situations in which occupations are undertaken to influence successful occupational performance.

A basic belief of the model is that people are naturally motivated to explore their world and demonstrate mastery within it. Their success in doing so is a measure of how successfully they have adapted. Adaptation can be viewed as a process whereby individuals meet the challenges they confront in daily living by using the resources (personal, social, and material) available to them. If they possess the necessary emotional maturity and problem-solving skills, people are able to set and achieve goals that contribute to their development throughout life.

A second important belief of this model is that settings in which people experience success help them feel good about themselves. This motivates them to face new challenges with greater confidence. The model proposes that through their occupations, people develop their self-identity and derive a sense of fulfillment. Fulfillment comes from feelings of mastery as well as from the accomplishment of goals that have personal meaning. Over time, these meaningful experiences permit people to develop an understanding of who they are and what their place is in the world.

BENEFITS OF THE MODEL

We propose that organizing knowledge for occupational therapy practice using a Person-Environment Occupational Performance Model offers several advantages over more tra-

Bibliographic citation of this chapter: Christiansen, C. & Baum, C. (1997). Person-environment occupational performance: A conceptual model for practice. In C. Christiansen & C. Baum (Eds.), *Occupational therapy: Enabling function and well-being* (2nd Ed.). Thorofare, NJ: SLACK Incorporated.

ditional reductionistic approaches to practice. First, this perspective helps us to identify and consider the many factors that influence performance, as well as the many dimensions of occupation. It presents the viewpoint that in order to understand performance, we must consider the characteristics of individuals, the unique environments in which they function, and the nature and meaning of the actions, tasks and roles to the person. Second, the model allows us to incorporate existing ideas and traditions within occupational therapy in a framework that is based on research and accepted information, and easy to understand.

Finally, it provides a framework for viewing and studying human behavior that combines knowledge about the impairments that impede performance, the environments that support performance, and the individual needs, preferences, styles and goals. Models which focus on the individual's needs and goals rather than his or her impairment are called client-centered models. The Person-Environment Occupational Performance Model is thus a client-centered model. It focuses on the individual and that person's daily occupations which are limited as the result of a health condition or disability.

This model requires that information from disciplines outside of occupational therapy be sought, used, recognized and respected. The complexity of occupation, the uniqueness of individuals and the diversity of environments makes this necessary, since no single discipline is sufficiently broad to encompass the knowledge required for all these areas. Delivered effectively, health care is the product of teams, which include people who produce knowledge and understanding (basic and social scientists) and people who apply that knowledge (health care providers and patients). From occupational therapy's perspective, the purpose of the partnership is to facilitate the health and function of the person whose occupational performance is threatened or impaired.

ORIGIN OF THE MODEL

The ideas underlying the Person-Environment Occupational Performance Model are not new. In many ways, the framework is similar to a model (called the Ecological Systems Model) proposed by occupational therapists Howe and Briggs (1982). It also shares characteristics in common with self-determination theory, formulated by Deci & Ryan (1991). Each of these models view performance as the result of complex relationships between the individual as an open system and the specific environments in which tasks and roles occur.

The Person-Environment Occupational Performance and the Ecological Systems Models consider the importance of stages of development as they influence motivation, skills and roles. Moreover, they each draw from a view of health that emphasizes the interaction of biological, psychological and social phenomena (Engel 1977; Mosey, 1974; Reilly, 1962). Finally, both frameworks view occupational therapy as a means for facilitating adaptation (in the broadest sense) when performance deficits are identified that interfere with daily occupations.

The model in this book builds on previous work to include scientific knowledge provided by scientists studying occupation and rehabilitation. In this framework, intervention is not viewed as a process of selecting purposeful activity in order to elicit an adaptive response in the manner described by King (1978). Rather, occupational therapy is viewed as a collection of strategies that engage the individual to develop or use resources which enable successful performance of the necessary and meaningful occupations in their lives. These strategies may or may not involve the individual's direct engagement in occupation. Nor do they necessarily involve a neurological response, since in some cases (such as environmental modification), the patient's active involvement may be working with the therapist to identify goals and strategies.

Because the desired outcome of therapy is the individual's ability to live a satisfying or productive life, an appropriate strategy may include teaching a patient to supervise others in the performance of tasks. A severely disabled individual, for example, might require (or request) a personal care attendant to assist with dressing and hygiene activities so that his or her time and energy can be saved for work, study, or other more personally satisfying occupations. The view of practice emphasized here is that occupational therapy almost never does things *to* people; it more frequently does things *with* people, sometimes requiring their active physical involvement and sometimes requiring only their interest, attention and cooperation.

In the following section, we will introduce each of the principal elements of the Person-Environment Occupational Performance Model, with an overview of some of the major points that are pertinent to these individual parts of the framework. Figure 3-1 provides a graphic overview of the Model. Note that many elements correspond to individual chapters found in the book.

THE PERSON AS AN OCCUPATIONAL BEING

An understanding of the model should begin with an examination of the influences that affect motivation and how an individual views him or her self. The need to demonstrate our selfhood becomes progressively stronger as we mature. From our earliest days in school, we proclaim our individual identities by putting our names on our work. The graffiti displayed in public places by gangs can be viewed as a group

statement of identity, and the personalized license plates owned by drivers of all generations are examples of the need to express our individuality. The assertion of identity is very much an important part of adolescence and continues throughout life as we express our unique selves through our dress and our productive occupations.

The developmental theorist Erik Eriksson (1968) emphasized the importance of self-identity in his important work, *Identity, Youth and Crisis*. Eriksson identified the challenges of various stages of life, portraying each as an opportunity to demonstrate competence and to contribute to a self which is viewed by ourselves and others as worthy.

MOTIVATION

While most people have routines that provide predictability and a degree of sameness to their lives, each day also holds possibilities for choosing among different things to do, particularly for discretionary or free time. The decision to choose one activity over another, or for initiating an activity at all, is an expression of motivation.

Over the past 50 years, theories of motivation have tended to fall into two groups. The first group, called intrinsic theories of motivation, emphasizes internal drives and needs. A second group, called cognitive theories of motivation, focuses on the role of thought processes which influence goal setting and self-control. Each group will be discussed in the following paragraphs.

Intrinsic Theories of Motivation

Intrinsic theories of motivation emphasize that behavior can occur as a result of free choice without any apparent external reward. The need for effectance described by White (1959), and the need for satisfaction gained from optimal experience or flow described by Csikszentmihalyi (1975, 1988) are two examples of intrinsic theories relevant to understanding the importance of occupation to everyday living.

Robert White (1959) believed that people have a competence motive, which he described as an innate drive to influence the environment. According to White, this drive provides the motivation for exploring, manipulating and acting, and is an important component in developmental learning.

Csikszentmihalyi (1988), a psychologist at the University of Chicago, has conducted research aimed at understanding the types of daily activities that bring satisfaction and happiness. He proposes that people are motivated to engage in pursuits that bring them pleasure without any particular goal in mind other than the doing of the activity itself, which is its own reward. These experiences are described as *flow*, a condition which constitutes a balance between perceived challenges and an individual's skills. Csikszentmihalyi describes

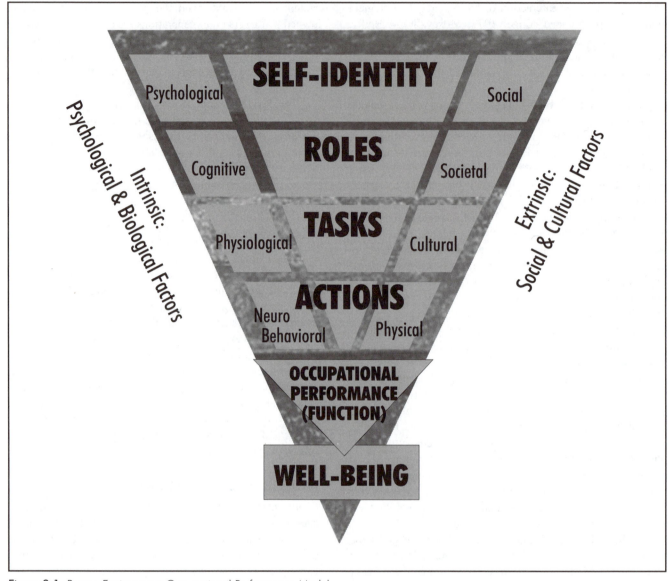

Figure 3-1. Person-Environment Occupational Performance Model.

the optimal flow experience as timeless, intensely satisfying, and absorbing. Maintenance of the flow experience requires increasing the complexity of the challenge and developing new skills, in a continuing pattern of development toward greater skills and competence.

Studies have shown that the experience of flow increases the perceived quality of life experiences (LeFevre, 1988) and can contribute to self-esteem (Wells, 1988). Studies of the relationship of flow to job satisfaction (Allison & Duncan, 1988; Jacobs, 1994) have shown inconclusive results. The concept of flow shares characteristics with conditions viewed as best for intervention in occupational therapy, elsewhere described as "the just right challenge" (Carlson & Clark, 1991).

Cognitive Theories of Motivation

Cognitive theories of motivation explain that people motivate themselves by formulating goals, and planning and regulating their actions to attain them. Rotter (1960), DeCharms (1968) and Bandura (1977) are three psychologists whose work has influenced our understanding of how experiences shape self-perceptions, which in turn influence behaviors. Cognitive influences on motivation include our individual explanations for what causes things to happen the way they do (attributions), our expectations of success or failure in tasks (known as expectancies), and our goals, which are the desired outcomes or consequences toward which our actions are directed. We begin our discussion of cognitive motivation with the theories of Rotter and DeCharms, whose work has been influential to understanding internality. *Internality* is the term given for describing the extent to which people feel that their actions can influence their environment.

INTERNALITY

Beginning in the earliest stages of development, people observe the consequences of their actions and begin to form perceptions of what causes things to happen. Rotter (1960) used the term *locus of control* to explain how these perceptions influence beliefs about cause and effect. Some people believe that events are mostly the result of chance, fate, luck or circumstances outside the person's control. These people are said to have an external (outside themselves) locus of control. Others perceive that events are influenced by their own actions, and people in this category are described as having an internal locus of control.

DeCharms (1968) offered a theory (called personal causation) which proposed that behavior is influenced by beliefs about what causes events to happen. This theory proposes two categories with their labels taken from the game of chess. The first category consists of persons who believe in their ability to act on the environment and influence their own destiny. People in this category are said to demonstrate origin-like behavior. In the second category, persons who believe that outcomes are the result of external forces are said to demonstrate pawn-like behaviors. These concepts are similar to the internal and external locus of control described by Rotter.

Burke (1977) was one of the earliest occupational therapists to recognize the importance of these theories for occupational therapy. She observed that patients with an external locus of control (pawn-like in the terminology of DeCharms) are less likely to perceive that their own actions contribute to their rehabilitation or recovery. Such individuals might require more encouragement, guidance or supervision than that required by patients with greater belief that their actions can influence events (internality).

SELF-EFFICACY

Another important psychological researcher, Albert Bandura (1977, 1986) studied the influence of past success on later success and used the term "self-efficacy" to describe our views of ourselves as competent. Research has shown that people who perceive themselves as competent tend to view their overall well-being as more favorable and are more likely to continue working on tasks despite early setbacks (Gage & Polatajko, 1994).

In contrast, people who experience repeated failure may develop a negative view of self and little confidence in their ability to influence events. The term "helplessness" has been used to describe people whose failures have led to low feelings of self-efficacy (Seligmann, 1975; Maier & Seligman, 1976). A severe traumatic event which results in loss of physical or cognitive ability (such as spinal cord injury or stroke), can give rise to feelings of helplessness. Helplessness is frequently accompanied by depression, a pessimistic outlook toward the future, and considerable anxiety.

Self-efficacy is an important concept for occupational therapists because a person's feelings of competence can be influenced by success in task-related experiences. Studies have shown that when people receive training designed to improve their sense of competence, they later show significantly greater success on new tasks than individuals who have not received such training (Kilpatrick-Tubak & Ross, 1978; Wool, Siegal & Fine, 1980). It is not the training that leads to later success, but rather the belief in oneself as an effective, competent person that provides the motivation to continue working at the task until one succeeds (O'Leary, 1985).

PERSONALITY

Another significant influence on occupational performance is personality. In the course of a typical day, we shift our attention from one goal to another, and as a result the nature of our occupations change. If we want to relax, we can select among several occupations to fulfill this goal. We may listen to music, watch television, read, or take a walk in the park. Our choice of occupation depends on several factors, one of which is our personality.

Personality can be described as the interests, values and attitudes of an individual that influence their attention, behavior, and interpretation of new events. Two types of theory have developed from personality research. The first is concerned with personality traits and the second with personality types. Traits affect a person's stable tendencies (such as how outgoing, responsible and even-tempered he or she is) and help explain purposeful behavior by indicating the reasons that motivated actions (Hogan, DeSoto & Solano, 1977).

Much psychological research has shown that personality traits influence activity preferences and levels in both children and adults (Buss & Block 1980; Frese, Stuart & Hannover, 1987; Furnham, 1981; George, 1978). Personality psychologists agree that five major trait domains account for the consistent tendencies that influence human behavior (Digman, 1990; John, 1987). These five major dimensions of personality relate to problem-solving skill, emotional adjustment, interactions with others, acceptance of group values and norms, and activity levels.

John Holland's Theory of Personality and Vocational Choice	
Overview	**Types and Preferences**
The theory of personality and vocational choice proposed by John Holland (1959, 1973) demonstrates the relationship between personality traits, types and occupations. Holland's theory is based on six types of personality, each reflecting a defined cluster of traits. For each personality type, Holland has proposed a type of environment with characteristics that support the interests and needs of its corresponding personality type. Holland suggests that personality type and environments interact to influence vocational choice, stability and satisfaction. Thus, for example, an artistic person in a highly structured vocational setting is in a mismatched environment and would have a low level of satisfaction. Holland's theory is quite powerful as a means for relating specific values and interests to occupation. The six personality types of the theory can be matched with every job in the U.S. Department of Labor's *Dictionary of Occupational Titles*. Holland's classification of personality types is also used to organize information on prominent measures of vocational interest, and more recently has been applied to leisure preferences.	**REALISTIC** Outdoor and technical interests Examples: farmer, technician **INVESTIGATIVE** Scientific and inquiring interests Examples: chemist, biologist **SOCIAL** Helping and people oriented interests Examples: psychologist, therapist **ENTERPRISING** Persuasive, political and power oriented interests. Examples: manager, executive **CONVENTIONAL** Organizational and clerical interests Examples: accountant, banker, tax expert **ARTISTIC** Dramatic and self-expressive interests Examples: musician, writer, actor

Figure 3-2. John Holland's Theory of Personality and Vocational Choice.

Research has shown that traits tend to occur together, forming trait clusters. These groups of traits are the basis for theories of personality type. Theories of personality type have been useful as ways to predict the kinds of environments or activities best suited to different individuals. For example, a theory by John Holland (1959) is widely used to help people determine vocational and leisure interests (Figure 3-2).

Personality differences influence activity choice and satisfaction, and also predict the types of working and living environments in which we feel most comfortable. Because an individual's preferences for occupation are an expression of his or her personality type, psychologists have shown increasing interest in studying the occupations of daily life as a means for understanding personality.

VALUES

Values are beliefs and interpretive sentiments that influence choice, conduct and meaning in daily life. Because they are enduring and influence thinking, doing and feeling in all domains of life, values are central to our understanding of occupation. Two theories are useful to review here. The first theory attempts to explain how values influence what people do and how they do it. The second theory offers a framework for understanding how people assign meaning to events.

Rokeach Theory of Values

A theory by Rokeach (1973, 1979) proposes that values function as standards that guide ongoing activities. According to this theory, there are two types of values. The first type defines what a person believes is the right thing to do, and these are called instrumental values. Instrumental values can be said to influence how we accomplish desired goals. Examples of instrumental values would be honesty or courage. The second type of values concerns desired goals or outcomes, and these were described by Rokeach as terminal values. Examples of terminal values (end-states) would be self-respect and wisdom (Figure 3-3).

According to Rokeach, values are organized according to their importance or strength as guiding principles in life. Values may be relevant to some types of activities, but not to others. For example, while courage might be an important value for work and play, it may be less applicable to personal care in the home. To the extent that values are viewed as applicable and important in more than one life domain, they will provide a connection between those domains.

Osgood's Semantic Differential

A second theory connects values with meanings and proposes that situations or ideas are interpreted along consistent dimensions. These interpretations of experiences naturally influence their meaning to us. An illustration from everyday life may help to explain the dimensions and illustrate the connection between values and meaning.

Suppose you have just seen a movie at the local cinema and someone asks you to describe the experience. Your reply might very well sound like this: "I thought it was good, it influenced my thinking a lot, but it was slow moving in parts."

This response illustrates the three evaluative dimensions of meaning, which are value, potency, and action (Osgood, 1962). Value concerns whether we have positive or negative feelings about an idea, object or situation. Potency concerns our perceptions of its power or magnitude, and action concerns the degree of energy or movement associated with whatever we are evaluating.

Research on Osgood's theory has been undertaken using a technique called the *semantic differential*. The semantic differential provides pairs of adjectives commonly used in language (such as good-bad, hot-cold, friendly-hostile) and asks persons to rate an idea, product, process or another person using these sets of paired adjectives. Analyses of studies using the semantic differential have yielded remarkably similar results throughout the world, consistently demonstrating that the meaning of persons, objects, ideas and experiences tends to be influenced by the factors described above.

David Nelson and his colleagues (Nelson, Thompson, & Moore, 1982) have used the semantic differential to study the perceived values (meaning) people attach to various occupations, often using selected craft activities. These studies have shown some evidence of shared meaning for occupations, but have also shown that individual meanings of occupations can change under varying situations.

MEANING

Meanings reflect our overall interpretations of life events. Most of our intentions and actions are filled with meaning. This meaning comes from the nature of a situation and how we interpret its significance based on our current goals, values and past experiences. There are individual meanings and collective or shared meanings.

Meaning is socially and culturally influenced. Our world is comprehensible to us only because our individual perceptions have been validated by others. Daily life is filled with signs and symbols that convey meaning. We find agreement in the names, purposes and shared meanings of events, objects and ideas. In a similar way, general agreement regarding the meaning of signs, symbols and sounds underlies everyday

Rokeach's Theory of Values	
Terminal Values	**Instrumental Values**
A comfortable life	Ambitious
An exciting life	Broadminded
A sense of accomplishment	Capable
A world at peace	Cheerful
A world of beauty	Clean
Equality	Courageous
Family security	Forgiving
Freedom	Helpful
Happiness	Honest
Inner harmony	Imaginative
Mature love	Independent
National security	Intellectual
Pleasure	Logical
Salvation	Loving
Self-respect	Obedient
Social recognition	Polite
True friendship	Responsible
Wisdom	Self-controlled

Note: Studies of this theory have confirmed its validity (Braithwaite & Law, 1985), while suggesting that physical well-being, individual rights, thriftiness, and carefreeness should be included to ensure that the value list is comprehensive.

Figure 3-3. Rokeach's Theory of Values.

language. Language, in turn, influences thought.

Signs are direct representations of conditions, objects or events, while symbols convey more complex and personal meaning. A coffee pot is recognizable to most people as a device for making coffee, but it can also have a personal meaning related to the particular experiences of an individual. For example, it might remind him or her of long talks over coffee in the kitchen of a deceased friend or relative. The field of anthropology has provided much useful information about the shared meanings of objects, events and activities. Symbols with spiritual meaning abound in our environment, and enrich our engagement in occupations (Campbell, 1962, 1988).

Berger and Luckman (1967) point out that the experience of reality is itself dependent upon social agreement. Both individual and shared meaning change over time. Our interest here is in the meaning of occupations. In general, occupations are made up of individual actions linked together in time and purpose. Like actions, occupations assume greater meaning if they can be identified as part of a larger situation or context.

The same is true for the meaning of actions or events in our own lives. As actions extend over time, their meanings are more identifiable. This has been demonstrated in research done by Goldman (1970) and by Vallacher and Wegner (1987). Their work has shown that when people are asked to describe what they are doing, acts of lesser significance are described in terms of process (how they are done), while actions of greater significance or meaning are described using motives and consequences (why they are done).

How people think about (and thus describe) their actions has significant implication for both performance and meaning. Actions linked to longer term goals and purposes are more likely to be maintained, and to contribute to one's self-concept. This is supported by research by Emmons (1986), who found that goals that were more abstract tended to have a greater influence on overall well-being than goals that were more concrete, and thus more likely to be shorter term.

One line of research has shown that goals become effective motivators and regulators of behavior because they are part of one's image of "possible selves" (Markus & Nurius, 1986; Markus & Ruvolo, 1980). A possible self is a personal image of the type of person we think we can become. This possible self serves as a motivator because it inspires the goal setting and actions necessary for achieving a desired identity.

SPIRITUAL MEANING

A very important part of the formulation of a self-identity during later adulthood includes appreciating one's life and deriving meaning from it. This aspect of existence goes beyond the typical categories of daily life, and is of universal concern yet intensely individual in its meaning. Perhaps best described as the spiritual dimension of occupations (Christiansen, 1997; Egan & DeLaat, 1994), it includes but is not synonymous with religion. Rather, it refers to an individual's sense of self and his or her beliefs about power, control and meaning in life, as these are formulated in thought and experience.

The late Joseph Campbell (1988) noted that spiritual concerns were more apparent in the daily lives of people living in simpler eras, and were evident in common symbols, in objects and in rituals. While many of these symbols, objects and rituals were associated with the influence of formal religions, others evolved from ancient cultures and represented the wisdom of the ages.

An occupation need not be a ritual, nor include special objects or symbols in order for it to have spiritual meaning. When a person pays special attention to the way in which an occupation is done and the place in which it is performed, it becomes an opportunity for having special meaning. Participating in expressive arts, visiting special or historic places, enjoying music, walking in nature, meditating, or gardening are among many specific occupations thought to nourish the soul by providing opportunities for creating meaning. It has been suggested that any occupation can be an activity of spirit if attention is given to its style and context (Kabat-Zinn, 1994).

OCCUPATIONAL PERFORMANCE

Occupational performance is the doing of occupation. As indicated in Chapter 1, we can describe the performance of occupation in terms of the types of occupations that people do, as well as according to their degree of complexity. We observe that recognizable actions form parts of tasks. The performance of selected tasks is an expectation of different roles, and our lifetimes (and lifestyles) are comprised of different combinations of roles.

Figure 3-4 illustrates an occupational performance hierarchy, reflecting increasing levels of complexity (and time). Using this hierarchy, a basic unit of occupational performance can be described as an action, such as lifting or walking, or grimacing the face. When actions are part of specific goal-oriented activities like lifting a basket, walking across a room to close a door, or folding a towel, they become tasks. Tasks are viewed as combinations of actions sharing some purpose recognized by the task performer.

A third level of occupational complexity in organizing the daily stream of behavior includes occupations. Occupations are segments of goal-directed behavior that are recognizable by others, and typically include a number of related tasks performed over time. Examples of recognizable occupations within each of the major domains described in Chapter 1 are dressing and grooming, housekeeping, report writing, keeping accounts, horseback riding, and tennis. Occupations are more complex than tasks. However, because of the ambiguity of terms used in the language describing daily endeavors, the difference between tasks and occupations reflects public agreement more than precise scientific demarcations of action. The question can be raised: "When does task performance become engagement in occupation?" The answer may very well be that task performance becomes engagement in occupation when we recognize that it is part of an identifiable stream of goal-directed behavior.

Roles typically involve the performance of many occupations. Roles can be defined as recognizable positions in society, each having a defined status and specific expectations for behavior. Roles can be occupational, familial or sexual; thus a person can have multiple roles at the same time (e.g., therapist, mother, wife). It is important to consider that a complete view of occupational performance must consider the actions, tasks, occupations and roles of individuals as they go about their daily lives.

As an illustration of the performance hierarchy we have described, consider that the category of work and productive occupations (AOTA, 1994) includes various occupations of home management. These include meal preparation and clean-up, shopping, money management, and household maintenance. These require a specific set of tasks such as planning a grocery list, and driving to the store. Actions to

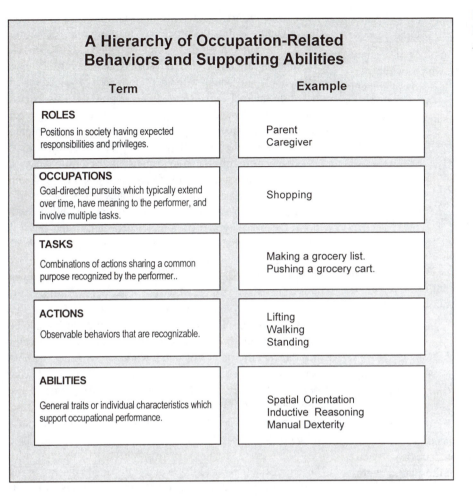

Figure 3-4. A Hierarchy of Occupation-Related Behaviors and Supporting Abilities.

support these tasks include pushing (a grocery cart), lifting and carrying (bags of groceries), and counting change. In turn, the actions required of shopping tasks can be analyzed in terms of their requisite abilities, such as near vision, flexibility, manual dexterity, and mathematical reasoning. Underlying these abilities are physiological, cognitive, psychological and neurobehavioral processes (described as intrinsic enablers of performance).

As discussed in Chapter 1, it has been traditional in occupational therapy to use the term *activity* in a general way to refer to all purposeful behaviors. Unfortunately, this general use does not lend itself to a clear description of the levels of complexity in performing the tasks, occupations and roles of everyday living. Nor does it assist us in describing understanding the many dimensions of occupational performance and the relationships among them.

Occupations as Structure

Occupations have a purpose. They are performed for work, pleasure, or self-maintenance. They usually entail social dimensions, such as whether they require cooperation or competition and whether they are public or private. An important characteristic of occupations is their temporal dimension. This pertains to how long they last and at which time(s) they are performed.

Adolph Meyer (1922) observed that occupations provide a necessary structure to our existence, noting that many persons in mental institutions at the time had lost the temporal order in their daily lives. Kielhofner (1977, 1978) provided a useful analysis of the temporal properties of occupation, noting that physical and mental illnesses frequently interfere with an individual's ability to manage time, either because his or her sense of time is distorted, or because the time required to accomplish necessary tasks has changed. He further suggested that role changes require a corresponding adjustment in the manner in which one organizes time. This phenomenon can be observed in retired persons who have not prepared for the increased amount of leisure time available in their lives. The term *temporal adaptation* has been used to describe the process of adjusting to changing temporal requirements in daily life or throughout the lifespan (Kielhofner, 1977).

Actions

Any observable behavior that is recognizable can be described as an "action", the basic building block of occupation. Actions often involve several steps which, when performed in a particular sequence toward the accomplishment of a goal, become part of task performance. Actions typically derive their meaning from the situations in which they are performed (or observed).

Tasks

Tasks are viewed as combinations of actions sharing some purpose recognized by the task performer. The nature of tasks can provide the motivation and context for learning skills and roles necessary for competent life performance. The performance of tasks can also reveal important information about the nature of emotional and cognitive disorders. A knowledge of the various dimensions of tasks is essential for the occupational therapist, who can use these dimensions in the selection of approaches to intervention.

Occupations

In Chapter 1, we defined occupations as "the ordinary and familiar things that people do every day" (Christiansen, Clark, Kielhofner et al., 1995, p. 1015). We suggested that occupations are identifiable and can be named by others. We also noted that they provide meaning and meet needs for self-maintenance, recreation, rest, creativity and productivity. Various patterns of occupations are characteristic of lifestyles. Patterns of occupations also characterize social roles.

Roles

Roles are important for occupational therapists to understand, because they outline the nature of occupational performance at various points in time. Thus, it can be asserted that occupational performance deficits have meaning principally in the context of an individual's role responsibilities. To speak of occupational dysfunction, then, is to refer to one's inadequate performance of social roles. In the following section, social roles are examined from the standpoint of their organizing properties and changing nature over the life span.

The concept of role emanates from social psychology and the symbolic interactionist school of thought, advanced principally by George Herbert Mead (1934) and Harry Stack Sullivan (1953). This view proposes that roles, defined as positions in society having expected responsibilities and privileges, form the very nucleus of social interaction. Smooth social interaction requires role-reciprocity, or the effective role performance of each member in a group. Roles affect development and personality through strong social approval when roles are enacted successfully, and equally strong sanctions when role expectations are not met. Socialization is thus the process of learning role behaviors.

Sarbin (1968) notes that within the boundaries of each role, expectations are formed by both society and the role occupant. Thus, one's satisfaction with the performance of valued roles is based on internal as well as external appraisals. This external influence is reflected in exemptions granted by society to persons who are experiencing difficult life events. An example is the "sick role," described eloquently by Parsons, which excuses persons from fulfilling role responsibilities during illness, as long as certain conditions are met, including seeking and complying with medical advice. Unfortunately, when the sick role is adopted by or ascribed to individuals with disabling conditions, the passivity and compliance expected in the sick role may conflict with the goals of the rehabilitation process. This is especially likely in situations where occupational therapy is appropriately practiced, since active participation and independence are valued (Burke, Miyake, Kielhofner & Barris, 1983).

Roles are dynamic in that throughout the lifespan, they are being acquired or replaced. For example, during adolescence, a major concern is occupational choice, or determining the specific nature of one's worker role. Later, parental roles may be acquired, subsequently to be replaced when one's children reach adolescence and leave home. These developmental transitions are especially important, since they involve the development of new skills or the integration of skills previously learned.

When persons cannot perform roles to satisfaction, either because of deficits in abilities and skills due to disease or disability, the conflicting demands of multiple roles (role conflict), or unclear role expectations, dysfunction is present. Such disruption in the roles of daily living, termed "occupational performance dysfunction" by Rogers (1983), constitutes the appropriate type of problem for occupational therapy intervention.

Abilities

The sense of self-respect and self-efficacy that define competence are gained through engagement in the tasks and roles required of daily living. Underlying the performance of life tasks are requisite abilities and skills. Although the terms *ability* and *skill* have often been used interchangeably in occupational therapy, it is useful to view them as distinct concepts.

Definitions provided by Fleischman (1975), a human factors scientist, are useful here. He defines abilities as general traits which are a product of genetic make-up and learning, much of which occurs during childhood and adolescence. Abilities (when abilities are impaired it is described as a functional limitation) are brought forth when one begins to learn a new task. As general factors, abilities may relate to performance on a variety of diverse tasks.

For example, an ability called *spatial orientation* is necessary for success at reading a road map and finding your way through a familiar room when the lights are out. *Reaction time*, another ability, is necessary for us to avoid snowballs hurled at us, return "slams" in a Ping-Pong match, and apply the brakes quickly when a dog suddenly decides to cross the road in front of our car. These examples are from a list of 52 abilities which have been derived from empirical studies over a number of years (Fleischman & Quaintance, 1984). A comprehensive list of these abilities with accompanying definitions can be found in Figure 3-5.

Abilities are the product of genetic factors and learning. Piaget and others have contributed immeasurably to our understanding of the processes through which cognitive and motor learning take place during early childhood. Thus, we know that abilities are developed very rapidly during the first years of life and that skill is attained in various age-related tasks in a complex spiral of maturation and interaction with the environment as the individual matures.

It has taken a great deal of methodical research to demonstrate that a relatively small number of underlying general abilities can explain proficiency in a large number of tasks. Research has shown that knowledge of these abilities and how to measure them can be linked with knowledge about the nature of tasks to predict performance and design efficient training programs. This method for understanding the dimensions underlying task proficiency is known as the ability requirements approach, and seems to hold considerable promise for those concerned with occupational performance.

Skill

In contrast, the term *skill* pertains to the level of proficiency in a specific task. The assumption is that skill in complex tasks can be explained by the presence of various underlying general abilities. Driving a car can be used as an example here. A professional race car driver has much more driving skill than the average person. This level of skill is determined by reaction time, perceptual speed, rate control, and other abilities, such as peripheral vision and motor control.

It is presumed that there is a relationship between learning and abilities. An individual with a high number of abilities is more readily able to learn the skills necessary to become proficient at a variety of specific tasks. However, studies have shown that the combinations of abilities influencing proficiency change as an individual gains experience at a particular task.

For example, consider a person performing a task that requires visual discrimination and quick reactions in moving a joystick (as is commonly required in various video and computer games). In this activity, visual-spatial abilities may influence performance more during early learning of the task, but motor abilities may assume more importance as the person gains experience.

Such changes in the influence of abilities as one gains experience in a task have important implications for predicting performance and for training, particularly in the learning of complex tasks. Since the abilities required for different levels of skill may change during the course of learning, ability testing to predict performance should be based on those abilities required at later points. Thus, if we emphasize the abilities required for final proficiency in a task during the early stages of training, this should facilitate the learning of complex tasks. Experiments done on the training of pilots have shown that this principle is valid (Fleishman, 1972).

Exploration can be viewed as a developmental step toward the attainment of competent performance. Reilly (1974) and others (Robinson, 1977) have noted the exploratory nature of play and its contribution to the acquisition of knowledge and skills necessary for competent performance. Through their interactions with people and things, individuals form sets of internal rules which govern future actions. Learning these internal rules is instrumental to the development of competence (Bruner, 1972).

Although abilities can be developed throughout the life span, most ability development occurs during childhood and adolescence. In adulthood, existing abilities are called on in the mastery of new tasks. In Chapter 18, Matheson and Bohr present the complexities and challenges of achieving occupational competence as it influences occupational performance throughout the life span.

INTRINSIC ENABLERS OF PERFORMANCE

Underlying general abilities are various supporting elements which are referred to as *performance enablers*. In this text, intrinsic factors contributing to performance are organized into psychological, cognitive, neurobehavioral, and physiological categories. These categories are consistent with, but not identical to, categories outlined in the Uniform Terminology documents developed by the AOTA, and referred to there as performance components.

Neurobehavioral Factors

Various neurobehavioral factors must be considered for their potential to support or facilitate performance. The sensory (olfactory, gustatory, visual, auditory, somatosensory, proprioceptive and vestibular) and motor systems (somatic, cerebellum, basal ganglia network, thalamic integration) exhibit principles that underlie all neuromotor performance. The ability to control movement, to modulate sensory input, to

Definitions for Ability Categories

1. **Oral Comprehension** is the ability to understand spoken English words and sentences.

2. **Written Comprehension** is the ability to understand written sentences and paragraphs.

3. **Oral Expression** is the ability to use English words or sentences in speaking so others will understand.

4. **Written Expression** is the ability to use English words or sentences in writing so others will understand.

5. **Fluency of Ideas** is the ability to produce a number of ideas about a given topic.

6. **Originality** is the ability to produce unusual or clever ideas about a given topic or situation. It is the ability to invent creative solutions to problems or to develop new procedures to situations in which standard operating procedures do not apply.

7. **Memorization** is the ability to remember information, such as words, numbers, pictures, and procedures. Pieces of information can be remembered by themselves or with other pieces of information.

8. **Problem Sensitivity** is the ability to tell when something is wrong or is likely to go wrong. It includes being able to identify the whole problem as well as the elements of the problem.

9. **Mathematical Reasoning** is the ability to understand and organize a problem and then to select a mathematical method or formula to solve the problem. It encompasses reasoning through mathematical problems to determine appropriate operations that can be performed to solve problems. It also includes the understanding or structuring of mathematical problems. The actual manipulation of numbers is not included in this ability.

10. **Number Facility** involves the degree to which adding, subtracting, multiplying, and dividing can be done quickly and correctly. These can be steps in other operations like finding percentages and taking square roots.

11. **Deductive Reasoning** is the ability to apply general rules to specific problems to come up with logical answers. It involves deciding if an answer makes sense.

12. **Inductive Reasoning** is the ability to combine separate pieces of information, or specific answers to problems, to form general rules or conclusions. It involves the ability to think of possible reasons for why things go together.

13. **Information Ordering** is the ability to follow correctly a rule or set of rules to arrange things or actions in a certain order. The rule or set of rules used must be given. The things or actions to be put in order can include numbers, letters, words, pictures, procedures, sentences, and mathematical or logical operations.

14. **Category Flexibility** is the ability to produce many rules so that each rule tells how to group a set of things in a different way. Each different group must contain at least two things from the original set of things.

15. **Speed of Closure** involves the degree to which different pieces of information can be combined and organized into one meaningful pattern quickly. It is not known beforehand what the pattern will be. The material may be visual or auditory.

16. **Flexibility of Closure** is the ability to identify or detect a known pattern (like a figure, word, or object) that is hidden in other material. The task is to pick out the disguised pattern from the background material.

17. **Spatial Orientation** is the ability to tell where you are in relation to the location of some object or to tell where the object is in relation to you.

18. **Visualization** is the ability to imagine how something will look when it is moved around or when its parts are moved or rearranged. It requires the forming of mental images of how patterns or objects would look after certain changes, such as unfolding or rotation. One has to predict how an object, set of objects, or pattern will appear after the changes are carried out.

19. **Perceptual Speed** involves the degree to which one can compare letters, numbers, objects, pictures, or patterns, quickly and accurately. The things to be compared may be presented at the same time or one after the other. This ability also includes comparing a presented object with a remembered object.

20. **Control Precision** is the ability to move controls of a machine or vehicle. This involves the degree to which these controls can be moved quickly and repeatedly to exact position.

21. **Multilimb Coordination** is the ability to coordinate movements of two or more limbs (for example, two arms, two legs, or one leg and one arm, such as in moving equipment controls. Two or more limbs are in motion while the individual is sitting, standing, or lying down.

22. **Response Orientation** is the ability to choose between two or more movements quickly and accurately when two or more different signals (lights, sounds, pictures) are given. The ability is concerned with the speed with which the right response can be started with the hand, foot, or other parts of the body.

23. **Rate Control** is the ability to adjust an equipment control in response to changes in the speed and/or directions of a continuously moving object or scene. The ability involves timing these adjustments in anticipating these changes. This ability does not extend to situations in which both the speed and direction of the object are perfectly predictable.

continued

Figure 3-5. Definitions for Ability Categories. From Fleishman, E. & Quaintance, M. (1984). *Taxonomies of human performance: The description of human tasks* (pp. 461-464). Orlando, FL: Academic Press. Reprinted with permission.

24. **Reaction Time** is the ability to give one fast response to one signal (sound, light, picture) when it appears. This ability is concerned with the speed with which the movement can be started with the hand, foot, or other parts of the body.

25. **Arm-Hand Steadiness** is the ability to keep the hand and arm steady. It includes steadiness while making an arm movement as well as while holding the arm and hand in one position. This ability does not involve strength or speed.

26. **Manual Dexterity** is the ability to make skillful coordinated movements of one hand, a hand together with its arm, or two hands to grasp, place, move, or assemble objects like hand tools or blocks. This ability involves the degree to which these arm-hand movements can be carried out quickly. It does not involve moving machine or equipment controls like levers.

27. **Finger Dexterity** is the ability to make skillful, coordinated movements of the fingers of one or both hands and to grasp, place, or move small objects. This ability involves the degree to which these finger movements can be carried out quickly.

28. **Wrist-Finger Speed** is the ability to make fast, simple repeated movements of the fingers, hands, and wrists. It involves little, if any, accuracy, careful control, or coordination of movement.

29. **Speed of Limb Movement** involves the speed with which a single movement of the arms and legs can be made. This ability does not include accuracy careful control, or coordination of movement.

30. **Selective Attention** is the ability to concentrate on a task one is doing. This ability involves concentrating while performing a boring task and not being distracted.

31. **Time Sharing** is the ability to shift back and forth between two or more sources of information.

32. **Static Strength** is the ability to use muscle force in order to lift, push, pull, or carry objects. It is the maximum force that one can exert for a brief period of time.

33. **Explosive Strength** is the ability to use short bursts of muscle force to propel oneself or an object. It requires gathering energy for bursts of muscle effort over a very short time period.

34. **Dynamic Strength** is the ability of the muscles to exert force repeatedly or continuously over a long time period. This is the ability to support, hold up, or move the body's own weight and/or objects repeatedly over time. It represents muscular endurance and emphasizes the resistance of the muscles to fatigue.

35. **Trunk Strength** involves the degree to which one's stomach and lower back muscles can support part of the body repeatedly or continuously over time. The ability involves the degree to which these trunk muscles do not fatigue when they are put under such repeated or continuous strain.

36. **Extent Flexibility** is the ability to bend, stretch, twist, or reach out with the body, arms, and/or legs, both quickly and repeatedly.

37. **Dynamic Flexibility** is the ability to bend, stretch, twist, or reach out with the body, arms and/or legs, both quickly and repeatedly.

38. **Gross Body Coordination** is the ability to coordinate the movement of the arms, legs, and torso together in activities in which the whole body is in motion.

39. **Gross Body Equilibrium** is the ability to keep or regain one's body balance or to stay upright when in an unstable position. This ability includes maintaining one's balance when changing direction while moving or standing motionless.

40. **Stamina** is the ability of the lungs and circulatory systems of the body to perform efficiently over long time periods. This is the ability to exert oneself physically without getting out of breath.

41. **Near Vision** is the capacity to see close environmental surroundings.

42. **Far Vision** is the capacity to see distant environmental surroundings.

43. **Visual Color Discrimination** is the capacity to match or discriminate between colors. This capacity also includes detecting differences in color purity (saturation) and brightness (brilliance).

44. **Night Vision** is the ability to see under low light conditions.

45. **Peripheral Vision** is the ability to perceive objects or movement towards the edges of the visual field.

46. **Depth Perception** is the ability to distinguish which of several objects is more distant from or nearer to the observer, or to judge the distance of an object from the observer.

47. **Glare Sensitivity** is the ability to see objects in the presence of glare or bright ambient lighting.

48. **General Hearing** is the ability to detect and to discriminate among sounds that vary over broad ranges of pitch and/or loudness.

49. **Auditory Attention** is the ability to focus on a single source of auditory information in the presence of other distracting and irrelevant auditory stimuli.

50. **Sound Localization** is the ability to identify the direction from which an auditory stimulus originated relative to the observer.

51. **Speech Hearing** is the ability to learn and understand the speech of another person.

52. **Speech Clarity** is the ability to communicate orally in a clear fashion understandable to a listener.

Figure 3-5 (continued). Definitions for Ability Categories. From Fleishman, E. & Quaintance, M. (1984). *Taxonomies of human performance: The description of human tasks* (pp. 461-464). Orlando, FL: Academic Press. Reprinted with permission.

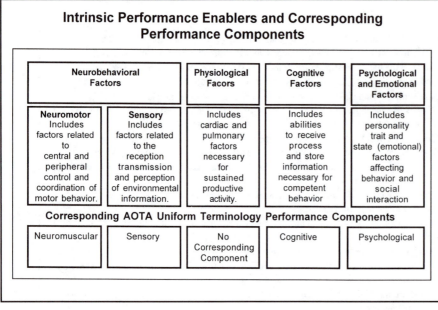

Figure 3-6. Intrinsic Performance Enablers and Corresponding Performance Components.

coordinate and integrate sensory information, to compensate for sensorimotor deficits, and to modify neural structures through behavior are all important characteristics that influence and support occupational performance.

The capacity of the sensory and motor system must be determined to facilitate adaptive and or compensatory responses. Interventions must be guided by basic neurobehavioral principles so that individuals can derive optimal benefit from therapy. The importance of the neuro-behavioral factors was anticipated early in the development of occupational therapy when Meyer (1922) challenged proponents of the field to observe the restorative benefits of engagement in occupation on the behavior of those receiving services.

Physiological Factors

Physical health and fitness are necessary requirements for those occupations requiring even moderate exertion or sustained effort. They are also key to preventing secondary problems. Abilities such as endurance, flexibility, movement, and strength must be considered in planning programs to help clients achieve personal goals and sustain health. Occupations can be used to engage individuals to use their motor and memory skills, which will in turn enhance their performance of tasks, and maintain both cognitive and physiological fitness. Physiological factors that influence performance are discussed in Chapter 10.

Cognitive Factors

Cognition involves the mechanisms of language comprehension and production, pattern recognition, task organization, reasoning, attention, and memory (Duchek, 1991). When these

mechanisms are intact, they support the person in learning, communicating, moving, and observing. When the mechanisms are deficient, they create functional limitations for the individual and his or her family. Rehabilitation services enable the individual to learn strategies to bypass the deficit and/or compensate for the loss.

The field of neuroscience is developing an understanding of how experiences generate changes in the nervous system that shape language, vision, coordinated movement, and cognition (Merzenich, Scheiner, Jenkins & Wang 1993). It should be the goal of occupational therapists to minimize the consequences of brain injury in the lives of those whose injuries adversely affect tasks of daily living, social interaction, family life, and vocational and educational pursuits. These issues are addressed in Chapter 11.

Psychological and Emotional Factors

Psychological factors describe the internal experiences, personal reactions and mechanisms through which the individual manages relationships between the environment and self. These factors, which include self-concept, self-esteem and emotional state (or affect) influence the individual's perception of self.

Psychological factors are basic to doing (Fidler & Fidler, 1973; Bonder, 1993). In addition to looking at how these factors contribute to effective performance, the occupational therapist is concerned with how a person's occupation contributes to his or her sense of well-being. Psychological factors may be more seriously impaired in some persons who have diagnosed psychological illness. However, psychological factors influence performance in all humans and must be considered (Figure 3-6).

ENVIRONMENT: THE CONTEXT OF PERFORMANCE

Occupational performance is always influenced by the characteristics of the environment in which it occurs. In noting this, Rogers (1983, p. 604) described the qualities of the environment as important "enablers of human performance." Perhaps because of the influence of medicine and its orientation toward the internal workings of the body, occupational therapists have given insufficient attention in the past to environmental factors and their influence on performance. Barris (1982) (Barris, Kielhofner, Levine & Neville, 1985) was one of the first writers in the field to attempt to organize dimensions of the environment within a conceptual framework, although the last decade has seen major advances in this area (Letts, Law, Rigby, Cooper, Stewart & Strong, 1994). Environmental theories are presented in Chapter 4.

Through a process identified by Berlyne (1960) as *arousal*, environments can influence our inclination to interact with or explore our environment. Arousal has both physiological as well as psychological characteristics related to one's level of alertness and has its most obvious affect on performance when persons are bored and inattentive (underaroused) or anxious (over-aroused). Three groups of environmental variables are associated with arousal. These include psychophysical characteristics such as loud noises and bright lights; ecological events which are related to one's well-being (such as a severe storm); and situations viewed as novel, surprising or ambiguous (called collative characteristics). The degree of match between the characteristics of the environment and our interests and values may have an impact on our inclination to explore or interact within that setting. Barris notes that the characteristics of settings which influence arousal must be carefully considered, so that an optimal level (producing neither boredom nor anxiety) is attained (Barris, 1982, p. 638).

The personality theorists Murray, Barrett & Hamburger (1938) were the first to recognize that characteristics of environments influence behavior by creating demands or expectations for behavior, either objectively or as perceived by the individual. Their term for this phenomenon was *press*. The concept of press has been refined and extended by other investigators, including Lawton (1980), and given prominence in the occupational therapy literature by Barris et al. (1985).

An individual's reaction to press is dependent upon his or her abilities as well as experience. As experience with new settings increases, an individual learns those behaviors which are expected, thus feeling competent within the chosen environment. This may encourage the individual to seek new settings which will provide novelty or challenge, thus providing motivation to acquire new skills.

Physical Properties of Environments

The physical properties of environments are the most obvious, and thus the most likely to be given consideration when environmental influences on performance are discussed. For many years, therapists have been doing pre-discharge home assessments, or surveying work sites in order to identify modifications necessary to accommodate persons with mobility limitations or other types of disability, such as sensory deficits.

Clearly, design is an important characteristic of the physical environment, and one that is deserving of even greater attention than it has received in the past. Physical environments must be considered for accessibility and arrangement, as well as for safety and aesthetics. Design considerations can and should accommodate all these issues if they are to support the individual's performance of occupations and provide for comfort and enjoyment. Both the suitability of personal living space to accommodate unique individual needs and the negotiability of public places are relevant to the analysis of physical environments.

The Cultural Environment

Culture refers to the values, beliefs, customs and behaviors that are passed on from one generation to the next. Culture affects performance in many ways, including prescribing norms for the use of time and space, influencing beliefs regarding the importance of various tasks, and transmitting attitudes and values regarding work and play (Altman & Chelmers, 1980; Hall, 1973). Culture also influences role expectations.

Each person has a cultural orientation that influences his or her choices regarding both what to do and how to do it. Cultural preferences must be respected and accommodated by therapy personnel as intervention is planned and delivered. Both knowledge and sensitivity to cultural influences on occupational performance are important to the effective delivery of care. These issues are discussed in Chapter 14.

Societal Factors

Human beings are group living, social animals whose relationships with others play a fundamental role in shaping behavior and attitudes toward the self. Societal acceptance is universally sought, and social rejection and isolation can have devastating psychological consequences. Prejudicial attitudes, stereotypes, and the intolerance of differences are products of ignorance and remain a part of the social environment.

People with observable differences must contend with the attitudinal barriers which inhibit their acceptance by others. Because these attitudinal barriers exist even among informed, educated persons (including health care professionals), the experience of disability must be studied and

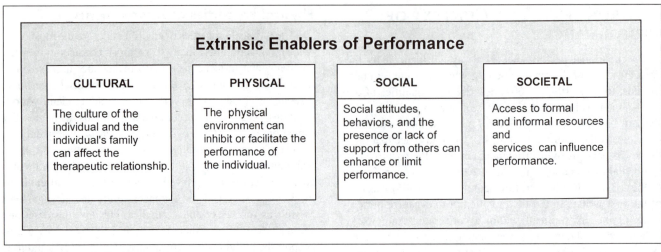

Figure 3-7. Extrinsic Enablers of Performance.

understood if such barriers are to be eliminated. Understanding these barriers is also relevant for persons with disability, since they must learn to recognize and contend with the stigma that accompanies them. This can be achieved through training in interpersonal techniques such as impression management (Goffman, 1963). Chapters 15 and 16 provide an in-depth discussion of these issues.

Social Support

People are social beings. What we do usually involves others. Social support affects occupation and contributes to health and well-being on several levels. Some individuals choose to have more social networks than others. When a disability occurs, how does one go about obtaining support for a network to support occupational performance? The occupational therapist must understand social support to use it effectively. The therapist must know about networks, types and sources of support and how to assess the patterns of social support used by his or her clients. These issues are presented in Chapter 17 (Figure 3-7).

APPLYING THE MODEL: OCCUPATIONAL THERAPY INTERVENTION

Client-centered practice is based on the principle that effective therapy begins with a careful understanding of the individual. An occupational therapy practice based on the concepts of client-centeredness is more likely to engage clients in the occupational therapy process and lead to increased cooperation and satisfaction with therapy (Law, Baptiste & Mills, 1995). The Person-Environment Occupational Performance Model provides a framework for

the clinician to organize information gained in interviews and formal assessments to form the basis for intervention that is collaborative and client-directed. Such an approach is better able to enlist the personal and spiritual resources necessary to facilitate the healing process (Matheis-Kraft, George, Olinger, & York, 1990).

In a client-centered approach, clients and therapists work together to identify problems of living related to the performance of occupations. Through collaboration, the focus and need for intervention and the preferred outcomes of therapy are determined (Baum & Law, 1997). The basic assumptions of a client-centered approach are: 1) clients and their families know themselves best, 2) all clients and families are different and unique, and 3) optimal client performance occurs within a supportive family and community context (Law, Baptiste, & Mills, 1995).

Using these assumptions, clients and therapists can jointly focus on their unique contribution and responsibilities. In such a partnership, clients expect to lead the decision-making process. To do this, clients require information that will enable them to make decisions about the services that will most effectively meet their needs. This information, when given in an understandable way, will ensure that clients can define occupational performance priorities for intervention and consider the risks and benefits of alternative strategies (Baum & Law, 1997). Clients expect to receive services in a timely manner and to be treated with respect and dignity during the occupational therapy process. The therapist encourages clients to use their own resources to help solve occupational performance problems. Clients will participate at different levels, depending on their capabilities, but all are capable of making at least some choices about how they prefer to lead their daily lives.

A client-centered approach encourages occupational therapists to assume responsibilities, such as encouraging client decision-making in partnership with other team members. The approach fosters a partnership with clients to enable them to identify their needs and individualize the services they perceive they will need in order to accomplish their goals. Client decisions are supported by therapists whenever possible. Otherwise, the therapist communicates clearly those reasons for not supporting a decision or choice. Therapists will also respect a client's values and visions as well as his or her style of coping without judging what is right or wrong. Clients are encouraged to recognize and build on their strengths, using natural community supports as much as possible (Baum & Law, 1997).

The occupational therapist, as well as the client, brings knowledge and experience to the therapeutic relationship. It is just as important for a client to understand why an occupational therapist is involved in his or her care and what the client can expect to achieve through occupational therapy as it is for the therapist to understand the issues and needs of the client. This facilitates the creation of an occupational performance history which includes information about the person, the environment, and the occupational factors that require occupational therapy intervention (Baum & Law, 1997).

The implementation of a Person-Environment Occupational Performance Model requires reexamination of how therapists access information to support a client-centered approach. Traditionally, occupational therapists have measured the components of function or the impairments of a person with a functional problem. A client-centered approach uses a top down approach (Trombly, 1995; Mathioweitz & Bass Haugen, 1994), in which the client determines what he or she perceives to be the important occupational performance problems which create difficulty in carrying out daily activities (work, self-maintenance, leisure, and rest).

The Person-Environment Occupational Performance Model offers a balanced model for viewing the client and jointly planning intervention. For a therapeutic relationship to evolve it is important for the client to understand the scope of the therapist's knowledge and the therapist's ability to access resources. Additionally, the client's knowledge of his or her condition and experience with the problem must become clear for the relationship to progress (Baum & Law, 1997). Occasionally, treatment planning must occur with a person who has a cognitive deficit, or because of age or intelligence does not have the capacity for independent decision-making. In this case, a family-centered approach is critical. A family-centered approach is based on the same principles as outlined above, with members of the family acting as the client's substitute or representative.

It is important for the occupational therapist to plan the first phase of the intervention to seek information from the client about his or her perception of the problem, needs, and goals. Information is shared to build the occupational perfor-

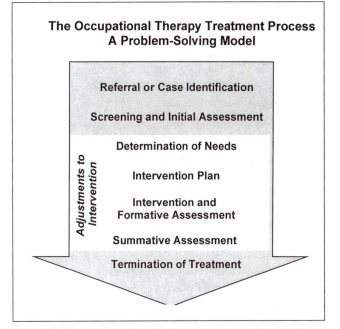

Figure 3-8. The Occupational Therapy Treatment Process: A Problem-Solving Model.

mance history, which includes information about the person, the environment, and the occupational factors that require occupational therapy intervention. Figure 3-8 identifies the steps the occupational therapist employs when using a Person-Environment Occupational Performance approach.

The goal of occupational therapy is to prevent, remediate or reduce dysfunction that impairs or limits occupational performance of an individual. In addressing occupational performance needs, therapists work with the individual, the family, other professionals, and perhaps citizens in the community to characterize the nature of the problem, develop an intervention plan, and deliver services or information. The success of intervention strategies must be determined through evaluation during and following the delivery of services. Together, these events constitute the approach taken in a problem-oriented process model.

While the individual elements of the occupational therapy process are discussed sequentially in the following sections, it is important to realize that the problem-oriented approach is not a linear process. Rather, it is a conceptual process during which the therapist continually moves back and forth between elements with the intent of crafting an approach tailored to the unique needs of a given patient. While an approximate treatment plan may be conceived during the initial phases of treatment, it is adjusted and refined in a series of successive therapeutic encounters, with the client taking more and more responsibility for independent problem-solving.

In some cases, the client will be referred for occupational therapy because a performance deficit exists due to a developmental condition, disease or injury. In other cases, referral may be made for the purpose of maintaining or improving the individual's occupational performance.

Assessment

Following referral, an initial phase involves the identification of the intrinsic and extrinsic factors that support and limit the activities, tasks, and roles of the client. One of the theoretical frameworks discussed in Chapter 4 can be used by clinicians to guide thinking about assessment and interventions. In collecting information, the therapist is attempting to characterize the nature of a patient's occupational performance status.

Assessment data should include details about the individual's assets as well as deficits, and should always reflect the environmental context in which the individual typically performs the activities, tasks and roles of daily living. Information on the person's past performance as well as environmental demands will be relevant, and should provide a sense of the client's interests, values and use of time. Analysis of these data will permit the identification of strengths and weaknesses. Based on this analysis, the therapist and client jointly are able to make an informed decision about the types of intervention which will be most effective in meeting the client's goals so they can be included in the occupational therapy plan.

Assessment is a process of collecting information to become fully informed about a client and his or her goals. It may include formalized approaches, such as standardized tests and structured interviews, as well as less obtrusive techniques, gained through informal interaction and skillful observation. It would be ideal if all assessment information could be gathered prior to developing a treatment plan and beginning intervention. However, in nearly every instance, intervention begins before the therapist gains a complete picture of the individual. In fact, it is misleading to characterize the assessment process as a discrete event which precedes intervention. In actual practice, experienced clinicians tend to make tentative inferences about patients before formalized assessment is completed. This process, termed "reflection-in-action" by Schon (1983), is viewed as instrumental to achieving the purpose of assessment, which is to frame the problem. These inferences represent informed guesses about individual problems and are based on experiences with similar patients.

As the therapist gains more experience (and thus more assessment information) with a particular individual, earlier inferences may be discarded or refined. Thus, information is gathered throughout the intervention process. In medical settings, a diagnosis has frequently been made on the patient prior to referral to occupational therapy. In such cases, this diagnosis may guide the therapist toward specific assessment tools and provide tentative expectations about the nature of performance deficits. But the medical diagnosis is a totally inadequate basis for planning interventions to address the occupational performance problems of the individual because it usually fails to provide any insight into the needs and expectations of the person. Furthermore, it says nothing about the assets of the patient, which are critical to forming a complete picture of the patient's occupational performance status and goals. For this reason, master clinicians typically use narrative reasoning to gain a complete understanding of the problem. Narrative reasoning involves understanding the client in terms of that person's unique life story (Mattingly & Fleming, 1994).

The diagnosis may also be accompanied by information from the physician's plan for medical management. This will be relevant to occupational therapy if it involves planned surgery, chemotherapy or other types of treatment which will create anxiety, influence attentional states, or otherwise diminish the patient's physical or mental capacity to plan and participate in treatment.

There are hundreds of existing assessment tools to assist the therapist in gaining a complete picture of the client and the intrinsic and extrinsic factors contributing to his or her occupational performance. Some provide information on specific enabling factors, such as psychological, cognitive, psychological, or neurobehavioral areas; while others are more global in their approach to environmental factors and actions, tasks and roles. Determining the utility and validity of assessments is a matter of importance to occupational therapists in all settings, since the objective is to select the combination of interviews and measures or data collection approaches that will provide the clearest and most complete picture of the individual's level of occupational performance with the least expenditure of time, energy and cost. Developing a sound approach to assessment requires a basic understanding of factors that contribute to occupational performance. Each factor is addressed in later chapters, including several devoted to a discussion of assessment and informed decision-making (Chapters 5, 6 & 7).

Planning Intervention Strategies

In addressing the needs of clients, competent occupational therapists draw upon their knowledge of the individual, the environment, and the assets and limitations which affect the quality of occupational performance. A careful consideration of this information and the possible treatment alternatives permits the selection of various strategies for meeting client-centered goals. In each case, the particular application of an intervention process will be unique, since individuals and their circumstances are unique.

Rogers (1982) cautions that a therapeutic program that is right for one patient is not necessarily right for another. She suggests that clinical inquiry be individualized and focus on three questions: 1) What is the client's current status in occupational role performance? 2) What could be done to enhance the client's performance? 3) What ought to be done to enhance the individual's occupational performance?

Take, for example, the performance challenges created by spinal cord injury. Even if two men of the same age from the same hometown were to sustain the same degree of quadriplegic paralysis, it is likely that their occupational therapy would vary considerably. This is because there would remain substantial differences in many individual (intrinsic) and environmental (extrinsic) factors which affected their performance, ranging from the physical characteristics of their usual living environment to their family and work roles, leisure interests and personalities. Thus, in competent practice, the same strategy will never be repeated in exactly the same manner with different individuals, since each will have a different configuration of circumstances (Figure 3-9).

It is the critical analysis of the intrinsic, extrinsic, and occupational factors and planning of intervention for the unique constellation of circumstances represented in each client that makes occupational therapy an immensely complex undertaking. Because of this complexity, treatment planning is one of the most challenging and critical skills for therapists to master. As Fleming and Mattingly (1994) point out, what occupational therapists do appears so very simple, but the process of determining what to do is so very complex. Despite its complexities, effective treatment planning can be accomplished if careful attention is devoted to the following elements of the process:

Summarizing the assessment data. In this initial component of the process, it is necessary to review the patient's strengths and weaknesses from the perspective of the Person-Environment Occupational Performance Model including the intrinsic, extrinsic and occupational factors.

Goal identification. Based upon the summary of strengths and weaknesses, a list of goals is developed with the client. These should directly relate from each identified problem or need. Short-term goals will often relate to problems identified in intrinsic enabling components. Long-term goals generally relate to the performance of functional daily living tasks related to role performance and must include strategies to manage environmental issues. The Canadian Occupational Performance Measure discussed in Chapter 5 can be used for this purpose.

Selecting intervention plans and methods. Here, specific methods and techniques for achieving goals must be determined. In achieving short-term goals, the emphasis may be on restoring ability and skills. However, means of re-engaging in meaningful occupations must be considered to foster the motivation of the individual and to use the engagement in the recovery process. Long-term goals may be more adaptive in nature, since tasks may need to be performed with restricted underlying ability and skill. As a consequence, compensatory techniques, special equipment, and environmental modification may be necessary to accommodate residual disability.

Pelland (1987) has observed that effective treatment plans are balanced, in that they address remedial and adaptive goals within and across treatment sessions. For example, in treatment of a grandmother who is recovering from CVA, one might devote time to compensating for a visual field deficit while encouraging her to bake cookies for her grandchildren—an activity which balances goals and strategies.

Planning for further data collection. Pelland also notes the importance of planning for further data collection, and documenting these intentions. By including assessment intentions within the overall intervention plan, the therapist assures that this important aspect of treatment is not neglected.

Developing priorities. Once each problem has an accompanying goal and plan, the vital task of determining priorities must take place. While the theoretical approach selected by the therapist can provide guidance, those interventions which are directed at reducing pain or preventing complications or deformities must be addressed. Another principle is that assessment must take precedence over intervention, since effective treatment is contingent on complete information. Principles of therapeutic management must involve the use of activities meaningful to the client that incorporate therapeutic principles to support recovery, e.g., encouraging trunk stability and arm positioning before focusing on fine motor skill. Simultaneously, the therapist can give early attention to goals and strategies which have clear implications for motivation and patient compliance.

Treatment planning includes a logical flow from identified problems to goals to intervention strategies. In essence, the treatment planning process, when performed by the clinician, can be likened to weaving. There is a clear design and guiding principles. The challenge is to combine the warp and weft in a way that captures opportunities for creativity and yet yields a satisfactory outcome.

The experienced weaver, like the clinician in providing treatment, executes the design with a shuttle that glides smoothly, wasting neither time nor energy in pursuit of the selvage that ends this effort and marks the beginning of yet another challenge. Critical to this analogy is to understand that the client is the loom, as he or she is the focus and the outcome or the fabric of the plan.

Implementing Treatment
Strategies for addressing occupational performance deficits tend to fall into five major categories, which are addressed in

Spinal Cord Injury: A Case Comparison of Occupational Therapy Intervention

Spinal cord injury (SCI) represents one of the major causes of death and disability among young adults. For those surviving, over half must contend with paralysis affecting sensation and voluntary motor control in all four extremities (quadriplegia). Acute medical intervention is designed to prevent further injury to the spinal cord and stabilize the body systems to assure satisfactory respiration, circulation and metabolism.

Once stabilization has occurred, the patient is ready for rehabilitation. Interdisciplinary teams, including the occupational therapist, strive to help the patient achieve as much independence as possible in all dimensions of life.

Patients with injuries at the level of the sixth cervical vertebra (C-6) are quadriplegic, maintaining only limited muscular control of their head and neck, upper trunk, and arms. However, they can attain high levels of independence. The following case summaries describe the circumstances and occupational therapy treatment of two 28-year-old men. The reader will find that although the diagnoses and ages of the patients may be the same, their therapeutic regimens are likely to vary significantly, based on their personalities, experiences, interests, motivations, social situations, and views of self.

Eric M.

Background: Eric was a 28-year-old law school graduate when he sustained his level C-6 spinal cord injury in an automobile accident on the way home from a family shopping trip. His wife, pregnant at the time, suffered a fractured arm, but recovered and delivered a healthy baby girl, their first child, three months later. Eric has worked as a staff assistant in the office of the county district attorney since receiving his law degree. As a child, he was an avid reader, who excelled in school. In his leisure time, he participated in team sports. He excelled in college and was active in student governance. Eric has remained very close to his parents and siblings. His father is a high school principal, and his mother is an English teacher. His three brothers and sisters live within a 50 mile radius of the old house Eric and his wife had begun restoring just months before their accident.

Intervention: During the early phases of treatment, Eric's occupational therapist provided passive range of motion of his joints to prevent deformities and introduced some activities to increase strength and endurance. Later, when he had gained the ability to sit upright without dizziness, he began learning how to pull himself to a sitting position without assistance. At first using a device called a mobile arm support, he was taught to eat and drink with a cuff designed to help him hold utensils. Once he gained sufficient strength, he began learning how to get into his wheelchair and propel it around the facility. He learned quickly because he was anxious to try new challenges, less afraid of failure because of the many experiences in his life where he had experienced success and mastery over challenges.

Eric's therapy team quickly involved his family in planning treatment and learning to provide needed assistance. A home visit by a member of the staff suggested that because of the nature of the old house they owned, it would be best to begin looking for a newer home without as many steps and architectural barriers.

After learning to use a special flexor hinge splint to allow independent grasp, he was quickly able to resume his professional activities on a part-time basis. Later, he was given training to drive a specially modified car, in which he can transport himself to work. Despite his impairment and disability, Eric has been able to return to active participation in the roles he previously occupied.

John R.

Background: John was also 28 when he crashed his motorcycle on the way home from a construction site where he worked as a house framer. John was living alone at the time of accident, saving money to attend a local technical school, where he intended to learn auto repair. He had previously attended a junior college for two years, but his academic performance suffered because he was unsure of his goals. His mother, a widow, died of cancer during this period. As an only child, John was not encouraged to be independent. He was an average student, who became interested in carpentry and mechanics during high school. He enjoyed working on his motorcycle and going on cross-country motorcycle outings as hobbies. John had a girlfriend at the time of his accident whom he had been dating for nearly twelve months, but had few other close friends.

Intervention: John's occupational therapists also provided passive range of motion of his joints to prevent contractures and introduced some activities to help build strength and endurance in his shoulders and arms for later parts of his therapy. John's acceptance of his condition was slow to develop. He was hostile toward staff and non-compliant. Although the nature of his work had provided him with sufficient strength in his upper arms to easily learn to transfer and propel his wheelchair, his progress was slow. He was depressed—especially after his girlfriend ended their relationship after learning of his permanent paralysis. He was fearful of attempting new skills and failing. Soon, he began attending group outings organized by the occupational therapy staff. His mood and interest in participating in his rehabilitation program improved somewhat after he began socializing with other patients who participated in these outings.

Nevertheless, John's progress was slow. His mechanical interests made him curious about the devices demonstrated by his occupational therapist to help him attain independence in self-care, but he remained reluctant to attempt new skills. Because of his physical limitations, pursuit of his previous vocational ambitions was not possible. After a series of tests, the vocational counselor recommended he study mechanical engineering, which he is now considering. He has become independent enough to be discharged to a group living facility, in which several former patients share attended apartments.

Figure 3-9. Spinal Cord Injury: A Case Comparison of Occupational Therapy Intervention.

Major Intervention Categories in Occupational Therapy				
Use of Occupation as a Therapeutic Medium	**Education and Training Strategies**	**Strategies for Sensory and Neuromotor Remediation**	**Modification of the Physical Environment**	**Application of Technological Aids and Devices**
Includes those strategies in which occupation, as activity, task, or role, is devised with therapeutic intent	Includes those strategies which employ education or training to enable acquisition of abilities or skills necessary for the performance of tasks or roles or use of remaining abilities to compensate for skill deficits	Includes strategies directed toward remediation of sensory and/or motor deficits. Frequently employs principles of reflex maturation and neurophysiology	Includes those strategies aimed at modifying aspects of the physical environment, either through attention to press or arousal or through changing physical and social properties	Includes the use of various devices and equipment which enable performance of tasks and roles despite limitations in ability or skill. Includes both low technology and high technology aids and equipment
Example: Group shopping trip to purchase party supplies by residents of nursing home	*Example:* A woman with multiple sclerosis learns energy conservation techniques	*Example:* Neuromotor techniques are used with a man who has left-sided paralysis following stroke	*Example:* Doors are widened in the home of a person who has paralysis due to spinal cord injury	*Example:* A child with cerebral palsy learns to communicate using a microcomputer with a special input device.

Figure 3-10. Major Intervention Categories in Occupational Therapy.

this text. Two major categories are related to modifying the environment, and include making changes in a person's physical environment and using technology in the form of various devices and aids. A third category is intrinsic in focus and includes various approaches to facilitating the recovery or adaptation of neurological, sensory and motor deficits. The remaining two categories have principles which warrant specific focus in the text. These include the means of delivering services and strategies that challenge the occupational therapist to take an active role in changing attitudes, policies and laws that shape the political and social environment (Figure 3-10).

SUMMARY

In this chapter we have summarized the elements of the Person-Environment Occupational Performance Model, including intrinsic (within the person) and extrinsic (within the environment) factors to be considered in planning intervention. Intrinsic factors relate to those psychological, cognitive, physiological and neurobehavioral influences on the performance of daily occupations. Extrinsic factors pertain to the interpersonal, societal, cultural and physical environments.

A summary of the principles of client-centered practice was also provided, including the importance of planning intervention around occupational performance goals identified by the client, and collaborating in the identification and selection of strategies based on an informed understanding of options. The process of intervention was described, summarizing various elements of the process, including data gathering, problem formulation and intervention selection. It was emphasized that understanding the client is fundamental to prudent and ethical delivery of therapeutic services.

STUDY QUESTIONS

1. Considering the major elements in the Person-Environment Occupational Performance Model, construct a visual diagram that conveys the relationships

between these elements.

2. Compare and contrast cognitive and intrinsic theories of motivation.

3. Define internality and describe how it can influence the occupational therapy process.

4. Explain relationships between personality and occupational choice.

5. Describe the elements in Osgood's theory of values.

6. Construct a hierarchy using the terms occupation, role, action, task, and lifestyle.

7. Identify several intrinsic enablers of performance.

8. Describe elements in the occupational therapy intervention process.

RECOMMENDED READINGS

Bandura, A. (1982). Self-efficacy mechanisms in human agency. *American Psychologist, 37*, 122-147.

Barris, R. (1982). Environmental interactions: An extension of the model of occupation. *American Journal of Occupational Therapy, 36*(10), 637-644.

Baum, C. M. & Law, M. (1997). Occupational therapy practice: Focusing on occupational performance. *American Journal of Occupational Therapy, 51*(4), 277-288.

Berlyne, D. E. (1960). *Conflict, arousal and curiosity.* New York: McGraw Hill.

Branholm, I. B. & Fugl-Meyer, A. R. (1992). Occupational role preferences and life satisfaction. *Occupational Therapy Journal of Research, 12*(3), 159-171.

Burke, J. P. (1977). A clinical perspective on motivation: Pawn versus origin. *American Journal of Occupational Therapy, 31*(4), 254-258.

Fleming, M. & Mattingly, C. (1994). *Clinical reasoning: Forms of inquiry in a therapeutic practice.* Philadelphia: F. A. Davis.

Hogan, R. (1982). A socioanalytic theory of personality. *Nebraska Symposium on Motivation, 30*, 55-89.

Pervin, L. A. (1968). Performance and satisfaction as a function of individual-environment fit. *Psychological Bulletin, 69*, 56-68.

Rowles, G. D. (1991). Beyond performance: Being in place as a component of occupational therapy. *American Journal of Occupational Therapy, 45*(3), 365-271.

Sarbin, T. R., & Allen, V. L. (1968). Role theory. In G. Lindsey & E. Aronson (Eds.), *Handbook of social psychology* (2nd ed.). Reading, MA: Addison-Wesley.

Smith, M. B. (1974). Competence and adaptation: A perspective on therapeutic ends and means. *American Journal of Occupational Therapy, 28*(1), 11-15.

White, R. W. (1971). The urge towards competence. *American Journal of Occupational Therapy, 25*(6), 271-274.

REFERENCES

Allison, M. & Duncan, M. (1988). Women, work and flow. In M. Cskiszentmihalkyi & I. Cskiszentmihalkyi (Eds). *Optimal Experience: Psychological Studies in Flow in Consciousness.* New York: Cambridge University Press; pp. 118-137.

Altman, &. Chelmers. (1980). *Culture and Environment.* Monterey, CA: Brooks/Cole.

American Occupational Therapy Association (1994). Uniform Terminology for Occupational Therapy (3rd Ed). *American Journal of Occupational Therapy, 48*, 1047-1059.

Bandura, A. (1977). Self-efficacy: Toward a unifying theory of behavioral change. *Psychological Review, 84*, 191-215.

Bandura, A. (1982). Self efficacy mechanisms in human agency. *American Psychologist, 37*, 122-147.

Barris, R. (1982). Environmental interactions: An extension of the model of occupation. *American Journal of Occupational Therapy, 36*(10), 637-644.

Barris, R., Kielhofner, G., Levine, R. E., & Neville, A. M. (1985). Occupation as interaction with the environment. In G. Kielhofner (Ed.), *A Model of Human Occupation: Theory and Application.* Baltimore: Williams & Wilkins; pp. 42-62.

Baum, C. M. & Law, M. (1997).Occupational therapy practice: Focusing on occupational performance. *American Journal of Occupational Therapy, 51*(4) 277-288.

Berger, P. L.& Luckman, T. (1967). *The Social Construct of Reality.* New York: Doubleday.

Berlyne, D. E. (1960). *Conflict, Arousal and Curiosity.* New York: McGraw-Hill.

Bonder, B. R. (1993). Issues in assessment of psychosocial components of function. *American Journal of Occupational Therapy, 47*(3), 211-216.

Braithwaite, V. A. & Law, H. G. (1985). Structure of human values: Testing the adequacy of the Rokeach Value Survey. *Journal of Personality and Social Psychology, 49*(1), 250-263.

Bruner, J. S. (1973). Organization of early skilled action. *Child Development, 44*, 1-11.

Bruner, J. S. (1990). *Acts of Meaning.* Cambridge: Harvard University Press.

Burke, J. P. (1977). A clinical perspective on motivation: Pawn versus origin. *American Journal of Occupational Therapy, 31*(4), 254-258.

Burke, J., Miyake, S, Kielhofner, G. & Barris R. (1983). The demystification of health care and demise of the sick role: Implications for occupational therapy. In G. Kielhofner (Ed.), *Health Through Occupation: Theory and Practice in Occupational Therapy.* Philadelphia: F.A. Davis; pp. 197-210.

Buss D., & Block, J. (1980). Preschool activity level: Personality correlates and developmental implications. *Child Development, 51*, 401-408.

Campbell, J. (1962). *The Hero with a Thousand Faces.* New York: Pantheon.

Campbell, J. (1988). *The Power of Myth.* New York: Doubleday.

Carlson, M., & Clark, F. (1991). The search for useful methodologies in occupational science. *American Journal of Occupational Therapy, 45*, 235-241.

Christiansen, C. H. (1981). Toward resolution of crisis: Research requisites in occupational therapy. *Occupational Therapy Journal of Research*, *1*(2), 115-124.

Christiansen, C. H. (1997). Acknowledging a spiritual dimension in occupational therapy practice. *American Journal of Occupational Therapy*, *51*, 169-172

Christiansen, C. H., Clark, F., Kielhofner, G. & Rogers, J. C. (1995). Position paper: Occupation. *American Journal of Occupational Therapy*, *49*, 1015-1018.

Costa, P. T. Jr. & McCrae, R. R. (1980). Still stable after all these years; Personality as a key to some issues in aging. In D. Baltes & O. G. Brim (Eds.) *Lifespan Development and Behavior, Vol 3*. New York: Academic Press.

Csikszentmihalyi, M. (1975). *Beyond boredom and anxiety*. San Francisco; Jossey-Bass

Csikszentmihalyi, M. & Csikszentmihalyi, I. (1988) *Optimal Experience: Psychological Studies in Flow in Consciousness*. New York: Cambridge University Press.

DeCharms, R. (1968). *Personal Causation: The Internal Affective Determinants of Behavior*. New York: Academic Press.

Deci, R. & Ryan, E. M. (1991). A motivational approach to self-integration in personality. *Nebraska Symposium on Motivation*, *38*, 237-288.

Digman, J. M. (198x). Personality structure: Emergence of the five factor model. *Annual Review of Psychology*, *41*, 417-440.

Duchek, J. (1991). Cognitive dimensions of performance. In C. Christiansen & C. M. Baum (Eds). *Occupational Therapy: Overcoming Human Performance Deficits*. Thorofare, NJ: SLACK Incorporated; pp. 283-303.

Egan, M. & DeLaat, M. D. (1994). Considering spirituality in occupational therapy practice. *Canadian Journal of Occupational Therapy, 61*, 95-101.

Erikson, E. H. (1968). *Identity, Youth and Crisis*. New York: W.W. Norton.

Emmons, R. A. (1986). Personal strivings: An approach to personality and subjective well-being. *Journal of Personality and Social Psychology*, *51*(5), 1058-1068.

Engel, G. (1977). The need for a new medical model: A challenge for biomedicine. *Science*, *196*, 129-136.

Fidler, G. S., & Fidler, J. W. (1973). Doing and becoming: Purposeful action and self-actualization. *American Journal of Occupational Therapy*, *32*, 305-310.

Frese, M. Stewart, J. & Hannover, B. (1987). Goal orientation and planfulness: Action styles as personality concepts. *Journal of Personality and Social Psychology*, *52*, 1182-1194.

Fleishman, F. E. (1972). On the relationship between abilities, learning and human performance. *American Psychologist*, *27*, 1017-1032.

Fleishman, E. A. (1975). Toward a taxonomy of human performance. *American Psychologist, 30*(12), 1127-1149.

Fleishman, E. A. &. Quaintance, M. K. (1984). *Taxonomies of Human Performance: The Description of Human Tasks*. Orlando: Academic Press.

Mattingly C. & Fleming, M. (1994). *Clinical Reasoning: Forms of Inquiry in a Therapeutic Practice*. Philadelphia: F. A. Davis.

Furnham, A. (1981). Personality and activity preference. *British Journal of Social Psychology*, *20*(1), 57-68.

Gage, M. & Polatajko, H. (1994). Enhancing occupational performance through an understanding of perceived self-efficacy. *American Journal of Occupational Therapy*, *48*(5), 452-462.

George, L. K. (1978). The impact of personality and social status upon levels of activity and psychological well-being. *Journal of Gerontology*, *33*, 840-847.

Goffman, I. (1963). *Stigma: Notes on the Management of a Spoiled Identity*. Englewood Cliffs, NJ: Prentice-Hall.

Goldman, A. (1970). *A Theory of Human Action*. Princeton, NJ: Princeton University Press.

Hall, E. T. (1973). *The Silent Language*. Garden City, NJ: Anchor Books.

Hogan, R., DeSoto, C. B. & Solano, C. (1977). Traits, tests and personality research. *American Psychologist, 32*, 255-264.

Holland, J. L. (1959). A theory of vocational choice. *Journal of Counseling Psychology*, *6*, 35-45.

Howe, M. C. & Briggs, A. K. (1982). Ecological systems model for occupational therapy. *American Journal of Occupational Therapy*, *36*, 322-327.

Jacobs, K. (1994). Flow and the occupational therapy practitioner. *American Journal of Occupational Therapy*, *48*, 989-995.

John, O. P. (1987). Towards a taxonomy of personality descriptors. In D. Buss & N. Cantor (Eds.) *Personality Psychology: Recent Trends and Emerging Directions*. New York: Springer-Verlag; 261-274.

Kabat-Zinn, J. (1994). *Wherever You Go, There You Are*. New York: Hyperion.

Kielhofner, G. (1977). Temporal adaptation: A conceptual framework for occupational therapy. *American Journal of Occupational Therapy*, *31*(4), 235-242.

Kielhofner, G. (1978). General system theory: Implications for the theory and action in occupational therapy. *American Journal of Occupational Therapy*, *32*, 637-645.

Kilpatrick-Tubak, B., & Roth, S. (1978). Attempt to reverse performance deficits associated with depression and experimentally induced helplessness. *Journal of Abnormal Psychology, 87*, 141-154.

King, L. J. (1978). Toward a science of adaptive responses. *American Journal of Occupational Therapy*, *32*, 429-437.

Lawton, M.P. (1980). *Environment and Aging*. Monterey, CA: Brooks-Cole.

Letts, L., Law, M., Rigby, P., Cooper, B., Stewart, D. & Strong, S. (1994). Person environment assessments in occupational therapy. *American Journal of Occupational Therapy*, *48*(7), 608-618.

Law, M., Baptiste, S., & Mills, J. (1995). Client-centred practice: What does it mean and does it make a difference? *Canadian Journal of Occupational Therapy, 62*, 250-257.

LeFevre, J. (1988). Flow and the quality of experience during work and leisure. In M. Csikszentmihalyi & I. Csikszentmihalyi (Eds.) *Optimal Experience: Psychological Studies in Flow in Consciousness*. New York: Cambridge University Press; pp. 307-318.

Maier, S. F., & Seligman, M. E. P. (1976). Learned helplessness: Theory and evidence. *Journal of Experimental Psychology (General)*, *105*, 3-46.

Matheis-Kraft, C., George, S., Olinger, M. J., & York, L. (1990). Patient driven healthcare works. *Nursing Management, 21*(9), 124-125, 128.

Markus, H., & Nurius, P. (1986). Possible selves. *American Psychologist, 41*, 954-969.

Markus H., & Ruvolo, A. (1980). Possible selves: Personalized representations of goals. In L. Pervin (Ed.), *Goal concepts in personality and social psychology* (pp 211-241). Hilldale, NJ: Lawrence Erlbaum Associates.

Mathiowetz, V. & Bass Haugen, J. B. (1994). Motor behavior research: Implications for therapeutic approaches to central nervous system dysfunction. *American Journal of Occupational Therapy, 48*(8), 733-745.

McRae, R. R., & Costa, P. T. Jr. (1996). *Toward a New Generation of Personality Theories: Theoretical Contexts for the Five Factor Model.* New York: Guilford Press.

Mead, G. H. (1934). *Mind, Self and Society.* Chicago: University of Chicago Press.

Merzenich, M. M., Scheiner, C., Jenkins, W., & Wang, X. (1993). Neural mechanisms underlying temporal integration, segmentation, and input sequence representation: Some implications for the origin of learning disabilities. *Annals of the New York Academy of Sciences, 682*, 1-22.

Meyer, A. (1922). The philosophy of occupation therapy. *Archives of Occupational Therapy, 1*(1), 1-10.

Mosey, A. C. (1974). An alternative: The biopsychosocial model. *American Journal of Occupational Therapy, 28*(3), 137-140.

Murry, H. A. , Barrett, W. G. & Hamburger, E. (1938). *Explorations in Personality.* New York: Oxford University Press.

Nelson, D. L., Thompson, G., & Moore, J. A. (1982). Identification of factors of affective meaning in four selected activities. *American Journal of Occupational Therapy, 36*, 381-387.

O'Leary, A. (1985). Self-efficacy and health. *Behavior Research and Therapy, 23,* 437-451.

Osgood, C. E. (1962) Studies on the generality of affective meaning systems. *American Psychologist, 17*, 10-28.

Pelland, M. J. (1987). A conceptual model for the instruction and supervision of treatment planning. *American Journal of Occupational Therapy, 41*(6), 351-359.

Reilly, M. (1962). Occupational therapy can be one of the great ideas of 20th century medicine. *American Journal of Occupational Therapy, 16,* 300-308.

Reilly, M. (1974). Preface. In M. Reilly (Ed.). *Play as Exploratory Learning.* Beverly Hills: Sage.

Robinson, A. L. (1977). Play: The arena for acquisition of rules for competent behavior. *American Journal of Occupational Therapy, 31*(4), 248-253.

Rokeach, M. (1973). *A Theory of Human Values.* New York: Free Press.

Rokeach, M. (1979). Some unresolved issues in theories of beliefs, attitudes and values. *Nebraska Symposium on Motivation, 27*, 261-304.

Rogers, J. C. (1982). The spirit of independence: The evolution of a philosophy. *American Journal of Occupational Therapy, 36*, 709-715.

Rogers, J. C. (1983). Clinical reasoning: The ethics, science and art. *American Journal of Occupational Therapy, 37*, 601-616.

Rotter, J. B. (1960). Generalized expectancies for internal versus external control of reinforcement. *Psychological Monographs: General Applications, 80*, 1-28.

Sarbin, T. R., & Allen, V. L. (1968). Role theory. In G. Lindsey &. E. Aronson (Eds.), *Handbook of Social Psychology* (2nd Ed). Reading, MA: Addison-Wesley.

Schon, D. (1983). *The Reflective Practitioner: How Professionals Think in Action.* New York: Basic Books.

Seligmann, M. E. P. (1991). *Learned Optimism.* New York: Alfred A. Knopf.

Sullivan, H. S. (1953). *Conceptions of Modern Psychiatry.* New York: W.W. Norton.

Trombly, C. A. (1995). Occupation: Purposefulness and meaningfulness and therapeutic mechanisms. *American Journal of Occupational Therapy, 49*, 960-972.

Vallacher, R. R., & Wegner, D. M. (1987). What do people think they're doing? Action identification and human behavior. *Psychological Review, 94*, 3-15.

Wells, A. (1988). Self-esteem and optimal experience. In M. Csikszentmihalyi & I. Csikszentmihalyi (Eds.) *Optimal Experience: Psychological Studies in Flow in Consciousness.* New York: Cambridge University Press; pp. 327-341.

White, R. W. (1959). Motivation reconsidered: The concept of competence. *Psychological Review, 66*, 297-333.

White, R. W. (1971). The urge toward competence. *American Journal of Occupational Therapy, 25*, 271-274.

Wool, R. N., Silegel, D., & Fine, P.R. (1980). Task performance in spinal cord injury: Effect of helplessness training. *Archives of Physical Medicine and Rehabilitation, 61*, 321-325.

Yerxa, E. J. (1967). Authentic occupational therapy. *American Journal of Occupational Therapy, 21*, 1-9.

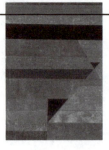

Chapter Content Outline

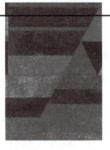

Abstract

This chapter focuses on the key theoretical ideas that underpin occupational therapy practice. Important concepts and assumptions about the person, the environment, and occupation are outlined. The dynamic nature of the person-environment-occupation relationship and its influence on occupational performance is reviewed. Ten theoretical models from environment-behavior studies which contribute significant ideas to the study of person-environment interactions are outlined. A discussion of historical approaches to the person-environment relationship is used to set the context for reviewing current and emerging occupational therapy models of practice that emphasize these concepts. Six occupational therapy models of practice which center on the person-environment-occupation relationship are explored to illustrate their theoretical foundations, key ideas, and implications for practice.

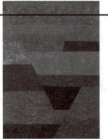

Key Terms

Environment

Environmental press

Occupation

Occupational performance

Person

Person-environment-occupation relationship

Person-environment fit

Theoretical model

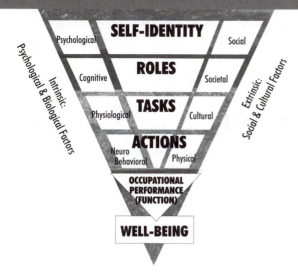

Theoretical Contexts for the Practice of Occupational Therapy

Mary Law, PhD, OT(C), Barbara A. Cooper, PhD, OT(C), Susan Strong, MSc, OT(C), Debra Stewart, BSc, OT(C), Patricia Rigby, MHSc, OT(C), Lori Letts, MA, OT(C)

OBJECTIVES

The information in this chapter is intended to help the reader:

1. understand the meaning and use of the term occupational performance in occupational therapy

2. review the complex nature and relationships between person, environment, and occupation

3. appreciate the contributions of environment-behavior theorists to the understanding of persons' occupational performance and person-environment fit

4. review the ways in which occupational therapy has historically considered the person-environment-occupation relationship

5. understand current and emerging theoretical models in occupational therapy practice that focus on the nature of the person-environment-occupation relationship

6. understand the implications of these current and emerging occupational therapy models for occupational therapy practice.

> *"People need to make use of their capacities through engagement in individually motivating and ongoing occupations, and if they are able, or encouraged to pursue this need, they will, apart from supplying sustenance for survival and safety, enhance their health."*
>
> Wilcock, 1991, p. 23.

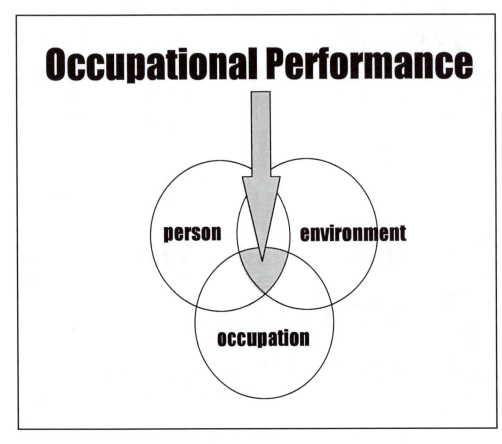

Figure 4-1. Person-environment-occupation relationship. Adapted with permission from Law, M., Cooper, B., Strong, S., Stewart, D., Rigby, P., & Letts, L. (1996a). The person-environment-occupation model: A transactive approach to occupational performance. *Canadian Journal of Occupational Therapy, 63,* 9-23.

KEY ISSUES IN THE STUDY OF PERSON-ENVIRONMENT-OCCUPATION RELATIONSHIPS

Occupational performance is the product of the dynamic relationship among persons, their occupations and roles, and the environments in which they live (Figure 4-1) (Law, Cooper, et al., 1996). The American Occupational Therapy Association supports this description of occupational performance, noting that occupational therapists use the term *function* interchangeably with occupational performance (AJOT, 1995).

Other professions also commonly use the term function. To others, the meaning of function may differ from that applied by occupational therapists; the term may apply to the function of human organs or to distinguish ability from lack of ability (AJOT, 1995). In contrast, the occupational therapist views function at a level which considers the dynamic transactional relationship of persons, occupations and environments, and assumes an inseparability of contexts, tempo-

ral factors, and physical and psychological phenomena (Law, Cooper, et al., 1996). Occupational therapists label the outcome of this relationship *occupational performance* to emphasize the distinctive meaning of function for occupational therapy.

Views of the Person

Persons can be viewed as individuals and as members of groups. Each individual possesses unique characteristics including those that are physical, emotional and spiritual, and each individual can assume a variety of roles such as parent, worker and friend, simultaneously. Roles vary across time and context in their importance, duration and significance (Law, Cooper, et al., 1996).

Attributes of the individual include self-concept, personality style, cultural background and competencies. How these attributes are expressed at any given time is influenced by personal factors, the occupation in which the person engages and the environmental context. Personal factors include general health, level of alertness, level of skill and past experiences. For example, a person may appear uncomfortable and make errors while playing piano to a large audience in a church hall, but play the piano at home with family members in a seemingly effortless manner. A person may appear to lack self-con-

Bibliographic citation of this chapter: Law, M., Cooper, B. A., Strong, S., Stewart, D., Rigby, P., & Letts, L. (1997). Theoretical contexts for the practice of occupational therapy. In C. Christiansen & C. Baum (Eds.), *Occupational therapy: Enabling function and well-being* (2nd ed). Thorofare, NJ: SLACK Incorporated.

fidence and skill engaged in occupation in one context, and in another context perform with skill and self-assurance. Each person brings expectations of success or failure to each occupational experience (Strong, 1995). Because of this, it is important to view the influences of person, environment and occupation on each person and his or her behaviours.

Values and beliefs shape how a person sees him or herself in relation to occupations and environments, and influences the way in which the world is observed and explored. They also influence the relationships persons have with other persons and group membership. In groups, the personal characteristics of individual members are displayed. Membership in groups can in turn shape behaviours. Groups are formed formally or informally based on factors including common interests such as photography; backgrounds such as religion; experiences such as Alcoholics Anonymous; views such as women's rights; and traits such as gender. A great deal can be learned about persons by identifying and observing the groups with which they associate.

DEFINITION AND CLASSIFICATION OF ENVIRONMENT

Environment is defined as those contexts and situations which occur outside the individual and elicit responses from him or her (Law, 1991). Environment is often narrowly described in terms of its physical characteristics, such as buildings, landscape and pollutants. Occupational therapists are broadening their consideration of environment to include social, political, economic, institutional and cultural considerations (Law, Cooper, et al., 1994).

Environments can be organized in a variety of ways. For example, environments can be classified by attributes such as privacy, safety and density (Windley and Scheidt, 1980); by functions such as home, work, school and retail businesses; or by scale such as room, building and community (Weisman, 1981). Occupational therapists and other healthcare professionals often consider enabling or disabling qualities of the environment (Law, 1991). No one classification method is more correct or more important than the other. The method chosen will depend upon the purpose for considering the environment.

A classification matrix which has been used in occupational therapy to acknowledge the transactional relationship of persons and environments organizes the environments by environmental factor (cultural, economic, institutional, physical, social) and by personal perspective (individual, family, neighbourhood, community, state, country) (Law, Cooper, et al, 1996). This matrix assists occupational therapists to consider the daily living experiences of their clients not only within the immediate environment, but also within the larger community.

The environment provides a context in which persons engage in occupations (Dunn, Brown and McGuigan, 1994). The context is shaped by the cues available in the environment, which in turn guide a person to choose to behave in certain ways. The cues, whether implicit or explicit, make evident the purpose for which the environment is expected to be used. For example, a church hall is most often used for events such as Sunday school class, musical concerts, political forums or wedding receptions. In this example, the cues may vary from the physical decor used, the social behaviours of persons in attendance, or from rules and expectations provided by the church. The cues may also be generated by the conditions of the environment at a given time. For example, a young woman may choose to take a taxi home from a shopping mall at night, rather than wait alone for a bus.

DEFINITION AND CLASSIFICATION OF OCCUPATION

In simple terms, occupation is what people do. Occupational therapists recognize that the experience of doing things is important to the health of individuals and societies. People engage in occupations for personal purposes and to meet societal needs and expectations. The specific knowledge and skills which occupational therapy practice brings to the study of occupation are unique.

Occupations can be described as groupings of functional tasks and roles in which persons engage over a lifetime for a variety of purposes such as self-maintenance, self-expression and fulfillment (Christiansen, 1991). These tasks are carried out in many environmental contexts to satisfy individual roles. The basic unit of occupation is action, which is defined as a singular pursuit in which a person engages. An example of an action is cutting vegetables. The purpose of cutting vegetables can be to accomplish a task such as preparing a casserole. Tasks involve grouping a set of actions for a specific purpose. Tasks are similarly grouped to fulfill the occupations persons pursue within various roles. For example, the occupation of meal preparation is comprised of a number of tasks such as preparing a casserole, a salad and a drink.

Occupations are pluralistic, complex and a necessary function of living (Law, Cooper, et al., 1996). A mother of a child with a disability may find that she juggles many occupations throughout a day to fulfill multiple roles as an employed worker, parent, spouse and advocate for her child. Engagement in meaningful occupation shapes our self-concept and identity. Through doing tasks and occupations, people draw upon their capabilities and test their competencies. Consequently, an occupational therapist may help a person with a recent impairment to experience success through the modification of activities and tasks. Experiences of success lead to views of self-efficacy, which help motivate a person to continue "doing things." Occupational therapy is guided by the belief that quality of life for any person is influenced by the performance of occupations within his or her lived environment.

Occupational Performance

Occupational performance is the outcome of the transactive relationship between persons, environments and occupations. It is the experience of a person engaged in purposeful tasks and occupations within an environment (Law et al., 1996). The transactive nature of the relationship between persons, occupation and environment acknowledges that all parts are inseparable, interwoven and interdependent. Transaction implies mutual influence—a dynamic situation in which individuals alter performance based on their perceptions of changing conditions in the environment. Transaction acknowledges the influence of roles, rules, norms and patterns of behaviour on occupation. Rather than viewing behaviours and events as static, they are seen as dynamic — shifting goals, purposes and motives that are part of the psychological and contextual properties of specific events. The goal of the occupational therapist is to understand the pattern and flow of particular events so that occupational performance can be enhanced (Altman & Rogoff, 1987). Change in one part of the relationship affects changes to the whole relationship. Occupational therapy intervention is focused on the person, the environment and the occupation together in a dynamic transactive manner, recognizing the inseparability of effect of these factors on occupational performance.

ENVIRONMENT-BEHAVIOUR STUDIES PERSPECTIVE

The environment and its influence on human behaviour has long captured the interest of professionals from many different disciplines, most notably architecture, anthropology, social science, environmental psychology and, more recently, occupational therapy. All these groups share the view that the relationship between people and environment is dynamic (i.e., constantly changing with time), complex and interdependent.

Following a broadly based appraisal of the environment-behaviour studies (EBS) literature, 10 models of particular interest to occupational therapy have been selected for presentation. These are: Baker and Intagliata (1982), Bandura (1986), Bronfenbrenner (1977), Gibson (1977, 1979), Gibson (1988), Kahana (1982), Kaplan (1983), Lawton (1986), Mandala of Health (Berlin, 1989; Hancock, 1985),

Moos (1980) and Weisman (1981). Each has a strong theoretical base and is well supported in the literature. Although the roots and purposes of the models vary, all address four common themes: how the person is conceptualized; the way in which the environment is conceived; the relationship between the person(s) and the environment; and the outcome or adaptive relationship that results. Most of the theoretical models are complementary and vary only in focus or emphasis rather than in conceptualization. Potentially all can be of use to occupational therapy practice (Table 4-1).

ENVIRONMENT-BEHAVIOUR MODELS

Baker and Intagliata

Baker and Intagliata's (1982) model resulted from their interest in issues related to quality of life and a desire to improve their understanding of how adults with long-term psychiatric illnesses perceived the quality of their lives. Within this model, the person possesses certain characteristics, physical and mental status, needs, knowledge, personal beliefs and attitudes. The person functions as the central filter and control through which the external environment is experienced. That is, the way in which the person perceives and interprets the environment is deemed paramount. Baker and Intagliata define the environment broadly, and believe that it consists of physical, social, economic, political, and cultural components. The relationship between the person and the environment is defined as the individual's satisfaction with the fit between his or her environmental experiences and personal needs. This fit is expressed subjectively as the person's measure of the quality of his or her own life and assessed objectively by observing the behaviour of the individual.

Baker and Intagliata's model can be useful to occupational therapists, providing a vehicle through which therapists can examine quality of life from the perspective of the various groups of people with whom they interact, in particular, clients with mental health problems. However, occupational therapists must recognize at all times that there may be important differences between the way they and their clients experience elements of the environment. Occupational therapists must be sensitive to clients' perceptions of the environment and be able to assess how these possibly divergent views influence their clients' stated needs. This model also suggests that important outcomes can be both behavioural and internal, influencing both satisfaction with and quality of life. Both of these issues are important for occupational therapists to consider when examining the outcomes of clinical interventions (Figure 4-2).

TABLE 4-1

Key Elements of Person-Environment Models

Theorist	How is the person conceptualized?	How is the environment conceived?	Person-environment interaction (adaptation)	OT application
Baker and Intagliata	Individual: • physical status • mental status • needs • knowledge • beliefs and attitudes	• the individual's perceived or experienced environment and the actual environment	The individual responds as: • an active participant; or • an instinctive responder	• focus on client perceptions of environments and quality of life • clients with mental health problems
Bronfenbrenner	Individual: • as a social agent seeks and creates meaning in the social environment	• social and cultural milieu of the individual	Interdependence: • change in one domain on social environment effects change in another domain	• emphasis on client's social environment (e.g., family interventions); paediatric practice, social development
Bandura	Individual: • six basic cognitive capacities	• the individual's perceptions of the environment are key	Perceived self-efficacy: • person's perceptions of his or her ability to be successful in an activity in a particular environment	• focus on environmental perceptions • encourages consultation with clients
Gibson and Gibson	Individual: • as a developing, curious, motivated learner • task oriented • perception	• the context or surroundings of the individual • supportive or constraining (affordance)	Interdependence: • personal activities matched to affordable of environment	•child development in the context of his or her surroundings
Mandala of Health	Community: • distinctive needs of community • social policy	• biological • physical • cultural • economic	• social and political implications of health • need to change environment not people	• community health • advocacy
Kahana	Individual: • needs • preferences	•the social characteristics of the residential setting	Congruence: •the well-being and function of the individual • individual choice of environment	• discharge planning, particularly with older adults • social environments
Kaplan	Individual: • the internal organization of incoming information about the environment	Individual: • opportunities • choices	Temporal flexibility: • to each experience one brings memories of past experiences which affect perception and anticipation	• general practice • psychiatric environments
Lawton	Individual: • the person possesses a set of abilities which constitute competence	Environmental press: • the forces in the environment in terms of their demand characteristics	Two possible responses: • adaptive behaviour whether + or − • affective response	• gerontology and frail individuals

TABLE 4-1 (continued)

Key Elements of Person-Environment Models

Theorist	How is the person conceptualized?	How is the environment conceived?	Person-environment interaction (adaptation)	OT application
Moos	Group of persons: • residing in an institutional setting • sociodemographics • self-concept • health factors • functional abilities	Environmental system consisting of: • physical factors • policy factors • suprapersonal factors • social climate factors	• stability and change within the institution for well-being of residents and staff	• assessing institutions and sheltered-care environments.
Weisman	Employees	Physical setting: • properties • components Organizations: • policy • objective	Congruence: • manipulation of the physical environment to ensure that the policies and objectives of the organization are met	• work environments

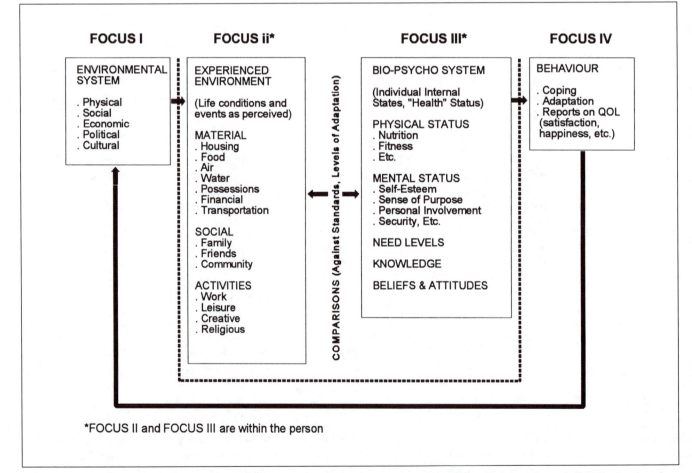

Figure 4-2. Baker and Intagliata's Quality of Life Model. Reprinted with permission from Baker, F., & Intagliata, J. (1982). Quality of life in the evaluation of community support systems. *Evaluation and Program Planning, 5,* 69-79.

Bandura's Perceived Self-Efficacy Model

The work of Bandura (1986) is rooted in social cognitive theory and identifies three main contributing concepts: The person, behaviour, and the outcome of the person's behaviour. These three areas are seen as interdependent and constantly interacting and have been organized by Bandura as the Model of Perceived Self-Efficacy. In the model, the person is conceptualized as having six basic capacities: symbolizing capacity, forethought capacity, vicarious capacity, self-regulatory capacity, change capacity, and self-reflective capacity. Perceived self-efficacy results from those personal attributes, and is defined as the individual's judgment about his or her own ability to perform specific activities successfully. Perceived self-efficacy is determined by the person's perceptions of his or her own skills and the characteristics of the environment. After assessing these factors, the person decides whether he or she is apt to be successful in performing a certain skill in a specific environment. Perceived self-efficacy is different from outcome expectancy, which is the anticipated outcome of a behaviour once it has taken place. Within the model, perceived self-efficacy is considered to be the result of transactions between the person, the environment and the behaviours occurring in the environment. Little description of the environment is provided by the model, as it views the perceptions of the individual as central to the relationship. Perceived self-efficacy can be influenced by past performance, observations of others, verbal persuasion and psychological cues.

This model can further the occupational therapist's understanding of clients' task performance within and outside the clinical environment. For example, therapists know that some clients are more willing than other clients to attempt new tasks in therapy. Perceived self-efficacy may provide the tool for therapists to analyze and interpret those differences; the client may simply feel that he or she will not be successful with the task. By applying Bandura's model, clinicians also may improve their understanding of why some clients seem unable to perform well in the community, yet appear to have the skills necessary to carry out similar tasks in a clinical environment. Perhaps the client's perceived self-efficacy may be high in the therapeutic environment, but low in what is seen as a more demanding or threatening milieu. In either case, the environment can be modified to support and build the perceived self-efficacy of clients.

The model suggests that there are many approaches to address self-efficacy, for example, having the client carry out the task, or watch someone else perform the task or discuss various approaches to performance. Finally, the model reinforces the need for therapists to ask clients how they perceive their own ability to accomplish functional tasks and to improve their understanding of how clients process informa-

tion. In the final analysis, observational strategies alone do not always provide a sufficient picture of client performance.

Bronfenbrenner

Bronfenbrenner's (1977) model emanated from his roots in developmental psychology and his perception of inadequacies and limitations in the available research on human development. Bronfenbrenner believed that identifying the interdependencies that existed between people and their social settings was important. In his model, the person is viewed as a social agent who interacts with all levels of the environment in order to develop him- or herself and bring understanding and meaning into his or her life. The environment is described in terms of the social and cultural milieu of the individual. It can be depicted as a series of nested circles radiating from the individual at the centre (the microsystem), next to a level that includes personal groupings, such as the family, work, and school (mesosystem), followed by a level of formal and informal social structures (exosystem), and last, to an outer layer of societal institutions (macrosystem). The relationship between the person and the environment is seen as fully interdependent, with the individual constantly interacting with all levels. Changes at any level of the environment will influence the individual's behaviour. Adaptation is seen as a process that the individual constantly initiates and participates in through this interaction with the environment.

Bronfenbrenner's work is of interest to occupational therapists for a number of reasons. Its emphasis on the social nature of the individual is relevant to practice because as clinicians we constantly interact with clients, and through this relationship become an intimate part of their social environment. Bronfenbrenner developed the model to describe human development and it can be used by occupational therapists as well to understand life span changes of clients within the context of their social systems. However, it may be especially useful in pediatric practice when developmental changes are so critical to treatment plans. The emphasis on the complex interdependence between individuals and their environmental surroundings is also important to note, and can assist therapists in recognizing the significance of expanding intervention strategies to include families and workplaces (Figure 4-3).

E. Gibson and J. Gibson's Model of Perceptual Development

E. Gibson (1988) and J. Gibson (1977, 1979), ecological psychologists, also stressed the interdependence of the person with his or her environment. These theorists believed strongly that a person's behaviour could only be understood in the context of the surroundings in which it occurs. In E. Gibson's

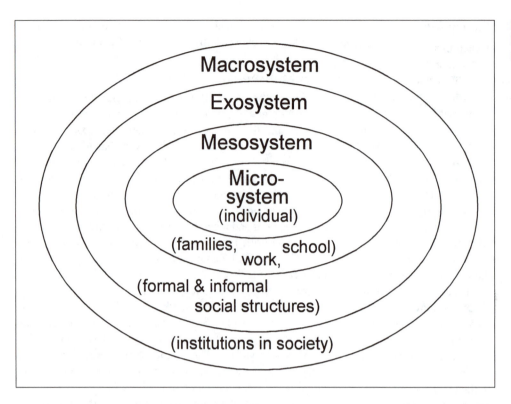

Figure 4-3. Bronfenbrenner's Ecological Systems Model (1977).

(1988) view, the individual is motivated to perform meaningful tasks and therefore constantly seeks to learn more about the various aspects of the environment that enable him or her to reach these goals. As conceptualized by the model, the environment can constrain or enhance the performance of tasks; J. Gibson (1977) calls this relationship *affordance*. The perceptual development of the person is guided and shaped by the process of learning personal parameters of affordance for different tasks in different settings and under different circumstances. Successful adaptation to the environment occurs when the person can match his or her activities to the affordance level of the environment or the environment can be modified to allow these activities to take place appropriately.

This developmental EBS model can be particularly useful to occupational therapists working with children. It emphasizes the importance of understanding a child's development in the context of the surroundings and of facilitating this by providing opportunities whereby the child can explore and learn about the environment in a manner suitable to achieving his or her goals. The child's lifelong perception of the environment and his or her motivation to function therein are influenced and shaped by these meaningful interactions. In the area of mental health, the model can be used to help therapists understand why limiting people's rights to self-determination may restrict their ability to make decisions, and consequently, to optimize life choices and opportunities. Under these circumstances, the therapist can facilitate the removal of environmental con-

straints and act as an advocate for his or her client.

Kahana

Kahana's (1982) model developed out of concerns for the suitability of new supportive residential environments developed for aging people. This model addressed the necessity of establishing a good fit between the needs and preferences of the individual and the social characteristics of the environment. In Kahana's model, the person is conceptualized as an individual who is able to clearly express views and preferences for his or her own residential requirements. The environment is considered in terms of press, i.e., the demand and enabling qualities of the setting. Kahana hypothesized that the preferences and needs of the individual would influence the type of residential environment selected, and that in turn, the environment would influence the well-being and functional behaviour of the individual. Ideally, the result of this interaction would be congruence, where the person would function at an optimal level within an environment that exactly matched his or her needs. Kahana placed particular attention on segregate versus congregate aspects of residential environments for older adults. There is no graphic representation of the model, which is based on the concepts of need-press theory that also form the basis for Lawton's work.

The model stresses the importance of the relationship between the person and the residential environment. This is important for occupational therapists to consider, particular-

Sources of Mental Activity	Type of Mental Activity	
	Images	Plans/Actions
Environment (external)	**1** environmental perception and knowledge	**2** required or necessary action
Person (internal)	**3** reflection	**4** purposive action and inclination

Figure 4-4. Kaplan's Model of Person-Environment Compatibility. Reprinted with permission from Kaplan, S. (1983). A model of person-environment compatibility. *Environment and Behavior, 15,* 311-332.

ly when undertaking home assessments or developing discharge plans for clients leaving the hospital. The physical needs of the person often form the focus of concern for ensuring supportive environments or exploring institutional placements. Kahana's model acts as a reminder that it is equally important to consider the social components of the environment and the less tangible demand and enabling qualities inherent in each setting when facilitating these moves.

Kaplan

Kaplan is an environmental psychologist whose definition of the environment emphasizes the person's subjective interpretation of the environment. Therefore, in this theoretical model, the critical component becomes the individual's cognitive interpretation and organization of environmental information, which in turn mediates how he or she uses that knowledge. Through this filter, the tangible qualities of the environment assume an additional layer of individualized symbolic meaning. Kaplan's model emphasizes the personal aspect of the person-environment interaction, and, since the interpretation of the image given by the environment and the person's related behaviour will depend on "the eye of the beholder," these outcomes are subject to great variability. Adaptation is defined as compatibility: A lack of environmental support, both perceived and tangible, will frustrate and impede goal achievement, whereas a supportive environment allows goals to be met and when optimal, becomes restorative.

By applying Kaplan's model, the occupational therapist can formulate a better understanding of why individuals interpret and react differently to the same environment. The model can be used to guide the choice of assessments used to determine the actual and perceived needs of the person. The therapeutic interventions developed should facilitate the per-

son's attainment of goals through the establishment of compatible surroundings that are supportive, address needs and reduce stress, thereby creating a restorative and healthy environment in which to live (Figure 4-4).

Lawton's Ecological Theory of Aging

Lawton (1982), an environmental psychologist, developed his Ecological Theory of Aging in conjunction with fellow gerontologist, Lucille Nahemow (Lawton & Nahemow, 1973). Their theory considered the person as an individual whose collective abilities, identified as biological, cognitive, motor skills and sensory/perceptual capacities, are defined as competence. Lawton and Nahemow conceptualized the environment in terms of press, or the forces present in the environment and their demand characteristics. Press can be negative, positive or neutral; a person's response can be adaptive or maladaptive. As competence declines, the person becomes more sensitive to the influences of the environment, both negative and positive. This is expressed theoretically as the environmental docility hypothesis. Outcome behaviours of competence, compared to observable norms, and self report of affect determine the degree of adaptation that the individual has been able to achieve. Figure 4-5 presents a graphic depiction of Lawton and Nahemow's theoretical ideas.

Although Lawton's model is most frequently applied by occupational therapists working in clinical gerontology, it lends itself to application with all individuals who lack competence in one or more of the four categories described by Lawton. Occupational therapy assessments can be used to measure the competence of the person; environmental assessments can determine the qualities of the environment that most influence the behaviours of interest. Interventions

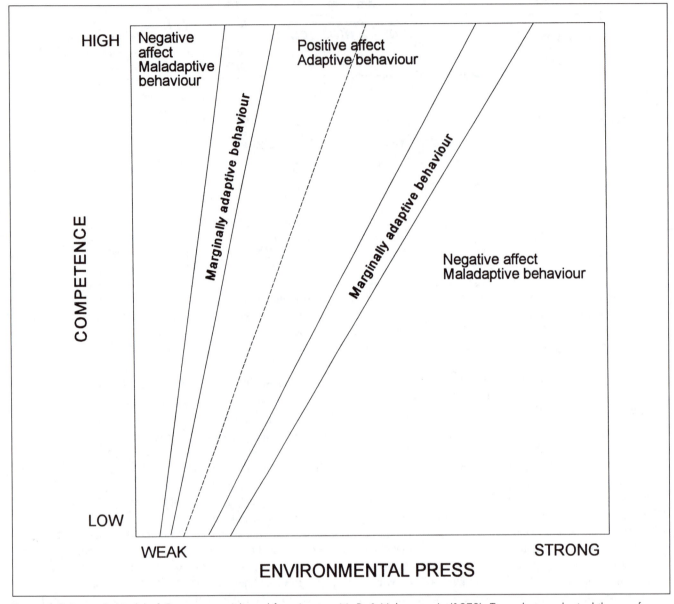

Figure 4-5. Lawton's Model of Competency. Adapted from Lawton, M. P., & Nahemow, L. (1973). Toward an ecological theory of adaptation and aging. In W. Preiser (Ed.), *Environmental design research* (pp. 24-32). Stroudsburg, PA: Dowden, Hutchinson & Ross.

that modify the environment can be matched to meet the needs of the frail individual who cannot change to manage the press of his or her environment.

Mandala of Health

The concept of a Mandala of Health (Berlin, 1989; Hancock, 1985) was developed by the healthy communities movement, which defined health as being more than the absence of disease and determined by a number of environmental factors. Proponents of this movement view communities as responsible for promoting healthy environments for

their citizens. The model conceptualizes the person as composed of three components: Body, mind and spirit. However, the individual is seldom considered in isolation of the family, which in turn acts as a mediator between the person and social institutions (Hancock, 1985). The environment is primarily conceptualized in terms of physical and psychosocial components, and these two components form the key determinants for producing healthy communities. The relationship between the person and the environment is viewed as constantly interacting. The model suggests that the health of individuals can be mediated by many personal and environmental factors.

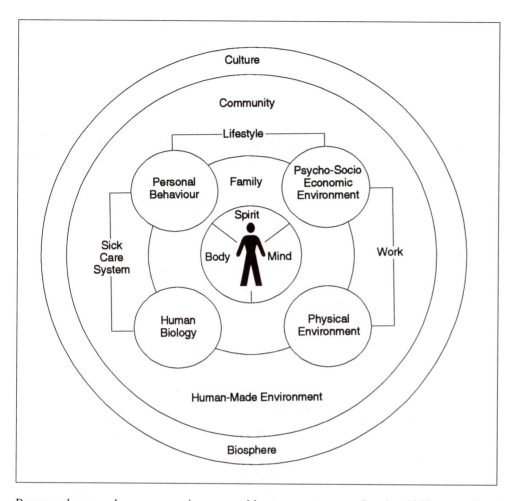

Figure 4-6. Mandala of Health. Reprinted with permission from Hancock, T. (1993). Health, human development and the community ecosystem: Three ecological models. *Health Promotion International*, 8, 41-47.

Power and money, key resources in communities, are seen as key determinants of health, resulting in social and political factors that can act as potential barriers or supports to health.

Because this model focuses on health as its main outcome, it is of great relevance to occupational therapists. As in Bronfenbrenner's model, the family is viewed as a major factor that influences the lives of individuals. In clinical practice, this should also be an important focus. The model provides many levels through which occupational therapists may intervene to promote health. Finally, because the model lends itself to considering social and political aspects of the environment, and how these influence health, it also provides a useful framework for occupational therapists involved in advocacy roles in communities (Figure 4-6).

Moos

As a clinical psychologist, Rudolph Moos (1980) became aware of the influence of the physical environment on the behaviour of his psychiatric patients, in particular, on their ability to cope. These observations formed the framework for a model he developed later with Sonne Lemke (Moos &

Lemke, 1979) to predict the ability of elderly people to live successfully in sheltered environments. Moos conceptualized the person as part of an aggregate or group; however, his model also permits a more individual application. He suggested that the personal system of the individual (socioeconomic factors, health, personality and coping skills) interacts in a reciprocal fashion with the environmental system to provide stability. Moos' framework conceptualizes the environment as a system made up of four components: The physical or architectural setting; institutional policy and program factors; the human aggregate; and social climate factors. The interaction between the environment and residents is mediated through a filter of cognitive appraisal, activation or arousal efforts and coping mechanisms. Successful adaptation to change and other environmental factors is reflected by a state of well-being, good morale, health, and activity levels.

This model would be useful to occupational therapists whose practice includes clients residing in sheltered care environments. The model may be most effective when used to address group needs as opposed to those of individuals, and is particularly useful for assessing facilities. In this capacity, Moos and colleagues have developed a set of reli-

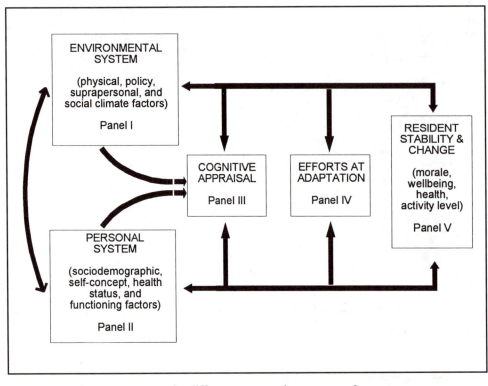

Figure 4-7. Environmental System—Moos. Adapted with permission from Moos, R. (1980). Specialized living environments for older people: A conceptual framework for evaluation. *Journal of Social Issues, 36,* 75-94.

able, valid self-report measures for different contexts that can be used to measure the four environmental components. The application of these determines the direction and focus of intervention for the residents of the facility (Figure 4-7).

Weisman

Weisman (1981) is an architect and psychologist. Of all the EBS theorists reviewed, he is the most concerned with the physical environment. Weisman conceptualizes the environment as a physical filter through which organizational and other environmental concerns are processed and considers the person as part of a group whose behaviour is motivated by the physical attributes of the building in conjunction with the policies and objectives of the organization. Adaptation is maximized when the physical environment is congruent with the policies and objectives of the organization and the goals of the people employed or residing there.

Weisman's model would be particularly useful to occupational therapists whose practice addresses the vocational needs of clients, working in the community. Like Moos' (1980) model, it is best used to address group needs as opposed to the needs of individuals. Unlike Moos, Weisman has not developed measures for either the environment or the users; these would need to be chosen from the common pool to suit the specific assessment requirements of the setting and its users. However, here too, the results of these measures determine the direction and focus for intervention for the users of the facility (Figure 4-8).

Summary

The models presented in this section propose ways of conceptualizing the person and the environment that are relevant for occupational therapists. The challenge is to apply these ideas in clinical practice. In doing this, the therapist will find that each model lends itself to different approaches to evaluation. For example, models that emphasize the individual's perception of the environment will require the use of self-report instruments, while other models may be better suited to the application of observational instruments. Interactional models that examine the person and environment as separate entities call for discrete person and environment measures. Those that are transactional in conceptualization consider the person and environment as an inseparable unit of measure, and require a combined approach to evaluation.

OCCUPATIONAL THERAPY PERSPECTIVE: VIEWS OF THE PERSON-ENVIRONMENT RELATIONSHIP

Before discussing current occupational therapy theoretical models that focus on the person-environment-occupation relationship, it is useful to consider how occupational therapy has viewed this relationship in the past. A review of North American occupational therapy journals over this century provides an historical picture of occupational therapy perspectives about the environment.

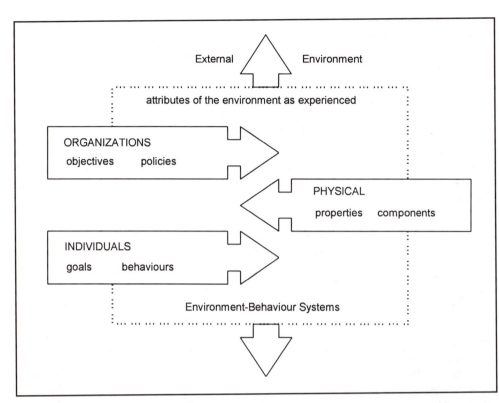

Figure 4-8. Weisman's Environment-Behaviour System Model. Reprinted with permission from Weisman, G. D. (1981). Modeling environment-behaviour systems: A brief note. *Journal of Man-Environment Relations, 1,* 32-41.

In the early part of the century, very little was written specifically about the environment. An article by Crane (1919) mentions how occupational therapy can bolster a patient's morale in hospital environments and recommends the establishment of "healthy hospital environments." By healthy hospital environments, Crane meant primarily physical aspects of the environment, such as colour and decorating. Other articles from this period discuss how occupational therapy can help a patient adjust to the hospital environment. From 1931 to 1940, there is still no mention of environmental theory in the occupational therapy literature. Only general ideas were put forward and these discussed the relationship of patients to the environment and suggested that occupational therapists could provide an environment conducive to recovery and skill development. The literature also discussed the establishment of outpatient occupational therapy clinics to assist patients in their readjustment to community life.

The literature from 1941 to 1950 largely focused on the central issue for occupational therapy during that decade, i.e., rehabilitation of soldiers during and after World War II. For the first time, several articles linked environmental theory and occupational therapy. For example, Boreman (1949) addressed the mental aspects of rehabilitation and stressed the importance of looking at the whole person in his or her physical and social environment. In 1942, Anderson discussed the environment as an interacting part of a person's behaviour.

By the 1950s and 1960s, there was an increased emphasis on the environment in the occupational therapy literature.

Because of the influence of the medical model at this time, an interactional approach to the discussion of the environment was predominant. For example, the environment was most often divided into two parts, physical and social. O'Reilly (1954), in an article about person-environment interaction, discussed how occupational therapy could fit the patient into an environment so that life could be resumed with minimal stress. She stated that an occupational therapy assessment should include a patient's ability or lack of ability as well as attention to the requirements of the environment. In the area of the physical environment, there was an increased emphasis on the use of equipment and assistive devices. It was during this time that terms such as "prosthetic environments," "milieu therapy" and "therapeutic communities" were put forward as means of establishing environments that would minimize the disabling factors of a disease (Pincus, 1968). In the area of occupational therapy with children, enrichment of the environment was viewed as one of many ways to modify behaviour. Occupational therapists began to view the environment as many different variables affecting patients. Reilly (1962) discussed the need of humans to master the environment, to alter or to improve it.

During the 1970s, there was a further expansion in the focus on the environment and person-environment interactions. For example, Takata (1971) stressed the importance of the environment in the development of play in children. Shaw (1971) wrote of the architectural barriers facing people with disabilities and the role of occupational therapy to change these barriers. Occupational therapy in the area of mental health began to focus more on social rehabilitation and less on personality reorganization. In 1972, Dunning, in an article on environmental occupational therapy, discussed how the patient should be viewed in his or her total environmental context. This decade ended with the introduction of a Model of Human Occupation (Kielhofner & Burke, 1980), which stressed the interaction between humans as living systems within the environment.

During the past two decades, tremendous growth and development of environmental theory in occupational therapy has occurred. Barris (1982) extended the view of the environment, discussing properties of the environment and how environments must provide an optimal level of arousal for each client. DiJoseph (1982) put forward the concept of mind, body and environment interacting through activity. Howe and Briggs (1982) proposed an ecological systems model for occupational therapy to study the relationship between organisms and their environment. Many articles were written about the Independent Living Movement (Bachelder, 1985; Baum, 1980) and the involvement of occupational therapists in different community projects. The importance of the environment as a way of influencing behaviour and the use of the environment as an intervention modality were also beginning to receive increased emphasis (Cooper, 1985; Washburn, 1986). The Canadian Association of Occupational Therapists and the Department of Health and Welfare (1983) published an application of the Model of Occupational Performance and Client-Centred Practice, which emphasized the constant interactions between people, their occupations and social, cultural and physical environments.

An outcome measure developed from the Canadian guidelines, the Canadian Occupational Performance Measure, was published (Law, Baptiste, et al., 1994) and implicitly includes the environment as a part of a person's occupational performance. Other authors (Christiansen & Baum, 1991; Law, 1991) began to discuss the complex interrelationships between individuals, their occupations and environments and challenged occupational therapists to use environmental intervention to facilitate occupational performance. The environment began to be viewed as an integral part of occupational performance which makes physical, psychological, social, spiritual and cultural demands on the individual but also provides resources that can be used to facilitate occupational performance.

OCCUPATIONAL THERAPY PERSPECTIVE: THEORETICAL MODELS

Several current and emerging theoretical models of practice in occupational therapy focus on the nature of the person-environment-occupation relationship and the implications of these ideas for occupational therapy practice. In this section, the following theoretical models will be reviewed:

Person Environment Occupational Performance (Christiansen & Baum, 1991), Ecology of Human Performance (Dunn, Brown, & McGuigan, 1994), Model of Human Occupation (Kielhofner, 1995), Person-Environment-Occupation Model (Law et al, 1996), Occupational Adaptation (Schkade & Schultz, 1992) and Contemporary Task-Oriented Approach (Mathiowetz & Bass Haugen, 1994; Bass Haugen & Mathiowetz, 1995). The development, key ideas, strengths and limitations of each model are summarized, and information about important concepts and the occupational therapy process can be found in Tables 4-2 through 4-6.

Person Environment Occupational Performance Model

Christiansen and Baum (1991) have developed a model for occupational therapy to facilitate therapists' understanding of occupational performance. Theoretical foundations of this model come from general systems theory, focused on open systems interacting with their environment, and from theories about person-environment interaction. The first version of this model was published as part of a book chapter that also discusses occupational therapy history and other models, so at times it was difficult to extract the key concepts and assumptions of the Person Environment Occupational Performance Model. The model has been revised (Christiansen & Baum, 1997) to reflect the transactional relationship between person, occupation and environment and the influence of intrinsic and extrinsic factors on occupational performance, health and well-being (Figure 4-9).

The strengths of this model lie in its focus on the complexity of person-occupation-environment relationships and the clear indication that occupational performance results from these transactions. With the revision to the figure representing the model, the authors have recognized the many factors which influence occupational performance. One limitation of the model is that the occupational therapy process which accompanies the Person Environment Occupational Performance Model appears quite linear in its focus. The model has not yet been subjected to extensive testing (Table 4-2).

Ecology of Human Performance Model

Ecology of Human Performance (Dunn et al., 1994) is a framework for occupational therapy practice and research which focuses on the impact of context. It provides occupational therapists with guidelines to include contextual features (physical, temporal, social, cultural, phenomenological) in their practice. Theoretical foundations stem from social sciences, in particular environmental psychology, and occupational therapy knowledge. In this framework, context and person are viewed as interactive. The person includes

TABLE 4-2

Person-Environment-Occupational Performance

Developers:	C. Christiansen and C. Baum
Origin:	Developed to emphasize a view of performance as an interaction between a person and his or her environment
Population:	All ages
Theoretical Foundations:	• General systems theory • Occupational Therapy theorists (Howe and Briggs, Kielhofner and Burke, Reilly, Reed) • Environmental theories • Neurobehavioural theories • Psychological theories (personality, motivation, values, agency)
Concepts and Assumptions:	• Performance results from complex interactions between person and the environments in which he or she carries out tasks and roles • Developmental stage influences performance • Performance is facilitated by intrinsic enablers (in person), environmental factors, and meaning of occupation • Occupational therapy intervention can facilitate a person's adaptation when he or she encounters problems in performance • A personal sense of competence influences performance
Client/Therapist Relationship:	Active patient involvement is important; therapist as "teacher-facilitator"
Expected Outcome:	Competence, occupational performance Development of "life performance skills" Improved health and well-being
Assessment:	Assess person's "assets, deficits" Pay attention to person's environment(s) Could be formal, standardized, observation, interview Outcomes should focus on well-being

Intervention:	• Uses a problem-asset oriented model
	• Produces a client/family centred plan
	• Should be unique to each person and be driven by client goals
	• Intervention principles:
	  1. Uses occupation as a therapeutic medium
	  2. Uses compensatory adaptive strategies to overcome intrinsic factors (psychological, cognitive, physiological, neurobehavioral)
	  3. Modifies physical environment within cultural parameters
	  4. Develops social networks
	  5. Works to remove barriers that limit occupational performance
	  6. Educates the client, family, and others (e.g., employers) in strategies to optimize performance, promote health, and prevent secondary conditions

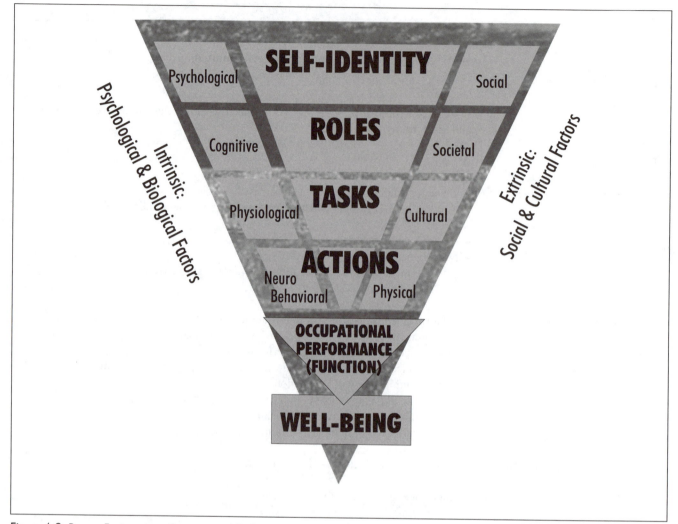

Figure 4-9. Person-Environment Occupational Performance Model.

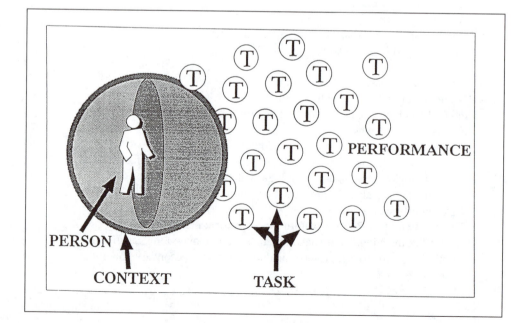

Figure 4-10. Ecology of Human Performance Model. Reprinted with permission from Dunn, W., Brown, C., & McGuigan, A. (1994). The ecology of human performance: A framework for considering the effect of context. *American Journal of Occupational Therapy, 48*, 595-607.

TABLE 4-3

Ecology of Human Performance

Developers:	W. Dunn and Occupational Therapy Faculty at University of Kansas
Origin:	Developed in response to the lack of consideration for complexities of context in occupational therapy
Population:	All ages
Theoretical Foundations:	• Environmental psychology • Occupational Therapy theorists (Kiernat, Barris, Howe and Briggs, Spencer)
Concepts and Assumptions:	• Ecology (the interaction between person and environment) affects human behaviour and performance • Performance cannot be understood outside of context • Context/environment includes physical, temporal, social, and cultural elements, and is considered to be broader than environment as it also includes the phenomenological experience of the person. • Relationships exist between the key variables of person, context, tasks, and performance • Environmental cues and features are used by a person to support performance of tasks
Client/Therapist Relationship:	Collaborative
Expected Outcome:	Performance of tasks Changes in context are used to support performance
Assessment:	Incorporate consideration of context New, contextually-relevant assessment tools are needed
Intervention:	Five alternatives described: 1. establish/restore (remediate) person's skills/abilities 2. alter the actual context in which persons perform 3. adapt contextual features and/or task demands to support performance in context 4. prevent the occurrence or evolution of maladaptive performance 5. create circumstances which promote more adaptable or complex performance in context

one's experiences, skills and abilities. Context is viewed as dynamic (non-linear) and interactional (Figure 4-10).

The strengths of this framework include its multidisciplinary theoretical foundations and clear definitions. Its generic perspective allows occupational therapists to apply it to clinical situations they encounter every day. The framework provides direction for the development of specific models of practice that recognize the interrelationship of the person and his or her context during task performance. It also recognizes the multifaceted nature of occupational therapy intervention.

The main limitation, as with other newly developed models, is the lack of evidence reported to date. Although it shows potential for clinical application, further work is needed to apply the theoretical constructs to everyday practice (Table 4-3).

Model of Human Occupation

The Model of Human Occupation is a conceptual model

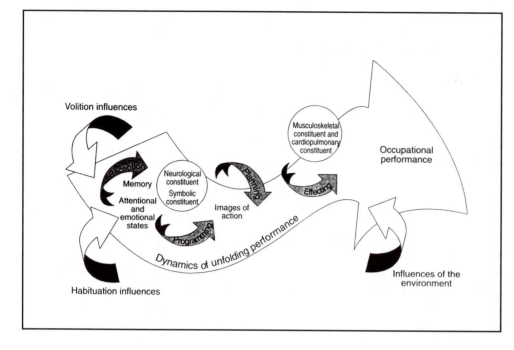

Figure 4-11. Model of Human Occupation. Reprinted with permission from Kielhofner, G. (1995). *A model of human occupation: Theory and application* (2nd ed.). Baltimore: Williams & Wilkins.

of occupational functioning that has been used to understand people's engagement in occupation and occupational dysfunction, and to guide practice in supporting change or reorganizing of occupational behaviour. It "focuses on the motivation for occupation, the patterning of occupational behaviour into routines and lifestyles, the nature of skilled performance, and the influence of environment on occupational behaviour" (Kielhofner, 1995, p. 2). The person is viewed as a complex, dynamic human system comprised of three subsystems influenced by his or her physical and social environments (Figure 4-11).

Of the models reviewed, this model is the most well-developed and most reviewed. Ideas written in 1985 have been updated with concepts of role theory and culture, and their application to occupational behaviour. Based on research findings and clinical review, concepts have integrated new information. The model articulates further development of self-organization through occupation whereby "occupational behaviour is self making" (Kielhofner, 1995, p. 22), and presents a more expanded concept of environment than its earlier version. The model adds to our understanding of: 1) the impact of chronic illness on occupational performance, and 2) the process of change in therapy. Therapists find particularly useful the suggestions about how to apply the model in practice through case illustrations, review of potential assessments, a detailed theoretical question list, and an explicit sample of a program development project.

At times, the use of jargon and creation of new terminology in the model obscures important concepts. Differences between task, activities, occupation, occupational forms, and

their relationship with the environment are at times unclear. The model would benefit from further development of how persons create and shape their occupations and their environments. The few suggested assessments which address the environment focus primarily on the presence or absence of supports and systems maintenance rather than clearly articulating disabling environmental barriers (Table 4-4).

Person-Environment-Occupation Model

The Person-Environment-Occupation Model represents a transactive approach to occupational performance. This model builds on concepts and assumptions from theorists such as Lawton and Nahemow (1973) and Csikszentmihalyi and Csikszentmihalyi (1988), and from current Canadian guidelines for occupational therapy practice and approaches to measurement, the Occupational Therapy Guidelines for Client-Centred Practice (CAOT, 1991) and the Canadian Occupational Performance Measure (COPM) (Law, Baptiste et al., 1994b). The model describes occupational performance as the product of a dynamic, interwoven relationship that exists among people, their occupations and roles, and the environments in which they live, work and play. In this approach, it is acknowledged that behaviour is influenced by and cannot be separated from contextual influences, temporal factors, and physical and psychological characteristics. A person's environments are continually shifting, and as these change, the behaviour necessary to accomplish a goal also changes. Occupational therapy intervention seeks to enable optimal occupational performance in occupations defined as important by the client (Figure 4-12).

TABLE 4-4

A Model of Human Occupation

Developer:	Gary Kielhofner
Origin:	Influenced from original occupational behaviour work at University of Southern California and Gary Kielhofner's master's thesis, which was refined/elaborated upon with Janice Burke & Cynthia Heard Igi for 1980 publication. Roann Barris and Anne Neville-Jan, together with many others, contributed to the first edition textbook. Twenty-two people contributed to the second edition.
Population:	All ages
Theoretical Foundations:·	• Occupational Therapy theorists (Reilly, Shannon, Nelson) • Systems theory; Cultural theory; Role theory • Environmental theories (Gibson, Lawton) • Personality theorists (Seligman, Allport, Maslow)

Concepts and Assumptions:·	• Human occupation: "doing culturally meaningful work, play, or daily living tasks in the stream of time and in the contexts of one's physical and social world" (Kielhofner, 1995, p. 3)
	• Change is a function of changes in the internal organization (e.g., growth, increased strength, skill acquisition) or new environmental conditions
	• Human system is a dynamic, changing, open system comprised of three subsystems: volition, habituation, mind-brain-body performance
	• These systems arrange themselves according to the demands of the situation in which they are performing; each contributes different but complimentary functions to the operation of the whole system
	• Environment influences occupational behaviour
	• Occupational performance: "meaningful sequences of action in which a person completes an occupational form" (Kielhofner, 1995, p. 113) using motor, process, communication, and interaction skills
	• Occupational dysfunction:
	  • disability results in breakdown of life's meaning or unable to place self in a "personal narrative" with possibilities and hope, loss/restrictions of habits and roles
	  • dysfunction occurs when people don't use their capacities in reasonable way to respond to reasonable societal expectations and when behaviour negatively affects integrity of human system

Client/Therapist Relationship:	Not explored in detail other than notation that data gathering is to be interactive.
Expected Outcome:	Develop a theory of the circumstances of the individual patient based on interview, structured assessments, and situated means. Enable an adaptive process and minimize the impact of impairments
Assessment:	Assessment process is interactive with client, analytical, and asks questions in three framework areas: Human System's Organization—clients' assets & liabilities; Environmental Influences—how it affords or presses occupational behaviour; and Systems Dynamics—examine skills demonstrated when engaged in occupations in their environment

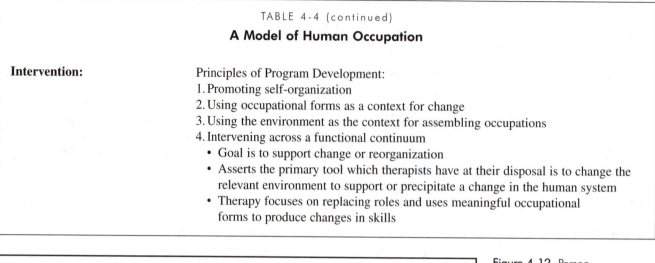

TABLE 4-4 (continued)
A Model of Human Occupation

Intervention:

Principles of Program Development:
1. Promoting self-organization
2. Using occupational forms as a context for change
3. Using the environment as the context for assembling occupations
4. Intervening across a functional continuum
   - Goal is to support change or reorganization
   - Asserts the primary tool which therapists have at their disposal is to change the relevant environment to support or precipitate a change in the human system
   - Therapy focuses on replacing roles and uses meaningful occupational forms to produce changes in skills

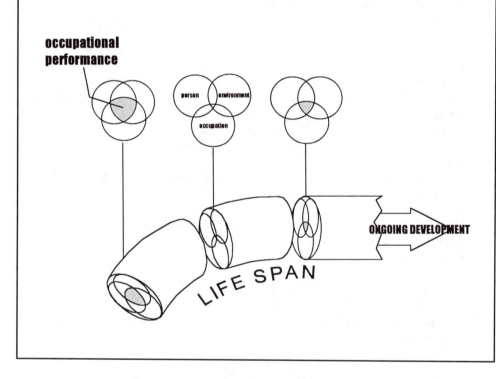

Figure 4-12. Person-Environment-Occupation Model. Reprinted with permission from Law, M., Cooper, B., Strong, S., Stewart, D., Rigby, P., & Letts, L. (1996). The person-environment-occupation model: A transactive approach to occupational performance. *Canadian Journal of Occupational Therapy, 63,* 9-23.

The key strength of this model is its focus on the transactional relationship between person, occupation and environment. Within the model, there is consideration of interventions that target the person, occupation and the environment in different ways. Thus, occupational therapists have options of using multiple avenues for eliciting change. In addition, the person's values and daily dilemmas underpin occupational therapy intervention. The authors of this model have also reviewed a wider repertoire of well-validated measures to assess the environment that have been developed by occupational therapy and other disciplines (Letts et al, 1994).

This model has undergone limited testing, primarily focused on the nature of the Person-Environment-Occupation relationships in clients with persistent mental health issues (Strong, 1995) and children with disabilities (Law, 1993). The Person-Environment-Occupation Model currently does not include much information on roles and their relationship with persons and occupation. The concept of occupational performance as described in the model could be developed further (Table 4-5).

TABLE 4-5

The Person-Environment-Occupation Model: A Transactive Approach to Occupational Performance

Developers:	M. Law, B. Cooper, S. Strong, D. Stewart, P. Rigby, L. Letts
Origin: Rehabilitation	Developed as part of an environmental research program in the School of Science, McMaster University
Population:	All ages
Theoretical Foundations:	• Canadian Guidelines for Occupational Therapy • Environmental theorists (Lawton and Nahemow) • Theory of "flow" (Csikszentmihalyi)
Concepts and Assumptions:	• The *person* is a unique being who assumes a variety of roles simultaneously. These roles are dynamic, varying across time and context in their importance, duration, and significance • *Environment is* defined broadly including cultural, socioeconomic, institutional, physical, and social considerations of the environment • *Occupation* is defined as groups of self-directed, functional tasks and activities in which a person engages over the lifespan. Time patterns and rhythms characterize the occupational routines of individuals over a day, a week, or longer • Occupational Performance is the outcome of the transaction of the person, environment, and occupation. It is defined as the dynamic experience of a person engaged in purposeful activities and tasks within an environment. Over a lifetime, individuals are constantly renegotiating their view of self and their roles as they ascribe meaning to occupation and the environment around them • The model assumes that its three major components (person, environment, occupation) interact continually across time and space in ways that increase or diminish their congruence. The outcome of greater compatibility is therefore represented as more optimal occupational performance
Client/Therapist Relationship:	Interdependent partnership to address occcupational performance issue defined by the client
Expected Outcome:	Improved fit between person, occupation, and environment will result in optimal occupational performance
Assessment:	The client, together with the therapist, identifies the client's occupational strengths and issues/problems in occupational performance. This can be done using a semi-structured interview (e.g., Canadian Occupational Performance Measure), or standardized assessment (e.g., Occupational Performance History Interview). Assessment of performance components, environmental conditions, and occupations helps to determine the focus and level of intervention
Intervention:	Interventions can target the person, occupation and the environment, offering multiple avenues for eliciting change. The goal is to facilitate changes which result in improved occupational performance

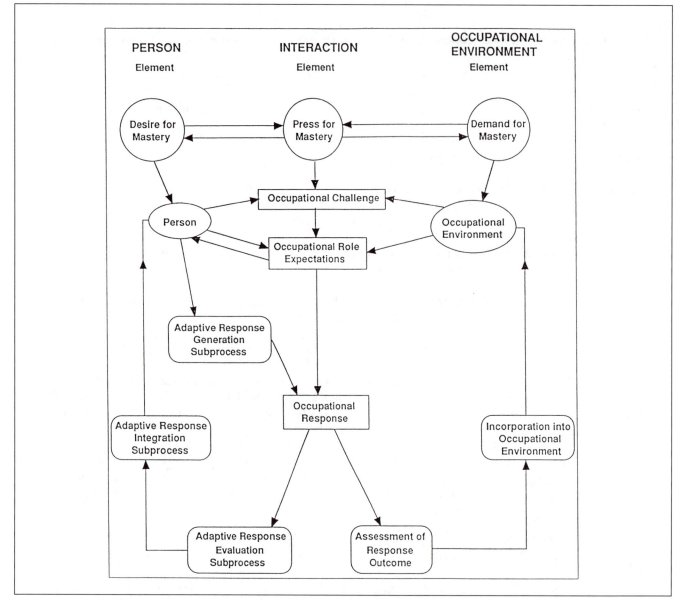

Figure 4-13. Occupational Adaptation Model. Reprinted with permission from Schkade, J. K., & Schultz, S. (1992). Occupational adaptation: Toward a holistic approach for contemporary practice, part 1. *American Journal of Occupational Therapy, 46,* 829-837.

Occupational Adaptation Model

Occupational adaptation (Schkade & Schultz, 1992) is a frame of reference for occupational therapy practice, education and research. A theoretical perspective of normal development, the model is intended to enhance our understanding of occupation and the benefits of occupational therapy. The framework outlines a process-based, non-hierarchical, non-stage-specific explanation of how occupation and adaptation become integrated into a single internal phenomenon within a person. Occupational adaptation is

viewed as both a state of occupational function and a normative process by which competence in occupational function develops (Figure 4-13).

The theoretical underpinnings of the Occupational Adaptation Model are congruent with current occupational therapy beliefs and the evolution of occupational therapy theory. The strengths of the framework are its generic perspective and detailed operational definitions and assumptions. The model adds a new perspective to occupational therapy practice by outlining a practice model (Schkade &

TABLE 4-6

Occupational Adaptation Model

Developers:	J. Schkade and S. Schultz
Origin:	Concept of occupational adaptation was selected by Texas Woman's University as a focus for research.
Population:	All ages
Theoretical Foundations:	• Occupational therapy theorists (Reed, Kielhofner, Nelson) • General systems theory
Concepts and Assumptions:	• Integrates constructs of occupation and adaptation into a single interactive construct • Occupation provides the means by which people adapt • Occupational adaptation is a normative process that is most pronounced in periods of transition • Person is made up of three systems: sensorimotor, cognitive, and psychosocial, as well as underlying subsystems • Occupational environments are those that call for an occupational response—they are contexts in which occupations occur (work, play and leisure, self-maintenance). • Occupations are activities characterized by three properties: active participation, meaning, and a product that is the output of the process • Adaptation is a change in the functional state of the person • Occupational adaptation is both a state (of competency in occupational functioning) and a process
Client/Therapist Relationship:	Interdependent/collaborative — Therapist functions as an agent of the patient's occupational environment, and the patient functions as the agent of his or her unique person systems
Expected Outcome:	• Improvement in the person's internal occupational adaptation process (self-initiation, generalization, and mastery) • Occupational adaptation as a state of competency in occupational functioning
Assessment:	• Identify the sources of dysfunction in the occupational adaptation process • Data gathering about the patient's occupational environments, role expectations, effect of presenting problem on the person's systems
Intervention:	• Focus is on the patient's internal adaptation process and the use of meaningful occupations • Directed at improving the patient's internal ability to generate, evaluate, and integrate adaptive responses in which relative mastery is experienced • The occupational environment is as important as the patient's condition • Activities, tasks, methods, and techniques must be centred on occupational activity that promotes satisfaction

Schultz, 1992) in a second article. The practice model guides therapists to view a person holistically, and gives equal weight to the person's internal processes and the environment.

The framework and practice model have not been formally tested yet, although the authors state that basic and applied research is currently taking place. A limitation in the practice model is the requirement that the therapists establish a close therapeutic relationship with the patient. This may not always be possible, particularly in some acute, community or consultation situations where patients are seen only once or twice. The detailed assumptions and relationships described by the authors may be difficult for many therapists and students to understand and apply to practice (Table 4-6).

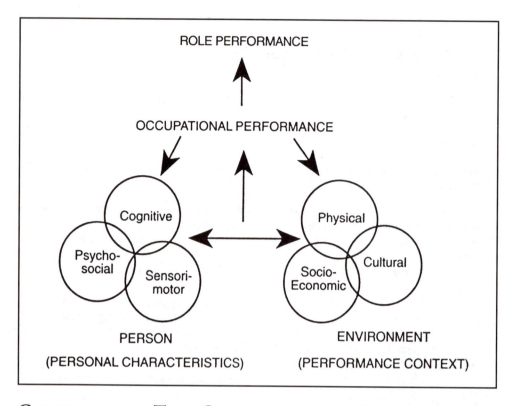

ROLE PERFORMANCE

OCCUPATIONAL PERFORMANCE

Cognitive

Psycho-social

Sensori-motor

Physical

Socio-Economic

Cultural

PERSON

(PERSONAL CHARACTERISTICS)

ENVIRONMENT

(PERFORMANCE CONTEXT)

Figure 4-14. Contemporary Task-Oriented Approach Model. Reprinted with permission from Mathiowetz, V., & Bass Haugen, J. (1994). Motor behavior research: Implications for therapeutic approaches to central nervous system dysfunction. *American Journal of Occupational Therapy, 48,* 733-745.

CONTEMPORARY TASK-ORIENTED APPROACH

Mathiowetz and Bass Haugen (1994) have developed the Contemporary Task-Oriented Approach to occupational therapy intervention, using concepts from a systems model of motor control, developmental theory and motor learning theories. In this model, a "top-down" approach to assessment and intervention is taken, with primary focus on the performance of functional tasks. Both personal characteristics (cognitive, psychosocial, and sensorimotor) and the performance or environmental context (physical, socioeconomic, cultural) are important factors in determining occupational performance and role performance. Concepts from motor learning theories such as knowledge of results and practice schedules are used to suggest appropriate learning strategies for clients as they relearn occupational performance tasks (Figure 4-14).

The strength of this model includes its use of contemporary motor theories to provide guidelines for occupational therapy intervention. The model acknowledges the complex interactions between persons and environment that affect occupational performance. Additionally, Bass Haugen and Mathiowetz (1995) have provided clear and detailed information about evaluation and intervention principles.

Similar to many other emerging models, the Contemporary Task-Oriented Approach is relatively new and has not been formally tested. The motor learning concepts that form the basis of recommended intervention have been developed and tested primarily with people without disabilities. It remains uncertain whether the same principles of motor learning will apply to people who have acquired disabilities. On a conceptual level, the Contemporary Task-Oriented Approach does not highlight the influence of occupation in the person-environment-occupation relationship. In this model, occupation is considered part of the environment (Table 4-7).

IMPLICATIONS FOR OCCUPATIONAL THERAPY PRACTICE

One of the most useful ways to illustrate the assessment and intervention approach which emanates from each model of practice is through a case illustration.

Paul is a man in his late 30s who sustained a closed head injury as a child. Residual impairments include a right hemiparesis and problems with speech articulation, short-term memory and perseveration. Paul received rehabilitation services when he was a child and adolescent. During his teen years, he held several summer jobs, including gas bar attendant, cleaner and filing clerk.

Paul fiercely values being independent. He lives an isolated life in a supervised boarding home with eight strangers who come and go. His family lives far away. Faced with large expanses of empty time, he often retreats to his bed or obsessively writes to organize his thoughts and ward off the encroachment of feelings of emptiness and loneliness.

TABLE 4-7

Contemporary Task-Oriented Approach

Developers:	Virgil Mathiowetz and Julie Bass Haugen
Origin:	Developed to emphasize that occupational therapy should focus on occupational performance and use contemporary motor theories as a basis for intervention
Population:	All ages, although primarily tested with adults
Theoretical Foundations:	• Systems model of motor control • Motor learning theory • Developmental theories
Concepts and Assumptions:	• Motor behaviour is facilitated and organized through performance of functional tasks • Performance of functional tasks is influenced by personal characteristics and the performance context • Personal characteristics and environmental factors are organized in a heterarchical fashion; control parameters which are personal characteristics or environmental factors are important in hindering or enabling performance • Use of motor learning strategies to practice a functional task will enhance the development of skilled performance
Client/Therapist Relationship:	Collaborative
Expected Outcome:	Improvement in task performance and role performance
Assessment:	• Assess functional tasks required to be performed by the person • Determine personal characteristics and environmental factors which are hindering performance • No specific recommendations about outcome measures

Intervention:	• Use an active learning approach
	• Client is an active participant in therapy intervention
	• Describe seven intervention principles:
	  1. Client identifies tasks of interest and importance
	  2. Client is encouraged to actively experiment with movements to achieve task performance
	  3. Therapist performs an analysis of client's movement strategies
	  4. Important personal characteristics and environmental factors which are hindering performance are changed
	  5. Outcome in terms of improved task performance is recorded
	  6. Further intervention can focus on developing more efficient movement strategies
	  7. Motor learning principles such as varying practice are used to enhance learning

Paul remembers riding a bicycle as a child and colliding with a car. Today, in his late 30s, he continues to negotiate daily activities with a mild right hemiparesis and problems with speech articulation, short-term memory and perseveration. Paul recounts growing up in a small town and particularly enjoying summer jobs helping other people as a gas bar attendant, cleaner and filing clerk. When he was 20 years old, he moved on his own to a large city, where he currently resides. He began experiencing mental health problems after his move, when he was in a stressful job. He experienced delusional thoughts, and was in and out of the hospital several times.

TABLE 4-8

Application of Occupational Therapy Models

Model	Client-therapist relationship	Assessment	Intervention	Outcome
Ecology of Human Performance (Dunn et al., 1994)	Collaborative among Paul, therapist, and staff	Evaluate Paul's performance of tasks within the context of the work setting—consider physical, social, cultural, and temporal features of the environment	Use a variety of interventions to alter the context of the work setting to enable Paul to perform tasks with his current skills (e.g., work in store to better match need for immediate gratification). Adapt contextual feature or task (e.g., arrange tables to promote social interaction). Remedial skills training to improve quality and quantity of his work	Enable functional performance to emerge at Paul's work, with the assigned tasks, and in his living situation. Improve match between Paul and the work setting
Person-Environment-Occupational Performance (Christiansen & Baum, 1991, 1997)	Active involvement of Paul in therapy process. Therapist acts as teacher –facilitator	Use a variety of measures to assess Paul's assets, deficits, and past performance. Assess work environment. Develop list of goals	Intervention is individualized and focuses on use of occupational tasks to improve Paul's skills in workplace (e.g., activities graded from immediate to less immediate gratification). Use compensatory techniques and environmental modifications as well. Explores options that fit his capabilities	Improvement in Paul's competence in performing targeted work skills or improve the fit of his skills to achievable tasks
Model of Human Occupation (Kielhofner, 1995)	Interactive, emphasizing Paul's individuality. Paul would take part in identifying problems and setting goals	Variety of assessment tools are used to evaluate Paul's assets, liabilities, performance, and influence of environment on occupational behaviour	Enable Paul to find a meaningful role in the work setting that he is able to perform well. Use occupational forms that have meaning to Paul to improve his skills and reorganize the work environment to facilitate his skill development	Enable person to develop, adapt, and make life transitions. Improved skills and development of new roles and habits

TABLE 4-8 (continued)

Application of Occupational Therapy Models

Model	Client-therapist relationship	Assessment	Intervention	Outcome
Person-Environment-Occupation (Law, Cooper, et al., 1996a)	Collaborative partnership between Paul, therapist and people in work site	Assess Paul's performance at work to identify personal, environmental, and occupational factors enabling or constraining occupational performance	With Paul, address factors that are decreasing fit between person, occupation, and environment (e.g., communication strategies; change physical layout; seek alternative living). Greater emphasis on changing occupation and environment than person	Optimal occupational performance as experienced by Paul. Improved fit between Paul, his work occupations, and the work environment
Occupational Adaptation (Schkade & Schultz, 1992)	Interdependent-therapist is agent of Paul's occupational environment; Paul is agent of his unique personal systems	Identify sources of dysfunction in Paul's occupational adaptation processes, including personal system and occupational environment; determine match with role expectations	Improve Paul's occupational adaptation through therapy using occupational readiness (e.g., development of strategies to delay gratification) and occupational activity (e.g., cleaning tasks that are more meaningful to him)	Improved in self-initiation, generalization (e.g., assuming other tasks at work), and relative mastery (e.g., satisfaction with work)
Contemporary Task-Oriented Approach (Bass Haugen & Mathiowetz, 1995)	Collaborative between Paul, therapist, and staff	Identify Paul's preferred movement strategies, along with personal and environmental characteristics which are hindering task performance; identify tasks which are important to Paul to perform	Intervene to change personal characteristics and environmental factors which are hindering task performance. Use varying practice conditions to enable Paul to practice task performance in different environments and under different performance conditions	Improvement in task performance. Development of efficient movement strategies.

In the past, Paul frequently participated in Industrial Therapy programs. A recent Vocational Assessment program suggested Paul was ready to work in a "transitional" setting. Anxious to work to feel useful and earn enough money to move to his own apartment, Paul agreed with his vocational counsellor's plans for him to work at a new cooperative business. Paul worked as part of a ceramics production line with 30 other people with persistent mental illness. After 6 months, Paul was referred to an occupational therapist for assessment and consultation, as he was not satisfied with working at the cooperative, and staff reported that he was not fitting in.

In Table 4-8, approaches to occupational therapy assessment, intervention, outcome and the client-therapist relationship are illustrated for each model.

A review of these five occupational therapy models indicates that they share many characteristics in the occupational therapy assessment and intervention process. For example, all acknowledge the important influence of the environment in shaping occupational performance. There are, however, some important differences between these models. The issues around roles are most well-developed by the Model of Human

Occupation, the Ecology of Human Performance Model and the Person-Environment-Occupational Performance Model. Distinguishing occupation from occupational performance conceptually is done in detail by the Person-Environment-Occupation and the Person Environment Occupational Performance models. Specific intervention guidelines that are linked to measurement procedures are included in the Model of Human Occupation and the Person-Environment-Occupation Model. In most of the models, the focus of primary intervention remains the person, while in the Ecology of Human Performance, Person-Environment-Occupation and the Person Environment Occupational Performance models, intervention can focus on enabling changes in the person, occupation and/or the environment.

Stating which model is more appropriate in certain clinical situations because the testing of the models is in its early stages. All of these models value occupation as a core concept of occupational therapy and occupational performances as a primary outcome. As more research studying the application of these models is completed, it will likely become more clear which is most appropriate in certain clinical situations. Clearly, the Model of Human Occupation has been subject to the most testing, but the revised model (Keilhofner, 1995) includes significant changes which have not been empirically tested. Perhaps the most important issue is not to determine which model is best, but to ensure that occupational therapists do use a model of practice to guide the occupational therapy assessment and intervention process so that it is clear to the client and to others that the primary focus is occupational performance.

In the development of occupational therapy models which focus on the person-environment-occupation relationship, several challenges for further theory development remain. One of the most important challenges is to investigate the nature of person-environment-occupation fit. For example, for persons at different ages and within different environments, what constitutes optimal occupational performance? How is optimal occupational performance best measured? If occupational performance is truly a person's dynamic experience with his or her daily life activities, then measurement of this experience would be best completed through qualitative or subjective assessment. The relationship between an individual's perceptions of occupational performance and objective measures of function remains unclear.

Another issue which requires further discussion and research is the specific person, environment and occupation factors that are necessary for completion of daily life tasks and activities. Information about the minimal level of performance components, the acceptable level of adaptation of an occupation, and/or the minimal level of environmental support is required to enable occupational therapists to target intervention in the most efficient and effective manner.

There is increasing evidence that occupation is an important determinant of health and well-being. Certainly one of the foundations underlying occupational therapy theory and practice is the belief that engagement in occupation will lead to enhanced health and well-being. Population health studies which have studied people's activities on a longitudinal basis have found a significant relationship between work, physical activity, leisure activities, social activities, and health and well-being (Law, Steinwender & Leclair, 1996). These relationships may be stronger for persons with disabilities who have fewer environmental resources. Research has also indicated that mediating factors of stress, control, and amount of free time have a significant influence on life satisfaction (Csikszentmihalyi & Csikszentmihalyi, 1988; Backman & Christiansen, 1996). Further research is required to determine the exact characteristics of occupation which are most influential in promoting health and well-being.

STUDY QUESTIONS

1. Define occupational performance. What are the major factors that influence a person's occupational performance?

2. Describe how occupational therapists use the term "function." How is this use different from the way "function" is defined and used by other health professionals?

3. Define environment and types of environmental factors. What environmental factors affect your current occupational performance?

4. Cite two examples of environment-behaviour theorists who emphasize the person's internal environment or perceptions of the world around them.

5. What is the common concept that all environment-behaviour theorists discuss in describing persons within their environment?

6. Review Bandura's concept of perceived self-efficacy. Identify examples in your life when self-efficacy has influenced the way in which you approached a challenging situation.

7. What are the primary changes in the way in which occupational therapy has defined and used the environment over the past 80 years?

8. Review the theoretical concepts and assumptions of the six current and emerging occupational therapy models of practice. What concepts are common to all models? What concepts are unique to only one model?

9. Think of an occupation which has been challenging for

you in the past. Use one of the occupational therapy models of practice to analyze that situation, including how you would assess the problem, and what you would recommend to enable you to meet the challenge.

REFERENCES

Altman, I., & Rogoff, B. (1987). World view in psychology: Trait, interactional, organismic and transactional perspectives. In D. Stokols & I. Altman (Eds.), *Handbook of environmental psychology* (Vol. 1). (pp. 7-40). New York: Wiley.

American Occupational Therapy Association (1995a). Position paper: Occupational performance. *American Journal of Occupational Therapy, 49*, 1019-1021.

Bachelder, J. (1985). Independent living programs: Bridges from hospital to community. *Occupational Therapy in Health Care, 2*, 99-107.

Backman, C., & Christiansen, C. (1996). *Personal projects and perceived wellbeing in working and retired adults.* Canadian Association of Occupational Therapists Conference, Ottawa, June, 1996.

Baker, F., & Intagliata, J. (1982). Quality of life in the evaluation of community support systems. *Evaluation and Program Planning, 5,* 69-79.

Bandura, A. (1986). *Social foundations of thought and action: A social cognitive theory.* Englewood Cliffs, NJ: Prentice-Hall.

Barris, R. (1982). Environmental interactions: An extension of the model of occupation. *Canadian Journal of Occupational Therapy, 36*, 637-644.

Bass Haugen, J. B., & Mathiowetz, V. (1995). Contemporary task-oriented approach. In C. A. Trombly (Ed.), *Occupational therapy for physical dysfunction* (4th ed.). Baltimore: Williams & Wilkins.

Baum, C. M. (1980). Independent living: A critical role for occupational therapists. *American Journal of Occupational Therapy, 34*(12), 773-774.

Berlin, S. (1989). The Canadian healthy community project: Shapes of the reality. *Plan Canada, 29*(4), 13-15.

Boreman, M. C. (1949). Mental aspects of rehabilitation. *Occupational Therapy and Rehabilitation, 23,* 68-73.

Bronfenbrenner, U. (1977). Toward an experimental ecology of human development. *American Psychologist, 32,* 513-531.

Canadian Association of Occupational Therapists (1991). *Client-centred guidelines for the practice of occupational therapy.* Toronto: Author.

Christiansen, C. (1991). Occupational therapy: Intervention for life performance. In C. Christiansen & C. Baum (Eds.), *Occupational therapy: Overcoming human performance deficits.* Thorofare, NJ: SLACK Incorporated.

Christiansen, C., & Baum, C. (1991). *Occupational therapy: Overcoming human performance deficits.* Thorofare, NJ: SLACK Incorporated.

Christiansen, C., & Baum, C. (1997). *Occupational therapy: Enabling function and well-being.* Thorofare, NJ: SLACK Incorporated.

Cooper, B. (1985). A model for implementing colour contrast in the environment of the elderly. *American Journal of Occupational Therapy, 39*, 253-257.

Crane, B. T. (1919). Occupational therapy. *Boston Medical and Surgical Journal, 181*, 63-65.

Csikszentmihalyi, M., & Csikszentmihalyi, I. S. (1988). *Optimal experience: Psychological studies in flow in consciousness.* Cambridge: Cambridge University Press.

DiJoseph, L. M. (1982). Independence through activity: Mind, body and environment interaction in therapy. *American Journal of Occupational Therapy, 36*, 740-744.

Dunn, W., Brown, C., & McGuigan, A. (1994). The ecology of human performance: A framework for considering the effect of context. *American Journal of Occupational Therapy, 48*, 595-607.

Dunning, G. (1972). Environmental occupational therapy. *American Journal of Occupational Therapy, 26*, 292-298.

Gibson, E. (1988). Exploratory behavior in the development of perceiving, acting and the acquiring of knowledge. *Annual Review of Psychology, 39*, 1-41.

Gibson, J. (1977). The theory of affordances. In R. Shaw & J. Bransford (Eds.), *Perceiving, acting and knowing* (pp. 67-82). Hillsdale, NJ: Erlbaum.

Gibson, J. (1979). *The ecological approach to visual perception.* Boston: Houghton-Mifflin.

Hancock, T. (1985). The mandala of health: A model of the human ecosystem. *Family and Community Health, 8*(3), 1-10.

Hancock, T. (1993). Health, human development and the community ecosystem: Three ecological models. *Health Promotion International, 8*, 41-47.

Howe, M. C., & Briggs, A. K. (1982). Ecological systems model for occupational therapy. *American Journal of Occupational Therapy, 36*, 322-327.

Kahana, E. (1982). A congruence model of person-environment interaction. In M. P. Lawton, P. G. Windley, & T. D. Byerts (Eds.), *Aging and the environment: Theoretical approaches* (pp. 97-121). New York: Springer.

Kaplan, S. (1983). A model of person-environment compatibility. *Environment and Behavior, 15*, 311-332.

Kielhofner, G., & Burke, J. (1980). A model of human occupation, part I: Conceptual framework and content. *American Journal of Occupational Therapy, 34*, 572-581.

Kielhofner, G. (1995). *A model of human occupation: Theory and application* (2nd ed.). Baltimore: Williams & Wilkins.

Law, M. (1991). The environment: A focus for occupational therapy. *Canadian Journal of Occupational Therapy, 58*, 171-179.

Law, M. (1993). *Planning for children with physical disabilities: Identifying and changing disabling environments through participatory research.* University of Waterloo, unpublished doctoral thesis.

Law, M., Cooper, B. A., Stewart, D., Letts, L., Rigby, P., & Strong, S. (1994). Person-environment relations. *Work, 4*, 228-238.

Law, M., Baptiste, S., Carswell, A., McColl, M. A., Polatajko, H., & Pollock, N. (1994). *Canadian occupational performance Measure Manual* (2nd ed.). Toronto, Canada: CAOT Publications ACE.

Law, M., Cooper, B., Strong, S., Stewart, D., Rigby, P., & Letts, L. (1996). The person-environment-occupation model: A transactive approach to occupational performance. *Canadian Journal of Occupational Therapy, 63*, 9-23.

Law, M., Steinwender, S., & Leclair, L. (1996). *Occupation, health and well-being: A review of research evidence*. Canadian Association of Occupational Therapists Conference, Ottawa, June, 1996.

Lawton, M. P., & Nahemow, L. (1973). Towards an ecological theory of adaptation and aging. In W. Preiser (Ed.), *Environmental design research* (pp. 24-32). Stroudsburg, PA: Dowden, Hutchison & Ross.

Lawton, P., Windley, P. G., & Byerts, T. O. (1982). *Aging and the environment: Theoretical approaches*. New York: Springer.

Lawton, P. (1986). *Environment and aging* (2nd ed.). Albany, NY: Plenum.

Letts, L., Law, M., Rigby, P., Cooper, B., Stewart, D., & Strong, S. (1994). Person-environment assessments in occupational therapy. *American Journal of Occupational Therapy, 48*, 608-618.

Mathiowetz, V., & Bass Haugen, J. (1994). Motor behavior research: Implications for therapeutic approaches to central nervous system dysfunction. *American Journal of Occupational Therapy, 48*, 733-745.

Moos, R., & Lemke, S. (1979). *The multiphasic environmental assessment procedure manual*. Palo Alto, CA: Social Ecology Laboratory, Stanford University and Veterans Administration Medical Center.

Moos, R. (1980). Specialized living environments for older people: A conceptual framework for evaluation. *Journal of Social Issues, 36*, 75-94.

O'Reilly, J. A. (1954). Occupational therapy in the management of traumatic disabilities. *Canadian Journal of Occupational Therapy, 21*, 75-80.

Pincus, A. (1968). New findings on learning in old age: Implications for occupational therapy. *American Journal of Occupational Therapy, 22*, 300-333.

Reilly, M. (1962). Occupational therapy can be one of the great ideas of 20th century medicine. *American Journal of Occupational Therapy, 16*, 1-9.

Schkade, J. K., & Schultz, S. (1992). Occupational adaptation: Toward a holistic approach for contemporary practice, part 1. *American Journal of Occupational Therapy, 46*, 829-837.

Shaw, J. A. (1971). Architectural barriers: A medical problem. *American Journal of Occupational Therapy, 25*, 13-15.

Strong, S. (1995). *An ethnographic study examining the experiences of persons with persistent mental illness working at an affirmative business*. McMaster University, unpublished master's thesis.

Takata, N. (1971). The play milieu—a preliminary appraisal. *American Journal of Occupational Therapy, 25*, 281-284.

Washburn, M. G. (1986). Designing environments for the elderly. *Occupational Therapy in Health Care*, 17-25.

Weisman, G. D. (1981). Modeling environment-behaviour systems: A brief note. *Journal of Man-Environment Relations, 1*, 32-41.

Windley, L., & Scheidt, R. (1980). Person-environment dialectics: Implications for functioning in old age. In L. Poon (Ed.), *Aging in the 1980's: Psychological issues* (pp. 407-423). New York: Academic Press.

Wilcock, A. (1993). A theory of the human need for occupation. *Occupational Science: Australia, 1*(1), 17-24.

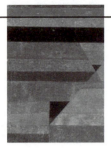

CHAPTER CONTENT OUTLINE

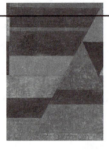

ABSTRACT

This chapter presents a review and analysis of assessment methods used to examine occupational performance and functional independence. Commonly used assessment instruments are discussed in terms of their ability to measure impairment, disability, and handicap as defined by the World Health Organization. The terminology and components of assessment in clinical and community environments are discussed with an emphasis on reliability, validity, and sensitivity. The therapists' role in assessment and clinical decision making is examined with a focus on how the information collected during the assessment process is used to facilitate development of programs of therapeutic intervention. The impact of assessment on program planning, cost effectiveness, and the establishment of prospective payment systems for rehabilitation services is explored.

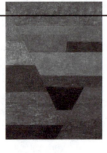

KEY TERMS

Evaluation

Measurement

Functional Assessment

Testing, Reliability

Validity

Sensitivity

Specificity

Scores

Standardization

Activities of Daily Living (ADL)

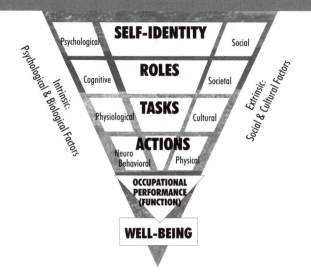

Occupational Performance Assessment

Kenneth J. Ottenbacher, PhD, OTR, FAOTA, Charles Christiansen, EdD, OTR, OT(C), FAOTA

OBJECTIVES

The information in this chapter is intended to help the reader:

1. understand the importance of assessment in identifying and resolving problems in human performance

2. recognize the elements associated with the development, application, and interpretation of human performance assessment

3. identify a conceptual model for categorizing the assessment of impairment, disability, and handicap

4. appreciate the importance of validity, reliability, and sensitivity in selecting and using assessment instruments

5. understand the relationship between assessment of occupational performance and the development of intervention programs

6. critically administer and analyze the results of occupational performance assessment instruments.

> *"The greater our understanding of occupations and how they maintain, enhance, and promote health and well being, the greater will be our ability to link this knowledge with practice and education of future students."*
>
> Johnson, 1996

OVERVIEW

The occupational therapy process can be divided into two stages according to Rogers and Holm (1991). The first stage involves identifying and defining the client's functional problems. This is accomplished through systematic assessment. Opacich (1991) noted in the first edition of this text that "without assessment, goal directed therapy becomes impossible" (p. 356). The second stage focuses on the resolution of the identified problems (Rogers & Holm, 1991). This stage includes the planning and implementation of intervention followed by reassessment. Rogers and Holm (1991) have used the term *occupational therapy diagnosis* to refer to the sequence of steps resulting in the formulation of problem statements describing the functional deficits toward which intervention is directed. The details of the occupational therapy diagnosis process are presented in the next chapter. This chapter focuses on the first stage of occupational therapy intervention defined by Rogers and Holm (1991), that is, the "identification of functional limitations through systematic assessment" (p. 234). The chapter begins with basic terminology and definitions emphasizing their importance in identifying a conceptual model for occupational performance assessment. The fundamental components of the assessment process are reviewed followed by descriptions of several instruments commonly used by clinicians to examine occupational performance. The chapter ends with a discussion of how recent trends in the development of managed care and prospective payment may affect occupational performance assessment.

DEFINITIONS AND TERMINOLOGY

The American Congress of Rehabilitation Medicine developed *Measurement Standards for Interdisciplinary Medical Rehabilitation* in 1992 (Johnston, Keith & Hinderer, 1992). These standards were designed "to be applicable to all members of the rehabilitation team — to physicians, physical therapists, occupational therapists, speech-language pathologists, nurses, psychologists, social workers, recreational therapists, rehabilitation engineers, and others" (Johnston et al., 1992, p. S-5).

One goal of developing and publishing the *Measurement Standards for Interdisciplinary Medical Rehabilitation* was to establish common definitions and terminology for assessment in medical rehabilitation. The American Occupational Therapy Association (1995a,b) has produced position papers and related documents describing the evaluation and assess-

ment process that are, at times, inconsistent with the terminology and definitions in the Measurement Standards for Interdisciplinary Medical Rehabilitation (Johnston et al., 1992). Students, clinicians, and researchers should be aware of these differences so that confusion in the assessment process is minimized. Confusion may occur as occupational therapy practitioners interact and share assessment results with other rehabilitation professionals in environments that emphasize team-oriented care and client-centered therapeutic programming.

The *Measurement Standards for Interdisciplinary Medical Rehabilitation* (referred to hereafter as the Interdisciplinary Standards, Johnston et al., 1992) define measurement as the "process implied whenever a number is attached to an observation" (p. S-5). No distinction is made in the Interdisciplinary Standards among the terms, measurement, assessment, and evaluation. Johnston et al. (1992) state that "the term measurement is used generically to denote assessment and evaluation procedures, tests, mechanical devices, observational procedures, and other procedures that are attached to a number, ordination, or categorization of an observation" (p. S-5).

In contrast, the Commission on Practice (COP) of the AOTA (1995) recently produced the following definitions for two commonly used measurement terms: "*Evaluation:* Evaluation will be used to refer to the process of obtaining and interpreting data necessary for intervention. This includes planning for and documenting the evaluation process and results. *Assessment*: Assessment will be used to refer to specific tools or instruments that are used during the evaluation process" (COP, 1995, p. 1072-1073).

In an article discussing the use of measurement terminology in occupational therapy entitled "A Proposal for Diverse Research Methods and Common Research Language," Short-DeGraff and Fisher (1993) observe that there is an ongoing debate in the occupational therapy literature regarding the use of research terms including measurement, assessment and evaluation. They proposed the following definitions: "*Assess*: To estimate or determine the significance, importance or value of. *Evaluate*: To judge or determine the worth or quality of; or to estimate. *Measure:* the process of determining quantitative differences in amount, based on the use of numeric units of like kind" (1993).

The American Physical Therapy Association (APTA) has published *Standards for Tests and Measurements in Physical Therapy Practice* (1991). These Standards are designed to provide the foundation for assessment in physical therapy and ensure the quality of practice. The APTA Standards include the following definitions: "*Assessment:* Measurement, quantification, or placing a value or label on something. *Evaluation*: A judgment based on a measurement; evaluations are judgments of value or worth of something. *Measurement:* The numeral assigned to an object, event, or person or the

Bibliographic citation of this chapter: Ottenbacher, K. J., & Christiansen, C. (1997). Occupational performance assessment. In C. Christiansen & C. Baum (Eds.), *Occupational therapy: Enabling function and well-being* (2nd ed.). Thorofare, NJ: SLACK Incorporated.

class (category) to which an object, event, or person is assigned according to rules" (APTA, 1991, p. 590).

In examining the various official definitions given to the terms assessment, evaluation, and measurement, one is reminded of the following exchange between Alice and Humpty Dumpty in Lewis Carroll's *Through the Looking Glass*. "When I use a word," Humpty Dumpty said in a rather scornful tone, "it means just what I choose it to mean—nothing more nor less." "The question is," said Alice, "whether you can make words mean so many different things." "The question is," said Humpty Dumpty, "which is to be the master — that is all" (1945, p. 219).

There is obviously no easy resolution to this semantic swamp. Nevertheless, terminology in the assessment process is important and needs to be brought to the attention of students and practitioners to minimize confusion. In this chapter, the terms *assessment* and *measurement* will be used to refer to the entire information gathering process, including the analysis and interpretation of data used to make treatment planning and intervention decisions for individuals or groups receiving occupational therapy services. This convention follows that used in the *Measurement Standards for Interdisciplinary Medical Rehabilitation* (Johnston et al., 1992). The reader will have to determine who is the "master" in using various measurement related terms in his or her individual clinical environment.

OCCUPATIONAL PERFORMANCE AND FUNCTIONAL ASSESSMENT

Another area of potential confusion for readers of this chapter (and the professional literature) involves the use of the terms *occupation, occupational performance, function* and *functional assessment*. Lawton (1971) originally described functional assessment as "any systematic attempt to measure objectively the levels at which a person is functioning in any of a variety of areas such as physical health, quality of self-maintenance, quality of role activity, intellectual status, social activity, attitude toward self, and emotional status" (p. 466). More recently, the definition of functional assessment proposed by Granger (1984) has been widely adopted and used in rehabilitation. According to Granger (1984), "functional assessment is a method for describing abilities and limitations and to measure an individual's use of the variety of skills included in performing tasks necessary to daily living, leisure activities, vocational pursuits, social interactions, and other required behaviors" (p. 24).

The AOTA position paper on occupation (1995a) refers to occupational performance "as the physical and mental abilities and skills required for satisfactory engagement in a given occupational pursuit" (p. 1015). The AOTA position paper notes that occupations have multiple dimensions including: performance, contextual, temporal, psychological, social, symbolic, and spiritual. In comparison, the term *function* denotes specifically the *performance* dimension of occupation. The AOTA has proposed that when occupational therapists use the term *function* they refer to an individual's performance of activities, tasks, and roles during daily living occupations (occupational performance).

This chapter focuses on the methods and strategies associated with assessment of occupational performance. The terms *functional assessment* and *occupational performance assessment* are used interchangeably in the remainder of this chapter. The phrase, "occupational performance assessment," is consistent, if not synonymous, with functional assessment, based on the definition proposed by the AOTA and common use in medical rehabilitation (1995a,b).

A CONCEPTUAL MODEL FOR OCCUPATIONAL PERFORMANCE ASSESSMENT

In describing the assessment process in medical rehabilitation, Coster and Haley (1992) note that the development of a conceptual framework is the most important step in the process of measurement. A conceptual framework is particularly important in occupational performance assessment because of the complexity of defining and measuring functional abilities. This complexity is frequently identified as one of the reasons for the slow progress in developing evaluation methods and conducting outcome studies in rehabilitation. DeJong (1987) has suggested that part of the difficulty in establishing evidence of effective clinical outcomes in rehabilitation is directly related to the "unit of analysis." The unit of analysis in rehabilitation generally, and occupational therapy in particular, is the individual and the individual's relationship with his or her environment. In contrast, the unit of analysis in many medical specialties is an organ, a body system, or a specific pathology. In fact, DeJong argues that traditional medical research and practice is organized around these organ systems and pathologies, e.g., cardiology, neurology, and orthopedics, among others. One consequence of this organizational structure is a focus on assessment and outcomes that emphasizes either an absence of pathology or the performance of a specific organ or body system; for instance, the use of an electrocardiogram (EKG) to evaluate the function of the heart. In contrast to these narrowly focused medical specialties, the goal of occupational therapy is to improve the person's ability to function as independently as possible in his or her natural environment. To achieve this goal requires instruments and assessment procedures that cover a liberal spectrum of activities and environments. DeJong (1987) suggests that "as the spectrum of functional activity broadens, it becomes more difficult to achieve a consensus on both conceptual and measurement issues" (p. 262). A common conceptual framework can help focus assessment efforts and reduce confusion in developing appropriate intervention strategies.

Granger (1984) originally proposed the World Health Organization's (WHO) *International Classification of Impairments, Disabilities and Handicaps* (ICIDH) as a model for discussing and organizing the assessment of functional performance. The ICIDH framework includes four levels: pathology, impairment, disability, and handicap. This model is briefly summarized below. The reader is referred to previous chapters for an in-depth discussion of the WHO model and its relation to other conceptual frameworks relevant to occupation (Wood, 1980; American Occupational Therapy Association, 1995b).

Impairment

In the context of health experience, an impairment is any loss or abnormality of psychological, physiological, or anatomical structure and function. (Note: "Impairment" is more inclusive than "disorder" in that it covers losses, e.g., the loss of a leg is an impairment, but not a disorder.)

Impairment is characterized by losses or abnormalities that may be temporary or permanent, and that include the existence or occurrence of an anomaly, defect, or loss in limb, organ, tissue, or other structure of the body, including the systems of mental function. Impairment represents exteriorization of a pathological state and, in principle, it reflects disturbances at the level of the organ or body system (World Health Organization, 1980).

Disability

In the context of health experience, a disability is any restriction or lack (resulting from an impairment) of ability to perform an activity in the manner or within the range considered normal for a human being. Disability is concerned with abilities, in the form of composite activities and behaviors, that are generally accepted as essential components of everyday life. Examples include disturbances in behaving appropriately, in personal care (such as excretory control and the ability to wash and feed oneself), in the performance of other activities of daily living, and in locomotor activities (such as the ability to walk) (World Health Organization, 1980).

Handicap

In the context of health experience, a handicap is a disadvantage for a given individual, resulting from an impairment or a disability, that limits or prevents the fulfillment of a role that is normal (depending on age, sex, and social and cultural factors) for that individual. Handicap is concerned with the value attached to an individual's situation or experience when it departs from the norm. It is characterized by a discordance between the individual's performance or status and the expectations of the individual or of the particular group of which he or she is a member. Handicap, thus, represents socialization of an impairment or disability and, as such, reflects the consequences for the individual — cultural, social, economic, and environmental — that stem from the presence of impairment and disability. Disadvantage arises from failure or inability to conform with the expectations or norms of the individual's universe. Handicap occurs when there is interference with the ability to sustain what might be designated as "survival roles" (World Health Organization, 1980).

Disablement

Disablement has been suggested as a collective descriptor designed to refer to experiences identified by the terms *impairment, disability* and *handicap* (Thuriaux, 1995). Disablement is widely used as an alternative to the awkwardness of repeating impairment, disability and handicap. It is important when using the term *disablement* to make a clear distinction from disability, as defined in the ICIDH. Disability is a condition related to level of impairment or pathology. Disablement is the state of the person with that condition.

It is also important to understand when using the ICIDH model that it is not a classification of individuals. What is being classified and defined are characteristics and attributes of the person, but not the person him- or herself. Although the three components of the WHO system (impairment, disability and handicap) are hierarchic in the sense that they represent increasingly complex activities, they are not a simple linear sequence. Inclusion at one level does not mean that difficulty will exist at the next level. For example, persons with below knee amputations have an impairment, but if they are able to accomplish all of their daily activities and remain employed and socially active with the use of a prosthesis, they may not have a disability or handicap.

The ICIDH model has also been proposed as providing a conceptual framework for assessing occupational performance (Mather, 1993; Townsend, Ryan & Law, 1990). Mathiowetz (1993) suggested that a deficit in role performance results in handicap (ICIDH definition); a deficit in occupational performance (e.g., the inability to dress) results in a disability; and a deficit in performance components (e.g., a loss in sensation) results in an impairment. Table 5-1 compares the ICIDH framework with commonly used occupational therapy terms.

The ICIDH has been integrated with the definition of functional independence proposed by Granger (1984) to provide a conceptual foundation for the measurement of functional abil-

TABLE 5-1

World Health Organization, *International Classification of Impairments, Disability and Handicap* as Compared to Occupation

Classification	Definition	Assessment Level
Impairment	Any loss or abnormality of psychological, physiological, or anatomical structure or function.	Performance Components
Disability	Any restriction or lack (resulting from impairment) of ability to perform an activity in the manner or within the range considered normal for a human being.	Occupational Performance
Handicap	A disadvantage for a given individual, resulting from an impairment or a disability, that limits or prevents the fulfillment of a role that is normal (depending on age, sex, and social and cultural factors) for that individual.	Role Performance

Adapted from Mathiowetz, V. (1993). Role of physical performance component evaluations in occupational therapy functional assessment. *American Journal of Occupational Therapy, 47*, 225-230, p. 227.

TABLE 5-2

Comparison of World Health Organization Model with Levels of Functional Assessment

	ORGAN LEVEL Pathology	PERSON LEVEL Behavioral	SOCIETAL LEVEL Role Assigment
Conditions	Anatomical, Physiological, Mental and Psychological Deficits determine ↓	Performance deficits within the Physical and Social Environments contribute to ↓	Environmental and Social Deficits Influenced by Social Norms and Social Policy create ↓
Key Terms	**Impairment** (Organic dysfunction)	**Disability** (Difficulty with Tasks)	**Handicap** (Social Disadvantages)
	Limitations in using Skills, Performing Activities, and Fulfilling Social Roles		
Analysis	Selected Diagnostic Descriptors	Selected Performance (Behavioral) Descriptors	Selected Role Descriptors
	Functional Assessment of Abilities and Activities		
Interventions	Medical and Restorative Therapy	Adaptive Equipment and Reduction of Physical and Attitudinal Barriers	Supportive Services and Social Policy Changes
	All Needing Long-range Coordination to Improve and Maintain Functioning		

From Granger, C. V. (1984). A conceptual model for functional assessment. In C. V. Granger & G. E. Gresham (Eds.), *Functional assessment in rehabilitation medicine* (pp. 14-25). Baltimore, MD: Williams and Wilkins.

ities. An adapted version of the conceptual framework for the measurement of functional abilities appears in Table 5-2.

This conceptual framework includes three levels: organ, person, and societal. The scheme provides a broad perspective regarding functional assessment that is consistent with the ICIDH model.

Measurement at the *organ* level focuses on anatomical, physiological, mental and psychological impairments. These impairments are evaluated using tests that examine strength, sensation, and range of motion, or psychological characteristics such as perception, memory and cognitive abilities.

At the *person* level, the focus is on performance deficits that are commonly referred to as activities of daily living (ADL). ADL include those skills that enable the person to interact independently with the physical and social environment. These skills include basic daily living skills such as dressing, eating, self-care and personal mobility. An extension of these activities is sometimes referred to as instrumental activities of daily living (IADL). IADL extend beyond basic self-care to include leisure, recreational and vocational activities. Specific skills such as shopping, managing money, and coordinating personal travel are examples of typical IADL skills. Many traditional functional assessment instruments focus on the measurement of individual performance at the person (disability) level.

The final stage in the conceptual model proposed by Granger (1984) is the *societal* level. Measurement at the societal level emphasizes the assessment of handicap. Measurement of handicap is complex and involves the evaluation of restrictions in the person's ability to fulfill meaningful social roles such as spouse, mother, father, worker, or student. The measurement of handicap requires the evaluation of complicated social and environmental interactions. Assessment at this level is broadly based and includes not only characteristics of the person, but the family, service providers, home environment, work setting, and leisure interests. Evaluation of social policy issues and practices is also part of the process of assessing handicap. Assessments at this level are often referred to as measuring "quality of life" and include the interaction of social roles, life satisfaction, health status, and personal independence.

The importance of clearly defining a conceptual framework for assessment of occupational performance is becoming increasingly important as the pressures for accountability and evidence for clinical effectiveness escalate. Health care reforms, including the introduction of managed care and prospective payment, have dramatically increased the demands for clinical accountability and patient-centered outcomes (DeJong & Sutton, 1995). In discussing the importance of patient centered outcomes in rehabilitation, Cope and Sundance (1995) recently observed that "outcome oriented rehabilitation fundamentally includes the identification of appropriate clinical outcomes to determine if they have been achieved" (p. 43). The identification of appropriate outcomes requires the development of a clear conceptual model to ensure that what is assessed is relevant when converted to a therapy outcome and examined by consumers, other professionals, and third party payors. In the past, therapists commonly evaluated performance at the level of impairment. For example, the muscle strength, range of motion, and sensation of a person with spinal cord injury were carefully examined at admission and discharge from rehabilitation. The outcomes that were desired and valued by the consumer, the client's family, and the payor, such as discharge to the home, the ability to complete self-care independently, and return to productive employment or familiar leisure and recreational pursuits, usually were not examined

or assigned a high priority in the therapeutic process. These outcomes occur at the disability (the person) and handicap (societal) levels of the ICIDH model (see Table 5-2). Thus, a discrepancy often existed between what was assessed by the therapist (impairment) and what was expected by the client, i.e., outcomes at the disability and handicap level.

Therapists assessing at the impairment level often assumed that a direct (linear) relationship existed between the ability to accomplish tasks at the organ/physiological (impairment) stage and the development of skills at the person (disability) or societal (handicap) level (see Table 5-2). For example, an occupational therapist examining range of motion and sensory perception in a person with hemiparesis from a stroke assumed that by evaluating this level of impairment, he or she could predict future ability to achieve skills at the person level, e.g., dressing. Current empirical evidence does not support this assumption. A comprehensive review of the literature on stroke rehabilitation revealed that gains in organ/physiological (impairment) skills are small, and did not automatically result in improved functional performance (Wagenaar & Meijer, 1991a; 1991b). Trombly (1995) recently reported the results of several studies in which correlations between motor impairment and ADL were aggregated. The findings indicated that the amount of variance in ADL accounted for by motor impairment was 31%. The majority, approximately 69%, of the variance associated with ADL performance was derived from other factors.

Clinical outcomes that are valued and desired by consumers, families, and payors will occur primarily at the person (disability) and societal (handicap) level. A clear conceptual framework can help guide assessment so that there is a direct and logical connection between what is assessed by therapists and what is expected as an outcome by consumers and their families. The conceptual framework developed by Granger (1984) and based on the ICIDH provides a logical way to integrate assessment, measurement, and functional performance with disablement. This framework will be used in the remainder of the chapter to examine aspects of the assessment process with an emphasis on functional/occupational performance assessment.

BASIC COMPONENTS OF ASSESSING OCCUPATIONAL PERFORMANCE

The assessment process in clinical environments involves four steps. These include: 1) identifying a concept or characteristic to be evaluated; 2) specifying an indicator of the concept or characteristic; 3) defining the information (data) necessary for assessment so that results can be quantified or classified; and 4) determining the reliability, validity and sensitivity of the assessment process.

The first step is identifying a concept or characteristic to be measured. A *concept* is a verbal or symbolic representation of the phenomenon in which the researcher (or clinician) is interested. The concept may refer to aspects of the rehabilitation process, the persons being served, therapist-patient interactions, or to ecological and environmental phenomena. Concepts are the building blocks of any language and are essential for professional communication and research. Some concepts are abstract and contain many ideas within them, e.g., quality of life, or community integration. Other concepts are concrete, e.g., degrees of range of motion (ROM) or walking.

The focus of this chapter is on assessments designed to provide information about the concepts associated with functional or occupational performance. As noted earlier, Granger (1984) describes functional independence as the person's ability to perform the tasks necessary to daily living, vocational pursuits, social interactions, leisure activities and related behaviors. A therapist interested in measuring functional performance needs some way to quantify or classify the abstract concept of functional independence. Without the ability to assign a quantity or classification to the abstract concept of functional performance, it is difficult to determine the extent of any functional limitation, how functional ability changes over time, or whether an intervention will be successful in maintaining or improving functional independence. To collect clinically useful assessment information requires that the concept of functional performance be made observable and recordable. Possible indicators of functional performance include an examination of a person's skill in selected ADL such as eating, dressing, grooming, toileting, and personal hygiene. It could also include IADL such as vocational or leisure pursuits. When a definition is made observable, it must include indicators that are used to collect information about the specific activity of daily living, and how the information was obtained, scored, and interpreted. For example, the Functional Independence Measure (FIM[SM]) (Guide, 1993) is one widely used method of defining functional abilities in operational or observable terms (Hamilton, Granger, Sherwin, Zielezny, & Tashman, 1987). The FIM includes 18 items divided into motor and cognitive domains. Each level of scoring (1 through 7) is defined, for example, 7 = complete independence, 3 = moderate assistance, and 1 = total assistance. The FIM score represents a measure of overall performance in daily living skills and provides a concrete indication of functional ability. Use of the FIM is one way to provide an operational definition for the concept of functional independence. There are many other possible operational definitions of functional or occupational performance. These operational definitions are reflected in the instruments discussed in later sections of this chapter. Different operational definitions focus on different aspects of complex conceptual variables. For example, the Barthel Index (Mahoney &

Barthel, 1965) is also a widely used instrument to examine activities of daily living. In many ways it is similar to the FIM. The Barthel Index, however, does not assess function in the areas of communication and cognition. Therefore, it provides an operational definition of functional performance that is different than the one provided by the FIM. Operational definitions are not inherently right or wrong; they render different orientations and perspectives on concepts that are difficult to define. Operational definitions make concepts observable and recordable. They also facilitate communication, replication, comparison, and the ability to accumulate a scientific knowledge base. It is important to remember that multiple operational definitions are necessary to define a complex concept like occupational performance.

The utility of an operational definition is reflected in the reliability, validity and sensitivity of the information obtained. Imprecise definitions (instruments) that cannot be used consistently (poor reliability) or that are not related to the concept being examined (poor validity and sensitivity) are useless, and contribute to confusion in clinical decision making. Estimates of reliability, validity, and sensitivity indicate whether or not there is a shared understanding of the concept. The ability to develop reliable, valid, and sensitive measures of occupational/functional performance is a high priority for occupational therapy researchers and clinicians. The remainder of this chapter examines issues associated with achieving this goal.

LEVELS OF MEASUREMENT AND VARIABLES

A *variable* is a measurable aspect of a concept (for example, dressing as a dimension of functional independence). A variable is translated into a measurable commodity by means of a definition that provides information at one of four basic levels of measurement. These levels of measurement are nominal, ordinal, interval, or ratio. The four levels are referred to as *scales of measurement* and form a continuum based on different types of information. Table 5-3 summarizes the properties and provides examples for each level of measurement.

The simplest level of measurement is that of *classification*, the nominal scale. This level contains two or more categories that are mutually exclusive and exhaustive. For example, a person may be classified as right-handed, left-handed or ambidextrous (mixed). *Mutually exclusive* means that the person can be assigned to only one category. *Exhaustive* refers to inclusiveness of the possible range of responses, i.e., everyone must fit into one of the three categories: right-handed, left-handed, or ambidextrous.

Ordinal measurement scales contain the properties of

TABLE 5-3
Levels of Measurement Commonly Found in Rehabilitation Investigations

Level of Measurement	Properties	Examples
Nominal	Classification in categories	Male; Female. left-handed; right handed. Republican; Democrat.
Ordinal	Order or ranking among categories	Social class. Degree of burns (1st, 2nd, 3rd degree).
Interval	Equal distance between points or numbers but no absolute zero	Temperature in degrees Fahrenheit. Calendar time.
Ratio	Equal distance between points or categories and the existence of an absolute zero	Degrees of range of motion. Cost for 1 hour of therapy.

nominal scales plus the additional characteristic that the scores can be rank ordered. For example, a therapist might examine a person with post-polio syndrome and rate the muscle strength in a lower extremity muscle group as trace, poor, fair, good, or normal. These five categories may be assigned numbers, with trace = 0 and normal = 4. The assignment of numbers to these ordered categories, however, does not designate equal distances between each category. That is, the difference between 1 and 2 is not necessarily the same as the distance between 3 and 4. Other symbols (a, b, c, or I, II, III, etc.,) can be used to convey the order of the classification and indicate what some researchers and clinicians regard as qualitative information.

Interval measurement scales include the properties of ordinal scales plus that of distance, i.e., equal distance between adjacent categories. In assessing a client with a spinal cord injury, a therapist may be interested in the number of social contacts the person has had outside the home over the period of a week. The number of social contacts is an interval-level variable (assuming, of course, that a consistent method of recording frequency of social contacts over time is used). Ratio measurement scales contain the properties of interval scales plus that of a natural origin, i.e., a fixed or absolute zero point. Calendars, for instance, have arbitrary origins. The point at which you start recording events is arbitrary. There is no absolute zero point where time does not exist. Thus, the variable of social contacts described previously is associated with an arbitrary zero point and does not have a natural origin (absolute zero).

The distinction between interval and ratio scales is a relatively minor one for practical purposes. Values from interval and ratio scales can be added and averaged. Values from nominal and ordinal scales do not have arithmetic properties; in

other words, they cannot be added, subtracted, multiplied, or divided. Controversy has developed recently regarding the appropriate methods to analyze ordinal level information collected in occupational performance assessments (Merbitz, Morris & Grip, 1989). Many of the most popular methods of evaluating functional capabilities use data that are ordinal in nature. For example, the items on the FIM rate a person's performance using an ordinal scale that ranges from complete dependence (assigned a score of 1) to complete independence (assigned a score of 7). One version of the Barthel Index discussed earlier also uses a four level ordinal scale (Granger, Hamilton, Gresham, & Kramer, 1989). The numeric values from these ordinal scales are frequently averaged and comparisons made using a variety of statistical procedures. Merbitz, Morris, and Grip (1989) have argued that functional assessment instruments based on ordinal level information produce scores that are easily misinterpreted and often misapplied in rehabilitation settings. Other authorities have argued that the nominal, ordinal, interval, and ratio classification system is inherently flawed and that decisions regarding how data should be analyzed must be based on the nature of the research question and not the level of data (Anderson, 1961). For example, Velleman and Wilkinson (1993) suggest that scale types (nominal, ordinal, interval, and ratio) are not attributes of the data, but rather depend upon the research questions the data are intended to address. They provide several examples demonstrating that scale type can change as a result of data transformation, or the scale can change as a function of the question the researchers choose to ask.

The issue of whether ordinal data collected in a structured manner can be used to make statistical inferences is complex. One approach adopted by several investigators in rehabilitation and occupational therapy has been to transform ordinal data using methods of Rasch analysis (Fisher, 1993; Wright & Linacre, 1989). Rasch analysis assumes that the consequence of any encounter between a person and a test item is governed by the difference between the ability of the respondent and the difficulty of the item on a latent trait dimension. A latent trait dimension is the abstract continuum associated with a construct (e.g., strength). Ability scores for persons are computed by transforming raw scores (total number of items completed correctly) to the natural logarithmic latent trait scale used to measure item difficulty. The Rasch model produces measures on a logit scale. The logit unit of measurement is the natural log of the odds of a correct response. The process of Rasch scaling transforms raw score data from items and persons into log units. This transformation allows the researcher to interpret the person and item information using the same units of measure. Once the scores for the persons and items have been transformed using Rasch scaling, other information about the persons and items can be obtained using a variety of statistical methods. The Assessment of Motor and Process Skills (AMPS) is one instrument developed by an occupational therapist to assess functional abilities based on the Rasch model (Fisher, 1993). The AMPS is described in a subsequent section of this chapter.

Rasch analysis and interpretations have also been reported for the Functional Independence Measure (Heinemann, Linacre, Wright, Hamilton, & Granger, 1993) and the Patient Evaluation and Conference System (PECS) (Silverstein, Fisher, Kilgore, Harley, Harvey & Harvey, 1992).

RELIABILITY IN OCCUPATIONAL PERFORMANCE ASSESSMENT

Reliability is a key component of the assessment process. Portney and Watkins (1993) state that "reliability is fundamental to all aspects of clinical research, because without it we cannot have confidence in the data we collect, nor can we draw rational conclusions from those data" (p. 53). Reliability refers to the extent to which there is consistency in responses on repeated applications of the measurement instrument. Repeated applications may be obtained over time (test-retest reliability), or by different raters (interrater reliability). Johnston et al. (1992) identify three types of reliability commonly encountered in clinical research: *interrater reliability* (agreement), *test-retest reliability* (also referred to as stability) and *internal consistency*.

Interrater Reliability

Interrater reliability refers to the extent to which two or more independent observers of the same phenomenon agree in their observations. For example, newborn infants are rou-

tinely evaluated to assess their physical activity, muscle tone, color and reflex responses immediately after birth. This rating is referred to as the Apgar score. The interrater reliability of the method used to obtain an Apgar score could be determined by having two raters independently score a group of infants using the Apgar criteria. The interrater reliability (agreement) would be obtained by computing the appropriate reliability statistic using the scores for both raters.

Test-Retest Reliability

The second type of reliability, test-retest, provides the researcher or clinician with information on the consistency of scores over time. Hand held pinch gauges are frequently used by therapists to measure finger pinch strength at pre- and post-intervention for persons with hand dysfunction receiving occupational therapy. The scores from two (or more) administrations can be analyzed to determine consistency (stability) over a specific period of time. An important issue in establishing test-retest reliability is the time between testing. The duration between first and second administration of the test will depend on the nature of the variable being assessed. In the finger pinch example, it would be reasonable to assume that pinch strength should not change over a period of 1 to 2 days and would be an appropriate retest interval.

Information on test-retest reliability (stability) is particularly important in investigations where the purpose is to analyze change over time. If there is a change in performance from the beginning of intervention to the end of treatment, we would like to believe that the change reflects a true improvement in ability and is not the result of measurement error. If the test-retest reliability for the instrument is high, then the probability that change in performance was due to measurement error will be small. This situation, of course, does not ensure that the change was due to treatment, but a reliable instrument can reduce the possibility that improvement was due to measurement error.

Internal Consistency

The final type of reliability discussed in the Measurement Standards for Interdisciplinary Medical Rehabilitation (Johnston et al., 1992) is internal consistency. Internal consistency refers to the degree to which items in an assessment instrument are related to each other. High internal consistency means that the items are closely related and presumably measuring the same construct. For example, an assessment of ADL might include 10 items assessing dressing, 10 items examining feeding, and 10 items evaluating ability to communicate. A test for internal consistency would examine the correlation among all individual items and the correlation among individual items and subgroups of items. The results should indicate that the 10 dressing items are more closely

---

TABLE 5-4

Illustration of Reliability and Agreement Using Sample Set of Data for Two Raters (Interrater).

The data reflect good reliability (co-variation), but poor agreement (consensus).

Subject	Scores for Rater 1	Scores for Rater 2
1	10	100
2	20	200
3	30	300
4	40	400
5	50	500
6	60	600
7	70	700
8	80	800
9	90	900
10	100	1000
Mean (SD)	**50 (10)**	**500 (100)**

Pearson Product Moment Correlation (*r*) = 1.00

---

related to each other than they are to the items evaluating communication. Specialized test statistics are available to provide a quantitative index of the internal consistency of items and subsets of items. Measures of internal consistency are often important in determining if the test is measuring the appropriate construct (concept) or if individual items should be revised or eliminated.

The term *reliability* is frequently used interchangeably with *agreement*. There are technical differences between these two terms that are important for the clinician to understand. Reliability indicates the degree of association or co-variation between two variables. Measures of reliability will be high if there is relative or proportional agreement between two variables. Agreement, in contrast, is a term that refers to the extent to which measurement procedures yield the same results across individuals or over time. Agreement requires that the values between two variables (raters or time) be the same. The data presented in Table 5-4 illustrate the distinction between reliability and agreement. Table 5-4 includes data for two raters. The scores for these two raters are not the same, but the relative ordering (co-variation) does not change across the raters. That is, the performance rated highest by rater one is also rated highest by the second rater, and the performance rated lowest by rater one is also rated lowest by rater two. There is no exact agreement between the two sets of scores, however, if we compute a Pearson product moment correla-

tion coefficient (*r*), we find that the *r* value is 1.00, indicating perfect reliability across the two raters. The Pearson *r* value is high because there is excellent co-variation across the two raters even though the exact agreement is poor. Several investigators have argued against the continued use of statistical procedures such as the Pearson product moment correlation (*r*) to examine reliability (Dunn, 1989; Ottenbacher & Tomcheck, 1993). Other methods, including the intraclass correlation approach, are becoming the preferred approach for determining reliability and agreement in clinical research (Shrout & Fleiss, 1979). Students, clinicians and researchers should be cautious in interpreting the results of reliability studies, particularly those using statistics (e.g., Pearson *r*) that examine covariation, but not agreement among scores.

VALIDITY IN OCCUPATIONAL PERFORMANCE ASSESSMENT

Validity is the degree of correspondence between the concept or characteristic being measured and the way in which it is represented in the natural environment. An instrument is valid when the test measures what it is intended to measure. Validity implies accuracy as well as relevance of response. The more concrete the concept being examined, the easier it is to obtain valid responses because the correspondence between the concept or characteristic and the way it is represented is usually clear. For example, collecting information on the age or height of clients can be easily verified by comparing the information with an official document or medical record. In contrast, a concept such as "community integration" is more abstract and, therefore, more difficult to verify. Definitions of community integration may contain large differences. These differences reflect the fact that what constitutes community integration is not consistently or uniformly agreed upon by researchers or clinicians.

Validity can be divided into two different forms: content validity and empirical validity. Content validity reflects the validity of the items and subscales of an instrument to accurately portray the concept. The content of the instrument should relate logically to the concept, that is, items should be relevant and represent all possible areas associated with the concept. For instance, a valid functional assessment instrument will include items that examine all areas of activities of daily living and the items will range from easy to difficult. A functional assessment instrument that does not include any items evaluating dressing ability would have poor content validity.

Empirical validity is the second broad component of validity. Empirical validity refers to the verification of predictions based on measurement of the concept. Empirical validity is often divided into concurrent validity, predictive validity, and construct validity. Some authors combine concurrent and predictive validity and refer to these two as crite-rion oriented validity (Johnston et al., 1992).

Concurrent Validity

A therapist measuring pain in a person with rheumatoid arthritis using an ordinal scale (mild, moderate, or severe pain), may compare the results with information concerning the amount of pain medication consumed over a specific period. The correlation derived from comparing the values obtained using the ordinal level scale with the amount of pain medica-tion taken provides a quantitative index of concurrent validity.

Predictive Validity

Predictive validity is verification of a relationship between the variable and an external criterion in the future. If children who score poorly on the Miller Assessment for Preschoolers (MAP) (Miller, 1986) when they are 2 years old are later found to have difficulty in school, as indicated by poor grades and below average teacher performance reports, then support is provided for the predictive validity of the MAP. A quantitative index of predictive validity is frequent-ly obtained by computing correlation coefficients between two sets of scores separated by the required time interval.

Construct Validity

Construct validity is the degree to which an instrument measures the theoretical construct (concept) it was designed to measure. Construct validity assumes that the concepts of interest are embedded in theory. Establishing construct valid-ity involves piecing together a network of relationships. As a simple example, a theory of quality of life may lead to the hypothesis that a positive relationship exists between quality of life and functional ability. That is, the better the quality of life, the more likely a person is to have a high level of func-tional independence. The verification of the hypothesis would add to the validity of the variable measuring the con-cept: quality of life. The process of establishing construct validity is complex because there are a large number of the-oretical predictions associated with most constructs, and it may be impossible to verify all of them for a particular vari-able. The development of construct validity is a continuous process and often requires numerous studies examining vari-ous theoretical predications.

ASSESSMENT SENSITIVITY

One indicator of sensitivity is the number of values that can be reliably discriminated for a given trait or characteris-tic. In a nominal scale, the reliable discrimination of three categories is more sensitive than the reliable discrimination

of two categories. For a variable such as depression, the cat-egories of none, mild, moderate, and severe provide more information than the categories of depressed versus not depressed. Generally, ordinal scales are more sensitive than nominal scales, if they are reliable, because ordinal scales are able to discriminate rankings of importance among cate-gories as well as the categories themselves. The key compo-nents of sensitivity are reliable discrimination and the num-ber of categories or values for a variable. A rating scale for quality of life with 10 levels (or values) is not more sensitive than a rating scale with three levels, unless there is evidence that the person can reliably discriminate among the 10 levels. The notion of sensitivity is especially important when thera-pists are measuring change in performance over time. If the variable is not sufficiently sensitive, it may not register any change when, in fact, real change has occurred.

TYPES OF ASSESSMENT

There are several classes of occupational performance assessment. Common ways to categorize occupational perfor-mance assessments include norm referenced versus criterion reference, standardized versus informal, quantitative versus qualitative, and performance-based versus self-assessments. These classification schemes are briefly discussed below.

Opacich (1991) observed that occupational therapists have long been familiar with informal assessment mecha-nisms. These are usually "home grown" or intuitive methods of delineating problems. Although these methods may be inherently valuable, the items and methods of administration and interpretation are generally not clearly defined. The analysis and interpretation of data yielded by these methods tends to be idiosyncratic or, at least, highly contingent upon the theoretical understanding and clinical experience of the practitioner using the informal method.

Standardizing assessment strategies or instruments entails defining what is to be examined, how it will be exam-ined, the manner in which data will be communicated, and how the information will be applied in clinical problem solv-ing. Formal standardized assessments represent a therapeutic advancement in terms of developing a common understand-ing of what is assessed. One advantage of standardized tests is that they lend themselves to critical analysis and duplica-tion. Standardized assessments describe performance in quantifiable terms, and they provide normative (or criterion-referenced) data as a standard of comparison. Statistical coefficients regarding validity and reliability of the instru-ment are provided to guide clinical decisions. Although stan-dardization does not ensure the high quality of an instrument, it does improve the ability to communicate results and com-pare findings across different examiners, settings and clients.

Two extensively standardized instruments authored by occupational therapists are the Miller Assessment for Preschoolers (MAP) (Miller, 1986) and the Sensory Integration and Praxis Tests (SIPT) (Ayres, 1989).

Norm-referenced tests imply that an individual's performance will be compared and/or ranked relative to a broad typical sample to which the test has previously been administered (the normative sample). Normative data are expressed numerically, so the interpretation of norm-referenced tests requires quantitative analysis using tables and graphs representing usual or "normal" performance. These comparisons are generally made using standardized scores that are interpreted in relation to a distribution of scores derived from the normative sample. In contrast, criterion-referenced tests employ descriptive standards by which to measure performance. Rather than comparing individual performance to a sample group, performance is judged in terms of a desired outcome. Since few norm-referenced tests address behaviors and characteristics of unique concern to occupational therapists, use of criterion-referenced tests in clinical practice is common. Criterion referencing is particularly useful when the therapist is evaluating performance competency or mastery. For instance, if an established performance criterion states that "functional dressing" is defined as successfully putting on a shirt, pants, shoes and socks and appropriately closing all fasteners in a period of fifteen minutes, then the client is measured against this criterion.

The distinction between performance-based assessments and self-assessments is particularly relevant for examining functional abilities (Guccione, 1991). Performance based assessments rely on the observations of client behaviors, usually by therapists or other professionals. The client is observed during the performance of an activity and the ability to accomplish the task is rated by the observer. Self-assessments are completed by the client or by a trained interviewer who solicits verbal information regarding the ability to perform certain activities.

During the administration of performance-based assessments, each activity is presented to the client and he or she is requested to complete the task. Generally the client is provided only verbal instruction to complete the task. In contrast, self-assessment solicits the information directly from the client. The success of self-assessments relies heavily on providing clearly worded questions and concise directions for completing the questions. Motivation to complete the questions is often an issue in developing, administering and completing self-assessments.

In administering and interpreting both performance based and self-assessments it is important to distinguish between questions that reflect a person's ordinary or habitual performance (for instance, "Do you do all of your own food shopping?"), and those that identify a person's perceived capacity to accomplish a task ("If you had to, could you do all of your own shopping for food?"). Understanding the difference between what a person actually does on a daily or routine basis and what he or she is potentially capable of doing is an essential element in developing functional goals and in determining the amount of assistance needed by the person. An individual with a spinal cord injury may have the capacity to prepare all of his or her meals. If, however, he or she never cooks and always relies on others to prepare meals, then this has obvious implications concerning the need for support resources and assistance.

OCCUPATIONAL PERFORMANCE/FUNCTIONAL ASSESSMENT INSTRUMENTS

The analysis of occupational performance focuses on the measurement and classification of functional activities and the individual's ability to successfully engage in these activities. The essence of occupational performance assessment is the measurement of how a person does certain tasks or fulfills roles in various dimensions of living. In a recent article titled "Functional Assessment and its Place in Health Care," Ikegami (1995) identified four uses of functional assessment: First, functional assessment information can be used as an indicator of patient outcomes; second, functional assessment can be used to provide baseline data in planning intervention; third, functional assessment information can be used to help determine payment for services; and, fourth, the results of functional assessment may be used for prediction to help drive programs aimed toward prevention. The specific instruments presented below were selected because they can be used to achieve the purposes identified by Ikegami (1995).

FUNCTIONAL ASSESSMENT INSTRUMENTS FOR ADULTS — COMPREHENSIVE

Five main domains relevant to occupational performance assessment are frequently used to evaluate the clinical usefulness of functional assessment instruments. These five domains are: mobility, communication, self-care, occupation, and social relations, and they correspond to the first five handicap codes of the ICIDH (WHO, 1980).

In the past decade, a large number of health measurement instruments designed to evaluate functional abilities have been developed. In a review, Feinstein, Josephy, and Wells (1986) identified more than 40 distinct ADL and functional assessment instruments. Fifteen of the most widely used instruments are briefly summarized in Table 5-5. In developing this list, the following criteria were used to select instruments for inclusion: 1) comprehensiveness with regard to the five ICIDH domains referred to previously; 2) use of interval or ordinal level scales; 3) ease and flexibility of administration (performance-based and self-assessment); 4) influence of assistive devices and aids; and 5) published information on reliability, validity and sensitivity.

More detailed information on selected instruments associated with the assessment of disability is presented below. The instruments discussed in the remainder of this chapter were chosen based on their widespread use or particular relevance to occupational therapy practice.

Functional Independence Measure (FIM)

The FIM is one of the most widely used methods of assessing functional status in persons with a disability (Guide, 1993). In discussing the measurement of functional status in rehabilitation, Johnston and colleagues noted that "the FIM is currently the most widely used measure of disability, being used in several hundred medical rehabilitation hospitals" (Johnston, Findley, DeLuca, & Katz, 1991, p. S115). Along similar lines, Grey and Kennedy (1993) observed that "in recent years the Functional Independence Measure has emerged as a standard assessment instrument for use in rehabilitation and therapy programs for disabled persons" (p. 458) A study of facilities in the United States specializing in care for patients with spinal cord injury/disease substantiated this claim. Seventy-two percent of the facilities surveyed reported using the FIM (Watson, Kanny, White & Anson, 1995). The FIM instrument was developed by a national task force co-sponsored by the American Academy of Physical Medicine and Rehabilitation and the American Congress of Rehabilitation Medicine (Guide, 1993; Hamilton et al., 1987). The original work of this task force was expanded by grants from the National Institute on Disability and Rehabilitation Research to the Department of Rehabilitation Medicine at the State University of New York at Buffalo. The FIM instrument is now part of the Uniform Data System for Medical Rehabilitation (UDSMR) and is widely used in the United States and internationally. There are currently more than 700 subscribers to the UDSMR data management service. Approximately 500 of these facilities are fully credentialed in the data collection process (Guide, 1993). Credentialing is achieved by meeting predefined quality control standards. These standards are described below.

The FIM is a minimal data set designed to assess functional independence. The FIM includes 18 items, each with a maximum score of 7 and a minimum score of 1. Total possible FIM scores range from 18 to 126. Each level of scoring is defined. For example, a score of 7 equals "complete independence," a score of 1 equals "complete dependence," and 3

equals "moderate assistance." The areas examined by the FIM include: self-care, sphincter control, transfers, locomotion, communication, and social cognition. These areas are further divided into motor and cognitive domains (Granger, Hamilton, Linacre, Heinemann & Wright, 1993). The motor domain includes the items in the areas of self-care, sphincter control, transfers, and locomotion subscales. The cognitive domain includes items from the subscales of communication and social cognition. The domains, subscales and items included in the FIM are presented in Table 5-6.

The FIM is intended to serve as a basic indicator of the severity of disability. It is designed to measure what the patient actually does, rather than what he or she is capable of doing. The underlying rationale for rating items on the scale relates to the amount of assistance needed by the person to complete the activities being measured. This permits the FIM to provide data that reflect both the social as well as economic costs of disability. Those facilities using the FIM and subscribing to the Uniform Data System for Medical Rehabilitation follow a protocol in administering the FIM and subsequent submission of the data to the UDSMR. Following the UDSMR protocol, the FIM is administered to persons receiving inpatient medical rehabilitation within 72 hours of admission and discharge, and 80 - 180 days post discharge. The FIM was designed primarily for inpatient acute rehabilitation populations and follow-up, but may also be appropriate for subacute rehabilitation and some home health programs. Many facilities have added items to the FIM for their own programs, but these items are not included in the UDSMR data set. The UDSMR is currently aggregating approximately 200,000 records annually, and there are more than 1 million records in the UDSMR database.

The UDSMR has developed a two-phase credentialing process to ensure maximum reliability of FIM ratings, and accurate and complete submission of facility data (Guide, 1993). Phase I involves the training and credentialing of all clinical staff in the use of the FIM (interrater reliability). Phase II involves a technical review of 6 months of facility data for errors or incomplete records, coding inconsistencies, and significant variations (> 2 SD) from the profile of other providers. The UDSMR provides regional training seminars on the FIM in collaboration with the American Rehabilitation Association. The interrater reliability of fully credentialed subscriber facilities is reported as ICC = 0.96 for total FIM scores with Kappa values from 0.66 to 0.83 for individual items. Detailed information regarding previous reliability studies is reported below. Investigations using Rasch analysis have examined the scaling properties, precision, unidimensionality, weighting and fit of the FIM items in two domains: Motor and Cognitive (Granger et al., 1993).

Several studies have been conducted to examine the reliability and validity of the FIM. In a recent publication, Hamilton, Laughlin, Fiedler, and Granger (1994) examined

TABLE 5-5

Comparison of Commonly Used Functional Assessment Instruments

(Using selected categories from the *International Classification of Impairment, Disability and Handicap.*)

Name*	Communication	Mobility	Self-care	Occupation	Social Relations
PECS	Comprehension Expression	Transfer Ambulation Environ. barriers	Feeding Grooming Dressing Continence	Home manage. Work Sports Recreation	Family
SIP	Communication	Walking Ambulation Transfer	Eating Body care	Home manage. Work Recreation Pastimes	Social interaction
FSRS	Comprehension Expression	Transfer Ambulation Stairs Environ. Surfaces Wheelchair Community mobility	Eating Grooming Dressing Bathing Continence		Family Social contacts
RDRS	Expression Hearing Sight	Walking Traversing outside	Eating Grooming Dressing Toileting Bathing Continence	Shopping	
LORS-3	Comprehension Expression	Wheelchair manage. Ambulation	Feeding Grooming Bathing Toileting Dressing		
FIM	Comprehension Expression	Transfer Walking Stairs Wheelchair	Feeding Grooming Dressing Bathing Toileting Continence		Social Interaction
Barthel	Transfer Walking Level	Feeding Grooming Dressing Washing Continence			
Katz	Transfer	Feeding Dressing Bathing Toileting Continence			

TABLE 5-5 (continued)

Comparison of Commonly Used Functional Assessment Instruments

Name*	Communication	Mobility	Self-care	Occupation	Social Relations
FSI		Transfer Walking inside Stairs Driving	Dressing Washing	Home manage. Work	Family Attending Meetings
FASQ		Sitting Standing Climbing ladders Driving Public transport.	Grooming Dressing	Home manage. Leisure	
FSQ		Walking inside/outside	Eating Dressing Bathing	Home manage. Work Recreation	Friends

* PECS = Patient Evaluation Conference System
SIP = Sickness Impact Profile
FSRS = Functional Status Rating System
RDRS = Rapid Disability Rating System
LORS-3 = Level of Rehabilitation Scale-3
FIM = Functional Independence Measure
FSI = Functional Status Index
FASQ = Functional Assessment Status Questionnaire
FSQ = Functional Status Questionnaire

interrater reliability by having two or more pairs of clinicians assess 863 patients undergoing inpatient medical rehabilitation at 74 UDSMR subscribing facilities. The ICC value for total FIM scores was 0.96. The ICC values for subscale scores ranged from 0.88 to 0.93. Ottenbacher, Mann, Granger, Tomita, Hurren and Charvat (1995) recently reported similar ICC values for interrater and test-retest reliability of the FIM for a sample of community-based elderly persons with disabilities.

The sensitivity of the FIM has also been examined. Dahmer, Shilling, Hamilton, Bonthe, Englander, Kerutzer, Ragnarsson, and Rosenthal (1993) examined 309 people with traumatic brain injury (TBI) admitted to five TBI Model System hospitals in the United States. The admission FIM average score was 59 with a 95% confidence interval of ± 3.2. The discharge FIM average score was 100 with a 95% confidence interval of ± 2.8. The results of this and other investigations (see following) indicate that the FIM is sensitive to change in functional skills that occur during rehabilitation.

In 1989, Merbitz, Morris, and Grip published a paper critical of many existing ADL assessments because they were based on ordinal level scales and the resulting data were frequently manipulated using parametric statistical techniques. Merbitz et al. (1989) argued that this practice results in mis-inferences regarding functional performance. Wright and Linacre (1989) proposed a Rasch transformation of ordinal (ranked) functional status scores into a linear scale so that mathematical operations could be conducted.

Using Rasch-transformed measures permits statistically valid comparisons of individuals based on aggregate scores. Rasch (latent trait) analysis of FIM data from 14,799 patients receiving rehabilitation revealed that the 13 motor items and 5 cognitive items can be converted into two unidimensional, interval measures: Motor and Cognitive (Heinemann et al., 1993). FIM motor and cognitive logit-transformed (Rasch) measures in a sample of 256 traumatic brain-injured adult persons admitted to rehabilitation at five TBI model systems hospitals correlated significantly with duration of post-traumatic amnesia (construct validity), and the Rancho Los Amigos Level of Cognitive Functioning Scales and the Disability Rating Scale (concurrent validity) (Granger, Divan, & Fiedler, 1995).

TABLE 5-6

Components of the *Functional Independence Measure* (FIM)

FIM (motor)

Self-care
    A. Eating
    B. Grooming
    C. Bathing
    D. Dressing upper body
    E. Dressing lower body
    F. Toileting

Sphincter control
    G. Bladder management
    H. Bowel management

Transfer
    I. Bed, chair, wheelchair
    J. Toilet
    K. Tub, shower

Locomotion
    L. Walk/Wheelchair
    M. Stairs

FIM (cognitive)

Communication
    N. Comprehension
    O. Expression

Social cognition
    P. Social interaction
    Q. Problem solving
    R. Memory

Levels of Scoring

Independence:
    7 - complete independence (timely, safely)
    6 - modified independence (device)

Modified dependence:
    5 - supervision
    4 - minimal assistance (subject 75%+)
    3 - moderate assistance (subject 50%+)

Complete dependence:
    2 - maximal assistance (subject 25%+)
    1 - total assistance (subject 0%+)

In addition, the 13 FIM motor items have been found to be the best predictors of rehabilitation length of stay for nearly all impairment groups (Stineman, 1994).

The Barthel Index

The Barthel Index was published in 1965 (Mahoney & Barthel, 1965) as a weighted scale for measuring basic daily living skills in persons with chronic disability. The original Barthel Index included 10 ADL variables: feeding, transfers, personal grooming and hygiene, bathing, toileting, walking, negotiating stairs, and bowel and bladder control. Each item is scored using a numerically weighted scoring system that assigns values based on degree of independence or need for assistance. The original Barthel Index item scoring weights are presented in Table 5-7. The total score ranges from zero to 100. A Barthel Index of 100 documents sufficient independence in self-care and mobility to eliminate the need for assistance in basic activities of daily living. The Barthel Index scoring system has been modified by several investigators. Granger, Albrecht, and Hamilton (1979), and Granger, Hamilton, Gresham, and Kramer (1989) developed an adapted version of the Barthel consisting of 15 items rated on a four-point scale. This instrument was an early precursor of the FIM. Shah, Vanclay, and Cooper (1989) have also published a modified version of the Barthel Index designed to improve its sensitivity by increasing the number of categories used to record function.

The Barthel Index has been widely used in rehabilitation environments for many years and has been the object of extensive research. Murdock (1992) has provided a comprehensive review and critical examination of the research on the reliability, validity and sensitivity of the Barthel Index. One of the criticisms of the Barthel Index, and other traditional measures of ADL, is the narrow focus on physical self-care abilities (Law, 1993). The popularity of traditional ADL assessments, such as the Barthel Index, is related to their usefulness in the management of nursing care, the assessment of progress in patient recovery and treatment effectiveness in basic ADL skills. More recently, the focus on occupational assessment and functional performance has expanded to include items evaluating psychosocial, cognitive, communication and social skills. The expanded focus is the result of changes in health care delivery, for example, more community and home-based interventions. The independent living movement has also played a role in facilitating the expansion of functional assessment. The independent living movement is a social movement including a constituency of persons with disabilities and other advocates striving to obtain full integration and participation in society for persons with a disability. As the trend toward com-

TABLE 5-7

Components of the *Barthel Index*

Items	With Help	Independent
1. Feeding (if food needs to be cut = help)	5	10
2. Moving from wheelchair to bed and return (includes sitting up in bed)	5-10	15
3. Personal toilet (wash face, comb hair, shave, clean teeth)	0	5
4. Getting on and off the toilet	5	10
5. Bathing self	0	5
6. Walking on level surface (or, if unable to walk, propel wheelchair) * score only if unable to walk	0	5
7. Ascend and descend stairs	5	10
8. Dressing (includes tying shoes, fastening fasteners)	5	10
9. Controlling bowels	5	10
10. Controlling bladder	5	10

A patient scoring 100 BI is continent, feeds himself, dresses himself, gets up out of bed and chairs, bathes himself, walks at least a block, and can ascend and descend stairs. This does not mean that he is able to live alone; he may not be able to cook, keep house, and meet the public, but he is able to get along without attendant care.

From Mahoney, F. I., & Barthel, D. W. (1965). Functional evaluation: The Barthel Index. *Maryland State Medical Journal, 14*, 61-65.

munity-based and client-centered care expands, instruments that are narrowly focused on basic ADL or too specialized in other ways will become less popular.

Patient Evaluation and Conference System (PECS)

The PECS was developed in a clinical setting for the purpose of structuring team conferences (Harvey & Jellinek, 1983). The main aims are recording the patient's progress and defining treatment goals. The PECS is a broad ranging instrument comprising 115 items divided into 16 different disciplinary sections. Each section is completed by the discipline that is primarily responsible for that specific aspect of care. The 16 discipline sections are listed in Table 5-8.

A 7-point ordinal scale is used for most items, with 1 representing "most dependent" and 7 indicating "full independence." The use of aids lowers the score. The 7-point scale makes the instrument sensitive to minor changes in functional level. The PECS has been used to predict the level of care needed after discharge from the hospital (Harvey, Silverstein, Venzon, Kilgore, Fisher, Steiner & Harley, 1992). The clinical validity has also been assessed by determining the relations between the predictive value of a CT scan and the

PECS score (Jellinek, Torkelson & Harvey, 1982). The results revealed a high correlation.

The interrater reliability for different sections of the PECS ranges from ICC = 0.68 to 0.80 (Chaudhuri, Harvey, Sulton, & Lambert, 1988). Silverstein, Kilgore, Fisher, Harley and Harvey (1991) have conducted extensive factor analyses of the structure of the PECS to assess the potential for unidimensional measurement of the construct of disability. A computerized graphic profile has been developed based on this research and is used to display the client's progress and goals using the information in the PECS sections (see Table 5-8). This profile is specifically designed to facilitate team conferences and can be used in research to predict which individuals will be most successful in reaching goals associated with independent function (Harvey & Jellinek, 1983).

ASSESSMENT PROCEDURES DEVELOPED BY OCCUPATIONAL THERAPISTS

The Assessment of Motor and Process Skills (AMPS) is an observational evaluation used to simultaneously examine the ability to perform IADL and the underlying motor and process

TABLE 5-8

Disciplinary Sections Included in the *Patient Evaluation and Conferencing System* (PECS)

Rehabilitation Medicine

Rehabilitation Nursing

Physical Mobility

Activities of Daily Living

Communication

Medication

Nutrition

Assistive Devices

Psychology

Neuropsychology

Social Issues

Vocational-Education Activity

Therapeutic Recreation

Pain

Pulmonary Rehabilitation

Pastoral Care

capacities necessary for successful performance (Fisher, 1994). The AMPS is an assessment system that requires a clinician to observe a person performing IADL as he or she would normally perform them. The person chooses to perform two or three familiar tasks from among more than 50 possibilities described in the AMPS manual. After the observation, the clinician rates the person's performance in two skill areas: IADL motor and IADL process. The motor and process areas are presented in Table 5-9. Motor skills are observable operations or actions that are thought to be related to underlying postural control, mobility, coordination, and strength. The AMPS motor skill items represent an observable taxonomy of actions used to move the body and objects during actual performance. Process skills are the actions used to organize and adapt a series of actions over time in order to complete a specified task. Process skills are thought to be related to a person's underlying attentional, conceptual, organizational, and adaptive capabilities. Like the AMPS motor skill items, the AMPS process skill items represent a universal taxonomy of actions that can be observed during any task performance.

During each IADL task performed for the assessment, and for each of the 16 motor and 20 process skills (see Table 5-9), the person is rated on a four-point scale: 1 = deficit, 2 = ineffective, 3 = questionable, and 4 = competent. The raw ordinal scores are analyzed using the Rasch approach referred to as many-faceted Rasch analysis. The approach is based on a mathematical model of likelihood that the person will receive a given score on each of the motor and process skill items. The observed counts of the raw scores of IADL motor and process skill items constitute ordinal (ranked) data. These counts are converted by logistic transformation into additive, linear measures. Once the raw scores are computer analyzed, the derived person ability measures (motor and process) are the estimates of the person's position on the two AMPS scales (Fisher, 1994). That is, the AMPS motor and process scales represent continua of increasing IADL motor or process skill ability, and the person's estimated position on the AMPS motor and process scales, expressed in logits, represents his or her IADL motor and process skill ability (Fisher, 1993; 1994).

The many-faceted Rasch analysis used in the AMPS allows simultaneous calibration of three aspects of performance: item easiness, task simplicity, and rater leniency. Each of these item characteristics is determined by using a probabilistic model. The ability measure produced by the Rasch analysis is the estimated person ability plotted on a linear scale and is defined by the skill item easiness and task simplicity but adjusted for the rater who scored the task performance (Fisher, 1993; 1994).

Because the person ability measures on the AMPS are adjusted for task simplicity, a clinician can use the ability measure to predict whether a person possesses the motor and process skills necessary to perform tasks that are more difficult than those the person was observed performing. Also, since the AMPS includes a large number of possible IADL tasks (50) and each person is observed performing only two or three, the number of possible alternative task combinations is very large. Regardless of how many different tasks the individual performs, however, the ability measure will always be adjusted to account for the ease and simplicity of those particular tasks, so direct comparisons can be made among persons even though they performed completely different tasks.

Fisher and colleagues have conducted a series of investigations using the AMPS with persons who have psychiatric, orthopedic, neurologic, cognitive and developmental disabilities (Fisher, 1993, 1994; Fisher, Liu, Velozo & Pan, 1992; Nygård, Bernspang, Fisher, & Winbald, 1994; Park, Fisher, & Velozo, 1994). Studies have also been conduced using the AMPS with older adults living in the community (Fisher, 1994). These investigations have established the preliminary reliability and validity of the AMPS. The AMPS is a new instrument and approaches the assessment of occupational performance in a nontraditional manner, that is, using many-faceted Rasch analysis. This approach has advantages for a field such as occupational therapy, but it also has disadvantages. The logic of the Rasch approach is not familiar to many therapists and the mathematical modeling used to develop the scoring system is complex. For these reasons, its

TABLE 5-9

Assessment of Motor and Process Skills (AMPS) Motor and Process Skill Areas

Motor		**Process**	
Stabilizes	Transports	Paces	Sequences
Aligns	Lifts	Attends	Terminates
Positions	Calibrates	Chooses	Searches/Locates
Walks	Grips	Uses	Gathers
Reaches	Endures	Handles	Organizes
Bends	Paces	Heeds	Restores
Coordinates		Inquires	Navigates
Manipulates		Initiates	Notices/Responds
Flows		Continues	Accommodates
Moves		Adjusts	Benefits

From Park, S., Fisher, A. G., & Velozzo, C. A. (1994). Using the Assessment of Motor and Process Skills to compare occupational performance between clinic and home settings. *American Journal of Occupational Therapy, 48*, 699.

widespread use may be impractical. However, the AMPS and other Rasch-based instruments are alternatives to traditional assessment approaches and represent an important new dimension in the evolution of functional assessment.

Canadian Occupational Performance Measurement (COPM)

The COPM is a criterion measure developed in consultation with the Department of National Health and Welfare and the Canadian Association of Occupational Therapists (Law, Baptiste, McColl, Opzoomer, Polatajko, & Pollock, 1990; Pollock, 1993). The COPM reflects a client-centered practice philosophy of measurement and incorporates roles and role expectations within the client's own environment. By client-centered, it is meant that the assessment incorporates roles and role expectations from within the client's living environment using a semi-structured, individualized interview approach.

The COPM encompasses the areas of self-care, productivity and leisure as the primary outcomes being measured, but can also include an assessment of performance components in order to gain an understanding of why the client may be having difficulty in a particular functional area. The COPM was designed to help therapists establish occupational performance goals based on client perceptions of need and to measure change objectively in defined problem areas (Law, Baptiste, McColl, Opzoomer, Polatajko & Pollock, 1990).

The COPM measures the client's identified problem areas in daily functioning. In those instances where a client is unable to identify problem areas (e.g., a young child, an individual

with dementia) a caregiver may respond to the measure. The COPM considers the importance, to the person, of the occupational performance areas as well as the client's satisfaction with present performance. The instrument takes into account client roles and role expectations and, in focusing on the client's own environments and priorities, ensures the relevance of identified areas in the assessment process.

The COPM can be used to measure a client outcome with different objectives for treatment, whether it is developmental, maintenance, restoration of function, or prevention of future disability. Because it is generic (not diagnosis specific) and can be used across different age groups, it is has wide applicability. The instrument is administered in a five step process using a semi-structured interview conducted by the therapist together with the client and/or caregiver. The five steps in the process include: problem identification/definition, initial assessment, occupational therapy intervention, reassessment and calculation of change scores. The original version included a procedure whereby rated importance was used as a weighting factor in calculating performance and satisfaction scores. However, this has been eliminated in the second edition based on findings from pilot studies that indicated the equivalence of scores whether or not importance weights are included.

First, problems are defined jointly with the client and appropriate caregivers. Once the problem areas are defined, the client is asked to rate the importance of each activity on a scale of 1 to 10. The client (or caregiver) is also required to rate his or her ability to perform the specified activities and his or her satisfaction with performance on the same 1 to 10 scale. These scores are then compared across time. There are two scores:

BARBARA

Barbara is a 56-year-old woman who was admitted to hospital because of depression. She lives with her husband and does occasional bookkeeping for a local business. They have two sons who are grown and have their own families. Barbara stated that she couldn't cope and was spending entire days in her room reading and worrying about everything. She avoided leaving the house so identified comfort with going out to shop and doing other activities as important. Barbara also wanted to explore what she could do for leisure as well as go on outings with her husband. Her trips with her husband had become difficult for her because he often shouted at or criticized other drivers.

During her initial assessment, Barbara's occupational therapist provided a description of occupational therapy, followed by a discussion of the three occupational performance areas of self-care, productivity and leisure. During the interview, the therapist probed to identify activities and performance problems in each area, along with potential environmental barriers. This provided the identification of problem statements to be used for assessment of the client's initial and follow-up ratings of performance and satisfaction. Additionally, it provided important guidance on the identification of intervention strategies aimed at performance components. At reassessment, Barbara was very satisfied with her performance on her goals, so occupational therapy was discontinued.

The COPM findings for Barbara were as follows:

COPM Findings

Problems	Importance	Time 1 Perfor.	Satisfaction	Time 2 Perfor.	Satisfaction
1. Ability/comfort to get out to shop/do other activities.	10	3	1	8	8
2. Finding activities to do during my days.	10	2	1	7	8
3. Pursue outings with husband.	10	1	1	7	9

Performance 1 = 6/3 = 2.0   Satisfaction 1 = 3/3 = 1.0
Performance 2 = 22/3 = 7.3   Satisfaction 2 = 25/3 = 8.3

Figure 5-1. Case study illustrating application of COPM. Adapted with permission from a case study by Jo Clarke in Canadian Occupational Performance Measure (2nd ed). Copyright 1995 by Mary Law, Sue Baptiste, Anne Opzoomer, Mary Ann McColl, Helene Polatajko and Nancy Pollock. Published by the Canadian Association of Occupational Therapists, Ottawa, Canada.

one for performance and one for satisfaction. Administration time takes about 30 to 40 minutes on average (see Figure 5-1).

The authors reported findings on an extensive pilot study of the COPM which involved administration of the instrument to 256 clients in many facilities across Canada and in other countries, including New Zealand, Greece and Great Britain (Law, Polatajko, Pollock, McColl, Opzoomer, & Baptiste, 1994). Data gathered during this multi-phase study included feedback from therapists and clients about the clinical utility of the COPM, data on the sensitivity of the instrument to change, and descriptive statistics on identified problems and client scores. The findings indicated that the average change scores for performance and satisfaction were approximately 1.5 times the standard deviation of the scores, indicating sensitivity of the instrument to perceived changes in occupational performance by clients. Comments by therapists involved in

the pilot studies were generally favorable regarding the clinical utility of the measure. Because the assessment involves an interview with clients who are often unaccustomed to participating in the identification of their own problems, some awkwardness with administration has been reported by therapists during their initial attempts at administration. Also, due to its reliance on client participation in the assessment process, it is viewed as unsuitable for use with clients having significant cognitive impairment. The perceived clinical utility of the COPM seems to be related to its flexibility, the use of client-centered approaches in practice, and support by administrators who value the philosophy underlying the instrument (Toomey, Nicholson & Carswell, 1995).

Research continues on the COPM, with particular attention to its validity as a bona fide measure of real changes in occupational performance. Although it is a new instrument, the

COPM has potential to provide useful and important information regarding occupational performance. One unique feature of the COPM is the quantitative emphasis on client satisfaction.

ASSESSMENT OF HANDICAP/QUALITY OF LIFE

Craig Handicap Assessment and Reporting Technique (CHART)

The CHART is one of the first instruments developed to assess handicap in rehabilitation practice as defined in the International Classification of Impairments Disabilities and Handicaps (ICIDH) (World Health Organization, 1980). The dimensions of handicap defined by the WHO were purposely used in constructing the CHART to ensure that it would assess performance at the handicap level and not overlap with instruments designed to examine impairment or disability. The goal of the CHART is to measure deviation from roles generally fulfilled by persons without disability or impairment. The scoring system was developed so that a maximum score of 100 for each dimension of handicap indicates that roles within the dimension have been fulfilled at a level equivalent to that of most persons without a disability.

The CHART includes six dimensions of handicap: 1) orientation, defined as an individual's ability to orient himself to his surroundings; 2) physical independence; 3) mobility; 4) occupation, defined as an individual's ability to occupy time in the manner customary to the person's age, sex, and culture; 5) social interaction; and 6) economic self-sufficiency, defined as an individual's ability to sustain customary socioeconomic activity and independence (Whiteneck, Charlifue, Gerhart, Overholser, & Richardson, 1992). The CHART is composed of 27 simple objective questions developed to assess an individual's activities in the six dimensions of handicap. The domains included in the CHART and sample questions are presented in Table 5-10.

The 27 questions comprising the CHART are administered as a semi-structured interview to the client or to a family member or caregiver familiar with the client. Reliability and validity studies have been conducted using the CHART on samples of persons with spinal cord injury (Whiteneck, Charlifue, Gerhart, Overholser, & Richardson, 1992). Test retest reliability ranged from r = 0.80 to 0.95 for the five dimensions. Subject proxy correlations were adequate for the total CHART score (r = .83), but low for the dimensions of economic self-sufficiency (0.69) and social integration (0.28). The results of the CHART have also been examined using Rasch analysis which revealed good item separation and item fit (Whiteneck, et al. 1992).

Studies using the CHART have examined reimbursement

patterns for SCI (Tate, Forchheimer, Daugherty, & Maynard, 1994), the relationship between severity of SCI patients' pressure ulcers and handicap (Fuhrer, Garber, Rintala, Clearman, & Hart, 1993), depression and handicap status in SCI (Fuhrer, Rintala, Hart, Clearman, & Young, 1992), and the relationship between handicap and functional abilities in persons who have had a stroke (Segal & Schall, 1995). The CHART is becoming one of the most widely used measures of handicap in rehabilitation practice environments. The instrument is based on the WHO dimensions of handicap and focuses on objective criteria that are easily quantifiable. The CHART assesses the extent of handicap for individuals living in the community, regardless of the number of years since their inpatient rehabilitation or the extent of their involvement with the health care system. Most of the initial research using the CHART has involved persons with spinal cord injury. Additional research is needed to extend the findings to persons in other disability categories.

Community Integration Questionnaire (CIQ)

The Community Integration Questionnaire (CIQ) was originally developed to assess the social role limitations and community interaction of persons with acquired brain injury (Wilier, Linn & Allen, 1993). The CIQ includes 15 items divided into three domains: home integration, social integration and integration into productive activities. Home integration includes five items associated with domestic activities, housework, caring for children, shopping, etc. Social integration includes six items related to visiting friends and engaging in leisure activities with others. The productive activities domain contains four items examining work, school, volunteer activities and the use of transportation.

The CIQ is normally completed by the person being evaluated (self-report). An interviewer may be present to assist with interpretation of specific items. In certain instances, the individual being assessed may not be able to complete the questionnaire because of expressive or receptive language deficits, memory impairment, or cognitive disability. In these cases a person familiar with the individual may complete the assessment. A computerized version of the CIQ is available to assist persons who may have difficulty with paper and pencil assessments. A version of the CIQ that can be administered over the phone has also been developed. The entire assessment can usually be completed in less than 15 minutes. The domain areas and sample questions are included in Table 5-11.

Twelve of the 15 items on the CIQ are scored on a three-point scale. Three items related to employment, school and volunteer activities (productivity scale) are scored on a six-point scale. The overall CIQ score represents a summation of the scores for individual questions and ranges from 0 to 29. A higher score indicates a higher level of community involvement. The reliability and validity of the CIQ have been exam-

---

TABLE 5-10

Domains and Sample Items for the *Craig Handicap Assessment and Reporting Technique* **(CHART)**

Physical Independence Scale (3 questions)

Sample questions:

1. How many hours in a typical 24-hour day do you have someone with you to provide assistance? (hours paid/hours unpaid)

2. Not including any regular care as reported above, how many hours in a typical month do you occasionally have assistance with such things as grocery shopping, laundry, housekeeping, or infrequent medical needs like catheter changes?

Mobility Scale (9 questions)

Sample questions:

1. On a typical day, how many hours are you out of bed?

2. Can you enter and exit your home without any assistance from someone? (yes/no)

Occupation Scale (7 questions)

Sample questions:

1. How many hours per week do you spend working in a job for which you get paid?

2. How many hours per week do you spend in recreational activities such as sports, exercise, playing cards, or going to movies? Please do not include time spent watching TV or listening to the radio.

Social Integration Scale (6 questions)

Sample questions:

1. Do you live alone or with: a spouse or significant other; children (how many); other relatives (how many); roommate (how many); attendant (how many)?

2. How many friends (nonrelatives contacted outside business or organizational settings) do you visit, phone or write at least once a month?

Economic Self-Sufficiency Scale (2 questions)

Sample questions:

1. Approximately what was the combined annual income of all family members in your household? (Consider all sources including wages and earnings, disability benefits, pensions and retirement income, income from court settlements, investments and trusts from relatives, child support and alimony, contributions from relatives, and other sources.)

2. Approximately how much did you pay last year for medical care expenses? (Consider any amounts paid by yourself or the family members in your household and not reimbursed by insurance or benefits.)

---

ined for persons with brain injury (Wilier, Rosenthal, Kreutzer, Gordon, & Rempel, 1993). The test retest reliability for the three subscales ranged from ICC = 0.83 to 0.91. Reliability for proxy assessment has also been shown to be high (ICC = 0.93). Scores on the CIQ have been shown to statistically differentiate among subjects with acquired brain injury living independently, living in a supported community situation, and living in an institution (Wilier, Ottenbacher, & Coad, 1994).

ASSESSMENT OF HEALTH STATUS

The assessment of functional ability and occupational performance is well established in many rehabilitation disciplines including occupational therapy. Functional performance measures have been developed to determine level of disability and improve clinical management of direct service delivery. While rehabilitation has been advancing and refining the measurement of functional status, the field of health service research has been developing measures that can be used for health policy decision making, program evaluation, resource allocation,

and clinical research. In contrast to rehabilitation, where assessment grew out of the needs of practicing clinicians, health status determination has focused on research (Keith, 1994). The work on health status measurement warrants the attention of occupational therapists and other rehabilitation providers. Over the past 20 years there have been large-scale projects devoted to the conceptual and methodological development of health status measurement and these instruments are being extensively used in health services research (Stewart & Ware, 1992). Descriptions of two widely used measures of health status, the *Medical Outcomes Study Short Form-36* (SF-36) (Stewart & Ware, 1992), and the *Sickness Impact Profile* (SIP) (Bergner, Bobbit, Carter, & Gilson, 1981) are presented below.

Short Form 36 (SF-36)

The Short Form 36 is used extensively in the United States to determine general health status in health service and health policy research and practice (Jenkinson, Wright, & Coulter, 1994). The SF-36 was originally developed from the *Medical Outcomes Study (MOS) Questionnaire*, which included 113 items related to all aspects of a person's general health and well-being (Stewart & Ware, 1992). The MOS was designed to examine the relationship between physician practice styles and patient outcomes. The MOS has provided important data on the functional and health status of adults with chronic conditions and on the well-being of patients with various diseases and disorders (Ware, Kosinski, Bayliss, McHorney, Rogers, & Raczek, 1995). The SF-36 is sometimes referred to as the MOS-36 or the *Health Status Questionnaire* (HSQ) 2.0. The SF-36 is usually completed as a self-report questionnaire, but can also be administered by a trained interviewer. The SF-36 includes eight core domains involving 35 items. The final (36th) item is a supplementary question related to change in health status during the past year. The eight domains assessed by the SF-36 include: general health, physical functioning, mental health, role limitations (physical), role limitations (emotional), bodily pain, energy/tiredness, and social functioning. The domains, number of items and topics covered are presented in Table 5-12.

Items in the SF-36 are scored on nominal (yes/no) or ordinal scales. Each possible response to an item on a scale is assigned a number of points. The total points for all items within a scale are then added and transformed mathematically to yield a percentage score, with 100% representing optimal health. The SF-36 has demonstrated very good reliability and validity. Test-retest values have ranged from r = 0.81 to 0.88 (Stewart, Hays, & Ware, 1988). Concurrent validity with other measures of physical and mental function has been established (Ware, Kosinski, Bayliss, McHorney, Rogers, & Raczek, 1995). As health care delivery continues to migrate to the community and increasingly emphasizes prevention and health promotion, measures of health status, such as the SF-36 will become a standard part of routine assessment.

Sickness Impact Profile (SIP)

Another commonly used health status evaluation instrument is the *Sickness Impact Profile* (SIP) (Bergner, Bobbit, Carter, & Gilson, 1981). The SIP was constructed in 1972 by Bergner, Bobbit, Pollard, Martin, and Gilson (1976) based on descriptions of "sickness related dysfunctions" that were obtained from individuals who were directly or indirectly involved in "sickness episodes." The SIP was revised in 1981 (Bergner, Bobbit, Carter, & Gilson, 1981) and is widely used in rehabilitation and health services research. The SIP is a measure of perceived health status providing a descriptive profile of the changes in a person's behavior due to sickness. Sickness is defined as "the individual's own experience of illness perceived through the effect on daily living activities, feeling and attitudes" (Bergner, Bobbit, Carter, & Gilson, 1981, p. 788). The SIP has been designed to be used with all categories of disability and is not associated with any specific impairment.

TABLE 5-11

Domains and Sample Questions from the *Community Integration Questionnaire* (CIQ)

Home Integration (5 questions)
Sample questions:

1. Who usually does shopping for groceries or other necessities in your household?

2. In your home who usually does normal everyday housework?

Social Integration (6 questions)
Sample questions:

1. Who usually looks after your personal finances, such as banking or paying bills?

2. Can you tell me approximately how many times a month you now usually participate in the following activities outside your home?
   A. Shopping
   B. Leisure activities such as movies, sports, restaurants, etc.

Integration into Productive Activities (4 questions)
Sample questions:

1. How often do you travel outside the home?

2. Please choose the answer below that best corresponds to your current (during the last month) work situation:
   Full-time employment (>20 hours per week)
   Part-time employment (<20 hours per week)
   Not working, but actively looking for work
   Not working, not looking for work
   Not applicable, retired due to age
   Volunteer job in community

The SIP includes 136 items, divided into 12 domains of activities: sleep and rest, eating, working, home management, recreation and pastimes, ambulation, mobility, body care and movement, social interaction, alertness behavior, emotional behavior, and communication. Every item is a statement of behavior and respondents are asked to check items that both apply to their situation on the day they fill out the assessment and as they are related to their health status in general. For example, items in the mobility control domain include: "I do not walk up and down hills," and "I dress myself but do so very slowly." A score is obtained by adding the number of items checked. The items are weighted by the category to which they belong. The use of assistive devices lowers the final score. The questionnaire may be self-admin-

TABLE 5-12

The Domains, Number of Items and Areas Covered by the *Medical Outcomes Study - Short Form* (SF-36)

Domain	No. of Items	Topics Covered
Self-reported general heath	5	Rating own health compared with other peoples' health
Physical functioning	10	Extent to which health limits ten levels of physical activity, e.g., walking, stair climbing
Mental health	5	Degree of nervousness/calmness, happiness/sadness
Role limitations - physical	4	Limits that physical health puts on range and extent of work
Role limitations - emotional	3	Limits that emotional problems put on range and extent of work
Bodily pain	2	Severity of pain and impact on activities
Energy tiredness	4	How energetic/tired
Social functioning	2	Impact of physical health or emotional problems on normal social activities
Supplementary question		
Change in health in past year	1	Single unscored item comparing health now with 12 months ago

Adapted from Dixon, P., Heaton, J., Long, A., Worburton, A. (1994). Reviewing and applying the SF-36. *Outcomes Briefing, 4*, 3-20.

istered or administered by a trained interviewer. To complete all SIP domains required 20 to 30 minutes. Recently, a short version of the SIP has been developed containing 68 items (Bruin, Diederiks, de Witte, Stevens, & Philipsen, 1994). Initial research suggests that the reliability of the shortened SIP(68) is as good as the longer version (Bruin, Buys, de Witte, & Diederiks, 1994).

Reliability for the standard SIP has been examined by several authors and reported to be high: r = 0.92 for test retest and 0.94 for internal consistency (Bergner et al, 1981; Pollard, Bobbit, Bergner, Martin & Gilson, 1976). The clinical validity of the SIP has been examined by determining the relationship between clinical measures of disease and the SIP score (Bruin, Buys, de Witte & Dierderiks, 1994). The SIP is a popular measure and has been used as the gold standard to examine new instruments of disability and health status (Bergner, 1984).

OCCUPATIONAL PERFORMANCE ASSESSMENT IN CHILDREN

Assessment of children has traditionally focused on the achievement of developmental milestones. Using this approach, the motor, sensory-perceptual, language, and social skills of children with disabilities are compared to those of children without disabilities matched on gender and age. The limitations of developmental assessments have been widely discussed and include factors such as the lack of standardization on children with disabilities, inadequate sampling of functional and adaptive skills, and poor sensitivity to change (Allen, 1987; Garwood, 1982). Haley, Coster and Fass (1991) identify two main conceptual advantages associated with the use of functional outcomes over traditional developmental tests: 1) functional assessment and outcomes are more consistent with the goals of parents, teachers and therapists; and 2) functional measures emphasize independence, not normality. Two instruments have recently been developed that focus on the assessment of functional abilities (occupational performance) in children: *The Pediatric Evaluation of Disability Inventory* (PEDI) (Haley, Coster, Ludlow, Haltiwanger, & Andrellos, 1992), and the *Functional Independence Measure for Children* (WeeFIM) (Guide, 1994).

Pediatric Evaluation of Disability Inventory (PEDI)

The PEDI is a comprehensive clinical assessment instrument that examines functional abilities in three content domains: self-care, mobility, and social function. The PEDI is designed for children with functional skills in the age range of 6 months to 7 years, 6 months. Administration time ranges from approximately 45 to 90 minutes depending on method of administration. The instrument may be completed by structured interview with the parent, teacher, or other

---

TABLE 5-13

Domains and Content Areas of the *Pediatric Evaluation of Disability Inventory* (PEDI)

DOMAINS	SUBSCALES		
	Functional Skills	Care Giver Assistance	Modifications/ Adaptive Equipment
Self-Care	15 skill areas 73 items	8 skill areas	8 skill areas
Mobility	13 skill areas 59 items	7 skill areas	7 skill areas
Social Function	13 skill areas 65 items	5 skill areas	5 skill areas
	Total score_____	Total score _____	Total score _____

---

caregiver familiar with the child, or based on observation of the child performing individual items.

The content domains in the PEDI are divided into skill areas and items. For example, the self-care domain includes a total of 73 items divided into 15 skill areas. Examples of skill areas in the self-care domain include: use of utensils (5 items), use of drinking containers (5 items), hair brushing (4 items), washing body and face (5 items). The various domains, skill areas and number of items for the PEDI are presented in Table 5-13.

Each of the domains and skill areas are scored on three separate scales: Functional Skills, Caregiver Assistance, and Modifications/Adaptive Equipment (see Table 5-13). In the Functional Skills Scale each item is scored as unable or limited in capability to perform in most situations (score = 0), or capable of performing the item in most situations (score = 1). The Care Giver Assistance Scale measures the amount of assistance required to complete a task and is scored on a six-point scale from independent to total assistance. The Modifications/Adaptive Equipment scale provides a frequency count of the type and extent of environmental modifications that the child requires to complete functional tasks. The PEDI manual provides detailed descriptions regarding the scoring for each scale.

Normative values are provided in the manual based on a standardization sample and the psychometric properties of the PEDI have been carefully examined. Internal consistency and item reliabilities are high (alpha coefficients 0.95 to 0.99). The interrater reliability and test-retest reliability of the PEDI have been examined and found to be adequate for all three scales (Reid, Boschen, & Wright, 1993). The Social Functions Modifications/Adaptive Equipment Scale has demonstrated the lowest reliability and the authors have

made some modifications to this scale. The validity of the PEDI has also been examined in several studies and found to be good (Haley, Coster, & Fass, 1991; Feldman, Haley, & Coryell, 1990). The PEDI is a well-developed instrument that has numerous clinical and research applications in assessing functional abilities in children.

Functional Independence Measure for Children (WeeFIM)

A version of the Functional Independence Measure, known as the WeeFIM (Guide, 1994), has been developed for children from the ages of 6 months through 7 years. The WeeFIM duplicates the FIM in terms of content and scoring protocol except that the social cognition and communication items have been modified to address the performance of children rather than adults (see Table 5-6 for a list of the FIM items and scoring protocol). Like the FIM, the WeeFIM includes 18 items divided into six subscales: self-care, sphincter control, transfers, locomotion, stairs, communication, and social cognition. The key components of the WeeFIM are similar to those of the FIM and include its minimal data structure, emphasis on consistent actual performance, and discipline free observations in diverse settings. Since the WeeFIM measures disability, not impairment, the focus of measurement is on the degree of task performance, not what caused the disability. For example, the WeeFIM measures motor performance by scoring mobility and other motor items in relation to predetermined criteria, regardless of the cause of the neuromotor dysfunction or whether the neuromotor typography is diplegic, hemiplegic, paraplegic or quadriplegic. As a minimal essential data set, the WeeFIM is not meant to replace comprehensive motor, communicative, or cognitive assessments. Rather, the WeeFIM allows developmental therapists, educators, rehabilitation professionals, and families to describe consistent basic performance in daily routine using a common language.

The developers have standardized the instrument for specific age groups, so that the measure of disability yielded by the WeeFIM is age-appropriate (Guide, 1994; Msall, DiGaudio, Duffy, LaForrest, Braun, & Granger, 1994). Reliability and validity studies have been reported and suggest good test-retest and interrater reliability. ICC values for test retest of the WeeFIM subscales range from 0.83 to 0.99 and interrater ICC values are similar (0.81 to 0.98) (Msall, DiGaudio, & Duffy, 1993). Rasch modeling of WeeFIM scores has revealed five strata of functional independence, the progression of items from easiest to hardest, and close clustering of domain subitems (McCabe & Granger, 1990). Validity studies have compared WeeFIM scores with amount of care taker assistance required to complete basic ADLs (Msall, DiGaudio, & Duffy, 1993). The WeeFIM has been applied to several pediatric populations to examine functional skills and provided useful information in program planning, communication with parents and family members, and assessing child progress (Msall, Monti, Duffy, & LaForrest, 1992; Msall, Roehmholdt, DiGaudio, & Duffy, 1992).

One of the strengths of the WeeFIM is that, like the FIM, it is not simply an evaluation instrument, but a functional assessment data management system. Data collected using the WeeFIM can be submitted to the Uniform Data System for Medical Rehabilitation (UDSMR). The UDSMR was described in an earlier section of the chapter examining the FIM. Data submitted to the UDSMR are being aggregated to form a national data base on functional performance in children across the United States. The WeeFIM data base is relatively small (several thousand records) at this time since the instrument only became available as a UDSMR service in January of 1995. As the data base expands it will provide a valuable resource for research, program evaluation and policy development regarding the delivery of services to children with disabilities and their families.

IMPLICATIONS AND CONCLUSIONS

In describing the importance of interdisciplinary assessment in rehabilitation, Johnston, Keith and Hinderer (1992) note that, "we must improve our measures to keep pace with the development in general health care. If we move rapidly and continue our efforts, we can move rehabilitation to a position of leadership in health care" (p. S-5). This statement also applies to the profession of occupational therapy. Numerous authorities in the field have emphasized the importance of assessing occupational performance to the continued viability of the field (Christiansen, 1993; Fisher & Short DeGraff,

1993; Trombly, 1993). The ability to develop new assessment instruments and understand existing tests will be absolutely critical to the evolution of occupational therapy in the coming decade. Without assessment expertise practitioners will be unable to meet the demands for efficiency, accountability, and effectiveness that are certain to increase in managed care environments. The interaction between the assessment process and professional accountability has been operationalized by Hamilton and colleagues (1987). They have proposed a model for estimating what they refer to as "care efficiency" in rehabilitation. The model of care efficiency is based on recovery of function following disease or injury and is presented in Figure 5-2. Care efficiency is determined by two factors: degree of improvement in functional skill (y-axis) and the cost of rehabilitation service as estimated by time spent in a rehabilitation program (length of stay) represented on the x-axis. The trajectory of the line, beginning at the y-axis, represents optimal function, which is interrupted by the onset of disease, accident, or injury. Following the onset of injury, for example, spinal cord trauma, the person's functional independence (occupational performance) is dramatically impaired. This reduction in functional independence is indicated by the sharp drop in the line representing functional ability. During the period of hospitalization and rehabilitation, the person's level of functional independence gradually returns. The rate of return is dependent on many factors, one of which is the effectiveness of the rehabilitative intervention provided. Eventually, the person's level of functional independence begins to plateau and the person is discharged (hopefully to the community). Using this model, care efficiency is estimated by dividing the increase in functional independence (depicted by values on the y-axis) by the rehabilitation cost/length of stay (the cost per day of hospitalization and rehabilitation) as depicted on the x-axis. The care efficiency index obtained from this analysis is dependent on the reliability, validity, and sensitivity of the measure of functional performance (y-axis). Without valid, reliable, and sensitive measures of functional ability, the care efficiency index will be impossible to accurately determine and the effectiveness and efficiency of rehabilitation services, including occupational therapy, will remain unknown.

The development of a prospective payment system for medical rehabilitation has served to further emphasize the importance of functional assessment in determining the cost-effectiveness of rehabilitation services (Stineman, Escarce, Goin, Hamilton, Granger, & Williams, 1994). The system currently under investigation and review by the Health Care Financing Administration (HCFA) is based on the use of Function Related Groups (FRGs). The system, referred to as the Functional Independence Measure - Function Related Groups (FIM-FRGs), uses admission scores from the FIM and other demographic and clinical data (rehabilitation

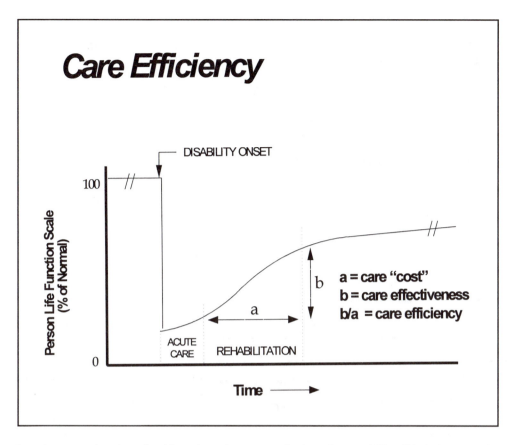

Figure 5-2. Determining care efficiency. Adapted with permission from Hamilton, B. B., Granger, C. V., Sherwin, F. S., Zielezny, M., & Tashman, J. S. (1987). A uniform data system for medical rehabilitation. In M. J. Fuhrer (Ed.), *Rehabilitation outcomes: Analysis and measurement* (pp. 139). Baltimore, MD: Paul H. Brookes.

impairment and age) to classify patients into categories based on (projected) length of stay (LOS) (Stineman, Hamilton, Granger, Goin, Escarce, & Williams, 1994). The FIM-FRG categories were developed using the large data base available from the UDSMR. Data used to develop the initial FRGs included records from a total of 36,980 patients who met specific selection criteria. The data for these patients were analyzed using a recursive partitioning algorithm, Classification and Regression Trees (CART) to form groups of persons based on LOS as recorded in the UDSMR data base. The initial FIM-FRGs included 53 distinct Function Related Groups for various rehabilitation impairments and explained 31.1% of the variance in LOS in a validation data set. A sample of a FIM-FRG classification tree for a person with stroke is presented in Figure 5-3.

The primary purpose of establishing FIM-FRGs is for use in developing a prospective payment system for medical rehabilitation (Stineman, 1994). By including functional performance and other clinical characteristics in a prospective payment system, it is hoped that reimbursement will be distributed among rehabilitation providers in a way that is conducive to high quality service delivery. The development of FIM-FRGs also makes it possible to identify "normative" length of stay benchmarks for patients in different rehabilitation impairment categories and with different degrees of dis-

ability. Work is currently underway by the federal government (HCFA) to validate the FIM-FRG process. A revised version of the FIM-FRGs are being developed using a larger and more recent data set from the UDSMR. The FIM-FRG II system will include new applications for continuous quality improvement (CQI) and program evaluation with a focus on functional performance as the primary outcome (Stineman, Goin, Hamilton, & Granger, 1995).

In the rapidly changing health care environment there are many variables related to service delivery and cost containment that occupational therapists cannot control. The interpretation of assessment procedures and the development of treatment programs, however, are still the direct responsibility of practitioners. Information concerning occupational performance assessment instruments and their clinical strengths and weaknesses will help practitioners to meet this professional responsibility and ensure that consumers of occupational therapy services receive the best available evaluation and treatment.

STUDY QUESTIONS

1. Explain how the results of occupational performance can be used to improve the clinical decision making

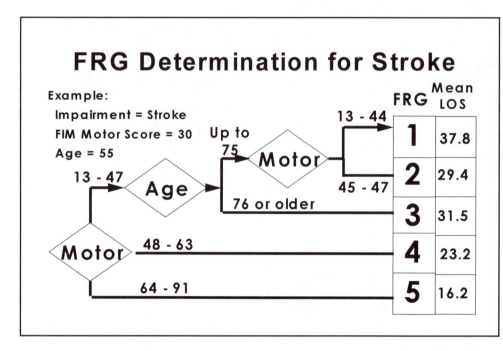

FRG Determination for Stroke

Example:

Impairment = Stroke

FIM Motor Score = 30

Age = 55

FRG	Mean LOS
1	37.8
2	29.4
3	31.5
4	23.2
5	16.2

Figure 5-3. Sample FIM-FRG Classification Tree. Adapted from Stineman, M. G., Hamilton, B. B., Granger, C. V., Goin, J. E., Escarce, J. J., Williams, S. V. (1994). Four methods for characterizing disability in the formation of function related groups. *Archives of Physical Medicine and Rehabilitation, 75,* 1277-1283.

process and select the most effective and appropriate intervention.

2. Discuss the differences in measuring impairment, disability, and handicap and provide examples of instruments that can be used to measure at each of theses levels.

3. Imagine that you are describing the results of an assessment to a client and his or her family. How do you explain that the test results are valid, reliable, and sensitive in terms that the client and the family members will understand?

4. Explain the difference between a test that is norm-referenced and one that is criterion-referenced.

5. Identify five basic activities of daily living included in the majority of occupational performance assessments.

6. Conflict results if assessment occurs at the impairment or disability level, while the expectation regarding therapeutic outcome is at the level of handicap or social role. Explain how careful assessment planning can reduce this conflict.

7. Discuss some advantages and disadvantages of performance based versus self-administered assessments of occupational performance.

8. Describe how assessment information might be used to establish a method of prospective payment for rehabilitation services. What are the implications for the practice of occupational therapy?

9. Identify similarities and differences in occupational performance assessment for adults and for children. Provide one example of an instrument designed to examine functional abilities in children.

REFERENCES

Allen, D. (1987). Measuring rehabilitation outcomes for infants and young children: A family approach. In M. J. Fuhrer (Ed.), *Rehabilitation outcomes: Analysis and measurement.* (pp. 45 - 57). Baltimore, MD: Paul H. Brookes.

American Occupational Therapy Association. (1995a). Position paper: Occupation. *American Journal of Occupational Therapy, 49,* 1015-1018.

American Occupational Therapy Association. (1995b). Position paper: Occupational performance: Occupational therapy's definition of function. *American Journal of Occupational Therapy, 49,* 1019-1020.

American Physical Therapy Association. (1991). Standards for tests and measurements in physical therapy practice. *Physical Therapy, 71,* 589-621.

Anderson, N. H. (1961). Scales and statistics: Parametric and nonparametric. *Psychological Bulletin, 58,* 305-316.

Ayres, A. J. (1989). *Sensory integration and praxis tests manual.* Los Angeles, CA: Western Psychological Services.

Bergner, M. (1984). The Sickness Impact Profile (SIP). In N. Wenger (Ed.), *Assessment of quality of life in clinical trials of cardiovascular therapy.* (pp. 152-159). New York: Le Jacq.

Bergner, M., Bobbit, R. A., Carter, W. B., & Gilson, B. S. (1981). The Sickness Impact Profile: Development and final revision of a health status measure. *Medical Care, 19,* 787-805.

Bergner, M., Bobbit, R. A., Pollard, W. E., Martin, D. P., & Gilson, B. S. (1976). The Sickness Impact Profile: Validation of a health status measure. *Medical Care, 14*, 57-67.

Bruin, A. F., Buys, M., deWitte, L. P., & Diederiks, J. P. M. (1994). The Sickness Impact Profile: SIP68, a short generic version, first evaluation of the reliability and reproducibility. *Journal of Clinical Epidemiology, 47*, 863-871.

Bruin, A. F., Diederiks, J. P., de Witte, L. P., Stevens, F. C. J., & Philipsen, H. (1994). The development of a short generic version of the Sickness Impact Profile. *Journal of Clinical Epidemiology, 47*, 407-418.

Carroll, L. (1945). *Through the looking glass: Alice's adventures in wonderland.* New York: Dell.

Chaudhuri, G., Harvey, R. F., Sulton, L. D., & Lambert, R. (1988). Computerized tomography head scans as predictors of functional outcome of stroke patients. *Archives of Physical Medicine and Rehabilitation, 69*, 496-498.

Christiansen, C. H. (1993). The issue is: Continuing challenges of functional assessment in rehabilitation: Recommended changes. *American Journal of Occupational Therapy, 47*, 260-264.

Commission On Practice. (1995). Clarification of the use of the terms assessment and evaluation. *American Journal of Occupational Therapy, 49,* 1072-1073.

Cope, D. N., & Sundance, P. (1995). Conceptualizing clinical outcomes. In P. Landrum, N. Schmidt, & A. McLean (Eds.), *Outcome-oriented rehabilitation: Principles, strategies, and tools for effective program management* (p. 43-56). Gaithersburg, MD: Aspen Publications.

Coster, W. J., & Haley, S. M. (1992). Conceptualization and measurement of disablement in infants and young children. *Infants & Young Children, 4*, 11-22.

Dahmer, E. R., Shilling, M. A., Hamilton, B. B., Bonthe, C. F., Englander, J., Kerutzer, J. S., Ragnarsson, K. T., & Rosenthal, M. (1993). A model system database for traumatic brain injury. *Journal of Head Trauma Rehabilitation, 8*, 12-25.

DeJong, G. (1987). Medical rehabilitation outcome measurement in a changing health care market. In M. J. Fuhrer (Ed.), *Rehabilitation outcomes: Analysis and measurement,* (p. 261-272). Baltimore, MD: Paul H. Brookes.

DeJong, G., & Sutton, J. P. (1995). Rehab 2000: The evolution of medical rehabilitation in American health care. In P. Landrum, N. Schmidt, & A. McLean (Eds.), *Outcome-oriented rehabilitation: Principles, dtrategies, and tools for effective program management* (pp. 3-42). Gaithersburg, MD: Aspen Publications.

Dunn, G. (1989). *Design and analysis of reliability studies: Statistical evaluation of measurement error.* New York: Oxford University Press.

Feinstein, A. R., Josephy, M. S., & Wells, C. K. (1986). Scientific and clinical problems in indexes of functional disability. *Annals of Internal Medicine, 105*, 413-420.

Feldman, A. B., Haley, S. M., & Coryell, J. (1990). Concurrent and construct validity of the Pediatric Evaluation of Disability Inventory. *Physical Therapy, 70*, 602-610.

Fisher, A. G. (1993). The assessment of IADL motor skill: An application of the many-faceted Rasch analysis. *American Journal of Occupational Therapy, 47*, 319-329.

Fisher, A. G. (1994). *Assessment of motor and process skills* (Research ed. 7.0). Fort Collins, CO: Department of Occupational Therapy, Colorado State University.

Fisher, A. G., Liu, Y., Velozo, C. A., & Pan, A. (1992). Cross-cultural assessment of process skills. *American Journal of Occupational Therapy, 46*, 876-885.

Fisher, A. G., & Short-DeGraff, M. A. (1993). Nationally speaking: Improving functional assessment in occupational therapy: Recommendations and philosophy for change. *American Journal of Occupational Therapy, 47*, 199-201.

Fuhrer, M. J., Garber, S. L., Rintala, D. H., Clearman, R., & Hart, K. A. (1993). Pressure ulcers in community-resident persons with spinal cord injury: Prevalence and risk factors. *Archives of Physical Medicine and Rehabilitation, 74*, 255-260.

Fuhrer, M. J., Rintala, D. H., Hart, K. A., Clearman, R., & Young, M. E. (1992). Relationship of life satisfaction to impairment, disability, and handicap among persons with spinal cord injury living in the community. *Archives of Physical Medicine and Rehabilitation, 74*, 255-260.

Garwood, S. G. (1982). (Mis)use of developmental scales in program evaluation. *Topics in Early Childhood Special Education, 1*, 61-78.

Granger, C. V. (1984). A conceptual model for functional assessment. In C. V. Granger & G. E. Gresham (Eds.), *Functional assessment in rehabilitation medicine* (p. 14-25). Baltimore, MD: Williams & Wilkins.

Granger, C. V., Albrecht, G. L., & Hamilton, B. B. (1979). Outcome of comprehensive medical rehabilitation: Measurement by the PULSES Profile and the Barthel Index. *Archives of Physical Medicine and Rehabilitation, 60*, 145-151.

Granger, C. V., Divan N., & Fiedler, R. C. (1995). Functional assessment scales: A study of persons after traumatic brain injury. *American Journal of Physical Medicine and Rehabilitation, 74*, 107-113.

Granger, C. V., Hamilton, B. B., Linacre, J. M., Heinemann, A. W., & Wright, B. D. (1993). Performance profiles of the Functional Independence Measure. *American Journal of Physical Medicine and Rehabilitation, 72*, 84-89.

Granger, C. V., Hamilton, B. B., Gresham, G. E., & Kramer, A. A. (1989). The stroke rehabilitation outcomes study: part II. Relative merits of the total Barthel index score and a four-item subscore in predicting patient outcome. *Archives of Physical Medicine and Rehabilitation, 70*, 100-103.

Grey, P., & Kennedy, N. (1993). The Functional Independence Measure: A comparative study of clinician and self-ratings. *Paraplegia, 31*, 457-461.

Guccione, A. A. (1991). Physical therapy diagnosis and the relationship between impairment and function. *Physical Therapy, 71*, 499-504.

Guide. (1993). *Guide for the Uniform Data Set for medical rehabilitation* (Adult FIM). Version 4.0 Buffalo, NY: State University of New York at Buffalo.

Guide (1994). *Functional Independence Measure for children* (WeeFIM). Outpatient Version 1.0. Buffalo, NY: State University of New York at Buffalo.

Haley, S. M., Coster, W. J., Ludlow, L., Haltiwinger, J. T., & Andrellos, P. J. (1992). *Pediatric Evaluation of Disabilities Inventory* (PEDI). Version 1.0. Boston, MA: New England

Medical Center Hospitals, Inc.

Haley, S. M., Coster, W. J., & Fass, R. M. (1991). A content validity study of the Pediatric Evaluation of Disability Inventory. *Pediatric Physical Therapy, 3*, 177-184.

Hamilton, B. B., Granger, C. V., Sherwin, F. S., Zielezny, M., & Tashman, J. S. (1987). A uniform national data system for medical rehabilitation. In M. J. Fuhrer (Ed.), *Rehabilitation outcomes: Analysis and measurement*. Baltimore, MD: Paul H. Brookes.

Hamilton, B. B., Laughlin, J. A., Fiedler, R. C., & Granger, C. V., (1994). Interrater reliability of the 7-level Functional Independence Measure. *Scandinavian Journal of Rehabilitation Medicine, 26*, 115-119.

Harvey, R. F., & Jellinek, H. M. (1983). Patient profiles: Utilization in functional performance assessment. *Archives of Physical Medicine and Rehabilitation, 64*, 268-271.

Harvey, R. F., Silverstein, B., Venzon, M. M., Kilgore, K. M., Fisher, W. P., Steiner, M., & Harley, J. P. (1992). Applying psychometric criteria to functional assessment in medical rehabilitation: III. Construct validity and predicting level of care. *Archives of Physical Medicine and Rehabilitation, 73*, 887-892.

Heinemann, A. W., Linacre, J. M., Wright, B. D., Hamilton, B. B., & Granger, C. V. (1993). Relationship between impairment and physical disability as measured by the Functional Independence Measure. *Archives of Physical Medicine and Rehabilitation, 74*, 566-573.

Ikegami, N. (1995). Functional assessment and its place in health care. *New England Journal of Medicine, 332*, 598-599.

Jellinek, H. M., Torkelson, R. M., & Harvey, R. F. (1982). Functional abilities and distress levels in brain injured patients at long-term follow-up. *Archives of Physical Medicine and Rehabilitation, 63*, 160-162.

Jenkinson, C., Wright, L., & Coulter, A. (1994). Criterion validity and reliability of the SF36 in a population sample. *Quality of Life Research, 3*, 7-12.

Johnston, M. V., Keith, R. A., & Hinderer, S. R. (1992). Measurement standards for interdisciplinary medical rehabilitation. *Archives of Physical Medicine and Rehabilitation, 73*, 12-S.

Johnston, M. V., Findley, T. W., DeLuca, J., & Katz, R. T. (1991). Research in physical medicine and rehabilitation: XII measurement tools with application to brain injury. *American Journal of Physical Medicine and Rehabilitation, 70* (suppl), S114-S130.

Keith, R. A. (1994). Functional status and health status. *Archives of Physical Medicine and Rehabilitation, 75*, 478-483.

Law, M. (1993). Evaluating activities of daily living: Directions for the future. *American Journal of Occupational Therapy, 47*, 233-237.

Law, M., Baptiste, S., McColl, M. A., Opzoomer, A., Polatajko, H., & Pollock, N. (1990). The Canadian Occupational Performance Measure: An outcome measure for occupational therapy. *Canadian Journal of Occupational Therapy, 57*, 82-87.

Law, M., Polatajko, H., Pollock, N., McColl, M., Opzoomer, A., & Baptiste, S. (1994). Pilot testing of the Canadian Occupational Performance Measure: Clinical and measurement issues. *Canadian Journal of Occupational Therapy, 61*(4), 191-197.

Lawton, M. P. (1971). The functional assessment of elderly people. *Journal of the American Geriatric Society, 14*, 465-481.

Mahoney, F., & Barthel, D. W. (1965). Functional evaluation: The Barthel Index. *Maryland State Medical Journal, 14*, 61-65.

Mather, J. H. (1993). The problem of functional assessment: Political and economic perspectives. *American Journal of Occupational Therapy, 47*, 240-246.

Mathiowetz, V. (1993). Role of physical performance component evaluations in occupational therapy functional assessment. *American Journal of Occupational Therapy, 47*, 227.

McCabe, M., & Granger, C. V. (1990). Content validity of a pediatric functional independence measure. *Applied Nursing Research, 3*, 120-122.

Miller, L. J. (1986). *The Miller Assessment for Preschoolers* (MAP). Littleton, CO: Foundation for Knowledge in Development.

Merbitz, C., Morris, J., & Grip, J. C. (1989). Ordinal scales and foundations of misinference. *Archives of Physical Medicine and Rehabilitation, 70*, 308-312.

Msall, M. E., DiGaudio, K. M., & Duffy, L. C. (1993). Use of functional assessment in children with developmental disability. *Physical Medicine and Rehabilitation Clinics of North America, 4*, 517-527.

Msall, M. E., DiGaudio, K. M., Duffy, L. C., LaForrest, S., Braun, S., & Granger, C. V. (1994). WeeFIM: Normative sample of an instrument for tracking functional independence in children. *Clinical Pediatrics, 44*, 431-438.

Msall, M. E., Monti, D., Duffy, L. C., & LaForrest, S. (1992). Measuring functional independence in children with spina bifida. *Pediatric Research, 31*, 12A (Abstract).

Msall, M. E., Roehmholdt, S. J., DiGaudio, K. M., & Duffy, L. C. (1992). Functional independence of school age children with Down syndrome. *Pediatric Research, 31*, 13A (Abstract).

Murdock, C. (1992) A critical evaluation of the Barthel Index: Part 1. *British Journal of Occupational Therapy, 55*, 109-111.

Nygård, L., Bernspang, B., Fisher, A. G., & Winbald, B. (1994). Comparing motor and process ability of persons with suspected dementia in home and clinical settings. *American Journal of Occupational Therapy, 48*, 689-696.

Opacich, K. J. (1991). Assessment and informed decision making. In C. Christiansen & C. Baum (Eds.), *Occupational therapy: Overcoming human performance deficits* (pp. 354-372). Thorofare, NJ: SLACK Incorporated.

Ottenbacher, K. J., Mann, W. C., Granger, C. V., Tomita, M., Hurren, D., & Charvat, B. (1995). Interrater agreement and stability of functional assessment in the community based elderly. *Archives of Physical Medicine and Rehabilitation, 75*, 1297-1301.

Ottenbacher, K. J., & Tomchek, S. D. (1993). Measurement in rehabilitation research: Consistency versus consensus. In C. V. Granger & G. E. Gresham (Eds.), *New developments in functional assessment. Physical medicine and rehabilitation clinics of North America* (pp. 463-474). Philadelphia, PA: W.B. Saunders.

Park, S., Fisher, A. G., & Velozo, C. A. (1994). Using the Assessment of Motor and Process Skills to compare occupational performance between clinic and home settings. *American Journal of Occupational Therapy, 48*, 697-709.

Pollard, W. E., Bobbit, R. A., Bergner, M., Martin, D. P., & Gilson, B. S. (1976). The sickness impact profile: Reliability of a health status measure. *Medical Care, 14*, 146-155.

Pollock, N. (1993). Client-centered assessment. *American Journal of Occupational Therapy, 47*(4), 298-301.

Portney, L. G., & Watkins, M. P. (1993). *Foundations of clinical research: Applications to practice*. Norwalk, CT: Appleton & Lange.

Reid, D. T., Boschen, K., & Wright, V. (1993). Critique of the Pediatric Evaluation of Disability Inventory (PEDI). *Physical and Occupational Therapy in Pediatrics, 13*, 57-87.

Rogers, J. C., & Holm, M. B. (1991). Occupational therapy diagnostic reasoning. A component of clinical reasoning. *American Journal of Occupational Therapy, 45*, 1045-1053.

Segal, M. E., & Schall, R. R. (1995). Assessing handicap of stroke survivors: A validation study of the Craig Handicap Assessment and Reporting Technique. *American Journal of Physical Medicine and Rehabilitation, 74*, 276-286.

Shah, S., Vanclay, F., & Cooper, B. (1989). Improving the sensitivity of the Barthel Index for stroke rehabilitation, *Journal of Clinical Epidemiology, 42*, 703-709.

Shrout, P. E., & Fleiss, J. L. (1979) Intraclass correlations: Uses in assessing rater reliability. *Psychological Bulletin, 86*, 420-428.

Silverstein, B., Fisher, W. P., Kilgore, K. M., Harley, J. P., Harvey, J. P., & Harvey, R. F. (1992). Applying psychometric criteria to functional assessment in medical rehabilitation II. Defining interval measures. *Archives of Physical Medicine & Rehabilitation, 73*, 507-518.

Silverstein, B., Kilgore, K. M., Fisher, W. P., Harley, J. P., & Harvey, R. F. (1991). Applying psychometric criteria to functional assessment in medical rehabilitation: I. Exploring unidimensionality. *Archives of Physical Medicine & Rehabilitation, 72*, 631-637.

Stewart, A., Hays, R. D., & Ware, J. E. (1988). The MOS short general health survey: Reliability and validity in a patient population. *Medical Care, 26*, 724-730.

Stewart, A., & Ware, J. E. (1992). *Measuring functioning and well-being: The medical outcomes study approach*. Durham, NC: Duke University Press.

Stineman, M. G. (1994). Function based classification for stroke rehabilitation and issues of reimbursement. *Topics in Stroke Rehabilitation, 2*, 40-50.

Stineman, M. G., Escarce, J. J., Goin, J. E., Hamilton, B. B., Granger, C. V., & Williams, S. V. (1994). A case mix classification system for medical rehabilitation. *Medical Care, 32*, 366-379.

Stineman, M. G., Goin, J. E., Hamilton, B. B., & Granger, C. V. (1995). Efficiency pattern analysis for medical rehabilitation. *American Journal of Medical Quality, 10*, 190-198.

Stineman, M. G., Hamilton, B. B., Granger, C. V., Goin, J. E., Escarce, J. J., & Williams, S. V. (1994). Four methods for characterizing disability in the formation of function related groups. *Archives of Physical Medicine and Rehabilitation, 75*, 1277-1283.

Tate, D. G., Forchheimer, M., Daugherty, J., & Maynard, F. (1994). Determining differences in post discharge outcome among catastrophically and noncatastrophically sponsored patients with spinal cord injury. *American Journal of Physical Medicine and Rehabilitation, 73*, 89-97.

Thuriaux, M. C. (1995). The ICIDH: Evolution, status and prospects. *Disability and Rehabilitation, 17*, 112-118.

Toomey, M., Nicholson, D, & Carswell, A. (1995). The clinical utili-

ty of the Canadian Occupational Performance Measure. *Canadian Journal of Occupational Therapy, 62*(5), 242-249.

Townsend, E., Ryan, B., & Law, M. (1990). Using the World Health Organization's International Classification of Impairments Disabilities and Handicaps in occupational therapy. *Canadian Journal of Occupational Therapy, 57*, 16-25.

Trombly, C. A. (1993). The issue is: Anticipating the future: Assessment of occupational function. *American Journal of Occupational Therapy, 47*, 258-259.

Trombly, C. A. (1995). Occupation: Purposefulness and meaningfulness as therapeutic mechanisms. 1995 Eleanor Clarke Slagle Lecture. *American Journal of Occupational Therapy, 49*, 960-972.

Velleman, P. F., & Wilkinson, L. (1993). Nominal, ordinal and ratio topologies are misleading. *The American Statistician, 47*, 65-72.

Wagenaar, R. C., & Meijer, O. G. (1991a). Effects of stroke rehabilitation (1): A critical review of the literature. *Journal of Rehabilitation Science, 4*, 61-73.

Wagenaar, R. C., & Meijer, O. G. (1991b). Effects of stroke rehabilitation (2): A critical review of the literature. *Journal of Rehabilitation Science, 4*, 97-109.

Ware, J. E., Kosinski, M., Bayliss, M. S., McHorney, C. A., Rogers, W. H., & Raczek, A. (1995). Comparison of methods for the scoring and statistical analysis of the SF-36 health profile and summary measures: Summary of results from the medical outcomes study. *Medical Care, 33*, AS264-AS279.

Watson, A. H., Kanny, E. M., White, D. M., & Anson, D. K. (1995). Use of standardized activities of daily living rating scales in spinal cord injury and disease services. *American Journal of Occupational Therapy, 49*(3), 229-234.

Whiteneck, G., Charlifue, S. W., Gerhart, K. A., Overholser, J. D., & Richardson, G. N. (1992). Quantifying handicap: A new measure of long-term rehabilitation outcomes. *Archives of Physical Medicine and Rehabilitation, 73*, 519-526.

Willer, B., Linn, R., & Allen, K. (1993). Community integration and barriers to integration for individuals with brain injury. In M. Finlayson, & S. Garner, (Eds.), *Brain injury rehabilitation: Clinical considerations* (pp. 355-375). Baltimore, MD: Williams & Wilkins.

Willer, B., Ottenbacher, K., & Coad, M. L. (1994). The community integration questionnaire: A comparative examination. *American Journal of Physical Medicine and Rehabilitation, 73*, 103-111.

Willer, B., Rosenthal, M., Kreutzer, J., Gordon, W., & Rempel, R. (1993). Assessment of community integration following rehabilitation for traumatic brain injury. *Journal of Head Trauma Rehabilitation, 8*, 75-87.

World Health Organization (1980). *International classification of impairments, disabilities, and handicaps: A manual for classification relating to the consequences of disease*. Albany, NY: World Health Organization Publication Center.

Wright, B. D., & Linacre, J. M. (1989). Observations are always ordinal: Measurements, however, must be interval. *Archives of Physical Medicine and Rehabilitation, 70*, 857.

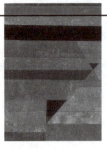

CHAPTER CONTENT OUTLINE

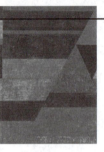

ABSTRACT

Before therapists can identify occupational therapy interventions that are appropriate for a client, the problems that these interventions are to alleviate or resolve must be identified and described. The process of problem identification and description is called diagnostic reasoning. Diagnostic reasoning, the beginning point of clinical reasoning, is a complex process involving multiple and diverse cognitive operations. The endpoint or product of this process is a descriptive statement called the occupational therapy diagnosis. To assist the reader in understanding diagnostic reasoning and the occupational therapy diagnosis, this chapter begins with a case scenario, which is then further developed throughout the chapter to illustrate the major concepts presented.

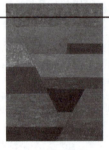

KEY TERMS

Cue

Diagnostic hypothesis

Heuristic

Occupational status

Occupational therapy diagnosis

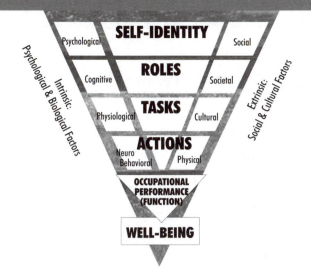

CHAPTER 6

Diagnostic Reasoning

The Process of Problem Identification

Joan C. Rogers, PhD, OTR/L, FAOTA, Margo B. Holm, PhD, OTR/L, FAOTA

OBJECTIVES

The information in this chapter is intended to help the reader:

1. define the occupational therapy diagnosis

2. understand the importance of the occupational therapy diagnosis for planning intervention

3. analyze the structure of occupational therapy diagnostic statements

4. understand the cognitive operations that underlie the diagnostic process

5. delineate the factors that guide the search for data needed to make an occupational therapy diagnosis

6. know strategies for preventing errors in diagnostic reasoning

7. articulate the ways in which the diagnostic reasoning of experts differs from that of novices.

"It is better to know some of the questions than all of the answers."
James Thurber

Mrs. Stub is a 76 year old widowed female of Northern European descent, who has lived by herself in a senior apartment since her husband died 5 years ago. Yesterday she was admitted to the short-term rehabilitation unit of Serenity Long Term Care Center (SLTC) directly from City Hospital's acute psychiatric unit, where she was treated for major depression during a 7-day stay. Mrs. Stub had been admitted to the psychiatric unit immediately following discharge from the neurology unit of the hospital, following a 6-day hospitalization for a right cerebrovascular accident (R CVA). The social worker's admission note to SLTC states that Mrs. Stub's expected discharge disposition is her home, however, because she is not independent in activities of daily living (ADL) she has been admitted to the SLTC rehabilitation unit near her daughter's home.

Figure 6-1. Background information for the case scenario.

INTRODUCTION

The scheme used to organize the chapter focuses first on the occupational therapy (OT) diagnosis and then shifts to highlight the cognitive operations therapists use to formulate it. In the first part of the chapter, the occupational therapy diagnosis is defined and its role in the occupational therapy process is delineated. Although occupational therapy presently lacks a uniform system for naming and classifying clients' problems in occupational status, the benefits that could be derived from developing a system are presented. To advance the development of a system, a structure for phrasing occupational therapy diagnostic statements is outlined. In the second part of the chapter, the cognitive operations of cue acquisition, analysis, and interpretation and hypothesis generation, refinement, and verification are discussed and illustrated with case data. Important intrinsic (i.e., client-related) and extrinsic (i.e., environmental) factors that influence diagnostic reasoning are identified as are common diagnostic errors and ways of preventing their occurrence. The chapter concludes with a discussion of differences in diagnostic reasoning between new and experienced therapists and suggestions for improving diagnostic reasoning (Figure 6-1).

As the Serenity Long Term Care Center (SLTC) occupational therapist reviews the medical chart of the new client, Mrs. Stub, she reads the physician's hospital discharge summary shown in Figure 6-2. While reviewing the chart she also learns that with each subsequent admission, Mrs. Stub presented new or revised pathologies, impairments, and disabili-

ties. The notes of the occupational therapist on the neurology unit indicated that he treated Mrs. Stub for deficits in left upper extremity (LUE) weakness and motor control secondary to the left hemiplegia. The documentation of the occupational therapist on the psychiatric unit indicated that, in addition to introducing compensatory strategies for LUE weakness and motor control impairments, she also addressed deficits in motivation and self-efficacy. Based on their assessments, the neurologic and psychiatric therapists made decisions about the nature of the problems to be addressed in occupational therapy. Rogers and Holm (1989, 1991) labeled the outcome of these decisions, the occupational therapy diagnosis.

The aim of this chapter is to foster an understanding of the occupational therapy diagnosis and the cognitive operations occupational therapists perform when formulating it. A better understanding of the cognitive operations that support the occupational therapy process can assist students and therapists to learn how to use them more effectively in making clinical decisions.

DEFINITION AND ROLE OF THE OCCUPATIONAL THERAPY DIAGNOSIS

The occupational therapy process, operationalized in the Standards of Practice (American Occupational Therapy Association [AOTA], 1994a) encompasses the series of actions that therapists undertake from the receipt of a referral through discharge and follow up. Initially, according to Rogers and Holm (1989, 1991) these actions focus on problem sensing and framing, and conclude with a problem definition (i.e., an occupational therapy diagnosis). Once the nature of the clinical problem or problems is clearly defined, action shifts to determining desired and feasible outcomes of inter-

Bibliographic citation of this chapter: Rogers, J. C., & Holm, M. B. (1997). Diagnostic reasoning: The process of problem identification. In C. Christiansen & C. Baum (Eds.), *Occupational therapy: Enabling function and well-being* (2nd ed.). Thorofare, NJ: SLACK Incorporated.

Pt is a 76 yowf, 14 days S/P RCVA with L hemiparesis. She has a h/o early macular degeneration, obesity, and hypertension. Pt. exhibits weakness in the LUE and shoulder musculature. Proprioception, light touch, deep pressure, and hot/cold discrimination are intact, but 2-point discrimination is impaired. LLE sensation is intact, and Pt. ambulates independently with the use of a quad cane. Evaluations indicate possible cognitive (MMSE= 24/30), but no perceptual impairments. Pt. remains mild/moderately depressed (Hamilton= 18), but mood is improved from admission. Pt. displays passivity when asked about her goals for rehabilitation, and is doubtful of her ability to return home.

Medication at discharge: Nortriptyline™ 50 mg qhs and Verapamil™ 240 mg qam

Mobility status at discharge: Pt. independently ambulates with a cane.

ADL status at discharge: Pt. is dependent in bathing and dressing, Independent in toileting and grooming.

IADL status at discharge: IADL not assessed.

Figure 6-2. Physician's discharge note in Mrs. Stub's medical chart.

vention in collaboration with clients, formulating and implementing problem solutions, and evaluating their effectiveness for achieving the established target outcomes. The former actions comprise occupational therapy assessment, i.e., the systematic collection and interpretation of client data regarding occupational status. The latter actions comprise occupational therapy intervention or the therapeutic procedures and techniques used to influence occupational status in a favorable way (Holm & Rogers, 1989). Occupational status is a collective term that incorporates all three occupational therapy performance dimensions—occupational role performance, the three occupational performance areas (i.e., activities of daily living, work/productivity/home management, play/leisure), and the three broad occupational performance components (i.e., sensorimotor, cognitive, affective).

OT Diagnosis

The occupational therapy diagnosis is strategically positioned at the interface between problem definition and problem solution. The occupational therapy diagnosis is a descriptive problem statement that succinctly describes actual or potential occupational status dysfunctions that are amenable to intervention with occupational therapy procedures and modalities. As the transition point between problem definition and problem solution, the occupational therapy diagnosis is the critical element in determining the accuracy and utility of occupational therapy intervention.

Problems must be thoroughly and accurately defined, and identified as important by clients, before they can be solved effectively and efficiently (Rogers & Holm, 1989, 1991).

A diagnosis establishes the hypothesized cause or nature of a condition, situation, or problem (Rogers & Holm, 1989, 1991). Diagnosis is usually considered in reference to medical or psychiatric conditions. The diagnosis of major depression, for example, means that in addition to either depressed mood or loss of interest or pleasure of two weeks duration or more, at least four of the following characteristics must be present: significant weight loss or gain or an increased or decreased appetite, insomnia or hypersomnia, psychomotor agitation or retardation, fatigue or loss of energy, feelings of worthlessness or inappropriate guilt, diminished ability to think and make decisions, and recurrent thoughts of death or suicide or suicide attempts or plans (American Psychiatric Association, 1994, p. 327). In making a diagnosis of major depression, the psychiatrist first examines the patient to ascertain if he or she has the distinguishing features of the condition. If these features are present, the diagnosis is positive. The "label," major depression, summarizes these signs and symptoms and suggests a range of medical interventions appropriate for managing the condition, such as electroconvulsive therapy, antidepressant medications, or interpersonal therapy.

When the term *diagnosis* is applied to the outcome of the occupational therapy assessment, it refers to a conclusion about the nature or cause of a problem that requires occupational therapy intervention (Rogers & Holm, 1989, 1991). The occupational therapy diagnosis describes the actual or potential effects of disease, trauma, development disorders, psychological maladaptation, age-associated changes, environmental deprivation, or other etiologic agents on occupational status. An active diagnosis refers to an occupational status problem that is present and requires intervention (Doenges, Moorhouse, & Burley, 1995). A potential diagnosis refers to a problem that has not yet occurred but may develop because risk factors that typically lead to the problem are present (Doenges et al., 1995). Preventive actions are needed to ward off problem development. Contractures are an example of an actual problem, while being at-risk for restrictions in joint range of motion following a traumatic brain injury resulting in a comatose state, reflects a potential problem. For an active diagnosis, the signs and symptoms characteristic of a diagnosis are evident, whereas for a potential diagnosis the signs and symptoms are likely to occur because the conditions that often cause it are present.

In applying the term diagnosis to occupational therapy, we intended to derive the same benefits from its use as is experienced in medicine. Specifically, that the occupational therapy diagnosis will provide an accurate description of a client's occupational status and that this description, in turn, will suggest strategies for occupational therapy interventions. Diagnostic judgments and causal attributions, however, must be carefully constructed if they are to perform these functions.

THE OT DIAGNOSTIC STATEMENT

Diagnosis is essentially a process of classifying and labeling. The characteristics of a particular occupational status dysfunction are recognized by the occupational therapy diagnostician, in consultation with a client, and labeled. The label is used to guide treatment. Assume, for example, that all dressing dysfunctions could be classified as Dressing Dysfunction A, B, or C. Dressing Dysfunction A is characterized by an inability to dress the upper body only and Dressing Dysfunction B is characterized by an inability to dress the lower body only. The distinguishing feature of Dressing Dysfunction C is the inability to dress both the upper and lower body. This rudimentary scheme would enable therapists to classify clients according to the site of their dressing dysfunction. The only guide that it provides for intervention, however, is to focus attention on occupational performance area and site of the occupational status dysfunction that requires intervention, namely, upper body dressing, lower body dressing, and both upper and lower body dressing respectively. Driessen, Dekker, Lankhorst, and van der Zee (1995) have demonstrated the reliability of occupational therapy diagnoses made at various levels of occupational status.

Suppose, however, that the occupational therapy diagnostic classification scheme was refined to take into account the nature of the impairment presumed to be causing the dressing dysfunction, with a 1 assigned to a dysfunction caused by a sensorimotor impairment, a 2 assigned to a dysfunction caused by a cognitive impairment, a 3 assigned to a dysfunction caused by an affective impairment, and a 4 assigned to a dysfunction caused by the environment. Figure 6-3 presents this refined diagnostic classification scheme. Inclusion of the nature of the impairment that is likely causing the dressing dysfunction substantively improves the meaning of the diagnostic label for intervention. For example, Dressing Dysfunction A.1 suggests restorative neuromotor interventions, such as range of motion, strengthening activities, and motor control techniques, or adaptive/compensatory strategies. Dressing Dysfunction A.2 suggests cognitive interventions, such as exercises to improve memory for task sequencing or a dressing notebook to substitute for deficits in procedural memory. Dressing Dysfunction A.3 suggests motivational interventions, such as organizing all clothing to be put on each morning onto a hanger, thus simplifying the decisions associated with dressing, and making the task seem possible to achieve with little effort. Dressing Dysfunction A.4 suggests environmental interventions such as increased lighting, so that clothes can be seen more easily, or lowering the bar in the closet, so that clothes can be reached. Obviously, a more refined diagnostic scheme would provide more specific guidance for occupational therapy interventions. The diagnoses themselves would be based on occupational therapy knowledge of task performance dysfunctions and the clustering of signs and symptoms into meaningful patterns.

Unfortunately, occupational therapy lacks standardized labels for describing the problems treated through its services. While the Uniform Terminology for Occupational Therapy, Third Edition (American Occupational Therapy Association, 1994b) specifies and define concepts essential to occupational therapy practice, it does not define the distinguishing features of occupational status dysfunctions or provide summary names or labels for them (e.g., problems with safety, independence, quality of outcome, etc.). In lieu of a standardized diagnostic scheme, occupational therapists either create their own unique descriptions or use terms from various occupational therapy theories or frames of reference (e.g., sensory-integration deficit, volitional disorder). Until a standardized system of diagnostic nomenclature is devised for the profession that is readily understood within the profession and among the other disciplines with which we interact, occupational therapists will need to rely on descriptive problem statements.

STRUCTURE OF THE OT DIAGNOSIS

To advance the development of occupational therapy diagnosis, Rogers and Holm (1989, 1991) suggested a structure for

Diagnostic Label	Characteristics
Dressing Dysfunction A.1	Inability to dress upper body related to sensorimotor impairment
Dressing Dysfunction A.2	Inability to dress upper body related to cognitive impairment
Dressing Dysfunction A.3	Inability to dress upper body related to affective impairment
Dressing Dysfunction A.4	Inability to dress upper body related to environmental limitations
Dressing Dysfunction B.1	Inability to dress lower body related to sensorimotor impairment
Dressing Dysfunction B.2	Inability to dress lower body related to cognitive impairment
Dressing Dysfunction B.3	Inability to dress lower body related to affective impairment
Dressing Dysfunction B.4	Inability to dress lower body related to environmental limitations
Dressing Dysfunction C.1	Inability to dress upper and lower body related to sensorimotor impairment
Dressing Dysfunction C.2	Inability to dress upper and lower body related to cognitive impairment
Dressing Dysfunction C.3	Inability to dress upper and lower body related to affective impairment
Dressing Dysfunction C.4	Inability to dress upper and lower body related to environmental limitations

Figure 6-3. Sample scheme for dressing dysfunctions in hypothetical occupational therapy diagnostic nomenclature.

phrasing descriptive problem statements (Figure 6-4). The DESCRIPTIVE (DE) part of the diagnostic statement describes the problem that the client is experiencing in occupational status. Clients are referred to occupational therapy primarily because of current or potential problems in role performance or activities of daily living (ADL), work/productive activities, or play/leisure activities (Holm & Rogers, 1989). At this step, describing the problem in performance with accuracy and specificity is necessary because this functional performance ultimately must change with occupational therapy intervention. The EXPLANATORY (EX) part of the diagnostic statement puts forth the presumed or probable cause of the problem. A problem may have several suspected causes, hence, more than one explanation may be given for any occupational status dysfunction. The explanatory phrase is a very critical part of the diagnostic statement because intervention strategies may vary based on the etiology of the occupational status dysfunction. For this reason, the presumed cause should be something that is amenable to occupational therapy interventions. The third part of the diagnostic statement briefly outlines the EVIDENCE (EV) that led to the conclusion that a problem existed, in other words, it gives the signs and symptoms for the problem description and explanatory cause. The fourth part of the diagnostic statement includes DIAGNOSTIC INFORMATION (DI), and names the pathologic agent that is the likely cause of the occupational status dysfunction. The SLTC occupational therapist used this structure to outline the OT diagnosis shown in Figure 6-4.

This structure satisfies the diagnostic requirements of describing the problem and suggesting strategies for occupational therapy intervention. In regard to causal attributions, it focuses on the more immediate causes of the dressing dysfunction (i.e., sensorimotor, cognitive, and affective impairments or environmental factors) while acknowledging the pathologic agents (i.e., stroke, depression, macular degeneration, hypertension, obesity). Although medical or psychiatric diagnoses may be the ultimate cause of problems in occupational performance, their influence on daily living activities is mediated by factors intrinsic and extrinsic to clients. These factors rather than the medical or psychiatric pathologies *per se* define the nature and cause of occupational status dysfunctions. When medical and psychiatric diagnoses are severe enough, they cause sensorimotor, cognitive, or affective impairments (World Health Organization [WHO], 1980). Spasticity, attention deficits, and apathy are examples of sensorimotor, cognitive, and affective impairments respectively. When impairments are severe enough, and compensatory actions are not instituted or are inadequate, task skills break down and disabilities result (WHO, 1980). Difficulty performing or an inability to perform ADL, work, home management, or play/leisure tasks are examples of disability. With the accumulation of disabilities, social role performance may become inadequate, resulting in handicap (WHO, 1980). Terminating a volunteer position at the art museum due to a lack of endurance for standing and waiting for public transportation illustrates handicap. Hence, impair-

Part of OT Diagnosis	Occupational Performance Terminology	Mrs. Stub's OT Diagnosis
DESCRIPTIVE	Occupational Performance	Unable to initiate or complete dressing tasks without verbal cues or physical assistance
EXPLANATORY	Performance Components	L hemiparesis, apathy
EXPLANATORY EVIDENCE (Cues from observation or assessment)	(Sensorimotor)	• Grade 3 (fair) mm. strength in L wrist flexors/extensors (R=WNL) • Grade 3 (fair) mm. strength in L elbow flexors/extensors (R=WNL) • Grade 3+ mm. strength in L shoulder flexors and abductors, elevators, and upward rotators (R=WNL) • Intact proprioception, light touch, and deep pressure • Hot/cold discrimination intact • 2-point discrimination absent on L & R digits (palmar/volar) • Uses magnifying glass to read newspaper, phone book, & bills, and moves head from side to side when reading • No apparent L visual field cut • Ambulates with a quad cane
	(Cognitive)	• Follows 1 and 2 step directions, but only after repetition, encouragement, and verbal and physical cues • MMSE score = 24
	(Affective)	• Expresses no interest in former activities, or learning compensatory strategies for independent dressing • Expresses doubts and fears about returning home alone • Hamilton score = 18
DIAGNOSTIC INFORMATION		R CVA, Major Depression, Macular Degeneration, Obesity, Hypertension

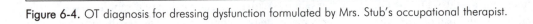

Figure 6-4. OT diagnosis for dressing dysfunction formulated by Mrs. Stub's occupational therapist.

World Health Organization Model's Negative Consequences of Pathology	World Health Organization Model Adapted to Reflect Positive Attributes	Occupational Performance Model
Handicap (non-fulfillment of societal roles)	Role fulfillment	Role performance
Disability	Ability	Occupational performance
Impairment	Skill	Performance components
Pathology	Health	—

Figure 6-5. Comparison chart of models used to organize occupational status data.

ments, disabilities, and handicaps are the immediate causes of the problems addressed by occupational therapists. To rephrase these concepts using the occupational performance model terminology, the consequences of a medical or psychiatric diagnosis can lead to dysfunctions in the occupational performance components, occupational performance, and occupational role (Figure 6-5) (Rogers & Holm, 1989, 1991). Rather than medical or psychiatric diagnoses, the three levels of occupational status should be used to explain occupational status dysfunctions, because they constitute the phenomenon influenced directly by occupational therapy interventions. Occupational therapists, for example, seek to manage low vision (i.e., impairment/performance component dysfunction) and difficulties in reading utility bills and cooking (i.e., disabilities/occupational performance dysfunction) caused by it, rather than the pathology of macular degeneration (i.e., medical diagnosis), which is appropriately treated by the ophthalmologist. Occupational status dysfunctions may be caused by environmental factors as well as impairments, disabilities, and handicaps. Hence, factors like architectural barriers and dependency-enhancing attitudes of caregivers may also be identified as explaining dysfunction.

A salient requirement of the occupational therapy diagnosis is that it be formulated in a manner that suggests interventions appropriate for managing the problem. A refined and detailed description of a clinical problem is pointless unless it helps to elucidate possible appropriate interventions. The explanatory and evidence parts of the statement are designed to serve this purpose. Based on the evidence, obvious appropriate interventions for Mrs. Stub's dressing dysfunction would focus on restoration of function, or compensation for the left hemiparesis that is the presumed cause of the performance problem. Restorative interventions would aim at improvements in LUE motor control and dexterity, and improved grasp and pinch strength, while compensatory interventions would seek to increase the skill and use of the right upper extremity and to provide a socially and physical-

ly supportive environment. In either case, progress would be determined by the extent to which problems in dressing performance are resolved. Although not as obvious, the occupational therapy diagnosis also suggests two other factors that must be accounted for in the intervention plan: possible cognitive impairment (i.e., needs cues to follow directions), and affective impairment (i.e., apathy). Interventions for Mrs. Stub's dressing dysfunction, using either restorative or compensatory strategies, may need to be adapted to address possible cognitive limitations. Additionally, if Mrs. Stub's apathy is of such magnitude that she is not motivated to dress herself, the therapist will have to adjust her approach to Mrs. Stub so that she can simultaneously be supportive and elicit Mrs. Stub's active participation in the OT interventions that will improve her occupational status.

The term *diagnosis* emphasizes the problematic aspects of a situation because if there is no occupational status dysfunction or risk for its development, there is no need for occupational therapy. When problems can be remediated, for example, motor control can be restored, memory retrained, or motivation revitalized, a problem-oriented diagnostic formulation is adequate for suggesting interventions. However, whenever full remediation is not possible and compensatory interventions need to be used, a client's strengths as well as deficits must be reflected in the problem formulation because the former may be useful in compensating for the latter (Rogers & Holm, 1989, 1991). The resources and limitations of a client's environment would be included in the identification of strengths and deficits. One limitation of the WHO model is that it focuses only on the negative consequences of pathology. The occupational performance model can be adapted to reflect the continuum of dysfunction to function. To complete the conceptual scheme in the WHO model, in Figure 6-5 we propose terminology that reflects clients' strengths as well. Thus, in regard to Mrs. Stub, the occupational therapy diagnostic evidence section includes data on Mrs. Stub's skills as well as impairments. The therapist might also supplement the diagnostic formulation with a prognostic statement like: "Mrs. Stub exhibits good rehabilitation potential as evidenced by her learning to dress her left hemiparetic extremity before her right normal extremity after one demonstration, and without additional instruction repeating the technique the following morning."

Unlike medical or psychiatric diagnoses, which remain the same regardless of the severity of the pathology, occupational therapy diagnoses may change over the course of intervention. As Mrs. Stub's dressing and bathing dysfunctions are alleviated, home management dysfunctions may be diagnosed. With another client, for example, the occupational therapy diagnosis of "(DE) At risk for contractures which could limit functional movements (EX) related to immobility and high flexor tone, (EV) as evidenced by flexor patterns in all joints (DI) due to comatose state associated with traumatic brain injury" changed to "(DE) Unable to assume or maintain a functional sitting position (EX) related to fluctuating tone and imbalance of strength in trunk musculature, (EV) with low tone on the R, high tone on the L, concave sitting posture to the L, (DI) following resolved coma associated with traumatic brain injury" as the client's medical and occupational performance status improve. As clients learn to perform easy tasks, progression to tasks of greater complexity becomes feasible, and the occupational therapy diagnosis changes accordingly.

OT Diagnostic Reasoning

Diagnostic reasoning, one component of clinical reasoning, refers to the cognitive operations used to formulate a diagnosis. When patients are not feeling well and go to a physician for help, they begin the appointment by relating their symptoms. Mr. Jem commented, for example, that he had severe pain in his back, a fever of 102 degrees, and chills so bad that he was shaking. Given these symptoms, the physician made a tentative diagnosis of kidney infection, ordered a urinalysis to confirm the tentative diagnosis, prescribed an antibiotic, and told the family to call if Mr. Jem's fever went higher or he was not better within 24 hours. The detailing of symptoms by the patient and the collection of laboratory data enabled the physician to describe and identify the medical problem. The pattern of signs and symptoms was meaningful to the physician because of the physician's medical knowledge. Recognizing (i.e., problem sensing) and naming (i.e., problem identification or diagnosing) the problem were pivotal steps leading to appropriate intervention (i.e., problem resolution).

This example is meant to illustrate that clinical problems do not define themselves. Rather, the diagnostician formulates them. The expertise of the diagnostician (i.e., physician, occupational therapist, physical therapist, nurse) is needed to select and acquire relevant data, organize it in a meaningful way, recognize and interpret patterns, and name the problems. The cognitive operations of selecting, acquiring, organizing, recognizing, interpreting, and naming are fundamental to diagnostic reasoning and support the interactive diagnostic processes of cue acquisition and hypothesis generation, refinement, and verification. These cognitive operations constitute the core of the information-processing model of diagnostic reasoning (Elstein & Bordage, 1988; Elstein, Shulman, & Sprafka, 1978, 1990). Although we will discuss them sequentially, they are interactive in the clinical context.

Diagnostic Reasoning: Cue Acquisition

For occupational therapists, the diagnostic process begins with the collection of data, or cues, about clients' occupational status. Cue acquisition includes the systematic collection and organization of client data. Decisions are made about the kind of data to collect (i.e., role performance; ADL, work, play/leisure performance; sensorimotor, cognitive, affective components), the extent of each kind of data to be collected, and the methods and tools to be used to collect the data. These data are then used by occupational therapists to construct clinical images or profiles of clients' occupational status that are sufficiently clear and detailed to yield accurate descriptions of their problems in the context of their life situations (Chapparo & Ranka, 1995; Rogers & Holm, 1989, 1991).

Types of Cues

Two types of assessment data about occupational status are generally acquired: subjective and objective. Subjective data, also called symptoms, are obtained directly from clients, or proxies (e.g., family members, advocates) if clients are unable to provide information. Subjective data represent clients' perceptions or beliefs about their occupational status. Responses to questions about the importance or value of independence in doing a task, the level of difficulty of task performance, the amount of pain experienced during task performance, the extent of fatigue that follows task performance, and recent changes in task performance are examples of subjective data. Objective data, also called signs, are obtained through direct observation and testing. Scores on standardized tests, like the Movement Assessment of Infants (Chandler, Andrews, & Swanson, 1980), the Miller Assessment for Preschoolers, (Miller, 1982), the Functional Independence Measure (FIM) (Uniform Data System for Medical Rehabilitation, 1993) and the Jebsen-Taylor Hand Function Test (Jebsen, Taylor, Trieschmann, Trotter, & Howard, 1969) are examples of objective data. Some data can be obtained through either subjective or objective means. For instance, therapists can ask clients if they are able to perform bathtub transfers or they can observe clients doing this. For other data, one method of data gathering may be impossible or impractical to implement. For example, although observation of dressing performance is feasible, the observation of recent changes in dressing performance is not generally feasible because it requires repeated observation over time. Hence, a history-taking interview using self-report would be the preferred data-gathering method for information about changes in occupational status. Concepts such as task-related values, pain or fatigue are also difficult to measure objectively.

Factors Impacting Cue Acquisition

Data gathering is not haphazard, but proceeds according to a plan. Some of the most important factors influencing the initial direction of the plan are: 1) client's medical or psychiatric condition; 2) referral question; 3) client's goals; 4) targeted discharge environment; 5) client's demographic characteristics; 6) clinical practice setting; 7) reimbursement; and 8) the therapist's frame of reference for practice. These factors provide shortcuts to diagnostic reasoning. Once they are called into play, they automatically bring to mind client images, realistic intervention timelines, and feasible frames of reference. The factors in turn limit or focus the search for data (Holm & Rogers, 1989; Rogers & Holm, 1989, 1991). They inherently define some data as clinically relevant and other data as clinically irrelevant. By narrowing the search for relevant clinical data, the process of information gathering is made more manageable and efficient.

Client's Diagnosis. A client's medical or psychiatric diagnosis provides a powerful tool for anticipating the influence of pathology on occupational status (Holm & Rogers, 1989; Rogers & Holm, 1991). Based on Mrs. Stub's diagnosis of R CVA, the occupational therapist anticipates problems in left upper extremity motor control and dexterity secondary to hemiparesis or hemiplegia, possible mobility deficits, and consequent problems in performing ADL, home management, and leisure activities. Similarly, her diagnosis of major depression suggests that apathy may prevent Mrs. Stub from using some of her retained task abilities and skills. Each of these diagnoses sets up a different clinical image and puts into motion a search for different data. The diagnosis itself may trigger use of a disease-based data collection protocol that outlines the most critical data to be collected for that diagnosis and may even specify the order in which these data are to be gathered. Past health problems may also play a role in the occupational therapy diagnosis.

Evidence suggests that pathology influences both data gathering and information processing. Rogers and Masagatani (1982) ascertained that diagnosis had such a powerful influence on clinical reasoning among occupational therapists that it overrode observable client cues. May and Dennis (1991) found that orthopedic physical therapists tended to use a receptive data-gathering style, marked by sus-

pending judgment until all data were gathered, while neurologic physical therapists preferred a perceptive data-gathering style, characterized by searching and responding to cues obtained from clients. In terms of information processing, the orthopedic therapists performed an ordered and systematic search for cues, while the neurologic therapists were more intuitive and considered alternative explanations simultaneously while keeping the total problem in mind.

The accuracy and richness of the information elicited from memory by a medical or psychiatric diagnosis is highly dependent on a therapist's knowledge of and experience with a particular diagnosis. The length of the experience, as well as the recency of the experience must be considered. Experience molds diagnostic impressions gleaned from textbooks into a continuum of occupational status dysfunctions associated with each diagnosis. These dysfunctional states may be qualified based on whether the diagnostic modifier is acute, chronic, severe, minimal, progressive, regressive, recurrent, exacerbation, remission, or intermittent. The memory image of clients with severe chronic rheumatoid arthritis would be quite different than that of clients with minimal involvement.

Reason for Referral. Referrals to occupational therapy may come from physicians but are also generated by other health care professionals or clients themselves. Typically, the referral sets minimum parameters for data acquisition (Holm & Rogers, 1989; Rogers & Holm, 1991). For example, Mrs. Stub's physiatrist referred her for physical assessment and treatment, her psychiatrist for coping skills, and her internist for problems in daily living activities. Thus, the data search was focused differentially as guided by the need to respond to the referral question. The search may be broadened as the pervasiveness of a client's problems in occupational status become apparent, but minimally it must cover the content suggested in the referral. An exception to this generalization is when, after consultation from the occupational therapist, the physician changes the focus of the referral.

Client's Goals. Unlike a medical diagnosis, for which a client's choices have no bearing on the diagnosis (e.g., I prefer a diagnosis of Lyme disease rather than arthritis), client's goals must be considered when formulating the occupational therapy diagnosis. Clients may have distinct preferences for the goals they wish to accomplish (e.g., toileting independence, self-feeding, using the telephone), as well as the sequence in which they wish to accomplish them. Moreover, clients may exclude goals that are common in rehabilitation, for example, dressing may be excluded because caregivers are planning to dress them. Once a client's goals are known, if there is a discrepancy between the client's goals and what can realistically be accomplished given the client's level of impairment and timeline for achieving the goals, the therapist and client must reach agreement on what is possible to achieve. After the therapist helps the client understand what can realistically be achieved, and the projected developmental sequence of accomplishments, the client and therapist collaborate in the setting of realistic target outcomes, and the data gathered will reflect the client's goals.

Targeted Discharge Environment. If the occupational therapy practice setting is inpatient, the question of discharge disposition becomes relevant to cue acquisition (i.e., to the type of data collected). If the client is a child, adolescent, or middle-aged adult who has severe impairments, and the family has the resources to manage the client's care at home, discharge from acute care might be to a rehabilitation center, and then to the home with continuing outpatient rehabilitation. Initial cue acquisition, therefore, would be for short-term intervention and to provide occupational status information to the rehabilitation facility staff. If clients are older adults, without family or kinship support, or financial resources for private care, the discharge environment may be to a nursing home. Because nursing home placement and associated costs are based on the level of care needed, cue acquisition would primarily focus on ADL and, perhaps, the special interests of clients, which could serve to motivate them to achieve more independence.

Client's Demographic Characteristics. Demographic characteristics are also important determinants of data selection and acquisition. Expectations for occupational performance change throughout the life span, based on developmental level as well as changes in the configuration of ADL, home management, work, and play/leisure activities associated with age level and role demands. Different information would be sought from a toddler with traumatic brain injury than from an adolescent with the same diagnosis. For example, it would be important to ascertain if the toddler could manage finger foods, extend arms and legs when being dressed, and manipulate building blocks to allow for play. It would be significant to know if the adolescent could manage utensils, don and doff upper and lower body clothing, use a pencil to complete a job application, and place a tape into and adjust a tape player. Like age, gender may also interact differentially with occupational status. Although tasks are not gender specific by nature, cultural norms have traditionally allocated some tasks by gender. Many men, for example, shy away from cooking, cleaning house, and doing the laundry, while many women avoid managing finances, changing oil in a car, or tacking down roof shingles. Recent cultural trends have tended to blur the distinction between tasks traditionally seen as men's or women's work, however, these impressions continue to be strong for many ethnic cultures, families, age levels, and clients, as well as for many occupational therapists.

Clinical Practice Setting. Occupational therapy clients may be seen in a variety of practice settings. These range from wellness (e.g., schools, stress management clinics,

developmental centers) to acute and chronic health care facilities (e.g., hospitals, outpatient clinics, home health), and encompass enhancing, restorative, preventive, remedial, and compensatory services. Each setting by virtue of its mission may dictate the parameters of occupational status that are to be managed in that setting. Acute rehabilitation facilities concentrate on impairments and their consequences for ADL, hand clinics highlight upper extremity dysfunction, and 13 school systems single out skills and behaviors that enable academic achievement.

Practice settings may also influence assessment decisions in more subtle ways. Use of the team approach in multidisciplinary settings may restrict the functional diagnoses seen in occupational therapy. Deficits in mobility, such as bed and toilet transfers, may be the sole purview of physical therapy in some settings. Similarly, restrictions on data gathering may be imposed by the resources that settings make available to therapists. If the Purdue Pegboard (Purdue Research Foundation, 1969) or a similar standardized tool is not available, therapists must come up with other means of measuring dexterity. If support has not been provided for the training necessary to administer the FIM or other assessment tools, the measures may be used incorrectly and test results may be invalid.

Reimbursement. A realistic plan for gathering data includes the client's health care coverage. If reimbursement for occupational therapy services includes a specific number of sessions, the plan for gathering data must be restricted to a reasonable proportion of those sessions to allow enough sessions for adequate intervention to occur. If the number of sessions is not restricted, but discharge is due to take place within a set number of days (e.g., acute care hospital), the data gathered must be restricted to that which will enable short-term intervention or help determine rehabilitation potential or future placement in the least restricted environment. Reimbursement sources may also establish the number of hours from admission that assessment data must be gathered and an intervention plan must be in place. Furthermore, some insurance coverage allocates a flat rate of reimbursement for a specific injury, impairment, or diagnosis which also impacts on the time that can be allocated for assessment (Holm & Rogers, 1989).

Therapist's Frame of Reference for Practice. Equally as significant as client and setting characteristics for selecting and acquiring client data are the characteristics of the information processor (i.e., the occupational therapist diagnostician). Although all occupational therapists meet the minimum educational standards for entry-level practice, each therapist approaches the diagnostic task with a unique repertoire of clinical experience, practice pattern preferences, professional values, and diagnostic expertise. It is unlikely that the therapist with a total caseload of clients with strokes will approach the assessment in the same manner as the therapist who rarely sees clients with strokes. During entry-level education, and more particularly during the initial years of practice, therapists organize didactic and experiential knowledge into a cognitive structure that is more directly usable in practice. One result of this knowledge organization is the development of a frame of reference for practice. This frame of reference includes the core concepts of occupational status as well as the relationships between these concepts. The occupational therapist's frame of reference, or conceptual structuring of the occupational therapy process, may also guide what data are selected and gathered (Holm & Rogers, 1989).

Cue Acquisition: General to Specific

The diagnosis, referral, goals of the client, discharge environment, client demographic characteristics, practice setting, reimbursement coverage, and therapist's frame of reference can expedite data gathering by providing ready-made parameters for the data to be gathered. Initially, data collection is general and moves to specifics. The therapist is trying to move from a vague clinical image of a client's occupational status to one that is more comprehensive and detailed. Thus, data acquisition quickly moves from a generic to a focused assessment, i.e., one where data gathering concentrates on information regarding a problem suspected by the therapist or noted by the client. For example, after Mrs. Stub indicated that she could feel her hand but could not move it the way she wanted, the therapist might perform a sensory evaluation to ascertain if Mrs. Stub was receiving and interpreting sensory input necessary for the motor control she desired.

Diagnostic Reasoning: Cue Analysis and Interpretation

During assessment a large amount of data are collected about a client. Some of these data are relevant to problem formulation and some are not. An occupational therapy diagnosis can only be as accurate as the data cues on which it is based. A flawless diagnostic reasoning process cannot correct for faulty data. Hence, a critical aspect of diagnostic reasoning is cue analysis. Cue analysis is a cognitive operation during which cues are checked for clarity, salience, completeness, reliability, and validity (Collier, McCash, & Bartram, 1996). During cue clarification, the meaning of cues is verified. For example, a client may state that she can bathe herself. By inquiring about the meaning of bathing to the client, however, the therapist may discover that "bathing" means "sponge bathing at the sink" because the client is unable or prefers not to use either the shower or bathtub. Determining the salience of cues involves appraising their significance to

the client database. As a personal care activity, bathing clearly fits within the parameters of occupational performance. If sponge bathing results in adequate cleansing of the body, bathing would be viewed as a performance ability rather than a disability. When cues are checked for completeness, the therapist questions whether more cues are needed to evaluate the significance of the data that are already available or respond to the reason for referral. In reference to bathing, for example, the therapist would want to know if this was accomplished safely as well as adequately and independently.

Cue Analysis: Reliability of Cues

Reliability of cues refers to the consistency of the collected cues (Holm & Rogers, 1989). Reliability evaluation can be approached in numerous ways (Collier et al., 1996). First, based on a client's physical and mental status, the therapist appraises the client's potential for being a reliable reporter. Clients who are lethargic, intoxicated, or demented may not be able to give accurate information about their occupational status; thus, data sources other than self-report would need to be used for data to be accurate. Second, the database is searched for inconsistencies. For example, a client might indicate that she lives alone in a six-room house, while her medical record indicates that she resides with her daughter and three grandchildren. These discrepancies would need to be clarified so that the context in which the client functions can be understood. Third, therapists use their clinical judgment to question the logical coherence of the cues. Hence, a therapist should question the presence of incontinence in a client with Alzheimer's disease who was still capable of independent dressing, because the incontinence is occurring out of the normal sequence of functional deterioration for this condition (Reisberg, Ferris, & Franssen, 1985), and is thus inconsistent with the clinical image for this client.

Cue Analysis: Validity of Cues

Cue validity refers to the extent to which a cue represents the concept that is being measured. For example, a diagnosis such as dressing dysfunction cannot be known directly because it is an abstract concept. Rather, the presence of a dressing dysfunction is inferred from cues such as the inability to don a cardigan or socks. Cue validation involves a confirmation or substantiation that the cue adequately reflects the concept; in other words, that donning a cardigan and socks is an adequate test of dressing ability. Methods of validation include obtaining multiple cues for the same concept (e.g., unable to don cardigan or socks on three occasions) and confirming data obtained from one data-gathering method with data obtained from a second method, as in checking self-report data with performance-based testing or self-report data with proxy-report data.

DIAGNOSTIC REASONING IN ACTION: CASE SCENARIO

Cue Acquisition: Initial Interview

After introducing herself and interacting with Mrs. Stub for several minutes, the SLTC therapist had gathered the following cues:

1. 76-year-old female, widowed, homemaker.
2. Mother of 2 daughters and 1 son, all living within 50 miles of client.
3. Grandparent of 4 grandchildren.
4. Has many friends in her apartment complex and doesn't believe she can continue to help the neighbor next door, who has Parkinson's disease.
5. Doesn't see how she can do her own cooking and laundry. Daughter has taken her grocery shopping every Sunday because she is having more trouble reading the labels. Daughter helps her carry groceries to her apartment. Doesn't think daughter can also cook and do laundry for her.
6. Doesn't see how she can play solitaire anymore.
7. Has been able to read the newspaper with her magnifying glass—likes to read the obituaries.
8. Can operate her radio — daughter brought it for her to have in her room.
9. Used to attend church with her son's family on Saturday evening, but had stopped going because it took too much effort.
10. When asked about problems with dressing, bathing, grooming, or oral hygiene, stated "I can't do anything."
11. "I have no interest in doing anything. I want to sleep all day."
12. "I know I can't even cook my grandchildren's favorite things anymore. I used to weigh 240 pounds, but I've lost 30 pounds over the last 3 months because I just wasn't interested in cooking anymore."

Cue Acquisition: Assessment

Based on the initial interview, the SLTC occupational therapist knew the occupational roles that Mrs. Stub had valued in the past, those that she could still accomplish, and those that she perceived she would no longer be able to fulfill. Based on the interview with Mrs. Stub and the data in the medical chart, the occupational therapist scheduled Mrs. Stub for two 2-hour assessment sessions. During these sessions she collected over 70 cues related to occupational status. The selection of cues to acquire was based on the client's valued roles, the abilities (i.e., ADL, home management, leisure) and skills (i.e., sensorimotor, cognitive, affective) necessary to

support those roles, the referral (i.e., evaluate and treat), and the targeted discharge environment (i.e., home).

Cue Analysis and Interpretation

To facilitate interpretation of cues acquired from the medical chart, the interview, and the assessment sessions, the therapist organized them into a meaningful cognitive structure. In Figure 6-6, we have clustered the cues concerning Mrs. Stub's performance under the concepts of occupational performance components, occupational performance, and occupational role. Cue clustering provides direction for focused cue acquisition and analysis. In reviewing Mrs. Stub's database (i.e., all cues/data specific to Mrs. Stub), the therapist might note that no data had been collected regarding the use of a shower or tub, grooming, or emergency telephone use. Hence, these data might be gathered next. Cue clustering also simplifies the database by arranging cues into meaningful units, or chunks, and reducing the number of items that one has to think about. For Mrs. Stub, the therapist arranged the cues under each occupational status concept. For example, under ADL, the 24 cues pertaining to specific tasks are arranged into five meaningful units. This process of arrangement, called chunking, facilitates thinking about the occupational status profile and identifying functional and dysfunctional patterns. For example, Mrs. Stub's cues in the ADL category suggest that upper extremity functions involving hand use at the front of the trunk or below the waist are intact, as long as they do not involve resistance (i.e., support hose) or finger manipulation (i.e., tying shoes), while those requiring hand use to the upper body (i.e., bra, overhead garment), excluding her mouth, are dysfunctional.

A second type of clustering interrelates cues to assist in exploring linkages between the DESCRIPTIVE and EXPLANATORY factors of the occupational therapy diagnostic statement. In regard to Mrs. Stub, a therapist might reason that donning and fastening shoes are related to obesity as evidenced by the inability to bend far enough at the waist to permit the hands to reach the feet. This rationale attributes the deficit in dressing to excess weight (i.e., restricted range of motion because of excess adipose tissue in the abdominal region) and in so doing uses a performance component dysfunction (restricted range of motion) to explain an occupational performance dysfunction (inability to reach, don, and tie shoes).

DIAGNOSTIC HYPOTHESIS GENERATION

From cue acquisition, diagnostic reasoning proceeds to hypothesis generation. Hypothesis generation is a cognitive operation familiar to all of us. As we go about our daily lives,

Occupational Performance Components

Sensorimotor

Left hemiparesis -- Fair+ mm. strength in L shoulder flexors/abductors/elevators, and upward rotators (Normal in R). Fair mm. strength in elbow flexors/ extensors, wrist flexors/ extensors (Normal in R).

Weak cylindrical grasp on L, Normal on R. L 3 point palmar pinch = 3 lb. (R = 8 lb) L Lateral pinch= 4 lb. (R = 9 lb)

Pt. uses a quad cane for ambulation. Pt. occasionally veers to the R.

Proprioception, light touch, deep pressure, hot/cold discrimination intact.

Pt. moves head from side to side when reading, and requires a magnifier for small print. No apparent L visual field cut.

Cognitive

Mini-Mental Status Examination (MMSE) score of 24, indicative of mild cognitive impairment.

Requires multiple verbal and physical cues to complete ADL tasks.

Affective

Hamilton Depression Scale (Hamilton) score of 18, indicative of a mild/moderate depression.

Pt. states "I have no interest in doing anything. I want to sleep all day."

When Pt. had difficulty manipulating fasteners during dressing, stated "I can't do anything."

Pt. states "I know I can't even cook my grandchildren's favorite things anymore."

Requires continuous encouragement to initiate tasks or conversations.

Occupational Performance

Activities of Daily Living (ADL)

Feeds self -- swallows solids and, manages utensils, cup, & glass without assistance.

Performs oral hygiene -- cleans teeth without assistance and dentures using a suctioned denture brush in the sink.

Performs toileting without assistance.

Dons underpants and slacks with loose elastic waistbands without assistance. Unable to don bra, overhead garments, fasteners, elastic stockings, or shoes without encouragement, verbal directions, manual guidance, or physical assistance.

Refuses to shower, bathes at the sink, but unable to adequately cleanse back, peroneal area, R shoulder, or feet without physical assistance.

Work/ Productivity/ Home Management

Pt. made soup, salad, and muffins, and cleaned up afterwards. Required continuous encouragement to continue the activity. Rechecked directions on can and box numerous times. Required physical assistance when opening the soup can and muffin box. Used magnifier to read directions.

Pt. used washer and dryer to launder clothes. Required continuous encouragement to initiate and complete the task. Verbal directions were provided about operation of the dials, and needed to be repeated X2.

Play/ Leisure

Refused to attempt Solitaire, even though this has been a favorite pastime.

Listened to a recording of a weather forecast, but was unable to repeat it, claiming "it didn't matter, because she wasn't going anywhere."

Occupational Roles

Family member roles
Parent [+]
Grandparent [-]
Friend [+]
Neighbor [-]

Self-carer/ Home-maintenance roles
Self-carer [-]
Cook [-]
Housekeeper [-]
Launderer [-]

Leisure roles
Game player (cards) [-]
Reader (newspaper) [+]
Reflector (listens to the radio) [+]

Organizational roles
Religious (attends church) [-]

[-] = Pt. anticipated problem fulfilling this role
[+]= Pt. did not anticipate problem fulfilling this role

Figure 6-6. Data cues acquired and organized by Mrs. Stub's occupational therapist in preparation for analysis, interpretation, and hypothesis generation.

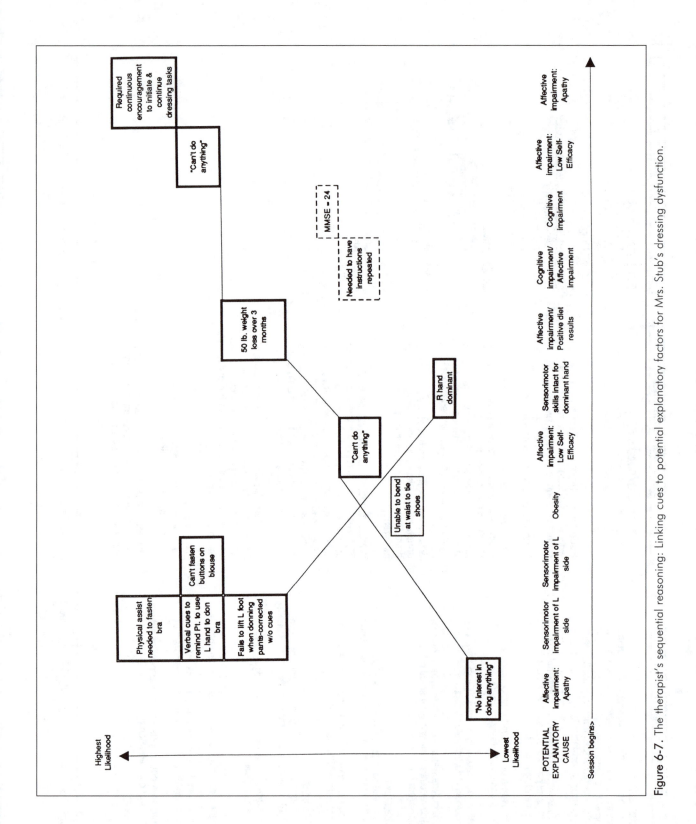

Figure 6-7. The therapist's sequential reasoning: Linking cues to potential explanatory factors for Mrs. Stub's dressing dysfunction.

we constantly develop ideas about how physical (e.g., tornadoes, floods) and social (e.g., outcome of presidential election) phenomena happen, how equipment (e.g., microcomputer) works, and how events will turn out (e.g., marriage of a friend, results of an anatomy test). *For example, an occupational therapy student was working with a nonverbal adult male client with developmental delay, who was being considered for transfer from a congregate care facility to a group home that required independence in ADL. As the student's supervisor observed the session, the student asked the client to demonstrate how he brushed his teeth each morning, using the new toothbrush and toothpaste placed on the sink. The client hung his head and then glanced furtively at the student supervisor several times. When the student asked the client if he needed assistance, the client shook his head from side to side, and looked again at the student supervisor, then hung his head — still making no attempt to initiate the task. Based on the cues, the student hypothesized that the client's failure to initiate the task was not a skill deficit, but an attention deficit — the client was distracted by the supervisor's observation of the process.* In clinical practice, hypothesis generation is used to structure clinical problems. By definition, a hypothesis is a tentative explanation of the nature of a clinical problem or situation. Hypotheses provide a conceptual framework for gathering, organizing, and interpreting clinical data (Elstein et al., 1978, 1990). They serve as guides for the clinical data that are relevant to acquire and for interpreting the significance of the data obtained. *To investigate his hypothesis, the student therapist asked the supervisor if she would mind leaving them alone for a few minutes until the task was completed. He reasoned that without the distraction of the supervisor, the client would attend to the task and demonstrate how he usually brushed his teeth. The client's response would affirm or reject the student's hypothesis and suggest the next steps in the assessment process.* Hypotheses provide a context, or frame, for clinical problem-solving. Their value lies in directing attention to some aspects of occupational status, and diverting it from others, so that sufficient data will be gathered to support, revise, or reject the hypothesis under consideration.

Hypotheses are generated early in the diagnostic process, often even before clients are seen by therapists, from data taken from medical records, conversations with other professionals, or referrals (Elstein et al., 1978, 1990). Cues are instrumental in formulating or evoking diagnostic hypotheses. The factors previously identified as expediting data collection (i.e., client's diagnosis, reason for referral, etc.) can also be used in the generation of hypotheses. Generally, hypotheses are derived from multiple rather than single cues. Predictions about occupational status dysfunction based on diagnosis and age, for example, are likely to be more accurate than those based on diagnosis or age alone. Sometimes cues are so internally consistent that one diagnostic hypothesis is sufficient. Usually this is not the case, however, and multiple hypotheses are offered and considered simultaneously. Initial diagnostic hypotheses reflect tentative inferences about occupational status dysfunction. They are likely explanations based on the assessment data.

DIAGNOSTIC REASONING IN ACTION: CASE SCENARIO

Simultaneous Consideration of Multiple Hypotheses

During the assessment session with Mrs. Stub, the therapist is trying to ascertain the reasons for her inability to dress herself (see cues on dressing in Figure 6-6) so that effective intervention can be planned. Critical elements of the therapist's sequential reasoning process on Mrs. Stub's dressing dysfunction are outlined in Figure 6-7. This figure portrays the collection and interpretation of cues, in the time sequence in which they were gathered, interpreted, weighted, and related to other cues. Although Mrs. Stub told the therapist during the initial interview that she had "no interest in doing anything," the therapist considered it a low likelihood that apathy could be a major cause of dressing dysfunction. Given Mrs. Stub's diagnosis of stroke, the sensory and motor impairments associated with her residual left hemiparesis emerged early as the causative factors. The following cues increased the likelihood that sensorimotor impairments were the explanatory cause: inability to don or fasten her bra, failure to lift the left foot when donning her slacks, inability to button the blouse, and the need for physical assists to continue task performance. Almost simultaneously, albeit at a lower level of likelihood, obesity is also considered. The therapist notes that Mrs. Stub becomes flushed as she leans over to don her shoes, and that she has difficulty reaching her feet because abdominal adipose tissue limits her range of motion in the trunk. When Mrs. Stub again repeats that she "can't do anything," after only her first try at reaching her shoes, apathy and low self-efficacy rise in likelihood as a negative influence on Mrs. Stub's motivation to independently dress herself. The therapist now sees this hypothesis as more likely than obesity, but less likely than sensorimotor impairment. Exploration of the most likely hypothesis, sensorimotor impairment, leads to the finding that Mrs. Stub is right-hand dominant. This cue reduces the likelihood of the sensorimotor hypothesis in the therapist's mind because the function of the hand used for skilled activity remains intact. The therapist finds support for an affective explanation for dressing dysfunction in the 50-pound weight loss, most of which occurred before her stroke. Additionally, although the need to have directions repeated is consistent with a cognitive impairment, as is an MMSE score of 24, both are also associated with depression and apathy. The continued insistence by Mrs. Stub that she "can't do anything" as well as the continuous encouragement that was needed for her to initiate and continue the dressing task further elevates the likelihood of apathy as an explanatory cause of her dressing dysfunction.

Thus, at this point, the therapist is entertaining four likely explanations of Mrs. Stub's dressing dysfunction: sensorimotor impairment, obesity, apathy and impaired self-efficacy, and cognitive impairment. As shown in Figure 6-7, as cues accumulate or are recalled, the likelihood of these early hypotheses rises and falls. The exact nature of the occupational performance dysfunction remains unclear, but the therapist has reasoned four possible hypotheses.

STRATEGIES FOR REFINING DIAGNOSTIC HYPOTHESES

As the diagnostic process continues to unfold, and assessment data accumulate, these early hypotheses are maintained, refined or discarded. *If the student's hypothesis about the presence of the supervisor interfering with task performance was accurate, then once the supervisor had left and the directions were repeated, the client would proceed with the oral hygiene task. If not, the student would be compelled to discard this hypothesis, put forth another explanation, and seek new cues.* To strengthen the diagnostic formulations, data acquisition becomes very focused with the intent of obtaining the cues that permit one to "rule in" or "rule out" each of the early hypotheses. The therapist reasons that if a client has a particular occupational status dysfunction, certain characteristics should be found and other characteristics should be absent. Diagnostic refinement involves interpreting new cues in the light of existing ones and examining all cues for their coherence. When new cues are consistent with a hypothesis, it remains credible and may be refined. When new cues are inconsistent with a hypothesis, it is abandoned, set aside for later consideration, or revised. New cues may also evoke new hypotheses. Hypothesis refinement then is a sequential, iterative process of cue acquisition and interpretation. It continues until one or more diagnostic hypotheses satisfactorily explain the available data (Elstein et al., 1978, 1990).

Because cue acquisition during hypothesis refinement follows no preordained pattern, it has been called unstructured problem-solving. Nonetheless, cue acquisition is guided by early hypotheses, and the efficiency of the diagnostic process depends on obtaining the data that are most likely to reduce diagnostic uncertainty. When cues are sought that are expected to support or enhance a hypothesis, this is called a confirmation data gathering strategy (Kassirer & Kopelman, 1991). When cues are sought that are expected to eliminate or reduce the plausibility of a hypothesis, that is called an elimination strategy (Kassirer & Kopelman, 1991). At the point where only a few hypotheses remain, a discrimination strategy may be employed, where the intent is to collect only those data that enable one to know which hypothesis provides the best clinical image (Kassirer & Kopelman, 1991).

As cues accumulate, the clinical image of a client's occupational status becomes more coherent and detailed. This image is compared to others stored in memory to provide further guidance for diagnosis and intervention, thus making the cognitive representation of an occupational status dysfunction in memory a critical element of diagnostic and clinical reasoning. Two fundamental theories about how new case profiles are compared to images in memory exist. One theory assumes that a new case is compared to a single, prototype model stored in memory. This prototype model evolves from clinical experience with clients having the same or similar performance problems. The prototype model is broad enough to encompass a vast range of problem manifestations (Bordage & Zacks, 1984; Elstein et al., 1990; Kassirer & Kopelman, 1991). The other theory holds that a new case is compared mentally to actual client cases recalled by the therapist. Accordingly, multiple cases are stored in memory for comparison with new cases. As therapists interact with new clients, they may find that a new client closely resembles a prior client. This resemblance entices therapists to think that the assessment and intervention approach used with the prior client would be equally appropriate for the present client. Rather than devising a new plan for the current client, the plan used with the client with similar characteristics is implemented (Fisher & Fonteyn, 1995).

DIAGNOSTIC REASONING IN ACTION: CASE SCENARIO

Refining the Diagnostic Hypothesis (OT Diagnosis)

In attempting to come to closure about the cause of Mrs. Stub's dressing dysfunction, the therapist reviews the cues supporting each of the four likely causes—sensorimotor impairment, obesity, apathy and impaired self-efficacy, and cognitive impairment. The therapist reasons that if Mrs. Stub was independent in dressing before her stroke, obesity could be eliminated as a cause of her dressing problems, because her recent 50-lb. weight loss should make dressing easier not harder. Mrs. Stub's ADL history reveals a premorbid rating of "independent" for dressing, leading the therapist to set aside the obesity hypothesis. In reviewing the cues suggestive of cognitive impairment, the therapist reasons that they could fit equally as well as evidence of depression, simultaneously raising the likelihood of the affective hypothesis and reducing that of cognitive impairment. Additional testing indicated that Mrs. Stub required only encouragement to complete a medication management task. Because medication management is among the first ADL tasks in which cognitive impairment is manifested, and Mrs. Stub completed this without instruction, the therapist gave further credence to the affective hypothesis. The therapist also reasons that if sensorimotor impairment is related to dressing dysfunction, then Mrs. Stub will have difficulty with bilateral tasks other than those involved in dressing. The therapist provides Mrs. Stub with the opportunity to perform cooking tasks and observes the anticipated bilateral skill dysfunction. Hence, both the affective and sensorimotor impairments remain viable alternatives.

DIAGNOSTIC VERIFICATION

The final step in diagnostic reasoning is to confirm the leading diagnostic hypothesis or hypotheses. Before an occupational therapy diagnosis can be accepted as the basis for intervention, it must be validated. The desired outcome of the diagnostic process is an accurate diagnosis. The ability to identify relevant cues is highly related to diagnostic certainty. Validation requires a final check on the coherence of all assessment data and of the congruence of the client's occupational status image with a known pattern of occupational status dysfunction consistent with biological and behavioral science. The therapist must then come to a conclusion about the adequacy and relevance of the evidence to decide if it is sufficient to accept a hypothesis as a basis for intervention.

Diagnostic reasoning, then, is a complex process comprised of multiple and diverse cognitive operations. In the process of performing these operations, therapists use *heuristics*. Heuristics are reasoning strategies, or shortcuts, that simplify complex cognitive tasks. Although the types of heuristics used by occupational therapists have not been identified, the following heuristics are employed by other clinical diagnosticians, specifically, physicians (Elstein et al., 1990; Kassirer & Kopelman, 1991) and nurses (Fisher & Fonteyn, 1995). Prior to cue acquisition, a commonly used heuristic is listing, or using a mental list to take a cognitive inventory of available and needed data. During the data gathering process focused questioning, or the asking of clarifying questions, helps the interviewer to obtain richer details about occupational status. Pattern recognition occurs, as data are acquired, or when generating or verifying hypotheses. Pattern recognition, or the identification of relationships among data that are similar or different from other clients or typical impairment and disabil-

ity patterns, can be helpful in directing further cue acquisition (Robertson, 1996). Similar to pattern recognition, representativeness is a heuristic that leads to assessment and intervention strategies for a client based on that client's likeness to a well-defined clinical entity, such as all previous clients treated who had a diagnosis of R CVA. Attending describes the process of selecting the most relevant cues from all available data about a client, and anchoring is a shortcut used to project future status from initial clinical data, enabling the relevance of newly acquired cues to be checked against projected outcomes. Heuristics are particularly useful when therapists are reasoning about dysfunctions in occupational status with which they are highly familiar. Although heuristics are useful for facilitating efficient reasoning, they can result in reasoning errors and biases, specifically because they are shortcuts.

DIAGNOSTIC REASONING IN ACTION: CASE SCENARIO

Diagnostic Verification

The SLTC occupational therapist retains and combines the two alternative explanations of Mrs. Stub's dressing dysfunction into one OT diagnosis (see Figure 6-4). The interaction of apathy and the impairments associated with her left hemiparesis can account for all problems observed during dressing. Because dressing had been an automatic task prior to her stroke, it is all the more frustrating for Mrs. Stub. Likewise, unlike the cooking that gives her and her family pleasure, there is no inherent pleasure in dressing. The OT diagnosis therefore suggests a combination of restorative neuromotor interventions and adaptive/compensatory strategies. Concomitantly, it suggests the need for task simplification, such as organizing all clothing to be put on each morning onto a single hanger, and thus reducing the decisions associated with dressing, as well as the need for motivational strategies such as arranging participation in social activities with her grandchildren so that Mrs. Stub has a reason for wanting to get dressed. If the target outcome of independence in dressing is met, the accuracy of the OT diagnosis is verified again. If not, then the therapist must consider common errors in diagnostic reasoning, make adjustments accordingly, and generate other hypotheses, or revise the intervention strategies.

ERRORS IN DIAGNOSTIC REASONING

Errors may occur at any point in the diagnostic process. The most frequent errors are discussed below along with suggestions for preventing their occurrence.

Cue Acquisition: Too Little or Too Much

When insufficient data are collected, the diagnostician may fail to recognize the presence of a problem or the causal factors. The use of assessment protocols that outline the parameters of concern to occupational therapy practice are helpful for preventing this type of error, because they encourage the therapist to screen occupational status broadly. The collection of too much data, especially if it is unfocused and disorganized, may result in confusion rather than improved diagnostic accuracy. Interestingly, Elstein, Shulman, and Sprafka (1978) found that the comprehensiveness of data gathering and the accuracy of data interpretation were not related. Hence, more data does not necessary result in a more accurate problem statement or diagnosis. To avoid this source of error, diagnosticians should consciously decide what data are needed early in the diagnostic process. More importantly, they should determine the relevance of data "on-line," that is, as it is gathered, rather than waiting until all data are collected before actively thinking about its meaning.

Inaccurate Interpretation of Cues

Data may be misinterpreted by failing to recognize their significance to problem formulation at all, or by clustering cues under the wrong problems. Searching for cues consistent with a prototype model, reference case, or classic textbook case, and matching cues to these, are methods of reducing cue misinterpretation.

Failure to Generate and Refine Multiple Hypotheses

As we have seen, hypotheses guide both data collection and interpretation. The risk in failing to generate multiple hypotheses is that unless the initial hypothesis is accurate, significant data about occupational status will not be collected, and hence cannot influence the client image or diagnostic formulation. *For example, by adhering to the "attention deficit—supervisor as a distractor" hypothesis, the student therapist neglected to ascertain if his nonverbal client had any teeth to brush—which he did not!* This error is sometimes referred to as premature closure and it can be prevented by considering multiple diagnostic hypotheses concurrently. Using a fixed or standardized data-gathering protocol, such as the Occupational Therapy Uniform Evaluation Checklist (Terminology Task Force, 1994), or OT Fact (Smith, 1993) assists in generating hypotheses because they cover the boundaries of occupational therapy practice.

Favoring a Confirmatory Strategy

The adaptive value of hypotheses use lies in the guidance they provide for structuring and limiting data gathering.

Nonetheless, hypotheses are conceptual biases. In refining and testing hypotheses, therapists have a tendency to overemphasize the significance of confirmatory evidence and discount the significance of negative evidence (Sober, 1979). The net effect of this tendency is that salient data may not enter the problem formulation and an erroneous hypothesis may be confirmed. To correct this error, evidence that rejects hypotheses should be sought as rigorously as evidence that supports them.

EXPERT-NOVICE DIFFERENCES IN DIAGNOSTIC REASONING

Differences are known in the way in which expert therapists and novice therapists, including students, implement diagnostic reasoning. Compared to novices, expert therapists derive more meaning from fewer cues and are able to more readily detect significant relationships between cues as well as patterns among them. Novices have difficulty sorting relevant from irrelevant data, and hence are prone to give equal emphasis to all data (Benner & Wrubel, 1982; Kari & Kalscheur, 1989). Although the use of hypothesis testing itself does not distinguish experts from novices, experts do generate hypotheses earlier in the diagnostic process. Experts then proceed to test these hypotheses with cues from the client database or newly obtained cues, whereas novices often adhere to a routinized, non-hypothesis-specific-data gathering strategy. In other words, experts conjure up a more effective inquiry strategy that enables them to focus more expeditiously on the occupational status dysfunction. Interestingly, neither experts nor novices use the approach typically taught in school of refraining from interpreting data until all data are available (Elstein et al., 1978).

In large part, these differences in diagnostic reasoning between experts and novices can be attributed to clinical experience. With experience, it becomes easier to recognize critical cues and cue patterns and generate and validate hypotheses. For experts, hypotheses emerge essentially automatically in the context of a rich network of memory associations involving knowledge application. The knowledge base of experts is more extensive, more interrelated, and more highly organized, typically in hierarchical structures, than that of novices (Barrows & Feltovich, 1987; Elstein et al., 1990). Experience with numerous clients, with each client manifesting an image of occupational status that is at the same time unique and yet similar to prior clients, produces an enriched prototype or cadre of specific cases, for comparison with new cases. Detection of similarity between new cases and stored cases, in a process called *pattern recognition*, expedites the reasoning process because it fosters direct, automatic retrieval of stored information (Barrows & Feltovich, 1987; Elstein, Shulman, & Sprafka,

1990). In addition to structuring the knowledge base, experience provides practice in knowledge application so that heuristics (i.e., reasoning strategies) can be applied with facility. Novices, lacking this base of clinical experience, are constantly confronted with unfamiliar client problems that are outside of their range of experience. Until clinical experience accumulates, they are forced to rely on book knowledge and less automatic decision-making (Neistadt, 1987).

Expertise, then, lies in both the richness of a therapist's knowledge base and the skill in accessing and using this knowledge in caring for clients. It develops from intensive experience with certain types of occupational status dysfunctions. Hence, therapists may be both experts and novices depending on their experience with the particular occupational status dysfunction presented by a client. When a therapist is confronted with a familiar client problem, diagnostic reasoning takes place very rapidly and almost automatically. In this case, it closely approximates pattern recognition. However, when a therapist is confronted with an unfamiliar or particularly difficult client problem, diagnostic reasoning more closely follows hypothesis testing (Barrows & Feltovich, 1987; Elstein et al., 1990).

Techniques for improving diagnostic reasoning are of interest to all therapists so that they may become more effective managers of client problems. To build diagnostic skill, therapists, regardless of their experience level, should "call-to-mind" their reasoning processes and critically reflect on them. Observation of experts, which includes opportunity for the experts to share their reasoning with novices, is an excellent way to discover clinical expertise. Also beneficial is consulting with colleagues and having them evaluate diagnostic statements and the reasoning processes used to construct them.

SUMMARY

The effectiveness of occupational therapy interventions is dependent on the accuracy of the OT diagnosis. If the problem in occupational status dysfunction is unclear, hypothesized causal factors are inaccurate, or supporting evidence is lacking or uninterpretable, decisions about occupational therapy interventions will be based on faulty data. Diagnostic reasoning, however, is an uncertain process. Requiring the therapist to proceed based on educated and experience-based inferences. The aim of this chapter was to foster an understanding of the structure of an OT diagnosis, and the cognitive operations occupational therapists perform when formulating it, as a means of decreasing the uncertainty. Diagnostic reasoning, hypothesis generation, strategies for refining diagnostic hypotheses, and diagnostic verification were presented with an accompanying case scenario

from clinical practice. Common errors in diagnostic reasoning were also explained, along with strategies to avoid them. Finally, expert-novice differences in diagnostic reasoning were discussed. While the diagnostic reasoning process may seem laborious at first, with practice and experience the cognitive operations become more efficient and accurate, thus increasing the accuracy of decisions about occupational therapy interventions.

STUDY QUESTIONS

1. How are diagnostic reasoning and clinical reasoning related?

2. What is the relationship between an OT diagnosis and an intervention plan?

3. Which factors that impact diagnostic reasoning can be influenced by the occupational therapist, and how?

4. What strategies can be used to prevent errors in diagnostic reasoning?

5. Using the evidence available to Mrs. Stub's therapist, structure a diagnostic statement and compare it to the one formulated by the authors. Are there differences? Are there similarities? Would the diagnostic statement result in a similar intervention plan for Mrs. Stub?

RECOMMENDED READINGS

Higgs, J., & Jones, M. (Eds.). (1995). *Clinical reasoning in the health professions*. Oxford, England: Butterworth-Heinemann.

REFERENCES

American Occupational Therapy Association. (1994a). Standards of practice for occupational therapy. *American Journal of Occupational Therapy, 48,* 1039-1043.

American Occupational Therapy Association. (1994b). Uniform terminology for occupational therapy (3rd ed.). *American Journal of Occupational Therapy, 48,* 1047-1054.

American Psychiatric Association. (1994). *Diagnostic and statistical manual of mental disorders* (4th ed.). Washington, DC: Author.

Barrows, H. S., & Feltovich, P. J. (1987). The clinical reasoning process. *Medical Education, 21,* 86-91.

Benner, P., & Wrubel, J. (1982). Clinical knowledge development: The value of perceptual awareness. *Nurse Educator, 7,* 11-17.

Bordage, G., & Zacks, R. (1984). The structure of medical knowledge in the memories of medical students and general practitioners: Categories and prototypes. *Medical Education, 18,* 406-416.

Chandler, L. S., Andrews, M. S., & Swanson, M. W. (1980).

Movement assessment of infants. Rolling Bay, WA: Infant Movement Research.

Chapparo, C., & Ranka, J. (1995). Clinical reasoning in occupational therapy. In J. Higgs & M. Jones (Eds.), *Clinical reasoning in the health professions.* Oxford, England: Butterworth-Heinemann.

Collier, I. C., McCash, K. E., & Bartram, J. M. (1996). *Writing nursing diagnoses: A critical thinking approach.* St. Louis: Mosby.

Doenges, M. E., Moorhouse, M. F., & Burley, J. T. (1995). *Application of nursing process and nursing diagnosis: An interactive text for diagnostic reasoning.* Philadelphia: F. A. Davis.

Driessen, M., Dekker, J., Lankhorst, G. J., & van der Zee, J. (1995). Inter-rater and intra-rater reliability of the occupational therapy diagnosis. *Occupational Therapy Journal of Research, 15,* 259-273.

Elstein, A. S., & Bordage, G. (1988). Psychology of reasoning. In J. Dowie & A. Elstein (Eds.), *Professional judgment: A reader in clinical decision making.* Cambridge, MA: Harvard University Press.

Elstein, A. S., Shulman, L. S., & Sprafka, S. A. (1978). *Medical problem solving: An analysis of clinical reasoning.* Cambridge, MA: Harvard University Press.

Elstein, A. S., Shulman, L. S., & Sprafka, S. A. (1990). Medical problem solving: A ten-year retrospect. *Evaluation & the Health Professions, 13,* 5-36.

Fisher, A., & Fonteyn, M. (1995). An exploration of an innovative methodological approach for examining nurses' heuristic use in clinical practice. *Scholarly Inquiry for Nursing Practice: An International Journal, 9*(3), 263-276.

Holm, M. B., & Rogers, J. C. (1989). The therapist's thinking behind functional assessment, II. In C. Royeen (Ed.), *Assessment of function: An action guide.* Rockville, MD: American Occupational Therapy Association.

Jebsen, R. H., Taylor, N., Trieschmann, R. B., Trotter, M. J., & Howard, L. A. (1969). An objective and standardized test of hand function. *Archives of Physical Medicine and Rehabilitation, 50,* 311-319.

Kari, N., & Kalscheur, J. (1989). *Clinical decision making: An educational model.* Paper presented at the annual meeting of the American Occupational Therapy Association. Baltimore, MD.

Kassirer, J. P., & Kopelman, R. I. (1991). *Learning clinical reasoning.* Baltimore, MD: Williams & Wilkins.

May, B. J., & Dennis, J. K. (1991). Expert decision making in physical therapy: A survey of practitioners. *Physical Therapy, 71,* 190-202.

Miller, L. J. (1982). *Miller assessment for preschoolers.* Littleton, CO: Foundation for Knowledge in Development.

Neistadt, M. E. (1987). Classroom as clinic: A model for teaching clinical reasoning in occupational therapy education. *American Journal of Occupational Therapy, 41,* 631-637.

Purdue Research Foundation. (1969). *Purdue pegboard.* Chicago, IL: Science Research Associates, Inc.

Reisberg, B., Ferris, S. H., & Franssen, E. (1985). An ordinal assessment tool for Alzheimer's-type dementia. *Hospital & Community Psychiatry, 36,* 593-595.

Robertson, L. J. (1996). Clinical reasoning, part 1: The nature of problem solving, a literature review. *British Journal of Occupational Therapy, 59*(4),178-182.

Rogers, J. C., & Holm, M. B. (1989). The therapist's thinking behind functional assessment, I. In C. Royeen (Ed.), *Assessment of function: An action guide.* Rockville, MD: American Occupational Therapy Association.

Rogers, J. C., & Holm, M. B. (1991) Occupational therapy diagnostic reasoning: A component of clinical reasoning. *American Journal of Occupational Therapy, 45,* 1045-1053.

Rogers, J. C., & Masagatani, G. (1982). Clinical reasoning of occupational therapists during the initial assessment of physically disabled patients. *Occupational Therapy Journal of Research, 2,* 195-219.

Smith, R. O. (1993). Computer-assisted functional assessment and documentation. *American Journal of Occupational Therapy, 47,* 988-992.

Sober, E. (1979). The art of science of clinical judgment: An informational approach. In H. T. Engelhardt, S. F. Spicker, & B. Towers (Eds.), *Clinical judgment: A critical appraisal* (pp. 29-44). Dordrecht, Holland: D. Reidel Publishing Co.

Terminology Task Force. (1994). Uniform terminology (3rd ed.). Application to practice. *American Journal of Occupational Therapy, 48,* 1055-1059.

Uniform Data System for Medical Rehabilitation. (1993). *Guide for the Uniform Data Set for Medical Rehabilitation (Adult FIM)* Version 4.0. Buffalo, NY: Author.

World Health Organization. (1980). *International classification of impairments, disabilities, and handicaps.* Geneva: Author.

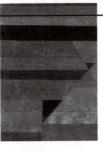

CHAPTER CONTENT OUTLINE

ABSTRACT

Clinical reasoning forms the basis of clinical practice. The therapist's confidence is based on his or her knowledge and is important in reducing uncertainty and ensuring that clinical decisions are defensible and can be clearly articulated. The nature of clinical reasoning in occupational therapy practice is explained. This is contrasted with the biomedical model of practice which has been the dominant model of practice in the health care setting. Clinical reasoning is broken down into its various subcomponents and discussed in terms of interdependent primary abilities such as knowledge, adult cognition and metacognition. This analysis is intended to show how a variety of factors can shape the reasoning strategies selected by a therapist in attempting to sense, understand and treat client problems. The chapter concludes with strategies that are designed to facilitate critical analysis and reflection.

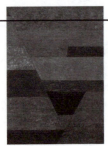

KEY TERMS

Clinical reasoning	Metacognition
Knowledge	Hypothesis
Cognition	Functional performance

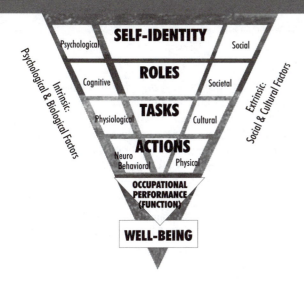

CHAPTER 7

Clinical Reasoning

Informed Decision Making for Practice

Catherine E. Bridge, BAppSc, MCogSc, Robyn L. Twible, Dip OT, MA

OBJECTIVES

The information in this chapter is intended to help the reader:

1. explain clinical reasoning

2. know why knowledge about theory is important for occupational therapy clinical reasoning in practice

3. understand classifications and terminology relating to reasoning content and process

4. identify the roles of knowledge, cognition and metacognition in expertise and clinical reasoning

5. identify the role of cues, context, task and skill in determining outcome

6. discuss the impact of personal values and beliefs on practice

7. view the clinical reasoning process via the use of selected case studies.

"They know enough who know how to learn."
Henry Brooks Adams, 1907 (*The Education of Henry Adams*)

INTRODUCTION

Clinical reasoning underpins all client-related thinking and decision-making in occupational therapy. From the moment a client is referred through all the treatment phases to the termination of intervention, the clinician is faced with a plethora of problem-solving and reasoning tasks. Professional practice demands that this cognitive ability is undertaken in a competent and defensible manner (Higgs & Jones, 1995a). Our knowledge of clinical reasoning and how it works, how we research and teach it, is still in its infancy.

The idea that clinical reasoning can be taught rests on two key assumptions: firstly, that clinical experiences are regular and repeatable enough that one can learn from experience, and secondly, that these regularities can be distinguished from random events and expressed in an understandable form (Harris, 1993). The terminology is new, but the attempt to both capture and teach regularities goes back to the beginnings of occupational therapy practice. Two approaches need to be considered in understanding and communicating how clinical reasoning occurs. The first is a content-oriented approach which relates to the idea that knowledge and reasoning are interdependent; the second is a process-oriented approach where the focus is on the nature of clinical reasoning and the development of expertise—in other words reasoning styles and stages. Both approaches are important in understanding and facilitating competent practice (Fonteyn, 1995; Higgs & Jones, 1995b).

Occupational therapists assess problems that are complex and not clearly delineated. The reasoning skills required of competent clinicians are dependent on well-developed critical and analytical reasoning abilities. The development of analytical reasoning skills as a means of improving clinical decision-making has been advocated by many sources (Barrows & Pickell, 1991; Fonteyn, 1995; Kassirer & Kopelman, 1991). Analytical skills can be developed by provision of guidelines, tool development and contextualisation using case studies. Assisting learners to use reasoning tools in a supportive and reflective environment is necessary for learners to make the cognitive shift from basic dualism (right versus wrong) to a more flexible, postformal cognitive stance in which it is legitimate to acknowledge uncertainty and to describe and reflect on differences.

The process of clinical reasoning is associated with, but different from, the notion of the occupational therapy treatment process, the series of steps that are advocated as part of the client-therapist interaction. These generic steps are part of the problem-oriented process model (Christiansen, 1991) and are referred to in all teaching programs and in evaluations of practice (Australian Association of Occupational Therapists, 1992). These steps provide a linear framework for action but are not reflected by reasoning in practice which is clearly not a linear process (Barris, 1987; Fleming, 1994; Mattingly, 1991; Mattingly & Fleming, 1994). Thus when discussing clinical reasoning it is important to be aware of the factors that shape the process and determine the reasoning processes that have been used. The reasoning processes are themselves not unique to occupational therapy practice but reflect adult cognitive development, which in turn is shaped by occupational therapy knowledge and the development of occupational therapy expertise. It is the knowledge and expertise that are unique to occupational therapy practice and determine the orientation to problem-solving and decision-making that are characteristic of occupational therapy practice.

ALTERNATIVE PERSPECTIVES AND DEFINITIONS

Clinical Reasoning

In examining both the content and process of clinical reasoning it is important to recognise that a number of definitions exist in clinical reasoning and occupational therapy literature. Some of the similarities and differences are highlighted to help the learner understand the implications for practice. For example, Cohn describes clinical reasoning as "a complex process dependent upon years of experience" (Cohn, 1989, p. 241). Inherent in this description are two key notions: 1) that expertise is associated with clinical experiences over time, and 2) that it is a complex process.

In describing the process, Cohn goes on to say that it is "based on our knowledge of procedures, interaction with patients, and interpretation and analysis of the evolving situation" (Cohn, 1989, p. 241). This implies that clinical reasoning is knowledge dependent and that relevant knowledge includes interviewing and facilitation skills. The fact that knowledge is divided into procedures and skills is also important. Implicit in this is the neuropsychological distinction between declarative and procedural knowledge; declarative knowledge being the "know that" aspect (i.e., knowledge of procedures) versus procedural knowledge which is the "know how" or skill component. The last part of Cohn's definition relates to the idea of conscious cognitive processes and our ability to reflect on them (i.e., metacognition).

A slightly different but fundamentally similar definition by Higgs defines clinical reasoning as "the process of using thinking, interpersonal and clinical skills and knowledge in

Bibliographic citation of this chapter: Bridge, C., & Twible, R. (1997). Clinical reasoning: Informed decision making for practice. In C. Christiansen & C. Baum (Eds.), *Occupational therapy: Enabling function and well-being* (2nd ed.). Thorofare, NJ: SLACK Incorporated.

order to acquire, evaluate and make sense of the mass of clinical information available to the health carer during interactions with clients" (Higgs, 1990, p. 13). Similarities are in terms of the value placed on knowledge and the declarative and procedural distinction. However, there are two additional notions of importance in this definition. Firstly, there is a clearer emphasis on the problem-oriented process model as indicated by the words "acquire" and "evaluate." Secondly, there is specific emphasis on making sense of clinical information. This is an important notion which directly relates to the underlying cognitive abilities that allow us to encode and organise our knowledge so we can filter out "noise" and interpret salient clinical cues.

Barris's definition, on the other hand, is fundamentally different. Barris defines clinical reasoning as a phenomena that "is elusive because it is an ongoing, interactive process of decision making, involving art, science and ethics, and because it is private — individuals rarely voice the steps they follow during decision making" (Barris, 1987, p. 148). The focus here is on the nature of the reasoning process, aspects of which imply both a non-linear and a tacit process. In fact, it is characteristic of the development of clinical expertise that as skills become automatic, the ability to verbalise about them is also increasingly difficult. Demonstrating ability but being unable to verbalise it is a phenomenon indicative of tacit knowledge structures. In this case, the word "tacit" just means knowledge that is not accessible to conscious introspective processes.

Unlike the two earlier definitions, knowledge is not referred to directly. Instead Barris includes similar terminology to that of Rogers in that explicit reference is made to science, ethics and art (Rogers, 1983). When Rogers originally introduced these terms to discussion of clinical reasoning, they were presented as entwined strands that filtered and influenced clinical understanding. The notion of knowledge is implicit in all three aspects, but the emphasis is not on a procedural or declarative distinction, but on the development of a personal and individual viewpoint that is situated in an environmental context. In other words, our ability to perform as clinical reasoners cannot be viewed outside a person-environment framework. Reasoning performance is determined by our need to meet environmental or work-related demands which are determined by physical, cultural and social contexts. Traditionally, scientific reasoning is often equated to logical problem-solving and reasoning abilities and is typical of the approach which underpins the biomedical model. Ethics relates to moral reasoning, which is both socially and culturally embedded, while art refers to how the processes of science and ethical reasoning come together and how complexity and uncertainty are managed.

Occupational Therapy versus Biomedical Practice

Occupational therapy problem-solving can be conceived of as ill-structured (not clearly delineated) in that the nature of the problem, intermediate steps and goal state are often unknown at the referral and initial interview stages. The problem space becomes defined through the process of assessment, intervention, and evaluation. The nature of the problem and thus the potential occupational goals only unfold as the client-therapist interaction develops. The problem space itself is a search for meaningful roles and role disruptions. This search is conducted in terms of a client's ability to undertake the activities and tasks that underpin successful role performance. Moreover, the search is framed in terms of environmental considerations (i.e., physical, social and cultural factors) and client-determined notions of acceptable role balance.

The fact that acceptable role balance can only be client determined is a crucial factor because it means that in occupational therapy interventions the client needs to be included in the decision-making process. Definition of the goal state thus involves mutual participation in decision-making between the client and the occupational therapist. Some would argue that this mutual participation in decision-making is not characteristic of biomedical practice, which tends towards either an active-passive or guidance cooperation continuum (Thomas, Wearing, & Bennett, 1991). In fact, mutual participation in decision-making is dependent on a shared knowledge base. In Australia, a study conducted by the law reform commission of Victoria revealed that 47% of doctors indicated that they would withhold information about risks of treatment from clients under certain circumstances (Thomas et al., 1991). This implies that the biomedical practitioner holds two basic beliefs about client involvement in decision making. Firstly, clients sometimes will not make "good" decisions. Secondly, knowledge of treatment implications may be harmful to some clients. What is important here is not whether these beliefs are valid, but how they affect the reasoning process and level of client involvement.

Biomedical reasoning is also in a sense ill-structured, but unlike occupational therapy it is centred around a medical diagnosis (Elstein, 1995). In other words, the biomedical goal is to isolate the malfunctioning body part and link this to a causal explanation. In this sense a biomedical diagnosis involves knowledge of clinical signs and symptoms. The reasoning process in biomedical terms has been characterised as a hypothetical-deductive one (Elstein, Shulman & Spafka, 1978). The notion of hypothetical-deductive thinking is a combination of both inductive and deductive reasoning and is typical of but not unique to medicine. Indeed in clinical reasoning studies undertaken in occupational therapy it was

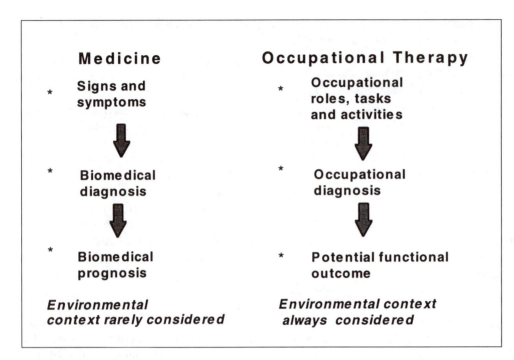

identified as part of routine diagnostic reasoning (Mattingly 1991; Rogers, 1982). Fleming labelled this process *procedural reasoning* to indicate it was only one of several reasoning processes used by occupational therapists, unlike biomedical practice where it is the dominant mode of clinical reasoning (Fleming, 1991a; 1991b).

Other key differences between biomedical and occupational reasoning relate to differences in the knowledge bases between the two professions and the nature of the inquiry undertaken. Both professions share some basic science, social science and anatomical knowledge, but the scope, depth and emphasis in terms of this knowledge are fundamentally different. The biomedical approach is a reductionistic one where the reasoning is bottom up, and its emphasis is on the identification of dysfunctional body parts in terms of abnormalities of structure. Viewing the body as a set of interrelating parts is a reductionistic viewpoint, and as such is characteristic of biomedical practice reasoning (Christiansen, 1991).

In contrast, the reasoning process in occupational therapy is holistic and top down. Meaningful roles are identified and only then are the tasks and activities that underpin them examined. Performance components or body parts are examined only as appropriate, and always in relation to the tasks and activities that they enable. Figure 7-1 provides an overview of the differences and similarities between medicine and occupational therapy.

Treating the Person as a Whole

Part of the rhetoric of occupational therapy practice is the notion of holism and holistic practice. Reductionism, as we have seen, is characteristic of biomedical practice and can be seen to equal a mechanistic view of body, but holism does not equate to a single part. The very essence of the notion of holism is the combination of mind and body, not a dichotomy between the two.

Many people have conceptual difficulty grasping the concept of holism. In holistic terms, a person is greater than and different from the sum of his or her parts. The "whole" person is a result of a mixture and interaction between *all* of the parts (i.e., body and mind). A good analogy is cake baking (Corcoran & Tanner, 1988). A cake can be conceived of as being composed of a number of parts (i.e., flour, sugar, leavening agent, etc.) but in the process of baking these parts are heated and combined. As a result, you cannot retrieve individual ingredients because they have been transformed. Examination of one of the ingredients or cake parts, such as the quality of the flour, will help predict the texture of the cake. However, as only one part, it cannot indicate the overall quality of the cake. In human terms, occupational roles can also be thought of as being composed of a number of parts. Like the cake, they are greater than the sum of their parts, exactly because they rely on a mixture of parts that dynamically interact in an interdependent way. For instance, a client with peripheral neuropathy will continue to be independent in self-maintenance as long as he or she can compensate for tactile deficits by visual and cognitive means.

A holistic viewpoint includes reduction, i.e., reduction in terms of examination of parts is a subset or component of the higher order concept of holism. This means that holism can be applied in most or all of the same contexts as reductionism. However, reductionism cannot be applied to explain the overall quality of a role or a person.

Occupational therapists do indeed attempt to define problem spaces and implement interventions within a framework where consideration is given to all aspects of the whole person. One way this is done is considering a client's role performance in terms of its environmental context (Rogers, 1983). Areas of interest to occupational therapists that commonly appear in the literature as reported by Denton (1987, p. 44) are:

- Living situation and responsibilities
- Self-care and personal hygiene
- Work
- Play and leisure
- Self-esteem and self-concept
- Self-expression and self-control
- Cognitive functioning
- Situational coping
- Neuromuscular functioning
- Sensory integration
- Interpersonal relationships
- Environmental constraints and resources.

Denton makes it clear that assessment of each of these areas would generate more data than could be used, so boundaries are drawn by the selection of a theoretical basis that organises areas in the domain of concern in different ways.

HOW DO I MAKE SENSE OF ALL THE DATA?

The novice or student reasoner is confronted with the problem of taking an ill-defined clinical problem and making sense of it. This is a complex and "messy" process. In the progress from an ill-defined to a well-defined problem, the nature of the problem itself is decomposed or broken down into subproblems or components of the larger or more general problem definition. It is characteristic of this stage that a number of questions are posed. Figure 7-2 indicates some of the basic questions that need to be answered in order to proceed.

The questions are the basis for breaking up the general problem area into more manageable subproblems. In dealing with the first question, which is where to start, guidance is provided by the problem-oriented process model, which indicates that the focus should be on referral and occupational therapy criteria (Denton, 1987).

Exactly what to look for in terms of occupational therapy criteria becomes the next subproblem. This is a particularly tricky one because the reasoner has to focus on what is salient and separate relevant data, as opposed to background noise. Knowledge is the crucial factor here without knowledge key data are overlooked and irrelevant data processed.

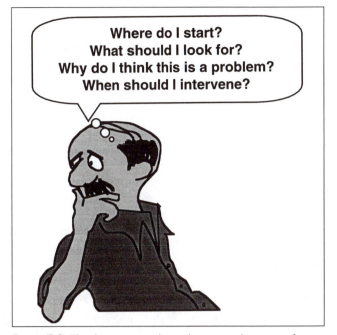

Figure 7-2. The therapist pondering how to make sense of clinical data.

What is noise and what is useful information is dependent on the ability to relate input to prior knowledge and to place the problem in context. Knowledge is what determines if the input is meaningful. Determining what is noise and what is meaningful data is like the saying about gardening: "a weed is anything that grows that isn't what you want" (Giarratano & Riley, 1989, p. 65).

In other words, data only becomes meaningful when it is transformed by knowledge into information. Information becomes knowledge when it is encoded and added to the existing knowledge base. Identifying knowledge gaps and acquiring knowledge is the basis of adult learning and curriculum-based initiatives like problem-based learning (Boud, 1981; Dressel & Thompson, 1973). That learners experience difficulties with this is not surprising. For example, a study conducted by Ryan indicated that inexperienced therapists only extracted 27% of key data from the same medical charts as more experienced therapists (Ryan, 1995, p. 248).

Extracting data is not a neat linear process. As additional data becomes available or as gaps and uncertainties are discovered, the therapist has to go back and reorganise the incoming data and reinterpret it. If a therapist can identify what knowledge is needed and develop a strategy for locating relevant knowledge, then the basis for a reasoning process dealing with this substep is in place. Knowing when you do not know implies an ability to reflect on both the knowledge itself and the reasoning process or steps in its transformation. This is a crucial aspect of developing competence and has been advocated by many people (Boud & Walker, 1991; Engel, 1991;

TABLE 7-1

Occupational Therapy Model Descriptor Form (Twible et al., 1993)

OCCUPATIONAL THERAPY MODEL DESCRIPTOR (OTMD)

Purpose: The purpose of this tool is to facilitate understanding of the various components of a theoretical model. It provides a framework by which a model can be described, analysed and evaluated. The process of model development is dynamic and results in the generation of new knowledge. This process begins with a set of ideas which are then translated into a guiding set of concepts and constructs. This evolves into a set of hypothesised relational statements which then form the basis for research into the validity of the model's propositions. This tool is not intended to be used to judge a model in terms of being "good" or "bad," rather, it assists in identifying the model's features. A complete description of the dimensions of a model requires an investigation of the literature and, if possible, consultation with both the model developers and those who have used it.

SECTION A: MODEL CONCEPTUAL FOUNDATIONS

Title of Model *What is the name of the model? Is it consistently referred to by this name?*

Date of Last Revision *What is the most recent version of the model?*

Model Developers *Indicate the authors of the current model.*

Origin of Model *Indicate the original author(s) and source. When did this model first appear? Did it evolve out of another model? Trace the historical development of this model, and the factors that influenced its modification.*

Philosophical & Theoretical Foundations *What is the philosophical underpinning of this model? What is the theory base of the model? What view does it take of humans? How does it view the world?*

Concepts & Constructs *What are the key terms used by this model? Are they defined and understandable? Are they comprehensive?*

Assumptions *What does this model assume to be true?*

Purpose *What is the purpose of the model? Identify specific goals and objectives.*

Suitable Populations *What client group is this model intended for?*

Category *What type of "model" is this? Is it a paradigm, a frame of reference, a professional or generic model or a practice model?*

SECTION B: STRUCTURE, PROCESS & OUTCOME

Client/Therapist Relationship *What is the therapist's role and what is the client's role? How and by whom are decisions made concerning the nature of the therapy process?*

Assessments, Procedures *Outline the model's assessment procedures and/or protocols, and list any standardised tools suggested for use.*

Intervention Strategies *What are the intervention strategies within this model, are they clearly described and is there any research evidence to suggest that they are effective?*

Precautions *Are there any precautions which must be taken into account when using this model? List any other factors likely to impact adversely on its implementation.*

Expected Outcomes *What are the expected outcomes and how are they evaluated?*

TABLE 7-1 (continued)
Occupational Therapy Model Descriptor Form (Twible et al., 1993)

SECTION C: ONGOING RESEARCH AND DEVELOPMENT

Evidence of Use in Practice
Does the literature describe the use of this model in practice? This would indicate whether or not the model has been translated from a theoretical perspective into the practice domain. How have research findings affected modification or acceptance of this model?

Evidence of Use in Related Areas
Is there any evidence that this model has been applied to areas outside of Occupational Therapy (i.e., management or education)? This indicates that the scope of the model is broader than Occupational Therapy practice.

SECTION D: PERSONAL VIEWS

Strengths
What are the advantages of the model? What is its scope? How has this viewpoint been shaped by your personal values and beliefs?

Limitations
What are the limitations of the model? How has this viewpoint been shaped by your personal values and beliefs?

References
What resources have been used in your description, analysis and evaluation of the model?
(numbered and supporting text as numerical citations)

Schon, 1987). Teaching critical and analytical thinking strategies and skills is one means of fostering this reflective stance. It is also useful in helping learners learn how to narrow the general problem area and deal with the uncertainties linked to a non-linear and ill-defined problem-solving process.

Answering the questions associated with when and how to intervene is also a knowledge-dependent activity. In this case, answers can be derived by selection of an appropriate occupational therapy frame or model. This step is contingent on knowledge of what models or frames exist and the ability to choose one that is valid for the general problem area and problem-solving context. Learning to critically evaluate a range of frames and models is important in both knowing and choosing between what is available. It is also critical in assisting learners to more deeply process ideas and thus develop their own personal isomorph. A personal isomorph is the internalised interpretation acquired by the therapist of a frame or model in the process of encoding and interpreting it into an existing knowledge base (Kortman, 1994). In other words, a personal isomorph is an internalised reflection of the original model but not an exact duplicate. The process of reflecting about and analysing models and frames can assist the novice or beginning clinician when faced with a decision about what model or frame to use. Table 7-1 is a critical analysis form called the "Occupational Therapy Model Descriptor" (Twible, Bridge, Ranka, Beltran, & Bye, 1993), which was developed for the purpose of teaching critical analysis and encouraging reflective practice.

KEY COMPONENTS IN CLINICAL REASONING

The idea that knowledge, cognition and metacognition are interdependent is not new (Higgs & Jones, 1995a). Their interdependence allows the clinician to reflect on practice and it is this process that provides the feedback to change our perceptual and behavioural responses. Moreover, it is this feedback loop over time that allows us to acquire new information and transform this into clinical expertise and clinical skill. This idea is congruent with the notion of clinicians as a special class of individuals engaged in clinical performance of activities and responding as open systems to their environments. The three interdependent cognitive components and the environmental components that are important in both influencing and interacting with tasks such as communication with clients are illustrated in Figure 7-3.

Along with the three key cognitive components of knowledge, cognition, and metacognition, there are also four variables that dynamically interact and thus have a significant effect in determining reasoning outcomes.

The term *cues* relates to the notion that the environmental context (via metacognition) will determine to some extent what is perceived. Cues are environmental triggers or prompts to memory that guide memory search. They are situated between cognition and metacognition because they are influenced by attention, vigilance and individual per-

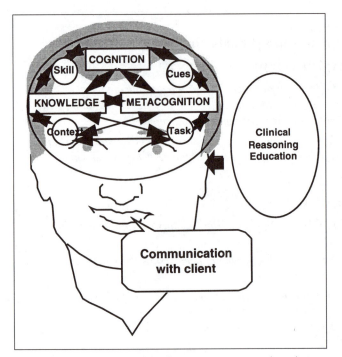

Figure 7-3. An overview of the factors important to clinical reasoning.

ceptual styles. Conscious attention to environmental cues is necessary to make sense of them, i.e., to filter out noise and transform environmental cues into useful information.

The term *skill* relates to the procedural versus declarative knowledge distinction made in the discussion of definitions of clinical reasoning; in other words it is the "know how" that mediates motor actions. It is situated between knowledge and cognition because it is the by-product of knowledge in action and requires direct cognitive input. For example, in Figure 7-3, the therapist needs to use interviewing skills to communicate with the client. Interviewing skills are learned and relate to knowledge stored in long-term memory, but also require cognitive skills to mediate motor functions.

The term *context* relates to the physical, social and cultural setting in which the reasoning is taking place. The context affects our ability to be reminded and affects our choice of tasks and tools. For instance, in an acute hospital ward setting, you are more likely to be reminded of lessons learned in that context and would be constrained in the types of tasks you could choose to engage in with the client, e.g., you would have to decide to the ward to observe road crossing or cooking performance.

Lastly, reasoning about *tasks* and task selection is influenced by context and prior knowledge. Task choice influences (via metacognition) the type and quality of clinical cues available. For example, in deciding to observe a client move from sit to stand, the environmental context is important because it

determines physical barriers such as low chairs. Knowledge is also important because otherwise you would not be reminded that low chairs require greater dynamic balance and increased hip flexion. The conscious ability to check for *context* and *knowledge* inconsistencies means that the reasoner is able to pick up on and interpret *cues*.

Knowledge

Because occupational therapists serve a wide range of individuals, the knowledge they need for practice is by definition also extensive. Knowledge is presented and conceptualised as concepts, constructs, principles and theories. The ability to articulate clinical reasoning and confidence in decisions made is directly proportional to the ability to notice and organise client-related phenomena in terms of their conceptual significance. Over the last 15 to 20 years, there have been major developments in occupational therapy theory and the scientific knowledge that supports interventions. Thus knowledge is important in shaping clinical reasoning by providing a means for therapists to understand what to attend to, how to attend to it and the relationships between phenomena that cause order and disorder (Kielhofner, 1992). Occupational therapy theories are loosely grouped in terms of their explanatory power and focus into paradigms, frames of reference and models (Hagedorn, 1992).

Occupational therapy theory is part of our unique body of knowledge. Theory serves to determine how problems are conceived and provides guidelines for the reasoning process in terms of what clients to accept into our programs and what assessment and intervention strategies to apply. At present there is no universal agreement within the profession about exactly what our domain of concern should be. However, the focus is in the process of shifting back to the construct of occupation and occupational dysfunction in the broadest sense (McColl, Law & Stewart, 1993). The fact that many experienced clinicians trained prior to the late 1970s is also important to note because they missed out on the opportunity to learn theory as undergraduates and therefore have difficulty verbalising their expertise in theoretical terminology (Wittman, 1990).

Theories about occupational behaviour help therapists to explain and predict events, or as Kielhofner (1992) would say, to "name and frame" problems. But it is important to understand and accept that despite using theory to name and frame problem areas, because there are so many variables involved, theory itself cannot lead to a single clear and right solution. Moreover, the present state of occupational therapy theoretical knowledge is still evolving (McColl et al., 1993). Characteristic of this early stage is that diversity is encouraged this is a natural and healthy process, but can be an uncomfortable position for learners.

Students also have difficulties in examining and describing the literature relating to theoretical knowledge development. This is due to the confusion among practitioners and academics about the exact definitions of terms and how the terms interrelate (Christiansen, 1991; Hagedorn, 1992; Kortman, 1994; McColl et al., 1993).

Although it is tempting trying to avoid definitions because of the current confusion, it cannot be avoided if an understanding of how knowledge guides occupational therapy practice and reduces uncertainty is to be reached. Knowledge can be conceived of hierarchically as a pyramid-type structure, with each layer being developed and refined from the one preceding it (Figure 7-4). At the most basic level, reasoning and decision-making are guided by personal values and beliefs that have been acquired over time and reflect the physical, cultural and social environment in which development occurred. In situations where other more specific knowledge is missing or inadequate, this is the level to which the therapist resorts. Everyone at some time has been confronted with choices about which little information is known; under these circumstances, decisions will be made on personal value and belief structures. For example, when choosing accommodation in a foreign city without a guidebook, your choice will depend on factors that relate to your personal values and beliefs. For some, this will mean the cheapest accommodation available, and for others cleanliness and an in-suite bathroom will be deciding factors. Figure 7-4 provides a view of how occupational therapy knowledge can be conceived of as a layered hierarchy. Like the problem-oriented process model, the hierarchy is best conceived of as a conceptual organiser rather than a strictly linear model. Precisely because real clinical reasoning is complex and needs to be broken down into numerous sub-problems, knowledge will be blended from a number of levels in even a relatively simple and apparently straightforward problem-solving activity.

The second layer of the model includes the notion of a professional paradigm. The word *paradigm* was chosen because unlike core or basic skills it has an inherent notion of change over time, reflecting the fact that the profession, like the individual, is influenced by its physical, social and cultural environment. A philosophically loaded word, it brings with it the Kuhnian notion of scientific revolution. This reflects the current trend in occupational therapy where there has been a paradigm shift away from both the behavioural and physiological reductionist perspectives. The new paradigm includes a shift toward a statement of fundamental principles and a philosophy on which a progression is built, i.e., "occupation" to "occupational science" (Wilcock, 1991). Many believe that developing a universally accepted group of basic or core skills is not possible and may not even be desirable. In the most general sense, a paradigm can be seen as the professional values and beliefs

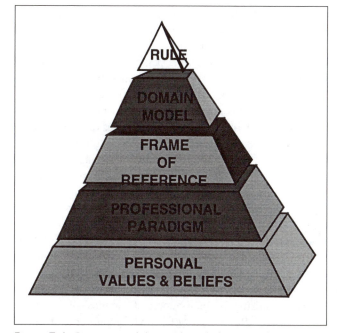

Figure 7-4. Occupational therapy knowledge viewed as a layered hierarchy.

which are learned and internalised throughout our professional novitiate. Common constructs that guide reasoning at this level are the professional values placed on independence or client-centred practice, for instance.

The third level includes frames of reference. This reflects a more rigorously tested and validated system of relationships than the more general professional values and beliefs. Frames of reference provide a framework that draws together the unifying theories and hypothesis of an area (Young & Quinn, 1992). In professional practice, a frame of reference specifies the nature, aims and procedures of the work and distinguishes it from other forms of practice (Young & Quinn, 1992). In this sense, a decision to select a specific frame of reference assists the therapist to attend to certain features and starts to predict outcomes. For instance, adopting the spatio-temporal framework proposed by Gilfoyle, Grady and Moore (1980) shapes how the therapist senses dysfunction and intervenes to correct it. Unlike practice models, it is less concrete and specific in determining how actions should be performed and in what sequence.

The fourth level is that of models. This represents the most organised and synthesised body of knowledge in occupational therapy and clearly demonstrates relationships between elements (Young & Quinn, 1992). Models of occupational therapy practice provide guidelines for naming and framing clinical problems. Kielhofner (1992) talks about them as the conceptual lens that focuses our practice. In this sense, they represent validated systems of relationships among carefully defined and measured constructs. Examples in this area include a model of human occupation (Kielhofner, 1985), the person-environment interaction model (Law et al., 1994), the person-environment occupational performance model (Christiansen & Baum, 1997), the sensory integration model (Ayres, 1980), etc.

The top level is that of rules. This is where relationships are so clearly defined that a correct answer or action can be identified. In occupational therapy no clear rules to guide action exist, so reasoning is almost always uncertain. The only exception to this might be in environmental reasoning where access standards apply. For example, in Australia, Canada, the United Kingdom and the United States, key concepts such as height of grab rails are specified and are mandatory for all new public buildings. Reasoning and decision-making about where to place a hand rail in a public building can be calculated in relation to the standard and is thus either correct or incorrect.

The acquisition, organisation and complex interrelationships between these layers of knowledge are crucial in the development of expertise and clinical mastery. As learners acquire theoretical knowledge they relate it to what they already know and what rings true for them in terms of their existing value and belief set.

Cognition

Adult cognitive skills are what determine our reasoning, problem-solving strategies and decision-making abilities. Cognitive abilities are usually taken for granted. As Craik points out, "the better they work the less we are conscious of them...it is only a fault which draws our attention to the existence of a mechanism at all." (Craik, 1943). Cognition can be viewed as a number of mental abilities such as encoding, reminding, forgetting and problem-solving, which together form a complex system of interdependent mental processes.

Cognition underpins our ability to acquire and develop roles; for instance, in a learner role, mental abilities such as memorisation, information ordering and reasoning allow tasks such as making sense of this book chapter possible (Christiansen, 1991). Adult cognition has important features which are characteristic and differentiate it from cognition at other stages of life. These features are individuality, the development of formal and post formal thought in a Piagentian sense and apparent age-related changes. In terms of individuality, adolescents and adults have characteristically unique knowledge and abilities (Rybash, Hoyer & Roodin, 1986). This is a result of the combination of environmental opportunities, learning preferences and individual choice. It is important to remember, however, that choices are often not conscious or deliberate.

Knowledge of Piaget's development stages suggests that during adolescence or young adulthood most people arrive at "the formal operations stage." People at this level demonstrate the ability to execute a logical, rational and deductive approach to problem-solving (Rybash et al., 1986). Rybash, Hoyer and Roodin (1986) argue that it is the next level, or postformal stage, that is truly characteristic of adult cognition. Postformal thought is context and knowledge dependent and is cyclic and interactive in nature. More importantly, reasoning is relative in that knowledge is viewed as something diverse that will change in relation to incoming information rather than an absolute truth (Nadien, 1986; Rybash et al., 1986).

When confronted with new or different problems, problem-solving skill relies on fluid intelligence or logical reasoning ability, which includes both inductive and deductive strategies. Inductive reasoning is also sometimes referred to as *hypothetical reasoning* or *generate and test*. The generation of hypotheses or best guesses for cause and effect relations is typical of classical scientific reasoning. Deductive reasoning, on the other hand, uses a process where solutions or outcomes are derived from prior knowledge when two premises or pieces of knowledge are assumed to be true, and new knowledge is derived by developing a new premise that is a logical development of the old knowledge. Regardless of whether inductive or deductive reasoning is used by adult reasoners, fluid intelligence, i.e., the ability to adapt to novel problem scenarios, decreases proportionally as crystallised intelligence increases (Hayslip & Panek, 1993; Nadien, 1986). This shift is linked to the growth of specialised expertise and is typical of adult age-related cognition (Rybash et al., 1986).

Adult reasoning and decision-making rely heavily on prior experience or analogical reasoning, such as when you are reminded of a similar case and lessons learned in that context. The ability to store and retrieve information in the form of extensive case libraries is a factor that contributes to what is sometimes referred to as crystallised intelligence, which increases with the accumulation of experience over time (Hayslip & Panek, 1993). The accumulation of experience over time is closely linked to the notion of the development of expertise. The growth of expertise is characteristic of adult development and consequent specialisation of skills and abilities.

Expertise can be defined as "knowledge about a particular problem domain, understanding of domain problems and skill at solving some of those problems" (Hayes-Roth, Waterman & Lenat, 1983, p. 4). Growth in expertise is accompanied by a hierarchically organised knowledge base that includes knowledge of domain interdependencies and the development of cognitive constructs that relate facts and information (Slater & Cohn, 1991). It appears that with the growth of expertise, memory is not expanded *per se*, but that chunks of information retrieved from memory are larger and richer and experts appear to be able to encode incoming data faster (Gilhooly, 1988).

Both analogical and logical reasoning rely on a well-organised knowledge base and a useful problem representation. Problem representation and organisation are critical because unless aspects of the problem can be broken down appropriately and knowledge is well-organised, the ability to retrieve information in a timely manner is next to impossible (Higgs & Jones, 1995a). Problem representation and knowledge organisation is facilitated by active engagement with the material to be learned. Organisation is also enhanced by learning and using verbal labels to categorise objects in order to better sort, index and retrieve them. If categorisation is poor then the ability to retrieve information becomes inefficient and unreliable. Therefore terminology and language are important to the retrieval of information. Familiarisation with professional concepts and constructs is part of the growth of expertise.

Metacognition

Metacognition is the ability to reflect on one's cognitive processors and mediate those processes (Flavell, 1976). In other words metacognitive skills include awareness of one's thought processes and introspection about one's actions or inactions (Nadien, 1986). Metacognition has been linked to the facilitation of learning and improvement of problem-solving skills (Biggs & Telfer, 1987; Carnevali, 1995). One means of encouraging reflective practice so cognitive processors can be mediated is for the learner to actively engage with new material by asking questions. Questioning arises from the learner's prior experience and knowledge (Marshall & Rowland, 1991). Questioning, therefore, enhances integration of new material with old material and thus leads to a richer knowledge base.

Metacognition is not a static ability but a developmental process that starts in childhood and matures in late adulthood (Nadien, 1986). Without metacognition, there is no means of scrutinising knowledge for accuracy, consistency or completeness. Reasoning and knowledge can be flawed for many reasons, and reasoning is usually combined with actions and can happen so fast that it is not always easy to bring current thought into consciousness (Fleming & Mattingly, 1994). All reasoning styles are prone to error of some type and degree. Use of analogical reasoning strategies, for instance, can mean that prior experience may limit the generation of new solutions in that it can lead to "functional fixedness" (Dunckner, 1971). This means that there is overgeneralisation of knowledge and a resultant mental block in perceiving new solutions (Mayer, 1992). Inductive reasoning, on the other hand, can be flawed because of the tendency to ignore falsifying data, whereas deductive reasoning can be flawed because it is easy to misinterpret premises or task demands (Gilhooly, 1988). Clearly, some checks on both cognitive processors and knowledge invoked are useful in gaining a sense of gaps or in understanding the probability of error. Because clinical reasoning is always reasoning in uncertainty, metacognition is a means of checking both process and knowledge.

FACILITATING REASONING BY USE OF A REFLECTIVE FRAMEWORK

Metacognition by itself is limited in that it requires additional cognitive resources and requires a self-critical stance, which can be very daunting, especially when trying to come to grips with unfamiliar concepts. Typically, learners and novices make errors because cues are missed and/or underpinning knowledge is missing. Individuals have difficulty identifying what is wrong when cues and/or knowledge are incomplete or lacking. Having some means to check current knowledge and understanding is essential, because in clinical practice it is not acceptable to interact with a client without any idea of what the client's potential dysfunctions might be. Figure 7-5 provides a means of conceptualising the relationship between the level of knowledge invoked, and the confidence in knowledge validity. The higher the level of knowledge invoked the greater the confidence and the smaller the degree of uncertainty.

Many people have advocated the enhancement of self-monitoring skills as a means of enhancing clinical reasoning (Barrows & Pickell, 1991; Boud & Walker, 1991; Carnevali, 1995; Corcoran & Tanner, 1988; Kassirer & Kopelman, 1991; Refshauge and Higgs, 1994; Ryan, 1995; Schwartz, 1991; Thomas et al., 1991). One means of achieving this is to apply a systematic set of questions or an explorative framework in order to facilitate metacognition or conscious reflection. It appears that the two most problematic areas are "problem sensing" or "noticing" and "problem validation" or "intervening." Interestingly, the terms problem sensing and problem validation come from the clinical reasoning literature (Neistadt, 1992; Rogers & Holm, 1990a; 1990b; 1991), whereas the terms noticing and intervening come from the adult learning literature (Boud & Walker, 1991). Both sets of terms describe and focus on the same things: the therapist or learner's interaction and reflections on the incoming data. They can be conceived of as two stages that follow each other in a cyclic pattern. They are interrelated and although presented in a linear form, in real everyday clinical interactions, follow so fast on each other that they are difficult to separate. The point of separating the two is solely to simplify and order the messy clinical data so as to make knowledge and process explicit and amenable to conscious reflection.

In stage one, *problem sensing*, attention is being paid to incoming data and reflection is based around that. Problem sensing or noticing is an active process that requires selective attention and assists the encoding and categorisation of incom-

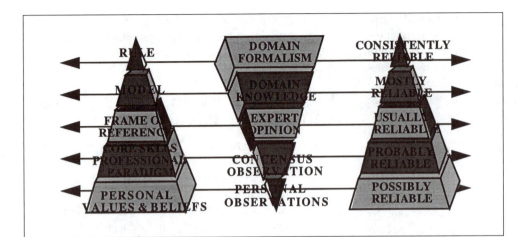

Figure 7-5. Relationship between knowledge levels and confidence.

TABLE 7-2

Prompts for Key Word Identification

Referral Data	Potential Information
Name	Ethnicity, sex and/or age.
Sex	Sex stereotyped occupational tasks and roles in relation to self-maintenance, productivity and leisure.
Date of birth	Developmental status and likely occupational tasks and roles in relation to self-maintenance, productivity and leisure.
Address	Socioeconomic status, dwelling type, proximity to services, pollution level or other environmental contaminants.
Diagnosis	Component problems likely to result in occupational contaminants.
Prognosis	Future occupational task and role dysfunctions.

---

ing data. The development of the ability to notice and attend to cues appropriately in the clinical scenario is crucial in learning discrimination. Discriminative abilities enable cases and case lessons such as those extracted from the clinical scenario to be stored and retrieved most efficiently. Attention to language, knowledge and knowledge extrapolation all assist in the development of an accurate clinical image.

Client referral data is an important factor in how problems are sensed and in deciding what aspects of incoming data to notice (Rogers & Holm, 1990b). Making the novice or student aware of these aspects and their relevance to occupational therapy hypotheses is an important step in assisting students to notice and to reflect on certain aspects. Some of the routine client referral information which can shape the

clinical image, and that is thus likely to impact on initial occupational hypotheses, are outlined in Table 7-2. Making students aware of how referral information can lead to occupational performance hypotheses is important because referral cues can affect what cues are attended to, how ambiguous cues are interpreted, and the relative importance and resulting certainty of cue interpretation (Rogers & Holm, 1990b).

As Niestadt (1992) points out, the original image of the client is formed automatically as incoming data from the occupational therapy referral and practice setting is processed. This processing happens in relation to current values and beliefs and includes predictions extrapolated from theory. Figure 7-6 is an attempt to assist the novice to more thoroughly reflect on and consciously process incoming data and to relate this to hypothesis generation in occupational therapy.

In stage two, *problem validation*, the focus is on the examination of discrepancies between the original clinical image and the real and gradually unfolding clinical scenario. Intervening is an ongoing interactive process that commences with the initial evaluation or interview. This is the part that Fleming & Mattingly refer to as "thinking in action" (1994, p.322). The notion of thinking in action is congruent with Boud and Walker's view of "intervening" being the "conscious action flowing from and influenced by a reflective process" (1991, p. 26). Problem validation requires overt action in extending and testing understanding. This can be done directly by observing or testing the client undertaking the actual task specified as the initial hypothesis, or indirectly by observing the client doing other activities which demand similar performance requirements (e.g., if a client has difficulty getting off of a chair, then you can suppose that the client will have difficulty getting off of a toilet).

Actions change the situation and create new experiences that influence how a situation will unfold. Asking a certain question or requesting a certain response from a client will in fact determine what happens next. Because other people are involved, relationships developed both with the client and

Key Words	Key words are found in the information presented to you prior to you seeing the client. This information can be presented verbally or in written form. It may be extensive giving lots of details about the client or extremely limited. Key words give you clues to the important/vital/significant factors of the client's condition, problems and situation. Key words help you identify the aspects of the case that you may need to find out about or just think about prior to seeing the client. This process of finding out information and/or thinking about the information that you already have enables you to work out what you will do, when to do it, and how best to do it when you first contact the client. More importantly why you are doing it based on some type of rationale.
Source and Level of Knowledge	What exactly do you know about the keyword and how confident are you that what you know is adequate? Explanations terms are as follows: 1. Source is where and/or, who and how you go about finding out more information about a specific factor (key word). The source can be a written (text, journal article, leaflet, catalogue etc), dialogue with one or more people (expert, peers, other health professional, relative etc) or it can be drawn from your past experience and observations. 2. Level of knowledge refers to the relationship between 'hierarchies of knowledge and decision confidence' as outlined in Figure 7-5.
Related Knowledge	This encompasses all additional related knowledge about the keyword. This may include information related to other professions and their practice. For example if the keyword is medical it will encompass all medical and nursing knowledge about diagnosis, intervention and likely outcomes for specific pathologies. This knowledge is the end result of your prior experience, reflection on the adequacy of this knowledge and consequent additional information search. Reflections on knowledge allow the reasoner to identify gaps. • the knowledge I already have on the subject • the knowledge I need to find out on the subject Related knowledge is essential basic information that you must have before you can make any further judgements about the client, their condition, situation and management.
Functional Implications	This is the information you infer about how the clients functional performance will be affected as a result of your understanding of the keyword and your related knowledge. Here you need to list the functional implications of the client's status and management. (This may encompass a physiological, psychological, functional, and social point of view).
Occupational Therapy Hypothesis	Your occupational therapy hypothesis is based on: _ Related knowledge _ Management implications _ Knowledge of occupational therapy models and frames of reference The outcome of your thinking about these factors is your occupational therapy hypotheses about the client. Each hypothesis comprises has two parts: 1. Diagnostic hypothesis or your initial/provisional Occupational Therapy problem. (eg. difficulty getting off toilet) 2. Prognostic hypothesis or expected outcome (eg. will become increasingly difficult over time).

Figure 7-6. A reflective framework for problem sensing (Bridge, Twible & Beltran, 1995).

with co-workers will affect what you do and say. Indeed an act such as asking a client to move from sit to stand, will bring about a change to the clinical situation and the type of data that can be extracted from it. Depending on the results of actions, hypotheses will be validated or denied. If hypotheses cannot be supported by incoming data, then either the problem does not exist for that client or you need to engage in the process of redefining the problem by reprocessing the data to identify alternative explanations for the problem. Expert reasoners usually select actions that are designed to provide disconfirmatory cues, because confirmatory cues can sometimes have competing explanations. For example, difficulty in moving from sitting to standing could be due to low seat height, stiff joints, poor endurance, unsuitable footwear or a slippery/unstable floor surface.

Reflection on stage two is important because it assists the process of evaluation, and because the evaluations are made explicit, assists in presentation of options and potential risks to the client, employer and funding bodies. When you are able to articulate and present a logical rationale for your occupational therapy treatments, you are more likely to achieve engagement, cooperation and professional credibility. Figure 7-7 is an attempt to assist the novice to reflect on actions and to make the most of possibilities.

Following are two case studies where the reflective frameworks previously discussed are used to better demonstrate how they might be applied. The cases themselves are simplified and information staged so as to reduce the information overload that can result. Awareness of all the factors and influences can be inhibiting, especially when confidence and experience are limited.

Case Example 1: Mrs. Sarah Williamson (Aged care)

You are working as a member of the occupational therapy team at a large public teaching hospital. Currently, you are providing occupational therapy services to the geriatric unit. When you go up to the ward, the charge sister informs you that Mrs. Williamson, a new client, was admitted overnight and requires occupational therapy services. You decide to find out more about Mrs. Williamson's needs, so you locate her case records and find out that last night Mrs. Williamson had a fall at home which resulted in a fracture to the neck of her left femur. You also note from the file that Mrs. Williamson is 78 years of age and a widow living in a home unit in a nearby middle-class suburb. The medical notes also indicate some osteoporosis.

At this stage, you might start to fill in the stage one reflective framework (Figure 7-8). You probably identified "fracture to the neck of her left femur" as a key word statement. You probably also feel fairly confident that you understand this term, but decide to look in an orthopaedic textbook to find out what medical interventions are most likely. The closest book is in the occupational therapy library and you

note that it was published in 1976. As a medical textbook, it represents expert opinion and this is usually reliable, but it is over 10 years old and medical management has changed much. So on reflection, you may decide that this knowledge source should be validated. You also may decide that further reading of the case notes or a quick question to the resident medical officer is all that is needed. Because you have been able to verify the type of surgery, you can now draw on your prior experience to recall potential functional implications and develop some occupational therapy hypotheses.

Because you have already developed some hypotheses, you can now start to consciously reflect on them using the stage two reflective framework (Figure 7-9). You therefore go to Mrs. Williamson's bedside, remembering to take an easyreacher, stocking gutter and long-handled shoehorn. Note how you have now moved to the stage two reflective framework, and movement between the two frameworks is iterative depending on validation and selection. While you are conducting your physical assessment and demonstrating the use of the easyreacher, Mrs. Williamson gets quite teary, stating that she doesn't know how she will be able to manage at home, especially with toileting since the doctor has just told her she needs to be careful of her hip for the next 3 months.

You could now add "female toileting" as a key word, and start to reflect on what you know about this. This reflection may prompt you to think about tasks associated with toileting, such as "normal sit to stand." You have just had to write an essay about this for your course in biomechanics, so you are aware that this has a high dynamic balance component and is more difficult for older persons. As you start to reflect on this you may decide that a home visit will be of value, and so on.

Case Example 2: Mr. Giovanni Bortelli (Community care)

Mrs. Bortelli, Giovanni's mother, has applied to the local department of housing for financial assistance to modify the family bathroom. The department of housing has contacted you as the local community therapist to carry out an assessment of Giovanni and Mrs. Bortelli's modification needs. The referral information indicates that Giovanni is 13 years of age and is currently living in the family home with his mother, who is divorced. During the day Giovanni attends a special school and has a diagnosis of arthrogryposis multiplex congenita (AMC).

At this stage you might start to fill in the stage one reflective framework for Giovanni (Figure 7-10). You almost certainly identified "arthrogryposis" as a key word statement. At this stage, you may never have encountered the word before, but from your current medical knowledge base you suspect that "arth" may indicate some sort of bone problem. You still have very limited knowledge and certainly have no idea what the functional implications might be. You therefore ask a fellow therapist on your team and she informs you that it may be a form of arthritis. You still have some doubt, so you decide to check this with Giovanni's local medical officer. The answer he

LOOK (magnifying glass icon) **Hypotheses Validation**	You need to identify critical features of the task or critical cues that could confirm or deny your initial hypotheses, e.g., _ poor dynamic balance _ poor static balance _ limited knee/hip extension _ uses/grabs onto objects for support _ unusually low toilet pan _ states cannot manage this task
Generate options	Within the context of your choice of models(s) you need to ask what can be done by you? _ Brainstorm or list as many options as possible. Having many ideas gives a wider range of options. It improves your chances of finding the 'best fit' for that person and context. It also gives you several options to fall back on, if for any reason you first choice is not accepted or isn't as effective as you had hoped.
Consider implications	For each option you have generated you need to consider factors likely to affect its suitability for the occasion and purpose, e.g., _ Where should it be done? (type of environment) _ Are there any sequencing issues to consider in how I structure my interventions? _ Are there cost factors (money, time, personnel) that will constrain choices _ What resources can be used? _ What are the time constraints and time factors I need to consider? _ What restrictions influence choices? (What is realistic?)
Assess Risks	Every intervention always carries some risk, although some may be very minor considerations. Risk factors range from physical to emotional and social. For example asking a client to stand up may carry the risk of both physical injury and psychosocial impacts such as confronting the client with the level of their disability. Therefore it is important to ensure you have considered all potential risk factors prior to selecting a specific intervention, e.g., _ Is there any potential of harm to the client via implementation of my intervention options? _ What is the chance of this occurring? _ How serious for the client might this be? If risk factors are identified you then need to decide what strategies you will put in place to reduce, manage or eliminate potential problems.
Select	This is a crucial decision point where you commit to a specific course of therapeutic actions or inaction. In considering what you will do or not do, your first priority is to prioritise the potential outcomes from the clients point of view, e.g., _ Which outcomes are mandatory? _ Which outcomes are desirable but not mandatory? _ What is the relative importance between the two?

Figure 7-7. A reflective framework for intervening (Bridge, 1993).

gives you is different from the one your fellow therapist gave, but more likely to be correct, so unless discrepancies appear while interacting with Giovanni, you will probably be content with this level and source of knowledge.

Again, identification of key words has assisted you to develop some hypotheses so you can now start to consciously reflect on them

using the stage two reflective framework (Figure 7-11). The use of the reflective framework helps you to pay attention or to notice any devices already in use, and to ask about how much physical assistance is required and at what times. On your home visit, you note that Giovanni is of average height but is considerably overweight. Giovanni is however able to mobilise independently using long leg

Figure 7-8. Use of a reflective framework for problem sensing with Mrs. Williamson.

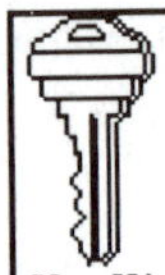 Key Words	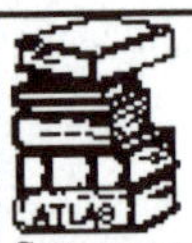 Source and Level of Knowledge	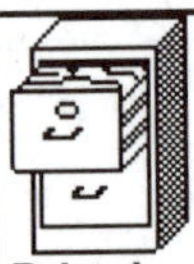 Related Knowledge	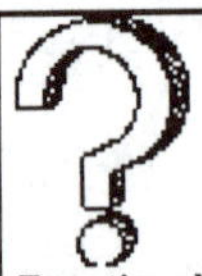 Functional Implications	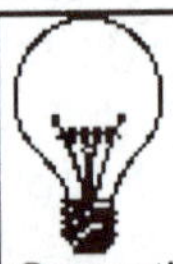 Occupational Therapy Hypothesis
fracture to the neck of her left femur	Medical textbook- (Adams, 1976) -usually reliable but now quite old so may question whether information is still valid	Medical intervention likely to be arthrodesis of the fracture i.e., a Pin and plate as elderly. Major surgery involved. – general anesthetic – associated edema in affected lower limb – open wound	– Partial weight bearing on affected side as a result of post-operative precautions – Bone and hip joint hypersensitive, pain on jarring, knocks, etc.	1. Will need assistive device to improve standing balance while mobilising. 2. Will benefit from increase in seat height. 3. Will have difficulty donning lower limb garments in standing
female toileting	Personal experience & knowledge of normative cultural custom -probably reliable	– Defecation seated on pan – Urination seated on pan – Genital cleansing seated on pan	– Need to shift weight on pan – Need to reach toilet paper while seated – Desirable to operate flush mechanism in stable position.	4. May benefit from grabrail on left side 5. Toilet roll holder needs to be within zone of comfortable reach 6. May need to be taught new technique
normal sit to stand	Biomechanical research articles - (Wheeler et al, 1983; Schultz, Yoshida, Iwakura & Inoue, 1983; Alexander & Ashton-Miller, 1992; Alexander, Schultz & Warwick, 1991) -mostly reliable	– Older persons find this more difficult – Large forces on lower joints – High dynamic balance component – Centre of gravity moves over feet in order to enter vertical standing phase	– Need for supportive assistive device – Preferably permanent placement	7. May benefit from armrests or bilateral grabrails.

callipers and forearm crutches, and he appears to be quite strong in the upper limbs. Giovanni already has a mobile shower commode chair and has a personal care assistant come each morning to assist with showering, as Mrs. Bortelli has a long history of sciatica. Giovanni tells you he can toilet independently at school while wearing his long leg callipers and using forearm crutches, and this is why he and his mother have asked for bathroom modifications. At this stage, you may add some more key words to your problem sensing framework while starting to validate your earlier hypotheses. For instance, you may decide to visit Giovanni at his school to observe how he manages to independently get on and off the toilet there, and so may discuss this possibility with Giovanni and his family.

Hypothesis Validation	Generate options	Consider implications	Assess Risks	Select
Hypothesis 3- difficulty donning lower limb garments _ patient states difficulty _ evidence of surgery etc.	1. Provision of assistive devices 2. Teach alternative technique 3. Physical assistance, etc.	1. Cost, Durability, Appearance, Availability, Training required etc. 2. Time, Cognitive capacity, etc. 3. Availability and willingness of person to take on additional tasks.	1. Equipment breakdown, Product liability, Client acceptance, Negligence 2. Likelihood of forgetting, Risk of re-injury, etc. 3. May require temporary relocation, Loss of privacy, Sense of dependence etc.	_ Mandatory- Minimise (L) hip flexion & extension _ Desirable- Early discharge _ Desirable- Return home _ Desirable- Independence etc.

Figure 7-9. Use of a reflective framework for intervening with Mrs. Williamson.

SUMMARY

In becoming a competent occupational therapist, you need to be aware of the factors that will shape how you reason clinically. Knowledge of alternative perspectives and definitions in clinical reasoning research is helpful in trying to understand what the key components might be and how they relate to each other. Precisely because occupational therapy reasoning is top down, not bottom up, and is focused on occupational role and task fulfillment, it involves active collaboration with the client. Knowing how and when to intervene and what boundaries to draw are tricky questions that are dependent on knowledge and information. In terms of knowledge content, occupational therapy students in the course of their education generally follow a wide ranging syllabus, which covers behavioural and biological sciences in addition to occupational therapy subjects. The content of all of these subjects is based on current knowledge and theory, all directed at capturing and explaining regularities and underlying principles that impact on occupational therapy practice. The ability to integrate, articulate and evaluate this information is crucial in developing competence.

As a therapist, it is your responsibility to present an adequate and logical rationale for each decision made. Your ability to do this and to integrate new knowledge can be facilitated by the adoption of a reflective and self-critical approach.

Active, self-directed learning will improve knowledge organisation and retention and thus facilitate the growth of expertise. However, it is important to remember that as adult thinkers, the type of knowledge and experience that each of you brings to each clinical scenario is based on a similar curriculum and professional value and belief base, but is processed, stored and integrated with existing knowledge, values and beliefs, and so is unique to each person.

Because each person brings different knowledge, values and beliefs to each clinical encounter, it is important to understand that reflective exercises are designed to make tacit thinking conscious, not to indicate a right or wrong way of viewing things. When reflective frameworks are applied to cases as part of small group learning experiences, students have commented that the opportunity to actively reflect and then to discuss and process differences within a group setting has been useful in highlighting alternate viewpoints, extending abilities to notice, and in refining articulation and rationalisation.

STUDY QUESTIONS

1. Explain clinical reasoning.

2. Describe the key differences between biomedical practice and occupational therapy practice.

Key Words	Source and Level of Knowledge	Related Knowledge	Functional Implications	Occupational Therapy Hypothesis
arthrogryposis	Visiting medical officer -usually reliable	Genetic instability of weight bearing joints.	– Unable to stand or mobilise without assistive devices	1. Will need assistive device to mobilise. 2. Will need physical assistance or mechanical devices to transfer.
male toileting	Personal observation & knowledge of normative cultural custom -probably reliable	– Defecation seated on pan – Urination in vertical stand position – Genital cleansing seated on pan for defecation	– Need to shift weight on pan – Dynamic balance challenged while standing to adjust clothing – Need to reach toilet paper while standing and while seated – Need to reach cistern button seated & standing	3. May benefit from supportive device 4. Toilet roll holder needs to be within zone of comfortable reach 5. May need to be taught new technique
abnormal sit to stand	Personal observation -possibly reliable	– Large forces on upper joints – Cannot bend hips and knees in order to enter vertical standing phase – High dynamic balance component	– Need good range of movement and muscle strength in upper limbs – Likely to require physical assistance or assistive devices – Greater risk of falling	6. May benefit from overhead support that can be used bilaterally 7. May require pan clearance for a shower - commode chair

Figure 7-10. Use of a reflective framework for problem sensing with Giovanni.

3. Describe the role of knowledge in clinical reasoning.

4. Explain how occupational therapy theory shapes clinical reasoning.

5. Name the five levels of the knowledge hierarchy.

6. Describe the relationship between knowledge and your confidence in the knowledge invoked.

7. Explain how a reflective framework is a useful tool to improve metacognition.

Figure 7-11. Use of a reflective framework for intervening with Giovanni.

Hypothesis Validation	Generate options	Consider implications	Assess Risks	Select
Hypothesis 1- Will need assistive device to mobilise _ Giovanni tells you what has been prescribed _ You observe aids in use _ etc.	1. Modify existing bathroom 2. Reassess existing equipment 3. Increase amount of Physical assistance etc.	1. Cost, Eligibility, Space required, Space available, Structural soundness, Accessibility, Prognosis, disruption to family etc. 2. Cost, durability, appearance, availability, training required etc. 3. Cost, availability, eligibility, willingness of person to take on additional tasks.	1. Negligence, Product liability, Municipal council approval, Funding approval, Confronts family with degree of disability, Client & family acceptance. 2. Equipment breakdown, Product liability, Client acceptance and Negligence 3. Continued loss of privacy, Sense of dependence etc.	_ Mandatory- Ensure toilet pan has unobstructed access for overtoilet shower-commode chair _ Desirable- Installation of supportive device to permit independence while wearing long leg callipers, etc.

8. Select some referral data from a case that you have been exposed to and try the reflective framework for yourself. Compare and discuss the results with your peers, what similarities or differences were there? Why do you think they occurred?

RECOMMENDED READINGS

Hagedorn, R. (1992). *Occupational therapy: Foundations for practice*. Edinburgh: Churchill Livingstone.

Higgs, J., & Jones, M. (Eds.). *Clinical reasoning in the health professions*. Oxford: Butterworth-Heinemann Ltd.

Kielhofner, G. (1992). *Conceptual foundations of occupational therapy*. Philadelphia: F. A. Davis Co.

Marshall, L. A., & Rowland, F. (1991). *A guide to learning independently*. Melbourne: Longman Cheshire.

Mattingly, C., & Fleming, M. H. (1994). *Clinical reasoning: Forms of inquiry in a therapeutic practice*. Philadelphia: F.A. Davis Co.

McColl, M. A., Law, M., & Stewart, D. (1993). *Theoretical basis of occupational therapy*. Thorofare, NJ: SLACK Incorporated.

REFERENCES

Australian Association of Occupational Therapists. (1992). *Competency standards for entry-level occupational therapists* (Penultimate draft): Author.

Ayres, J. (1980). Southern California Sensory Integration Tests. Los Angeles, California: Western Psychological Services.

Barris, R. (1987). Clinical Reasoning in psychosocial occupational therapy. *Occupational Therapy Journal of Research, 7*(3),

147-161.

Barrows, H., & Pickell, G. (1991). *Developing clinical problem-solving skills.* New York: W. W. Norton.

Biggs, J. B., & Telfer, R. (1987). *The process of learning* (2nd ed.). Sydney: Prentice Hall.

Boud, D. (Ed.). (1981). *Developing student autonomy in learning.* London: Kogan Page.

Boud, D., & Walker, D. (1991). *Experience and learning reflection at work.* Geelong, Victoria: Deakin University.

Bridge, C. (1993). *Shaping clinical reasoning using theory.* Unpublished lecture material. School of Occupational Therapy, Faculty of Health Sciences, The University of Sydney. NSW: Australia.

Bridge, C., Twible, R., & Beltran, R. (1995). *Stage one: Reflective framework for clinical reasoning.* Unpublished lecture material. School of Occupational Therapy, Faculty of Health Sciences, The University of Sydney. NSW, Australia.

Carnevali, D. L. (1995). Self-monitoring of clinical reasoning behaviours: Promoting professional growth. In J. Higgs & M. Jones (Eds.), *Clinical reasoning in the health professions* (pp. 347). Oxford: Butterworth-Heinemann Ltd.

Christiansen, C. (1991). Occupational therapy: Intervention for life performance. In C. Christiansen & C. Baum (Eds.), *Occupational therapy: Overcoming human performance deficits* (pp. 1-43). Thorofare, NJ: SLACK Incorporated.

Cohn, E. S. (1989). Fieldwork education: Shaping a foundation for clinical reasoning. *The American Journal of Occupational Therapy, 43*(4), 240-244.

Corcoran, S., & Tanner, C. (1988). Implications for clinical judgement research for teaching. In National League for Nursing (Ed.), *Curriculum revolution: Mandate for change* (pp. 159-176). New York: Author.

Craik, K. (1943). *The nature of explanation.* Cambridge: Cambridge University Press.

Denton, P. L. (1987). *Psychiatric occupational therapy: A workbook of practical skills.* Boston: Little, Brown and Company.

Dressel, P. L., & Thompson, M. M. (1973). *Independent study.* San Francisco: Jossey-Bass.

Dunckner, K. (1971). *On problem solving.* Westport, CT: Greenwood.

Elstein, A. S. (1995). Clinical reasoning in medicine. In J. Higgs & M. Jones (Eds.), *Clinical reasoning in the health professions* (pp. 347). Oxford: Butterworth-Heinemann Ltd.

Elstein, A. S., Shulman, L. S., & Spafka, S. A. (1978). *Medical problem solving: An analysis of clinical reasoning.* Cambridge, MA: Harvard University Press.

Engel, C. E. (1991). Not just a method but a way of learning. In D. Boud & G. Feletti (Eds.), *The challenge of problem-based learning* (pp. 23-33). London: Kogan Page.

Flavell, J. H. (1976). Metacognition aspects of problem solving. In L. B. Resnick (Ed.), *The nature of intelligence.* Hillsdale, NJ: Lawrence Erlbaum Associates.

Fleming, M. H. (1991a). Clinical reasoning in medicine compared with clinical reasoning in occupational therapy. *The American Journal of Occupational Therapy, 45*(11), 988-996.

Fleming, M. H. (199lb). The therapist with the three-track mind.

The American Journal of Occupational Therapy, 45(11), 1007-1014.

Fleming, M. H. (1994). The therapist with the three track mind. In C. Mattingly & M. H. Fleming (Eds.), *Clinical reasoning: Forms of inquiry in a therapeutic practice.* Philadelphia: F.A. Davis Co.

Fleming, M. H., & Mattingly, C. (1994). Action and inquiry. In C. Mattingly & M. H. Fleming (Eds.), *Clinical reasoning: Forms of inquiry in a therapeutic practice.* Philadelphia: F.A. Davis Company.

Fonteyn, M. E. (1995). Clinical reasoning in nursing. In J. Higgs & M. Jones (Eds.), *Clinical reasoning in the health professions* (pp. 347). Oxford: Butterworth-Heinemann Ltd.

Giarratano, J., & Riley, G. (1989). *Expert systems: Principles and programming.* Boston, MA: PWS-KENT Publishing Co.

Gilfoyle, E. M., Grady, A. P., & Moore, J. (1980). *Children adapt.* Thorofare, NJ: SLACK Incorporated.

Gilhooly, K. J. (1988). *Thinking: Directed, undirected and creative* (2nd ed.). U.K.: Academic Press.

Hagedorn, R. (1992). *Occupational therapy: Foundations for practice.* Edinburgh: Churchill Livingstone.

Harris, I. B. (1993). New expectations for professional competence. In L. Curry & J. Wergin (Eds.), *Educating professionals: Responding to new expectations for competence and accountability* (pp. 17-52). San Francisco: Jossey-Bass.

Hayes-Roth, F., Waterman, D. A., & Lenat, D. B. (Eds.). (1983). *Building expert systems.* Reading, MA: Addison-Wesley.

Hayslip, B., & Panek, P. E. (1993). *Adult development & aging* (2nd ed.). New York: HarperCollins College Publishers.

Higgs, J. (1990). Fostering the acquisition of clinical reasoning skills. *New Zealand Journal of Physiotherapy,* (December), 13-17.

Higgs, J., & Jones, M. (1995a). Introduction. In J. Higgs & M. Jones (Eds.), *Clinical reasoning in the health professions* (pp. 347). Oxford: Butterworth-Heinemann Ltd.

Higgs, J., & Jones, M. (1995b). Clinical reasoning. In J. Higgs & M. Jones (Eds.), *Clinical reasoning in the health professions* (pp. 347). Oxford: Butterworth-Heinemann Ltd.

Kassirer, J., & Kopelman, R. (1991). *Learning clinical reasoning.* Baltimore: Williams and Wilkins.

Kielhofner, G. (Ed.). (1985). *A model of human occupation: Theory and application.* Baltimore, MD: Williams and Wilkins.

Kielhofner, G. (1992). *Conceptual foundations of occupational therapy.* Philadelphia: F. A. Davis Company.

Kortman, B. (1994). The eye of the beholder: Models in occupational therapy. *Australian Journal of Occupational Therapy, 41*, 115-122.

Law, M., Cooper, B., Letts, L., Rigby, P., Stewart, S., & Strong, S. (1994). *A model of person-environment interactions: Application to occupational therapy.* Hamilton, Canada: McMasters University.

Marshall, L. A., & Rowland, F. (1991). *A guide to learning independently.* Melbourne: Longman Cheshire.

Mattingly, C. (1991). What is clinical reasoning? *The American Journal of Occupational Therapy, 45*(11), 979-986.

Mattingly, C., & Fleming, M. H. (1994). *Clinical reasoning: Forms of inquiry in a therapeutic practice.* Philadelphia: F.A. Davis Co.

Mayer, R. E. (1992). *Thinking, problem solving, cognition* (2nd ed.). New York: W. H. Freeman and Company.

McColl, M. A., Law, M., & Stewart, D. (1993). *Theoretical basis of occupational therapy.* Thorofare, NJ: SLACK Incorporated.

Nadien, M. (1989). *Adult years and aging.* Dubuque, IA: Kendall Hunt Publishing Company.

Neistadt, M. E. (1992). The classroom as clinic: Applications for a method of teaching clinical reasoning. *The American Journal of Occupational Therapy, 46*(9), 814-819.

Refshauge, K., & Higgs, J. (1994). Teaching clinical reasoning in health science curricula. In J. Higgs (Ed.), *Clinical reasoning in the health professions* (pp.105-116). Oxford: Butterworth-Heinemann Ltd.

Rogers, J. C. (1982). Clinical reasoning of occupational therapists dunng the initial assessment of physically disabled patients. *Occupational Therapy Journal of Research, 2*(4), 195-219.

Rogers, J. C. (1983). Clinical reasoning: The ethics, science and art. *The American Journal of Occupational Therapy, 37,* 601-616.

Rogers, J. C., & Holm, M. B. (1990a). *The therapist's thinking behind functional assessment: Part one.* Rockville, MD: The American Occupational Therapy Association Inc.

Rogers, J. C., & Holm, M. B. (1990b). *The therapist's thinking behind functional assessment: Part two.* Rockville, MD: The American Occupational Therapy Association Inc.

Rogers, J. C., & Holm, M. B. (1991). Occupational therapy diagnostic reasoning: A component of clinical reasoning. *The American Journal of Occupational Therapy, 45*(11), 1045-1053.

Ryan, S. (1995). Teaching clinical reasoning to occupational therapists during fieldwork education. In J. Higgs & M. Jones (Eds.), *Clinical reasoning in the health professions* (pp. 246-257). Oxford: Butterworth-Heinemann Ltd.

Rybash, J. M., Hoyer, W. J., & Roodin, P. A. (1986). *Adult cognition and aging: Developmental changes in processing, knowing and thinking.* New York: Pergamon Press.

Schon, D. (1987). *Educating the reflective practitioner.* San Francisco: Jossey-Bass.

Schwartz, K. B. (1991). Clinical reasoning and new ideas on intelligence: Implications for teaching and learning. *The American Journal of Occupational Therapy, 45*(11), 1033-1037.

Slater, D. Y., & Cohn, E. S. (1991). Staff development through analysis of practice. *The American Journal of Occupational Therapy, 45*(11), 1038-1043.

Thomas, S., Wearing, A., & Bennett, M. (1991). *Clinical decision making for nurses and health professionals.* Marickville, NSW: Harcourt Brace Jovanovich Ltd.

Twible, R., Bridge, C., Ranka, J., Beltran, R., & Bye, R. (1993). *Occupational Therapy Model Descriptor (OTMD),* Unpublished lecture material. School of Occupational Therapy, Faculty of Health Sciences, The University of Sydney. NSW: Australia.

Wilcock, A. A. (1991). Occupational science. *The British Journal of Occupational Therapy, 54*(8), 297-300.

Wittman, P. P. (1990). The disparity between educational preparation and the expectations of practice. *The American Journal of Occupational Therapy, 44*(12), 1130-1131.

Young, M. E., & Quinn, E. (1992). *Theories and principles of occupational therapy.* London: Churchill Livingstone.

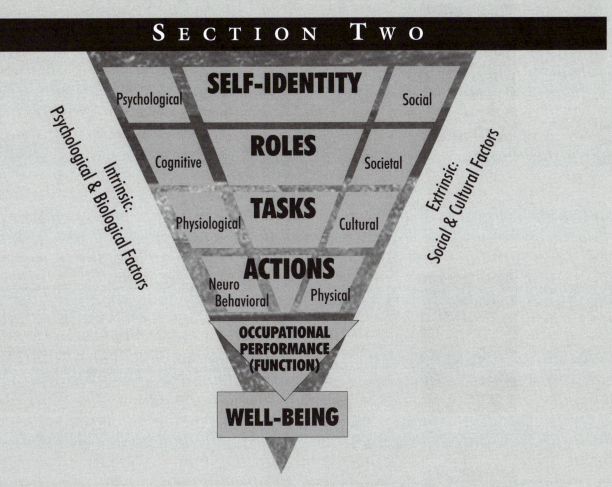

Intrinsic
Psychological and
Biological Factors

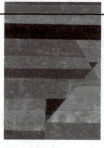

Chapter Content Outline

Abstract

This chapter reviews the basic systems and functions of the central nervous system. After providing overviews of each system, the chapter also provides methods for interpreting the meaning of behaviors from a neuroscience point of view.

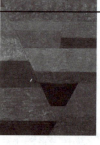

Key Terms

Autogenic facilitation

Autogenic inhibition

Balance of power

Centrifugal control

Convergence

Divergence

Plasticity

Release phenomenon

Suppression

Excitation

Inhibition

Intersensory integration

Compensatory action of the CNS

Corporal potentiality

Topographic

Tonotopic

Somatotopic

Habituation

Sensitization

Poor registration

Sensitivity to stimuli

Sensation seeking

Sensation avoiding

Homonymous hemianopia

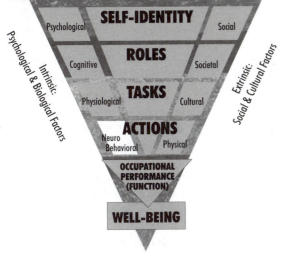

CHAPTER 8

Implementing Neuroscience Principles to Support Habilitation and Recovery

Winnie Dunn, PhD, OTR, FAOTA

OBJECTIVES

The information in this chapter is intended to help the reader:

1. appreciate the importance of various brain functions in the performance of life tasks

2. identify the basic neurological mechanisms which support performance

3. describe the similarities and differences among systems within the central nervous system

4. understand the roles of attentional, motivational and emotional systems in support of performance

5. recognize examples of release phenomena within the CNS

6. identify a range of contextually relevant interventions to support performance in persons with brain involvement in their disability

7. interpret the meaning of behaviors from a neuroscience point of view, as a contributing factor in intervention planning.

"...the demonstration that learning is accompanied by changes in the effectiveness of neural connections suggests a new view of the relationship between social and biological processes in the generation of behavior."
—Eric R. Kandel, 1991

BASIC NEUROLOGICAL PRINCIPLES THAT SUPPORT PERFORMANCE

Neurological principles enable us to understand how the nervous system operates to support performance. They are important because they subserve all the functions of the central nervous system (CNS) and are one of the key intrinsic factors that support occupational performance (see Person-Environment Occupational Performance Model in Chapter 3). The occupational therapist can select and design activities compatible with central nervous system functions, and take full advantage of their impact to support or facilitate performance.

Centrifugal Control

Centrifugal control, the most basic principle of CNS operations, is the brain's ability to regulate its own input. The CNS ensures that the information it receives and processes is the most useful for its own functioning. Four types of centrifugal control: suppression, balance of power, divergence and convergence (Noback & Demerest, 1987) will be discussed.

Suppression

Suppression is the CNS' ability to screen certain stimuli so that other stimuli receive more careful attention. Persons are bombarded with an array of sensory stimuli throughout the day; through suppression, the brain determines which stimuli warrant attention and response and which stimuli can be ignored safely. People who are distractible are likely to have poor suppression; they have difficulty engaging in purposeful behavior because they are constantly attending to all the other stimuli available in the environment. Those with poor suppression often have difficulty screening out appropriate stimuli. If the wrong stimuli are screened out or if stimuli are screened based on rigid or ritualistic patterns rather than in response to specific environmental demands, the person may engage in inappropriate or even dangerous behaviors.

Balance of Power

The balance of power refers to the complementary functions of the various parts of the brain. For example, certain parts of the brain are responsible for increasing activity level, while other parts provide inhibitory control. Some parts of the brain initiate movement and other parts stop or control the amount of movement that occurs. Normally, there is a balance of power, enabling the CNS to finely tune responses to meet all environmental demands.

When the balance of power is disrupted as in brain injury,

Bibliographic citation of this chapter: Dunn, W. (1977). Implementing neuroscience principles to support habilitation and recovery. In C. Christiansen & C. Baum (Eds.), *Occupational therapy: Enabling function and well-being* (2nd ed.). Thorofare, NJ: SLACK Incorporated.

the CNS experiences a *release phenomenon*. With injury in higher cortical centers, arousal mechanisms are released from inhibitory control, which can lead to hyperactivity and distractibility. These behaviors do not reflect dysfunction in the arousal mechanisms themselves (i.e., the reticular activating system), but rather represent a disassociation of arousal systems from control usually provided by modulating centers (i.e., a release). A release phenomenon can occur in any part of the CNS related to any function. Many of the abnormal behaviors observed and documented by occupational therapists can be attributed to a release phenomenon, or poor maintenance of the balance of power in the CNS.

Divergence

Divergence is the CNS's ability to send information it receives from one source to many parts of the CNS simultaneously. For example, if the brain receives a stimulus signaling potential harm, that information needs to get to many areas simultaneously to generate "fight or flight" responses. Divergence also ensures that an entire muscle is engaged in action when a movement is required, rather than a small number of muscle fibers.

Convergence

Convergent neurons require input from a variety of sources before a response will be generated. For example, a specific neuron may activate only if it receives three or more types of input. Convergent neurons enable the CNS to temper responsiveness to specific stimuli thus preventing a person from reacting inappropriately when only partial stimuli are available. Without this convergent neuronal network, the individual would respond to every stimulus, demonstrating poor integration of the convergent neuronal network.

Balance of Excitation and Inhibition

Excitation

Excitation is the depolarization of neurons that moves them closer to the activation threshold. Temporal patterns occur when a neuron is repeatedly stimulated, enabling the neuron to either be slowly depolarized or to continue sending a message over and over again as is required to maintain muscle tone for postural control. Spatial neuronal patterns occur simultaneously over many areas of the brain when engaging many CNS components at once is important, such as when noticing a sound, recognizing it as a baby's cry, determining it is a hungry cry, and proceeding to fill that need.

Inhibition

Inhibition is the hyperpolarization of neurons that makes it more difficult for the neurons to activate. Inhibition is the

CNS's ability to decrease its responsiveness to specific stimuli at any given moment. Although neuroscientists frequently discuss descending inhibition (i.e., higher centers having an effect on lower centers), the CNS is rich with interneuron networks that can inhibit neighboring cells (i.e., lateral inhibition). Lateral inhibition helps make target stimuli stronger and clearer, which contributes to organization and integration of information for the CNS.

Feedback and Feedforward Mechanisms

Feedback is the CNS's ability to send information back to itself as a check and balance. This enables the person to judge whether actions already initiated need to be modified for the future. Noback & Demerest (1981) describe two general types of feedback: local feedback and reflected feedback. Local feedback inhibition occurs when small interneurons within a neighboring circuit form connections that stop a stimulus that has been occurring in a large neuron. This mechanism helps keep activity from continuing beyond its useful period. For example, a local feedback circuit can stop the ongoing firing of a motor neuron by sending an inhibitory signal to the motor nerve, thus allowing a person to relax the muscle and stop the movement. This inhibition, however, occurs only if the local circuit neuron information is stronger than other messages on that large motor neuron. Reflected feedback occurs when higher CNS centers send descending fibers to influence the sensory or motor neurons. These higher centers can send excitatory or inhibitory messages making it either easier or more difficult to activate the neurons.

Feedforward circuits exert influence in a forward direction coinciding with the information flow of the neurons. This most frequently occurs in ascending sensory system pathways to either alert higher centers about incoming information or inhibit some areas in order to strengthen the focus of more important parts of the environmental stimuli. Feedforward inhibition is critical for task performance, because people always are confronted with more stimuli than are needed to complete the task successfully.

Intersensory Integration

Intersensory integration is a critical feature of the CNS. Interneurons in the spinal cord participate in primitive intersensory integration, however the brain stem is a primary site for this activity. Nuclei in the brain stem receive input from several sensory sources, allowing organization and integration of information at this level. For example, the vestibular nuclei receive input from the vestibular organ, the visual system and the proprioceptors. This intersensory integration supports the development of a multidimensional map of self and environment and a map of how self and environment interact appropriately.

Plasticity

Plasticity is the CNS's ability to adapt structurally or functionally in response to environmental demands. Previously, neuroscientists believed that plasticity was most evident during the prenatal stage and childhood; now researchers have found that there are various types of internal and external environmental alterations that support or inhibit the manifestations of plasticity (Lund, 1978). When individuals participate in interventions that require more functional patterns of movement, they receive organized patterns of sensory feedback that may alter the internal environment, creating opportunities for axon reorganization, altered synaptic activity, or dendritic branching, just as enriched environments support these actions during the developmental periods (Bach-y-Rita, 1980; Moore, 1980). Such findings challenge innovative rehabilitation practice.

Compensatory Action of the CNS

Parts of the CNS are interdependent (Moore, 1980). When damage occurs to one or more portions of the system, the interdependency relationships are disrupted; the resulting observable behaviors and performance are hypothesized to be compensating for the loss of information from one of its members. This compensatory model suggests that the CNS centers do not function on their own to initiate action, but work as part of a network in the CNS to enable a particular action. When data are not available to the system because of damage, the network is disrupted, making it difficult for a particular action to occur. Destructive behavior is the result of an incomplete and compensating CNS.

Summary

The principles of centrifugal control, balance of excitation and inhibition, plasticity, and compensatory action are basic and must be used to design interventions that support occupational performance. Interventions that conflict with these basic principles compromise the person by not enabling them to profit from the therapeutic experience.

THE SENSORY SYSTEMS

The olfactory (smell) and gustatory (taste) systems are primitive, chemically-based sensory systems signaling the CNS about odors and tastes. The somatosensory, proprioceptive and vestibular systems enable an individual to develop an accurate map of self and how one interacts with the environment. Finally, the visual and auditory systems are responsible for mapping environmental variables so that interaction with the environment can be accurate and reliable.

General Principles of Sensory System Operations

Although each sensory system is unique, there are some basic similarities in the way all sensory systems develop and function:

1. *Input mechanisms.* Each sensory system is responsible for bringing information from the environment to the nervous system for processing.
2. *Processing levels.* Each sensory system processes its own special brand of information at a variety of central nervous system levels including the receptor site, spinal cord, brain stem, thalamus (except for olfactory), and higher cortical centers.
3. *Multidimensional information.* The sensation from each sensory system is complex and multidimensional.
4. *Purposes for processing information.* Each sensory system processes information for two primary purposes: a) to identify stimuli in the environment, making the CNS aware of these stimuli, determining which require attention and which are potentially harmful (i.e., arousal or alerting mechanisms) and b) gathering information to construct maps of self and environment to be used by the CNS for organization and planning (i.e., discrimination or mapping).

When the CNS is functioning normally, the arousal/alerting and discrimination/mapping components complement each other to form a balance of power. This allows the individual to interact with the environment and gather information for discrimination and mapping under most conditions, while always having the capability to notice potentially harmful stimuli. This balance of power is delicate and requires constant assessment of environmental stimuli so that all potentially important stimuli are noticed without interfering with ongoing purposeful activity.

The components of arousal/attention and discrimination/mapping will be discussed in each sensory system section. As a guide to understanding the sensory systems, Tables 8-1, 8-2, and 8-3 summarize key information that can be used therapeutically. Table 8-1 lists the descriptors for each sensory system; the descriptors are divided into columns to correspond to the arousal/alerting and discrimination/mapping functions that each descriptor tends to support. For example, light touch is an arousal/alerting stimulus in the somatosensory system, while touch pressure is a discrimination/mapping stimulus. It also contains a brief definition of each descriptor, with a simple daily life example to aid in application.

Table 8-2 uses the same descriptor words and organizing columns and provides a brief rationale for using each sensory descriptor in a therapeutic manner. Remembering that each type of sensation is important can be therapeutic when selected and applied appropriately. For example, light touch

can be a therapeutic input if a provider needs to increase alertness in a person who is lethargic; the additional arousal/alerting input could establish a more optimal biobehavioral state for engaging in a functional task. In a later section we will consider ways to use these sensory stimuli in relation to the arousal and attentional mechanisms.

Table 8-3 contains examples of observable behaviors which might indicate difficulties with sensory processing during daily life tasks. Information from this table could be used to construct a referral or observational checklist for interdisciplinary team members and assist team members (including family members) in learning how to consider the impact of sensory processing on performance.

The Chemical Senses

The gustatory system is responsible for our sense of taste. Early in evolution, the differentiation between the gustatory and olfactory systems was minor because primitive organisms lived in the sea. When they moved to land, these two systems differentiated to serve the organism in very different ways. The gustatory system became the final checking system for food that was to enter the body, whereas the olfactory system became the chemical sense that could determine the location or direction of stimuli (e.g., food or predators) from a distance. The olfactory system became important for mapping the environment for survival (Coren, Porac, & Ward, 1984). From a neuroanatomical standpoint, senses of smell and taste travel by very different routes to inform the cerebral cortex about environmental events.

The Gustatory System

Taste is determined by an items' solubility, intensity, and amount. There is general agreement that taste can be labeled with language: sweet, salty, sour, and bitter (Coren, Porac, & Ward, 1984). Tastes are discriminated both by the types of molecules found and by the way they are broken down by the chemicals within the system. Taste buds are the receptor organs for the gustatory system. As many as 10,000 taste buds are available to young people; this amount decreases during the aging process.

Gustatory information travels from the sensory receptors in the tongue to the brain stem where the information is relayed to the thalamus. The thalamus sends information to the cortical taste area in the sensory homunculus or the parietal lobe and enables us not only to have an accurate map of the tongue but also to allow conscious sensation of taste (Heimer, 1983). Because taste is part of the cranial nerve network, its functions are jeopardized by brain stem trauma. Additionally, gustatory information reaches both the hypothalamus and the cortical taste area in the inferior frontal gyrus. Degenerative neurological diseases that affect these areas have a corresponding effect on taste and subsequent food intake. The hypothalamus connections are important because of their believed contributions to feeding behaviors which drive the organism to ingest food (Bellingham, Wayne, & Barone, 1979).

The characteristic taste patterns of the tongue have been mapped by many authors. Although the separation of function is important from a neuroscience standpoint, from a functional standpoint the overall appeal of food is the major consideration. An individual's response to taste are very unique and seem to rely not only on experiential information but also on the genetic makeup of the individual. Some researchers have reported groups of people as being immune to tastes for certain substances. One of these substances is caffeine. Studies have shown that there are those who taste caffeine and those who do not (Blakeslee & Salmon, 1935; Coren, Porac, & Ward, 1984; Hall, Bartoshuk, Cain, & Stevens, 1975). From testing various substances, researchers hypothesize that there is a genetic mechanism that either allows or does not allow responsiveness to specific chemical changes that the substances produce.

Because of the deterioration process with aging, elderly persons often complain about blandness of food. Halpern and Meiselman (1980) found that salting food is in part a person's attempt to reach that person's specific threshold for taste. Recovery from stimulation in the gustatory system occurs within 10 seconds after the stimulus, so a slower eating process or a process of mixing bites of salty food with bites of unsalty food is likely to produce less continuous seasoning of food during the meal.

Olfactory Sense

The olfactory system responds to odors in the environment. The process of smell is a complicated one, beginning with the intake of substances by the olfactory epithelium in the top portion of the nasal cavity. The internal cells of the olfactory system project directly to portions of higher centers and bypass the thalamus, unlike all other sensory systems.

The olfactory system is a very sensitive system, even more sensitive than its chemical counterpart, the gustatory system. However, unlike the taste system, researchers have been unable to discover basic categories of smell. The system is so complex and capable of responding to so many types of odors, that classification becomes extremely difficult.

Humans tend to underrate the role and effects of the olfactory system on performance and functioning in daily life. With specific connections to the limbic system, the olfactory system has the potential to establish memories and associations of our roles as children and adults as well as memories of recent events. Because of the direct connections with arousal networks, the olfactory input also can increase our level of responsiveness quickly. Use of strong odors to arouse people in semi-comatose states points out the powerful role of olfactory input.

Clinicians must remain aware of the olfactory sensory system in the planning and provision of services. Because individuals emit specific odors, persons may recognize their therapist not only from visual, auditory, and somatosensory cues, but also from olfactory cues. This factor may contribute to disorientation and agitation when substitutions occur. Additionally, therapists must be very careful about the additions of odors such as shampoos, perfumes, and laundry detergents. Although these factors go unnoticed by the normally functioning nervous system, a vulnerable system may react in unpredictable ways. Therapists must consider all possibilities when unusual behaviors present themselves as observable behavior provides a window to CNS activity.

Olfactory input is also important in the environments where persons are served. The sterile environment of the hospital provides a type of olfactory sensory deprivation (Moore, 1980). In the familiar home environment, the olfactory system can contribute to orientation by familiar odors.

Persons who have difficulty with the olfactory system often begin to complain about the taste of foods. Even though the smell of food does not contribute directly to its taste, people seem to associate the smell of food with the taste. Because both taste and smell relate to individuals' food preferences, therapists should be curious regarding interpretations of food complaints.

Somatosensory System

The somatosensory system responds to stimuli from the skin surface. The unique placement of these receptors senses where the body ends and where the world begins. The combined input from various somatosensory receptors form a multidimensional picture of skin stimulation.

Receptive fields are the location on the surface of the skin that is innervated by one neuron; they contribute to multidimensional maps. Accurate somatosensory perception requires not only that the receptive fields function accurately, but that they function in concert with each other. Receptive fields overlap a great deal on the head, hands, and arms (Figure 8-1), whereas they overlap very little on the back (Figure 8-2). This is functionally significant because human beings identify the exact location of the touch experience on body surfaces that have overlapping receptive fields because the various neurons from several receptive fields that share that location report information to the brain simultaneously, but can only identify the general area being touched on the back. Multiple input from various sources enables the brain to narrow the possible locations until it can identify the one spot on the surface of the skin that is shared by all of the activated neurons.

TABLE 8-1

Arousal/Alerting and Discrimination/Mapping Descriptors of the Sensory System

Sensory System	Arousal/Alerting Descriptors*	Discrimination/Mapping Descriptors**
For all systems	**Unpredictable:** The task is unfamiliar; the child cannot anticipate the sensory experiences that will occur in the task.	**Predictable:** Sensory pattern in the task is routine for the child, such as diaper changing—the child knows what is occurring and what will come next.
Somatosensory	**Light touch:** Gentle tapping on skin; tickling (e.g., loose clothing making contact with skin). **Pain:** Brisk pinching; contact with sharp objects; skin pressed in small surface (e.g., when skin is caught between chair arm and seat). **Temperature:** Hot or cold stimuli (e.g., iced drinks, hot foods, cold hands, cold metal chairs). **Variable:** Changing characteristics during the task (e.g., putting clothing on requires a combination of tactile experiences). **Short duration stimuli:** Tapping, touching briefly (e.g., splashing water). **Small body surface contact:** Small body surfaces, as when using only fingertips to touch something.	**Touch pressure:** Firm contact on skin (e.g., hugging, patting, grasping). Occurs both when touching objects or persons, or when they touch you. **Long duration stimuli:** Holding, grasping (e.g., carrying a child in your arms). **Large body surface contact:** Large body surfaces include holding, hugging; also includes holding a cup with the entire palmar surface of hand.
Vestibular	**Head position change:** The child's head orientation is altered (e.g., pulling the child up from lying on the back to sitting). **Speed change:** Movements change velocity (e.g., the teacher stops to talk to another teacher when pushing the child to the bathroom in his wheelchair). **Direction change:** Movements change planes, such as bending down to pick something up from the floor while carrying the child down the hall. **Rotary head movement:** Head moving in an arc (e.g., spinning in a circle, turning head side to side).	**Linear head movement:** Head moving in a straight line (e.g., bouncing up and down, going down the hall in a wheelchair). **Repetitive head movement:** Movements that repeat in a simple sequence (e.g., rocking in a rocker).
Proprioception	**Quick stretch:** Movements that pull on the muscles (e.g., briskly tapping on a muscle belly).	**Sustained tension:** Steady, constant action on the muscles pressing or holding on the muscle (e.g., using heavy objects during play). **Shifting muscle tension:** Activities that demand constant change in the muscles (e.g., walking, lifting, and moving objects).
Visual	**High intensity:** Visual stimulus is bright (e.g., looking out the window on a bright day). **High contrast:** A lot of difference between the visual stimulus and its surrounding environment (e.g., cranberry juice in a white cup). **Variable:** Changing characteristics during the task (e.g., a TV program is a variable visual stimulus).	**Low intensity:** Visual stimulus is subdued (e.g., finding objects in the dark closet). **High similarity:** Small differences between visual stimulus and its surrounding environment (e.g., oatmeal in a beige bowl). **Competitive:** The background is interesting or busy (e.g., the junk drawer, a bulletin board).

TABLE 8-1 (continued)

Arousal/Alerting and Discrimination/Mapping Descriptors of the Sensory System

Sensory System	Arousal/Alerting Descriptors*	Discrimination/Mapping Descriptors**
Auditory	**Variable:** Changing characteristics during the task (e.g., a person's voice with intonation). **High intensity:** The auditory stimulus is loud (e.g., siren, high volume radio).	**Rhythmic:** Sounds repeat in a simple sequence/beat (e.g., humming; singing nursery songs). **Constant:** The stimulus is always present (e.g., a fan noise). **Competitive:** The environment has a variety of recurring sounds (e.g., the classroom, a party). **Noncompetitive:** The environment is quiet (e.g., the bedroom when all is ready for bedtime). **Low intensity:** The auditory stimulus is subdued (e.g., whispering).
Olfactory/ gustatory	**Strong intensity:** The taste/smell has distinct qualities (e.g., spinach).	**Mild intensity:** The taste/smell has nondistinct or familiar qualities (e.g., cream of wheat).

*Arousal/alerting stimuli tend to generate "noticing" behaviors. The individual's attention is at least momentarily drawn toward the stimulus (commonly disrupting ongoing behavior). These stimuli enable the nervous system to orient to stimuli that may require a protective response. In some situations, an arousing stimulus can become part of a functional behavior pattern (e.g., when the arousing somatosensory input from putting on the shirt becomes predictable, a discriminating/mapping characteristic).

**Discriminatory/mapping stimuli are those that enable the individual to gather information that can be used to support and generate functional behaviors. The information yields spatial and temporal qualities of body and environment (the content of the maps), which can be used to create purposeful movement. These stimuli are more organizing for the nervous system.

From Dunn, W. (1991). The sensorimotor systems: A framework for assessment and intervention. In F. P. Orelove & D. Sobsey (Eds.), *Educating children with multiple disabilities: A transdisciplinary approach* (2nd ed.). Baltimore, MD: Paul H. Brookes. Reprinted with permission.

When the receptors send information to the central nervous system, the neurons travel into the spinal cord to ascend to higher centers. In certain ascending pathways of the somatosensory system, synapses occur immediately upon entrance to the spinal cord, while others travel to the brain stem before their first synapse occurs (Figure 8-3). Traditionally, the somatosensory pathways have been divided into two systems: the posterior columns for touch-pressure and proprioception, and the lateral spinothalamic for light touch, pain, and temperature reception. Recent evidence suggests that a broader view of somatosensory processing is required to interpret clinical observations accurately. When studying brain systems, attempting to explain the very complex actions of the CNS in an oversimplified way is common. As research techniques and technology become more sophisticated, scientists and practitioners gain knowledge and achieve a better understanding of the complexity of the CNS.

Heimer (1983) reports that the ascending sensory pathways can be divided into three categories, each showing an important role to the understanding of performance.

1. The first category is the *anterolateral system*. This is located in the anterior (front) and side portions of the spinal cord and appears to be responsible for processing pain and temperature information. This includes the spinothalamic tract, the spinoreticular and spinotectal tracts. Because they are very closely related anatomically, damage to one often involves damage to the others as well.

The anterolateral pathways synapse at the spinal cord level that corresponds to the receptor input location, the second neuron crosses over to travel in the anterior or lateral aspect of the spinal cord to the thalamus, and then to the sensorimotor cortex. Collateral fibers synapse with the reticular cells in the brain stem en route to the thalamus. The spinoreticular tract also synapses in the reticular cells of the brain stem. Reticular connections are important when examining the characteristics of arousal.

2. The second category includes pathways for touch-pressure, vibration, and proprioception. Although the *dorsal columns* have been seen classically as the pathways that carry out these functions, recent studies have shown that the *dorsolateral fasciculus* (which lies just laterally to the dorsal columns and the posterior horn of the gray matter) also carries this information, especially from the lower extremities. Researchers have also shown weak processing of touch-pressure input via anterolateral pathways.

TABLE 8-2

Reasons for Incorporating Various Sensory Qualities into Integrated Intervention Programs

Sensory System	Arousal/Alerting Descriptors	Discrimination/Mapping Descriptors
For all systems	**Unpredictable:** To develop an increasing level of attention to keep the child interested in the task/activity (e.g., change the position of the objects on the child's lap tray during the task).	**Predictable:** To establish the child's ability to anticipate a programming sequence or a salient cue; to decrease possibility to be distracted from a functional task sequence (e.g., use the same routine for diaper changing every time).
Somatosensory	**Light touch:** To increase alertness in a child who is lethargic (e.g., pull cloth from child's face during peek-a-boo). **Pain:** To raise from unconsciousness; to determine ability to respond to noxious stimuli when unconscious (e.g., flick palm of hand or sole of foot briskly). **Temperature:** To establish awareness of stimuli; to maintain attentiveness to task (e.g., use hot foods for spoon eating and cold drink for sucking through a straw). **Variable:** To maintain attention to or interest in the task (e.g., place new texture on cup surface each day so child notices the cup). **Short duration:** To increase arousal for task performance (e.g., tap child on chest before giving directions). **Small body surface contact:** To generate and focus attention on a particular body part (e.g., tap around lips with fingertips before eating task).	**Touch pressure:** To establish and maintain awareness of body parts and body position; to calm a child who has been overstimulated (e.g., provide a firm bear hug). **Long duration:** To enable the child to become familiar, comfortable with the stimulus; to incorporate stimulus into functional skill (e.g., grasping the container to pick it up and pour out contents). **Large body surface contact:** To establish and maintain awareness of body parts and body position; to calm a child who has been overstimulated (e.g., wrap child tightly in a blanket).
Vestibular	**Head position change:** To increase arousal for an activity (e.g., position child prone over a wedge). **Speed change:** To maintain adequate alertness for functional task (e.g., vary pace while carrying the child to a new task). **Direction change:** To elevate level of alertness for a functional task (e.g., swing child back and forth in arms prior to positioning him or her at the table for a task). **Rotary head movement:** To increase arousal prior to functional task (e.g., pick child up from prone [on stomach] facing away to upright facing toward you to position for a new task).	**Linear head movement:** To support establishment of body awareness in space (e.g., carry child around the room in fixed position to explore its features). **Repetitive head movement:** To provide predictable and organizing information; to calm a child who has been overstimulated (e.g., rock the child).
Proprioception	**Quick stretch:** To generate additional muscle tension to support functional tasks (e.g., tap muscle belly of hypotonic muscle while providing physical guidance to grasp).	**Sustained tension:** To enable the muscle to relax, elongate, so body part can be in more optimal position for function (e.g., press firmly across muscle belly while guiding a reaching pattern; add weight to objects being manipulated). **Shifting muscle tension:** To establish functional movements that contain stability and mobility (e.g., prop and reach for a top; reach, fill, and lift spoon to mouth).

TABLE 8-2 (CONTINUED)

Reasons for Incorporating Various Sensory Qualities into Integrated Intervention Programs

Sensory System	Arousal/Alerting Descriptors	Discrimination/Mapping Descriptors
Visual	**High intensity:** To increase opportunity to notice object; to generate arousal for task (e.g., cover blocks with foil for manipulation task). **High contrast:** To enhance possibility of locating the object and maintaining attention to it (e.g., place raisins on a piece of typing paper for prehension activity). **Variable:** To maintain attention to or interest in the task (e.g., play rolling catch with a clear ball that has moveable pieces inside).	**Low intensity:** To allow the visual stimulus to blend with other salient features; to generate searching behaviors, since characteristics are less obvious (e.g., kind own cubby hole in back of the room). **High similarity:** To establish more discerning abilities; to develop skills for naturally occurring tasks (e.g., scoop apple sauce from beige plate). **Competitive:** To facilitate searching; to increase tolerance for natural life circumstances (e.g., obtain correct tools from equipment bin).
Auditory	**Variable:** To maintain attention to or interest in the task (e.g., play radio station after activating a switch). **High intensity:** To stimulate noticing the person or object; to create proper alerting for task performance (e.g., ring a bell to encourage the child to locate the stimulus).	**Rhythmic:** To provide predictable and organizing information for environmental orientation (e.g., sing a nursery rhyme while physically guiding motions). **Constant:** To provide a foundational stimulus for environmental orientation; especially important when other sensory systems (e.g., vision, vestibular) do not provide orientation (e.g., child recognizes own classroom by fan noise and calms down). **Competitive:** To facilitate differentiation of salient stimuli; to increase tolerance for natural life circumstances (e.g., after child learns to look when his or her name is called, conduct activity within busy classroom). **Noncompetitive:** To facilitate focused attention for acquiring a new and difficult skill; to calm a child who has been overstimulated (e.g., move child to quiet room to establish vocalizations). **Low intensity:** To allow the auditory stimulus to blend with other salient features; to generate searching behaviors since stimulus is less obvious (e.g., give child a direction in a normal volume).
Olfactory/ gustatory	**Strong intensity:** To stimulate arousal for task (e.g., child smells spaghetti sauce at lunch).	**Mild intensity:** To facilitate exploratory behaviors; to stimulate naturally occurring activities (e.g., smell of lunch food is less distinct, so child is encouraged to notice texture, color).

From Dunn, W. (1991). The sensorimotor systems: A framework for assessment and intervention. In F. P. Orelove & D. Sobsey (Eds.), *Educating children with multiple disabilities: A transdisciplinary approach* (2nd ed.). Baltimore, MD: Paul H. Brookes. Reprinted with permission.

TABLE 8-3

Examples of Observable Behaviors That Indicate Difficulty With Sensory Processing During Daily Life Tasks

	Personal Hygiene	Dressing	Eating	Homemaking	School/Work	Play
Somatosensory	• withdraws from splashing water • pushes washcloth/towel away • cries when hair is washed & dried • makes face when toothpaste gets on lips, tongue • tenses when bottom is wiped after toileting	• tolerates a narrow range of clothing items • prefers tight clothing • more irritable with loose-textured clothing • cries during dressing • pulls at hats, head gear, accessories	• only tolerates food at one temperature • gags with textured food or utensils in mouth • winces when face is wiped • hand extends & avoids objects & surfaces (finger food, utensils)	• avoids participation in tasks that are wet, dirty • seeks to remove batter that falls on arms	• cries when tape or glue gets on skin • overreacts to pats, hugs; avoids these actions • only tolerates one pencil, one type of paper, only wooden objects • hands extend when attempting to type	• selects a narrow range of toys, textures similar • can't hold onto toys/objects • rubs toys on face, arms • mouths objects
Proprioception	• can't lift objects that are heavier such as a new bar of soap • can't change head position to use sink & mirror in same task	• can't support heavier items, e.g., belt with buckle, shoes • fatigues prior to task completion • misses when placing arm or leg in clothing	• uses external support to eat (e.g., propping) • tires before completing meal • can't provide force to cut meat • tires before completing foods that need to be chewed	• drops equipment (e.g., broom) • uses external support such as leaning on counter to stir batter • has difficulty in pouring a glass of milk	• drops books • becomes uncomfortable in a particular position • hooks limbs on furniture to obtain support • moves arm, hand in repetitive patterns (self-stimulatory)	• unable to sustain movements during play • tries before game is complete • drops heavy parts of a toy/game
Vestibular	• becomes disoriented when bending over the sink • falls when trying to participate in washing lower extremities	• gets overly excited/distracted after bending down to assist in putting on socks • cries when moved around a lot during dressing	• holds head stiffly in one position during mealtime • gets distracted from meal after several head position changes	• avoids learning to obtain cooking utensil • becomes overly excited after moving around the room to dust	• avoids turning head to look at persons; to find source of a sound • after being transported in a wheelchair, more difficult to get on task • moves head in repetitive pattern (self-stimulatory)	• avoids play that includes movement • becomes overly excited or anxious when moving during play • rocks excessively • craves movement activities
Visual	• can't find utensils on the sink • has difficulty in spotting desired item in drawer • misses when applying paste to toothbrush	• can't find buttons on patterned or solid clothing • overlooks desired shirt in closet or drawer • misses armhole when donning shirt	• misses utensils on the table • has trouble getting foods onto spoon when they are a similar color to the plate	• can't locate correct canned item in the pantry • has difficulty finding cooking utensils in the drawer	• can't keep place on the page • can't locate desired item on communication board • attends excessively to bright or flashing objects	• has trouble with matching, sorting activities • has trouble locating desired toy on cluttered shelf

TABLE 8-3 (CONTINUED)

Examples of Observable Behaviors That Indicate Difficulty With Sensory Processing During Daily Life Tasks

	Personal Hygiene	Dressing	Eating	Homemaking	School/Work	Play
Auditory	• cries when hair dryer is turned on • becomes upset by running water • jerks when toilet flushes	• is distracted by clothing that makes noise (e.g., crisp cloth, accessories)	• is distracted by noise of utensils against each other (e.g., spoon in bowl, knife on plate) • can't keep eating when someone talks	• is distracted by vacuum cleaner sound • is distracted by TV or radio during tasks	• is distracted by squeaky wheelchair • is intolerant of noise others make in the room • overreacts to door closing • notices toilet flushing down the hall	• play is disrupted by sounds • makes sounds constantly
Olfactory/ gustatory	• gags at taste of toothpaste • jerks away at smell of soap	• overreacts to clothing when it has been washed in a new detergent	• tolerates a narrow range of foods • becomes upset when certain hot foods are cooking	• becomes upset when house is being cleaned (odors of cleansers)	• overreacts to new person (new smells) • intolerant of scratch-n-sniff stickers • smells everything	• tastes or smells all objects before playing

The dorsal column fibers take a somewhat different route to the thalamus and cortex. The neuron at the receptor site travels into the spinal cord and directly up through the posterior columns to the medulla (the lowest portion of the brain stem). At this point, a synapse occurs and the new fibers cross to the other side of the brain stem and travel to specific parts of the thalamus (ventrobasal complex of thalamus). This set of neurons synapses in the thalamus and then the next neutron carries information on to the sensorimotor cortex, specifically the postcentral gyrus of the parietal lobe. The postcentral gyrus contains the map of an individual's body from a sensory point of view. It is frequently referred to as the sensory homunculus.

The fibers that travel in the dorsolateral fasciculus synapse at the cervical level and the spinal cord. The new neuron crosses to the other side of the spinal cord and travels with the spinothalamic tract to the thalamus and on to the cortex. The source of some of the earlier confusion about the function of the ascending pathways is due to the mixed anatomical and functional relationship of the dorsolateral fasciculus with the dorsal columns and the anterolateral system.

3. The third functional category reported by Heimer (1983) includes the *unconscious proprioceptive pathways*. The spinocerebellar tracts serve the very specific function of providing the cerebellum with direct accurate sensory information before it is processed at higher levels of the brain. These pathways travel directly from the receptor side through the spinal cord and into the cerebellum. Pathways such as these allow the cerebellum to orchestrate motor activity through access to the sensation that stimulates a response. The higher motor centers also send processed information to the cerebellum, and so a comparison takes place between the original stimulus and this processed information in order to plan the motor event correctly. One can experience the action of the unconscious proprioceptive pathways when attempting to correct one's own movements. The cerebellum compares the plan and the sensation to determine whether an alteration must occur. It is this process that allows one to avoid knocking a glass over by picking it up correctly.

Acknowledging the functional significance of the anatomical relationships among these pathways is important. Some somatosensory sensations are ipsilateral to the pathways that

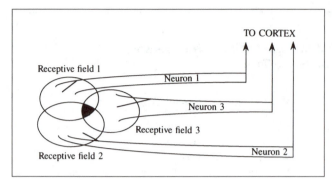

Figure 8-1. Three overlapping receptor fields send information to the cortex. This shared information helps localize the touch sensation.

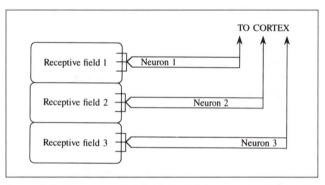

Figure 8-2. Three receptive fields that do not overlap. Separate pieces of information make it difficult to determine exactly where the touch occurred.

carry the input while others are contralateral to their corresponding pathways in the spinal cord. When there is damage in the spinal cord, pain and temperature loss is contralateral to the lesion while touch-pressure loss is ipsilateral to the lesion site. However, once nerve fibers reach the brain stem level all the sensory losses being contralateral to the lesion site.

Vestibular System

Structure and Function

The vestibular system makes a unique contribution to the multidimensional maps that enable individuals to interact with the environment effectively. The other sensory systems primarily provide information about self or environment. By providing constant and ongoing information about how the body interacts in the environment (i.e., person-environment fit); the vestibular system enables the individual to remain oriented in space and time.

In the final analysis, one may have a well-developed sensory map of the external world and a well-

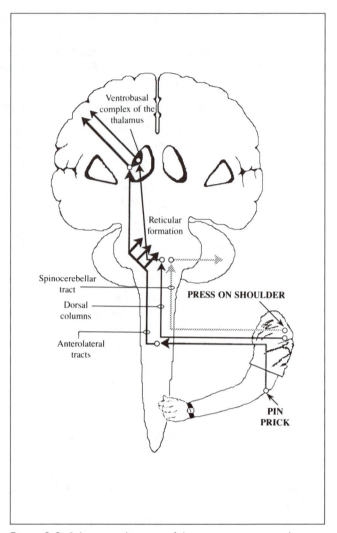

Figure 8-3. Schematic diagram of the somatosensory pathways.

developed motor map of movement from one place to another, but if one does not know where they are with respect to that map, they are virtually incapable of using that spatial mapping information. And the vestibular system appears to be the system that gives information about the individual's location in the overall spatial map (Cool, 1987, p. 3).

The vestibular organ is comprised of five components: three semicircular canals and two chambers. Collectively, they respond to type, direction, angle, and speed of movement, and head position. Information from these receptor sites combines within the CNS to determine the exact orientation of the head. Receptors in the three semicircular canals are most sensitive to angular movements, whereas the receptors of the chambers are responsible for linear movement (Heimer, 1983; Kornhuber, 1974; Goldberg & Fernandez,

1984). Gravity provides a major source of information for the vestibular receptors.

Three *semicircular canals* are located in each inner ear. The three semicircular canals are oriented at right angles to each other just like the three surfaces that meet in the corner of a room. If one would place one semicircular canal on each wall and the floor of the corner this would provide a good visual image of how the semicircular canals are related to each other anatomically. The structure of both sets of semicircular canals allows the brain to determine all head positions and movements. Corresponding canals on the right and left side respond in a complementary way so that the brain can determine which direction the head is moving. When the head moves in one direction, the canals on one side will produce an excitatory response while the corresponding canal on the other side will be inhibited. This causes a differential effect in central connections between the two sides and allows the brain to interpret the direction of head movement.

To fire the vestibular nerve, there must be a change in head position, rate (acceleration or deceleration), or direction in which the head is moving. When a person is engaged in a continuous angular movement (such as spinning at a constant speed and direction), the vestibular nerve does not fire. The two chambers are called the *utricle* and the *saccule*. The chambers respond to linear movement, especially along and against the force of gravity. Jumping up and down, running, and riding a wheeled toy or in a car provide linear stimulation.

Direct input from the vestibular organ travels to the vestibular nuclei (at the pontomedullary junction of the brain stem) and to a specialized portion of the cerebellum dedicated to vestibular processing (the flocculonodular lobe). The vestibulocerebellar connections are critical for postural control. Both the vestibular nuclei and cerebellum receive vestibular, proprioceptive, somatosensory, and visual input. This multisensory information is organized to produce basic background movements necessary for postural control.

Postural Control Network

The postural control network is comprised of three primary descending motor pathways that work together to create background movements, enabling an individual to engage in other activities. The *lateral vestibulospinal tract* is the largest of the tracts; it facilitates the extensor muscles, especially in the upper trunk and neck (Heimer, 1983; Noback & Demarest, 1981). The *medial vestibulospinal tract* is a small tract that facilities flexor tone while inhibiting extensor tone. The third pathway establishes the balance of power within the system; the *reticulospinal tract*, provides additional support for excitation of flexion and inhibition of extension. These pathways work together to modulate body posture (Figure 8-4). The vestibulocerebellar connections are well-documented pathways which also have an important role in the mainte-

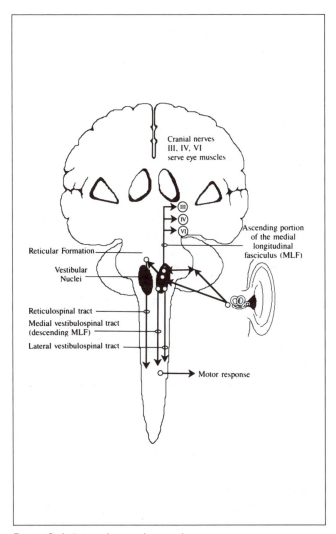

Figure 8-4. Postural control network.

nance of posture and orientation. As stated above, the cerebellar connections with the vestibular nuclei provide the inhibitory control necessary for maintenance of posture.

Postural control is a basic, primary functional behavior. Even in controlled studies where the vestibular organ has been removed, there is a serious initial change in postural stability but within a short period of time compensatory action reinstates some of the functions that have been lost (Darian-Smith, 1984). It is believed that other reflexive and sensory systems which contribute to postural control as well take over the orientation functions. Dependence on visual and proprioceptive input seems to occur when vestibular input is no longer available. The interrelationships among the sensory systems form the core of the multidimensional maps that allow appropriate interaction of self in the environment. As Jongkees (1974) states:

The vestibular organ is only one of the organs that inform us about our position in space. It cooperates with visual and kinesthetic sensations from muscles, joints, etc. As long as the information from these various sources is the same, we are well-informed about our position and our movements and everything is balanced. But as soon as they do not agree our balance is lost and we are subject to the frightening sensation of having lost contact with the world around us (p. 414).

The vestibular system acts as the silent partner during task performance, actively contributing postural control while the person's attention is focused on something else (Kornhuber, 1974). When an individual is carrying out a task, attention must be focused intently on the cognitive and perceptual components of that task. As other systems are providing information to the brain about the task, the vestibular system must automatically maintain the body's dynamic orientation in space to support task performance. If one were to have attention directed away from cognitive tasks every time vestibular stimulation were provided, human beings would be unable to engage in purposeful activity. deQuiros and Schrager (1978) use the term *corporal potentiality* to describe the ability to screen out vestibular and postural information at conscious levels in order to enable the cortex to engage in higher cognitive tasks. When individuals must expend a lot of energy processing vestibular information for postural control, cognitive processing may be disrupted.

Vestibulo-ocular Pathways

The vestibulo-ocular pathways enable the individual to coordinate head and eye movements. The medial longitudinal fasciculus (MLF) travels within the brain stem connecting the vestibular nuclei with the cranial nerve nuclei that serve the eye muscles (specifically cranial nerves III, IV, and VI, the oculomotor, trochlear, and abducens nerves, respectively). This ability to distinguish the source of the movement is necessary to maintain orientation in space. When there is a conflict between expected and obtained sensory information from eyes, eye muscles, and/or vestibular organ, connections with the autonomic nervous system generate a reaction (e.g., nausea, sweating); these reactions are usually classified as "motion sickness." Kornhuber (1974) related motion sickness to limbic system functions; it establishes the relationships among patterns of stimuli and particular autonomic reactions. The individual's control of motion and spatial orientation is threatened when the various sensory inputs simultaneously demand mutually incompatible postural adjustments.

Connections and Higher Cortical Connections

Physiological studies have demonstrated that certain brain centers produce short latency (quick) responses after vestibular stimulation. For example, through the collateral connections with the reticular cells, it is thought that vestibular information reaches higher centers of the brain for arousal and alerting responses. Reticular cells connect with the limbic system and would thus be associated with emotional feelings related to the movement experience.

Some evidence shows connections to the thalamus which is the major integrating structure for the cortex. Simple animal experiments show that various portions of the thalamus may respond to vestibular stimulation including the ventral posterior-inferior nucleus (a sensory relay area) of the thalamus, the ventral lateral nucleus (although its primary role is motor relay) and the medical geniculate body (an auditory relay area) (Abraham, Copack & Gilman, 1977; Buttner & Henn, 1976; Deecke, Schwartz, & Fredrickson, 1974; Liedgren & Rubin, 1976; Magnin & Fuchs, 1977; Wepsic, 1966). Several authors have postulated that collateral vestibular fibers enter the lateral geniculate body (a visual relay area) to signal the visual system to prepare for potential head movement, so that visual images can coincide with head and eye movement and the individual can maintain orientation in space and time (Kornhuber, 1974). None of these authors cite specific locations as solely vestibular relays, but conclude that vestibular information is integrated with other types of information at the brain stem and higher levels (Darian-Smith, 1984). This hypothesized pervasive influence is compatible with clinical observations of disorientation when a child or adult has vestibular dysfunction.

Connections to cortical regions are also being studied (Darian-Smith, 1984). Two regions in the parietal lobe have been sited as the most likely locations for vestibular processing: the inferior temporal lobe and a portion of the primary sensory areas of the parietal lobe. Darian-Smith (1984) hypothesizes that the first region is related to one's perception of the body in space, while the second area seems to relate vestibular input to the motor output that is generated by the motor cortex.

Muscular Afferents (Proprioception)

Muscular afferents, usually discussed as part of the motor system, are receptors housed within the muscle belly, tendons, and joints to provide ongoing information to the CNS about the integrity of the muscle. Most people are familiar with these receptors as the *muscle spindles* and *Golgi tendon organ* (GTO). These receptors provide an excellent example of the intimate relationship between sensory and motor functioning within the neuromusculoskeletal system.

The muscle spindle is a small muscle fiber surrounded by connective tissue that is housed within the fleshy part of the muscle belly. These encapsulated fibers are dispersed throughout the muscle belly so that they may respond to any changes in muscle integrity. The muscle spindles are responsive to the length and changes in length of the muscle.

The muscle spindles contribute to a function called *autogenic facilitation*, which is the ability to stimulate one's own muscle to contract. For example, when the muscle belly is stretched, the muscle spindle fibers are also stretched and send an impulse into the spinal cord. The spinal cord interneurons and the motor neurons can then fire to facilitate contraction of the actual muscle belly fibers themselves. When the muscle belly contracts, the spindle is no longer stretched and the action can stop (Crutchfield & Barnes, 1984). The muscle spindle may play an important role in initial learning or relearning of motor movements by supporting the tension of those muscles as the individual experiments with the movements (Crutchfield & Barnes, 1984).

Although spinal cord action is the focus when studying the muscle afferents, this information is also traveling to the cortex via ascending sensory pathways and interacting with descending motor influences. When the descending influences are altered because of trauma or disease, the balance of power is upset at the spinal cord level leading to a release phenomenon. The inhibitory control from higher centers is lost, "releasing" the muscle spindle from this modulating influence. When the muscle spindle acts continuously without inhibitory modulation, autogenic facilitation predominates the muscle action, producing spasticity (Crutchfield & Barnes, 1984).

The Golgi tendon organ is located within the tendons at the end of each muscle belly. The GTO is interwoven within this collagenous fiber so that when changes in tendon tension occur, the GTO can notice and respond to these changes. This can occur both when muscle contraction pulls on the nonelastic tendon or during the extreme ranges of passive stretching. The GTO functions through a process known as *autogenic inhibition*. Autogenic inhibition is the process of inhibiting the muscle which generated the stimulus while providing an excitatory impulse to the antagonist muscle. This process prevents the individual from overusing or damaging the muscle and the corresponding joints.

Through this mechanism, the GTO seems to contribute to cramp relief. During muscle cramping, the muscle is shortened and contains a high degree of tension. When the individual stretches the cramped muscle, the tendon stretches, firing the GTO. When the GTO impulse reaches the spinal cord, an inhibitory impulse is produced (autogenic inhibition) allowing the muscle with the cramp to relax (Crutchfield & Barnes, 1984).

Because the GTO inhibits its own muscle and excites the antagonist, the two sets of GTOs in complementary muscles maintain a balance of power across joints. The stability that is produced across a joint by complementary muscle action is called co-contraction. Weight-bearing positions rely on co-con-traction, as do goal-directed movements which are supported by a stable joint or body area. Stability can be provided both proximally and distally. Movement of extremities is supported by trunk stability (e.g., reaching for a glass on the counter), while movement in the trunk can be supported through stability in the extremities (e.g., when an individual stabilizes with arms and hands to move the trunk to perform a handstand).

By understanding the concepts of autogenic facilitation of the muscle spindle and autogenic inhibition of the GTO, the therapist can better control the sensory and motor environment when planning intervention. For example, a quick stretch activates muscle spindles (changes in muscle length) engaging autogenic facilitation of the stretched muscle, whereas a maintained stretch past the tension state of the muscle is more likely to fire the GTO-producing autogenic inhibition, relaxing the muscle being stretched.

The Visual System

The visual system is one of the most advanced sensory systems in the human organism. Although cell clusters form early in fetal life, this system becomes most functional in the postnatal period. Vision is the most prominent sensation; there are more fibers in the optic nerve than in all the sensory tracts in the entire length of the spinal cord (Kandel & Schwartz, 1985). Because of its anatomical organization from the front to the back of the cortex, it also provides an excellent vehicle for localization of CNS problems.

Retina

The retina is the receptor mechanism of the visual system. The retinal cells have been studied extensively because they are an extension of the CNS. When the CNS environment has been altered in a way that might affect the nerve cells or supporting structures, these changes can be observed in the retina. The retinal cells operate to maximize the reception of both light and color. Additionally, the complex interneuron network is set up to facilitate the transmission of the clearest visual image through lateral inhibition of neighboring cells. Specific retinal cells activate a specific optic nerve cell; this pattern of organization continues to the occipital lobe. This *topographic* or retinotopic organization allows the cortex to construct an accurate and reliable map of the visual environment.

Visual Pathways

The pathways for visual input travel from the front of the cortex (behind the eyeball) to the back (occipital lobe); the other sensory systems ascend from the receptor site to the cortex. This makes the visual system quite vulnerable to all types of cortical damage, but also provides a consistent source of diagnostic data for localizing the injury site. As with other

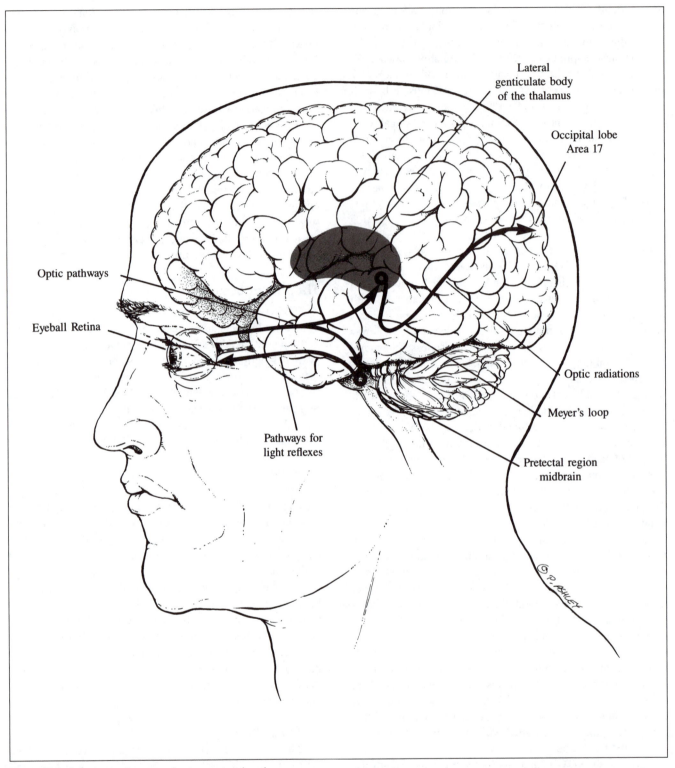

Figure 8-5. Schematic diagram of primary visual pathways.

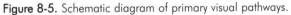

sensory systems the visual system has two subsystems that enable both alerting and mapping to take place efficiently. Figure 8-5 provides a diagram of the visual pathways.

The first visual system is referred to as the geniculocalcarine or geniculostriate system (Noback & Demarest, 1981). The nerve cells exit the eyeball, having obtained input from the retina and course backward toward the occipital lobe. The first segment, the *optic nerve*, covers the region from the eyeball to the converging point for all the optic nerve cells, called the *optic chiasm*. Complete severing of the optic nerve results in total blindness of the eye served. At the optic chiasm, central vision is carried through nerve cells that do not cross. These cells remain in the lateral aspects of the convergence point. Peripheral vision is carried through nerve cells that cross over at the optic chiasm, therefore if the crossed fibers are damaged, the individual loses peripheral vision; this is commonly known as *tunnel vision.*

After passing through the optic chiasm region, the fiber pathway is known as the *optic tract*; these fibers travel to the lateral geniculate body (a nucleus of the thalamus). The optic tract carries all information from the contralateral visual field. Just after exiting the lateral geniculate body, the fibers travel forward and out before coursing backward; this curved portion of the optic radiations is called Meyer's loop. This curve is necessary so that the fibers can travel around the lateral ventricles. This new bundle of fibers is called the optic radiations. As with the optic tract, the optic radiations carry information about the contralateral visual field. The optic radiations travel back to the occipital lobe, specifically, the calcarine sulcus (area 17), hence the name geniculocalcarine pathways.

The geniculocalcarine system seems to provide answers to the question "What is it?" by gathering information about the characteristics of the objects in the environment. The maps that are formed in the primary and association visual areas allow the individual to determine the identity and function of objects.

The second visual system is called the *tectal system*. The tectal system seems to answer the question "Where is it?" by identifying presence and location of stimuli (i.e., orienting) for the individual. The fibers that serve this function pass through the optic nerve, chiasm and tract, but synapse in the tectal region of the midbrain (Schiller, 1984). (Remember that the midbrain is the highest portion of the brain stem and the tectum is made up of the superior and inferior colliculi.) Although the superior colliculus is considered a primary relay station for visual input through tectal system connections, it is also a relay station for somatosensory and auditory input (Kandel & Schwartz, 1985), allowing a coordination of these inputs for proper orientation to the arousing stimulus. An individual with cortical brain damage may alert to visual stimuli because the tectum is operating at the brain stem level, but will be unable to follow through with a goal-directed behavior related to the stimulus because the pathways that lead to the cortex are disrupted.

Visual System Functions and Therapeutic Interventions

The visual system is designed to recognize contrasts (Kandel & Schwartz, 1985). When the visual environment is diffuse or homogeneous, the cells of the visual system have difficulty responding. They search for the highest contrast possible, attempting to make this area distinct. The eyes continuously change position with very tiny movements to activate new retinal cells. In this way, the brain gets ongoing information about the object and can keep the image clear. Busy visual environments can be difficult for the visual system to handle. With too many competing images, the visual system cannot isolate significant high-contrast locations to generate the nerve impulses. For example, think of how difficult it is to find something in the "junk drawer" in the kitchen. This is because there are many overlapping objectives of varying shapes, sizes and colors; the competition is so great that clarity is frequently lost.

Altering the sensory environment to increase the chances for success in task performance enables the individual to actively engage the environment. This in turn increases accurate and reliable sensory feedback that can be stored and used for future tasks. Therapists can improve orientation in a visually disoriented individual by providing a high-contrast visual environment. For example, one could place a dark cloth or board on the countertop to help distinguish light-colored food items when preparing food. Contrast between the bed covering and the nightstand in the bedroom would facilitate getting on the bed. Therapists can advise clients of ways to minimize problems with visual competition by organizing cabinets, shelves, and drawers into sections for predetermined items or placing tool outlines (shadows on walls or racks to show which utensils or tools belong in each location). This not only provides a high contrast foreground-background for the items, but also minimizes stacking or cluttering of objects on top of each other.

The most common visual field defects that therapists encounter are tunnel vision (loss of peripheral vision) and *homonymous hemianopia* (loss of one side of the visual field). Figure 8-6 demonstrates where these problems occur in the pathways. Because visual field loss is often permanent, it can have a significant impact on task performance. Consider the risks that are present when peripheral vision is not available to an individual. Many stimuli to which people attend are first noticed in the peripheral field, and much of one's body orientation relies on peripheral field input. Therapeutic intervention must incorporate patterns of movement that compensate for the loss of peripheral vision. For example, one can set

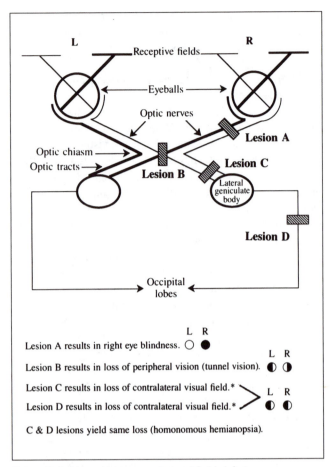

L
R
Receptive fields
Eyeballs
Optic nerves

Lesion A

Optic chiasm
Optic tracts

Lesion C
Lesion B
Lateral
geniculate
body

Lesion D

Occipital
lobes

L   R
Lesion A results in right eye blindness. ○ ●
                                                        L   R
Lesion B results in loss of peripheral vision (tunnel vision). ◐ ◑

Lesion C results in loss of contralateral visual field.*   L   R
                                                                                       ◐ ◑
Lesion D results in loss of contralateral visual field.*

C & D lesions yield same loss (homonomous hemianopsia).

Figure 8-6. Neural lesions and visual field deficits.

up activities that require the individual to move the head from side to side, minimizing the effects of peripheral loss, and facilitating routine use of head movement to obtain visual input from a wider area (e.g., placing important stimuli to the side). Automatic use of head turning and body repositioning will contribute greatly to independence.

Homonymous hemianopsia is the loss of one side of the visual field. This can impair a person's independence because the individual can miss important cues from nearly half of the visual environment. Individuals with a homonymous hemianopsia frequently complain that objects are missing, when in fact they may be present but outside of the remaining visual field. Therapeutic intervention for these individuals must incorporate new head positioning to maximize use of intact visual fields and minimize the effects of the lost visual field. This can be achieved by turning the head toward the lost visual field which places the retained visual field in front of the individual and moves the lost field over the shoulder. This new position facilitates more awareness of the immediate visual environment., The therapist must design methods that make this postural change an automatic

one. For example, one can place items that are most important to the individual in the lost visual field to increase head turning to look for them, or play a card game and place the deck in a position to facilitate head turning. Auditory cues such as "look to the left, Mr. Jones" can be helpful initially, but there is a danger that the individual will become dependent on cues from others and never internalize this adaptation for independent task performance. Family education is also important to balance emerging adaptive behavior with safety.

Auditory System

Structure and Function

The auditory system is also one of the newer sensory mechanisms in the CNS. The auditory system processes sound primarily for communication, but also as a means of environmental orientation. Direction, distance, and quality of sound all contribute to the ability to orient within our environment from an auditory perspective (Kiang, 1984). Although other professionals specialize in working with problems of the auditory system, occupational therapists must also be aware of the basic mechanisms within the auditory system so that therapeutic approaches and environmental adaptations can accommodate functional difficulties that might arise from dysfunction in this system.

The auditory receptor is divided into three sections: the outer, middle, and inner ear. Through these three components, airwaves are transformed into pressure waves within a fluid system. The pressure waves displace hair cells located in the inner ear and this action fires the nerve cells. The outer ear consists of the auricle (the part of the ear visible to us), the ear canal, and the eardrum or the *tympanic membrane*. The outer ear is vulnerable to obstructions in the canal or perforations of the eardrum, both of which diminish hearing on that side.

The middle ear is a chamber that contains three small bones (*malleus, incus,* and *stapes*) and two small muscles (*tensor tympani* and *stapedius*). When the ear drum vibrates, the small bones vibrate, which then emits pressure on the surface of the inner ear (*cochlea*). The Eustachian tube connects this self-contained chamber with the throat to provide a passageway to equalize pressure in the middle ear. The Eustachian tube is frequently the site of infection because bacteria or viruses can easily get trapped within its small diameter. This blocks the passageway into the middle ear making the pressure increase. Ear infections such as these occur frequently with young children, partly because their Eustachian tubes are less angled, allowing for less efficient drainage. This is a major reason why many children have plastic tubes placed in their ears during early childhood. The tube is inserted through the eardrum and provides an alternate means for pressure maintenance in the middle ear.

The cochlea is shaped like a snail with several chambers inside. The movement of the fluid within these chambers allows displacement of the hair cells. When the hair cells are displaced, the auditory nerves fire. Specific hair cells are responsible for specific sounds, and fire specific nerve cells. This process is known as *tonotopic* organization and is the mechanism by which the CNS can identify the sounds heard.

The central connections of the auditory system are unique in comparison to other sensory systems. Figure 8-7 illustrates the auditory pathways. The ascending pathways of the auditory system are bilateral in nature; this is significant because loss of the input on one side will not completely stop the information processing to both sides of the brain. In terms of functional performance, the individual experiences inability to localize sounds from the environment with loss of hearing to one ear or auditory nerve. Under normal conditions, the brain is able to compare the loudness of the sounds from the two ears to determine from which direction the sound is coming. When one ear has lost its ability to transmit information, the brain no longer can locate the direction, hence the person can hear the sound clearly, but has more difficulty finding it. Clinically, these individuals respond to sounds by changing posture or looking around to search for the origin of the sound.

These bilateral connections in the ascending auditory system extend throughout the brain stem. The inferior colliculus is a major relay point for auditory fibers (remember it is in the midbrain and is part of the tectum as described in the visual section). The inferior colliculus functions to alert the individual to auditory stimuli in the environment. From the brain stem, information travels to the medical geniculate body (in the thalamus) and the temporal lobe.

The auditory system also has a feedback mechanism that performs an important function. This feedback system follows a similar course as the ascending pathways but in a more unilateral pattern. This fiber pathway inhibits hair cells carrying extraneous or unimportant background noise from the environment, thus allowing the individual to attend to important sounds. This process is called auditory figure-ground perception. This is the mechanism which allows students to filter out such noises as rustling paper and shuffling feet in the classroom so they can hear the teacher's voice more clearly.

Auditory System Intervention Approaches

Although other professions may test the auditory system in more detail and may work on specific auditory components in their intervention plans, the occupational therapist is responsible for the effects of auditory deficits on task performance. Therapists must decide whether intervention should be set up in a quiet isolated place to avoid noisy environ-

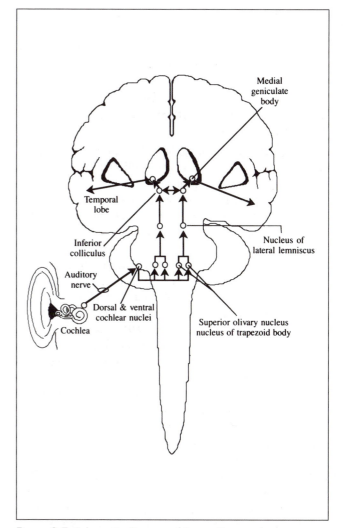

Figure 8-7. Schematic diagram of the auditory pathways.

ments and decrease the amount of effort required by the auditory system or in a more natural environment in which the individual must develop inhibitory skills. Both choices are therapeutically sound, but must be actively chosen as part of the intervention goals. For example, the therapist may choose to work in quiet environments early in the intervention process so that other areas of concern such as postural control can be addressed without competition. The therapist might choose a simpler postural task while working in a more competing auditory environment to help the individual learn to screen out the extraneous noises that will always be part of the natural environment. A portable tape recorder and earphones are helpful to introduce controlled auditory stimuli, which can later be incorporated into other activities. The therapist can control the type of sound (e.g., clinic noise, classroom noise, neighborhood noise, music, talking) and the volume on the tape so that as the client adjusts to one condition, it can be altered slightly. Therapists monitor performance in relation to task difficulty and the amount of environmental competition for attention, as this is another subtle variable that certainly can affect task performance.

Principles for Designing Therapeutic Interventions Based on Sensory System Functions

Although understanding how the sensory systems are organized and function, this is not sufficient information for planning effective therapeutic interventions using neuroscience principles. Therapists must also have a framework for applying the neuroscience knowledge they have acquired to solve the actual problems that persons with performance needs face each day. Dunn, Brown, and McGuigan (1994) offer a pragmatic approach to making this link in their *Ecology of Human Performance* (EHP) framework. In this framework, the person is considered within the context of daily life, and the focus of intervention is on the interaction between person and context. The EHP framework suggests that providers must consider not only the person's skills and abilities, but also what the person needs and wants to do, and in addition, where the person will be performing these daily life tasks. In this spirit, it is insufficient to consider only a person's sensory processing abilities without also looking at what sensory events are either occurring or available in the person's performance context.

One way to consider the sensory aspects of context is to complete a Sensory Task Analysis. Table 8-4 provides a blank form, and Table 8-5 contains an example of a completed form for washing one's face. The terminology on the form matches the terms and explanations provided in Tables 8-1 and 8-2, so they can be used as a reference. The analysis requires several steps. First, analyze the task as any person would experience it; in this case, there would be sensory experiences from the sound of the water, the splashing, the cloth, etc (refer to the "what the task routine holds" column). Next, add information about the context (refer to the "what the context holds" column), items on the school sink that would be a different visual experience than at home. In the final column, the team members can brainstorm about possible intervention alternatives. For example, if the splashing water (e.g., light touch) is distracting the person from completing the task, an intervention would be to turn off the water while applying the soap. Table 8-5 lists examples of interventions to change each of the sensory experiences that might occur during face washing. As the team considered possibilities, they would select one option, and try it within the functional task. This would enable the team to learn which interventions were successful; if multiple options were implemented simultaneously, knowing which option contributed to the success would be difficult.

The Motor Systems

The motor systems are a network of internal motor circuitry and exiting pathways that process incoming sensory messages, organize plans for movement in response to stimuli and desired actions and transmit the messages to the motor neurons that serve the body. The motor system components are part of the overall integrated schema which enables the nervous system to receive, interpret and respond to life demands.

The Somatic Motor System

The somatic motor system serves the voluntary muscles. A network of descending motor pathways modulate the output to the lower motor neurons that generate the desired movements. The descending motor pathways originate in several places in the CNS and transmit messages to specific places in the body. The most critical thing to remember about the somatic motor system is that these pathways cannot operate without sensory input and processing. Figure 8-8 illustrates the sensory cortical areas that provide input to the motor centers of the cortex to generate the activity for the somatic motor output.

Three categories of motor output pathways exist in the CNS: finely tuned movement, postural control and limb control. Figure 8-9 illustrates these pathways.

Finely Tuned Movements

Two pathways oversee the finely tuned movements of the body. The *corticospinal pathway* controls finely tuned movement of the hands; this pathway travels from the motor cortex to the spinal neurons that serve the hand muscles. The *corticobulbar pathway* serves the motor neurons in the cranial nerve system to support finely tuned movement of the face and head (via the motor cranial nerves). This pathway travels from the motor cortex into the brain stem; different parts of this pathway terminate on the various motor cranial nerves so a person can smile, wink, move the eyeballs, chew and turn the head.

Postural Control

The second category of motor output pathways serves postural control. The descending pathway that serves this function is the *corticoreticulospinal pathway* (i.e., from the cortex to the reticular formation, and then through subsequent pathways to the spinal cord). This pathway along with output from the cerebellum (see below) modulates the descending postural control pathways that exit the brain stem to serve spinal level neurons for postural control. Specifically, the three pathways involved in postural control are the *medial and lateral vestibulospinal tracts* and the

ROUTINE/TASK SENSORY CHARACTERISTICS		WHAT DOES THE TASK ROUTINE HOLD?			WHAT DOES THE PARTICULAR ENVIRONMENT HOLD?	WHAT ADAPTATIONS ARE LIKELY TO IMPROVE FUNCTIONAL OUTCOME?
		A	B	C		
Somatosensory	light touch (tap, tickle)					
	pain					
	temperature (hot, cold)					
	touch-pressure (hug, pat, grasp)					
	variable					
	duration of stimulus (short, long)					
	body surface contact (small, large)					
	predictable					
	unpredictable					
Vestibular	head position change					
	speed change					
	direction change					
	rotary head movement					
	linear head movement					
	repetitive head movement (rhythmic)					
	predictable					
	unpredictable					
Proprioceptive	quick stretch stimulus					
	sustained tension stimulus					
	shifting muscle tension					
Visual	high intensity					
	low intensity					
	high contrast					
	high similarity (low contrast)					
	competitive					
	variable					
	predictable					
	unpredictable					
Auditory	rhythmic					
	variable					
	constant					
	competitive					
	noncompetitive					
	loud					
	soft					
	predictable					
	unpredictable					
Olfactory/ Gustatory	mild					
	strong					
	predictable					
	unpredictable					

Task _____
Components: A = _____
B = _____
C = _____

Table 8-4. Sensory components of task performance. From Dunn, W. (1991). The sensorimotor systems: A framework for assessment and intervention. In F. P. Orelove & D. Sobsey (Eds.), *Educating children with multiple disabilities: A transdisciplinary approach* (2nd ed.). Baltimore, MD: Paul H. Brookes. Reprinted with permission.

Table 8-5. Sample completed form for analyzing sensory characteristics of face washing.

ROUTINE/TASK: Washing face — SENSORY CHARACTERISTICS	WHAT DOES THE TASK ROUTINE HOLD? A	B	C	WHAT DOES THE PARTICULAR ENVIRONMENT HOLD? (classroom sink)	WHAT ADAPTATIONS ARE LIKELY TO IMPROVE FUNCTIONAL OUTCOME?
Somatosensory					
light touch (tap, tickle)	X				Turn water off to decrease splashing
pain					
temperature (hot, cold)	X				Try alternative water temperatures
touch-pressure (hug, pat, grasp)	X				Pat face instead of rubbing cloth on face
variable	X				Pat large face area
duration of stimulus (short, long)	L				
body surface contact (small, large)	L				Try washing one part only; begin with chin area
predictable	X				(NOTE: make sure routine is consistent day to day)
unpredictable					Alter water source so don't have to bend head down (e.g., in a pan or tub)
Vestibular					Keep head up so don't have the down-up pattern
head position change	X				
speed change					Keep head up; if need arousal, place items on counter to encourage more head turning
direction change	x				
rotary head movement					
linear head movement	X				
repetitive head movement - rhythmic					
predictable					
unpredictable					
Proprioceptive					
quick stretch stimulus	X				Move objects to decrease head control requirements
sustained tension stimulus	X				
shifting muscle tension					
Visual					
high intensity					
low intensity					
high contrast					
high similarity (low contrast)	X			X Other objects	Use dark wash cloths & light soap; use dark containers on light counter; remove extra items from counter
competitive	X			X on sink	
variable				X Counter changes day to day	
predictable	X			X	If arousal is needed, vary placement of items
unpredictable					
Auditory					
rhythmic	X				Prepare wet cloth; don't have running tap water
variable	X				Use tub of water instead of running water
constant					
competitive					
noncompetitive	X			X Other students	Have child to the bathroom alone
loud					
soft	x				
predictable				X Teacher's voice	Provide physical prompts and decrease talking
unpredictable					
Olfactory/Gustatory					
mild	x			X Unplanned	If arousal is needed, use strong-smelling soap
strong	x				
predictable	X				
unpredictable					

Task ____
Components: A = ____
B = ____
C = ____

From Dunn, W. (1991). The sensorimotor systems: A framework for assessment and intervention. In F. P. Orelove & D. Sobsey (Eds.), *Educating children with multiple disabilities: A transdisciplinary approach* (2nd ed.). Baltimore, MD: Paul H. Brookes. Reprinted with permission.

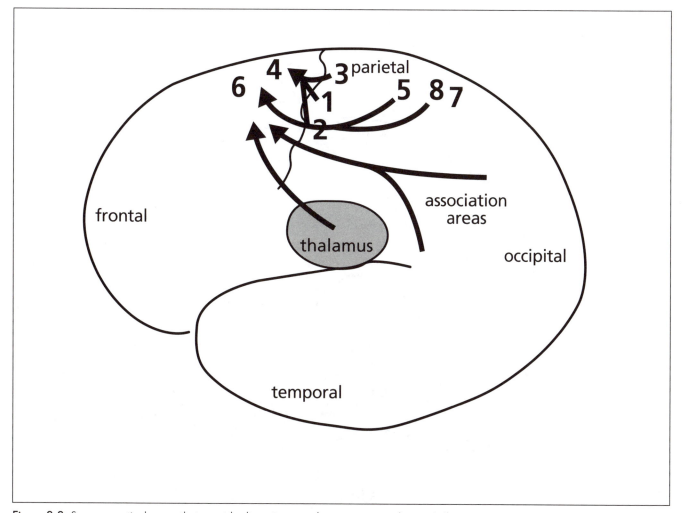

Figure 8-8. Sensory cortical areas that provide direct input to the motor cortex (areas 4,6).

reticulospinal tract. The coordination of excitation and inhibition of these pathways enables persons to hold and shift posture with and against gravity.

Limb Control

The third category of motor output pathways serves limb control. The descending pathway that serves this function is the *corticorubrospinal pathway* (i.e., from the motor cortex through the red nucleus in the brain stem and onto the spinal cord).

Understanding the organizational structure of the descending pathways is important, because many times persons who have had brain injury will have differing levels of function for each category of movement. This happens because brain injury can affect these pathways differently due to their anatomical locations. For example, some persons will have a harder time moving the limbs, but can perform finely tuned movement in the hands when they can rest the wrist on a surface, thereby avoiding the limb control issue.

Another person may have difficulty with postural control, but can turn the head to interact with others or bite and chew during a meal if the body can be stabilized in supported seating. Occupational therapy personnel can design more effective adaptations when these subtle movement differences from a nervous system perspective are understood.

The Cerebellum

The cerebellum is a fascinating internal structure of the CNS whose job is to orchestrate motor activity. The cerebellum is located just behind the brain stem and just under the occipital lobe of the cortex. The cerebellum is able to orchestrate motor activity by monitoring the ongoing sensory input that contributes to the need to move, and by comparing that input with the early drafts of one's plan about moving. This comparison enables the cerebellum to make adjustments in the motor plan before the message to execute the motor action is activated.

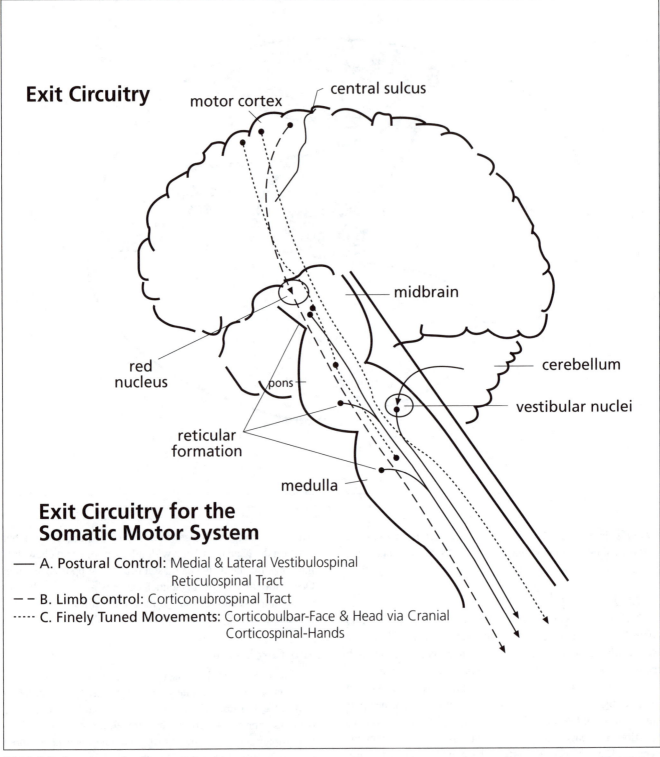

Exit Circuitry

motor cortex

central sulcus

midbrain

cerebellum

red nucleus

pons

vestibular nuclei

reticular formation

medulla

Exit Circuitry for the Somatic Motor System

— A. **Postural Control:** Medial & Lateral Vestibulospinal
    Reticulospinal Tract
– – B. **Limb Control:** Corticonubrospinal Tract
···· C. **Finely Tuned Movements:** Corticobulbar-Face & Head via Cranial
    Corticospinal-Hands

Figure 8-9. Exit circuitry for the somatic motor system.

The internal structure of the cerebellum is very intricate, and an explanation of this structure is beyond the scope of this chapter. However, understanding the utility of this intricate set of neurons and connections is important. The internal architecture is composed of neurons that bring information into the cerebellum, internal neurons that process the information, and neurons that send the processed information out of the cerebellum to other parts of the brain. This internal architecture works on an elaborate set of excitatory and inhibitory connections among the neurons to make sure that the right amount of information gets transmitted to the rest of the CNS.

There are two key areas of influence for the cerebellar output. First, the cerebellum has direct connections with the vestibular nuclei in the brain stem. The purpose of these connections is to provide modulation to the pathways that provide support for postural control. Figure 8-4 illustrates the relationship among the vestibular nuclei, the cerebellum and the descending pathways to support postural control (also read the vestibular section of this chapter, above). We believe that the cerebellum provides inhibitory control over these pathways.

The second key connection for the output of the cerebellum is the motor nuclei of the thalamus. The cerebellum sends the preprogrammed message about the motor plan (i.e., the "here's how to do it" message) to the ventral lateral nucleus of the thalamus; it is in this nucleus that the cerebellar information joins with information from the basal ganglia (the "let's go" message, see next section), and the new message is sent onto the motor cortex. The ability to move in intricate ways and so accurately in response to environmental demands is due to the convergence of cerebellar and basal ganglia information for use by the higher cortical centers. Figure 8-10 illustrates the interaction among the cerebellar output, basal ganglia output and the motor nuclei of the thalamus; this internal motor circuitry of the CNS prepares the motor cortex for action.

When the cerebellum is disrupted, the person experiences a loss of control over voluntary movements. This is because the rest of the motor circuitry is released from the modulated planning the cerebellum can provide. The classic signs of cerebellar dysfunction are ataxia (i.e., a drunken gait) and intention tremors (i.e., the tremor only occurs when the person tries to do something).

The Basal Ganglia Network

The basal ganglia is also an intricate internal motor circuitry of the CNS. The primary structures of the basal ganglia are the caudate nucleus, the putamen (i.e., the input structures) and the globus pallidus (i.e., the output structure). They are located above and to the side of the thalamus, which is in the center of the brain (Figure 8-11) and are separated from the thalamus by the internal capsule. This anatomic relationship is important when one considers trauma to the brain in which

adjoining structures might be affected. For example, if a person suffered an aneurism, lost blood supply or had a tumor in the center of the brain, the basal ganglia, internal capsule and thalamus could be affected together, even though they would not necessarily have a functional relationship to each other.

The basal ganglia network is primarily responsible for initiating movement and for regulating stereotypic movements. The basal ganglia accomplishes these tasks through excitatory and inhibitory connections among the primary and support structures of the basal ganglia. These connections are very complex, and rely on various neurotransmitters within these neural networks to operate properly. Scholars and practitioners have written a lot about these connections; let us consider just the basic principles of their operation here.

The input structures of the basal ganglia (i.e., the caudate nucleus and putamen) are modulated by a structure called the subthalamus. When this modulation is disrupted, the basal ganglia must try to work with poorly organized information; this results in movements that are poorly organized as well. The classic problem that occurs when the subthalamus is dysfunctional is called ballisms; ballistic movements are explosive movements that occur without apparent warning or provocation.

The output structure of the basal ganglia (i.e., the globus pallidus) is modulated by a structure called the substantia nigra. When the output of the basal ganglia is disrupted, a different problem occurs. The information cannot flow out of the basal ganglia, and so the "let's go" message that the brain expects from the basal ganglia cannot be sent (or is sent at a very low rate). This results in the person having a problem initiating movements, and so appears to get stuck in positions, or ends up in poor postural positions, because shifting posture requires additional movement initiation.

The classic disorder associated with this problem is Parkinson's disease. The reason that the drug L-Dopa reduces this aspect of the movement problem is that the substantia nigra operates heavily with the neurotransmitter dopamine, and L-Dopa creates a substitute for the reduction of dopamine that occurs in Parkinson's disease. The effects are reduced over time as the brain somehow gets accustomed to the levels, and increasing dosages have to be used. There are also side effects of long-term use of drugs such as this; other parts of the brain also use dopamine, and are affected by the introduction of L-Dopa. These other areas may get overused, resulting in abnormal signs from these other centers (i.e., a release phenomenon).

Whenever the balance of power is disrupted in the CNS, one sees a *release phenomenon*, and too much or too little needed behaviors occur as a result. Many clinical signs of disruption in the basal ganglia are the result of the release phenomenon. Slowness of movement (i.e., bradykinesia), resting tremors, choreiform (rhythmic, involuntary), athetoid (i.e., writhing) and ballistic (i.e., explosive, involuntary) movements

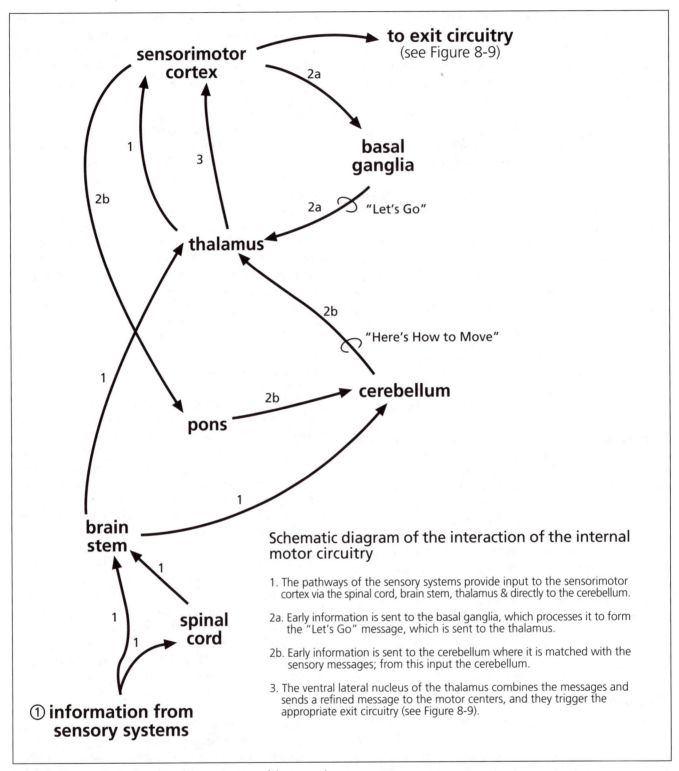

Figure 8-10. Schematic diagram of the interaction of the internal motor circuitry.

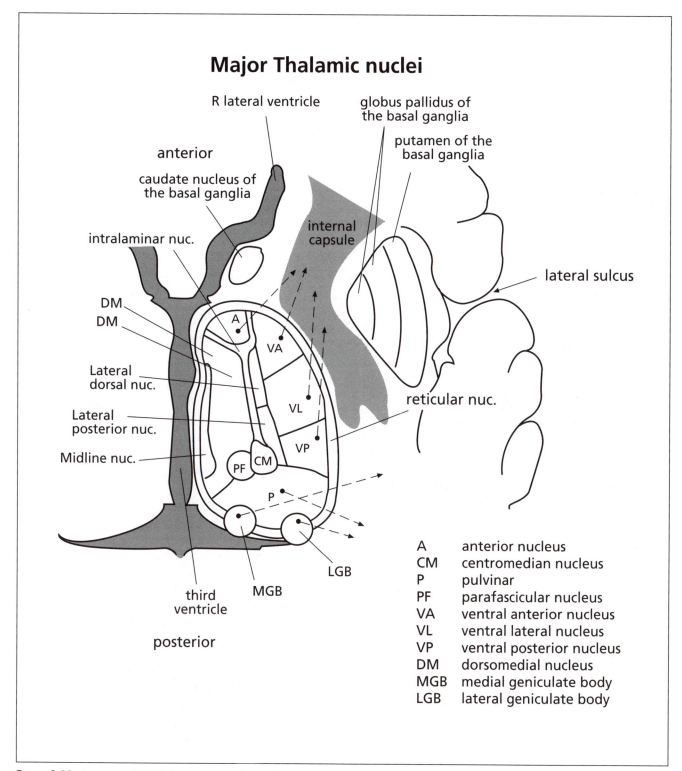

Figure 8-11. Anatomy of the thalamus, internal capsule and basal ganglia.

TABLE 8-6

Functions of the Major Nuclei of the Thalamus

Thalamic Nucleus	Cortical Connection	Function Supported
Anterior	limbic system	emotional tone
Dorsomedial	prefrontal lobe	judgement/reasoning
Centromedian Intralaminar Midline	reticular system	generalized arousal
Ventral Anterior Ventral Lateral	posterior frontal lobe	motor functions
Pulvinar	association areas	higher cognitive thought

Ventrobasal Complex
   *VP Lateral
 	
   *VP Medial
   *VP Inferior
	parietal lobe	sensory mapping (i.e.,
		somatosensory,
		somatosensory,
		vestibular)

Lateral Geniculate Body	occipital lobe	visual system functions
Medial Geniculate Body	temporal lobe	auditory system functions

are all indications of a loss of the balance of power in the basal ganglia and associated structures. These clinical signs can be disruptive to functional performance by interrupting ongoing activity, or making it hard to engage in the activity at all.

INTERACTION AMONG SENSORIMOTOR SYSTEMS TO SUPPORT PERFORMANCE

Many believe it is erroneous to consider the function of the sensory and motor systems separately, and thus refer to these networks as the sensorimotor system (e.g., Moore, 1980; Dunn, 1991a; Kandel, Schwartz & Jessell, 1991). The CNS receives information from the sensory organs, processes the sensory information, creates possible responses, filters them through the internal motor circuitry, and produces a motor response, which is executed by the motor neurons and musculoskeletal system. The motor systems cannot operate without sensory information, either during the current event requiring a response, or from memories of prior events which helped to construct maps of the body and the environment.

Thalamic Integration

The thalamus is an integrating structure that sits in the center of the brain (Figure 8-11). It is a critical structure because **every single stimulus that goes to and from the brain** (except olfaction) **must travel through the thalamus**. This gives the thalamus a big responsibility, that of organizing input and output so that it serves an optimal purpose in

helping the organism to respond properly. Table 8-6 contains a summary of the major nuclei of the thalamus, their system connections and the general function each nucleus supports.

Motor Control

Motor control is the ability to manage one's body for movement (Dunn, 1991b), but is different from praxis (see cognitive section below). We use movement schema that we have created from experience or practice to make our movements more efficient. The motor cortex supports the sequencing, timing and maintenance of control over movements; all the motor centers of the brain rely on sensory information to activate the desired movements. There are several questions that therapists can ask themselves to identify motor control issues that may be interfering with performance (Dunn, 1991c); Table 8-7 contains these questions.

Principles for Designing Therapeutic Interventions Based on Motor System Functions

The EHP framework outlines five intervention approaches that can be used to provide therapeutic supports. The five interventions acknowledge the ways that therapists can address not only person-related variables, but also task and context variables that can affect performance. *Establish/restore* interventions address person variables; the therapist identifies the person's skills and abilities, and designs interventions to improve them. When therapists

---

TABLE 8-7

Questions That Enable Professionals to Consider Factors That Affect Motor Control

- Can the individual carry out discrete movements (those with a clear beginning and end)?

- Can the individual carry out movements that are in a clear sequence with each other?

- Can the individual carry out movements that are continuous (e.g., steering a car, holding onto a cup of water)?

- Can the individual carry out predictable sequences of movement?

- Can the individual carry out movements when the environment is unpredictable?

- Is the individual's reaction time appropriate for the situational demands?

- Can the individual sustain performance for continuous tasks?

- Can the individual continue a repetitive movement pattern?

- Can the individual anticipate movement demands?

- Can the individual create the correct amount of force, velocity, and control to carry out effective movements?

- Are there differences in performance between the finely tuned movements of the hands, limb movements, trunk control and face/head control?

From Dunn, W. (1991). Assessing human performance related to brain function. In C. Royeen (Ed.), *Neuroscience foundations of human performance*. Rockville, MD: AOTA. Used with permission.

---

move cooking supplies to higher shelves so that the person who has spasticity will have to stretch muscles and increase range of motion, they are using a restorative intervention.

Adaptive interventions address task and context variables; the therapist identifies what the person wants and needs to do, and considers the person's skills, the characteristics of the task and the context in which it needs to be performed. If a person wanted to eat a meal, but only had one hand available for eating, the therapist would design adaptive interventions by placing dycem under the plate, attaching a plate guard and teaching the person to use a rocker knife for cutting.

The *Alter* interventions require the therapist to understand the person's skills and abilities and the possible contexts for performance. Alter interventions occur when the therapist identifies the best possible match between the person's skills and a particular performance context. Most important to remember about the alter intervention is that one does not change the person or the context, but rather finds the best match between them. For example, if a person has a cerebellar disorder, which results in the person having intention tremors and ataxia (i.e., lots of extra movements whenever the person tries to move), a therapist might identify a political marketing firm for employment, because all the workers wear headsets, and this person could have extraneouos movements without this affecting the ability to talk to people on the phone about the candidates. The person's tremors do not go away from the intervention, and the firm is not asked to make any changes in the job for the person.

Preventative interventions occur when therapists use their expertise to anticipate problems in the future, and design interventions to keep negative outcomes from occurring. When the motor systems are disrupted, persons commonly have problems with decubitus ulcers (i.e., skin breakdowns) on bony prominences due to their inability to move easily to shift posture or position during the day. Therapists anticipate that this might occur, and design interventions with the person to provide cues throughout the day to remember to move body parts away from weight-bearing surfaces.

The *Create* interventions address the larger contextual needs of communities. Occupational therapists have expertise that can make daily life more available, interesting and enjoyable for everyone, not just those who have performance needs. We use create strategies when we apply occupational therapy expertise to make a context better for everyone, without concern for disabilities. For example, serving on a commission to design the community's day care environments, or playgrounds would be a create intervention. Working with a corporation to make the office building easier for everyone to work in (e.g., signage, "friendly" work stations, chair height and work surface height options), or designing a community living neighborhood for elders employs a create intervention. Knowledge of the entire CNS is useful in identifying "creative" interventions in this category.

THE COGNITIVE SYSTEMS

Cortical Supports for Cognitive Performance

The CNS is organized so that information can be integrated for complex thinking and problem-solving tasks. Integrating diverse information enables persons to address more difficult dilemmas than are possible with the more singular processing that is observable in less-evolved organisms. General questions that providers can ask to determine the role of cognition in performance are provided in Table 8-

---

TABLE 8-8

Questions That Enable the Professional to Consider Factors That Affect Cognition

- Are basic sensory experiences intact?
- Can the individual interpret incoming sensory information in a reliable manner?
- Can the individual organize and integrate complex configurations of stimuli?
- Can the individual create a plan to act on the interpretations and configurations identified?
- Can the individual use memory to support cognitive activity?
- Can the individual use resources to make effective decisions?
- Are there indications of somatic motor disruptions that would interfere with the manifestations of cognition?
- Are drugs affecting the individual's ability to demonstrate cognitive abilities?
- Do times of day affect cognitive performance?
- Are there any indications of disruptions in biological rhythms that would diminish cognitive abilities?

From Dunn, W. (1991). Assessing human performance related to brain function. In C. Royeen (Ed.), *Neuroscience foundations of human performance*. Rockville, MD: AOTA. Used with permission.

---

8. Three key features of the cognitive systems in people are the arousal and attentional mechanisms, the language and communication systems and the systems that support praxis.

Arousal and Attentional Mechanisms

DeMoja, Reitano and Caracciolo (1985) describe the relationship between arousal and performance as a complex matrix affected by three variables: the structure of the individual's personality, the difficulty of the task, and the structure of the situation in which the task is to be performed. Vinogradova (1970) described several events which must occur in order for the CNS to register a stimulus. First, the appropriate receptors must recognize that a change has occurred in the environment. Second, the CNS must determine whether such a stimulus has occurred before. Third, the CNS must decide whether or not to act on the stimulus. Finally, the CNS must carry out the decision. Further, it appears that under normal conditions the CNS tends to investigate stimuli that are not familiar and inhibit conscious awareness of familiar stimuli (McGuinness & Pribram,

1980). Table 8-9a provides a worksheet that enables providers to consider the aspects of attention that may be affecting performance.

As an example, think about yourself as a student in a theoretical astronomy class. Although you might have an inherent ability to initiate and hold attention to the typical features of the classroom learning environment (e.g., the teacher's voice, the writing on the overhead, the pencil and paper for notetaking), the subject matter content may force you to expend an extreme amount of effort. The heightened effort might reduce your capacity, making it less possible to tolerate distractions in the class. Table 8-9b contains a completed form about this example to show you how this might look as a task is analyzed from an attentional perspective.

DeGangi and Porges (1991) describe the neural mechanisms that support arousal and attention. The sensory systems must be able to register that a stimulus is occurring to begin the processes. Specifically, the arousal/alerting aspects of each sensory system (see Tables 8-1, 8-2, and 8-3) send collateral fibers to the reticular formation, a center for arousal in the brain stem. The reticular formation then sends excitatory information to higher centers in the brain, including the limbic system (i.e., the hippocampus and the amygdala if you are interested in the structures' names), the thalamus and the cortex. The reticular mechanisms provide excitation for the centers they connect with, making it easier for those centers to activate in response to additional input. It is a "pay attention" message for the other centers as more focused information comes their way.

The factors described above are all part of the functioning arousal and attentional system. Each of these processes can be disrupted when the CNS is not functioning properly; when arousal and attention are disrupted, a person's performance is also placed in jeopardy.

Dunn (1997) describes the interaction between the neurological mechanisms that enable a person to notice and respond to sensory stimuli and the behavioral responses possible as a model for understanding a person's repertoire of behaviors from a neurological point of view. Table 8-10 provides a summary of their proposal about this interaction.

A person's neurological thresholds refer to the amount of stimuli necessary to reach a point of noticing or reacting to the stimuli. Those who have high thresholds take a longer time to react; some neurological and social science authors refer to this condition as *habituation*. When habituation is operating, the CNS is responding to the stimulus as if it is familiar, requiring little attention. Low thresholds, on the other hand, trigger more readily, and therefore cause the person to react more frequently to stimuli in the environment. This heightened reactivity is sometimes referred to as *sensitization*.

When addressing persons who have performance needs, providers must observe behavior. The model in Table 8-10

———— *Sensory Features* ————

	Touch	Motion	Smells	Taste	Temperature	Sounds	Sights	Surprise/ Novelty	Complexity	Conflicting Information	Intensity	Other
A. Attention What gets the individual's attention for functional tasks?												
What holds the individual's attention for functional tasks?												
What interrupts the individual's attention within functional tasks?												
								Sameness	Predictability	Task completion	Innocuousness	
What enables the individual to release attention?												
B. Effort What level of effort does the individual demonstrate to hold attention on functional tasks?	Nearly effortless			A moderate amount of effort			Extreme effort					
Which tasks/ environmental factors contribute to the level of effort necessary to perform functional tasks?	Difficulty of info that must be processed	Amount of info that must be processed	Amount of time that the task requires	Necessity for continuous/sustained effort	Amount of interfering conditions in the environment	Need for ongoing environmental support	Other factors:	Other factors:	Other factors:	Other factors:	Other factors:	Other factors:

Table 8-9a. Worksheet to review the attentional features of an individual's performance. From Dunn, W. (1991). Assessing human performance related to brain function. In C. Royeen (Ed.), *Neuroscience foundations of human performance.* Rockville, MD: AOTA. Reprinted with permission.

Sensory Features

	Touch	Motion	Smells	Taste	Temperature	Sounds	Sights	Surprise/ Novelty	Complexity	Conflicting Information	Intensity	Other
A. Attention What gets the individual's attention for functional tasks?						Teacher's voice						
What holds the individual's attention for functional tasks?		Class demonstration					Notes on board					
What interrupts the individual's attention within functional tasks?						Bell at end of class				Neighbor talking		
								Sameness	Predictability	Task completion	Innocuousness	
What enables the individual to release attention?										*		
B. Effort What level of effort does the individual demonstrate to hold attention on functional tasks?	Nearly effortless			A moderate amount of effort			Extreme effort *					
Which tasks/environmental factors contribute to the level of effort necessary to perform functional tasks?	Difficulty of info that must be processed *	Amount of info that must be processed *	Amount of time that the task requires *	Necessity for continuous/ sustained effort *	Amount of interfering conditions in the environment *	Need for ongoing environmental support	Other factors:	Other factors:	Other factors:	Other factors:	Other factors:	Other factors:

Table 8-9b. Worksheet to review the attentional features of an individual's performance. From Dunn, W. (1991). Assessing human performance related to brain function. In C. Royeen (Ed.), *Neuroscience foundations of human performance.* Rockville, MD: AOTA. Reprinted with permission.

TABLE 8-10

Relationship Between Behavioral Responses and Neurological Thresholds and the Behavioral Repertoire that is Likely to be Present with Each Interaction

Neurological Thresholds	Behavioral Responses	
	respond in accordance with threshold	**respond to counteract threshold**
high (habituation)	poor registration	sensation seeking
low (sensitization)	sensitivity to stimuli	sensation avoiding

proposes two distinct methods of responding in relation to one's neurological thresholds. First, persons can *respond in accordance with their thresholds*; this suggests that their behavioral repertoire mimics their thresholds. In this case, persons with high thresholds would appear to respond to very few stimuli, while persons with low thresholds would tend to respond to many stimuli. Secondly, persons can *respond to counteract their thresholds*; suggesting that persons' behavioral repertoires try to offset the impact of their neurological thresholds. In this case, persons with high thresholds would exert a lot of energy seeking stimuli to try to meet their thresholds, while persons with low thresholds would exert energy to keep from triggering their thresholds.

All of these factors fall on a continuum related to the intensity of response. For example, persons can have a slight tendency to register stimuli poorly, or can have a great deal of trouble registering stimuli. Similarly, persons could tend to counteract the effects of their thresholds, or aggressively act to counteract their thresholds. Also likely is that persons have variability within their CNS on particular days and within particular sensory systems (e.g., the somatosensory system being more sensitive than the vestibular system). Let us consider the general categories of each behavioral repertoire, its potential effects on performance and how to construct effective interventions for persons demonstrating these behaviors.

Poor Registration

When persons have difficulty registering stimuli due to high thresholds and act in accordance with those thresholds, they tend to have a dull or uninterested appearance. We know from this model that their nervous systems are not providing them with adequate activation to sustain focus on tasks or contextual cues. When serving persons who have poor registration, it is important to find ways to enhance the task and contextual experiences so that there is a greater likelihood that thresholds will be met. One can increase the contrast and reduce the predictability of cues in the task; for example, make objects heavier, change the color of items (e.g., put pink food coloring in the milk), add rotary movement or bending to the task routine. With these persons, always think

of how to make the experience more dense or intense with stimuli. The more they have the opportunity to trigger their thresholds, the more they are likely to be able to develop adaptive responses.

Sensitivity to Stimuli

When persons have sensitivity to stimuli due to low thresholds and act in accordance with those thresholds, they tend to seem hyperactive or distractible. They have a hard time staying on tasks to complete them or to learn from their experiences because their low neurological thresholds keep directing their attention from one stimulus to the next whether it is part of the ongoing task or not. When serving persons who have sensitivity to sensory stimuli, emphasize the discriminating/mapping features of sensory systems (see Tables 8-1, 8-2, and 8-3), because these aspects of sensory input do not increase arousal. These persons need organized input limiting distractions to draw them away from the task at hand. For example, use touch-pressure to make contact rather than light touch; organize tasks to have linear movement rather than rotary movement. The more discriminating/mapping input these persons can obtain, the better their chances for completing tasks and learning from them.

Sensation Seeking

When persons have high thresholds, but develop responses to counteract their thresholds, they engage in behaviors to increase their own sensory experiences. These persons add movement, touch, sound and visual stimuli to every experience. They might sing to themselves, dance in their seat, touch everything, hang on objects or people or chew on things a lot in an attempt to meet their high thresholds. When serving persons who seek sensation, it is important to first observe them carefully to obtain information about what sensations they add to their behavioral repertoire. The most effective interventions for these persons incorporate the sensations the persons need into their functional life repertoires. For example, if a person seeks movement input, but this is interfering with functional life performance, tasks can be reconstructed tasks to include more movement, so persons get the input they require as part of the daily life routine. In this example, we can move clothing items to different parts of the room, so it will require more walking, bending and reaching to get ready for the day. Honoring the input they seek can also reduce anxiety and assist with attentional focus.

Sensation Avoiding

When persons have low thresholds and develop responses to counteract their thresholds, they try to avoid activating their thresholds; they might appear to be resistant and unwilling to participate. There may be something about meeting their neurological thresholds that is uncomfortable, and therefore persons try to circumvent this event by reducing their activity, many times through withdrawal. This may be a way to discriminate these persons from those who have poor registration. Persons with poor registration may not appear to notice what is going on, while persons who are avoiding would display behaviors that indicate noticing and withdrawal from the situation. Another strategy persons in this category use is to develop rituals for conducting their daily life; it is possible that these rituals serve to provide a pattern of neural activity that is familiar and acceptable. When serving these persons, we must also honor the discomfort they experience. Observing their rituals and analyzing the features of the rituals provides a wealth of information. It is often successful to begin intervention with one of the rituals, expanding it in some small way, so that there is a blending of familiar and new stimuli. This enables the person to incorporate the new stimuli into a comfortable pattern. When providers try to disrupt the rituals too aggressively, this only leads to more avoidance behaviors, and functional performance declines even more.

Language/Communication

The process of communicating includes consideration of all facets of transmitting and receiving information. Reading, writing, speaking and listening have been traditionally considered forms of communication. However, we must also consider nonverbal communication, such as body posture, gesturing and eye contact, and other features of communication such as tone of voice or nonword sounds as part of the communication process. This more inclusive view brings in more CNS structures and systems to the process of having successful communication, but also provides more avenues for adaptation to support communication. Table 8-11 provides a listing of the primary areas of the brain involved with language, and summarizes the communication functions present or lost with damage to these centers.

As with all cognitive functions, communication is dependent upon adequate sensorimotor processing. For higher cortical functioning to occur (in this case, communication), the brain must integrate information. Oetter, Laurel, and Cool (1991) suggested that four major integration centers support communication. The *posterior parietal lobe* organizes spatial data for "object localization"; when a person can organize data to map the environment, communication about the environment's makeup is possible. The *inferior temporal lobe* combines information to create a map of the characteristics of places and things, or "object identification"; one example of this is facial recognition. *Wernicke's area* is located at the intersection of the parietal, occipital and temporal lobes, and processes information to enable the brain to interpret language (i.e., receptive language). In the left hemisphere, Wernicke's area processes speech communication, while in the right hemisphere Wernicke's area processes information to interpret nonverbal communication. *Broca's area* is located in the frontal lobe, and through connections with Wernicke's area, integrates information for expressive language.

Praxis

Praxis is a conceptual process by which the individual creates, organizes and plans new motor acts. Praxis is a conceptual process, and not a motor act. Praxis is supported by several higher cortical centers, making it part of the cognitive processes of the brain. Evidence suggests that praxis is closely related to the information available from the sensory systems; the more a task requires sensory input and feedback, the more task performance is adversely affected in conditions of dyspraxia and apraxia. Figure 8-12 contains a diagram of the sensorimotor links to the key motor cortex structures that support praxis. The dilemma for professionals is that we must observe outward behaviors to make our interpretations about a person's abilities; assuming that difficulty with movement is automatically a motor problem is an error. Table 8-12 contains a list of questions that professionals can ask when considering praxis as a factor in performance. When considering the praxis aspects of performance, Ayres (1985) suggested that we consider three aspects of the process: ideation, planning and motor execution.

Ideation is the formation of ideas about what a person might want to do. It is an internal process in which the nervous system either gathers information from stimuli in the environment or recruits information from memory stores (i.e., stimuli from past experiences) to formulate an idea about what to do. When individuals have ideational deficits, they do not have the capacity to figure out what can be done. Individuals with ideational difficulties display very simplified or repetitive patterns of movement, illustrating their inability to formulate ideas for action. When serving persons who have ideational praxis problems, we have to be very systematic in designing intervention activities. Intervention must build on the person's repertoire of skills; making a task too complex too soon can immobilize the person from engaging in the

	Wernicke's Area	Broca's Area	Anterior Border (Zone Watershed)	Posterior Border (Zone Watershed)	Supramarginal Gyrus	Angular Gyrus	Right Hemisphere
Can the individual understand spoken information (listen)?	No	Yes	Yes	No			
Can the individual understant written information (read)?	No	Yes	Yes	No			
Can the individual write legibly? With coherent thoughts?	No	No	No	No			
Can the individual vocalize? Convey coherent thoughts?	No	No					
Can the individual repeat what someone else has said?	No	No	Yes	Yes			
Can the individual read aloud?	No	No	Yes		No	No	
Does the individual use/understand intonation?	Yes	Yes			No	No	No
Can the individual spell? (Be sure to check premorbid ability.)	Yes						
Can the individual use gestures to communicate?	Yes	Yes					No
Does the individual recognize nonverbal cues (e.g., facial expressions, body postures)?	Yes	Yes					No
Can the individual understand/create proper syntax/grammar?	No	No					
Is the individual's speech fluent (rate, rhythm okay)?	Yes	No	No	Yes			
Is the individual aware of own errors in talking, writing?	No	Yes					
Can the individual "find" the right word when talking?	No	No		No			

Table 8-11. Areas of the brain involved with language functions (if the brain is damaged, can the individual perform the specified task?). From Dunn, W. (1991). Assessing human performance related to brain function. In C. Royeen (Ed.), *Neuroscience foundations of human performance*. Rockville, MD: AOTA. Reprinted with permission.

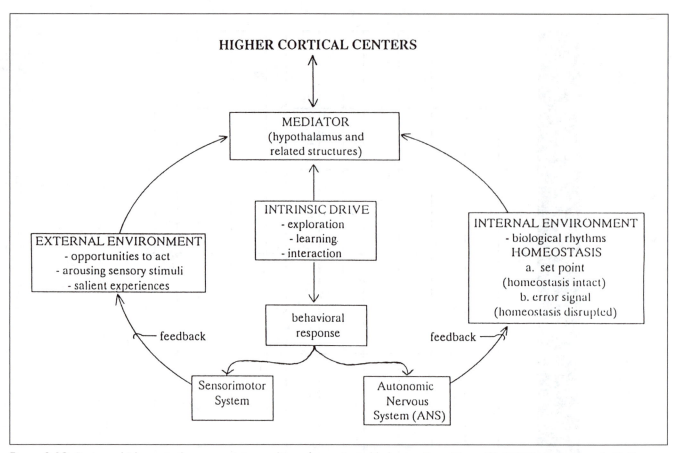

Figure 8-12. Factors which create the appropriate conditions for motivated behavior. From Dunn, W. (1991). Motivation. In C. B. Royeen (Ed.), *AOTA Self Study Series on Neuroscience*. Rockville, MD: AOTA. Used with permission.

environment. We must also create interventions which enhance the sensory information available to the person, to build maps of self and environment for use in idea generation. For example, we might make objects heavier in a routine, to increase the proprioceptive feedback for the person. We might also start with a routine that is in the person's repertoire, and embellish the routine one part at a time. This allows the person to experience increasingly complex sensorimotor actions to build neuronal models for engaging the environment. Increasing complexity leads to more advanced body and environmental maps which can be used for future idea generation.

Planning is the process of organizing information to design a method for responding to environmental demands. Planning is also an internal process which uses sensorimotor information to figure out an efficient and effective way to move. The motor plan is not the movement itself. When a person has difficulty with motor planning, he or she has the information needed to create the ideas, but has difficulty figuring out how to get his or her body to implement ideas about moving. When persons have planning problems, they display several types of movement difficulties. First, they

will be very clumsy; because they are unable to make a good plan, their efforts to move in response to environmental demands are inaccurate. Secondly, it is common for persons with planning problems to be able to verbally describe what needs to be done; they have good ideas, but they are unable to create a plan for doing it themselves. This characteristic can extend to being bossy and directive; this is likely to be a coping strategy for completing the task effectively, while reducing the possibility of errors that will occur if they try to carry out the task themselves. Sometimes persons with planning problems destroy objects more easily than others; this may be related to their poor modulation of movements, which can lead to holding something too tightly, dropping objects, bumping into objects, etc.

Providing intervention for persons with planning problems is challenging. Since they make a lot of errors, it is common for persons with planning problems to either quickly refuse to try new things, or to make many mistakes, adding to their misperceptions about how to move. We must build intervention scenarios that provide a motor planning challenge; but we must also design the activity so that we can pre-empt failure by intervening *before* the person makes an error. When one lets the person perform incorrectly and then corrects it with them, we allow incorrect patterns to form and we erode the person's already tenuous confidence about moving.

The third factor in the process is motor execution. **This is not part of praxis**. Motor execution is the act of carrying out the movement that has been conceived and planned during praxis. It is what one observes, but it is not praxis. When persons have motor execution problems without praxis problems, they may also look clumsy. However, persons who only have a motor execution problem will profit from their movement experiences, i.e., they will be able to adjust their performance based on internal and external feedback about performance. Practice helps motor execution to improve; routine and repetitive practice does not help persons with praxis problems.

Principles for Designing Therapeutic Interventions Based on Cognitive System Functions

Remembering to address the cognitive aspects of performance as we design therapeutic interventions is always challenging. A main reason for this is that we are still observing sensorimotor behaviors as we are determining cognitive abilities and needs. In order to get you started, Table 8-13 provides examples of therapeutic interventions (using the EHP framework) that an occupational therapist might design for selected cognitive problems that are interfering with performance.

THE AFFECTIVE SYSTEMS

Emotional System

Structure and Function of the Limbic System

The limbic system is an older, more primitive part of the CNS. It evolved from the "smell" brain in other species; this smell brain was responsible for primitive instincts and drives (Moore, 1976). The primary structures of the limbic system are the limbic lobe (i.e., the cingulate gyrus), the hippocampus and the amygdala. The hippocampus is involved with storage and retrieval of memory, and is implicated in dementia as tangles and placques form to reduce its function. The amygdala is involved with the ability to register sensory input, and contributes to the arousal/alerting mechanisms described earlier.

Moore (1976) describes the functions of the limbic system using the acronym "MOVE!" The word itself is important, because the limbic system supports our instincts to survive; however, she also used the letters to remind us of the primary functions of the limbic system. The "M" stands for memory;

TABLE 8-12

Questions That Enable the Professional to Consider Factors That Affect Praxis

- Is the individual aware of body parts and their capabilities?
- Does the individual demonstrate awareness of environmental features that may affect performance needs?
- Does the individual have experiences to draw from to create an idea?
- Can the individual express or demonstrate awareness of ideas about how to accomplish a task?
- Can the individual adapt performance to match task demands?
- Does the individual profit from observations and demonstration or physical prompts?
- Does the individual notice errors in performance?
- Can the individual use common objects as they were intended to be used?
- Does the individual create functional adaptations for the use of common objects?
- Can the individual combine separate movements into a functional sequence?
- Are there specific areas of problem performance (e.g., postural, oral)?

From Dunn, W. (1991). Assessing human performance related to brain function. In C. Royeen (Ed.), *Neuroscience foundations of human performance*. Rockville, MD: AOTA. Reprinted with permission.

---

this includes the instinctual, genetic memories and the more cognitively oriented short- and long-term memory systems. The circuitry that is involved with the hippocampus establishes ways to store and retrieve memories effectively. Each person constructs individualized ways to use this system.

The "O" stands for the olfactory functions of the system. The olfactory system is a major input for the limbic circuitry, and contributes to the rich memories persons have related to the smells of their lives (e.g., being in grandma's kitchen while bread was baking; standing in the hay fields just after the harvest). The direct neural connections make these memories very intense and available even if they are old memories. Providers can take advantage of these connections with persons who are confused by providing more familiar smells in the environment for orientation; the odors can trigger memories when more traditional cognitive strategies cannot. For example, a daughter can wear her traditional perfume when visiting her mother, or spray the perfume on pictures of herself, so the mother will

TABLE 8-13

Examples of Therapeutic Interventions from the Ecology of Human Performance Framework for Selected Cognitive System Disruptions

Performance Need and Neuro Correlate	Problems That Are Occurring	Restorative Interventions	Adaptive Interventions	Alter Interventions	Preventative Interventions
Sarah is a school aged girl whose parents want her to participate in her classroom activities; she has high sensory thresholds	Sarah seeks auditory, movement and touch stimuli throughout the day, which interrupts seatwork and class participation	Swing and sing with Sarah on the playground at arrival to provide additional input so she can focus her attention when she goes to class. During seatwork, place Sarah's supplies around the room so she can move about to get them as she works	Provide seatwork directions on tape, so Sarah can listen to them as needed to complete assignments	Work with parents and Sarah to get her involved in the community center dance club, which has both active, freestyle dancing and karaoke	Have Sarah join the choral group at church to prevent social isolation that may occur
Lana, an older woman who wishes to cook for her grandchildren; has apraxia	Lana can tell you what needs to be done, but has trouble carrying out the movements herself; this sometimes causes frustration	Provide physical prompts and hand over hand guidance to open containers; pour and stir ingredients so she can learn how movements feel during the task	Purchase ready made meals that can be heated up with the grandchildren	Go to restaurants with grandchildren as an alternative eating environment for socializing with children	
Presley, a young adult who wishes to have friends; R hemisphere damage affects nonverbal language centers	Presley doesn't understand intonation, gestures, facial expressions; doesn't use gestures properly to communicate	Watch movies together and talk about the gestures, facial expressions, intonation; practice having the same interaction as the movie	Find a buddy to go to book club with him; buddy will intervene to support his interactions	Identify an email bulletin board for socialization so that there is not a requirement for using or interpreting gestures, intonation	Locate job possibilities and necessary job skills for employment to prevent restricted living options due to financial restraints

REMEMBER: the Create intervention is applied within the community to benefit all persons in the community of interest, and does not specifically address disabilities.

have this additional cue about who is in the picture.

The "V" stands for visceral connections. The limbic system coordinates visceral responses with cognitive, emotional and sensorimotor responses. Eating engenders all of these systems, as persons make decisions about what, when and how to eat, along with where and with whom to eat (adding the cognitive and emotional features into the story). When providers can include all aspects of these systems into occupational performance, there is a much better chance of supporting performance in the natural environment.

The "E" stands for emotional tone, or drive. These drives include the drive to "feed," or nurture oneself, the drive to fight or flight and the drive to reproduce. These drives in humans go beyond mere physical survival; in humans the drive to survive includes being loved. When persons do not have attachments, they fail to thrive physiologically, and in young children and elders, this can result in death. We must "feed" the body and the spirit in order to survive.

Perspectives about Affect and Emotion

DeGangi and Greenspan (1991) provide an excellent discussion about the theoretical and application constructs related to affect and emotion. They propose that "emotional expression provides a window into an individual's internal experience of the world" (p. 4). They describe five major elements related to the function of emotion in performance. First, the person engages in *cognitive appraisal*, by evaluating the contextual features before, during and after the emotional experience. This involves assessing the impact of each factor on the event as well. Secondly, *physiological responses* are linked to emotions, demonstrating the link between the biological and affective systems in the CNS. Third, the person must display a *readiness to act* (i.e., a motivational state); attentional state and emotional capacity contribute to this factor (see section on motivation in this chapter). Fourth, there must be a *motor expression* of the emotion through the internal and somatic motor circuitry of the CNS. Finally, persons have *subjective experiences* related to their emotions; memory and imagination are important factors in how a person experiences emotions. These are critical factors to consider when interacting with persons who need occupational therapy and their families; remember that as the therapist you also have these issues happening for yourself during your professional interactions. Table 8-14a contains a worksheet to discover the affective and emotional tone aspects of a person's performance.

Let us work through a simple example. When an adolescent faces meeting a girlfriend's parents for the first time, issues of affect and emotional tone become salient. The adolescent has some general skills that will be useful in this situation, but they must be applied in a new way. For example, the adolescent understands the meaning of being with one's family and how to greet and engage in basic conversation. Modulating these factors during this new situation may be extremely challenging due to the high autonomic nervous system activity (e.g., dry mouth, sweating), while having low somatic motor system output (e.g., movements choppy or restrained) (Dunn, 1991a). This may lead to overreactions, like laughing too loudly, or missing important cues, such as passing food at the right time. Table 8-14b contains a completed form related to this example.

Motivational System

Motivation is a complex process; to understand it, we must study both neuroscience and social science (Dunn, 1991a). Stellar and Stellar (1985) explain that the modern concept of motivation has developed from the need to account for two behavioral conditions: noticing stimuli and selecting responses. Kelly (1985) acknowledged the importance of motivation by including motivation as one of the three basic functional systems of the CNS (the sensory and motor systems are the other two). Table 8-15a contains a worksheet to discover the motivational aspects of performance.

Dunn (1991a) provides an application of these general motivational features to daily life. As a therapist, you might attend a workshop in which you learn a new intervention alternative, which you are anxious to share with your colleagues at work. If you have not conducted an inservice before, you might be both nervous about presenting and excit-

ed about learning some teaching skills. On the day of the event, you might awaken early due to your excitement, and get ready faster than usual. When you get to work, others tell you about their excitement over your inservice because of not only the content, but your pleasant personal style. Just before the inservice time, you might begin to feel warm, and so get something cool to drink before going to the room to check things over one more time. The inservice goes well, and leads to many questions, invitations to plan interdisciplinary interventions based on your new information and other positive feedback, thus reinforcing you to try this again. Table 8-15b contains a summary of the motivational features of this event.

Neural and Behavioral Science Principles Underlying Motivation

Professionals tend to think of a person's internal state as the primary determinant of motivation. However, there are other factors that must also be considered when determining a person's motivation (Stellar & Stellar, 1985). The external environment must provide adequate cues and supports to enable the desired performance and the person must have had opportunities to understand the relationship between the cue to perform and the desired performance. Difficulty with any of these factors can affect a person's motivation (Dunn, 1991a). For example, a mother's usual pattern of waking her son so he can get ready for his baseball game (i.e., something the son *wants* to do) is to walk into the room and call his name (i.e., the son understands the meaning of the stimulus). However, she knows that he may be overly tired because of getting to bed late the night before (i.e., she recognizes that he may have a depleted internal state), so she turns on the light, flips on the radio and touches his shoulder to wake him (i.e., adding external environmental stimuli to increase the chances for the motivated behavior to occur). Just as in this example, when serving persons with disabilities, providers must give attention to all the factors that influence motivation.

Persons need the motivational system to not only initiate, but to sustain behavior. There is a great deal of interdependence among the elements. The primary CNS mediator for motivation is the hypothalamus. The hypothalamus provides mediation at several levels of operation within the CNS. One level of mediation occurs as the hypothalamus organizes information from the internal and external environments. The hypothalamus oversees the CNS operations that regulate biological rhythms and homeostasis (which are primary factors in the internal environment), and receives information about the external environment from the sensorimotor systems. With the objective being to maintain or reinstate homeostasis, the hypothalamus modulates the amount and type of information that travels to higher centers to produce responses. Remember, from a CNS perspective, there are only two types of output: somatic motor output through the sensori-

Questions regarding affect/emotional tone

Ratings: Mark the box that best represents performance (optimal performance is shaded)

Questions regarding affect/emotional tone	1	2	3	4	5
Does the individual have information that enables decision making?	No resources		Some resources		Sufficient resources
Does the individual have memory of past events and experiences?	No memory		Some memory		Sufficient memory
Is the individual aware of the impact of own behavior on others?	No awareness		Some awareness		Sufficient awareness
Does the individual follow "display rules" (cultural norms) in situations?	Follows no "display rules"		Follows some "display rules"		Always follows "display rules"
Do somatic motor expressions (facial expressions and body postures) and ANS output match?	No match		One is more prominent than the other		Somatic and ANS output match
Does the individual use a range of facial expressions, posture, gestures?*	Extremely limited		Some		Wide range
	1 (-)	2 (-)	3	2 (+)	1 (+)
Does the individual respond appropriately to nonverbal cues (facial expressions, body postures, gestures) of others?	Underreactive responses		Appropriate responses		Overreactive responses
Do emotional reactions match situations?	Emotions weaker than situational demands		Emotions match situational demands		Emotions stronger than situational demands
Does the individual display appropriate amount of: a. ANS output	Too little		Appropriate		Too much
b. Somatic output In relation to situational demands?	Too little		Appropriate		Too much
Is the individual's mood consistent with emotional responses?**	Mood unchanging; situations do not affect mood		Mood consistent with emotions		Mood highly variable; inconsistent with situation, emotional responses

* Describe facial expressions, postures, gestures that are typical of this individual:

** Describe the individual's typical mood(s):

Table 8-14a. Worksheet to review affect/emotional features of an individual's performance. From Dunn, W. (1991). Assessing human performance related to brain function. In C. Royeen (Ed.), *Neuroscience foundations of human performance.* Rockville, MD: AOTA. Reprinted with permission.

Questions regarding affect/emotional tone	Ratings: Mark the box that best represents performance (optimal performance is shaded)				
	1	2	3	4	5
Does the individual have information that enables decision making?	No resources		Some resources *		Sufficient resources
Does the individual have memory of past events and experiences?	No memory		Some memory	*	Sufficient memory
Is the individual aware of the impact of own behavior on others?	No awareness		Some awareness *		Sufficient awareness
Does the individual follow "display rules" (cultural norms) in situations?	Follows no "display rules"		Follows some "display rules"	*	Always follows "display rules"
Do somatic motor expressions (facial expressions and body postures) and ANS output match?	No match		One is more prominent than the other *		Somatic and ANS output match
Does the individual use a range of facial expressions, posture, gestures?*	Extremely limited		Some *		Wide range
	1 (-)	2 (-)	3	2 (+)	1 (+)
Does the individual respond appropriately to nonverbal cues (facial expressions, body postures, gestures) of others?	Underreactive responses	*	Appropriate responses		Overreactive responses
Do emotional reactions match situations?	Emotions weaker than situational demands		Emotions match situational demands		Emotions stronger than situational demands *
Does the individual display appropriate amount of: a. ANS output	Too little		Appropriate		Too much *
b. Somatic output In relation to situational demands?	Too little	*	Appropriate		Too much
Is the individual's mood consistent with emotional responses?**	Mood unchanging; situations do not affect mood		Mood consistent with emotions	*	Mood highly variable; inconsistent with situation, emotional responses

* Describe facial expressions, postures, gestures that are typical of this individual:

** Describe the individual's typical mood(s):

Table 8-14b. Worksheet to review affect/emotional features of an adolescent who is meeting a boyfriend's or girlfriend's family for the first time. From Dunn, W. (1991). Assessing human performance related to brain function. In C. Royeen (Ed.), *Neuroscience foundations of human performance.* Rockville, MD: AOTA. Reprinted with permission.

Questions regarding motivational state	Ratings: Mark the box that best represents the individual's performance (optimal performance is shaded)		
	Low	**Medium**	**High**
What is the individual's overall level of motivation for functional performance?			
How does the internal environment interact with level of motivated behavior?	Conflicts with need to perform functional tasks	Neither supports nor conflicts	Supports functional performance
How does the external environment interact with level of motivated behavior?	Conflicts with need to perform functional tasks	Neither supports nor conflicts	Supports functional performance
How much experience has the individual had with the functional task to develop relationships between salient stimuli and appropriate responses?	None	Some experience	A sufficient amount
What are the characteristics of the individual intrinsic motivation? a. need to assert oneself	Very low need	Moderate need	Very high need
b. need to interact with others	Very low need	Moderate need	Very high need
c. need to feel competent/successful	Very low need	Moderate need	Very high need
d. need to obtain reinforcement	Very low need	Moderate need	Very high need
How is motivated behavior manifested? a. ANS output	Too little	Appropriate	Too much
b. Somatic motor output	Too little	Appropriate	Too much

	Difficulty of information needed in the task	Amount of information that needs to be processed	Amount of time the task requires	Necessity for continuous/ sustained effort	Highly interfering environment	Environment that provides ongoing support
Which task/enviromental factors interact with this individual's level of motivation to perform functional tasks? a. contribute to motivated behavior						
b. interfere with motivated behavior						

Table 8-15a. Workshhet to review the motivational features of an individual's performance. From Dunn, W. (1991). Assessing human performance related to brain function. In C. Royeen (Ed.), *Neuroscience foundations of human performance.* Rockville, MD: AOTA. Reprinted with permission.

Questions regarding motivational state	Ratings: Mark the box that best represents the individual's performance (optimal performance is shaded)		
	Low	Medium	High
What is the individual's overall level of motivation for functional performance?			*
How does the internal environment interact with level of motivated behavior?	Conflicts with need to perform functional tasks	Neither supports nor conflicts	Supports functional performance *
How does the external environment interact with level of motivated behavior?	Conflicts with need to perform functional tasks	Neither supports nor conflicts	Supports functional performance *
How much experience has the individual had with the functional task to develop relationships between salient stimuli and appropriate	None *	Some experience	A sufficient amount
What are the characteristics of the individual intrinsic motivation? a. need to assert oneself	Very low need	Moderate need *	Very high need
b. need to interact with others	Very low need	Moderate need	Very high need *
c. need to feel competent/successful	Very low need	Moderate need *	Very high need
d. need to obtain reinforcement	Very low need	Moderate need	Very high need *
How is motivated behavior manifested? a. ANS output	Too little	Appropriate	Too much *
b. Somatic motor output	Too little	Appropriate *	Too much

Which task/environmental factors interact with this individual's level of motivation to perform functional tasks?	Difficulty of information needed in the task	Amount of information that needs to be processed	Amount of time the task requires	Necessity for continuous/sustained effort	Highly interfering environment		Environment that provides ongoing support
a. contribute to motivated behavior	*	*	*	*			*
b. interfere with motivated behavior						*	

Comments:

Table 8-15b. Completed worksheet to review the motivational features of a therapist who is giving her first inservice. From Dunn, W. (1991). Assessing human performance related to brain function. In C. Royeen (Ed.), *Neuroscience foundations of human performance.* Rockville, MD: AOTA. Reprinted with permission.

TABLE 8-16

Questions that Elucidate the Contributions of Various Motivational Factors to Task Performance

Factor in motivation	Definition	Questions that service providers ask to determine the contribution of this factor to motivated performance
Incentive	The person needs or values the goal object	What does this person want to do? What does this person need to do to function in life? What behaviors or activities do family values support? What types of rewards does this person respond to?
Expectancy	The person: 1. Understands that the task is relevant to goal attainment 2. Believes that the act will lead to the goal	Have I made a clear link between the activities we are doing in therapy and the person's desired goals? Does the person accept that what we are doing will lead to goal attainment? Are there ways for me to provide external support (e.g., task adaptation or environmental modification) to make the relationship to goals more apparent?
Success	The person selects the task based on the need to complete the task correctly	What is the person's level of frustration tolerance? Does the person seem to care/notice when a task is incomplete or incorrect? Are task adaptations acceptable to the person, or does the person insist on one particular pattern of performance?

From Dunn, W. (1991). Motivation. In C. B. Royeen (Ed.), *AOTA self study series on neuroscience.* Rockville, MD: AOTA.

motor systems and autonomic nervous system (ANS) output. Somatic motor output is any output in which the voluntary muscles move; ANS output includes actions such as secretion of the glands, activation of the digestive system, or alteration of heart rate and breathing.

Let's consider an example. When persons are hungry, homeostasis is disrupted. The hypothalamus "notices" this disruption and (through higher brain centers) triggers a sensorimotor response (e.g., opening the refrigerator to pull out a leftover vegetable dish). As the person consumes the food, the ANS is triggered to act in the digestive process, and all of the subsequent feedback to the hypothalamus via the internal and external environments leads the hypothalamus to recognize that homeostasis is reinstated. In service provision, one takes advantage of understanding this process by designing strategies that either disrupt or facilitate attainment of homeostasis. We wait until a person is cold to work on pulling up the covers; we work on eating skills when the person is hungry; we address reciprocal interactions when the person needs something. By taking advantage of the biological and contextual supports available, providers and the persons they serve have more opportunities to be successful.

Brody (1983) characterizes these biological processes in behavioral terms. He describes three factors that determine a person's tendency to perform a task, the incentive, the expectancy and the need for success. Incentive refers to the person valuing the goal, creating an 'incentive' to perform. Expectancy refers to the person's ability to understand that the particular task they are performing will help to reach the goal. Success refers to the person's need to complete the task correctly; those who place a higher value on correctness will select simpler tasks. Table 8-16 contains a summary of these factors and a list of questions that providers can ask to ensure they have addressed these factors in intervention planning. Table 8-17 contains a case example using these factors.

Motivational Aspects of Common Disorders

Applying the knowledge from the literature about motivation to the day-to-day needs of persons who have performance needs is challenging (Dunn, 1991a). It is also disrespectful to consider that one perspective can ever explain or solve the challenges persons face. The purpose of this discussion is to help the reader consider the possibility of a motivational dysfunction as a component of each condition (Dunn, 1991a).

Attention Deficit Hyperactivity Disorder (ADHD). Barkley (1990) proposed a controversial hypothesis that children with ADHD have an underlying motivational disorder. He argues that the inconsistent situational behaviors of these children, and if this is indeed a factor, opens up both behav-

CASE INFORMATION: Mr. Cassandra has had a stroke. He has a history of being self-reliant and independent. He has indicated to the therapist that he would like to carry out personal hygiene, dressing, and bathing tasks for himself. The therapist decides he will work with Mr. Cassandra twice a day. He will visit Mr. Cassandra in the morning to provide input and assistance during his morning routine, and then will work on coordination and endurance to support self-care tasks later in the morning. Mr. Cassandra works very hard during the morning routine. He also expresses appreciation for the adaptations the therapist creates to enable him to participate in self-care tasks. However, Mr. Cassandra does not sustain performance during the late morning session; he complains and gives up easily, frequently collapsing on the mat to rest. Mrs. Cassandra begins spending full days with her husband as he prepares for discharge. Although Mr. Cassandra has developed adapted skills and endurance for self-care tasks, Mrs. Cassandra persistently provides so much help that he does not have to use his skills.

ANALYSIS: Intrinsic Factors	Situation: Therapist and Mr. Cassandra during the morning routine	Situation: Therapist and Mr. Cassandra during the late morning session	Situation: Mrs. Cassandra helping during morning routines**
Incentive	Mr. Cassandra expressed a desire to take care of his own personal hygiene and self-care.	Mr. Cassandra expressed a desire to take care of his own personal hygiene and self-care.	Mrs. Cassandra feels guilty that her husband has had a stroke; her role as caretaker of the family is her incentive to be persistent in providing 'too much help'.
Expectancy	Mr. Cassandra sees the relevance of the therapist's input to his desired goal; demonstrates highly motivated behaviors to engage in tasks.	Mr. Cassandra does not see the relationship between learning to prop on extended arm and hand as a means to develop background postural control for dressing; 'expectancy' is poor. Mr. Cassandra is, therefore, noncompliant with propping activities even though the desire to get dressed is great.*	Mrs. Cassandra knows how important it is to Mr. Cassandra to be well-groomed; she believes that by helping him, which speeds up the process, he will be ready for the day.
Success	Mr. Cassandra is challenged by the problems he faces, and wants to participate in the learning/ skill acquisition process	Although Mr. Cassandra is challenged to develop self-care skills, his inability to see the 'expectancy' relationship to his goal leads to discouragement; success at these skills is not important.	Mrs. Cassandra wants to avoid seeing Mr. Cassandra struggle; it reminds her that he has a disability.

*The therapist has not made a clear connection between postural control activities and self-care. It is likely that Mr. Cassandra will actively participate in these activities (demonstrate motivation) when he understands their importance in supporting self-care.

**Mrs. Cassandra does not recognize that Mr. Cassandra is challenged by his endeavors to reestablish self-care skills. She incorrectly presumes that the outcome (being 'ready') is the most important feature. She is also unaware of the risk that Mr. Cassandra may learn 'helplessness' if he stops being challenged to succeed.

Table 8-17. Case analysis of individual intrinsic motivation factors. From Dunn, W. (1991). Motivation. In C. B. Royeen (Ed.), AOTA self study series on neuroscience. Rockville, MD: AOTA.

ioral and medical interventions. From a behavioral perspective, children with ADHD are more in control when they participate alone with an adult (e.g., less inattention, less impulsivity); in groups, misbehavior escalates. In returning to the model proposed above, perhaps dysfunction with the internal mechanisms that support motivation can be overridden by greater external environmental supports (Dunn, 1991a).

From a medical perspective, considering the motivational system in the CNS offers different medication regime alternatives. Barkley (1990) discriminates children who have hyperactivity from those who do not within the attentional deficit population. He proposed that children who have hyperactivity (i.e., are aggressive, disinhibited and disruptive) may have a problem in the dopamine system that serves the prefrontal and limbic systems in the CNS. Children who are more lethargic may be more likely to have difficulties in the posterior association cortex, the hippocampus and the feedback mechanisms from higher to lower CNS centers; norepinephrine is a more likely neurotransmitter to be involved in these centers. These possible neurological differences point out the importance of understanding the underlying mechanisms in functions like motivation as interdisciplinary teams collaborate to identify the best possible intervention options (Dunn, 1991a).

Addiction. Addiction might be considered a vigorous motivational state (Dunn, 1991a). Scientists have had to change both the internal and external environments to mimic addiction in animal models; for example, prestimulation of parts of the hypothalamus enhances the expected external performance in animals (Stellar & Stellar, 1985). Some persons are more prone to addiction than others; perhaps in their systems, there is a difference in the optimal conditions for responding, in which certain chemical inducements more easily trigger responses. Additionally, in the more primitive CNS systems many connections are reciprocal, such that once the cycle of responding begins, it continues for a longer time that would be desirable. Thus, an interaction between internal state conditions and the external environment sustain the behaviors of addiction. There are certainly other factors that contribute to the patterns of addiction; this is one additional perspective.

Schizophrenia. The two phases of schizophrenia (i.e., positive and negative symptoms) suggest different neurological disruptions related to the motivational systems (Dunn, 1991a; Sachar (1985b). During positive symptom phases, the person has delusions and hallucinations; we believe that overactivity of the dopamine neurons in the limbic system contribute to this biobehavioral state (the limbic system is a key structure in the motivational connections of the CNS with the hypothalamus). Antischizophrenic drugs block this extra dopamine transmission and reduce these positive symptoms; this drug intervention may reduce the overactive status of this

aspect of the motivational system. Negative symptoms include low motivation, shallow affect and social incompetence; researchers believe that diffuse brain damage has occurred when these symptoms are present. Drug regimes are not helpful with diffuse brain damage. Some functional life interventions supplied by occupational therapy may provide additional external environmental input to counteract the effects of a diminished internal state, enabling some level of motivated performance, particularly for activities of daily living.

Depression. Depression might be considered a dormant motivational state; persons display loss of interests and an inability to derive pleasure from situations. Brain stem, limbic system and hypothalamic connections with noradrenaline and serotonin neurotransmitters are suspect with depression (Sachar, 1985a). When these pathways are disrupted, input to key motivational structures may be diminished, leading to an inability to sustain an internal state that can support motivated performance. Drug interventions are extremely effective, suggesting that this internal state can be reestablished, providing opportunities for responding to the environment more appropriately.

Brain Trauma. Key structures of the motivational system form the walls of the brain ventricles. When trauma leads to enlargement of the ventricles (e.g., bleeding into the ventricles), these key structures can be disrupted due to the pressure from the enlarging ventricles. A person can demonstrate a change in motivational capacity or status due to internal anatomical and physiological changes such as this; careful review of available records can alert a provider about this possibility. Changes in motivational status can be marked by increased agitation, aggression or a shutdown in responsiveness. In persons who do not have an identified brain trauma, these changes must trigger further investigation through referrals.

Principles for Designing Therapeutic Interventions Based on Affective System Functions

Affect and emotional tone can either provide strong supports or create barriers to performance. The worksheets outlined in Tables 8-14 and 8-15 provide a good beginning framework for therapists to design therapeutic interventions. Table 8-18 provides examples of therapeutic intervention planning for an adolescent who wishes to work, but who displays poorly modulated internal motivation as identified from Table 8-15.

SUMMARY

The CNS is a complex that supports life and its activities. The occupational therapist's challenge is to use its principles

TABLE 8-18

Ways to Design Therapeutic Interventions for a High School Boy Who Wants to Work But Has Poorly Modulated Internal Motivation System

Performance Need and Neurological Correlate	Possible Problems (data from Table 8-17)	Restorative Interventions	Adaptive Interventions	Alter Interventions	Preventative Interventions
Ryan wants to work; disruption in connections of the hypothalamus are leading to poorly modulated internal motivation (see Table 8-17)	Ryan displays a high need to assert himself				Work with Ryan and manager to identify stocking plans for sections of the store
	Ryan displays a high need to interact with others	Schedule work during peak traffic times to improve number of chances for Ryan to have contact with others			
	Ryan displays a low to moderate need to feel competent and successful		Assign a prescribed pattern for the stocking task		
	Ryan displays a low need to obtain reinforcement			Locate a large grocery store for Ryan's employment	

to help persons whose CNS is disrupted to use activity in context. This is the essence of occupation.

This chapter only addressed a few of the key features of CNS operations that support or create barriers for performance; there are many neuroscience texts that provide information on these topics in more depth (e.g., Kandel, Schwartz & Jessel, 1991). As a closing exercise, let us look at one constellation of neurological problems and the intervention possibilities that emerge with that neurological status. Table 8-19 provides a summary of the CNS structures that are affected when the middle cerebral artery is infarcted (we are using the right middle cerebral artery in this example). The Table summarizes the possible clinical problems that would emerge from this insult, and then offers functional life interventions using the restorative (i.e., remedial) and adaptive (i.e., compensatory) approaches. Using this process, the provider can make links between the neurological correlates and behavioral implications, and expand thinking about

intervention options for persons who have performance needs to help them achieve their objectives by tapping the exquisite potential of the CNS as they live fruitful lives.

STUDY QUESTIONS

1. Explain why the arousal/alerting and discrimination/mapping are necessary for normal performance.

2. Why is centrifugal control a critical feature of sensory processing?

3. Describe differences in performance difficulties with disruptions in the motor systems.

4. Design one of each intervention for a cognitive difficulty using the EHP framework.

5. Identify three intervention strategies for someone who is a "sensation seeker."

CNS Structure	Possible Problems	Possible Adaptations (Compensatory Approach)	Possible Remedial Strategies (Remedial Approach)
Right precentral gyrus, primary motor	Weakness or clumsiness on the left side, particularly of the face, arm, and hand	Use large-handled utensils to make it easier to grasp; use light containers so weakness is not a barrier; find one-handed alternative for tasks	Place objects so the individual can prop with the left arm while performing tasks with the right hand and arm
Right postcentral gyrus, primary sensory cortex	Sensory loss on the left side, particularly of the face, arm, and hand; sensory loss tends to involve touch pressure and proprioception more than pain and temperature	Create activities that require more activity with the right side, to minimize the effects of sensory loss on the performance of specific tasks	Use lighter-fitting clothing during the day to increase touch pressure and proprioceptive input to the limbs during activity
Fibers leaving the lateral geniculate body: Meyer's loop Optic radiations (These fibers run deep within the temporal lobe en route to the occipital lobe)	Visual field loss; possibly a full homonomous hemianopsis	Place all objects in the right visual field so the individual does not have to manage the visual field loss	Create opportunities for the individual to reposition the head to maximize use of intact visual field (e.g., turn head to the left)
Association cortex (Parieto-occipito-temporal region)	Impaired spatial perception, which manifests in difficulty copying, finding the way in the building, or putting clothes on properly—may neglect the left body side	Provide a higher level of supervision to maintain safety Alter placement of personal hygiene materials on sink to minimize confusion (e.g., only one thing on the sink at a time) Adapt clothing to provide cues	Systematically increase the number and amount of objects to deal with at the sink for personal hygiene Provide verbal cues to prompt correct donning of clothing
Posterior limb of the internal capsule (contains the sensory and motor projections)	Same as sensorimotor areas above		
Basal ganglia structures (deep in the cortex of the middle cerebral artery region)	Difficulty with movement; apraxia along with sensorimotor losses	Provide environmental cues to prompt the individual in movement routines	Provide rich sensorimotor experiences to reestablish body schema and ability to organize body movements

Table 8-19. Completed worksheet to analyze the neuroscience and intervention issues for an infarction to the right middle cerebral artery. From Dunn, W. (1991). Assessing human performance related to brain function. In C. Royeen (Ed.), *Neuroscience foundations of human performance.* Rockville, MD: AOTA. Reprinted with permission.

REFERENCES

Abraham, L., Copack, P. B., & Gilman, S. (1977). Brain stem pathways for vestibular projections to cerebral cortex in the cat. *Experimental Neurology, 55*, 436-448.

Ayres, A. J. (1985). *Developmental dyspraxia and adult onset apraxia.* Torrance, CA: Sensory Integration International.

Bach-y-Rita, P. (Ed.). (1980). *Recovery of function: Theoretical considerations for brain injury rehabilitation.* Baltimore: University Park Press.

Barkley, R. (1990). *Attention deficit hyperactivity disorder: A handbook for diagnosis and treatment.* New York: The Guilford Press.

Bellingham, W. P., Wayne, M. J., & Barone, F. C. (1979). Schedule-induced eating in water deprived rats. *Physiology and Behavior, 23*, 1105-1107.

Blakeslee, A. F., & Salmon, T. H. (1935). Genetics of sensory thresholds: Individual taste reactions for different substances. *Proceedings of the National Academy of Sciences of the U.S.A., 21*, 84-90.

Brody, N. (1983). *Human motivation.* New York: Academic Press.

Buttner V., & Henn, V. (1976). Thalamic unit activity in the alert monkey during natural vestibular stimulation. *Brain Research, 103*, 127-132.

Cool, S. J. (1987). A view for the "outside": sensory integration and developmental neurobiology. *Sensory Integration Newsletter, 10*(2), 2-3.

Coren, S., Porac, C., & Ward, L. M. (1984). *Sensation and perception.* Orlando: Academic Press.

Crutchfield, C. A., & Barnes, M. R. (1984). *The neurophysiologic basis of patient treatment: Volume III, Peripheral components of motor control.* Atlanta: Stokesville Publishing Co.

Darian-Smith, I. (1984). The sense of touch: Performance and peripheral neural processes. In I. Darian-Smith (Ed.). *Handbook of physiology, Section 1: The nervous system, Volume II: Sensory processes, part 2* (pp. 739-788). Bethesda: American Physiological Society.

Deecke, L. D., Schwartz, W. F., & Fredrickson, J. M. (1974). Nucleus ventroposterior inferior (VPI) as the vestibular thalamic relay in the rhesus monkey. *Experimental Brain Research,* 20, 88-100.

DeGangi, G. A., & Greenspan, S. I. (1991). Affect/Interaction Skills. Neuroscience foundations of human performance. *AOTA Self Study Series, 6.*

DeGangi, G. A., & Porges, S. W. (1991). Attention/Alertness/Arousal. Neuroscience Foundations of Human Performance. *AOTA Self Study Series, 5.*

DeMoja, C. A., Reitano, M., & Caracciolo, E. (1985). General arousal and performance. *Perceptual and Motor Skills, 61*, 747-753.

Dunn, W. (1997). The impact of sensory processing abilities on the daily lives of young children and their families: A conceptual model. *Infants and Young Children, 9*(4), 23-35.

Dunn, W. (1991a). Motivation. Neuroscience Foundations of Human Performance. *AOTA Self Study Series, 7.*

Dunn, W. (1991b). Assessing Human Performance Related to Brain Function. Neuroscience Foundations of Human Performance. *AOTA Self Study Series, 12.*

Dunn, W., Brown, C., & McGuigan, A. (1994). The ecology of human performance: A framework for considering the effect of context. *American Journal of Occupational Therapy, 48*(7), 595-607.

Goldberg, J. M., & Fernandez, C. (1984). The vestibular system. In I. Darian-Smith (Ed.). *Handbook of physiology, Section 1: The nervous system, Volume II: Sensory processes, Part 2* (pp. 977-1022). Bethesda: American Physiological Society.

Hall, M. J., Bartoshuk, L. M., Cain, W. S., & Stevens, J. C. (1975). PTC taste blindness and the taste of caffeine. *Nature (London), 253*, 442-443.

Halpern, B. P., & Meiselman, H. L. (1980). Taste psychophysics based on a simulation of human drinking. *Chemical Sense, 5*, 279-294.

Heimer, L. (1983). *The human brain and spinal cord.* New York: Springer-Verlag.

Jongkees, L. B. W. (1974). Pathology of vestibular sensation. In H.H. Kornhuber (Ed.), *Handbook of sensory physiology, Volume V1/2, Vestibular system Part 2: Psychophysics, applied aspects and general interpretations* (pp. 413-450). New York: Springer-Verlag.

Kandel, E. R., & Schwartz, J. H. (1985). *Principles of neural science.* New York: Elsevier.

Kandel, E. R., Schwartz, J. H., & Jessell, T. M. (Eds.). (1991). *Principles of neural science* (3rd ed.). New York: Elsevier Science Publishing Co.

Kelly, J. (1985). Principles of the functional and anatomical organization of the nervous system. In E. Kandel & J. Schwartz (Eds.), *Principles of neural science* (2nd ed.) (pp. 211-221). New York: Elsevier.

Kiang, N. Y. S. (1984). Peripheral neural processing of auditory information. In I. Darian-Smith (Ed.), *Handbook of physiology, Section 1: The nervous system, Volume II: Sensory processes, Part 2* (pp. 639-674). Bethesda: American Physiological Society.

Kornhuber, H. H. (1974). The vestibular system and the general motor system. In H. H. Kornhuber (Ed.), *Handbook of sensory physiology, Volume V1/2, Vestibular system Part 2: Psychophysics, applied aspects, and general interpretations* (pp. 581-620). New York: Springer-Verlag.

Liedgren, S. R., & Rubin, A. M. (1976). Vestibulo-thalamic projections studied with antidromic techniques in the cat. *Acta Oto-laryngology, 82*, 379-387.

Lund, R. D. (1978). *Development and plasticity of the brain: An introduction.* New York: Oxford University Press.

Magnin, M., & Fuchs, A. F. (1977). Discharge properties of neurons in the monkey thalamus tested with angular acceleration, eye movement, and visual stimuli. *Experimental Brain Research, 28*, 293-299.

McGuinness, D., & Pribram, K. (1980). The neuropsychology of attention: Emotional and motivational controls. In W. Hiack (Ed.), *The brain and psychology* (pp. 95-139). Orlando: Academic Press.

Moore, J. (1976). Behavior, Bias and the Limbic System. *American Journal of Occupational Therapy, 30*(1), 11-19.

Moore, J. (1980). Neuroanatomical considerations relating to recovery of function following brain lesions. In P. Bach-y-Rita (Ed.), *Recovery of function: Theoretical considerations for brain injury rehabilitation* (pp. 9-90). Baltimore: University Park Press.

Noback, C. R., & Demarest, R. J. (1987). *The human nervous system.* New York: McGraw-Hill.

Oetter, P., Laurel, M. K., & Cool, S. J. (1991). Sensorimotor Foundations of Communication. Neuroscience Foundations of Human Performance. *AOTA Self Study Series, 10.*

deQuiros, J. B., & Schrager, O. L. (1978). *Neuropsychological fundamentals in learning disabilities.* San Rafael, CA: Academic Therapy Publications.

Sachar, E. (1985a). Disorders of feeling: affective diseases. In E. Kandel & J. Schwartz (Eds.), *Principles of neural science* (2nd ed.) (pp. 717-726). New York: Elsevier.

Sachar, E. (1985b). Disorders of thought: The schizophrenic syndromes. In E. Kandel & J. Schwartz (Eds.), *Principles of neural science* (2nd ed.) (pp. 704-716). New York: Elsevier.

Schiller, P. H. (1984). The superior colliculus and visual function. In I. Darian-Smith, *Handbook of physiology, Section 1: The nervous system, Volume II: Sensory processes, Part 2* (p. 457-506). Bethesda, MD: American Physiology Society.

Stellar, J., & Stellar, E. (1985). *The neurobiology of motivation and reward.* New York: Springer-Verlag.

Vinogradova, O. S. (1970). Registration of information and the limbic system. In G. Horn & R. A. Hinde (Eds.), *Short-term changes in neural activity and behavior* (pp. 95-139). Cambridge University Press.

Wepsic, J. G. (1966). Multimodal sensory activation of cells in the maguocellular medial geniculate nucleus. *Experimental Neurology, 15,* 299-319.

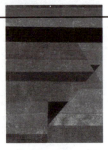

Chapter Content Outline

Abstract

Traditionally, control of movement was considered to be hierarchical in which higher cortical and subcortical areas of the nervous system inhibited the lower brainstem and spinal cord structures. Thus, therapy for individuals with movement-related problems, focused on decreasing primitive patterns and abnormal reflexes and providing sensory input and feedback to produce desired "normal" movement. Recent research has challenged the assumptions upon which the traditional treatments were based. Contemporary models have emerged in which the musculoskeletal and central nervous systems interact with the environment, as well as the intent or goal of an individual, to determine how a task is performed and the degree of neuromotor control necessary. This chapter will introduce readers to contemporary models of motor control and compare traditional and contemporary approaches to movement problems. The chapter will also discuss how these approaches guide assessment of occupational performance in individuals with movement-related problems. In addition, principles for intervention using client-centered occupations are described that incorporate current advances in motor learning and control.

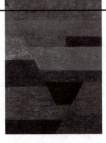

Key Terms

Affordance

Blocked practice

Bradykinesia

Control parameter

Degrees of freedom

Dysdiadochokinesia

Dysmetria

Dyssynergia

Perceptual trace

Random practice

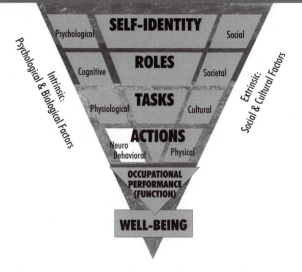

Movement Related Problems

Janet L. Poole, PhD, OTR

OBJECTIVES

The information in this chapter is intended to help the reader:

1. compare the assumptions of traditional rehabilitation treatments and the contemporary models related to the treatment of individuals with movement related problems

2. describe the contemporary models of motor control

3. identify assessments of individuals with movement related problems at both the occupational performance and component levels

4. incorporate intervention principles based on contemporary models and client-centered occupations into treatment of clients with movement related problems.

"Coordination of movement is the process of mastering the redundant degrees of freedom of the moving organism."

N.A. Bernstein, 1967

INTRODUCTION

> *My name is Virginia Chavez and I am 75 years old. I had a stroke 2 months ago. I am able to walk a little. My left arm is weak; I can move my shoulder a little and bend my elbow. My fingers bend a little and I can hold a cup. In therapy, I practice lifting my arm up and trying to keep my elbow straight, dusting, and holding cups. I wish I could try to use my arm more. I keep trying to move it but the therapist says I must be careful not to move it abnormally, whatever that means. I just want my arm to move better so I can go home and cook and make cookies for my grandchildren. I know my husband will help me, but I love to cook. I do not care if my arm does not move normally, if I could just hold a rolling pin or a bowl.*

Movement provides the means by which the individual interacts with the environment; it is the visible behavior that supports occupation. In this role, it also supports the neural development of emotions, cognition, socialization, and communication (Cech & Martin, 1995). A movement-related impairment may interfere with the development or maintenance of skills needed for daily living—as in the case of Mrs. Chavez. The environment, acting as the external stimulus, as well as the intent or goal of the individual will determine how a task is performed and the degree of neuromotor control necessary. The purpose of this chapter is to discuss the identification of assessments and interventions to address occupational performance deficits in individuals with movement-related problems. The chapter will contrast traditional and more contemporary approaches to movement problems and suggestions will be made as to how to incorporate current advances in motor learning and control in the use of client-centered occupations for the process of recovery.

TRADITIONAL AND CONTEMPORARY VIEWS ON MOTOR LEARNING, MOTOR CONTROL, AND MOTOR DEVELOPMENT

Assumptions of Traditional Views

1. The control of movement was considered to be hierarchical. In a hierarchical system, higher cortical and subcor-

tical areas of the central nervous system direct and inhibit the lower brainstem and spinal cord structures (Walsche, 1961). The lower structures were thought to modulate more primitive and automatic behaviors. Thus, early theorists viewed the development of motor control as a relationship between the developing brain and the emergence of motor behavior in the infant (Gesell, 1954; McGraw, 1945).

2. Primitive reflexes seen early in motor development were thought to correspond to the neuromaturation of the spinal cord and brainstem. As higher centers of the central nervous system matured, reflex behavior decreased and righting and equilibrium reactions emerged in conjunction with the neuromaturation of midbrain and cortical structures.

3. Voluntary movement was thought to emerge only when reflex behavior was integrated (Walsche, 1961). When damage occurred to the higher centers of the central nervous system, a regression to lower levels of motor control was thought to occur because primitive reflexes and stereotypic movements were observed (Bobath, 1985; Denny-Brown, 1950).

The hierarchical model has been the basis for the neurofacilitation treatment techniques used today in the treatment of persons with central nervous system disorders (i.e., Rood, Bobath, proprioceptive neuromuscular facilitation, Brunnstrom). Treatment based on this model focuses on decreasing primitive patterns and abnormal reflexes and providing sensory input and feedback to produce desired "normal" movement. A basic assumption of the neurofacilitation approaches was that practice and repetition of normal movement would result in permanent changes in the central nervous system. This concept of practice and repetition with feedback was also supported by early motor learning theorists (Adams, 1971; Kottke, 1980).

The focus of early motor learning research was on changes in performance observed during practice and/or by varying feedback. Errorless practice of specific movements (blocked practice) and parts of tasks were considered to be more effective than practicing variations of movements (random practice) or whole tasks (Adams, 1971; Kottke, 1980). Physical and verbal guidance provided individuals with a "feel" of the correct movement (Kottke, 1980) and immediate precise feedback was recommended (Adams, 1971). According to the hierarchical model, sensory input is required for motor output. This assumption was also supported by early motor learning theorists. In Adams' closed loop theory (1971), an individual compares feedback from an ongoing movement to the memory of past movements. The memory for past movements, or *perceptual trace*, was considered to be an internal reference for the correct response. This trace becomes stronger with practice. Thus, if errors

Bibliographic citation of this chapter: Poole, J. L. (1997). Movement related problems. In C. Christiansen & C. Baum (Eds.), *Occupational therapy: Enabling function and well-being* (2nd ed.). Thorofare, NJ: SLACK Incorporated.

occur, an incorrect perceptual trace was developed. According to Adams' theory, individuals with sensory impairments would not be able to correctly learn a motor task unless other feedback such as vision was available. This concept of feedback has been refuted by recent research.

When the afferent sensory nerves of insects and animals are cut, movements can be produced in the absence of sensory feedback (Grillner, 1975). Based on these results, a motor program or open loop theory was proposed in which muscle commands for action are prepared prior to the movement sequence and the entire sequence is carried out without peripheral feedback (Brooks, 1986; Keele, 1968; Schmidt, 1988). Thus, the concept of feed-forward replaced the idea of feedback dependent movement. Feed-forward control was also seen in preparatory movements incorporating postural balance (Nashner & McCollum, 1985). The motor program theory was based on a hierarchical model of motor control. Higher centers were considered to have executive functions for organizing programs and storing the rules for the lower structures such as specifying which muscles participate, the order of contractions, and the temporal phasing of the muscle contraction.

Review of Traditional Rehabilitation Treatment for Individuals with Central Nervous System Dysfunction

The traditional theorists, including Rood, Brunnstrom, Bobath, and Knott and Voss, based treatment on the hierarchical model of motor control. In the Rood approach, treatment consisted of facilitating an individual through the developmental sequence using sensory stimulation to inhibit or facilitate a motor response (Rood, 1954, 1956; Stockmeyer, 1967). Specific sensory stimulation such as fast brushing, quick stretch, and tapping facilitated a motor response while neutral warmth, joint compression, and maintained stretch were used to inhibit motor responses.

Proponents of proprioceptive neuromuscular facilitation (PNF) treatment viewed proprioception as the key sensory system to promote recovery (Knott & Voss, 1968; Voss, Ionta, & Meyers, 1985). According to this approach, normal movement and posture were dependent on a balanced interaction of antagonist and agonist muscles. To promote agonist/antagonist interaction, diagonal and spiral patterns were used, as these patterns paralleled functional movement.

Brunnstrom's movement therapy (Brunnstrom, 1970; Sawner & LaVigne, 1992) was designed exclusively for the treatment of individuals with hemiplegia. The major premise of the Brunnstrom intervention was the use of guided sensory input and positive reinforcement to promote voluntary control of muscle synergies that occur after the stroke. To facilitate voluntary movement, the client was encouraged to use selected postural reflexes such as the asymmetrical tonic neck, tonic labyrinthine, and tonic lumbar reflexes. The therapist guided the client's hemiparetic limbs to move first in synergy patterns, then in patterns that deviated from the synergies, and finally in patterns seen in individuals with no impairment.

The neurodevelopmental treatment (NDT) approach viewed neuromotor dysfunction as a deficit in the "normal postural reflex mechanisms" with abnormal tone and reflexes interfering with normal movement (Bobath, 1967, 1990). Treatment focused on inhibiting abnormal reflexes and associated reactions by using "handling" and sensory facilitation to guide motor output. Because spasticity was seen as the major cause of the neuromotor deficit, the focus of treatment was reduction of spasticity in preparation for movement. This approach specifically applied to treatment of individuals with stroke and cerebral palsy.

These theories have been challenged by new research, which has demonstrated that movement is supported by a blending of voluntary and reflex behavior rather than hierarchical control as was previously thought (Gordon, 1987; Horak, 1991). Contemporary models propose to incorporate new knowledge of neurophysiology and musculoskeletal systems interactions with the environment as a means for an individual to organize functional movement. This approach is consistent with occupational therapists' principles of engaging individuals in activities that are important to them.

Assumptions of Contemporary Models

Contemporary models of motor control view the central nervous system as a heteroarchical organization involving the interaction of many systems (Bernstein, 1967; Kelso & Tuller, 1984). Movement is distributed among a number of anatomical structures resulting in controlled action which is influenced by development, training, or changing environmental conditions (Turvey, Fitch, & Tuller, 1982). Because normal movement is goal-directed, functional tasks performed by an individual are thought to be a therapeutic way to achieve motor control.

Contemporary views on motor learning focus on how feedback and practice affect permanent changes in motor behavior (Jarus, 1994; Poole, 1991; Schmidt, 1991). Current research has documented the effectiveness of feedback and practice on skill acquisition and the retention of these skills. The results of these studies suggest that feedback is more beneficial to the learner when: 1) it is given less frequently, 2) after multiple trials, and 3) as a summary of the individual's performance. Additionally, 4) feedback is most effective when given for responses outside a given error range or bandwidth. For example, when working with a client who would like to dress himself faster, the therapist may only provide feedback when he takes longer than the pre-agreed time of 30 minutes.

TABLE 9-1

Motor Learning Principles Applied to Occupational Therapy

Concept	Jarus (1994)	Poole (1991)	Sabari (1991)
Feedback	Less frequent feedback	Frequent feedback in early learning Less frequent feedback in later learning	Feedback to augment impaired sensation
Practice	Blocked practice in early learning Random practice in later learning Vary context of task	Blocked/constant practice in very early learning Random practice in later learning Vary context Task dependent in later learning	Dependent on task type if environment/object moves and is unpredictable Vary context
Type of task practiced	Open tasks in which environment/object move and are unpredictable	Functional tasks determined by client's interests and capabilities	Functional tasks determined by client's interests and capabilities

Once the skill is acquired, retention of the skill is needed to maximize function. To facilitate generalization or transfer of a learned movement, contemporary research has found that practice should stimulate the real-life environment in which performance will take place. *Random practice*, in which tasks practiced during a therapy session change randomly, has been found to be more effective than *blocked practice*, in which one task is practiced repeatedly before practicing another task (Shea & Morgan, 1979). Likewise, practice of an entire task is better than practice of part of a task, especially with tasks in which timing is a crucial variable such as driving or walking (Newell, 1981). Jarus (1994), Poole (1991, 1995), and Sabari (1991) have applied contemporary motor learning concepts to occupational therapy practice (Table 9-1).

Contemporary motor development theorists consider development the result of the interaction of many systems rather than the neuromaturation of the infant or child (Heriza, 1991; Thelen, Fisher, & Ridley-Johnson, 1984). For example, progression in motor patterns such as primitive kicking and moving from supine to stand have been attributed to anthropometric characteristics and environmental demands (Thelen et al., 1984; VanSant, 1988). Development is thought not to follow a fixed sequence of cephalo -> caudal or proximal -> distal direction, but to occur simultaneously in many directions. Therefore, behaviors seen after central nervous system damage are now seen as attempts at functional movement which may be the most appropriate, efficient, and effective strategy available to the individual. Following stroke, individuals' abilities to reach targets within and outside Brunnstrom's (1970) synergy patterns followed no sequential

order. Biomechanical demands of the task rather than stereotyped linkages of muscles dictated which muscles were activated (Trombly, 1992, 1993). Several newer models of motor control have been proposed to explain the interaction among the environment, musculoskeletal system, and nervous system for mastery of functional tasks. The following models will be discussed: 1) systems theory, 2) dynamical systems theory, and 3) ecological approach.

Systems Theory

Systems theory views control of movement as being distributed throughout many interacting systems (Bernstein, 1967). These systems include the musculoskeletal, sensorimotor, perceptual/cognitive and emotions, as they interact with the environment. Bernstein (1967) noted that individuals have multiple *degrees of freedom* available in joint actions that need to be controlled to produce movement. To solve the degrees of freedom problem, Bernstein proposed that muscles are constrained in groups to act together in conjunction with the skeletal system as a unit. These units of movements were called synergies and later referred to as coordinative structures. The synergies used are determined by environmental conditions and functional goals (Turvey et al., 1982). For example, the sequence of muscles activated to maintain balance differs depending on how large the perturbation or challenge to balance is and the width of the individual's base of support (Horak & Nashner, 1986). The systems model can be used to account for variability and flexibility necessary to provide movement specifically tailored to the task and the environment.

Dynamical Systems Theory

The dynamical systems theory stresses the interactions of many systems to control movement (Kelso & Tuller, 1984; Kelso, Tuller, & Harris, 1987). Dynamic systems are self-organizing. Patterns of movement organize from subsystems working cooperatively for a specific function; patterns change or emerge into new behaviors as the functional demands change. For example, changes in muscle mass, bone length, and fat concentration in an adolescent gymnast force the gymnast to try new movements to accomplish routine stunts.

There are four basic assumptions of the dynamic theory (Kelso & Tuller, 1984):

- The first assumption: complex behaviors are constrained into simplicity by compressing degrees of freedom. Similar to the systems theory, the dynamic theory suggests that the multiple muscles and joints in the body are organized into functional groups or synergies.

- The second assumption: self-organizing patterns of movement are formed by the interaction of a large number of subsystems inherent in the organism itself. Thus, the controlling system changes depending on the task and context and is not predetermined (Heriza, 1991).

- The third assumption: organisms tend to settle into preferred but not obligatory coordinated movement patterns. When the system is challenged, a return to the preferred or stable movement pattern is observed.

- The fourth assumption: changes within each subsystem are not linear. When one subsystem or a component is altered and reaches a critical value, the system shifts into a whole new behavior pattern. For example, in quadruped animals, as speed of gait is altered, the animal shifts from walk to trot to pace to gallop. The transition periods are characterized by periods of increased variability, then less variability, and finally points at which new behaviors are observed. A variable that causes a transition is a control parameter. Control parameters may be the environment, weight, strength, size, texture, speed, and/or degrees of freedom. Scholz and Kelso (1990) suggest that manipulating control parameters, observing whether the behavior is stable or unstable, and identifying points of transitions in behavior will assist in understanding movement.

Ecological Approach

In the ecological approach (Gibson, 1979; Reed, 1982), movement is organized and coordinated specific to the task and the environment in which the task is being performed. Gibson (1979) uses the term *affordance* to describe the physical properties of the environment that allow or constrain movement. For example, the height of a step determines whether that step is climbable; a surface above the ground at knee height may be determined as sit-on-able such as a chair, but an empty cardboard box turned upside down is not. Babies learn what items in the environment afford pulling up to standing, such as a chair or a coffee table. Although an empty laundry basket does not afford pulling to standing due to the unstable base, the baby does not learn this until he or she has fallen several times. According to the ecological theories, an individual learning or acquiring a skill uses many muscle combinations to yield a functional outcome. For example, babies learn to come to standing in several ways: a baby can move from kneeling to half kneeling and push up with one leg, or from a kneeling position a baby can pull on a secure piece of furniture and extend both knees simultaneously. Despite the method used, the same outcome of standing is achieved. The ecological theory also addresses tool use by an individual. Tools allow individuals to interact with the environment by extending their perceptions of possible motor outcomes. Toddlers use tools to obtain objects beyond their reach, such as using a toy shovel to move an object on a countertop closer. In addition, movement generated by the individual is adapted according to the intended use of the tool. For example, a fork is held one way to feed oneself but is held very differently when used to stabilize food that will be cut with a knife.

CONTEMPORARY TREATMENT MODELS FOR INDIVIDUALS WITH CENTRAL NERVOUS SYSTEM DYSFUNCTION

Motor Relearning Programme (MRP)

Carr and Shepherd (1987) incorporated concepts from the motor learning literature to the treatment of clients with motor impairment after stroke. According to the MRP, movements should be goal-directed and related to the environment to maximize recovery of function. The four steps in the MRP are: 1) analysis of the task and client performance, 2) practice of poorly performed components, 3) practice of the entire task, and 4) transfer of training. Carr and Shepherd (1987) advocate identifying the goal, practicing tasks in their entirety, providing feedback, and practicing at the client's peak of performance. Practicing tasks in their entirety has been emphasized because research has shown that isolated exercises do not always transfer to a functional task (Winstein, Gardner, McNeal, Barto, & Nicholson, 1989). However, individual components initially may need to be practiced separately if a client is having difficulty with a particular component. Practice of the component should be followed immediately by practice of the whole task. In the MRP, therapist guided movements are kept to a minimum to allow the client to be an active participant in solving movement problems. Clients are encouraged to use visual feedback while the therapist gives verbal feedback regarding what is correct or incorrect about the client's performance. Furthermore, practice under different environmental conditions is advocated to encourage transfer and generalization of the learned movement strategies to new situations (Carr & Shepherd, 1987). In summary, the motor learning program views treatment as a process of teaching and learning. Although the program recognizes the importance of tasks and environmental context, the guidelines provided to improve motor control emphasize practice of essential components of tasks. The client is viewed as an active participant encouraged to develop problem-solving skills regarding his or her movement problems.

Task-Oriented Model of Neurologic Facilitation

The task-oriented model is based on the idea that the central nervous system must solve problems to accomplish motor tasks (Green, 1972; Horak, 1991). The model assumes that movement control is organized around goal-directed functional behaviors rather than specific muscle or movement patterns. Recognizing that the same task may be accomplished in more than one way, clients are encouraged to learn alternative movement patterns that can be used in a variety of environments. For example, one can stand from a supine position by using the abdominal muscles to attain long sitting, then bend the knees to move the center of mass forward to a squat position, and then stand. Or one can roll from a supine position to one side and push up to side sitting, rotate to an all fours position, and then push up to standing. Both methods yield the same outcome of standing (VanSant, 1988). The therapist's role is to provide feedback from a wide variety of sources while manipulating environmental and musculoskeletal demands to allow the emergence of efficient and functional behaviors (Horak, 1991). The task-oriented approach has been applied to occupational therapy practice by Bass Haugen and Mathiowetz (1995) and Flinn (1995). Bass Haugen and Mathiowetz suggest that the therapist collaborate with the client to identify tasks of importance, provide practice in varying contexts, and manipulate factors internal and external to the individual for optimal task performance. Flinn (1995) applied the task-oriented approach to the treatment of a client with left hemiplegia. The client wanted to resume her roles as homemaker and caregiver for her children. In therapy, she practiced using her affected arm to stabilize herself in standing while doing meal preparation and clean-up and carrying items. The therapist manipulated the musculoskeletal demands of tasks by having the client stabilize some joints involved in a task and by decreasing the amount of movements required against gravity.

ASSESSMENT

Assessments for occupational performance are discussed in Chapter 5. In most of these assessments, performance is rated according to how much physical assistance is needed. There are few assessments at the disability level that identify how occupations are accomplished or the processing that is done. Furthermore, the importance of the occupation to the individual is often neglected. Traditional approaches to assessment of individuals with movement related problems have focused on the impairment or component level, particularly tone and developmental reflexes. More contemporary views on assessment would advocate testing at the disability or occupational performance area level to know what individuals want and need to do to function in their roles. Indeed, it is the accomplishment of tasks related to one's goals that drive motor behavior. But the demands placed upon the individual change as the task and context change and as the factors intrinsic and extrinsic to the individual change. Therefore, testing in different contexts is also important. If a disability is identified, assessment would continue at the impairment or component level to determine constraints to performance as motor control is viewed as the result of the interaction of many systems by contemporary theories. The following section reviews briefly assessments at the disability or occupational performance level and at the impairment or component level. In Chapter 5, Ottenbacher and Christiansen discuss occupational performance assessments in more detail.

Disability Level Assessments

The Canadian Occupational Performance Measure (COPM)
The COPM is a semi-structured interview that measures a client's self-perception of occupational performance, (Law, Baptiste, Carswell, McColl, Polatajko, & Pollock, 1991). The COPM takes about 30 to 40 minutes to administer. It is the client who identifies issues in performance, although the therapist may need to define occupational performance. For each basic occupational performance area (self care, productivity, leisure), clients are asked to first identify issues in performance and then rate on a scale from 1 to 10, the importance of each activity.

Performance Assessment of Self-care Skills (PASS)
The PASS (Rogers & Holm, 1994) simultaneously provides data concerning activities of daily living and types of person (i.e., demonstration, manual guidance), task (i.e., presentation of small units of information), and environmental (i.e., rearrangement of furniture) assists. The PASS consists of

26 tasks: 3 self-care, 5 mobility, and 18 instrumental activities of daily living. Three subscores are obtained: level of independence, safety, and outcome or quality of performance. The PASS is designed for use with adults with all types of diagnoses. It takes 1 1/2 to 3 hours to administer as it is a performance-based test focusing mainly on instrumental tasks of daily living.

Structured Observational Test of Function (SOTOF)

The SOTOF (Laver & Powell, 1995) assesses eating from a bowl with a spoon, washing hands, pouring and drinking a beverage, and dressing with a long-sleeved front-opening garment and the underlying neurological function for each activity. Language, hearing, cognition, motor function, vision, sensation, and several aspects of perception are observed as the client performs the activities of daily living tasks. The test is short and takes approximately 10 minutes per activity.

Assessment of Motor Process Skills (AMPS)

The AMPS (Fisher, 1992) allows the therapist to simultaneously assess motor and process skills and instrumental activities of daily living task performance that are important to the client. The motor skills are related to the underlying posture, mobility, coordination and strength capabilities of the client. The process skills are related to the underlying attentional, ideational (conceptual), organizational, planning, and adaptive capabilities of the person. The AMPS can be administered in any setting in 30 to 60 minutes.

The Arnadóttir OT-ADL Neurobehavioral Evaluation Instrument (A-ONE)

The A-ONE (Arnadóttir, 1990) simultaneously assesses function and neurobehavioral processes. Dressing, grooming and hygiene, transfers and mobility, feeding, and communication are included in the function section while specific impairments, such as sensory/perceptual dysfunction, cognitive disturbances, and emotional disturbances, are noted for each functional activity.

Pediatric Evaluation of Disability Inventory (PEDI)

The PEDI (Haley, Coster, Ludlow, Haltiwanger, & Andrellos, 1992) measures capability and performance in children from 6 months to 7.5 years of age in 3 domains: self-care, mobility, and social function. The self-care domain includes feeding, grooming and bathing, dressing and toileting. The mobility domain includes transfers and locomotion. The social domain includes comprehension, expression, problem solving, play, and safety. While this test does rate the degree of physical assistance needed for performance, it also identifies the type of caregiver assistance needed, modifications such as environmental modifications or adapted equipment needed to do different occupations, and the capability of the child to do the occupation with the adapted equipment.

Impairment Level Assessments

Range of Motion

Adequate joint range of motion allows body parts to move freely in space and maintains a balanced workload on the muscles, thus maintaining efficiency of movement. Joint range of motion is typically measured with a goniometer. There are two types of range of motion: passive range of motion (PROM) and active range of motion (AROM). PROM is the motion available in a joint when it is moved by an outside force, such as a therapist. This measurement informs the examiner about the extendibility of the joint capsule, associated ligaments, and muscles (Norkin & White, 1985). AROM is the range through which a client can move a joint using his or her own muscle power. This measurement provides the examiner with additional information about muscle strength and functional ability. Detailed instructions for placement of goniometers to measure each joint and average normal values for range of motion are provided in Trombly (1995) and Norkin and White (1985).

Muscle Strength

Muscle strength is assessed by the use of Manual Muscle Testing (MMT), a Cybex machine, or functional strength patterns. MMT is a test of static voluntary isometric strength. Manual resistance is provided by a therapist, who scores the strength of a muscle or groups of muscles based on whether the movement is against gravity and how much resistance a muscle group can take. Detailed instructions and scoring are provided in Daniels and Worthingham (1986), Kendall, McCreary, and Provance (1993), and Trombly (1995). A hand-held muscle dynamometer can also be used to test static muscle strength. The client pushes against the plate and piston of the dynamometer while the therapist applies a counter force. However, reliability of hand-held dynamometry is limited by the strength of the tester (Wadsworth, Nielsen, Corcoran, Phillips, & Sannes, 1992). In isokinetic testing, the velocity of a moving body part is kept constant while resistance that is directly proportional to the torque produced by a muscle is provided throughout the whole range of motion. Isokinetic testing provides a quantitative assessment of torque control, timing, and reciprocal muscle action. Isokinetic testing requires bulky and expensive instruments such as the Cybex, KINCOM, Biodex, and Orthotron. Functional strength of the lower extremities can be tested by the "Timed Stands" test (Csuka & McCarty, 1985). Subjects sit in an armless chair and are requested to perform 10 repetitions from sitting to standing. The score is the time to perform 10 repetitions to the nearest 10th of a second (Csuka & McCarty, 1985).

Tone

Muscle tone is a velocity-dependent response of a muscle to passive stretch (Gordon & Ghez, 1991). The assessment of tone is usually accomplished by passively moving the limb quickly throughout its available range of motion (Trombly & Scott, 1989). If the muscle contracts to resist the passive movement, that is a stretch reflex occurs, the muscle is said to be spastic. If the stretch reflex occurs during the last one-fourth of the range, the muscle is said to have mild spasticity. If the stretch reflex occurs midrange, the muscle is said to have moderate spasticity. If the stretch reflex occurs in the initial one-fourth of the range, the muscle is said to have severe spasticity. This method for assessing spasticity is subjective and attempts have been made to design a more quantifiable way of measuring tone. One attempt is the Modified Ashworth Scale (Ashworth, 1964; Bohannon & Smith, 1987) in which resistance encountered to passive movement is rated on a 5 point ordinal scale from no increase in muscle tone to rigidity in a position of flexion or extension. Another more objective device to measure dynamic and static aspects of tone at the wrist only was devised by McPherson, Mathiowetz, Strachota, Benrud, Ingrassia, and Spitz (1985). Law and Cadman (1988) provide a review of methods used to measure spasticity.

Developmental Reflexes and Reactions

Reflex testing has been an important part of assessment of individuals with movement related problems. Reflexes are normally present during gestation and infancy but become integrated by the central nervous system early in life. However, they have been observed to re-emerge in normal children and adults under conditions of fatigue or stress or following brain damage (Bobath, 1985; Hellebrandt, Houtz, Partridge, & Walters, 1956). Reflex testing procedures have been described in detail by Bobath (1985) and Fiorentino (1973).

Balance and Equilibrium

Balance can be assessed at the impairment level (strength, ankle range of motion, sensation), at the strategy level, and/or at a task performance level. The critical impairment factors related to balance appear to be ankle range of motion, lower extremity strength, and sensation (Woollacott & Shumway-Cook, 1995). Decreased ankle range of motion may limit an individual's ability to use an ankle strategy for postural control whereas decreased strength may affect appropriate recruitment of and timing of motor unit activation. However, other musculoskeletal impairments are important as well for alignment of the body in an upright position and use of available responses to control posture (Woollacott & Shumway-Cook, 1995).

Sensory loss can result in faulty feedback or perceptions regarding the environment. Evaluations that test at the strategy level include the Clinical Test for Sensory Interaction and Balance (CTSIB) and the EquiTest System. The CTSIB (Crowe, Dietz, Richardson, & Atwater, 1990; Shumway-Cook & Horak, 1986) is a clinical test to assess the ability of children and adults to maintain balance under five different sensory conditions: three visual and two support surface (Table 9-2). The EquiTest is a computerized system that quantifies balance strategies and sensory organization strategies under the same six conditions. The EquiTest can be interfaced with an EMG machine to determine onset latencies for various postural muscles. However, it is expensive and not easily available. Table 9-2 describes several commonly used balance assessments. Task performance tests, such as the Berg Balance Scale (Berg, Wood-Dauphinee, Williams, & Gayton, 1989), Functional Reach (Donahoe, Turner, & Worrell, 1993; Duncan, Weiner, Chandler, & Studenski, 1990), the Timed Get Up and Go Test (Podsiadlo & Richardson, 1991), and the Tinetti (Tinetti, 1986), assess balance during tasks such as walking, coming to standing, picking object from the floor, and reaching.

Dexterity

Numerous tests exist to measure fine motor dexterity and rapid manipulation of objects (see McPhee, 1987 for a review). Many were developed to aid in the selection of employees for jobs requiring fine dexterity. Table 9-3 lists common dexterity assessments. Both the Box and Block Test (Mathiowetz, Volland, Kashman, & Weber, 1985) and the Minnesota Rate of Manipulation Test (American Guidance Services, 1969) measure handling of large objects. Mathiowetz and Bass Haugan (1995) recommend the Box and Block test over the Minnesota Rate of Manipulation Test because it has a time limit, a broad range of normative data, and is administered with the client sitting. The Nine-hole Peg Test (Mathiowetz, Weber, Kashman, & Volland, 1985) and the Purdue Pegboard (Tiffen, 1968) measure finer manipulation skills. Mathiowetz and Bass Haugan (1995) recommend using the Purdue over the Nine-hole test. The Purdue has a time-limit, high test-retest reliability, was normed for a broader range, and has bilateral and unilateral subtests. The Crawford Small Parts Dexterity Test (Crawford & Crawford, 1956) and the Bennett Hand Tool Test (Bennett, 1965) measure tool usage. However, the Crawford involves small hand tools, such as tweezers and a small screwdriver, while the Bennett Hand Tool test evaluates the ability to remove and replace from an upright board, two sizes of nuts, washers, and bolts and one size of screws. The Jebsen Hand Function Test (Jebson, Taylor, Trieschmann, Trotter, &

TABLE 9-2

Balance Assessments

Test	Description	Population
CTSIB (Shumway-Cook & Horak, 1986; Crowe et al., 1990)	Stand both feet, eyes open and closed Stand both feet, dome, eyes open Stand foam, eyes open and closed Stand foam, dome, eyes open	Children and adults
Functional Reach (Duncan, et al., 1990 Donahoe, 1993)	Client reaches forward with extended arm parallel to a yardstick at shoulder level	Children and adults
Berg Balance Scale (Berg et al., 1992)	14 items which include: Get in and out of chair Transfer bed to chair Reach forward Pick up object from floor Unilateral stance and tandem Dynamic weight shift	Older adults
Tinetti Test (Tinetti, 1986)	13 items which include: Standing and sitting balance Arising from chair Turning balance Unilateral stance Reach object from high shelf Pick up object from floor	Older adults
Timed "Up and Go Test" (Podsiadlo & Richardson, 1991)	Client stands from chair with armrests, walks a short distance and turns around, returns to chair and sits down	Older adults

Howard, 1969) simulates dexterity tasks of daily living. Of all the tests classified as functional hand evaluations, only the Jebsen Hand Function Test has normative data and is standardized. However, each hand is tested separately because there are no items requiring bilateral hand use.

Coordination

Coordination is the ability to control movements smoothly and accurately. Coordination impairment is often, but not always, related to a particular part of central nervous system involvement. Therefore, the clinical symptoms that are observed are related to the location of damage or disease. Disturbances in coordination and their definitions are as follows. *Dysdiadochokinesia* is the inability to perform rapid alternate movements and results in irregular and unrhythmical movements. *Dyssynergia* or movement decomposition is a lack of smoothness of movement due to lack of reciprocal action in opposing muscle groups. The rebound phenomena of Holmes is the loss of the check reflex to stop forceful actions (Ghez, 1991). *Bradykinesia* is slowed or depressed movement resulting in difficulty initiating and stopping

movements and changing directions. *Dysmetria* is the inability to stop a movement at a desired position resulting in a client pointing past or stopping short of a goal. Dysmetria is more pronounced with vision occluded in a client with a posterior column lesion than with a cerebellar lesion. An *ataxic gait* is a wide-based and staggering gait. Ataxia is more pronounced when vision is occluded or in a poorly lit room in a client with a posterior column lesion. A client with a cerebellar lesion may veer toward the side of lesion during gait. A *tremor* is an involuntary oscillating movement. In cerebellar lesions, a tremor that occurs during voluntary movement and increases as the limb nears the goal is called an intention tremor. A resting tremor is observed in lesions of the basal ganglia in which the tremor decreases with purposeful movement but increases at rest. Coordination tests evaluate the ability or inability to reverse movements between opposing muscle groups, judge distance and speed of voluntary movements, or hold a limb or segment of a limb in one position. Table 9-4 describes the coordination tests, the deficit tested for, and the location of the lesion for the deficit.

TABLE 9-3

Dexterity Assessments

Test	Description	Population
Bennet Hand Tool Test (Bennett, 1965)	Test consists of board with 2 uprights at each end with 3 sizes of nuts, bolts, and washers on one end. Client removes all bolts from one upright and places them on corresponding rows on the other upright. Client is timed.	Adults
Box and Block Test (Mathiowetz et al., 1985)	Client transfers blocks one at a time over a partition and releases them for 15 seconds. Score is the number blocks transferred in 15 seconds.	Children ≥ 6 years Adults
Crawford Small Parts Dexterity Test (Crawford & Crawford, 1956)	Part I - client is given 3 minutes to use tweezers to pick up pins and collars and insert them in a metal plate one at a time. Part II - client picks up a screw, starts the screw into a threaded hole with the fingers and then uses a screwdriver and both hands to tighten the screw. Timed for 5 minutes.	Adults
Jebson-Taylor Hand Function Test (Jebson et al., 1969; Taylor et al., 1973)	Seven subtests which are timed and include: writing, card turning, picking up small objects, simulated feeding, stacking checkers, picking up large light objects, picking up large heavy objects.	Children ≥ 6 years Adults
Minnesota Rate of Manipulation Test (American Guidance Services, 1969)	Five subtests which are timed and performed on a form-board with round discs and include: placing, turning, displacing, one-handed turning and placing, and two-handed turning and placing.	Adults
Nine Hole Peg Test (Mathiowetz et al., 1985)	Client picks up 1/4" diameter pegs from a container one at a time and puts them into holes spaced 1-1/4" apart. Once the holes are filled, the pegs are removed one at a time. The score is the time to complete both placing and removing pegs.	Adults
Purdue Pegboard Test (Tiffan, 1968; Mathiowetz et al., 1986)	Client performs two operations: rapid placing of small pins in pegboard and assembly of pins, washers, and collars. For placing, client is timed for 30 seconds for each hand separately and then both hands together. For the assembly, client is timed for 1 minute.	Children ≥ 5 years Adults
O'Conner Finger Dexterity or Tweezer Dexterity Test (Hines & O'Connor, 1926)	Client picks up very small pins with either the fingers or tweezers and places them in small holes on a pegboard. Scoring is the number of seconds to fill the board with a pin in each hole.	Children ≥ 13 years Adults
Grooved Pegboard (Trites, 1977)	Client picks up pegs with a key along one side, rotates them to match holes with randomly positioned slots, and inserts them into the holes. There are 25 holes. Scoring is the number of seconds to fill the board with a peg in each hole.	Children ≥ 5 years Adults

TABLE 9-4
Selected Coordination Assessments

Test	Description	Deficit Tested for	Possible Lesion Site
Finger to Nose	Client's shoulder is abducted to 90,° with the elbow extended. Client flexes elbow to touch index finger to nose.	Dysmetria	Posterior column Cerebellum
		Intention tremor	Cerebellum
		Movement decomposition	Cerebellum
Alternate Nose to Finger; Toe to Therapist's Finger	Client alternately touches index finger or great toe to tip of therapist's index finger. The position of the therapist's finger can be altered during testing.	Dysmetria	Posterior column Cerebellum
		Dysdiadochokinesia	Cerebellum
		Intention tremor	Cerebellum
		Movement decomposition	Cerebellum
Pronation/ Supination	Elbows flexed to 90°, arm into side, client alternates pronating and supinating forearms	Dysdiadochokinesia	Cerebellum
Alternate Heel to Knee; Heel to Toe	Supine, client touches the heel of one lower extremity alternately to the knee and big toe of the opposite extremity.	Dysdiadochokinesia	Cerebellum
		Movement decomposition	Cerebellum
Finger Opposition	Client touches tip of thumb to tip of each finger in sequence	Dysdiadochokinesia	
Finger to Finger	Client's shoulders are abducted to 90,° with elbows extended. Client flexes both elbows simultaneously to approximate index fingers from both hands.	Intention tremor	Cerebellum
Rebound Test	Client resists elbow flexion while therapist suddenly releases the resistance. Opposing muscles should contract and "check" movement	Rebound phenomenon of Holmes	Cerebellum
Walking	Client walks on a straight line, at different speeds, and turns	Ataxia if wide base and unsteady	Posterior column if performance decreases with vision occluded
		Ataxia	Cerebellum if veers to side of lesion
		Bradykinesia	Basal Ganglia if shuf fling, no arm swing, difficulty initiating and changing direction

TABLE 9-5

Stroke Motor Function Assessment

Test	Areas of Assessment
Fugl-Meyer Assessment of Sensorimotor Recovery after Stroke (Fugl-Meyer et al., 1975)	Balance sitting and standing Lower extremity motor score (includes coordination) Upper extremity motor score (includes coordination) Sensation Joint range of motion Pain
Motor Assessment Scale (Carr et al., 1985)	Supine to side lying Supine to sitting over the bed Balance sitting Sitting to standing Walking Upper arm function Hand movements Advanced hand activities Muscle tone
Rivermead Motor Assessment (Lincoln & Leadbitter, 1979)	Gross Function - balance, transfers, gait Leg and trunk function Arm function
Action Research Arm Test (Lyle, 1981)	Grasp and lift items Grip Pinch Gross arm movements
Functional Test for the Hemiparetic Extremity (Wilson et al., 1984)	7 functional levels, tasks include: Stabilizing items with arm or hand Grasping small items In-hand manipulation tasks

Motor Function After Stroke

Because of the severe motor impairments often seen after a cerebrovascular accident, several motor assessments have been specifically designed to quantify motor deficits in the hemiparetic upper extremity (see Poole & Whitney, 1995 for a review). These include the Fugl-Meyer Assessment of Sensorimotor Recovery after Stroke (Fugl-Meyer, Jääskö, Leyman, Olsson, & Steglind, 1975), the Motor Assessment Scale (Carr, Shepherd, Nordholm, & Lynne, 1985), the Rivermead Motor Assessment (Lincoln & Leadbitter, 1979), the Action Research Arm Test (Lyle, 1981), and the Functional Test for the Hemiparetic Upper Extremity (Wilson, Baker, & Craddock, 1984). These tests are summarized in Table 9-5.

Sensation and Perception

The contributions of the sensory systems to movement are to receive input from the environment and provide the individ-

ual with updated information regarding the execution of movement (feedback). Sensation and perception affect the intent to move. If insufficient information is perceived from the body and the environment, correct motor responses will not be developed. A loss of input from one sensory system may or may not be compensated by input from another system. For example, an individual with proprioceptive loss in the lower extremities may rely on vision to maintain posture. However, if vision is diminished from a sensory loss or if the individual is in a dark room, it may be difficult to maintain a stable posture. Procedures for assessing sensation perception are described in detail in Trombly (1995) and Pedretti and Zoltan (1990).

Cognition

The cognitive processes that are important for learning motor tasks include pattern recognition, attention, memory, and problem solving (Poole, 1995). These processes affect a client's ability to perceive, organize, store, or retrieve information. Several tests assess occupational performance deficits that relate to processing information, including the AMPS (Fisher, 1992) and the Kitchen Task Assessment (Baum & Edwards, 1993). These are discussed further in Chapter 11.

INTERVENTION

The traditional approaches to treatment of individuals with movement-related problems included interventions based on the theories of Rood, Brunnstrom, Bobath, and Voss and colleagues. These theories proposed to normalize tone and recommend following a developmental sequence providing controlled sensory input. These approaches suggested that repetition and application cause habituation. The major principles of these approaches were discussed previously. The reader should refer to the original source for specific intervention techniques.

The assumptions underlying the traditional approaches are not consistent with what is now known about the central nervous system (Gordon, 1987; Horak, 1991). Therapists need to move beyond focusing on tone and decreasing primitive reflexes and abnormal movement patterns. Research has shown that normalizing does not necessarily yield normal movement (Dietz, Quintern, & Berger, 1981) and abnormal movement patterns are now viewed as the most appropriate, efficient and effective strategies for functional movement given the constraints of the damaged nervous system (Heriza, 1991). However, two of the traditional approaches, NDT and PNF, are still evolving through disciples of the Bobaths and Knott and Voss. Recent continuing education courses on NDT and PNF are promoting to a greater extent, active participation of the client in treatment and functional performance. Thus, for NDT and PNF, the contemporary approaches are being blended into the older traditional approaches.

In the contemporary approaches, both functional goals and environmental constraints are considered key to treating individuals with movement related problems. Spasticity is no longer considered the most significant impairment constraining function. For example, Sahrmann and Norton (1977), in examining whether flexor spasticity in the biceps prevented effective activation of the triceps, found that impairment in movement was not due to spasticity in the biceps but due to a timing problem that caused a delay in the biceps ceasing a contraction and limiting ability of the triceps to recruit motor neurons. Other studies have shown that teaching clients with stroke and cerebral palsy to reduce their own tone via biofeedback resulted in decreased tone but no improvement in functions for either the upper or lower extremity (Dietz et al., 1981; Nielson & McCaughey, 1982). Contemporary

---

TABLE 9-6

Occupational Therapy Intervention Principles Based on Contemporary Models of Motor Control

1. Use occupations that are important to the client for evaluation and treatment (a client-centered approach).
2. Consider neural and non-neural factors as possible influences on dysfunction.
3. Manipulate critical personal and environmental systems (control parameters) to cause changes in motor behavior.
4. Two critical control parameters may be strength and controlling degrees of freedom.
5. Provide active participation in practice appropriate to client's status but which encourage experimenting with solutions to motor problems.
6. Structure practice for optimal retention and generalization.
7. Provide feedback.

---

approaches view impairments in movement as difficulty in controlling degrees of freedom and/or problems with motorneuron firing. The following are principles for intervention based on the contemporary models (Table 9-6).

1. Use occupations that are important to the client for evaluation and treatment (a client centered approach). Functional goals are motivators to move. The COPM can be used to identify occupations important to the client. If performance is not satisfactory to the client, then consider the components that may affect performance (range of motion, strength, sensation, coordination). One caution with using functional outcomes is that there may be a ceiling effect which fails to capture fine aspects of recovery so a therapist may also have to use a finer measure, such as time, as an outcome measure.

2. Consider neural and non-neural factors as possible influences on dysfunction. If a soft tissue contracture or bony constriction exist, myofascial release, joint mobilization, surgery, and/or serial casting may be appropriate. If a muscle has shortened, it will need to be lengthened to get normal movement. For example, a client with a shortened gastrocnemius muscle will not be able to achieve heel strike during gait, and a client with a shortened rhomboid muscle will not be able to achieve full shoulder flexion.

3. Manipulate critical personal and environmental systems (control parameters) to cause changes in motor behavior. Observe how the client approaches a task. When a client

has good motor recovery his or her movements are stable yet flexible. However, in the acute stage of recovery, clients use movement patterns that show little stability as is observed in early learning, so task performance is not effective. These clients are in a period of transition which is a good time to facilitate new movements (Kamm, Jensen, & Thelen, 1990). If the client performs a task in only one way, that way may only work in one context. For example, is a flexor synergy pattern used for all reaching tasks? Can the client adapt to different demands? With these clients, it is more difficult to change these movement patterns and clients will revert back to these learned behaviors. To assess how stable the pattern is, first observe what fluctuates and quantify the collective variables (reaction time, movement time, rate, variability). Then observe what happens if the pattern is challenged by changing some critical factor (person or environment). The critical factor will differ according to the task, environment, and person. These critical factors or control parameters could be weight, size, texture, different culture, splint, positioning, speed, accuracy, degrees of freedom, or the environment. For example, if a client demonstrates increased wrist flexion and difficulty in hand grasp and release, the difficulty might be due to decreased strength, increased tone, or an inability to control two joints simultaneously. How could the therapist determine which is the critical factor? By reducing the degrees of freedom with a wrist splint, the client may achieve finger flexion and extension for grasp and release. In this solution, wrist stability (i.e., decreased strength and inability to control two joints) is deficient. Therefore, the focus of therapy would be to strengthen the wrist extensors. However, if a wrist splint is applied and the client still has difficulty with grasp and release, then the finger muscles may need strengthening.

4. Two critical control parameters may be strength and controlling degrees of freedom. The strengthening program may consist of active functional tasks, active-assistive exercises, or resistive exercises. Isolated muscle exercises should be used as an adjunct to the active functional activities. Active functional activities could first be performed in the direction of gravity, such as pushing objects into a drawer or pushing the brake on the wheelchair. The activities could be graded to be performed next with gravity eliminated and finally against gravity. Ostendorf and Wolf (1981) and Wolf, Lecraw, Barton, and Brigitte (1989) provide graded functional tasks for clients post stroke.

Motor function in clients after stroke was shown to improve with active engagement of the hemiparetic arm in occupations. Taub (1980) coined the term "learned non-use" of the impaired limb to refer to observations that even rehabilitated clients after stroke rarely used their impaired limb for functional tasks. To address this issue, several studies, using a "forced use paradigm" (Taub, Miller, Novack, Cook, Fleming, Nepomuceno, Connell & Crago, 1993; Wolf, Lecraw, Barton, & Brigitte, 1989) in which the unimpaired arm is restrained, resulted in documented improvements in the impaired arm. Subjects practiced tasks that required upper limb function (eat, write, throw ball, push button, manipulate checkers) for 6 to 7 hours a day for 2 weeks. Significant improvements in speed and force of movements were observed in these clients. The most compelling finding was that the improvement was sustained for 1 to 2 years post intervention and the subjects felt improvements significantly enough to want to do it again (Wolf et al., 1989).

When using active-assistive exercises, concentric and eccentric motions in straight planes followed by isometric contractions at the end of the movement are used (Flinn, 1995). Resistive exercise with different grades of theraband could be done for strengthening exercises. Theraband is particularly effective for individuals without active grip control.

Another control parameter to manipulate is the degrees of freedom required for a task. Degrees of freedom in the extremities can be reduced by stabilizing or eliminating some joints or by decreasing movement against gravity. One approach would be to have the client rest the elbow or forearm on a surface for activities involving the wrist and/or grasp and release. Another solution could be to have the client hold the arm against body with the shoulder adducted for activities requiring elbow, wrist and hand motions. A third solution might be to have the client substitute a flat hand for grasp to stabilize objects such as a pillow to put on a pillowcase or the pants while fastening or unfastening them. The effect of gravity can be reduced by having the client stand rather than sit or by moving the task to a lower surface.

Erhardt's (1982) sequence for developing release involves adding degrees of freedom as a client progresses in movement control. A client is able to release objects that are externally stabilized on a support surface, such as a table, before he or she can release objects in space. For example, releasing a soda pop can on a table would be easier than releasing the can into a trash receptacle.

The environment is another control parameter that can be manipulated to enhance motor performance. Clients with movement control problems may have lost the ability to adapt quickly to changes in environmental conditions. Since it would be impossible to teach every movement pattern, clients may have to learn adaptations. When adaptation is impossible, some clients may have to avoid certain conditions such as walking to the bathroom at night without turning on a light. Other clients may only be independent in a sheltered or familiar environment. When evaluating the environment, consider whether the environment is stable and predictable or in motion and unpredictable (Gentile, 1987). The majority of occupations involve some element of unpredictability. For example, one uses many different types of tools for drinking, such as a mug, tea cup, glass, can, glass or plastic bottle, paper cup, etc. Thus, one may have to learn to adapt to different weights, sizes, textures, and spatial placement of these drinking tools. Occupations in which the environment is in motion, such as driving, propelling a wheelchair, and working on an assembly line, require ongoing monitoring of the environment and oneself. In structuring practice of these types of occupations, the therapist should systematically change environmental conditions.

5. Provide active participation in practice appropriate to client's status but which encourage experimenting with solutions to motor problems. Flinn (1995) recommends that a client with hemiparesis be encouraged to incorporate the impaired limb into one new task every day. She encourages clients to do homework and practice motor tasks at home or in the hospital room. As soon as a client has an idea of a task expected of him or her, practice should consist of variations of the task in random order. When clients are presented with tasks in an unpredictable fashion, they are forced to engage in more active processing because the solution that had been developed for the previous task is no longer successful without some modification (Lee & Magill, 1983). In constructing and reconstructing the motor solution, the client is developing problem-solving strategies.

6. Structure practice for optimal retention and generalization. Tasks should also be practiced in their entirety rather than in parts. Whole practice has been found to generalize or transfer better than part practice, especially if timing is an element. However, the advantage of part practice is that the client does not have to constantly repeat the steps that have been mastered.

For some clients with cognitive as well as motor impairments, task-specific training or nongeneralizable solutions may need to be developed. A blocked practice schedule of doing the same tasks over and over within the actual environmental context may be necessary.

7. Provide feedback. Cueing and feedback should be used more frequently in early learning so the client develops an ideal of correct and incorrect performance. However, feedback should gradually be withdrawn. Verbal and physical guidance interfere with long-term learning as the client depends on the therapist instead of him- or herself. However, visual feedback is important in making corrections for accuracy so the client can watch the extremities to receive feedback and be less dependent on the therapist. Slower movements make it easier for a client to process internal feedback or feedback from a therapist. However, the client will need to learn to modulate forces so speed should be varied.

Case Study 1: Hemiplegia Due to Cerebral Vascular Accident

Mrs. Chavez, who was introduced at the beginning of the chapter, had a right hemisphere middle cerebral artery infarction 2 months ago. She can actively abduct her left shoulder to 45 degrees. She can actively flex her elbow fully but simultaneously abducts her shoulder. She can actively flex and extend her wrist and fingers through partial range of motion. Tone is moderately increased in the biceps and rhomboids. In the left lower extremity, Mrs. Chavez can actively flex her hip. She lacks knee flexion during gait and can bear weight partially on her left lower extremity. Sitting balance is fair. As stated earlier, Mrs. Chavez would like to resume her homemaker role.

Traditional Intervention

Intervention according to traditional neurofacilitation methods would focus on reducing tone in the biceps and rhomboids and promoting normal movement. To decrease tone, the client would sit or stand and practice bearing weight on the left upper extremity with the elbow and wrist and fingers in extension and the shoulder in external rotation. Another technique to decrease tone is scapula mobilization in which the client is supine and the therapist moves the scapula into elevation, depression, abduction, and adduction (Bobath, 1990). To increase active movement, the client would start in the supine position initially to practice controlling shoulder and elbow movements. Other techniques to increase active movement might be to tap or vibrate the muscle bellies or tendons (Rood, 1954, 1956) or resist different muscle groups in the uninvolved upper extremity (Brunnstrom, 1970). When Mrs. Chavez has control over several arm movements, she could perform some tasks with her left arm, such as dusting a table or wiping the kitchen counter. To incorporate her left arm in mobility occupations, such as rolling, coming to sitting and standing, and transfers, Mrs. Chavez could clasp her hemiparetic hand with her uninvolved hand while doing the mobility task.

Contemporary Intervention: An Occupational Performance Approach

Intervention according to more contemporary models would focus on functional tasks. Historically, spasticity was considered the major barrier to volitional control in clients with hemiplegia. However, today, biomechanical alignment and muscle weakness due to decreased number of agonist motor units, prolonged contraction time due to changes in the contractile properties of motor units, and disrupted recruitment order and decreased firing rates in agonist motor units are considered to be the primary motor problems

(Bourbonnais & Vanden Noven, 1989; Sahrmann & Norton, 1977). Furthermore, patterns of movements observed post stroke are considered to be the most effective and efficient attempts at functional movement given the neuromuscular constraints and difficulty in controlling the degrees of freedom following a stroke (Horak, 1991). Therefore, a more contemporary approach would focus on helping Mrs. Chavez regain homemaking skills. She could practice functional tasks such as lifting her left arm to put it into her apron sleeve, stabilizing a bowl or dishes with her left arm during meal preparation and/or cleanup, and sliding objects with her left arm on the countertop into a drawer. To control the degrees of freedom in her left arm, Mrs. Chavez could stand while performing the abovementioned tasks. To reduce the degrees of freedom in the left arm to practice grasp and release, Mrs. Chavez could rest her forearm on the countertop while stabilizing a container or dishes. As Mrs. Chavez exhibits more controlled movements in her left arm, she could sit while performing tasks with her left arm and begin to perform tasks involving grasp and release without resting her forearm on the countertop (i.e., increasing the degrees of freedom). The therapist could also test Mrs. Chavez's strength in her left arm to determine whether additional strengthening exercises are needed.

Case Study 2: Parkinson's Disease

Mr. Cohen is a 60-year-old male who was diagnosed with Parkinson's disease 3 years ago. He is experiencing difficulty maintaining balance during standing and ambulating. He has decreased range of motion and flexibility in the trunk and pelvis. His head, trunk, and center of mass are displaced forward during standing.

Traditional Intervention

Traditional treatment for Mr. Cohen would consist of initially using relaxation techniques such as slow rocking and rotation of the trunk before working on postural control (Rood, 1956). Segmental rolling using proprioceptive neuromuscular facilitation patterns could be used to decrease trunk rigidity and increase upper trunk extension (Knott & Voss, 1968). Equilibrium reactions in which the therapist perturbs Mr. Cohen's balance in standing and sitting might be used to facilitate recovery of balance. Mr. Cohen could practice self-initiated balance by rocking back on his heels while attempting to maintain his balance. He could also practice standing and balancing on different surfaces such as a mat, foam, or an equilibrium board.

Contemporary Intervention: An Occupational Performance Approach

Contemporary treatment would focus on postural control in the context of a task with an emphasis on anticipatory adjustments and flexibility. Motor problems in Parkinson's disease do not appear to be due to weakness or delayed onset of automatic postural responses but due to excessive contraction of muscle/antagonistic muscle recruitment, a decreased ability to modify movement patterns in

response to changing task demands and decrease in anticipatory postural control (Horak, Nashner, & Nutt, 1988; Rogers, 1991). To increase automatic and anticipatory postural adjustments, Mr. Cohen could work on maintaining his balance while performing a variety of upper extremity tasks such as reaching, lifting, pushing, pulling, and holding objects with one or both hands. Speed, effort, and task complexity could be graded to facilitate his ability to modify postural responses as the demands of the task change. He could pull open the medicine cabinet to get out supplies for shaving or brushing his teeth, perform the activity or activities, and then replace the items. Mr. Cohen could practice opening doors and walking in areas where the surface varies, such as walking from the floor to a carpet or from the sidewalk to grass or gravel. Environmental adaptations could consist of sitting in a rocking chair at home so he can use momentum to initiate coming to standing.

Case Study 3: Cerebral Palsy

Adam is a 6-year-old boy who was diagnosed with left spastic cerebral palsy at 6 months of age when his parents observed his inability to reach with his left hand for toys in his environment. Passive range of motion is generally within normal limits. However, when actively reaching with his left arm, he is able to reach overhead with shoulder flexion and abduction to 120 degrees. He reaches for objects on a table during play with his elbow flexed, his forearm in pronation, his wrist in neutral, and his thumb adducted into his palm with accompanying finger flexion into a fisted hand position. He lacks 40 degrees of full active elbow extension. With cylindrical toys 3 inches in diameter, Adam is able to grasp the toy; however, the thumb remains subluxed at the metacarpophalangeal joint. He is unable to actively release the object once he grasps it. He is unable to grasp smaller objects such as buttons or shoelaces due to poor motor control.

Traditional Intervention

Traditional treatment would focus on decreasing spasticity and eliciting automatic reactions in the left upper extremity through movement provided by the therapist. Increased muscle tone in Adam's shoulder, elbow, and hand could be initially reduced through bearing weight on an open palm while side sitting (Bobath, 1967). He could use his right hand for play activities that are placed to his left side. Protective responses could be elicited while Adam is placed prone on the therapy ball and quickly moved forward to the floor to bear weight on both hands. Once the spasticity is decreased and his left hand is used for protective responses, therapy would focus on Adam using his left hand for holding objects during bilateral activities.

Contemporary Intervention: An Occupational Performance Approach

Contemporary treatment would focus on increasing active control in Adam's left upper extremity. Today, the primary motor problems in cerebral palsy are considered to be weakness in the antagonist muscles and difficulty with timing of muscle activation bursts such as prolonged contraction time and/or delayed onset of muscle activation (McCubbin & Shasby, 1985; Nielson & McCaughy, 1982). The focus in therapy could be to train Adam to actively control his left arm during reach and grasp and release activities. Adam could be given specific play activities to isolate elbow extension and forearm supination while grasping objects. One activity could be to grasp small cars with his left hand and place them in a tube placed at shoulder height in a vertical position. Once he has placed the car in the tube, he is asked to release it so it will fall down the tube into a container placed below. Different sized cars, animals, and action figures could be incorporated into the activity to increase in challenge to the activity and to aid in generalization to other grasp and release abilities. In addition, a small opponents splint, made of neoprene, could be used to reduce the degrees of freedom in the thumb, maintain the thumb in a neutral position, and correct metacarpophalangeal subluxation.

CONCLUSION

The assumptions underlying the traditional neurofacilitation theories for the treatment of clients with movement related problems are being challenged by more recent neurophysiological and biomechanical research. These findings have led to the development of different motor control theories that emphasize the interaction between the client and the environment and the interaction of many self-organizing systems. The newer theories have been based on findings with normal adults and children, but researchers are applying and testing these theories with clients with movement-related problems (Carr & Shepherd, 1987; Flinn, 1995; Horak et al., 1988; Rogers, 1991; Taub et al., 1993; Wolf et al., 1989). In general, these theories advocate using a client-centered approach with consideration of the environment in which the client functions for both evaluation and intervention. Assessment should address the client's goals and capabilities at a more global occupational performance or disability level. If a disability exists, more in-depth assessment of the components may be necessary. For intervention, more contemporary models suggest using functional tasks (occupations), considering biomechanical as well as neural factors as causes for dysfunction, manipulating personal and environmental systems to achieve changes in motor behavior, providing appropriate practice for retention and generalization, and providing feedback. Schmidt (1991), a noted motor learning theorist, suggests that therapists use the most effective techniques to increase learning in clients by challenging them by structuring random practice sessions and giving feedback infrequently. In therapy, these suggestions will result in the client's ability to retain and generalize performance in their everyday lives.

ACKNOWLEDGMENT

The author wishes to acknowledge the contribution of Patricia A. Burtner, PhD, OTR/L, who developed the case study on cerebral palsy and provided feedback on this chapter.

STUDY QUESTIONS

1. Compare and contrast traditional and contemporary treatment models for individuals with movement related problems.

2. List two ways to evaluate each of the following: range of motion, muscle strength, balance and equilibrium, dexterity, coordination, and motor control after stroke.

3. How would your assessment differ if using a contemporary task-oriented approach instead of a traditional neurofacilitation approach?

4. How does a client-centered approach relate to traditional neurofaciliation and contemporary approaches to movement-related problems?

5. Give two examples of control parameters and how they could be used in treatment.

6. How should practice and feedback be structured to enhance learning and retention of motor skills?

7. Give two examples of treatment using contemporary approaches to promote recovery in a client who has sustained a head injury with resultant hemiparesis in the left upper extremity. The individual has active motion in all joints in the left arm, except that he cannot achieve full shoulder flexion without simultaneously internally rotating the humerus and tends to flex the wrist when grasping items. He has some impairment in higher cortical functions. He wants to be able to bowl again (he was on his high school bowling team) and resume his part-time job as a cook at a local fast-food restaurant.

RECOMMENDED READINGS

Brooks, V. B. (1986). *The neural basis of motor control.* New York: Oxford University Press.

Burtner, P. A., & Woollacott, M. H. (1996). Theories of motor control. In C. M. Fredericks & L. K. Saladin (Eds.), *Pathophysiology of the motor systems: Principles and clinical presentations* (pp. 217-237). Philadelphia: F.A. Davis.

Gentile, A. M. (1992). The nature of skill acquisition: Therapeutic implications for children with movement disorders. In H. Forssberg & H. Hirschfeld (Eds.), *Movement disorders in children* (pp. 31-40). Basel, Switzerland: S. Karger.

Lister, M. J. (Ed.). (1991). *Contemporary management of motor control problems: Proceedings of the II Step conference.* Alexandria: VA: Foundation for Physical Therapy.

Malouin, F., Potvin, M., Prevost, J., Richards, C., & Wood-Dauphinee, S. (1992). Use of an intensive task-oriented gait training program in a series of patients with acute cerebrovascular accidents. *Physical Therapy, 72,* 781-789.

Mulder, T., & Hulstijn, W. (1988). From movement to action: The learning of motor control following brain damage. In O. G. Meijer & K. Roth (Eds.), *Complex movement behavior: The motor-action controversy* (pp. 247-259). New York: North Holland.

Poole, J. L. (1991). Motor control. In C. B. Royeen (Ed.), *AOTA self-study series: Neuroscience foundations of human performance* (Monograph No. 11, pp. 1-31). Rockville, MD: American Occupational Therapy Association.

Richards, C. L., Malouin, F., Wood-Dauphinee, S., Williams, J. I., Bouchard, J. P., & Brunet, D. (1993). Task-specific physical therapy for optimization of gait recovery in acute stroke patients. *Archives of Physical Medicine and Rehabilitation, 74,* 612-620.

REFERENCES

Adams, J. A. (1971). A closed loop theory of motor learning. *Journal of Motor Behavior, 3,* 111-150.

American Guidance Services. (1969). *The Minnesota Rate of Manipulation tests: Examiner's manual.* Circle Pines, MN: Author.

Àrnadóttir, G. (1990). *The brain and behavior: Assessing cortical dysfunction through activities of daily living.* St. Louis: C.V. Mosby Co.

Ashworth, B. (1964). Preliminary trial of carisoprodol in multiple sclerosis. *Practitioner, 192,* 540-542.

Bass Haugen, J., & Mathiowetz, V. (1995). Contemporary task-oriented approach. In C. A. Trombly (Ed.), *Occupational therapy for physical dysfunction* (pp. 510-527). Baltimore: Williams & Wilkins.

Baum, C., & Edwards, D. E. (1993). Cognitive performance in senile dementia of the Alzheimer's type: The kitchen task assessment. *American Journal of Occupational Therapy, 47,* 431-436.

Bennett, G. K. (1965). *Hand-tool dexterity test: Manual of directions.* New York: Psychological Corp.

Berg, K. O., Wood-Dauphinee, S. L., Williams, J. I., & Gayton, D. (1989). Measuring balance in the elderly: Preliminary development of an instrument. *Physiotherapy Canada, 41,* 304-311.

Bernstein, N. (1967). *The coordination and regulation of movement.* London: Pergamon Press Ltd.

Bobath, B. (1967). The very early treatment of cerebral palsy. *Developmental Medicine and Child Neurology, 9,* 373-390.

Bobath, B. (1985). *Abnormal postural reflex activity caused by brain lesions.* Rockville, MD: Aspen Systems Corporation.

Bobath, B. (1990). *Adult hemiplegia: Evaluation and treatment.* London: William Heinemann Medical Books Limited.

Bohannon, R. W., & Smith, M. B. (1987). Interrater reliability of a modified Ashworth scale of muscle spasticity. *Physical Therapy, 67,* 206-207.

Bourbonnais, D., & Vanden Noven, S. (1989). Weakness in patient with hemiparesis. *American Journal of Occupational Therapy, 43,* 313-319.

Brooks, V. B. (1986). *The neural bases of motor control.* New York: Oxford University Press.

Brunnstrom, S. (1970). *Movement therapy in hemiplegia.* New York: Harper and Row.

Carr, J. H., & Shepherd, R. B. (1987). *A motor relearning programme for stroke.* Rockville, MD: Aspen Publications.

Carr, J. H., Shepherd, R. B., Nordholm, L., & Lynne, D. (1985). Investigation of a new motor assessment scale for stroke patients. *Physical Therapy, 65,* 175-178.

Cech, D., & Martin, S. (1995). *Functional movement: Development across the life span.* Philadelphia: W.B. Saunders.

Crawford, J. E., & Crawford, D. M. (1956). *Manual: Crawford Small Parts Dexterity test.* New York: Psychological Corp.

Crowe, T. K., Dietz, J. C., Richardson, P. K., & Atwater, S. W. (1990). Interrater reliability of the pediatric clinical test of sensory interaction for balance. *Physical and Occupational Therapy in Pediatrics, 10,* 346-354.

Csuka, M., & McCarty, D. J. (1985). Simple method for measurement of lower extremity muscle strength. *American Journal of Medicine, 78,* 77-81.

Daniels, L., & Worthingham, C. (1986). *Muscle testing: Techniques of manual examination.* Philadelphia: W.B. Saunders.

Denny-Brown, D. (1950). Disintegration of motor function resulting from cerebral lesion. *Journal of Nervous and Mental Diseases, 112,* 1-45.

Dietz, V., Quintern, J., & Berger, W. (1981). Electrophysiological studies of gait in spasticity and rigidity: Evidence that altered mechanical properties of muscle contribute to hypertonia. *Brain, 104,* 431-449.

Donahoe, B. K., Turner, D., & Worrell, T. W. (1993). The use of functional reach as a measurement of balance in healthy boys and girls ages 5-15. *Physical Therapy, 73,* 71.

Duncan, P. W., Weiner, D., Chandler, J., & Studenski, S. (1990). Functional reach: A new clinical measure of balance. *Journal of Gerontology, 45,* 192-197.

Erhardt, R. P. (1982). *Developmental hand dysfunction: Theory, assessment and treatment.* Tucson, AZ: Therapy Skill Builders.

Fiorentino, M. (1973). *Reflex testing: Methods for evaluating central nervous system development.* Springfield, IL: Charles C. Thomas.

Fisher, A. G. (1992). *Assessment of motor and process skills manual.* Unpublished test manual. Colorado State University, Fort Collins.

Flinn, N. (1995). A task-oriented approach to the treatment of a client with hemiplegia. *American Journal of Occupational Therapy, 49,* 560-569.

Fugl-Meyer, A. R., Jääskö, L., Leyman, I., Olsson, S., & Steglind, S. (1975). The post-stroke hemiplegic patient. I. A method for evaluation of physical performance. *Scandinavian Journal of Rehabilitation Medicine, 7,* 13-31.

Gentile, A. M. (1987). Skill acquisition: Action, movement, and neuromotor processes. In J. H. Carr, R. B. Shepherd, J. Gordon, A. M. Gentile, & J. M. Held (Eds.), *Movement science: Foundations for physical therapy in rehabilitation* (pp. 93-154). Rockville, MD: Aspen.

Gesell, A. (1954). The ontogenesis of infant behavior. In L. Carmichael (Ed.), *Manual of child psychology* (pp. 335-373). New York: John Wiley & Sons Inc.

Ghez, C. (1991). The cerebellum. In E. R. Kandel, J. H. Schwartz, & T. M. Jessell (Eds.), *Principles of neural science* (pp. 626-646). New York: Elsevier.

Gibson, J. J. (1979). *An ecological approach to visual perception.* Boston: Houghton-Mifflin Co.

Gordon, J. (1987). Assumptions underlying physical therapy intervention: Theoretical and historical perspectives. In J. H. Carr, R. B. Shepherd, J. Gordon, A. M. Gentile, & J. M. Held (Eds.), *Movement science: Foundations for physical therapy in rehabilitation* (pp. 1-30). Rockville, MD: Aspen.

Gordon, J., & Ghez, C. (1991). Muscle receptors and spinal reflexes: The stretch reflex. In E. R. Kandel, J. H. Schwartz, & T. M. Jessell (Eds.), *Principles of neural science* (pp. 564-580). New York: Elsevier.

Green, P. H. (1972). Problems of organization of motor systems. In R. Rosen & F. M. Snell (Eds.), *Progress in theoretical biology* (pp. 304-348). San Diego: Academic Press.

Grillner, S. (1975). Locomotion in vertebrates: Central mechanisms and reflex interaction. *Physiological Reviews, 55,* 247-304.

Haley, S. M., Coster, W. J., Ludlow, L. H., Haltiwanger, J. T., & Andrellos, P. J. (1992). *Pediatric evaluation of disability inventory (PEDI): Developmental, standardization, and administration manual.* Boston: New England Medical Center Hospitals Inc.

Hellebrandt, F. A., Houtz, S. J., Partridge, M. J., & Walters, C. E. (1956). Tonic neck reflexes in exercises of stress in man. *American Journal of Physical Medicine, 35,* 144-159.

Heriza, C. (1991). Motor development: Traditional and contemporary theories. In M. J. Lister (Ed.), *Contemporary management of motor control problems: Proceedings of the II Step conference* (pp. 99-125). Fredericksburg, VA: Bookcrafters Inc.

Hines, M., & O'Connor, J. (1926). A measure of finger dexterity. *Personnel Journal, 4,* 379-382.

Horak, F. B. (1991). Assumptions underlying motor control for neurological rehabilitation. In M. J. Lister (Ed.), *Contemporary management of motor control problems: Proceedings of the II Step conference* (pp. 11-27). Fredericksburg, VA: Bookcrafters Inc.

Horak, F. B., & Nashner, L. M. (1986). Central programming of postural movements: Adaptations to altered support surface configurations. *Journal of Neurophysiology, 55,* 1369-1381.

Horak, F. B., Nashner, L. M., & Nutt, J. G. (1988). Postural instability in Parkinson's disease: Motor coordination and sensory organization. *Neurology Reports, 12,* 54-55.

Jarus, T. (1994). Motor learning and occupational therapy: The organization of practice. *American Journal of Occupational Therapy, 48,* 810-816.

Jebson, R. H., Taylor, N., Trieschmann, R., Trotter, M., & Howard, L. (1969). An objective and standardized test of hand function. *Archives of Physical Medicine and Rehabilitation, 50,* 311-319.

Kamm, K., Thelen, E., & Jensen, J. L. (1990). A dynamical systems approach to motor development. *Physical Therapy, 70,* 763-775.

Keele, S. W. (1968). Movement control in skilled motor performance. *Psychological Bulletin, 70,* 387-403.

Kelso, J. A. S., Holt, K. G., & Kugler, P. N. (1980). On the concept of coordinative structures as dissipative structures: II. Empirical lines of convergence. In G. E. Stelmach & J. Requin (Eds.), *Tutorials in motor behavior* (pp. 49-70). New York: Elsevier.

Kelso, J. A. S., & Tuller, B. (1984). A dynamical basis for action systems. In M. Gassaniga (Ed.), *Handbook of cognitive neuroscience* (pp. 321-356). New York: Plenum Publishing Corp.

Kelso, J. A. S., Tuller, B., & Harris, K. S. (1987). A dynamic pattern perspective on the control and coordination of movement. In P. F. McNeilage (Ed.), *Production of speech* (pp. 137-173). New York: Springer-Verlag Inc.

Kendall, F. P., McCreary, E. K., & Provance, P. G. (1993). *Muscle testing and function.* Baltimore: Williams & Wilkins.

Knott, M., & Voss, D. (1968). *Proprioceptive neuromuscular facilitation.* New York: Harper and Row.

Kottke, F. J. (1980). From reflex to skill: The training of coordination. *Archives of Physical Medicine and Rehabilitation, 61,* 551-561.

Laver, A., & Powell, G. (1995). *The Structured Observational Test of Function (SOTOF).* Berkshire, UK: NFER-NELSON.

Law, M., Baptiste, S., Carswell, A., McColl, M., Polatajko, H., & Pollock, N. (1991). *The Canadian Occupational Performance Measure.* Toronto, Canada: CAOT Publications.

Law, M., & Cadman, A. (1988). Measurement of spasticity: A clinician's guide. *Physical and Occupational Therapy in Pediatrics, 8,* 77-95.

Lee, T. D., & Magill, R. A. (1983). The locus of contextual interference in motor-skill acquisition. *Journal of Experimental Psychology, 9,* 730-746.

Lincoln, N., & Leadbitter, D. (1979). Assessment of motor function in stroke patients. *Physiotherapy, 65,* 48-51.

Lyle, R. C. (1981). A performance test for assessment of upper limb function in physical rehabilitation and research. *International Journal of Rehabilitation Research, 4,* 483-492.

Mathiowetz, V., & Bass Haugan, J. (1995). Evaluation of motor behavior. In C. A. Trombly (Ed.), *Occupational therapy for physical dysfunction* (pp. 157-185). Baltimore: Williams & Wilkins.

Mathiowetz, V., Federman, S., & Weimer, D. (1985). Box and block test of manual dexterity: Norms for 6-19 year olds. *Canadian Journal of Occupational Therapy, 52,* 241-245.

Mathiowetz, V., Rogers, S., Dowe-Keval, M., Donohoe, L., & Rennells, C. (1986). The Purdue Pegboard: Norms for 14-19 year olds. *American Journal of Occupational Therapy, 40,* 174-179.

Mathiowetz, V., Volland, G., Kashman, N., & Weber, K. (1985). Adult norms for the Box and Block test of manual dexterity. *American Journal of Occupational Therapy, 39,* 386-391.

Mathiowetz, V., Weber, K., Kashman, N., & Volland, G. (1985).

Adult norms for the Nine-Hole Peg Test of finger dexterity. *Occupational Therapy Journal of Research, 5,* 24-38.

McCubbin, J. A., & Shasby, G. B. (1985). Effects of isokinetic exercise on adolescents with cerebral palsy. *Adapted Physical Activity Quarterly, 2,* 56-64.

McGraw, M. B. (1945). *The Neuromuscular maturation of the human infant.* New York: Hafner Press.

McPhee, S. D. (1987). Functional hand evaluations: A review. *American Journal of Occupational Therapy, 41,* 158-163.

McPherson, J. J., Mathiowetz, V., Strachota, E., Benrud, C., Ingrassia, A., & Spitz, M. L. (1985). Muscle tone: Objective evaluation of the static component at the wrist. *Archives of Physical Medicine and Rehabilitation, 66,* 670-674.

Nashner, L. M., & McCollum, G. (1985). The organization of human postural movements: A formal basis and experimental synthesis. *Behavior and Brain Science, 8,* 135-172.

Newell, K. M. (1981). Skill learning. In D. H. Holding (Ed.), *Human skills* (pp. 203-226). New York: Wiley.

Nielson, P. D., & McCaughey, J. (1982). Self-regulation of spasm and spasticity in cerebral palsy. *Journal of Neurology, Neurosurgery & Psychiatry, 44,* 690-698.

Norkin, C. C., & White, D. J. (1985). *Measurement of joint motion: A guide to goniometry.* Philadelphia: F.A. Davis.

Ostendorf, C. G., & Wolf, S. L. (1981). Effect of forced use of the upper extremity of a hemiplegic patient on changes in function: A single case design. *Physical Therapy, 61,* 1022-1028.

Pedretti, L. W., & Zoltan, B. (1990). *Occupational therapy: Practice skills for physical dysfunction.* St. Louis: C.V. Mosby Co.

Podsiadlo, D., & Richardson, S. (1991). The timed "up and go": A test of basic functional mobility for frail elderly persons. *Journal of the American Geriatrics Society, 39,* 142-148.

Poole, J. L. (1991). Application of motor learning principles to occupational therapy. *American Journal of Occupational Therapy, 45,* 531-537.

Poole, J. L. (1995). Learning. In C. A. Trombly (Ed.), *Occupational therapy for physical dysfunction* (pp. 265-276). Baltimore, MD: Williams & Wilkins.

Poole, J. L., & Whitney, S. L. (1995). *Assessments of motor function post stroke: A review.* Manuscript submitted for publication.

Reed, E. S. (1982). An outline of a theory of action systems. *Journal of Motor Behavior, 14,* 98-134.

Rogers, J. C., & Holm, M. B. (1994). *Performance assessment of self-care skills (PASS)* (Version 3.1). Unpublished functional performance test, University of Pittsburgh, PA.

Rogers, M. (1991). Motor control problems in Parkinson's disease. In M. J. Lister (Ed.), *Contemporary management of motor control problems: Proceedings of the II Step Conference* (pp. 195-208). Fredericksburg, VA: Bookcrafters Inc.

Rood, M. (1954). Neurophysiological reactions as a basis for physical therapy. *Physical Therapy Review, 43,* 444-449.

Rood, M. (1956). Neurophysiological mechanisms utilized in the treatment of neuromuscular dysfunction. *American Journal of Occupational Therapy, 10,* 220-225.

Sabari, J. S. (1991). Motor learning concepts applied to activity-based intervention with adults with hemiplegia. *American Journal of Occupational Therapy, 45,* 523-530.

Sahrmann, S. A., & Norton, B. J. (1977). The relationship of voluntary movement to spasticity in the upper motor neuron syndrome. *Annals of Neurology, 2,* 460-465.

Sawner, K., & LaVigne, J. (1992). *Brunnstrom's movement therapy in hemiplegia.* Philadelphia: J.B. Lippincott.

Schmidt, R. A. (1988). *Motor control and learning: A behavioral emphasis.* Champaign, IL: Human Kinetics Publishers Inc.

Schmidt, R. A. (1991). Motor learning principles for physical therapy. In M. J. Lister (Ed.), *Contemporary management of motor-control problems: Proceedings of the II Step Conference* (pp. 49-63). Fredericksburg, VA: Bookcrafters Inc.

Scholz, J. P., & Kelso, J. A. S. (1990). Intentional switching between patterns of coordination depends on the intrinsic dynamics of the patterns. *Journal of Motor Behavior, 22,* 98-124.

Shea, J. B., & Morgan, R. (1979). Contextual interference effects on the acquisition, retention, and transfer of a motor skill. *Journal of Experimental Psychology: Human Learning and Memory, 5,* 179-187.

Shumway-Cook, A., & Horak, F. B. (1986). Assessing the influences of sensory interaction on balance. *Physical Therapy, 66,* 1548-1550.

Stockmeyer, S. A. (1967). An interpretation of the approach of Rood to the treatment of neuromuscular dysfunction. *American Journal of Physical Medicine, 46,* 900-956.

Taub, E. (1980). Somatosensory differentiation research with monkeys: Implications for rehabilitation medicine. In L. P. Ince (Ed.), *Behavioral psychology in rehabilitation medicine: Clinical applications* (pp. 371-401). New York: Williams & Wilkins.

Taub, E., Miller, N. E., Novack, T. A., Cook, E. W., Fleming, W. C., Nepomuceno, C. S., Connell, J. S., & Crago, J. E. (1993). Technique to improve chronic motor deficit after stroke. *Archives of Physical Medicine and Rehabilitation, 74,* 347-354.

Taylor, N., Sand, P. L., & Jebsen, R. H. (1973). Evaluation of hand function in children. *Archives of Physical Medicine and Rehabilitation, 54,* 129-135.

Thelen, E., Fisher, D. M., & Ridley-Johnson, R. (1984). The relationship between physical growth and a newborn reflex. *Infant Behavior and Development, 7,* 479-493.

Tiffin, J. (1968). *Purdue Pegboard: Examiner manual.* Chicago: Science Research Associates.

Tinetti, M. E. (1986). Performance oriented assessment of mobility problems in elderly patients. *Journal of the American Geriatric Society, 34,* 119-126.

Trites, R. L. (1977). *Neuropsychological test manual.* Ottawa, Canada: Royal Ottawa Hospital.

Trombly, C. A. (1992). Deficits of reaching in subjects with left hemiparesis: A pilot study. *American Journal of Occupational Therapy, 46,* 887-897.

Trombly, C. A. (1993). Observations of improvement of reaching in five subjects with left hemiparesis. *Journal of Neurology, Neurosurgery & Psychiatry, 56,* 40-45.

Trombly, C. A. (1995). *Occupational therapy for physical dysfunc-

tion. Baltimore: Williams & Wilkins.

Trombly, C. A., & Scott, A. D. (1989). Evaluation of motor control. In C. A. Trombly (Ed.), *Occupational therapy for physical dysfunction* (pp. 55-71). Baltimore: Williams & Wilkins.

Turvey, M. T., Fitch, H. L., & Tuller, B. (1982). The Bernstein perspective in human motor behavior. In J. A. S. Kelso (Ed.), *Human motor behavior: An introduction* (pp. 239-283). Hillsdale, NJ: Lawrence Erlbaum Associates, Inc.

VanSant, A. F. (1988). Rising from a supine position to erect stance: Description of adult movement and a developmental hypothesis. *Physical Therapy, 68*, 185-192.

Voss, D. E., Ionta, M. K., & Meyers, B. J. (1985). *Proprioceptive neuromuscular facilitation: Patterns and techniques.* New York: Harper & Row.

Wadsworth, C. T., Nielsen, D. H., Corcoran, D. S., Phillips, C. E., & Sannes, T. L. (1992). Interrater reliability of hand-held dynamometry: Effects of rater gender, body weight, and grip strength. *Journal of Sports Physical Therapy, 16*, 74-81.

Walsche, F. M. P. (1961). Contribution of John Hughlings Jackson to neurology. *Archives of Neurology, 5*, 99-133.

Wilson, D. J., Baker, L. L., & Craddock, J. A. (1984). Functional test for the hemiparetic upper extremity. *American Journal of Occupational Therapy, 38*, 159-164.

Winstein, C., Gardner, E. R., McNeal, D. R., Barto, P. S., & Nicholson, D. E. (1989). Standing balance training: Effect on balance and locomotion in hemiparetic adults. *Archives of Physical Medicine and Rehabilitation, 70*, 755-762.

Wolf, S. L., Lecraw, D. E., Barton, L. A., & Brigitte, B. J. (1989). Forced use of hemiplegic upper extremities to reverse the effect of learned nonuse among chronic stroke and head-injured patients. *Experimental Neurology, 104,* 125-132.

Woollacott, M., & Shumway-Cook, A. (1995). *Motor control: Theory and practical applications.* Baltimore, MD: Williams & Wilkins.

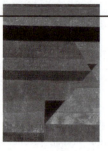

Chapter Content Outline

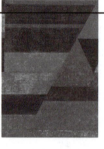

Abstract

This chapter provides an overview of the concept and components of health-related physical fitness and considers the integral position of these concepts in understanding human and occupational performance. Methods to assess components of physical fitness and to provide exercise and activity programs to produce positive adaptations are discussed. Potential effects of aging, disease, and inactivity on fitness and performance are presented as well as the impact of fatigue and economy of effort.

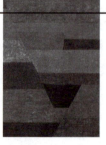

Key Terms

Physical fitness

Cardiorespiratory fitness

Muscular fitness

Body composition

Overload principle

Specificity principle

Physiologic adaptation

Physiologic capacity

Inactivity

Deconditioning

Exercise prescription

Physical fitness assessment

Physical activity and health

Fatigue

Economy of effort

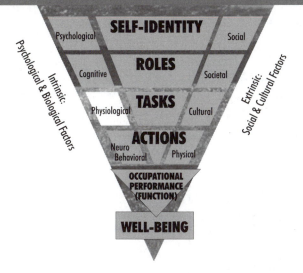

CHAPTER 10

Promoting Health and Physical Fitness

Marian A. Minor, PhD, PT

OBJECTIVES

The information in this chapter is intended to help the reader:

1. understand the concept of physical fitness as integral to the process of human and occupational performance
2. define the components of health related physical fitness
3. understand the principles of training and physiologic adaptation in enhancement of performance
4. identify potential causes and signs of diminished physical fitness and fatigue
5. assess the components of physical fitness
6. recommend exercise and activity to achieve health and fitness goals.

"The weakest and oldest among us can become some kind of athlete, but only the strongest can survive as spectators. Only the hardiest can withstand the perils of inertia, inactivity, and immobility."

J. Bland and S. Cooper: *Seminars in Arthritis and Rheumatism*, 1984

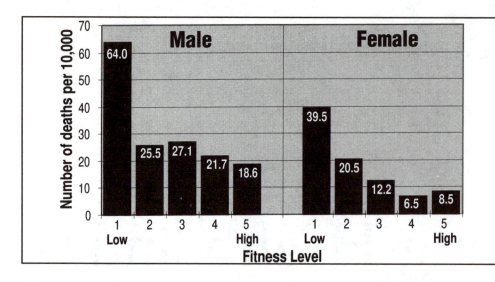

Figure 10-1. Physical fitness and longevity. From Blair, S. N., Kohl, H. W., & Paffenbarger, R. S. (1989). Physical fitness and all-cause mortality: A prospective study of healthy men and women. *Journal of the American Medical Association, 262,* 2395-2401.

INTRODUCTION

People who are physically active are healthier and live longer than people who are sedentary. Evidence from population-based surveys, epidemiologic studies, and controlled clinical trials indicates that regular physical activity is necessary for health. Inactivity is a major and independent risk factor for cardiovascular disease, hypertension, hyperlipidemia, adult-onset diabetes, and obesity. People who are inactive have more disease and die younger than people who engage in even moderate amounts of physical activity on a regular basis. This is important information for everyone (Figure 10-1).

Since the 1980s, efforts to increase physical activity levels have become major public health campaigns in most industrialized countries. In addition to recognizing that regular physical activity is important for promoting and maintaining the health of people without existing disease, it is now understood that people with a variety of diseases and disorders also benefit from regular physical activity (Blair, 1993). These benefits apply to general health promotion and disease prevention, as well as to achievement and maintenance of levels of cardiovascular and neuromusculoskeletal fitness necessary to support performance and occupational roles. Inactivity, in and of itself, produces disease. When disease or injury leads to inactivity, the consequences of the inactivity, often intertwined with advancing age and comorbid conditions, compound and amplify the potential cascade of impairment and diminished capacity, contributing to unnecessary functional burden and secondary disability (Figure 10-2).

Physical inactivity and the resulting poor fitness are major health problems across the life span. Reasons given for sedentary behaviors include: children and adults watch too much television, workers are too busy, and families are stressed with care of parents, maintaining employment or relocating. People who do not exercise regularly say it is too expensive, too time-consuming, too inconvenient, too uncomfortable, or they do not think that they can be successful. Other reasons given for not being physically active include a number of diseases and disorders such as arthritis, heart disease, hypertension, visual and hearing impairments, back pain and orthopedic impairments, asthma, nervous and mental disorders, diabetes, mental retardation, pulmonary diseases, and stroke. Table 10-1 lists the major health-related reasons for physical activity limitation in the United States.

The cure for inactivity is to increase physical activity. The modes and process of this cure are determined by the needs, status, and preferences of the individual, available resources, and therapeutic or health-related goals. Physical activity is defined as "any bodily movement produced by skeletal muscles that results in caloric expenditure" (Caspersen, Kriska, & Dearwater, 1985, p. 127). Exercise, a type of physical activity, is "planned, structured, repetitive physical activity that results in improvement or maintenance of one or more facets of physical fitness" (Caspersen, Kriska, & Dearwater, 1985, p. 127). Inactivity may be addressed both through the prescription of specific exercise routines and through recommendations for increasing the amount of physical activity performed during the course of the day.

The health professional may find him- or herself as an activity/exercise advocate within the context of a therapeutic program, or in a broader perspective of health promotion and disease/disability prevention. In either environment, the principles of minimizing functional loss and promoting health and physical fitness through physical activity are integral to

Bibliographic citation of this chapter:Minor, M. A. (1997). Promoting health and physical fitness. In C. Christiansen & C. Baum (Eds.), *Occupational therapy: Enabling function and well-being* (2nd ed.). Thorofare, NJ: SLACK Incorporated.

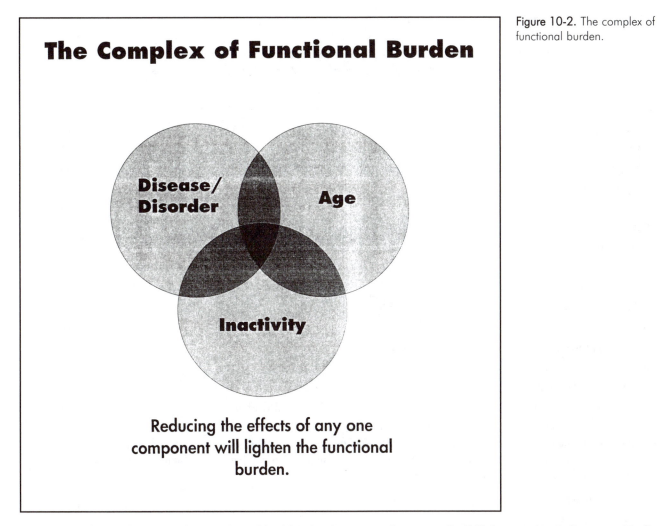

Figure 10-2. The complex of functional burden.

the process of rehabilitation and promotion of health-related quality of life.

PHYSICAL FITNESS IN REHABILITATION AND HEALTH PROMOTION

To perform activities and accomplish tasks, a person must be able to move body parts, manipulate objects, and move the body through space. The physical ability to perform these activities in a meaningful way depends upon a person's state of physical fitness.

What is physical fitness? According to exercise scientists and physical educators, health-related physical fitness is a multifactorial phenomenon consisting of: 1) cardiorespiratory function, 2) muscle strength, 3) muscle endurance, 4) flexibility, and 5) body composition. Physical fitness is determined by heredity, activity levels, age, and presence of pathology. Individuals often describe their fitness in terms of being able to jog three miles or perform a weight training routine. Often

people equate flexibility, strength or slimness with fitness. However, health-related physical fitness is not directly related to athletic performance or physique. Physical fitness can be defined in terms of the person and his or her environment as "the capacity to meet successfully the present and potential physical challenges of life" (Lamb, 1984, p. 5) or as "the ability to carry out daily tasks with vigor and alertness, without undue fatigue and with ample energy to engage in leisure time pursuits and to meet the above average physical stresses encountered in emergency situations" (President's Council on Physical Fitness and Sport, 1992). Every person can achieve the goal of optimal personal fitness to support individual performance. Regular physical activity, targeted at specific needs in the areas of cardiovascular and musculoskeletal status, is the path toward adequate fitness and satisfactory physical performance.

Physical and mental limitations do not exclude people from the possibility of being physically fit. It is often the ensuing consequences of inactivity which produce unnecessary impairment and limitations. In a rehabilitation program,

TABLE 10-1

Percentage of Persons with Activity Limitation Reporting Specified Causes of Limitation All Ages: United States, 1983-1985

Main Cause	%	All Causes	%
Orthopedic Impairments	16.0	Orthopedic Impairments	21.5
Arthritis	12.3	Arthritis	18.8
Heart Disease	11.5	Heart Disease	17.1
Visual Impairment	4.4	Hypertension	10.8
Intervertebral Disk Disorders	4.4	Visual Impairments	8.9
Asthma	4.3	Diabetes	6.5
Nervous Disorders	4.0	Mental Disorders	5.6
Mental Disorders	3.9	Asthma	5.5
Hypertension	3.8	Intervertebral Disk Disorders	5.2
Mental Retardation	2.9	Nervous Disorders	4.9
Diabetes	2.7	Hearing Impairments	4.3
Hearing Impairments	2.5	Mental Retardation	3.2
Emphysema	2.0	Emphysema	3.1
Cerebrovascular Disease	1.9	Cerebrovascular Disease	2.9
Osteomyelitis/Bone Disorders	1.1	Abdominal Hernia	1.8

Notes: Nervous disorders include epilepsy, multiple sclerosis, Parkinson's disease, and other selected nervous disorders. Mental disorders include schizophrenia and other psychoses, neuroses, personality disorders, other mental illness, alcohol and drug dependence, senility, and special learning disorders (mental deficiency [sic] is not included). Content of other condition categories is described in LaPlante, 1988.

Source: National Health Interview Survey, adapted from LaPlante, 1989.

it is important to consider physical fitness as the foundation on which functional capacity and skill learning are built. Improvement of physical fitness enables people to extend their capacities to successfully accomplish desired activities and maximize performance.

Physical Fitness as an Organizational Concept

The multifactorial concept of physical fitness can be applied as an organizational framework in the rehabilitation process and study of human performance. The five components of physical fitness—cardiorespiratory function, muscle strength, muscle endurance, flexibility, and body composition—encompass the physiologic bases of human performance. These five components have been quantitatively defined and can be measured to reveal differences over time and between individuals. The concept and the measurement tools are applicable to a wide range of ages, abilities, and fitness levels.

There are five major reasons to use physical fitness as an organizing concept to study human performance.

1. The components of physical fitness and occupational performance share a common outcome measure: the capacity to perform work and sustain effort to complete tasks.

2. There is a wealth of objective and valid measurement tools that require little or no conversion from their use as physical fitness measures (cardiovascular and musculoskeletal) to be used as assessment and outcome measures, guide treatment, and monitor progress. Normative data are available for many of these measures which allows comparison of individual results with the general population.

3. The five measurable physiologic components of physical fitness have the capacity to respond and adapt to demands, both acute and chronic, imposed by changes in physical activity. The ability to measure components separately provides specific information to both the individual and the health care provider to identify specific

deficits and direct interventions to areas of need.

4. The concept of physical fitness focuses on wellness and provides a mechanism for individual assessment and prescription of physical activity to promote health and support performance.

5. Physical fitness, particularly aerobic fitness, may be used as an outcome measure indicative of general health and well-being.

COMPONENTS OF PHYSICAL FITNESS

Cardiorespiratory Function

Cardiorespiratory fitness is dependent on pulmonary and cardiovascular (heart, blood vessels, and blood components) systems and specific cellular components, particularly in muscle, which enable the body to use oxygen. The respiratory and cardiovascular systems comprise the oxygen transport system which delivers oxygen to the working muscles and removes chemical waste products. Cellular metabolism within the muscles and liver replenishes energy supplies required by the working muscles. Cardiorespiratory fitness can be defined as the ability to take in, transport, and use oxygen. The cardiorespiratory functioning of our bodies is continuous, recognized externally by the signs of pulse, blood pressure, and respiration.

Cardiorespiratory function is amazingly sensitive and responsive to our needs, even to anticipation of need. At rest in the supine position, one might have a pulse of 60 beats per minute and a respiration rate of 12 breaths per minute. Sitting up puts a slightly greater load on the cardiorespiratory system by using greater muscle activity to support the head and trunk and to overcome the force of gravity on venous return of blood from the abdomen and lower extremities. In the seated position, pulse might increase to 65 beats per minute and breathing rate to 14 breaths per minute. As one stands up, there is more demand to supply oxygen to a greater number of recruited muscle fibers and to counteract a greater effect of gravity. Now one might have a pulse of 75 beats per minute and a breathing rate of 16. The gradual increase in these vital signs indicates the increasing work being performed by the cardiorespiratory system. In addition to the direct stimulation of cardiovascular response, psychological stress, anxiety or the anticipation of increased activity also cause heart rate and respiration to increase.

Stepping on a motor-driven treadmill, climbing onto a bicycle ergometer, or engaging in a lifting task that imposes a gradual increase in workloads results in incremental increases in heart rate, breathing and blood pressure as the work becomes harder. At the point of maximal capacity, a person's ability to respond reaches a plateau, and increasing work loads do not elicit increased responses. If demand continues at this intensity, the point of exhaustion soon occurs.

A common term in the lexicon of physical fitness is *aerobic*—aerobic fitness, aerobic training, and aerobic endurance. Aerobic means "with oxygen." Aerobic fitness includes cardiovascular capacity and the capacity of working muscle to use oxygen to replenish energy supplies (aerobic metabolism).

Pulmonary Factors

Pulmonary factors such as lung volume, vital capacity, breathing rate, and pulmonary ventilation normally do not limit physical activity unless the person has significant pulmonary disease or is at a high altitude. Even during intense exercise, ventilation is only about 60% to 85% of a healthy person's maximum capacity for breathing. Under most conditions, the arterial blood leaving the heart is 97% saturated with oxygen. Therefore, in the absence of pulmonary disease, most of the limitation to endurance performance depends not on our ability to inspire and diffuse oxygen into the blood, but on the ability of the heart and circulatory system to deliver oxygen, and cellular mechanisms to use the oxygen for energy production.

Pulmonary impairment may limit cardiorespiratory fitness both directly and indirectly. Cardiorespiratory fitness may be affected directly by inadequate pulmonary ventilation when the amount of oxygen in the blood does not satisfy the increased cellular needs of exercising muscles. Pulmonary impairment indirectly affects cardiorespiratory fitness by the increased energy required to breathe. In pulmonary disease, breathing itself may become exhaustive work and the oxygen supply may be greatly reduced to the nonrespiratory muscles, resulting in diminished performance. Studies investigating the effect of endurance or aerobic exercise training on people with chronic obstructive pulmonary disease (COPD) show that performance can be improved by participation in an endurance training exercise program even with no significant improvement in pulmonary function (Atkins, Kaplan, & Timms, 1984).

Cardiovascular Factors

The cardiovascular system is made up of: 1) the heart, which provides the force for blood flow and maintains circulation; 2) the arterial system, which conducts oxygen-rich blood to tissues; 3) the capillaries, which provide the medium for exchange between the blood and tissues; and 4) the veins, which return blood to the heart and serve as an active blood reservoir. The amount of blood that the heart pumps in a minute is the *cardiac output,* and is measured in milliliters per minute (ml/min). Cardiac output is the primary indicator of the ability of the heart to meet the demands of physical activity. Cardiac output is a product of the *heart rate* (beats per minute) and *stroke volume* (milliliters of blood ejected from the left ventricle with each stroke). The heart responds to a demand for increased blood flow with greater cardiac output by increasing both heart rate and stroke volume.

The aerobically trained and conditioned heart has a greater stroke volume and produces a greater cardiac output at the same heart rate as an untrained heart. Thus, the conditioned heart produces greater cardiac output at a lower heart rate than the untrained heart. Less work (fewer beats per minute) results in lowered oxygen demand by the heart muscle itself and longer periods of relaxation (diastole) in which the ventricles can fill. Longer filling time favors increased stroke volume. Stroke volume changes with body position and is greatest in the prone or supine position.

The presence of coronary artery or peripheral vascular disease may affect the ability of a person to be physically active because of compromised blood flow to the heart muscle and/or the exercising skeletal muscle. Insufficient blood flow to support the needs of the contracting heart muscle may result in exertional angina (angina pectoris), experienced as chest pain or pressure.

Muscle Strength

Muscle strength is the amount of force that can be exerted by one or a group of muscles in a single voluntary contraction. The force exerted in a voluntary contraction depends on a number of factors: 1) recruitment of muscle fibers and their contractile capacity, 2) mechanical advantage of the lever system, 3) neuromuscular mechanisms, and 4) motivation. Muscle size and strength are closely associated. The larger (cross-sectional area) muscle is generally the stronger one, but not necessarily the most successful in performance when factors of speed, power, coordination, or endurance are required.

The growth in the cross-sectional area of a muscle is due primarily to an increase in muscle fiber size (hypertrophy), rather than an increase in the actual number of fibers (hyperplasia). Current research indicates that the larger, fast-twitch muscle fibers that have a greater capacity to develop tension show a more pronounced hypertrophy in response to strength training than do the slow-twitch fibers. Adaptations in slow-twitch fibers occur primarily in response to muscle endurance training through changes in enzymatic content of the slow twitch fibers rather than increased fiber size.

Strength can be developed and measured as either static strength, developed in an isometric contraction, or dynamic strength, developed in an isotonic or isokinetic contraction. Dynamic strength measurements are more related to performance in sport and work than are isometric measurements. Isometric strength, however, is important in considerations of posture and balance. Isometric techniques allow precision in strength assessment and training when a specific muscle or muscle group is in question. Activities of daily life are accomplished by varying combinations of isometric and isotonic (both concentric and eccentric) work.

Isometric Strength

In isometric activities, there is little or no joint motion as the muscle exerts the necessary force to accomplish the task, such as sustaining a pinch, carrying a heavy package in your arms, or clenching your jaw. There are also isometric phases of most muscular activity. Isometric strength can be expressed in terms of muscle tension as a percentage of the *maximum voluntary contraction* (MVC) exerted under static conditions. At 15% to 20% MVC the contraction can be maintained for a considerable period. Tensions above 50% are fatiguing and maximum contraction can be maintained for only a few seconds to a few minutes. Maintaining a high intensity isometric contraction becomes an anaerobic activity: blood vessels supplying oxygen to the working muscle are occluded and aerobic metabolism becomes impossible. Training to improve static strength will not show comparable gains in dynamic strength of the same muscle. Furthermore, isometric strength is specific to the joint angle at which the strength training was performed.

Isotonic Strength

Isotonic strength is defined as the maximum weight that can be lifted at one time. Isotonic contractions may result from force generated as the muscle shortens (concentric) or from force exerted as the muscle lengthens (eccentric). Strength measured in a concentric contraction is really a measure of strength at the hardest part of the lift, and this may be at the beginning or the end of the range, depending on the muscle lever system and the length-tension ratio. Isotonic strength is often measured and expressed in terms of a *repetition maximum* (RM). One repetition maximum (1 RM) is the force that can be lifted one time only. Training regimens often are defined in multiple terms, that is 3 RM or 10 RM. To establish a valid 1 RM amount, at least three attempts should be performed to reach a plateau.

Muscle Endurance

Given the strength needed to perform an activity, additional improvement in performance requires muscle endurance. Endurance means the ability to persist. Muscular endurance is defined and measured as the repetition of submaximal contractions (isotonic) or submaximal holding time (isometric). The use of the term *muscular endurance* should not be confused with cardiovascular endurance. It is possible to develop considerable endurance in a small muscle, such as a finger flexor, without having any noticeable effect on cardiovascular endurance. The oxygen required for a small muscle mass to sustain activity over an extended period can be satisfied without stressing the cardiovascular system. Thus, most people can type, do needlework, or play the piano without raising their respiration, heart rate, blood pressure, or oxygen consumption above their usual sedentary levels. The active muscles have the endurance to persist to accomplish the activities without imposing a stress on cardiovascular performance. When there is a greater demand for larger muscle mass to perform an activity, for example, the repetitive contraction of the quadriceps required to pedal a bicycle, the magnitude of the oxygen requirement to sustain muscular activity increases dramatically. Also this more strenuous activity involving large muscles requires the work of the cardiorespiratory system to activate and sustain increased circulation to the active muscles.

When the size of the active muscle mass produces an increased demand for oxygen to sustain activity, and/or when the intensity of the muscular work produces an increased oxygen demand, then cardiorespiratory endurance and muscular endurance become interrelated. For example, a total-body activity of relatively low level of intensity, such as walking at a natural pace, will require certain levels of both cardiorespiratory and muscular endurance to sustain the activity for more than a few minutes. If the intensity increases from walking to jogging, increased demands are made on both the active muscles, to sustain the rhythmic activity, and the cardiorespiratory system, to maintain the increased circulation. The muscle mass/exercise intensity relationship is demonstrated by the differences in energy expenditure between bicycle and arm ergometry. The smaller muscle mass of the upper extremities engaged in arm ergometry requires less oxygen per unit of time than a comparable effort on the bicycle ergometer powered by the considerably greater muscle mass of the lower extremities.

Flexibility

Flexibility is the component of physical fitness that describes the range of motion of a joint or sequence of joints. Flexibility is determined by the following factors: 1) the elasticity of soft tissues surrounding the joint (skin, muscle, tendon, ligament, joint capsule, and other periarticular connective tissue); 2) conditions within the joint that may restrict motion, such as bony deformity, malalignment, or inflammation; and 3) excessive body fat or muscle mass that can be an external obstruction limiting range of motion. Pain, both acute and chronic, also may limit flexibility. Even in the absence of disease-related restrictions, range of motion varies with age, occupation, sex, and activity levels.

Tables of normal range of motion are widely used in clinical assessment even though there is disparity among published normal values. These normative tables seldom describe how the measurement was made, from what population the values were taken, or the standard deviations for the mean values. Without this information, normative data should be applied cautiously to individuals. The current use of radiologic and electronic technology may be helpful in gaining a clearer picture of ideal values and adequate ranges of joint motion.

Static Flexibility and Dynamic Flexibility

Static and dynamic flexibility are two important concepts relating to joint motion within the domain of flexibility. Static or extent flexibility refers to the actual arc of motion that a joint will allow. This is commonly referred to as joint range of motion. Clinically, we measure static flexibility with a goniometer and describe the joint angle achieved in degrees. Measurement of static flexibility may be achieved by either active or passive motion of the body segments surrounding the joint.

Dynamic flexibility refers to the ease of movement rather than the amount of movement produced by joint motion. Dynamic flexibility can be defined and measured as the amount of resistance of a joint to movement or the ability of a joint to make rapid and repeated flexing movements (Winnick & Short, 1985). Although dynamic flexibility is not commonly measured in a clinical setting, the ease or "looseness" of movement can be an important evaluation to make in assessing the functional consequences of impaired flexibility. In research settings, dynamic flexibility has been measured with arthrography (Byers, 1985) to determine the amount of resistance to passive motion of a joint. Another method is to simply count the number of repetitions of active joint motion that can be accomplished within a given time period. Both of these methods are subject to error introduced by active resistance to motion or by limitations in muscle strength and endurance.

Body Composition

Body composition refers to the fat and nonfat elements of the body or to the relative leanness/fatness of the individual. Height and weight tables can give us some idea of ideal total body weight for people of the same sex and similar age and frame size. These tables tell us who is overweight or underweight with respect to the general population. However, these tables are not valid for determining an individual's lean to fat proportions.

The total amount of body fat exists as either essential fat or storage fat. *Essential fat* is needed for normal physiologic functioning and is the fat stored in bone marrow, throughout the nervous system, and in all organs of the body. Without a certain amount of essential fat, body function deteriorates. In women, essential fat also includes sex-characteristic fat deposits in the breasts, uterus, hips, and thighs. *Storage fat* is the fat deposited in the adipose tissue throughout the body and serves as an energy reserve, insulator from cold, and protector of vital organs from physical trauma. Major storage fat deposits are located beneath the skin (subcutaneous fat) and around major organs such as the heart and kidneys. It is storage fat that is most subject to change with alterations in diet and exercise. Approximately 50% of body fat is subcutaneous storage fat.

Men and women have a similar recommended percent of storage fat, 12% for women and 15% for men. There is a much greater gender difference with regard to essential fat, which is approximately 3% for men and 12% for women. For young adults, the desired body fat percent is considered to be 13% to 15% for males and 25% for females.

Although body composition tables show an increasing percentage of body fat with advancing age, there is no particular reason to believe that this increased percent of body fat is an inevitable consequence of aging. The tendency of people to reduce physical activity with aging contributes to greater body fat in relation to lean body weight. This trend is neither necessary nor desirable.

The health risks of obesity are well known; however, being too lean may also have health risks. People with body fat measurements below the essential fat percentages of 3% for males and 12% for females often exhibit health problems. In women, adipose tissue is used for estrogen storage. Young women with extremely low body fat, such as those who perform strenuous physical training, sometimes experience amenorrhea and osteoporosis. This may be associated with insufficient essential body fat to support the normal physiologic functioning of the menstrual cycle or bone remodeling. Malnutrition and some chronic disease may also result in a wasting phenomenon in which lean body mass is reduced (cachexia). For example, persons with systemic inflammatory diseases, such as rheumatoid arthritis, often demonstrate an increased resting metabolism, reduced lean body mass, and muscle wasting.

RESPONSE AND ADAPTATION

Physiological systems respond to stimulation or physiologic stress. Repeated stress on a physiologic system leads to adaptations in the system. Physical activity can be an appropriate and positive stressor, leading to organ and organ system adaptations and resulting in improved fitness. The physiologic components respond to the stimulus of regular physical activity; changes lead to increased functional capacity and performance.

The Overload Principle

Application of the appropriate positive stress is referred to as overloading the system. The principle of overload states that repeatedly imposing a stress above that normally experienced will cause adaptations to occur in the physiological systems experiencing the overload. The only mechanism by which adaptive changes for improved function can occur is through the application of this overload principle. If there is no overload, there is no adaptation for improvement. Overload is a positive stressor that can be quantified. The appropriate overload for an individual is achieved through varying the intensity, duration, and frequency of the activity. The combination of intensity, frequency, and duration that constitutes an appropriate overload is dependent on the individual, the activity, the environment and the training objectives. A woman who normally runs three miles daily in 30 minutes will need to run more miles or at a faster pace to achieve overload. A sedentary woman recovering from an acute flare of rheumatoid arthritis in which she was in bed for 2 weeks, may very well be at appropriate overload with an activity program of 5 minutes of ambulation three times daily. A man who walks a 15-minute mile every day in Atlantic City may find that in Denver he can only do a half-mile or might slow down to a 20-minute mile to avoid becoming short of breath. For this man, the altitude in Denver has the effect of increasing the intensity of his exercise effort and producing an overload.

Application of overload is required for improved fitness. With individual assessment and activity prescription, people at all levels of function and fitness can be given the opportunity to engage in appropriate activities to improve fitness and function. Although any of the three exercise variables (intensity, duration, or frequency) can be adjusted to produce the desired overload, research shows that intensity is the most potent factor for producing adaptations. By correctly applying the principle of overload, we are able to prescribe and monitor activity programs that will result in improved fitness for even the most deconditioned or disabled individual.

The Specificity Principle

The principle of specificity refers primarily to the specificity of training or the specific adaptation that occurs in response to the overload. Training one body part or system does little to effect changes elsewhere. It is obvious that progressive resistance exercises for the triceps would not produce change in knee extension strength, nor would passive flexibility exercises for the low back improve abdominal wall strength.

Identifying specificity of training is not so obvious for increased muscle strength and/or endurance. In this instance, the specificity applies to the type of contraction (isometric or isotonic) and the joint angle or speed of shortening of the contraction. For example, isometric strength training for the biceps done at 90 degrees of elbow flexion will do little to improve strength or endurance measured during either dynamic elbow flexion or isometric contraction at 20 degrees.

Attention to the specificity of training for muscular fitness is crucial in the rehabilitation setting, where improved function often depends on maximization of limited resources. The activity of eating involves a combination of isometric and isotonic strength of the trunk, shoulder girdle and upper extremity in order to grip a utensil and produce the necessary stabilization and repetitive movements. Endurance is also needed for the movement to be repeated over the course of a meal. If the individual can accomplish the movement, then using the actual movement as the training exercise is usually the most effective path to improved function. However, if the individual is not able to accomplish the movement, it is necessary to identify the limiting factors—whether it is a deficiency in strength, endurance or a combination of both—and in which muscle groups the deficiency lies.

The principle of specificity states that the most effective training routine is one that most closely parallels the requirements of the desired performance. By knowing the muscular requirements of the activity and the muscular resources at hand, you can apply the principle of specificity of training to develop an effective training program. Using activities of daily living in training to improve performance in those activities is the most efficient and effective method. For example, when the goal of training is for the person to be able to rise from a sitting position in a chair, the more closely strengthening exercises for quadriceps and hip extensors can be sequenced to match the movement patterns of rising from a chair, the faster this functional performance will improve.

The Body's Reaction to Physical Activity

Physiologic reaction to physical activity can be divided into two types: response and adaptation. *Response* is immediate reaction to activity. Response involves the sudden, temporary changes that occur with a single bout of activity and which disappear shortly after the activity is over. Increased heart rate, respiration and oxygen consumption are examples of response to a brisk 10-minute walk.

Adaptation is a more or less persistent change in structure or function following repeated bouts of activity. It is adaptation, the consequence of training, which enables the body to eventually respond more easily to subsequent episodes of the same activity. The following are examples of adaptation: 1) muscle hypertrophy and increased strength following a 16-week program of progressive resistance exercise; 2) increased maximal oxygen consumption after 10 weeks of a walk/jog program; or 3) a change in body composition from 30% to 25% fat after a 6-month combined program of moderate dietary restriction and daily brisk walking.

Exercise Response and Overload

In rehabilitation and training for improved physical fit-

ness, we are generally interested in producing adaptations by imposing appropriate and positive stressors on the physiologic systems. Although adaptation for improved function is the goal, we regulate activity (training) stress by monitoring the immediate response to the activity. Careful monitoring of the responses to each episode of activity is necessary to make adjustments in the activity to ensure maximum safety and effectiveness.

For activity to produce adaptation, it must impose an increased load or stress on the system sufficient to produce change but not so great as to cause injury. Monitoring immediate response to activity will allow you to regulate the activity to stay within safe but effective limits. If the exercise objective is to improve endurance for walking and the method is a walking program, it is important to determine the appropriate level of overload (intensity and duration of the stimulus) to produce adaptations in aerobic systems. If the client, after being on his or her feet and walking for 5 minutes, has a heart rate of 180 beats per minute (bpm), respiration of 24, and feels that he or she is working as hard as possible, the session is too strenuous and needs to be modified. On the other hand, if after 10 minutes of walking activity, there is essentially no change in these measures above resting levels, there is insufficient stress to produce change. In this case, increasing the stimulus (speed, grade, duration) is necessary to progress toward the goal of increased endurance.

Exercise Response and Training Effects

Response to a single bout of exercise is also the method of evaluating progress toward adaptation. For example, if the goal is to increase the client's endurance for performing activities of daily living, the therapist might begin by developing a schedule for increasing ambulatory time periods in the course of preparing a meal. The goal is for the client to be able to sustain ambulation and meal preparation tasks without assistance or rest periods. The repeated bouts of activity will eventually produce adaptations in strength and endurance to help reach the goal of sustained performance. Monitoring response to the individual bouts of ambulatory activity will allow the therapist and the client to keep the activity within safe limits, to adjust the level of activity stress if needed, and to verify that adaptations are occurring. This can be done by measuring heart rate and respiration, and by keeping track of self-perceived exertion, fatigue, and pain.

Many adaptations brought on by exercise training tend to reduce the relative stress of exercise, and the response to the training periods will become less pronounced as adaptation occurs. Heart rate and respiration will decrease for the same amount of work, blood pressure will stabilize, perceived exertion will lessen, and fatigue will be delayed or reduced. Therefore, the positive changes in observable responses over time can be a method to evaluate change and provide positive feedback and reinforcement for the client and the therapist during the course of the program.

Physiologic Capacity Versus Performance

Physiologic adaptations and changes in observable performance are closely related but do not necessarily tell the same story. Although pure physiologic adaptations in cardiorespiratory function, muscular fitness, or flexibility are governed by the principles of overload and specificity, the variables affecting changes in performance are more diverse.

For example, a study is conducted with two young women, Helen and Anne, who can be tested in all the components of fitness. Tests show that they have the same measurements for maximal oxygen consumption, muscular strength and endurance, flexibility, and percentage of body fat. They are the same age, height, and weight, and are training for cross-country running. During the season, Anne usually wins or places among the first three finishers, whereas Helen is usually one of the last runners to finish or drops out. What is responsible for such differences in the performances of two people who appear to be so similar and capable of equal effort and outcomes? There is, of course, no one answer that applies in all cases. Possible explanations for differences in performance related to a complex and prolonged task can vary from motivation, self-efficacy, pain threshold, and fear of injury to differences in economy of effort, glycogen and lactic acid metabolism, or muscle fiber composition.

It is impossible in real life to have two people exactly the same; however, we often see people who appear to be very similar physiologically who exhibit differences in observed performance. In the clinical setting, it is common to observe patients with similar disease and impairments who demonstrate marked differences in function and disability. We even see changes in the same person's performance from one day to the next. Clinicians and trainers often think that if they could just uncover this secret of performance, they would have the key to success and be able to help people achieve their maximal performance. But there are undoubtedly many keys for unlocking this mystery of human performance, and they include not just physiological factors but psychological and social factors as well.

A methodical approach to the question of performance can yield valuable information and all possibilities related to physical fitness should be examined. This approach is relatively new to the rehabilitation process. In the past, clinicians often have focused on the clinical diagnosis or pathology as the primary explanation for performance levels. If a disease state or trauma did not provide the answers, then psychosocial variables such as motivation, depression, or helplessness

were considered. Rarely have health care professionals considered the underlying physiologic foundation of performance capacity. The recognition of physical fitness and exercise underlies the importance of evaluating physical fitness as part of the clinical assessment.

In the example of Anne and Helen, who were physiologically equal but whose performances varied, it was important to first measure fitness levels to determine that they were physiologically equal rather than just assuming equal fitness because the women appeared alike in age, height, weight, and involvement in the same training program. Differences that cannot be observed without proper testing, such as maximal oxygen consumption, percentage body fat, or muscular fitness, could certainly account for performance differences. Therapists all too often tend to overlook a thorough fitness examination and instead focus on age, sex and disease-related factors as the basis for performance deficits. To achieve optimal outcomes, a comprehensive evaluation of performance must include assessment of physical fitness and therapeutic intervention must address deficits.

REASONS FOR DIMINISHED FITNESS

Inactivity and Immobilization

The human body requires the stresses imposed by an upright posture and adequate levels of regular physical activity to maintain healthy functioning of all physiologic systems. Prolonged periods of inactivity produce an imbalance in the normal relationship between rest and physical activity, which causes a negative stress on every system in the body. Observation of the effects of weightlessness during space flight has stimulated research into the effects of inactivity and loss of postural stimuli on healthy subjects during bed rest and immobilization (Sandler & Vernikos, 1986). These studies allow us to separate the effects of inactivity from the effects of an existing illness. Prolonged periods of inactivity can be institutionally imposed or self-imposed, such as bed rest prescribed for the treatment of an acute illness or injury, neuromuscular inactivity due to paralysis, or a sedentary existence. Depending on the degree and duration of the inactivity, adaptations occur as the body responds to this situation. The result of these adaptations is a deterioration in all aspects of physical fitness, commonly known as deconditioning. Extreme forms of deconditioning are known as hypokinetic degenerative disease, the immobilization syndrome, or hypokinesia. As shown in Table 10-2, a number of chronic conditions are clearly associated with inactivity and poor physical fitness.

When evaluating a client and planning a therapeutic intervention, a therapist should consider the level of the person's regular physical activity before and after the onset of disease or injury. The greater the inactivity, the greater the amount of negative adaptation or deconditioning. For example, if two 75-year-old men come to the clinic for evaluation and rehabilitation following a right hemisphere cerebrovascular accident, evaluation of their physical fitness could provide insights into the differences in their performance levels. Even with a similar neurologic impairment, they may be quite dissimilar in their ability to perform activities of daily living. Evaluating prior activity habits and activity history since the cerebrovascular accident will reveal a great deal about the physiologic status that each brings to the rehabilitation setting.

Cardiorespiratory Deconditioning

Prolonged inactivity results in cardiorespiratory system changes that compromise its ability to adequately respond to changes in activity level and changes in body position. Prolonged, insufficient activity results in increased resting heart rate, loss of blood volume, decreased heart volume, stroke volume, cardiac output and coronary blood flow, impaired orthostatic response, and diminished aerobic capacity or maximal oxygen consumption. Clinical manifestations of cardiorespiratory deconditioning are: 1) reduced exercise tolerance, which is demonstrated by increased heart rate and respiration at low work loads, as well as diminished capacity; 2) early onset of fatigue; 3) exertional dyspnea; and 4) perception of doing heavy or maximal work at low to moderate workloads.

If the person has been at rest in the horizontal position, he or she may experience a marked rise in heart rate and drop in blood pressure upon standing up (orthostatic hypotension). Standing upright may also produce syncope and fainting if the hypotension is severe or if the person is particularly sensitive to the low pressure. Diminished cardiorespiratory fitness makes a person less capable of adjusting to the increased physiologic demands of strenuous activity, particularly exercise of sudden onset.

Muscular Deconditioning

Lack of muscle use leads to loss of muscle mass, commonly called disuse atrophy. It may take only 4 to 8 weeks of disuse for muscle to atrophy to one-half normal size. If activity is resumed within that time, full function usually returns. However, after 4 months of inactivity, a significant number of muscle fibers deteriorate, and full recovery is unlikely. In the case of loss of nerve supply (denervation), this process is more rapid and profound. Muscle fibers eventually will be replaced by fat and connective tissue; after 2 years this process is essentially complete.

During bed rest or immobilization, muscles necessary for upright posture (antigravity muscles) and muscles necessary for locomotion are the most affected and undergo proportional decreases in strength and actual muscle mass. Under normal conditions, the demands of muscle-loading and movement pro-

---

TABLE 10-2

The Relationship Between Physical Activity or Physical Fitness and Selected Chronic Diseases or Conditions, 1963-1993

Disease or Condition	Number of Studies	Strength of Evidence
All-cause mortality	>10	↓↓↓
Coronary artery disease	>10	↓↓↓
Hypertension	5-10	↓↓
Obesity	>10	↓↓
Stroke	5-10	↓
Peripheral vascular disease	<5	→
Cancer		
Colon	<10	↓↓
Rectum	>10	→
Stomach	<5	→
Breast	<5	↓
Prostate	5-10	↓
Lung	<5	↓
Pancreas	<5	→
Noninsulin-dependent diabetes	<5	↓↓
Osteoarthritis	<5	→
Osteoporosis	5-10	↓↓
Functional capability	5-10	↓↓

→ = No apparent difference in disease rates across activity or fitness categories;

↓ = Some evidence of reduced disease rates across activity or fitness categories;

↓↓ = Good evidence of reduced disease rates across activity or fitness categories, some evidence of biological mechanisms;

↓↓↓ = Excellent evidence of reduced disease rates across activity or fitness categories, evidence of biological mechanisms, relationship is considered causal.

From Blair, S. N. (1993). Physical activity, physical fitness, and health. *Res Q Exerc Sports, 64,* 365.

---

duce a balance between the synthesis and degradation of contractile proteins so that muscle mass is maintained or increased. With insufficient loading, there is greater degradation than synthesis. Products of muscle breakdown appear in the blood and urine, indicating that muscle atrophy is underway.

Loss of contractile proteins causes a decrease in cross-sectional muscle mass, which is directly proportional to loss of muscle strength. Decreased muscle endurance and maximal oxygen consumption are also a consequence of muscle atrophy.

TABLE 10-3

Clinical Manifestations of Prolonged Immobilization

Muscular
Decreased Strength
Decreased Endurance
Muscle Atrophy
Impaired Task Precision
and
Poor Coordination

Skeletal
Osteoporosis
Joint Fibrosis and Ankylosis

Cardiorespiratory
Increased Heart Rate
Decreased Cardiac Output/Reserve
Orthostatic Intolerance
Phlebothrombosis
Decreased Vital Capacity
Decreased Maximal Voluntary Ventilation
Impairment of Coughing Mechanism

Psychological
Depression
Apathy
Intellectual Dulling

Muscle disuse is typically associated with significant atrophy of the fast-twitch (Type II) muscle fibers and a decrease in the oxidative enzymes needed for energy production during endurance activities. In a study of morphological changes in muscle immobilized by casting, it was found that after 1 month in a cast, the proportion of Type II fibers decreased from 80% to 57%. Retraining after cast removal resulted in a return to precast values (Sandler & Vernikos, 1986). The oxidative energy systems in Type I and II fibers are needed to support sustained activity. A prolonged reduction in muscular work leads to a reduction in the volume and efficiency of these aerobic energy systems. Deconditioning in the aerobic energy systems diminishes the body's potential for maximal oxygen consumption. Thus, the decreased maximal oxygen consumption of inactivity that was mentioned as a cardiorespiratory adaptation is not only a consequence of the diminished capacity of the heart to deliver oxygen to working muscles, but also a result of diminished capacity of the muscles to use oxygen.

Adaptations in muscle tissue vary with the type and dura-

tion of the inactivity. Innervation is an important factor in the balance between synthesis and degradation of contractile proteins, as observed by the decrease in muscle protein content that occurs when the nerve supply to a muscle is interrupted. A completely denervated muscle may lose 90% to 95% of its normal bulk. In the case of immobilization by splinting, the degree of muscle atrophy is only 30% to 35%. Loss in strength is progressive over time. Some studies have shown a 20% loss of residual strength for each week of inactivity. Although muscle can adapt to increases in activity imposed by a retraining program, the rate of recovery is much slower than the rate of loss. The realistic expectation from a vigorous restrengthening program is probably no more than a 10% increase of initial strength per week.

Diminished Flexibility

Flexibility of connective tissue decreases rapidly with inactivity. In muscles and around joints where flexibility is required for normal motion, there is a loose meshwork of areolar connective tissue that allows a considerable and easy range of motion. When a body part is immobilized or the normal range of motion is restricted, the mere continuation of normal metabolic activity of connective tissue leads to diminished flexibility. When undisturbed by motion, the connective tissue network will shorten to the length to which the tissue is regularly asked to stretch.

Normal connective tissue adapts to the stress of imposed motion, reorganizing the meshwork to allow more or less flexibility as required. Significant shortening in the connective tissue meshwork can occur within 1 week of restricted motion. If motion is restricted due to imposed immobilization or because of edema, trauma, or impaired circulation, the connective tissue meshwork reorganizes to a shorter length, and also produces a dense connective tissue at the involved site. This dense connective tissue replaces the normal loose, areolar connective tissue and this dense fibrosis may start in as few as 3 days (Donatelli & Owens-Burkhart, 1981).

Increased Percentage of Body Fat

Inactivity results in an increased proportion of body fat to lean body weight not only because excess calories are stored as adipose tissue, but also because of the adaptive decrease in muscle mass. In addition to the well-known health risk factors associated with obesity such as coronary heart disease, hypertension, and Type II diabetes, high body fat percentage affects performance. The trade-off in body composition between fat and lean body weight occurs between secondary fat deposits (a storage compartment) and muscle mass (an active work-producing compartment). These are the two largest body compartments, and they are closely related metabolically.

Inactivity and immobilization affect all organ systems. This chapter addresses only those decrements related to physical fitness; however, prolonged inactivity leads to a myriad of other physical and mental conditions. Table 10-3 lists several clinical manifestations of prolonged immobilization. In fact, prolonged inactivity affects every organ in the body, disturbs hormonal and metabolic functions, and contributes to bone mineral loss and osteoporosis. The adaptations to prolonged inactivity may at times cause a greater degree of disability than the original incident that caused the person to become inactive.

Aging

There is no question that physiologic capacity and performance are to some extent age-dependent. Physiologic capacity tends to increase rapidly through childhood, peaks in the late teens to early thirties, and gradually declines with increasing age. However, results from research on aging point to more differences than similarities in both the processes of aging and the consequences for performance. Changes associated with aging occur at different rates in different people, and even at different rates within the same person. There are large differences between chronological age and biological age, even within age groups. Many changes traditionally associated with aging appear to be not so much age-dependent as activity-dependent.

The most universal change with age is a decreasing ability to respond to physiologic stress and an increasing time required to return to prestress levels (Weg, 1983). This is a diminished homeostatic capacity that may become manifest only when the current stressor is greater than that normally encountered. In general, resting values (heart rate, respiration, blood pressure, oxygen consumption) are less indicative of aging changes than response and recovery values. Conversely, the resting heart rate appears to be more sensitive to level of fitness than to age.

Cardiorespiratory Changes with Aging

A decrease in maximal heart rate occurs with age and is not related to gender or cardiorespiratory fitness. Age-predicted maximal heart rate can be estimated by the following formula: 220 - age = maximal heart rate (± 10 beats per minute). Conversely, the resting heart rate appears to be more sensitive to level of fitness than to age.

The clinical application of decreasing maximal heart rate with age is important in prescribing exercise intensity or level of exertion, and improved fitness is often reflected in a lower resting heart rate. Other cardiorespiratory changes that affect exercise capacity and training intensity are a decrease in cardiac output because of decreased maximal heart rate and diminished stroke volume, decreased maximal oxygen consumption because of lowered efficiency of the heart in pumping blood, and a decreased muscle mass. There seems to be little change in the ability of the oxidative ener-

gy systems to use oxygen. With advancing age there can be a reduction in respiratory efficiency, and pulmonary function may become a limiting factor, particularly for high intensity exercise.

Age-related changes in cardiorespiratory fitness are often compounded by the deleterious effects of inactivity and atherosclerosis. In the absence of coronary and peripheral vascular disease, people in their 80s have been able to engage in progressive cardiorespiratory training programs and exercise vigorously enough to produce physiologic adaptations and improved aerobic capacity (Smith & Gilligan, 1983). Any training program for older clients should be based on individualized prescription, well-supervised, gradually progressive, include a thorough warm-up period, and initiated only after a thorough medical assessment.

Muscle Changes with Aging

Muscle mass and measured muscle strength, both static and dynamic, diminish progressively with age. However, it appears that the effect of inactivity plays a large role in explaining this decline. Exercise programs may result in improvements in strength, oxidative capacity, and muscle hypertrophy.

A research finding of particular clinical interest is the discrepancy between performance of a brief arm-cranking test and measured muscle strength in 80-year-old subjects. When compared with values from younger subjects, the older subjects showed a 45% reduction in the work performed by arm cranking, but only a 28% decline in strength (Shephard, 1978). There are many possible reasons for this discrepancy: inadequate speed of contraction needed to generate enough power to perform the task, poor coordination resulting from fatigue, lack of practice at the motor skill, or inefficient muscle fiber recruitment. A manual muscle test indicating "good strength" in a muscle group may indicate little about the individual's ability to use that strength ability to generate adequate muscular power or skill to perform a task at a functional level. With aging, lack of sheer muscle strength is generally not the primary limiting factor in performance capability for activities of daily living.

Muscle biopsy studies of age-related changes in muscle fiber composition show that the greatest deterioration is in the fast-twitch (Type II) fibers, which are responsible for high intensity or velocity contractions. The primary metabolic systems of these muscle fibers are anaerobic, providing energy for muscle work that generate great force or power but cannot be sustained for more than a few seconds or minutes. Slow-twitch fibers (Type I) show less deterioration with aging. Type I fibers are the site of aerobic muscle metabolism and are responsible for supporting low to moderate muscular work for long periods of time.

It is still unclear how much of this selective fiber deterioration is explained by aging itself and how much is due to disuse. Because activity patterns tend to become less physically demanding with aging, it is possible that the change of muscle fiber composition is an adaptive response to lower level stress demands of activities that are low to moderate in intensity and speed. In general, older muscle tissue shows a slow decline in strength, tone, speed, and endurance. However, appropriate exercise regimens can result in physiologic adaptations and improved performance at any age). In fact, studies of people who have maintained vigorous exercise programs into their 80s show that physical activity is effective in delaying and reducing changes in muscle strength and endurance. Studies of resistance training in institutionalized persons over 70 demonstrate significant improvements in muscles strength and functioning in activities of daily living.

Changes in Flexibility

Problems with decreased flexibility and the risk of connective tissue injury increase with advancing age. Again, both biological aging and insufficient activity contribute to these problems. Studies done on connective tissue at the cellular level indicate that the aging process does result in loss of elastic tissue and alterations in the structure of the collagen molecule, reducing flexibility in muscle, tendon, ligament, and joint capsule. Age-related changes in the structure of articular cartilage appear to make it less resilient and more susceptible to injury. Loss of resiliency, thinning, and degenerative changes have been noted in articular cartilage as early as the second decade of life.

Changes in molecular structure and vascularization of connective tissue increase the risk of injury to muscle, tendon, and articular structures and decrease the ability of these tissues to repair themselves. During the aging process, there appears to be a progressive decrease in capillaries and an increase in tendon calcification. These changes, associated with the increased likelihood of tendon ruptures, are also known to accompany reduced physical activity.

For all of these reasons, the clinical approach to the older or deconditioned person with respect to flexibility goals and the need for flexibility during exercise should be one of caution. Gradual progression of exercise activities that include adequate warm-up and gentle, active static stretching, both before and after the conditioning period, will help reduce the incidence of sprain and strain injuries. The common features of the aging joint are often loss of both mobility and stability. Appropriate physical activity can have a preventive and a rehabilitative role in maintenance of good flexibility. Adequate flexibility of the trunk and lower extremities is extremely important for balance and the ability to successfully recover from a stumble.

Changes in Body Composition in Aging

In industrialized societies where there are adequate food supplies and socioeconomic pressures for retirement, population studies show that increasing age is associated with increased percentage body fat. Reported percentages for body fat average around 28% for elderly men and 38% for elderly women, in contrast to 15% and 25%, respectively, for young men and women. Although there is a normal degree of muscle wasting that begins between the fifth and seventh decades of life, the increase in percentage body fat is felt to be a consequence of inactivity rather than a natural phenomenon of aging. Studies of masterclass male athletes in their 70s, 80s, and 90s have shown no more than 14% body fat (Shephard, 1978).

An increase in percentage body fat with age is not always accompanied by an increase in body weight. In fact, body weight tends to climb from the mid-20s to mid-40s, and then begins a gradual decline while percentage body fat is increasing. This increase in body fat can be masking a gradual decrease in lean body tissue, primarily of skeletal muscle and bone. Decreased muscle mass, due to a reduced synthesis of muscle proteins, results in decreases in muscle strength, power and endurance, and lessened maximal oxygen consumption maxVO_2.

Osteoporosis or loss of bone mass is a major problem of aging, particularly in women, and is associated with age and inactivity. It is the loss of bone density and strength that occurs when more bone is resorbed than is formed in the remodeling process. If severe, osteoporosis can result in compression fracture of vertebrae and fractures in long bones. Osteoporosis is often a contributing factor to hip fractures in the elderly. Postmenopausal women are particularly at risk for severe osteoporosis. Other risk factors include: sedentary lifestyle, insufficient calcium intake, smoking, alcohol consumption, a slight build, and northern European lineage.

Therapeutic recommendations for the prevention and treatment of osteoporosis include supplementary dietary calcium, moderate-intensity weight bearing exercise such as walking, reduction of lifestyle risk factors, and often estrogen replacement therapy for postmenopausal women. When planning programs for a person at risk for osteoporosis, avoiding situations that produce increased pressure on the vertebrae is important. Spontaneous compression fracture is most common in the thoracic vertebrae. Fracture resulting from increased loading is most common in lumbar vertebrae. Therefore, in the treatment setting, avoid those postures that cause increased stress in the thoracic and lumbar regions such as extreme trunk flexion, slouched sitting posture, sudden forceful movements of the spinal column, and lifting heavy weights. It is also extremely important to observe all safety precautions to prevent falls.

When advanced age is a factor, it is important to look beyond body weight for measures of individual muscular and skeletal fitness. Trying to assess a client's habitual activity level through self-report can be risky. It has been noted that older people and obese people tend to overestimate their physical activity both in terms of time spent in activity and intensity. Most studies indicate that the general trend with age is toward less physical activity.

Disease

Whether the condition is acute or chronic, traumatic or insidious in origin, physiologic changes are produced that often alter capacity or performance. Rehabilitation deals with reversing or minimizing the effects of the pathology to maximize functional performance, promote health, and reduce unnecessary disability that may occur as the result of inactivity.

Consideration of physical fitness and the physiologic bases of performance suggests a clinical perspective with which to view alterations in performance that often accompany illness or injury. This perspective includes assessment of physical fitness in addition to the traditional evaluation measures that often are disease or function specific. The assessment of physical fitness gives crucial information whatever the cause of the performance deficit. Addressing fitness through the three component areas helps: 1) differentiate between disease specific and health-related fitness effects on performance, 2) describe and localize areas of ability and disability, and 3) supply important information for effective treatment planning.

When planning a treatment program it is important to know if the performance decrements are a direct consequence of the pathology or if they are confounded by other causes. A clinical approach that includes attention to physical fitness as a factor affecting performance is also a positive and optimistic approach. We know that the components of fitness are amenable to improvement with appropriate training at any age, any stage of deconditioning, and in the presence of disease.

It is rare that performance cannot be improved by appropriate training to improve some parameter of fitness. For example, cardiorespiratory conditioning programs are used for both primary prevention and rehabilitation of coronary heart disease. These same techniques also have been successfully used to improve performance in rehabilitation programs for people with diagnoses as COPD, chronic pain syndrome, and clinical depression. Individuals with paraplegia due to spinal cord injury can improve cardiorespiratory fitness and maintain healthy cardiac status through conditioning programs using upper extremity aerobic exercise such as arm cranks and self-propelled wheelchair exercise regimes.

Physical fitness and disease are not opposite ends of the health spectrum. They are both variables in the multifactorial paradigm of human performance. There are three important facts to remember for the therapist planning rehabilitation programs: l) the presence of illness or injury does not exclude the possibility of fitness or of improving health and fitness with appropriate physical conditioning; 2) the absence of sufficient physical activity on a regular basis leads to declining fitness, poor general health, unnecessary disability and secondary disease; and 3) assessment and individualized recommendations for conditioning exercise may be incorporated into a comprehensive rehabilitation program. Regular exercise and physical activity contribute to health, reduce unnecessary functional burden and minimize disability in diseases and disorders of both chronic and traumatic origin (Figure 10-3).

ASSESSMENT AND PRESCRIPTION OF PHYSICAL ACTIVITY TO PROMOTE HEALTH AND PHYSICAL FITNESS

Individualized Assessment and Recommendation

Herbert A. deVries (1980) defined the essential components of a scientific prescription of exercise. These general principles apply to all individualized health-related physical activity recommendations:

1. Determine the objectives of the exercise program. This requires assessment of the individual in the five components of health-related fitness and mutual goal-setting.
2. Choose the exercise modality appropriate to achieving the goals. The exercise programs for improving upper-extremity strength, increasing low-back flexibility, or improving cardiovascular endurance will be different and specific.
3. Develop the exercise program with specific recommendations for exercise intensity, duration of the exercise at each session, and frequency of the sessions. The intensity recommendations should be stated as ranges with established upper level values that the client should not exceed and lower level, "insufficient load" values.
4. Determine realistic expectations for rate of change and amount of improvement to be achieved. Change is a function of various factors in each individual, including initial fitness levels, intensity of the training, type of training, age, general health and psychosocial dimensions.

Assessment of Cardiorespiratory Fitness

Cardiorespiratory fitness—the capacity to take in, transport, and utilize oxygen—is assessed by monitoring heart rate, blood pressure, and cardiac function, and sometimes by direct measurement of oxygen consumption, while the person is performing known and progressively strenuous workloads. The most common methods of measuring this work (ergometry) are the motor-driven treadmill and bicycle ergometer. Other methods that also allow monitoring of both response

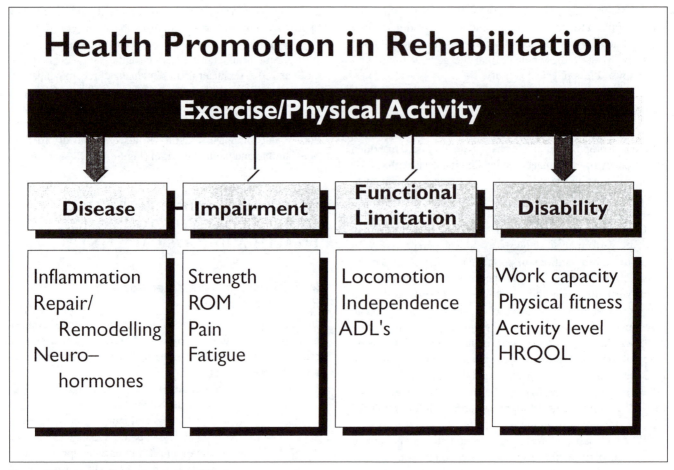

Figure 10-3. Health Promotion in Rehabilitation.

and workload are step tests and arm crank ergometry.

Oxygen consumption is the difference between the rate at which inspired oxygen enters the lungs and the rate at which expired oxygen leaves the lungs. The most common measurement used to assess cardiorespiratory fitness is maximal oxygen consumption ($maxVO_2$). $MaxVO_2$ is defined as the greatest amount of oxygen that the individual can use in a given amount of time. The better the cardiorespiratory fitness, the higher the maximal oxygen consumption. Oxygen consumption can be measured directly in an appropriately equipped exercise laboratory or estimated from measures of heart rate at known submaximal workloads. Other terms synonymous with maximal oxygen consumption are maximal oxygen uptake, maximal oxygen intake, aerobic power and aerobic capacity. $MaxVO_2$ can be expressed in absolute terms of milliliters of oxygen per minute (ml/min), or in relative terms of milliliters of oxygen consumed per kilogram of body weight per minute (ml/kg/min). By relating oxygen consumption to body size, it is possible to compare fitness levels of individuals of different sizes. In general, men tend to have higher $maxVO_2$ than women, even after correcting

for body weight. However, when oxygen consumption per kilogram of lean body mass is calculated, the gender difference becomes smaller.

Initial fitness levels and health status determine the intensity and duration of the work that a person is asked to perform in the cardiorespiratory assessment. For example, a conditioned long-distance runner who wants to assess the effects of a 3-month intensive training program might start with treadmill running at a speed of five miles per hour and increase the slope and speed every 1 or 2 minutes until exhaustion. A 75-year-old man who had a myocardial infarction 2 weeks earlier and is now ready to be discharged to home would be assessed by the cardiac rehabilitation team using a low-level exercise test that could start at 1.5 miles per hour with no slope and gradually increase slope or speed. Both procedures assess cardiorespiratory function and fitness.

The Need to Test Cardiovascular Status

In the past, exercise stress testing to diagnose cardiovascular disease was recommended prior to initiation of an exercise program for all persons over 40. Reassessment of the guidelines for clinical exercise testing has led to new recommendations that take into account both the health of the individual and the intensity of the exercise to be performed (Gordon, Kohl, Scott, Gibbons, & Blair, 1992) (Table 10-4). These guidelines allow a greater number of people without symptomatic cardiovascular disease to begin a low- to moderate-intensity exercise program without performing a physician-supervised exercise stress test. However, a brief medical history to identify the presence of cardiovascular risk and other exercise-related factors is necessary (Figure 10-4).

Exercise to Improve Cardiorespiratory Fitness

The following principles should guide activity programs aimed at improving cardiorespiratory fitness:

1. The physical activity should require rhythmic, dynamic contractions of large muscle groups.
2. The intensity, duration, and frequency of the activity should be based on current cardiovascular status and should be gradually progressive.
3. The activity should impose a demand on the cardiovascular system above accustomed levels. For a person who is markedly deconditioned, any regular program of activity that moderately elevates heart rate and breathing above resting levels for at least 30 minutes at least 3 days a week will lead to some aerobic endurance benefits. For a person who already has good cardiovascular endurance, the exercise must be more intense to provide the overload stimulus necessary to produce improvement. Activity that is too intense increases the risk of injury without concomitant training benefit.
4. The aerobic or training activity should begin gradually with adequate warm-up to prepare the cardiovascular and musculoskeletal systems for increased workloads.
5. An intensity range should be individually established based on age, medical status, and current activity level. An intensity that should not be exceeded should be set and steadfastly observed. Intensity may be monitored by heart rate or rating of perceived exertion.
6. Activities that require excessive upper-extremity use, particularly with arms elevated above chest height, or sustained isometric contractions tend to elevate blood pressure but produce no training effects for improved cardiovascular (aerobic) endurance. Heavy resistance weight training programs or aerobic routines that rely on arm movements are not appropriate methods to improve cardiovascular endurance. If elevated blood pressure is a risk factor, such activities can be dangerous.

Specifics of the Exercise Prescription

The exercise prescription, based on the principles of overload and specificity, delivers the appropriate exercise

---

TABLE 10-4
Guidelines for Exercise Testing

Purposes of Exercise Stress Testing:

- Screen for silent ischaemia
- Basis for exercise prescription

Cardiovascular Disease Risk Factors ($\geqslant$ 2 = at risk):

- Hypertension (BP $\geqslant$ 160/90 mmHg)
- Serum cholesterol $\geqslant$ 240 mg/dL (6.2 mmol/L)
- Cigarette smoking
- Diabetes mellitus
- Family history

Perform Supervised Exercise Stress Test for:

1. Apparently Healthy: men $\geqslant$ 40; women $\geqslant$ 50 for vigorous exercise only
2. Persons at Risk with no symptoms: all ages for vigorous exercise only
3. Persons at Risk with symptoms and disease: all ages for moderate and vigorous exercise

Moderate Exercise Intensity

- 40-60% max VO_2 = 60-75% age-predicted maximal heart rate; RPE= 11-13
- Well within current capacity; sustainable comfortably for 60 minutes
- Slow progression; noncompetitive activity

Vigorous Exercise Intensity

- > 60% max VO_2 = > 75% age-predicted maximal heart rate; RPE= 14-16
- Substantial challenge; fatigue within 20 minutes

Gordon, N. F., Kohl, H. W., Scott, C. B., Gibbons, L. W., & Blair, S. N. (1992). Reassessment of the guidelines for exercise testing. *Sports Medicine, 13*, 293-302.

---

dose through the choice of exercise mode, as well as duration, frequency and intensity of the activity. The latter three factors are interrelated and are varied within the prescription to provide an appropriate dose of exercise. Within training and safety guidelines, a higher intensity for a shorter duration will provide the same training effect as a longer duration of the activity at a lower intensity.

SAMPLE

PHYSICAL ACTIVITY READINESS QUESTIONNAIRE

Your answers to the following questions will help you decide about your exercise plan. Read them carefully and circle the appropriate answer. Common sense is the best guide in choosing your answer: If you have any doubt, circle "YES" or consult your instructor.

1.   Has your doctor ever told you that you have heart or lung problems?   YES   NO

2.   Have you ever had heart surgery?   YES   NO

3.   Have you frequently felt any chest discomfort or pain?   YES   NO

4.   Do you frequently feel dizziness and/or faintness?   YES   NO

5.   Has your doctor ever told you that you have high blood pressure?   YES   NO

6   Do you take medication to lower your blood pressure?   YES   NO

7.   Are you aware of any bone, back or joint problems that could be

     aggravated by exercise?   YES   NO

8.   Has exercise ever made you experience severe shortness of

     breath, wheezing or coughing?   YES   NO

9.   Have you ever been told by your doctor that you have diabetes?   YES   NO

10. Are you over age 60 and not involved in regular exercise?   YES   NO

11. Are you pregnant?   YES   NO

12. Can you think of any other reason why exercise might cause problems
     for you? (For instance, have you had surgery in the last six months?)   YES   NO
     Please explain:

     _____

     _____

If you have answered "YES" to any of these questions, please seek your doctor's help in determining the right exercise program for you.

_____   _____
Participant's signature   Date

Figure 10-4. Physical Activity Readiness Questionnaire Sample.

The most effective *exercise modes* engage as much of the total body muscle mass as feasible. Body orientation (upright or horizontal), weight bearing status (total, partial, or gravity eliminated) and muscle groups involved (upper, lower, and/or total) can be modified according to physical need. Choices such as exercise location (indoor, outdoor), social context (class, group, partners), and cultural acceptability also must be considered for these are important factors in the willingness of the person to adopt and maintain the exercise habit.

Duration is the prescriptive variable that defines the length of an exercise session or the total amount of exercise/activity accumulated during the exercise day. *Frequency* refers to the number of days per week that the activity is performed. *Intensity* describes the level of exertion or energy expenditure required to perform the activity. Intensity can be assessed in a number of ways. The most common methods are heart rate, perceived exertion (Noble, Borg, & Jacobs, 1983), and ability to speak normally. Moderate intensity exercise/activity is the safest and most effective. The ranges and relationships of heart rate, perceived exertion and exercise intensity are shown in Figure 10-5. An appropriate level of perceived exertion and the ability to speak normally are the most practical methods for an individual who is unaccustomed to taking a pulse to monitor exercise intensity and stay with a moderate range. Intensity is often expressed in terms of METs. This concept is useful in prescribing modes of activity within fairly broad intensity ranges, but does not give the individual the tools to monitor actual exertion. The definition of MET is given below (see boxed aside). A number of physical activities with equivalent MET values are shown in Table 10-5.

These variables of the exercise prescription can be manipulated to form a safe and effective beginning exercise dose for even the most deconditioned individual and progressed as endurance and capacity improve. For example, a beginning prescription might recommend 3 days of walking a week at a low to moderate level of intensity for a total of 15 minutes a day accumulated in three sessions. As the individual improves, the prescription is modified to include 4 days a week of moderately intense walk accumulated in three 10-minute bouts a day.

The specifics of a physical fitness prescription address the five components of physical fitness described in this chapter. A comprehensive prescription will be based on assessment and intervention in all five areas. Table 10-6 outlines a physical fitness assessment.

The recommended exercise program for physical fitness in the general population contains components that address cardiovascular and musculoskeletal conditioning. The exercise regimen for cardiorespiratory or aerobic fitness produces peripheral adaptations in the skeletal muscles involved in the physical activities and also central adaptations in cardiopulmonary function. Initial changes occur most often in the

---

Measuring Energy Expenditure: MET

MET (metabolic equivalent) is an expression of energy cost relative to the resting energy expenditure. Resting energy expenditure, considered to be approximately the same for all persons, is set at 3.5 ml of oxygen consumption per kilogram of body weight per minute. Therefore, one MET is oxygen consumption at rest and is considered to be 3.5 ml/kg/min. An energy expenditure of 5 METs is equal to oxygen consumption of 17.5 ml/kg/min (5 x 3.5 = 17.5). The rate of energy expenditure or oxygen consumption for an activity that requires 5 METs is 5 times that required to support the energy needs of the person at rest.

Individual differences in resting oxygen consumption and in energy expenditure for actual performance limit the usefulness of METs as a method for comparing actual energy expenditure between individuals. METs are primarily useful as a technique for assessing relative rates of energy expenditure between activities. Therefore, METs can be a general guide to exercise intensity and energy expenditure. The greater the METs, the more intense the activity and greater the energy expenditure required to support the activity. Excitement, anxiety, obesity, and poor economy of effort may produce excessive metabolic increases so that METs expended during the performance of an activity may be greater than expected.

---

peripheral compartment and improvements in muscular endurance may be observed first. Exercises for improvement of flexibility usually are included in warm-up and cool-down periods. Table 10-7 describes the American College of Sports Medicine recommendations for cardiovascular fitness (1990).

Physical Activity Recommendations for Health: How Much is Enough?

Information obtained since the late 1980s about the importance of even low levels of regular physical activity has prompted a new look at the traditional exercise prescription for cardiorespiratory fitness. Recent findings indicate that activity-related risk factors can be markedly reduced and health improved by adding a modest amount of physical activity to the daily routine. Current recommendations for a sedentary person who wishes to improve general health are shown in Table 10-7. This recommendation is less intense (low to moderate exertion) and allows the *accumulation* of 30 minutes of exercise in as short as 8- to 10-minute bouts throughout the exercise day. Frequency is suggested as most days of the week (Blair, Kohl, & Gordon, 1992).

The advantages of this recommendation are its adaptability to a variety of environments and physical abilities; the ease with which physical activity can be added to the course of

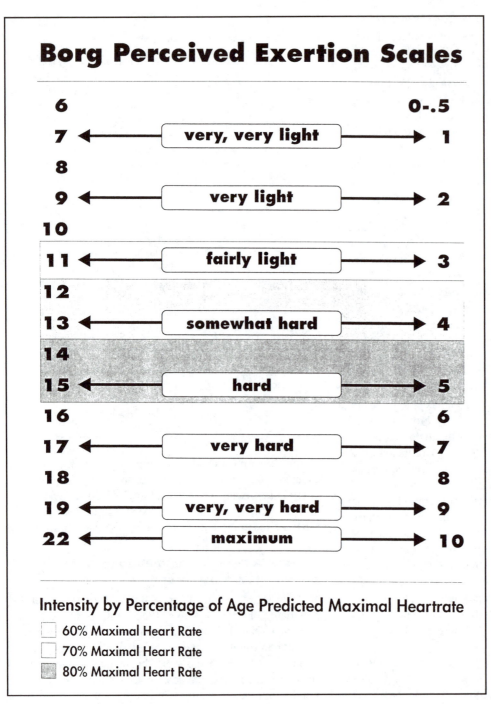

Figure 10-5. Borg Scales of Perceived Exertion.

current daily activities, and a low level of exertion and time commitment required of the beginning exerciser. For individuals with mobility limitations due to weakness, pain, limitations in motion, fatigue or biomechanical problems, this recommendation provides a method for meaningful, health-promoting physical activity in achievable bouts. Incorporation of these recommendations may be the goal of some persons. For others, achievement of this activity level may be the first step in a more vigorous conditioning program.

Evaluation of Muscle Strength and Endurance

In clinical practice, a test of muscle strength is often used in an evaluation of functional level. Because function depends to a great extent on ability to sustain activity for a desired period of time, muscle endurance should be assessed at a level of effort comparable to that required for the function in question. Adequate dynamic strength of the deltoid, shoulder external rotators, and scapular stabilizers is required to move

TABLE 10-5

Energy Expenditure for Work and Leisure Activities*

	WORK/SELF MAINTENANCE	PLAY/LEISURE		WORK/SELF MAINTENANCE	PLAY/LEISURE
1 ½ METs	Desk work	Walking (1 mph), standing, playing cards, driving car, sewing, knitting	6-7 METs	Shoveling (10 lbs)	Walking (5 mph), bicycling (11 mph), tennis singles, square dancing (folk), water skiing
2-3 METs	Auto repair Radio and TV repair Janitorial work Bartending	Walking (2 mph), billiards, bowling, golf (power cart), fishing (on bank), playing piano, shuffleboard, level bicycling (5 mph)	7-8 METs	Carrying (80 lbs) Digging ditches Heavy carpentry	Jogging (5 mph), bicycling (12 mph), basketball (social), touch football, downhill skiing, ice hockey
3-4 METs	Bricklaying Machine assembly Wheelbarrow (100 lbs) Cleaning windows Lawn mowing (power)	Walking (3 mph), horseshoe pitching, golf (pulling bag cart), bicycling (6 mph), archery, fly fishing (standing)	8-9 METs	Shoveling (14 lbs)	Running (5 ½ mph), bicycling (13 mph), handball (social), jump rope (60-80 skips/ min), fencing
4-5 METs	Painting Light carpentry Paper-handing Raking leaves Bicycling (8mph) Hoeing	Walking (3 ½ mph), table tennis, golf (carry bag), tennis (doubles), ballroom dancing	10 METs	Shoveling (16 lbs)	Running (6 mph)
			3 ½ METs	Climbing stairs with 25 pound load	Handball (competitive), jump rope (120/min), skiing, cross country (at >5 mph)
5-6 METs	Digging garden Light shoveling	Walking (4 mph), bicycling (10 mph), skating (recreational), badminton, fishing (in waders)			

* 1 MET = 3.5 ml O_2/kg/min = 1.25 kcal/min for 70 kg person

the upper extremity into a position necessary to brush teeth or comb hair. Adequate static strength is necessary to maintain the position momentarily. Endurance, both dynamic and static, must also be adequate for the task to be accomplished.

Exercise to Improve Muscle Strength

For the most part, the research that forms the rationale for the general principles for strength training has been per-formed with healthy, generally young, subjects with unim-paired musculoskeletal systems. Adherence to these princi-ples produces maximal strength gains in normal, healthy people; however, application of these principles in the reha-bilitation setting requires consideration of many additional factors, including musculoskeletal and neural pathology.

Principles underlying muscle strength training include the following:

1. Greatest strength gains are achieved by performing a reg-

TABLE 10-6

Physical Fitness Assessment

COMPONENT & DEFINITION	PRIMARY STRUCTURES INVOLVED	ASSESSED BY
Cardiorespiratory Function (ability to take in, transport and use oxygen)	heart vascular system lungs blood components cellular respiration	• oxygen uptake • cardiac output • heart rate • blood pressure • perceived exertion
Muscle Strength (maximum amount of force that can be exerted in one contraction)	Type II muscle fibers myoneural mechanisms muscle energy stores anaerobic enzymes	• isometric strength by make/break test • isotonic strength by 1 repetition maximum
Muscle Endurance (maintenance of activity at submaximal exertion)	Type I muscle fibers systemic energy stores mitochondria oxidative enzymes	• isometric endurance by holding time • isotonic endurance by number of repetitions to fatigue
Flexibility (range and ease of joint movement)	joint structures periarticular tissues	• static/flexibility using goniometry • dynamic flexibility by resistance testing
Body Composition (proportion of fat to lean body mass)	lean body mass (muscle, bone) body fat (storage & essential fat)	• skin fold measurement • bioimpedance • hydrostatic weight • total body counter

ular program of overload at maximal or near maximal resistance. The load must be progressively increased to keep pace with strength gains and to continue to provide an overload stimulus. High resistance exercise regimes are considered the most effective for producing strength gains.

2. Apply the overload to the specific muscle groups and in movement patterns and speeds that are congruent with performance goals. There is some indication that training at higher speeds improves strength gains.

3. To avoid early-onset fatigue in small muscle groups, start exercising large muscle groups before smaller ones.

4. Maximum strength gains are made when the muscle is overloaded at the same length (static) or at the same velocity (dynamic) in training as in testing or actual performance.

5. The rate of strength gain is greatest when the muscle is weakest in relation to maximal potential strength. Early gains in strength performance are due to neuromuscular learning rather than physiologic adaptation.

6. Allow adequate recovery between individual exercise sessions and between exercise bouts. Fatigued muscles are not able to respond and adapt to overload stress as well as muscles that have recovered from previous exercise. Frequency of strength training is prescribed for every other day to allow the muscle time to recover. Training adaptations occur during the recovery period.

7. There is no difference in the effectiveness of free weights or various resistance equipment in improving strength.

8. Heavy resistance exercise is not recommended for persons with hypertension.

Recommendations for Static Strengthening

1. Training contraction may be a "maximal" voluntary contraction held for 1 second, or a submaximal contraction

(two-thirds maximal) held for 6 seconds. Holding the contraction for a longer period increases the possibility of post-exercise pain and stiffness and produces no additional training benefit.

2. Optimal training effect is achieved by repeating contractions 5 to 10 times daily.

3. To improve functional strength, the isometric contractions should be performed at many joint angles through the range of motion.

4. Intense and/or sustained isometric contractions may produce an extreme rise in both diastolic and systolic blood pressure if held for more than a few seconds and should be avoided by people with cardiovascular disease or hypertension.

Recommendations For Dynamic Strengthening

1. Progressive resistance exercise (PRE) techniques are appropriate to a wide variety of settings and rehabilitation needs. PRE requires determination of 10 RM for the targeted muscle group and uses a graded series of 3 sets of 10 lifts each, either beginning or ending with a set of 10 RM. A traditional progression is grading resistance in sets from ½ 10 RM, to ¾ 10 RM to 10 RM. Determination of 10 RM must be performed periodically to adjust overload to increased muscle performance.

2. For a person who is just beginning a weight training program, it may be safest to begin lifting weights at 12 RM if the weight load is being kept constant across sets. After 2 to 3 weeks of training, load may be increased to 6 or 8 RM. Exercise between 3 and 12 RM is most efficient range for improving strength.

3. Frequency of training sessions should be two or three times a week.

4. Strengthening of muscles responsible for a complex movement should be accomplished with exercises designed to incorporate or imitate that movement. Strengthening contractions should be done through the full range of motion.

Another form of dynamic strengthening is isokinetic training. Isokinetic strengthening techniques rely on specialized equipment that is capable of producing variable resistance throughout the range of motion. Theoretically, isokinetic training assures a constant and peak activation of muscle fibers throughout the range of motion by matching resistance to available muscular force. There is a variety of isokinetic equipment with different methods of producing the isokinetic effect. The isokinetic training program will be determined by the equipment being used, training goals, and the abilities and needs of the trainee. The general principles of strengthening apply to isokinetic training. Special attention should be paid to the velocity of training contractions. For improvement of strength in a complex movement, the velocity of training con-

---

TABLE 10-7

Exercise Recommendations

Physical Activity for General Health

- Mode: whole body, dynamic activity
- Frequency: 4-7 days/wk
- Intensity: 40-60% max VO_2 = 60-75% max HR
- Duration: 30 minutes accumulation

Blair, S. N., Kohl, H. W., & Gordon, N. F. (1992). How much physical activity is good for health? *Annu Rev Public Health, 13,* 99-126.

Exercise for Cardiovascular Fitness

- Mode: dynamic, repetitive exercise of major muscle groups
- Frequency: 3-5 days/wk
- Intensity: 50-70% max VO_2 = 65-80% max HR
- Duration: 20-60 minutes continuous

Exercise for Physical Fitness (Cardiovascular and musculoskeletal)

Cardiovascular fitness program with flexibility exercise and resistive, strengthening program

- Mode: dynamic, resistance (upper & lower body)
- Frequency: 2-3 days/wk
- Intensity: 8-10 exercises at 60-80% 1RM (= to moderate fatigue)
- Duration: 8-12 repetitions of each

American College of Sports Medicine Position Stand. (1990). The recommended quantity and quality of exercise for developing and maintaining cardiorespiratory and muscular fitness in healthy adults. *Medicine and Science in Sports and Exercise, 22,* 265-274.

---

tractions should be as close as possible to the velocity of contractions used in the functional, unloaded motion. A disadvantage to isokinetic training is the limited ability of the equipment to be adjusted for individual variations in body structure.

Exercise to Improve Muscle Endurance

Muscle strength is measured as the maximum amount of force that a muscle can exert in a single contraction; muscle endurance depends on the capacity of a muscle to repeatedly perform submaximal contractions or to sustain force. Muscular endurance is measured by the number of repetitions that can be performed or the period for which activity can be sustained. Cardiovascular endurance is improved by whole-body activities that stress the oxygen delivery system, but muscle endurance is only improved by local, muscular activity that stresses the capacity of the muscle to use oxygen and produce energy. When a person jogs or cycles to improve cardiovascular endurance, muscle endurance of the active lower-extremity muscles will improve as well. However, there will be no improvement in muscle endurance in the upper extremities without specific activities to produce local adaptive changes.

Muscular endurance is related to muscular strength. Adequate strength must precede endurance training and adequate strength improves endurance. Endurance increases when a muscle group is able to work at a smaller percentage of maximal capacity. This occurs when either the muscle becomes stronger or the amount of force required to perform the motion decreases. If a person's muscular strength is deficient it may require a near maximal effort for that person to lift hand to mouth. Such a person would not be able to repeat this motion in a given amount of time as often as a person who performs this motion with less effort.

If muscular strength is constant, endurance decreases as the intensity of effort required to produce the movement increases. For example, level running at six miles an hour can be sustained for a much longer time than level running at ten miles an hour or running up a grade. Thus, when we talk about muscle endurance we must also consider the muscular strength and intensity of effort relevant to the activity being performed.

The following is a summary of principles related to improving muscle endurance:

1. The overload (resistance) principle applies to training for muscle endurance as well as to strength training. Although more repetitions are required in endurance training, overload is necessary for improvement to occur.
2. Appropriate overload for endurance training will generally produce improvements in both muscle strength and endurance.
3. Overload should be gauged so that the individual can perform at least 20 full-range repetitions of the motion and/or be able to sustain the activity for at least 30 seconds. If adding external resistance is not possible, overload can be achieved by gradual increases in the speed of the motion. If both strength and endurance are low, initial training may need to progress only by increasing the number of repetitions.
4. Constant attention to balancing resistance and repetitions in the exercise program is the key to achieving optimal improvement. Although "low resistance, high repetition" is the popular slogan for endurance training, too little resistance produces limited improvement.
5. In the absence of limiting factors, endurance training should occur three to five times per week and include two to three sets of 20 repetitions each while maintaining

appropriate overload. Most of the literature from exercise physiology deals with muscular training in terms of weight loads. However, the same principles can be applied to training programs that use activities of daily living, work-related tasks, or recreational activities. In the rehabilitation setting, it is possible to use these principles by adjusting the number of repetitions, speed of performance, frequency and duration of training sessions, and/or the application of external resistance.

Assessing Flexibility

What is adequate flexibility? Our definition of physical fitness as the capacity to successfully meet the present and potential physical challenges of life provides us with a framework for defining adequate flexibility. Assessing flexibility strictly in terms of the client's present needs is rather straightforward. For example, one might need to determine how much shoulder flexion is required to reach an upper cabinet or how much knee and hip flexion is necessary to descend stairs, or one might need to determine how much cervical rotation is needed to provide a safe field of vision for a person driving in reverse or merging into freeway traffic.

It is evident that flexibility required to perform most tasks of daily living does not make use of the full potential range available. Flexibility assessment should not be limited to merely meeting clients' present requirements, but should consider meeting potential physical challenges if the joint must move beyond its present range. Injuries occur when motion is forced beyond the existing range, so adequate flexibility must include range above that normally required. Currently, to evaluate flexibility deficits and determine reasonable expectations of flexibility, we must continue to rely on judicious interpretation of the existing normative tables and on the assessment of bilateral range of motion.

The rehabilitation process usually contains specific objectives and therapeutic exercise regimens designed to improve or maintain range of motion in the presence of disease or trauma. The goal of flexibility is achieved by applying various techniques, some of which may be specifically addressed to the underlying causes of the flexibility deficit, such as upper motor neuron lesion spasticity, the rigidity of Parkinson's disease, paralysis from peripheral nerve damage, or decreased flexibility associated with rheumatologic conditions. Therapeutic stretching techniques, based on Golgi body tendon functioning and reciprocal innervation, are typically employed when the restricted motion is associated with neuromuscular and contractile elements of the muscle.

In this discussion of flexibility, we will focus on the principles of achieving adequate flexibility of muscle and periarticular connective tissue in relation to the extensibility inherent in these structures, rather than therapeutic exercise regimens for specific diseases. In order to increase static or extent flexibility, exercise techniques are based on gradually producing minor distensions in connective tissue. The summation of these minor changes can produce major changes in overall extensibility of the periarticular structures and can result in gains in range of motion.

Techniques to Improve Flexibility

Some guidelines for improving flexibility are as follows:
1. Static stretching is preferable to ballistic stretching, because static stretching reduces the risk of injury from overstretching, requires less energy and tends to relieve rather than cause muscle soreness. A static stretch should be held from 10 to 30 seconds.
2. Increased flexibility is produced by overstretching, yet overstretching should not exceed normal muscle length by more than 10%.
4. More repetitions are required to increase flexibility than to maintain it.
5. Flexibility exercises should be performed both before and after endurance and/or strengthening activities.
6. Stretching exercises performed actively make the best use of neurophysiologic mechanisms favoring increased flexibility.

Passive Stretching Versus Active Stretching

The techniques employed to increase flexibility are classified in two ways: either by the source of the force producing the movement or stretch, or by the characteristic of the applied stretch, which is either constant or rebounding. Passive stretching is applied externally by either another person or gravity, and active stretching is performed when the movement occurs from one's own internal muscular force. Static stretching is holding the lengthened or stretched position without movement, while ballistic stretching is bouncing or repeated rhythmic movements intended to produce a rebound stretch at the outer limits of the range.

Current thought in both medical and sports literature appears to favor active, static stretching techniques. This active, static stretching has been found to be more beneficial because of less risk of overstretching and injury, post-exercise soreness, energy consumed, and opposing muscle activity to impede optimal stretching (Luttgens & Wells, 1982). Active, static stretching includes active movement to the outer limit of the current range, active effort to stretch slightly past this point, and holding the lengthened position from 10 to 30 seconds. The exercise should be repeated several times a day. The decision as to how far to stretch beyond current range must be an individual one. Some maintain that the stretch should not exceed 10% of the normal range. Others assert to stretch just to the point of increased tension.

Stretching that produces increased pain is probably counterproductive.

Flexibility can be overdone. Flexibility is excessive when it overcomes the natural supportive function of the periarticular connective tissue and surrounding muscle. Excessive flexibility (hypermobility) results in joint instability and increased risk of strain and injury. The protective supporting role of periarticular connective tissue and muscle is particularly important for weight-bearing joints that are subjected to repeated stress in the course of normal daily activities.

Assessment of Body Composition

The methods used to estimate body fat are hydrostatic weighing (underwater), bioimpedence measurement, and the skin-fold measurement technique. Hydrostatic weighing and bioimpedence require equipment and are most often used in research settings. The skin-fold technique, a practical method for body composition screening, can be applied in a wide variety of settings. Special calipers measure skin-fold thickness at specific body sites. The thicker the skin-fold, the more subcutaneous fat. Because subcutaneous fat is 50% of human body fat, thickness of skin-folds is a valid indicator of total body fat. Tables of normative values are used to estimate body fat from skin-fold thickness at designated sites.

Improving Body Composition

A healthy proportion of lean body weight to body fat is part of good physical fitness. Achieving and maintaining this balance is important because obesity is a risk factor in many diseases and an adequate lean body mass of muscle and bone is essential to support functional activity. The following principles summarize important relationships between exercise and body composition:
1. Participation in regular exercise can lead to a reduction in appetite. Several studies have shown that subjects who were physically active actually ate less than sedentary controls.
2. Moderate to vigorous exercise not only increases metabolic rate during the exercise itself, but also tends to elevate the metabolic rate for up to 24 hours following the exercise. An increased metabolic rate results in greater caloric expenditure.
3. Weight loss accomplished through exercise is almost entirely due to fat loss with a maintenance or gain in lean tissue/muscle.
4. Moderately intense exercise such as brisk walking, when sustained for more than 45 minutes, tends to stimulate the metabolism of stored fat (glycogen sparing) for energy to support the activity.
5. A program that includes moderate dietary restriction and regular exercise to create a negative energy balance is

---

TABLE 10-8

Clinical Indications of Fatigue

Muscular

Decreased strength

Decreased contraction time

Increased recovery time

Tremors with contraction

Increased muscle lengthening time

General

Decreased coordination

Decreased smoothness/rhythm of performance

Appearance of compensatory/extraneous movements

General slowing down

Loss of concentration

Loss of interest

Increased frustration

---

more likely to produce maintenance of weight loss than dietary manipulation alone.

6. An exercise program to increase muscle mass (a muscle strengthening program) is also an effective method to improve body composition and increase lean body mass. In some nutritionally compromised persons, increased caloric intake may be needed to offset the energy expenditure of exercise.

Other Factors Affecting Performance

Aging, inactivity, and disease may affect capacity and performance directly through the physiologic components of fitness. Fatigue and poor economy of effort are more likely to be signs of diminished fitness that appear during physical activity and affect performance.

Fatigue

The exercise physiologist defines fatigue as the inability to maintain a given exercise intensity. The clinician is familiar with fatigue as a symptom reported by the client and often associated with a particular disease. The experience of fatigue includes two concepts: exertional fatigue which is closely related to neuromuscular and cardiorespiratory activity, and the more global experience of fatigue. Fatigue implies a decrement in performance and includes both physiologic and psychosocial factors. In determining level of performance and impact of fatigue, the psychosocial variables of motivation, fear, pain tolerance, and general mental state may be as important as the physiologic variables, especially in low-intensity, sustained-duration activities encountered in vocational and leisure pursuits. Underlying disease must also be considered as contributing to fatigue.

Fatigue is often a symptom associated with conditions such as multiple sclerosis, inflammatory arthritis, post-polio syndrome, fibromyalgia, and Lyme disease. Management of fatigue can be an important issue in comprehensive care, and should be addressed from the standpoint of control of disease activity and possible depression, as well as through self-management strategies such as energy conservation, effective sleep habits, and exercise.

The physiology of exertional fatigue also is a complex phenomenon. There is active research and controversy regarding the anatomical site(s) and mechanisms of fatigue that implicate the central nervous system, peripheral nerves, myoneural junction, and the muscles as possible sources of fatigue. There is debate about whether fatigue is due to accumulation or depletion of specific metabolites or is a general homeostatic response. What is clear is that there is no one site or mechanism that explains fatigue in all cases. For example, fatigue occurring when a person attempts to maintain a tight grip for 20 seconds is due primarily to anaerobic mechanisms supporting contraction in the finger flexors and intrinsics of the hand; however, the possibility of changes at the neuromuscular junction cannot be disregarded. Fatigue occurring when a person begins a gait-retraining program could be due to inadequate oxygen transport or utilization by the active muscles, or a variety of neural and/or muscular causes.

Exertional fatigue is activity-specific for the intensity and duration of the activity and for the body parts involved in the activity. The physiologic status of the individual is a major determining factor in onset of fatigue. However, psychologic factors such as motivation and attention or distraction also are important. Fatigue is also influenced by environmental stressors such as heat, altitude, and humidity. The more complex and sustained the activity, the more difficult it is to determine specific causes of fatigue.

Fatigue is not always a negative factor. For physiologic adaptations to take place, some physiologic fatigue must occur. Activity that is strenuous enough to result in a sense of general tiredness or some fatigue is associated with improved sleep behaviors and improved sense of well-being and relaxation. There is an important distinction between exercise-induced fatigue and exhaustion. Exercise to the point of exhaustion is appropriate only in the most controlled laboratory testing procedures with on-site medical supervision. It is the therapist's or trainer's responsibility to monitor physical activity to provide overload that encourages adaptation without producing exhaustion.

It is necessary to be able to identify the onset of fatigue and understand its implications in the clinical setting. Clinical observation and client self-report should both be used to monitor fatigue. Table 10-8 lists observable signs and symptoms of fatigue. Client self-report also can be an important tool for monitoring fatigue from day to day, for assessing improvement over time, and for helping the client develop skills to monitor his or her own exertion and fatigue level outside the clinic.

Clinical observation to determine onset of fatigue can be systematic and is based on knowledge of a number of performance-related principles. The inability to maintain or repeat the production of a given force by muscular contraction, another definition of fatigue, describes the first observation of fatigue. The clinical onset of muscular fatigue will be evidenced by changes in muscular performance such as decreased strength, decreased time of contraction and/or increased time of recovery, increased time for muscle lengthening following contraction, tremors with contraction, and substitution and compensatory movements. If the fatigue is related to insufficient coronary circulation and/or insufficient oxygen delivery (hypoxia), the clinical signs may be shortness of breath, increased heart rate and respiration with no increase in workload, sweating, or general sense of tiredness, especially in the exercising muscles. General performance may slow down and attention may wander. (Symptoms such as chest pressure or pain, nausea, and numbness in upper extremities should be considered as a coronary event and emergency procedures should be followed). Heart disease may limit daily activity by actual fatigue of the heart muscle or by the inability of the heart to provide adequate cardiac output.

Fatigue results in muscular incoordination. This, an easily observable sign of fatigue, is a change in the smoothness, the rhythm, or the coordinated effort with which a task is performed. The key to this observation is the word "change." Poor coordination and extraneous movement often appear in the early stages of motor skill learning. The incoordination and extraneous movements must be a deviation from an established rhythm or pattern to be considered a sign of fatigue. Some people actually develop recognizable fatigue patterns that appear as they tire at a particular task. Normally the change in movement pattern that accompanies the onset of fatigue requires even more effort and speeds the fatigue process. Incoordination may appear as a general loss of rhythmic motion, or more specifically, as difficulty in performing movements that require rapid contraction and relaxation of antagonistic muscle groups or that require sequenced movement of body parts.

Loss of concentration is often a sign of fatigue. If activity continues past the point of appropriate overload, and fatigue becomes pronounced, harm can result. Pronounced

fatigue brings with it an increased susceptibility to injury as muscular control and protective tension are lost. Sprains and strains become more likely, and the ability of the muscle to respond to loading and to dissipate shock is reduced. Post-exercise muscle soreness increases with undue fatigue. This has been viewed as a possible reason for the poor exercise compliance rates associated with exercise regimes that are severely fatiguing to individuals.

Continuing activity past the point of fatigue is counterproductive for both motor skill acquisition and physiologic muscle fiber adaptation. Practice for motor learning is most effective when neuromuscular capacity to sense and respond to both internal and external stimuli is not diminished by fatigue, and when motivation and concentration on the task at hand are high. Muscle fiber adaptation to physiologic overload appears to occur during periods of rest when the muscle fibers are being repaired from the microinjuries incurred during vigorous exercise. This process occurs during both endurance training and strength training. However, it is felt that the injury-repair process is particularly crucial to muscle-strengthening programs involving the fast-twitch muscle fibers.

Exercise or activity may be adjusted to prevent undue fatigue by changing any of the three exercise parameters: intensity, duration, and/or frequency. The adjustments should be based on the type of fatigue that occurs. Intensity and duration of the exercise are the most commonly manipulated variables; however, the frequency of the activity can be of vital concern. Frequent, intense training can lead to a state known as overtraining. Overtraining, recognized as a serious concern by coaches and athletic trainers, is characterized by deterioration in performance and general conditioning and a loss of interest or motivation. Overtraining is most likely a combination of prolonged physical and psychological fatigue, and is probably an all-too-common and unrecognized impediment to continued progress in intensive rehabilitation programs. By recognizing overtraining as a potential difficulty and by manipulating activity type, intensity, duration, and frequency, the members of the team will be able to engage the client in safe and effective rehabilitation.

Fatigue can be symptomatic of the disease itself. Many of the systemic, rheumatologic disorders such as rheumatoid arthritis, systemic lupus erythematosus, and polymyalgia rheumatica include marked fatigue as a clinical sign of heightened disease activity. In these cases, effective disease control is generally accompanied by diminished fatigue.

In the case of multiple sclerosis, undue fatigue can have prolonged effects on performance. Traditionally, medical recommendations have been to avoid strenuous activity. However, too little physical activity and poor fitness can add to the debilitating effects of this disease. It may be that one of the difficulties people with multiple sclerosis have in determining appropriate levels of activity is the inability to recognize signs of muscular fatigue as early as a person without nervous system pathology. It is possible that the person with multiple sclerosis may be recognizing exhaustion rather than fatigue. Exercise programs for the person with multiple sclerosis must be carefully monitored and systematically progressed to provide opportunities for enhanced fitness without exacerbating the signs and symptoms of the disease. Similar safeguards should be observed in exercise programs for people with post-polio syndrome.

Economy of Effort

The cost of production applies to economics, automotive engineering, and exercise physiology. The amount of input (dollars, gasoline, or calories) required to produce a given product (profit, miles traveled, or useful work) is expressed proportionally (percentage of profit, miles per gallon, or calories per hour). In the field of human performance, this ratio of energy input to work output can be expressed in both mathematical and clinical terms. Mechanical efficiency is calculated as a percentage of the actual mechanical work accomplished divided by the input of energy. The term *work* is used in the physical science concept of force acting through a vertical distance and applies only to external work performed. The mechanical efficiency of the locomotor activities of walking, running, or cycling is between 20% and 30%.

The primary factor that affects efficiency is the energy required to overcome internal and external friction. In terms of the efficiency equation, this is wasted energy because it does not produce measurable work. Mechanical efficiency varies among individuals, activities, and speed of performance. To a point, mechanical efficiency can be improved with training. Economy of effort is used in a clinical sense to describe differences in energy requirements between individuals and individual performances over time. It is the more clinically useful concept, requiring only a gauge of the energy input or effort required to produce a given performance. Economy of effort is commonly based on the amount of oxygen consumed while performing a particular activity. Because heart rate during submaximal exercise is proportional to oxygen consumption, the more easily monitored heart rate during performance can be used to evaluate economy of effort for an individual over time. To compare individuals, it is necessary to evaluate effort as a percentage of predicted maximal heart rate achieved.

The less energy expended to produce a given amount of work, the greater the economy of effort. In most activities the goal is to produce the most work for the least cost. Efficiency of performance is most relevant to activities that require effort lasting more than a few minutes. Sustained performance relies on aerobic endurance that is affected by oxidative capacity, availability of energy stores, and the energy needed to perform the activity.

The strategy to improve endurance performance—that is, lengthen performance time—is to improve oxidative capacity, increase energy stores, or reduce the energy required to perform the activity. By reducing the energy requirement, there is less stress on oxidative capacity and less depletion of energy stores, and the onset of fatigue is delayed. Improving the economy of effort reduces the energy requirement. When sustained performance is the goal, adjustments that improve economy of effort translate into improved performance. Economy of effort relates to endurance performance just as writing checks relates to your bank balance at the end of the month; the more you use early, the less you have to get you through to the end. Economy of effort may be affected by a number of factors. Those most relevant to rehabilitation and training are fatigue, skill, speed of performance, and biomechanical factors including weight and posture.

Fatigue interferes with economy of effort. As muscular fatigue occurs, more and more motor units are recruited to produce or maintain tension. More active motor units require greater energy consumption. Consequently, for the same work output, greater input is required and efficiency is reduced. In the more general sense, as fatigue sets in, established skill levels may be reduced as rhythmical and sequenced movement patterns are disrupted. Extraneous and inefficient motions appear. Fatigue is often accompanied by loss of attention and motivation, both important factors in efficient performance.

Motor Skill Proficiency and Economy of Effort

As skill or proficiency in performing an activity increases, the economy of effort improves. Early motor learning or relearning is characterized by unnecessary muscular tension and extraneous, poorly coordinated movements. As skill improves with effective practice and training, observers can see the performance become smoother, less effortful, and more productive. The performer notes improvement as motions become more automatic, more comfortable, and less tiring. As skill improves, less energy is used to accomplish the task and economy of effort improves as well. Thus the task can be accomplished more satisfactorily and for longer periods. This relationship between motor skill proficiency and economy of effort is one of the most important aspects of the principle of specificity of training. It is only by practicing the activity itself that motor skill learning and increased efficiency can occur.

Speed of Performance and Economy of Effort

Speed of performance also affects mechanical efficiency and economy of effort. In a pure muscular contraction, increasing velocity of the contraction is associated with decreased tension production and reduced efficiency. In complex motor patterns required for ambulation and self-care, the association between speed and efficiency is not as straight-

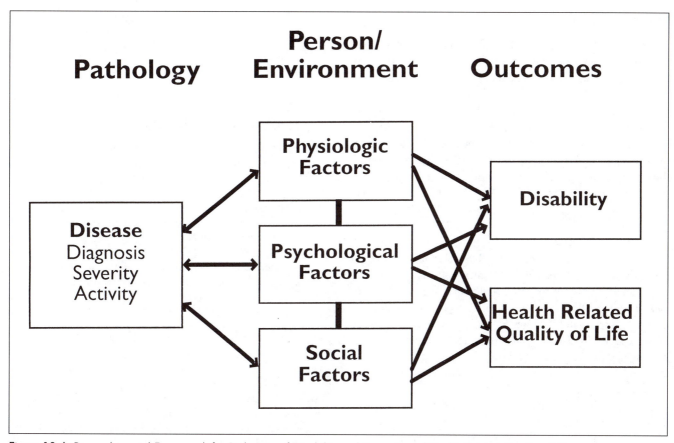

Figure 10-6. Biopsychosocial Framework for Reduction of Disability and Promotion of Health-Related Quality of Life.

forward. For any complex motor pattern, there appears to be a range of speed in which optimal efficiency occurs. Performance that is either much slower or faster than the optimal range results in poor economy of effort.

A great deal of research has been done regarding mechanical efficiency of running and walking speeds, and we can use this as an example to illustrate this concept of speed and efficiency. Gait analysis studies tell us that the most efficient walking speed for the nondisabled adult is approximately 2.4 miles per hour (4 kilometers per hour). Efficiency of walking is similar for healthy adults, and varies with speed and incline. Walking slower than 2 miles per hour requires more energy and is less efficient than walking at slightly faster speeds. When walking increases to speeds greater than about 5 miles per hour, it becomes more efficient to run than to walk. The techniques of race walking are aimed at reducing energy costs as much as possible while adhering to the requirements of maintaining a walking rather than a running pattern. For people who need to maximize endurance performance (marathon runners, production workers, freight loaders, and therapists), it is important to develop movement patterns and rhythms that expend less energy.

For people who are interested in producing an energy deficit or training overload, economy of effort may not be the goal. For example, to develop a greater caloric deficit in an exercise program, the individual may choose to walk at 5 miles per hour rather than to jog. In this way, he or she will be using more energy per distance covered. Walking or running on sand or with additional weight on the feet or ankles increases the workload. Although these actions reduce mechanical efficiency, they can be used to produce an overload for strength or endurance training.

Taking advantage of mechanical inefficiency to produce a training effect can benefit people who have an extremely low exercise tolerance. In a study of the energy cost of extremely slow walking in cardiac patients, Franklin and colleagues showed that walking speeds between .8 and 2 miles per hour imposed similar metabolic and cardiac demands, approximated 7 ml/kg/min oxygen consumption, and could be useful in exercise training for select individuals with coronary heart disease (Franklin et al., 1983). The clinical implication of these findings is that even extremely slow walking can be a conditioning activity.

CONCLUSION

There are many factors that affect performance other than physiologic variables. These other factors include motivation, fear, pain, self-efficacy, and sociocultural norms, and are discussed in depth elsewhere in this text. These factors can affect an individual's observed performance during functional assessment in the clinical setting. They can influence actual individual daily activity levels that in turn affect physical fitness. We must always remember that human performance is the product of physiologic and psychosocial variables that together influence individuals. Observable performance should never be assumed to be a clear indication of physiologic capacity.

Regular participation in adequate levels of physical activity are essential to health and physical fitness for everyone. Certain conditions and circumstances may limit an individual's ability to be active and health and physical fitness decline. Diminished physical capacity as a result of inactivity or immobilization is an important, often overlooked, factor in disease-related impairment, functional limitation, and disability. The framework of physical fitness can be used in client evaluation and planning comprehensive treatment.

The physiologic basis of an individual's ability to perform tasks and engage in meaningful activities and occupational roles may be assessed, described and changed within the organizational framework of physical fitness. It is essential to include fitness as an integral component of the rehabilitation process. Fitness information contributes to the understanding of disability and health-related quality of life. Physical fitness, as a measure of the physiologic basis of performance, must be assessed and addressed as a potentially modifying factor in the outcomes of disability and health-related quality of life (Figure 10-6).

STUDY QUESTIONS

1. Describe the five components of health-related physical fitness. How is physical fitness applicable to clinical assessment?

2. Why is cardiorespiratory fitness important? What are the effects of prolonged inactivity on cardiorespiratory fitness?

3. Discuss the aging versus inactivity question in relation to muscle strength and muscle endurance.

4. Can human performance be accurately predicted by objective measurements of physiologic performance? Why or why not?

5. Describe some of the manifestations of prolonged inactivity.

6. What is meant by the principles of overload and specificity?

RECOMMENDED READINGS

Blair, S. N., Kohl, H. W., Paffenbarger, R. S., et al. (1989). Physical fitness and all-cause mortality: A prospective study of healthy men and women. *Journal of the American Medical Association, 262,* 2395-2401.

McArdle, W. D., Katch, F. I., & Katch, V. L. (1996). *Exercise physiology, energy, nutrition and human performance* (4th ed.). Philadelphia: Lea and Febiger.

Pollock, M. L., Wilmore, J. H., & Fox, S. M. (1990). *Exercise in health and disease: Evaluation and prescription for prevention and rehabilitation* (2nd ed.). Philadelphia: W.B. Saunders.

REFERENCES

American College of Sports Medicine. (1996). *Guideline for Exercise Testing and Prescription* (4th ed.). Philadelphia: Lea and Febiger.

American College of Sports Medicine Position Stand: The recommended quantity and quality of exercise for developing and maintaining cardiorespiratory and muscular fitness in healthy adults. (1990). *Medicine and Science in Sports and Exercise, 22,* 265-274.

Atkins, C. J., Kaplan, R. M., Timms, R. M., et al. (1984). Behavioral exercise programs in the management of chronic obstructive pulmonary disease. *Journal of Consulting and Clinical Psychology, 52,* 591-603.

Blair S. N. (1993). Physical activity, physical fitness, and health. *Res Q Exerc Sports, 64,* 365-374.

Blair, S. N., Kohl, H. W., & Gordon, N. F. (1992). How much physical activity is good for health? *Annu Rev Public Health, 13,* 99-126.

Byers, P. H. (1985). Effect of exercise on morning stiffness and mobility in patients with rheumatoid arthritis. *Research in Nursing and Health, 8,* 275-281.

Caspersen, C. J., Kriska, A. M., & Dearwater, S. R. (1985). Physical activity, exercise and physical fitness: Definitions for health-related research. *Public Health Rep, 100,* 126-130.

deVries, H. A. (1980). *Physiology of exercise for physical education and athletics* (3rd ed.). Dubuque, IA: William C. Brown.

Donatelli, R., & Owens-Burkhart, H. (1981). Effects of immobilization on the extensibility of periarticular connective tissue. *Journal of Sport and Physical Training, 3,* 67-72.

Franklin, B. A., Pamatmat, A., Johnson, S. (1983). Metabolic cost of extremely slow walking in cardiac patients: Implications for exercise testing and training. *Archives of Physical Medicine and Rehabilitation, 64,* 564-565.

Gordon, N. F., Kohl, H. W., Scott, C. B., Gibbons, L. W., & Blair,

S. (1992). Reassessment of the guidelines for exercise testing. *Sports Medicine, 13,* 293-302. Lamb, D. R. (1984). *Physiology of exercise responses and adaptations.* New York: MacMillan Publishing Co.

Luttgens, K., & Wells, K. F. (1982). *Kinesiology: Scientific basis of human motion* (7th ed.). New York: CBS College Publishing.

Noble, B. J., Borg, G. A. V., & Jacobs, I. (1983). A category-ratio perceived exertion scale: Relationship to blood and muscle lactates and heart rate. *Medical Science and Sports Exercise, 15,* 523-528.

Sandler, H., & Vernikos, J. (Eds.). (1986). *Inactivity: Physiological effects.* Orlando, FL: Academic Press.

Shephard, R. J. (1978). *Physical activity and aging.* London: Crooms Helm Ltd., Publishers.

Smith, E. L., & Gilligan, C. (1983). Physical activity prescription for the older adult. *Physician Sports Medicine, 11,* 91-101.

Weg, R. B. (1983). Changing physiology of aging. In D. S. Woodruff & J. E. Birren (Eds.), *Aging, scientific perspectives and social issues* (2nd ed.). Monterey, CA: Brooks/Cole Publishing Company.

Winnick, I. P., & Short, F. X. (1985). *Physical fitness testing of the disabled.* Champaign, IL: Human Kinetics Publishers, Inc.

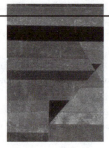

CHAPTER CONTENT OUTLINE

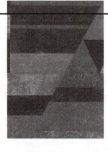

ABSTRACT

Cognition supports an individual's ability to perform the most basic and most complex activities of daily life. This chapter explores the basic cognitive mechanisms that support occupational performance (i.e., attention and memory), various approaches to the assessment of cognition, and the treatment of cognitive disabilities. Both bottom-up performance component (microlevel) and top-down functional (macrolevel) approaches to cognitive assessment are reviewed, as well as an integrative functional approach. Treatment strategies are presented which reflect an integrative functional approach. A case study illustrates these assessment and intervention principles.

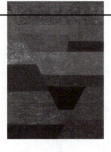

KEY TERMS

Adaptation

Attention

Awareness

Bottom-up Performance Component Approach

Contextual modifications

Episodic memory

Explicit memory

Implicit memory

Integrative Functional Approach

Micro-assessment

Satisfaction

Self-efficacy

Semantic memory

Top-down Functional Approach

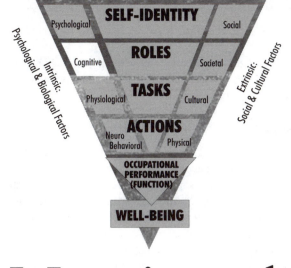

CHAPTER 11

Meeting the Challenges of Cognitive Disabilities

Janet M. Duchek, PhD, Beatriz C. Abreu, PhD, OTR, FAOTA

OBJECTIVES

The information in this chapter is intended to help the reader:

1. understand how cognition influences the performance of life tasks

2. identify fundamental components of attention and memory and deficits related to each

3. compare and contrast bottom-up vs. top-down approaches to cognitive assessment

4. identify various cognitive assessments within each of these approaches

5. understand the value of an integrative functional approach to cognitive assessment which combines bottom-up and top-down assessment

6. appreciate an integrative approach to the treatment of cognitive disability as a means of promoting client centeredness, satisfaction, and self-efficacy.

> *"I think, therefore I am."*
> Descartes

INTRODUCTION

What is cognition? How does cognition affect occupational performance? Cognition can be defined very broadly as the acquisition and use of knowledge (Neisser, 1967). Given such a definition, it is obvious that cognition represents a basic fundamental property of humans that supports an individual's self-identity, roles, tasks, and occupations. Nearly all aspects of occupational performance are guided in some way by cognition. Furthermore, cognition interacts with neurobehavioral, physiological, and psychological factors, as well as the existing physical, cultural, and social environment to ultimately affect occupational performance and the health of the individual.

In this chapter, we first discuss the basic cognitive mechanisms which support performance. This chapter focuses primarily on the cognitive components of attention and memory, keeping in mind that changes in the attentional and/or memory system will have an impact on higher order cognitive processes, such as language and problem-solving skills. Both bottom-up performance components (microlevel) and top-down functional (macrolevel) approaches to cognitive assessment are presented, as well as an integrative functional approach. Specific cognitive intervention strategies are reviewed and more general intervention approaches are discussed (bottom-up, top-down, and integrative). Finally, case studies illustrating these principles of assessment and intervention are presented.

BASIC COGNITIVE MECHANISMS THAT SUPPORT PERFORMANCE

Cognition is comprised of several components which underlie performance, such as attention, memory, pattern recognition, language comprehension and production, problem-solving and reasoning, decision-making, and intelligence. Each of these components of cognition also represents a broad area of study and can be further reduced to subcomponents (see Chapter 8 for information regarding neural substrates related to cognition). Clearly, most activities involve a complex interaction among many of these components, and performance can be easily affected by a deficit in any aspect of cognition. Several client populations with whom occupational therapists work suffer from cognitive disabilities, such as individuals with Alzheimer disease, learning disorders, traumatic brain injury, stroke, schizophrenia, etc. A basic understanding of the cognitive skills and mechanisms that

Bibliographic citation of this chapter: Duchek, J. M., & Abreu, B. C. (1997). Meeting the challenges of cognitive disabilities. In C. Christiansen & C. Baum (Eds.), *Occupational therapy: Enabling function and well-being* (2nd ed.). Thorofare, NJ: SLACK Incorporated.

are impaired and/or spared in such clients can enable more detailed analyses of occupational performance deficits and thus guide intervention.

Attention

Attention represents the basic initial stage of information processing. Attention needs to be directed at specific sensory input and sustained for some period of time before further processing can take place. Although we all have some common understanding of the term "attention," it has been difficult to precisely define, accurately assess, and successfully treat attentional deficits. Three components of attention have been defined as *alertness, selection*, and *allocation* (Posner & Boies, 1971). These three components of attention all represent different aspects of our attentional system and are not necessarily mutually exclusive.

A very basic component of attention is the alertness or preparedness of the individual. Alertness refers to both the physical and mental level of arousal that is necessary to respond. Furthermore, arousal can be tonic or phasic (Posner & Rafal, 1987). Tonic arousal refers to a general level of wakefulness from one time of the day to another and depends upon physiological indices. *Phasic arousal* refers to a specific level of alertness due to some kind of warning signal and depends upon the functioning of the appropriate brain structures (i.e., ascending reticular formation).

A second component of attention involves the ability to *selectively* attend to certain information. Clearly, an efficient processing system must be able to activate or select information from the environment that is relevant to the task at hand. At the same time, the system must be able to actively suppress or inhibit information that is not relevant to the task. Furthermore, the control of this selection and inhibition represents an important aspect of processing. There are times when one has to shift this focus of attention such that now the selected information must be inhibited and the inhibited information must be selected. A breakdown in inhibitory efficiency has been used as an explanatory construct for cognitive performance deficits in such diverse populations as children with attention deficit disorder (Tannock, Schachar, Carr, Chajczyk, & Logan, 1989), adult depressives (Posner, 1986), individuals with schizophrenia (Cohen & Servan-Schreiber, 1992), healthy older adults (Duchek, Balota, Faust, & Ferraro, 1995), and individuals with dementia of the Alzheimer type (Balota & Duchek, 1991).

Attentional capacity refers to the limited pool of cognitive resources available for allocation for any given cognitive task (Kahneman, 1973). A difficult cognitive task, such as driving in a rain storm during rush hour traffic, will require more capacity than a more simple cognitive task, such as driving on a deserted country road. In this example, the primary task of driving on the country road does not use as much attentional capacity as driving in rush hour traffic and attention can be divided between driving and another activity, such as carrying on a conversation. Thus, attention can be selective and shiftable, but it is limited to some degree.

With much practice a particular task can become automated, and thus require less attentional capacity from the reservoir. For example, as an adult, the task of reading is relatively automated compared to the reading done by a young child. Reading is a task which combines many component skills and is cognitively demanding for the young child. The child must first have extensive practice recognizing the features of letters so this skill becomes automatic, then he or she can focus attention on converting letters to sounds, and eventually extract meaning from the words. Through extensive practice, capacity-demanding tasks can become automatic (e.g., riding a bike, playing tennis), thus freeing attentional capacity for the processing of other information. Of course, it is also possible that complex tasks which were once automatic can become effortful with the onset of a cognitive disability (e.g., head injury, Alzheimer disease).

Attentional Deficits and Functional Performance

Attentional deficits are commonly seen in various clinical populations. For example, for brain-injured individuals, Ben-Yishay, Rattok, and Diller (1979) have listed insufficient alertness, inability to selectively attend to relevant information and inhibit irrelevant information, inability to sustain attention over a period of time, and response perseveration due to the inability to shift attention, as attentional deficits. Clearly, any of these deficits may impair learning and daily functioning in the brain-injured patient. Complaints of mild head injured individuals often relate to attention, concentration, and distractibility which may in turn affect an individual's ability to resume daily activities (e.g., work or school) and prior roles (e.g., parent or spouse). In fact, Vikki, Ahola, Holst, Ohman, Servo, and Heiskanen (1994) found that measures of cognitive flexibility involving the ability to shift attentional sets predicted psychosocial recovery after head injury.

It also has been suggested that some attentional deficits are associated with normal aging (Hartley, 1992). For example, Hasher and Zachs (1988) have presented a cognitive model describing how a deficit in inhibitory control could account for difficulties older adults have in language comprehension. They argue that with age, there is a breakdown in an inhibitory mechanism which serves to monitor or limit the contents of "working memory" at any given time. This inhibitory mechanism normally keeps the listener on the "goal path" of the conversation and a breakdown in inhibitory control allows more "nongoal path" ideas to enter consciousness, thereby impairing the comprehension of and memory for the conversation. In this case, the listener will have to rely more on the surrounding environment for cues to comprehend and retrieve the conversation.

Likewise, individuals with Alzheimer disease experience deficits in dividing attention, maintaining attention, selecting and shifting attention (Parasuraman & Nestor, 1991) and inhibitory control (Balota & Duchek, 1991). Such deficits can have serious implications for functional activities, such as driving. In fact, it appears that measures of visual attention are related to driving performance in Alzheimer disease (Duchek, Hunt, Bull, Buckles, & Morris, in press). We have found that some measures of selective attention differentiate safe vs. unsafe drivers who are in the early stages of the disease.

Thus it appears that some of the basic research on attentional deficits may have clear and important implications for working with various clinical populations with cognitive disabilities. The ability to control attentional processes serves to regulate various cognitive behaviors which clearly affect functional performance, such as the speed of processing information, the ability to maintain a cognitive set and persist toward a goal, the ability to anticipate consequences and self-correct actions, etc. In particular, the research on selective attention has implications for: a) structuring written and oral communication that is devoid of extraneous and irrelevant information; and b) structuring physical environments and structuring cognitive support mechanisms, such as verbal or visual cueing. Clearly, further research needs to be conducted which elucidates the important relationship between cognitive processing and functional activities which will ultimately lead to the cognitive functions underlying occupational performance.

Memory

Trying to remember what happened at the meeting last week, forgetting the phone number you just looked up, understanding the meaning of *edema*, and knowing how to play tennis, all involve some aspect of memory. Because memory is complex and multifaceted, memory theorists have provided us with distinctions among various types of memory which have proven useful for understanding disorders of memory and their impact on functional performance. Figure 11-1 displays a schematic of the relationship among the task environment, attentional control, various memory systems and behavioral output.

Short-term vs. Long-term Memory

Short-term memory (STM) is often referred to as "working memory" (Baddeley & Hitch, 1974) and is likened to our consciousness. It serves an important function by holding information in consciousness for further processing. For example, while reading this sentence, your working memory is combining sensory information from the page (i.e., the letters) with your stored knowledge base (i.e., the meanings of words and their relationships in the context of the sentence)

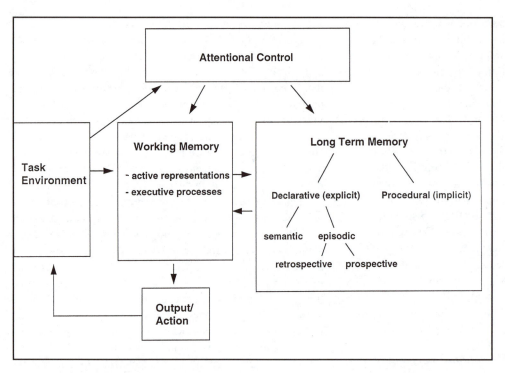

Figure 11-1. Relationship between attention and memory. Adapted from Bruer, J. T. (1993). *Schools for thought.* Cambridge, MA: MIT Press.

to aid in comprehension. However, since STM is limited in both duration and capacity, this limitation restricts our ability to simultaneously perform other cognitive tasks. Thus STM is closely tied to attentional processes as well. (The reader should see Andiel & Liu, 1995 for further information regarding the implications of working memory for assessment and intervention with older adults.)

Given the limited nature of STM, there must be a more permanent memory store for all the information we have. This more permanent store is long-term memory (LTM). Some memory theorists argue that information is never lost from LTM, but it may be inaccessible. It also has been suggested that LTM has no limitations in capacity. Because of the enormous amount of information stored in LTM, it must be organized in some meaningful way so that information is relatively easy to access. Otherwise, we would have to search the entire contents of our LTM every time we tried to remember something. In order to further specify the nature of LTM processing, other theoretical frameworks have been proposed. (The following distinctions are not necessarily mutually exclusive.)

Episodic vs. Semantic Memory

Tulving (1972) proposed a distinction between episodic memory (memory for personal episodes or events that have some contextual or temporal reference) and semantic memory (memory for general knowledge). An example of the difference between these two types of memory can be illustrated in trying to answer two questions: "Where did you go on

summer vacation last year?" and "Is a whale a mammal?" Both of these questions require a search of LTM, but they seem to tap different types of stored information. To answer the first question, one must retrieve a personal event that occurred in the past, but to answer the second question, one must retrieve the defining characteristics of a mammal and decide whether a whale fits those characteristics.

Although both episodic and semantic memories represent information that is stored in LTM, the type of information differs in important ways. Episodic memories have some personal and temporal reference, whereas semantic memories are stored as general knowledge without any personal or temporal reference. Thus, retrieval from episodic memory is guided primarily by the temporal or contextual tags stored with the relevant information. In contrast, semantic memory is organized as a complex network and retrieval can be guided by several dimensions such as meaning, associations, or rules.

Retrospective vs. Prospective Memory

One also can describe memory as being retrospective or prospective in nature. Retrospective memory refers to remembering information or events that occurred in the past (oftentimes what we think of as episodic memory). Of course, the "past" can refer to retrieving memories for an event from the recent past (e.g., 1 hour ago) to the remote past (e.g., 30 years ago). The retrieval of recent vs. remote memories poses an interesting contradiction in terms of memory loss with age. Many older adults will anecdotally report that their remote memory is better than their recent memory (i.e., one cannot remember where they put their glasses this morning, but can describe in great detail an event that occurred 30 years ago). The scientific literature has not always supported this contention (Craik & Jennings, 1992). It is important to keep in mind that: a) remote memories typically represent personally important and well-rehearsed events. (i.e., the same story has been repeated numerous times over the years and clearly the individual is not able to retrieve all events from 30 years ago); and b) the accuracy of such remote memories is sometimes questionable and difficult to verify.

Prospective memory refers to remembering to carry out some action in the future "remembering to remember." Remembering to make a phone call this afternoon and remembering to take your pills today represent the use of prospective memory. The efficiency of prospective memory will depend upon: a) the saliency of the to-be-remembered event; and b) the ability to plan forward and carry out self-initiated activities to remember the event (Craik & Jennings, 1992). When an individual is unable to self-initiate processing to remember the event, external cues in the environment will be needed.

Explicit vs. Implicit Memory

Explicit memory refers to memory which involves the deliberate and conscious retrieval of information, as in a typical recall or recognition test. Implicit memory refers to a facilitation in performance due to prior experience with the task, even though there may not be any conscious recollection of the task (Graf & Schacter, 1985). This distinction has received considerable attention in the memory literature because amnesics exhibit a dissociation in performance between these two types of memory tasks. For example, amnesic patients will show no explicit memory for learning a motor skill, but will show improved skill performance (e.g., Cohen & Squire, 1980). Furthermore, it has been suggested that implicit and explicit memory are associated with and perhaps mediated by different brain regions (Schacter, 1995).

The notion of implicit memory has been important in acknowledging the impact of prior experience on performance in the absence of the conscious recollection for that experience. In other words, one can potentially influence performance and produce changes in performance without the conscious recollection of the episode which changed performance. Thus, "memory" for some experiences can be expressed via performance without explicit remembering. Of course, this has important implications for occupational therapists who design interventions to affect performance.

Declarative vs. Procedural Memory

The distinction between declarative and procedural memory represents another useful distinction for stored memories. Declarative memory represents our knowledge for factual information, such as our knowledge of the visual system. This type of knowledge seems to be represented as a series of related statements and can be easily described verbally. The phrase "knowing that" is often used to describe declarative knowledge. Procedural knowledge represents our knowledge for the necessary procedures to perform some activity, such as our knowledge for riding a bike. This type of knowledge seems to be represented as a set of procedures and cannot be easily described verbally. The phrase "knowing how" is often used to describe procedural knowledge. There does seem to be some interaction between declarative and procedural knowledge. In other words, procedural knowledge may first start as declarative knowledge, but with much practice, the knowledge becomes procedural in nature and the skill eventually becomes automated (e.g., learning to play a musical instrument).

Memory Deficits and Functional Performance

Memory deficits can arise from several disorders such as head injury, chronic alcohol abuse, tumors, temporal lobe surgery, cerebral vascular accidents, etc. Memory loss is even a common complaint of older adults, however, this loss typically does not interfere with daily functioning. Studies have examined various aspects of memory processing in different clinical populations. For example, there have been reports of deficits in the strategic search of remote episodic memory in patients with frontal lobe lesions and Korsakoff's syndrome (e.g., Kopelman, 1989; Mangels, Gershberg, Shimamura, & Knight, 1996). Individuals with Multiple Sclerosis may experience deficits in working memory and the speed of information processing (D'Esposito, Onishi, Thompson, Robinson, Armstrong, & Grossman, 1996). Short-term and long-term memory deficits have been associated with head injury (e.g., Crossen & Wiens, 1988; Guilmette & Rasile, 1995; Reid & Kelly, 1993) and anterior communicating artery aneurysms (ACoA) (e.g., Alexander & Freedman, 1984; Simkins-Bullock, Brown, Greiffenstein, Malik, & McGillicuddy, 1994). Furthermore, as previously indicated, amnesics show a dissociation in performance on explicit and implicit memory tasks (e.g., Cermak, Verfaellie, & Chase, 1995; Graf & Schacter, 1985). Clearly, the literature indicates that memory functioning is best understood in dementia of the Alzheimer type (DAT).

Alzheimer disease is a degenerative disorder which affects approximately 10% of the population over 65 (Evans, Funkenstein, Albert, et al., 1989). It is the most common form of dementia, and memory impairment is often the initial hallmark clinical symptom of the disease. It is interesting to note that often the diagnosis of dementia of the Alzheimer type (DAT) is made in large part on the basis of change in functional performance which reflects the underlying memory impairment. For example, families will become concerned when they observe memory impairment in everyday activities, such as forgetting to transfer funds in the bank or getting lost when traveling to a friend's house. A substantial amount of research has been devoted to delineating the nature of these memory deficits as the disease progresses (see Nebes, 1992).

There is not much loss in the capacity of working memory early in Alzheimer disease, however, later in the disease, measures of digit span are greatly reduced (Botwinick, Storandt, & Berg, 1986). Furthermore, there is a deficit in retaining the contents of working memory, especially when there is interfering information (Baddeley, Logie, Bressi, et al., 1986). Long-term memory, especially episodic memory is clearly impaired in DAT. Explicit attempts to remember newly learned information over any substantial period are very difficult. Individuals with DAT are unable to use their own cognitive resources to reconstruct the context and temporality of an event. Contextual cues must be provided to help reconstruct the memory even in the early stages of the disease. Likewise, prospective memory is greatly impaired and can have serious safety ramifications (e.g., forgetting to take medications, forgetting to turn off the stove).

Although semantic knowledge may be relatively well preserved in the earlier stages of the disease, if the task involves effortful retrieval of semantic information, deficits may be observed (Knesevich, LaBarge, & Edwards, 1986; Botwinick, Storandt, & Berg, 1986). There is evidence for preserved implicit memory performance in early DAT (e.g., Knopman & Nissen, 1987; Moscovitch, Winocur, & McLachlan, 1986) when the task makes use of existing rather than new associations and skills (see Ferraro, Balota, & Connor, 1993). Likewise, evidence for preserved procedural knowledge (but not declarative knowledge) can often be seen in the earlier stages of DAT when an individual can still play the piano, yet cannot remember the name of the piece.

It is clear from the literature that memory deficits are pervasive in DAT and have a clear impact on one's ability to function in everyday activities. The cognitive support of a caregiver is essential as the disease progresses. Setting up new routines for DAT patients and expecting learning and memory to occur is not realistic. Furthermore, any activity which involves self-initiated cognitive processing will not be successful. Instead, the physical and cognitive environment needs to be carefully structured to guide cognitive processing and thus support performance (see Chapter 13 for information regarding the impact of the environment on occupational performance).

ASSESSMENT

Occupational therapists are often confronted with the issue of the cognitive status of their client. They are involved in assessing the integrity of the cognitive system in relation to the ability to function in everyday life. Therapists are called upon to assess cognition and design intervention accordingly, which often involves the family as part of the assessment and treatment process. A variety of methods are used by occupational therapists to assess cognition which include the use of standardized and nonstandardized tests, interview, and observation. Such techniques fall into two more general assessment approaches: a bottom-up performance component approach vs. a top-down functional approach.

Bottom-up Performance Component Approach

Given that cognition is composed of several different components, cognitive assessments often reflect the bottom-up approach. That is, cognitive assessments may include a battery of subtests each of which measures different components of cognitive functioning, e.g., attention, short-term memory, long-term memory, language comprehension, etc. This approach reflects a bottom-up performance component emphasis wherein cognition is reduced into subcomponents and the assessment of the subcomponents is used to create a fine grain analysis of specific deficit areas. In this light, the bottom-up approach reflects assessment at a micro or impairment level of analysis.

This approach to assessment closely mirrors the way neuropsychological assessment has been designed. Most neuropsychological assessments are designed to assess brain-behavioral relationships and are used for diagnostic, treatment, and research purposes (Lezak, 1983). Goldstein (1987) describes neuropsychological tests as either comprehensive or specialized. Comprehensive assessments include a battery of subtests which measure various components of cognition, psychomotor, and perceptual functioning. Specialized assessments include tests which measure aspects of a more specific cognitive component, such as attention or language. A list of some of the neuropsychological assessments is presented in Table 11-1 (also see Duchek, 1991; Lezak, 1983 for a more comprehensive review of neuropsychological assessment).

Clinicians have sometimes borrowed various elements of these well-known neuropsychological assessments to create cognitive assessments for occupational therapy or will use more specialized tests to evaluate specific deficit areas (e.g., digit span to examine working memory or trailmaking to examine visual motor sequencing; see Toglia, 1994a). The Lowenstein Occupational Therapy Cognitive Assessment (LOTCA) and the Rivermead Behavioral Memory Test (RBMT) are two cognitive tests which represent a more bottom-up performance component assessment approach.

The LOTCA was originally developed for use with brain-injured patients (Katz, Itzkovich, Averbuch, & Elazar, 1989) and is based upon the theoretical works of Luria and Piaget,

TABLE 11-1

Comprehensive and Specialized Neuropsychological Assessments

Sample Comprehensive Assessments

Wechsler Adult Intelligence Scale- Revised (WAIS-R): Designed as a test of general intelligence. Consists of verbal and performance subscales. Verbal scale includes six tests which measure verbal functioning and reasoning: vocabulary, comprehension, similarities, arithmetic, digit span. Performance scale includes five speeded tests which measure psychomotor and perceptual integrative skills: picture completion, picture arrangement, digit symbol, object assembly, block design (Wechsler, 1945a; Wechsler, 1981).

Halstead-Reitan Battery (HRB): Designed to answer questions regarding brain-behavior relationships and is used as a comprehensive neuropsychological assessment (although lengthy). Subtests include Halstead category, factual performance, speech perception, finger tapping, seashore rhythm, Reitan aphasia screening, trailmaking A and B, perceptual disorders (Halstead, 1947; Goldstein, 1984).

Luria Nebraska Neuropsychological Battery (LNNB): Designed as a general neuropsychological assessment of brain injury based on the work of Luria. Consists of 269 items representing 11 content areas or subscales: motor, rhythm, tactile, visual, receptive speech, expressive speech, writing, reading, arithmetic, memory, intellectual (Golden, Hammeke, & Purisch, 1978; Golden, 1981).

Sample Specialized Assessments

Stroop Test: Measure of selective attention and inhibitory control sensitive to brain damage. Test consists of words (e.g., RED) printed in colors (e.g., green). Under various conditions task requires individual to name the color and ignore the word (Stroop, 1935; MacLeod, 1991).

Paced Auditory Serial Addition Test (PASAT): Measure of attentional control sensitive to subtle effects of brain injury. A series of digits are continuously presented and task requires individual to add each presented digit to the previous digit. Speed of presentation is also varied across trials (Gronwall, 1977).

Wechsler Memory Scale (WMS): Commonly used memory battery designed to assess various aspects of memory. Consists of six subscales: personal and current information, orientation, mental control, logical memory, visual reproduction, associate learning (Wechsler, 1945b).

Wisconsin Neuromemory Battery: General memory battery which includes tests associated with components of memory processes. Consists of 14 tests: selective reminding, word recognition, face recognition, recurring figures, 7-24 test, visual sequential coding, word learning, sentence recall, tri-word recall, paired associate, story recall, word fluency, token test, famous events (Grafman, 1984).

Benton Visual Retention Test (BVRT): Designed as a test of visual memory sensitive to brain damage. Consists of a number of geometric designs which the individual must view for a defined period and then reproduce from memory (Benton, 1974).

Verbal Fluency Tests: Designed as tests of speech production and word-finding ability for brain damage. Test requires individual to produce a response to a question (e.g., name as many words as you can that start with "s") in a certain period of time (Wertz, 1979).

Wisconsin Card Sorting Test (WCST): Designed as a test of mental flexibility and ability to shift response sets. Consists of a card sorting task which requires the individual to sort according to a principle which must be deduced from the examiner's feedback (correct or incorrect) after each trial. Considered to be sensitive to frontal lobe damage (Grant & Berg, 1948).

Raven's Progressive Matrices: Designed as a visual-spatial reasoning task which is free from cultural bias. Visual patterns are presented with one part removed and the individual is required to choose the correct pattern from a number of alternatives to complete the pattern (Raven, 1960).

Porteus Maze Test: Designed as a test of planning and foresight. The test consists of a set of visual mazes through which the individual must trace the correct path without going down a blind alley (Porteus, 1965).

as well as the clinical experiences of the authors. The outcome of the LOTCA is intended as a starting point for further assessment and/or occupational therapy intervention, or as a measure of clinical change. The test consists of a number of subtests (20) which fall under four general cognitive processes/abilities: orientation, perception, visuomotor organization, and thinking operations. Each subtest is scored on a 4- or 5-point scale. The LOTCA places heavy emphasis on visual perceptual skills, such as shape identification and block design, relative to cognitive skills such as attention and memory. For example, attention is assessed via one item (attention and concentration) which is scored on a 4-point scale. The LOTCA represents an assessment that is more "neuropsychological" than "functional" in nature. In fact, some of the subtests on the LOTCA are closely based upon tests from various neuropsychological batteries (e.g., copying geometric figures, block design, pictorial sequence). Given the neuropsychological nature of the LOTCA, it is interesting to note that it is being used in occupational therapy for not only assessment and a measure of clinical change, but also to guide OT treatment. Inherent in this approach is the assumption that these subcomponents of cognition are related to functional performance. However, as Abreu, Duval, Gerber, & Wood (1994) point out, this relationship is not necessarily causal and unidirectional.

The Rivermead Behavioral Memory Test (RBMT) was originally developed to assess memory impairment in individuals with brain damage (Wilson, Cockburn, & Baddeley, 1985). It was designed to identify individuals who may experience problems in everyday functioning due to their memory impairment. Thus, the 11 items were chosen to represent everyday situations which involve memory functioning (e.g., remembering names, appointments, routes, etc.), as well as two conventional memory tests (paired associates and digit span). Like the LOTCA, the RBMT is intended for initial assessment, monitoring clinical change, and guiding treatment. In some ways, the RBMT appears to be more functional in nature than the LOTCA since various items are more directly related to everyday memory situations and complaints of brain-damaged individuals. However, some items are quite similar to neuropsychological tests (e.g., orientation, prose recall). Thus, the RBMT still represents a performance component approach to assessment since it assesses subcomponents of memory impairment (e.g., prospective, immediate, long-term memory), yet items are intended to reflect everyday memory situations.

The contextual memory test (CMT) (Toglia, 1993) and the Toglia Category Assessment (Toglia, 1994b) are examples of bottom-up components of cognitive subskill tests that operationalize the process of providing cues to determine the underlying reasons for an individual's difficulty with a task. These tests are designed to help in determining the individual's performance and analyze his or her strategy based on a dynamic assessment. Both tests were originally developed to assess memory and categorization abilities of adults with a variety of diagnoses including that of acquired brain injury, and schizophrenia. Dynamic assessment is based on Vygotsky's (1978) principles that assume that the use of guidance and cues during testing can identify and discriminate a learning potential not identified by static or non-guided tests which do not use cueing.

Allen's (1985) evaluation strategy is to analyze and score an individual's cognitive performance during crafts and activities. She has developed a screening tool (leather lacing) called the Allen Cognitive Level (ACL) and the Allen Diagnostic Module (ADM) designed to verify the ACL score on six cognitive levels (Allen & Reyner, 1996). Within the ADM, 24 craft projects have been standardized and rated using expanded rating criteria for modes of performance that constitute a decimal system added to the original six cognitive levels (Allen, Earhart, & Blue, 1992). Allen proposes that the cognitive levels are related to functional outcomes for clients who have cognitive disabilities. Allen argues that use of cognitive levels can provide a guideline for predicting and determining the amount and type of assistance that an individual will require while performing activities of daily living.

Top-down Functional Approach

In contrast to a bottom-up performance component approach, a top-down approach to assessment is focused at a macro or functional level of analysis. In other words, cognition is not reduced to subcomponents in order to identify specific deficit areas, but instead cognitive functioning is inferred from everyday activities in order to identify abilities and deficits in occupational performance. It has been argued that assessment at the functional level will more readily guide OT intervention than assessment at the impairment level (Dunn, 1993; Fisher & Short-DeGraff, 1993). Functional cognitive assessment is often addressed in more nonstandardized ways through the use of interview and observation. For example, information regarding the impact of cognitive functioning on daily life tasks may be gleaned from an interview which addresses the client's inability to engage in certain activities and/or roles (e.g., DePoy & Burke, 1992; Kielhofner & Henry, 1988). Given the lack of insight which often accompanies cognitive impairment, interviews with family members also may be imperative (e.g., the Functional Behavior Profile; Baum, Edwards, & Morrow-Howell, 1993). The integrity of cognitive functioning also may be inferred from the observation of a client performing a particular task or activity. The Routine Task Inventory (RTI) (Allen, 1985; Earhart & Allen, 1988) assesses the cognitive level of disability observed while a client engages in routine tasks, such as bathing, grooming, etc.

Activity or task analysis will often reveal underlying cognitive problems, as well as the interaction of cognitive abilities with the physical and/or social environment which ultimately affect performance. Although such functional approaches do not necessarily address the specific underlying cognitive deficit, they may still provide adequate information necessary for a functional treatment approach (Toglia, 1992).

Recently, various assessments have been developed in occupational therapy which better reflect the top-down functional approach to measuring cognition. The Assessment of Motor and Process Skills (AMPS) was developed to assess an individual's ability to perform a functional daily life task (Fisher, 1992). Functional tasks (e.g., making a bed, vacuuming, etc.) are self-selected by the client, and the therapist examines performance in reference to 15 motor and 20 process skills. Motor skills reflect those skills based upon movement (e.g., posture, mobility, coordination, etc.), whereas process skills reflect those skills based upon cognition (e.g., attention, organization, initiation, etc.). Therapists must be trained in the use of the AMPS and the scoring involves a complex statistical procedure (Rasch analysis) which takes into account subject ability, item difficulty, and rater severity. Although the AMPS has been used for research purposes (e.g., Nygard, Bernspang, Fisher, & Winblad, 1994; Pan & Fisher, 1994; Park, Fisher, & Velozo, 1994), the clinical utility of the tool may be somewhat limited for these reasons.

The Kitchen Task Assessment (KTA) represents another more functionally based standardized assessment of cognition (Baum & Edwards, 1993). The KTA was developed for use with individuals with Alzheimer disease and examines the cognitive support necessary to complete a functional task (i.e., a cooking task). Clients perform a cooking task (e.g., making pudding), and performance is rated in terms of initiation, organization, performing all steps, sequencing, judgment and safety, and completion. The therapist bases this rating on a 4-point scale which reflects the level of assistance necessary to successfully complete the task. The KTA is unique in that it not only provides an assessment of client performance but also provides information to caregivers regarding the cognitive support necessary for functional performance. The KTA is designed to directly guide treatment planning with the family.

In a similar vein, the Rabideau Kitchen Evaluation-Revised (RKE-R) was designed as a functional meal preparation task for adults with traumatic brain injury (Neistadt, 1992). Performance is scored as a function of the component steps involved in the task (making a cold sandwich and hot beverage) and the amount of assistance needed to complete the task. In all of the abovementioned assessments, subcomponents of cognition are still being measured, yet they are observed during the performance of an everyday task. Thus, these more performance-based assessments provide informa-

tion regarding functional activities, as well as some of the cognitive components underlying impaired performance. Also these assessments can be administered in the context of the client's home environment to better assess the interplay among cognition, function, and the environment which is often missing in other standardized tests (see Spencer, Krefting, & Mattingly, 1993). These and other OT-developed assessments which reflect the topdown functional approach are presented in Table 11-2.

An Integrative Functional Approach to Assessment

An integrative assessment approach interfaces the micro or bottom-up assessment of performance components with a macro or top-down functional assessment of occupational performance. One assumption underlying this approach is that a relationship exists between the micro and macro levels of performance, and that this relationship is neither unidirectional nor causal (Wood, Abreu, Duval, & Gerber, 1994). If one considers a client's micro-capacity to attend, for example, one can readily understand the connection between attention and the performance of a more macro function such as driving a car. One can also readily understand that the macro-challenge of driving might be a powerful motivator to a young male who attends to driving better than he does to any other task. The micro-macro relationship is thus conceptualized as multidimensional and complex; it requires that therapists combine various methods, from which a more effective and personalized assessment can emerge (Abreu, 1992; 1994).

A certain artificiality involved in describing any assessment approach. A therapist, for purposes of analysis or education, will break down a process and name its components. In reality, most assessments that occur clinically consist of a therapist's moving fluidly among the various components; the interaction appears seamless. During the integrative approach to assessment the therapist moves back and forth from the micro to the macro elements that characterize the performance of the client. Both the approach and its use of micro and macro elements can be illustrated by a more specific example relating to cognition.

Assessment of cognition at the micro level aims to identify and analyze the information processing strategies used by the individual during specific cognitive tasks. This analysis occurs through a process of observing and recording the effects of modifications made to both the task and the environment as the individual performs. In addition to the therapist's analysis, and perhaps more necessary for a full micro assessment, is the collaborative identification of those characteristics in the environment that seem to be environmental regulators for the individual. Environmental regulators are those parameters such as people, objects, and conditions sur-

---

TABLE 11-2

Top-Down Functional Assessments Addressing Cognition

Assessment	Purpose
Assessment of Motor and Process Skills (AMPS) (Fisher, 1992)	assesses motor and cognitive skills in functional daily life tasks
Kitchen Task Assessment (KTA) (Baum & Edwards, 1993)	examines the cognitive support necessary to complete a cooking task
Rabideau Kitchen Evaluation—Revised (RKE-R) (Neistadt, 1992)	assesses cognitive functioning and assistance needed in a meal preparation task
Arnadottir OT-ADL Neurobehavioral Evaluation (A-ONE) (Arnadottir, 1990)	examines the link between neurobehavioral deficits and functional performance in daily activities
Cognitive Performance Test (CPT) (Burns, 1990)	assesses cognitive capabilities and limitations in daily life tasks
Structured Observational Test of Function (SOTOF) (Laver & Powell, 1995)	examines the link between perceptual and cognitive deficits and functional performance in basic self-care tasks

---

rounding the individual that seem to have a positive and/or negative effect on his or her achieving success in the task (Abreu, 1995; Gentile, 1987; Schmidt, 1988).

Evaluating Attention

Consider, for example, a therapist's evaluation of attention. One attentional task designed to investigate visual attention is the visual cancellation test from the Quadraphonic Approach (Abreu, 1992). This test measures an individual's ability to detect the presence of a particular stimulus; it can also be used to identify visual neglect. The test consists of three subtests, each containing 60 targets in a field of 300 stimuli. The 60 targets are randomly distributed into four quadrants so that each quadrant has a total of 15 targets (Figure 11-2). Notice that each subtest is the same. The only difference is that each subtest changes one of the surface characteristics (either number, letter, or shape) of the target stimuli. In this manner the client is given the opportunity to repeat the same task three times and demonstrate the performance effects from the repeated experience. The client is not told that it is the same test with only one surface characteristic changed.

The therapist presents the subtests in a predetermined sequence, asking the individual to find the target stimuli. The individual's performance is measured by recording the accuracy of detection, the time taken, and the type of strategy used during the completion of each subtest. Additionally, the individual's response to the use of contextual modifiers is noted in order to estimate the degree to which the client's perfor-

mance can be modified or changed. This aided performance using guidance and cues constitutes a dynamic interaction among the therapist, client, and task. Not all clients with brain injury increase accuracy or time, or improve their organizational visual scanning strategy after three repetitions; the locus of lesion, the recovery stage, and the diagnosis seem to have an effect on the performance (Abreu, 1992).

Contextual Modifications

The therapist also notes the contextual modifications that must be made so that the individual can perform. Contextual modifications are cues that can originate from three primary sources—the therapist, the task/environment, and the client —and from an interplay among them that occurs during task performance. Although clinically these modifications interact closely, it is important to articulate and distinguish them for purposes of evaluation, treatment, and research.

Conducting a Micro-Assessment

When assessing at the micro level the therapist repeats the task in an attempt to observe and identify the individual's training or any performance effects (improvements or decrements due to repetition) that occur during task completion. The performance effects are also investigated through question and answer exchanges and through a form of therapist probing that uses verbal and nonverbal as well as general and specific cues. For example, the therapist might ask the individual a question such as, "Was it easier for you to do this

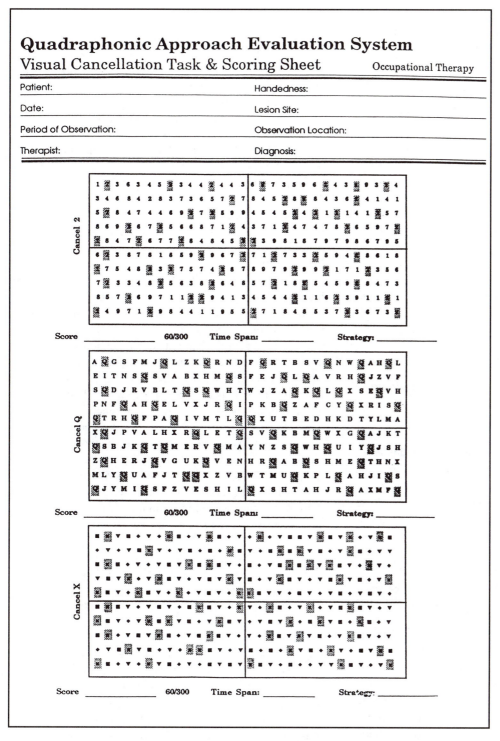

Figure 11-2. Visual cancellation task from the Quadraphonic Approach Evaluation. From Abreu, B. (1993). The quadrophonic approach: Supplemental handout to workshop sponsored by Therapeutic Service Systems. Reprinted with permission.

task?" The therapist then helps the individual become aware of his or her capacity for error detection and correction, knowledge of results and performance, impairments, and compensatory strategies. The results of this collaborative exchange establish the groundwork for developing an individualized treatment program. These contextual modifiers are documented in a narrative note because this type of information qualifies the individual's performance. Computer programs for qualitative data analysis are available to compare the status of the individual's performance upon admission with that upon discharge (Weitzman & Miles, 1995).

In order to rate and classify the micro-performance of an

individual, the therapist can define the skill being tested and specify a 100% performance level. One suggested method for determining such a performance level is to break the skill being tested (attention in this case) into equally or unequally rated/weighed parts. For example, attention to task at a 100% level may be defined as the ability to complete four attention tests (either standardized or nonstandardized), each valued at 25%. One nonstandardized example is: visual cancellation test (25%), modified stroop test (25%), auditory visual addition test (25%), and modified trail test (25%). The therapist can then rate performance in terms of a percentage. Further rating and categorization can then occur for purposes of placement in groups or measuring progress. Individuals who score 90% or above might be given a 7 on a scale of 7; those scoring 25% or below might be given a 1 on that same scale. These numerical assignments are documented because this type of information establishes the individual's program evaluation that compares admission and discharge status. Computer programs for quantitative data analysis are available to assess outcome goals (Statistical Package for the Social Sciences, 1992).

Conducting a Macro-Assessment

Assessment of an individual at the macro level turns to an examination of the individual's subjective sense of satisfaction and adaptation after a breach in health (Abreu, 1994; Trombly, 1993). For this element of the assessment, the therapist will rely on functional evaluations of the individual's real-life occupations and narrative communications from the individual and from family members. Through *interview* questions that prompt personal sharing, the therapist seeks to better understand the individual's personal story; the individual might be asked to bring personal documents, photographs, or meaningful objects that can enhance communication (Clark, 1993). Because brain injury can cause expressive and receptive disorders of communication, alternative methods of eliciting information are quite important. The use of narrative for the macro assessment helps to discover the way in which the individual makes sense of his or her life experiences (Polkinghorne, 1988; Riessman, 1993).

The integrative approach to assessment as it relates to cognition is thus a pulling together of the micro and macro aspects of performance in a way that reveals the individual's awareness of his or her cognition—whether in the realm of attention, decision-making, or problem-solving disability, use of adaptive and maladaptive strategies to process information, and use of compensatory strategies that replace a loss of function.

Because awareness of disability is an aspect of cognition, and because an individual's awareness of disability is important to this assessment approach and to any subsequent treatment, a more in-depth discussion of awareness is necessary.

Awareness

Most individuals are not completely aware of their individual strengths and weaknesses. However, if individuals are not adequately aware of their difficulties, their lack of awareness can result in poor life satisfaction, inadequate strategies for information processing and adaptation, and problems with communication, safety, and judgment (Abreu, 1981, 1992, 1993, 1994; Barco, Crosson, Bolesta, Werts, & Stout, 1991; Toglia, 1989, 1991, 1993, 1994). Some clinicians use the words *insight* and *anosognosia* to denote awareness of disability (Prigatano & Schacter, 1991; Weinstein, Friedland, & Wagner, 1994). Therapists must distinguish between awareness of disability and denial. In this chapter, denial refers to a conscious or unconscious reluctance to recognize deficits based on psychological factors (Barco et al., 1991; Lezak, 1978).

Awareness of disability refers more specifically to an individual's conscious or less conscious ability to recognize either his or performance deficits or those circumstances, people, or conditions that can cause danger, harm, or personal loss after a neurological injury. An individual's awareness of disability must be evaluated in all realms of intervention—whether rehabilitative, habilitative, or preventive—because an individual who is unaware of a deficit will do nothing to adapt to or compensate for the loss of function. The assessment of awareness of disability is documented in the literature on neuropsychology. One common method of assessing awareness is to have the individual complete a self-rating scale; the self-rating may relate to performances at both the micro and macro levels. The scores are then compared with those of the therapist and of a family member or caretaker. One therapist's way of rating awareness is presented in the awareness scale (Figure 11-3).

Individuals with cognitive impairments vary tremendously in their levels of awareness of disability. Because acquired brain injury includes such a variety of diagnoses as traumatic brain injury, stroke, brain tumor, encephalitis, anoxia, and Alzheimer disease, variance in levels of awareness might be predicted (DeLuca, 1992; Gasquoine & Gibbons, 1994; Prigatano, Altman, & O'Brien, 1990; Prigatano & Schacter, 1991; Seltzer, Vasterling, Hale, & Khurana, 1995; Vasterling, Seltzer, Foss, & Vanderbrook, 1995). Brain injury can lead to profound disturbances in performing daily routines. Perhaps the most disturbing consequence of neurological damage for some individuals is the cognitive awareness that once-effortless daily routines have become difficult or nearly impossible (Kihlstrom & Tobias, 1991). These individuals may communicate a great sense of despair. On the other hand, other individuals suffer from the opposite problem; they lack awareness of any difficulty. The level of awareness of an individual will affect treatment significantly.

AWARENESS SCREEN/MACRO---CLIENT'S ANSWERS

ID#:_____ Age:_____ [ ]Male [ ]Female DATE:_____

TEST: [ ] Initial [ ]Mid-Stay [ ]Discharge Therapist ID Code:_____

STATEMENT: "Today I am going to test your awareness of how well you feel you can....
[ ] Physically care for yourself [bathe, groom, dress, feed/eat, housekeeping, laundry]
[ ] Shop, cook, prepare meals
[ ] Find your way around your environment [your house, neighborhood, hospital proper]
[ ] Manage money or perform banking functions

IA: "Are you aware of any changes in your ability to perform this function since your injury?"
[ ] No [ ] Yes   Do you feel you will have a :
How well do you predict you will do?   [ ] Perfect score
                                                  [ ] Almost perfect score
[ ] 100% Accurate   [ ] Very good score
[ ] 75% Accurate   [ ] Slightly above average score
[ ] 50% Accurate   [ ] Average score
[ ] 25% Accurate   [ ] Below average score
[ ] Less than 25% Accurate.   [ ] Poor score

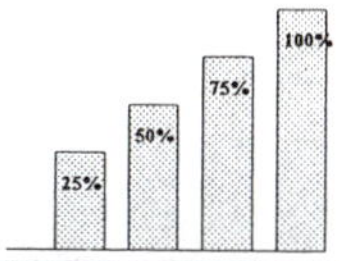

ADMINISTER THE TEST:

EA "How well do you think you did on the test?"   Do you feel your score was ...
[ ] 100% Accurate   [ ] Perfect score
[ ] 75% Accurate   [ ] Almost perfect score
[ ] 50% Accurate   [ ] Very good score
[ ] 25% Accurate   [ ] Slightly above average score
[ ] Less than 25% Accurate.   [ ] Average score
                                                  [ ] Below average score
                                                  [ ] Poor score

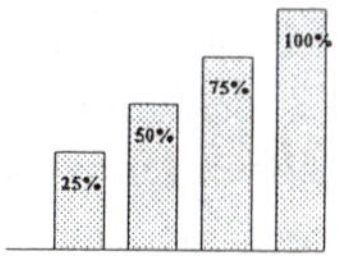

ACTUAL TEST RESULTS WERE:

AA :How do you think your performance might impact your ability to live independently, work and have fun?
[ ] I will be independent.
[ ] I will be independent if my environment is modified.
[ ] I will not need physical assistance but, need to be supervised about 20% of the time?
[ ] I will need actual assistance, from a person, for about 25% of my needs.
[ ] I will need actual assistance, from a person, for about 50% of my needs.
[ ] I will need actual assistance, from a person, for about 75% of my needs.
[ ] I will need actual assistance, from a person, for most of my needs.

Awareness is the ability of having or showing realization, perception or knowledge of disability."

Intellectual Awareness(IA): The client's ability to understand, at some level, that a particular function in impaired."

Does the client need explanation, coaching and demonstration of deficit areas during evaluation/treatment?

Emergent Awareness(EA): The client's ability to recognize a problem when it is occurring."

Anticipatory Awareness(AA): The client's ability to anticipate a problem will occur as a result of some deficit."

(Crosson, et al, 1989)

Figure 11-3. Awareness Scale. From Abreu, B. (1993). The quadraphonic approach: Supplemental handout to workshop sponsored by Therapeutic Service Systems. Reprinted with permission.

Treatment: Learning as Therapy

Although learning has been defined in broad terms, the process is not a single or all-or-none phenomenon (Schwartz, 1985). Learning can be conceptualized as either a series or family of functions that can create a relatively *permanent change* in an individual's behavior as a consequence of an experience (Kandel, 1976; Schmidt & Bjork, 1992).

Some therapists advocate a dichotomy of treatment—remedial vs. adaptive—stating that the decision to pursue one approach over the other is based on the individual's learning capabilities. The large assumption that supports this approach is that occupational therapists are able to precisely assess an individual's learning potential through a nontraditional technique called dynamic assessment (Toglia, 1989, 1991, 1992, 1993). The suggestion is that individuals should be treated differently based on their learning capacities.

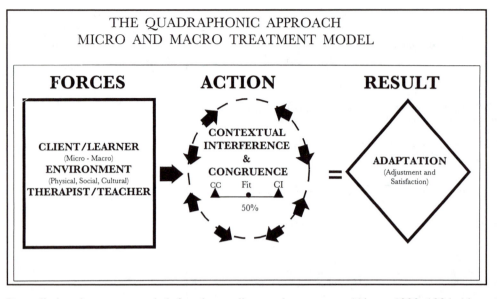

Figure 11-4. Environmental fit treatment model.

Remediation is recommended for those clients who can engage in abstract learning, whereas functional adaptation is suggested for those who rely on association or representational learning (Neistadt, 1993a, 1993b, 1993c, 1994; Toglia, 1991, 1992). This approach matches an individual's capacity to learn information with a preferred treatment.

Other clinicians advocate a more integrative approach that combines interventions that address both macro and micro levels of functioning (Abreu, 1992, 1994; Wood et al., 1994). The premise that underlies this approach is that the capacity to process information is not the sole determinant of treatment. Each individual's larger capacity to act, adapt, and use compensatory strategies, along with his or her own personal goals and satisfaction with various learning strategies, should factor into treatment. All of these variables need to be considered so that treatment consists of an intervention that is multidimensional and client-centered.

Porn's (1984, 1993) model for effective adaptation proposes that any learning of new behaviors, attitudes, and values occurs subsequent to a state of disequilibrium among three areas: the individuals' will/goals/agency, the individual's potential for action, and the opportunities for action (Abreu, 1994; Wood et al., 1994). Treatment based on this model aims to help the individual achieve effective adaptation and personal satisfaction. An individual's adaptation has been defined as those changes that make behaviors and attitudes more congruent with the new internal and external demands that follow disease, trauma, loss, or stress (Abreu, 1994). Satisfaction is defined as an individual's being in a state of equilibrium relative to his or her real and ideal capacity to function on the day to day.

Based on this approach, an integrative treatment plan will match the individual's capacities with opportunities for action in three types of environments: physical, social, and cultural. The matching process is called the environmental fit

(Abreu, 1992, 1994; Abreu & Hinojosa, 1992) (Figure 11-4). As an integral part of traditional task analysis, the therapist examines the physical characteristics of the environment. The analysis is done in order to create the most effective context within which the individual can generalize learning, make contextual modifications, and thus progress from training to function (Abreu, 1981; Abreu & Toglia, 1987). Because treatment is a collaborative process, the therapist will ask the individual to consider any proposed task to determine whether it is meaningful. A similar collaboration will include members of the family and community who will participate in a team approach to treatment alongside representatives from the professional disciplines involved in the case. The bottom-up or micro approach reflects a biomedical rehabilitation model in contrast to the top-down or macro approach that reflects a client-centered and community-based rehabilitation model of practice. The reader is referred to Chapter 21 for a review of these rehabilitation models. The case that follows represents the combination of bottom-up and top-down evaluations and intervention strategies that characterizes the integrative approach.

Case Example

Anna is a 50-year-old occupational therapist who suffered a traumatic head injury during a car accident. She is married, with two sons attending graduate school. Prior to this event, she jointly owned and managed a rehabilitation service company with her husband, a physical therapist, within a Jewish community in New York. Immediately after her injury, her husband assumed her managerial role in addition to providing direct care to clients in one of their offices. Her sons were out of state, John attending law school in California and Harry attending medical school in Texas.

Anna's acute care was received at a hospital where she

remained for 6 weeks while her medical conditions were stabilized. She was transferred to an inpatient rehabilitation unit where she remained for 8 weeks. She received occupational therapy services and became independent in the basic elements of self-care and was able to walk without devices. She was then transferred to a community re-entry center where her ability to fulfill her role as a business manager, wife, and community member were to be assessed and facilitated.

Information from Occupational Therapy Services

Anna's selective attention, speed of information processing, and vigilance or sustained attention were impaired. She showed failure to anticipate and to appreciate consequences, poor organization, narrowed attention, failure to maintain set, impersistence, and poor error recognition and correction; she benefited from feedback. The occupational therapist referred to the speech/language and the neuropsychology department reports for further information about her cognitive skills.

Information from Speech/Language Services

Prosody and speaking rate: prosody is the appropriate variation in pitch, loudness, duration, and rate during speech production. Anna displayed very minimal prosodic variations, characterized by both monopitch and monoloudness. Her typical conversational speaking rate was functional. Anna's reduced prosody could have been related to a relatively flat affect. She demonstrated near-normal prosodic variations when talking about topics of great interest to her. It was not likely that her volume would improve as Anna had always been soft-spoken. However, it did not affect her ability to communicate. She did not need speech language pathology services.

Information from Neuropsychology Services

Intellectual functioning: Anna obtained a full scale IQ score of 90 on the WAIS-R (verbal IQ 110; performance IQ 66), which placed her in the average range of intellectual functioning. However, there was a significant discrepancy between her verbal and performance IQ scores, suggesting a dissociation between verbal and nonverbal intellectual functioning. Memory and attention: Retrograde amnesia was estimated at several days. Anna was oriented to person, but not to place and time, misstating her location as well as the date, month, or day of the week. She was not able to name the current president. Immediate auditory attention was mildly defective. Anna was able to repeat a maximum of 5 digits forward and 3 digits backward. Simple mental control was quick and without errors. Rote verbal learning was severely defective, with no improvement in learning across several trials. Free recall of the same rote verbal material following an interference task was severely defective. Immediate cued structured recall was severely defective. Free delayed recall of the same material was severely defec-

tive. As with immediate recall, cued structured delayed recall yielded no significant improvement and was also severely defective. Presentation of the same material in a recognition format yielded only modest improvement in recall, suggesting compromised encoding of rote verbal information. Several intrusion errors were noted, suggesting a mild tendency to confabulate in the recall of previously learned material.

Immediate memory for meaningful verbal material was moderately defective. Delayed recall of the same material was severely defective with no memories recalled, suggesting decay. Immediate memory for simple drawings was average, while delayed recall of the same material was defective with no reproduced memories, suggesting decay. Copy of a complex geometric design was also defective, as were immediate and delayed reproduction of the same design, suggesting a decreased ability to reproduce and recall complex visual material.

In summary, at the microlevel of occupational functioning, Anna's capacity for action was limited due to disturbances in attention, memory, and executive functioning that included the capacity for anticipating consequences, establishing goals, planning, organizing, initiating, executing activities, and self-monitoring and correcting errors.

As soon as she was admitted to the transitional center, Anna began to ask when could she go home. Her rehabilitation team explained that she was unsafe alone, and Anna was given daily psychological counseling and support to help her process the information emotionally. Anna was concerned that she was at the rehabilitation unit, and although she thought that she would rather be at home, she decided to engage in the rehabilitation process, but for 2 months only.

Anna's goals were to be able to function independently and to be able to manage her business with her husband. Although the work goal was considered questionable by her family, the rehabilitation team decided to start training and to re-evaluate the results in 2 months. The usual timetable (or critical pathway) for independence in work training at this unit is 120 days.

The specific treatment environment used by Anna included: her semi-private apartment room complete with bathroom shower and kitchen, the group modules treatment room, the therapist's private office, the occupational therapy kitchen, the treatment unit's leisure room which included a pool table, and large-screen TV and stereo system, the unit patio, the grounds of the unit which included a greenhouse and a gardening and picnic area, two neighboring shopping malls, a neighboring church, and the unit's cars and vans. Anna's occupational therapy consisted of one-on-one treatment and group treatments with up to 6 other clients and a facilitator (therapist/certified assistant/aide) from the occupational therapy staff.

The center uses a variety of therapeutic interventions which in Anna's case included the opportunities for restoration and for alternating adaptation with prevention and with the creation of a range of performances in keeping with her will and goals (Dunn, Brown, & McGuigan, 1994; Dunn, Brown, McClain, & Westman, 1994). With respect to sociocultural environments, Anna had a very nurturing relationship with her husband and sons; they were a very supportive and caring family. She also had many friends, relatives, and colleagues who were available and provided support.

One Occupational Therapy Treatment Intervention

The following section presents a sampling of one treatment module addressing money management. Commentary inserted throughout this sampling illustrates the clinical reasoning of the therapist relative to the micro and macro elements of Anna's treatment. It is hoped that interspersing these comments within the description of the treatment module will communicate a sense of the fluid movement of a therapist's reasoning as it occurs during the intervention process. These comments represent the therapist's reflections on the frame of reference, the therapeutic techniques, and the therapist's attempts to personalize the occupational therapy program for the client. At this point, the reader may benefit from reviewing Chapter 7 on clinical reasoning.

Money management group occurred from 9:00 to 10:00 once a week. Money management issues were also handled in other one-on-one sessions in occupational therapy, neuropsychology, speech and language, and leisure therapy. To target cognitive deficits at both the micro and macro levels the group was occupation-based, having as its central focus a weekly trip to the bank.

> Remember that Anna is a real person confronting a complex adaptive challenge in her life. Although Anna shows specific impairments in cognitive components, these impairments are interfaced with many other components and dimensions in her life. Recognize that cognitive performance is integrated into Anna's actions within her physical, social, and cultural environments. Her expectations for performance and her control of her performance vary. As a team we must provide as many opportunities for adaptive and satisfying action as we can.

Daily documentation in occupational therapy used a 7-point scale to address the following cognitive issues: use of adaptive strategies, verbal and task initiation, organizational skills, and problem solving. Therapists recorded Anna's performance at admission (initial level or IL) and at discharge (discharge level or DL). This money management evaluation strip is a portion of the evaluation/discharge form that was added to Anna's chart.

7.0=Independent	100%
6.0=Modified Independence	90%
5.0=Supervised Assistance	80%
4.0=Minimal Assistance	75%
3.0=Moderate Assistance	50%
2.0=Maximum Assistance	25%
1.0=Dependent	0%

At the time of admission, the neuropsychology department on this unit provided all clients with a three-ring notebook to use as a functional memory tool. The notebook included a monthly calendar, a daily schedule, and a to-do list to enable weekly planning for leisure activities, shopping, basic need-satisfying activities, and meal preparation.

> Remember that Anna's budget is very complex and large because she was managing a very successful therapist placement agency and a private office. She owned the building within which the office was housed. The money management group was working out of her societal context.

The group began with introductions of the group's goals and a review of individual goals. There were 7 goals for individuals in this group: 1) demonstrate coin knowledge; 2) do mathematical calculations (mental, paper/pencil, and calculator); 3) make change; 4) reconcile a checkbook; 5) complete banking transactions; and 6) budget and develop compensatory strategies for money management.

> Anna benefits from compensatory external aids for memory, using checklists, outlines, calendar planners, and the memory notebook given by the neuropsychology department. She also benefits from the use of the pillbox organizer given by her case manager, labels and cue cards on the cabinet, the alarm clock, and her alarm watch which helps her orient to time, date, and appointments.

Anna's perceptual/cognitive capacities were simultaneously retrained and counterbalanced by providing environmental modifications to compensate for her micro impairments and to simultaneously attend to her more macro functional limitations in her physical, social, and cultural environments.

> Anna can benefit from metacognitive training. The training requires competency in communication, which Anna has. This technique is an interactive instructional training method used to increase a client/learner's introspection skills. The training uses questions, probes, and conscious verbal reflections about any money management issues that occur in reference to self (person), goal (task), and action (strategy.) These reflections intend to heighten awareness about specific and individual problems.

Anna was given the opportunity to make change, a task requiring coin knowledge and mathematical calculations.

> Divide your observations into those related to compensatory, behavioral management, and cognitive self-management strategies for better documentation of progress.

Anna had visual acuity problems: She required that all printed material be enlarged to a print size equivalent to 20/100 acuity on the Snellen chart. In addition, the lighting and illumination conditions were increased in both the OT unit and her apartment trial room. Anna used her glasses, and a variety of magnifiers were also available in the group.

> Remember that postural control and positioning can enhance performance in vision and cognitive skills.

Talking calculators with large numbers were also made available to her.

> Anna needs to bypass the deficit area and to use certain strategies for successful adaptation for living skills, work, and leisure.

Anna was given the opportunity to handle cash, a community checking account, and later, her own personal checking account. Banking tasks included check writing, checkbook reconciliation, and going to the bank to make her financial transactions. Anna got lost frequently in walking to the bank if she went unescorted. This problem would also negatively affect her driving skills.

> Anna cannot benefit from using "vanishing cues," a technique in which the individual tries to learn a specific task or skill through rote repetition. The task is practice and practice with the gradual fading of cues given.

Finally, this module provided opportunities for budgeting that included Anna's personal plan to adjust her weekly expenses at the center to the fixed income of $200.00 a month per client provided through the training module. Budgeted items included her personal needs such as shampoo, deodorant, and groceries for the week and funds for the weekend leisure activities.

> Anna's intensive-remedial training in this module is not generalizing to everyday life situations.

Anna's strategy of planning ahead and checking her mathematical calculations was not effective. She was unable to detect or correct errors spontaneously. Her performance in money management deteriorated when we decreased the structure or external cues for the task involved.

Anna was trained to do some planning and self-monitoring when cued. She was unable to use self-generated strategies. She was trained to group things together (chunk) and use association strategies such as relating item-place-price.

> Remember that although information-processing theory predicts that task difficulty is determined by the demands of the task on the nervous system, other theories need to explain the fact that Anna can process complex information in quilt-making (one of her favorite hobbies) but not in money management (one of her work roles). She seemed to put more personal effort in the quilt making than in the money management training.

Anna's visit to her office with the goal of role simulation of money management challenges was unsuccessful. She showed no awareness of errors or disability. Her husband and co-workers were supportive but were surprised to see the degree of cognitive impairments she had because she appeared physically healthy.

Clinical considerations relative to Anna's *restorative interventions* included the following questions:

1. Could Anna benefit from scaffolding? Scaffolding refers to the support the therapist provides so that the client can succeed in performing a task.
2. Could Anna benefit from constant feedback (100%) or less frequent feedback (50%)?
3. Could Anna benefit from knowledge of performance as well as from knowledge of results? Knowledge of performance refers to augmented feedback related to the nature of the movement patterns produced. Knowledge of results refers to the nature of the results produced in terms of environmental goals.
4. Could Anna benefit from cognitive self-management training strategies? This treatment uses an externally generated program of direct instructions and prompts for attention and memory and then leads to self-instructional training. It fosters self-talk or verbal self-regulation.
5. Could Anna benefit from behavioral management? This treatment strategy modifies specific behaviors with the use of adequate stimulus, reinforcement, and response cost to facilitate specific responses and/or inappropriate behaviors.
6. Could Anna benefit from compensatory strategies assuming her attention and memory functions are difficult or almost impossible to retrain?
7. Could Anna benefit from forward chaining or reverse chaining? These treatment strategies focus training on the sequence of a given task. Forward chaining trains the client to learn the steps of the task as they occur in their natural sequence. Reverse chaining refers to training the client to first learn the last step in the sequence.
8. She improved her performance in attention and memory drills only when she was given directed instructions or explicit prompts to use the previously trained memory strategies. Could Anna benefit from attention and memory drills with use of contextual modifications?
9. Anna showed limited evidence that she was able to apply the strategies independently in a novel situation. Her unawareness of disability was a factor in not achieving optimal re-training and compensatory strategies. Could Anna's unawareness of disability limit her ability to achieve optimal retraining and compensatory strategies?

At this treatment unit, when the rehabilitation process or trial period ends there is a graduation ritual. The trainees talk about their past, present, and future for 15 minutes. Anna prepared her speech with the neuropsychology and occupational therapy staff. When presenting at rehearsal she repeated her speech 3 times without realizing that she had repeated it. Because we videotaped rehearsal and she saw the video, on that day she was aware of her cognitive disability.

Anna was unable to return to her business in the same capacity. Her physical, social, and cultural environments were all a supporting factor in her rehabilitation. She was able to reconstruct her life with different roles and responsibilities. Anna continues to experience the chronic condition of cognitive disabilities after brain injury. She remains stable, and she is fairly satisfied with her performance and follow-up rehabilitation services that check on her compensatory and preventive strategies every 3 months.

This intervention with Anna is offered as a representative sampling of the manner in which the integrative approach occurs in one setting among individuals with acquired brain injury. Any therapist who has gained experience in this practice arena understands the need for caution in claiming a "best way" to approach the complexities of cognitive disability.

CONCLUSION

Ben-Yishay and Diller (1993) summarize their perspective in a review article:

Cognitive rehabilitation is both a theoretical concept as well as a body of remedial intervention techniques, and it is still evolving. It would be premature to draw definite conclusions regarding its validity and use for rehabilitation purposes based on the current evidence. (p. 204)

Occupational therapy is more than merely a process of learning strategies that allow one to adapt. Occupational therapy is also about *satisfaction, self-efficacy,* and *interdependent relationships* and functions. For this reason, occupational therapy practice, particularly in the area of cognitive disability, remains more of an art than a science. An integrative approach that moves back and forth between a consideration of the bottom-up and top-down performance of the individual is one way to enact the art as well as the science of practice.

STUDY QUESTIONS

1. Discuss the relationship between cognition and occupational performance.

2. Identify the three components of attention.

3. Compare and contrast: short-term vs. long-term memory, episodic vs. semantic memory, retrospective vs. prospective memory, explicit vs. implicit memory, declarative vs. procedural memory.

4. Describe the bottom-up performance component approach to cognitive assessment.

5. Identify three cognitive assessments which reflect the bottom-up approach.

6. Describe the top-down functional approach to cognitive assessment.

7. Identify three cognitive assessments which reflect the top-down approach.

8. Describe the integrative functional approach to assessment.

9. Describe the integrative functional approach to intervention.

10. Prepare a case study utilizing the integrative approach to assessment and intervention.

RECOMMENDED READING

Abreu, B., & Price-Lackey, P. (1994). Documentation and additional consideration. In C. B. Royeen (Ed.), *AOTA self-study series: Cognitive rehabilitation.* Rockville, MD: American Occupational Therapy Association.

Allen, C. K., Earhart, C. A., & Blue, T. (1992). *Occupational therapy treatment goals for the physically and cognitively disabled.* Rockville, MD: American Occupational Therapy Association.

Anderson, S. W., & Tranel, D. (1989). Awareness of disease states following cerebral infraction, dementia, and head trauma: Standardized assessment. *Clinical Neuropsychology, 3*, 327-339.

Arnadottir, G. (1990). *The brain and behavior: Assessing cortical dysfunction through activities of daily living (ADL).* St. Louis: C. V. Mosby Company.

Bisiach, E., Valler, G., Perani, D., Pagagno, C., & Berti, A. (1986). Unawareness or disease following lesions of the right hemisphere: Anosognosia for hemiplegia and anosognosia for hemianopia. *Neuropsychologia, 24*, 471-482.

Christiansen, C. (1994). *Ways of living: Self-care strategies for special needs.* Rockville, MD: American Occupational Therapy Association.

Christiansen, C., & Baum, C. (Eds.). (1991). *Occupational therapy: Overcoming human performance deficits.* Thorofare, NJ: SLACK Incorporated.

Cicerone, K. D., & Giacino, J. T. (1992). Remediation of executive function deficits after traumatic brain injury. *NeuroRehabilitation, 2*(3), 12-22.

Deaton, A. V. (1986). Denial in the aftermath of traumatic head injury: Its manifestations, measurement, and treatment. *Rehabilitation Psychology, 31*(4), 231-240.

Druckman, D., & Bjork, R. A. (Eds.). (1991). *In the mind's eye: Enhancing human performance.* Washington, DC: National Academy Press.

Druckman, D., & Bjork, R. A. (Eds.). (1994). *Learning, remembering, believing: Enhancing human performance.* Washington, DC: National Academy Press.

Giles, G. M., & Clark-Wilson, J. (1993). *Brain injury rehabilita-*

tion: A neurofunctional approach. San Diego, CA: Singular Publishing Group, Inc.

Graham, J. R., & Lilly, R. S. (1984). *Psychological testing.* Englewood Cliffs, NJ: Prentice-Hall, Inc.

Heaton, R. K., & Pendleton, M. G. (1981). Use of neuropsychological tests to predict adult patients' everyday functioning. *Journal of Consulting and Clinical Psychology, 49,* 807-821.

Ingvar, D. H. (1985). Memory of the future: An essay on the temporal organization of conscious awareness. *Human Neurobiology, 4,* 127-136.

Kaplan, C. P., & Corrigan, J. D. (1994). The relationship between cognition and functional independence in adults with traumatic brain injury. *Archives of Physical Medicine and Rehabilitation, 75,* 643-647.

Katz, N. (Ed.). (1992). *Cognitive rehabilitation: Models for intervention in occupational therapy.* Stoneham, MA: Butterworth-Heinemann.

Lam, C. S., McMahon, B. T., Priddy, D. A., & Gehred-Schultz, A. (1988). Deficit awareness and treatment performance among traumatic head injury adults. *Brain Injury, 2*(3), 233-242.

Levin, H. S., Eisenberg, H. M., & Benton, A. L. (Eds.). (1991). *Frontal lobe function and dysfunction.* New York: Oxford University Press.

Lister, M. J. (Ed.). (1991). *Contemporary management of motor control problems.* Alexandria, VA: Foundation for Physical Therapy.

Mattingly, C., & Fleming, M. H. (1994). *Clinical reasoning: Forms of inquiry in a therapeutic practice.* Philadelphia, PA: F. A. Davis.

McGlynn, S. M., & Schacter, D. L. (1989). Unawareness of deficits in neuropsychological syndromes. *Journal of Clinical and Experimental Neuropsychology, 11,* 143-205.

Neistadt, M. E. (1989). Normal adult performance on constructional praxis training tasks. *American Journal of Occupational Therapy, 43*(7), 448-455.

Neistadt, M. E. (1991). Occupational therapy treatments for constructional deficits. *American Journal of Occupational Therapy, 45,* 225-233.

Neistadt, M. E. (1992). Occupational therapy treatments for constructional deficits. *American Journal of Occupational Therapy, 46*(2), 141-148.

Nockelby, D. M., & Deaton, A. V. (1987). Denial versus distress: Coping patterns in post head trauma patients. *International Journal of Clinical Neuropsychology, IX*(4), 145-148.

Psathas, G. (1995). *Conversation analysis: The study of talk-in-interaction* (Vol. 35). Thousand Oaks, CA: Sage Publications.

Reber, A. S. (1993). *Implicit learning and tacit knowledge: An essay on the cognitive unconscious.* New York: Oxford University Press.

Sohlberg, M. M., & Mateer, C. A. (1989). *Introduction to cognitive rehabilitation: Theory and practice.* New York: Guilford Press.

Sunderland, A., Harris, J. E., & Baddeley, A. D. (1983). Do laboratory tests predict everyday memory? A neuropsychological study. *Journal of Verbal Learning and Verbal Behavior, 22,* 341-357.

Sunderland, A., Harris, J. E., & Gleave, J. (1984). Memory failures in everyday life following severe head injury. *Journal of Clinical Neuropsychology, 6,* 127-142.

Van Zomeren, A. H., Brouwer, W. H., Rothengatter, J. A., & Snock, J. W. (1988). Fitness to drive a car after recovery from severe head injury. *Archives of Physical Medicine and Rehabilitation, 69,* 90-96.

Weinstein, A. (1988). In W. H. Burke, M. Wesolowski, & W. F. Blackerby (Eds.), *Head injury rehabilitation: Management of memory disorders* (Vol. 8). Houston, TX: HDI Publishers.

Wilson, B. A. (1987). *Rehabilitation of memory.* New York: Guilford Press.

Wilson, B. A., & Moffat, N. (Eds.). (1984). *Clinical management of memory problems.* London: Aspen Systems Corporation.

Winstein, C. J., & Schmidt, R. A. (1990). Reduced frequency of knowledge of results enhances motor skill learning. *Journal of Experimental Psychology: Learning Memory Cognition, 16,* 677-691.

Ylvisaker, M., Szekeres, S. F., Henry, K., et al. (1987). Topics in cognitive rehabilitation therapy. In M. Ylvisaker & E. M. R. Gobble (Eds.), *Community re-entry for head injured adults* (pp. 137-220). Boston: Little, Brown.

Ylvisaker, M., & Szekeres, S. F. (1989). Metacognitive and executive impairments in head-injured children and adults. *Topics in Language Disorders, 9*(2), 34-49.

REFERENCES

Abreu, B. C. (1981). Interdisciplinary approach to adult visual perceptual function. Dysfunction continuum. In B. C. Abreu (Ed.), *Physical disabilities manual* (pp. 151-181). New York: Raven Press.

Abreu, B. C. (1992). The quadraphonic approach: Management of cognitive-perceptual and postural control dysfunction. *Occupational Therapy Practice, 3*(4), 12-29.

Abreu, B. C. (1993). *The quadraphonic approach: Supplemental handout to workshop sponsored by Therapeutic Service Systems.* New York: Therapeutic Service Systems.

Abreu, B. C. (1994). Perceptual motor skills. In C. B. Royeen (Ed.), *AOTA self-study series: Cognitive rehabilitation.* Rockville, MD: American Occupational Therapy Association.

Abreu, B. C. (1995). The effect of environmental regulations on postural control after stroke. *American Journal of Occupational Therapy, 49,* 517-525.

Abreu, B. C., Duval, M., Gerber, D., & Wood, W. (1994). Occupational performance and the functional approach. In C. B. Royeen (Ed.), *AOTA self-study series: Cognitive rehabilitation.* Rockville, MD: American Occupational Therapy Association.

Abreu, B. C., & Hinojosa, J. (1992). Process approach for cognitive-perceptual and postural control dysfunction for adults with brain injury. In N. Katz (Ed.), *Cognitive rehabilitation: Models for intervention in occupational therapy.* Stoneham, MA: Butterworth-Heinemann.

Abreu, B. C., & Toglia, J. P. (1987). Cognitive rehabilitation: An occupational therapy model. *American Journal of Occupational*

Therapy, 41, 439-448.

Alexander, M. P., & Freedman, M. (1984). Amnesia after anterior communicating artery aneurysm rupture. *Neurology, 34,* 752-757.

Allen, C. K. (1985). *Occupational therapy for psychiatric diseases: Measurement and management of cognitive disabilities.* Boston: Little, Brown and Company.

Allen, C. K., Earhart, C. A., & Blue, T. (1992). *Treatment goals for the physically and cognitively disabled.* Rockville, MD: American Occupational Therapy Association.

Allen, C. K., & Reyner, A. (1996). *How to start using the Allen diagnostic module: A guide to introducing Allen's theories into your practice.* Colchester, CT: S&S Worldwide.

Andiel, C., & Lui, L. (1995). Working memory and older adults: Implications for occupational therapy. *American Journal of Occupational Therapy, 49,* 681-686.

Arnadottir, G. (1990). *The brain and behavior: Assessing cortical dysfunction through activities of daily living (ADL).* St. Louis: Mosby.

Baddeley, A. D., Logie, R., Bressi S., Della Sala, S., & Spinnler, H. (1986). Dementia and working memory. *Quarterly Journal of Experimental Psychology, 38A,* 603-618.

Baddeley, A. D., & Hitch, G. J. (1974). Working memory. In G. H. Bower (Ed.), *The psychology of learning and motivation* (Vol. 8). New York: Academic Press.

Balota, D. A., & Duchek, J. M. (1991). Semantic priming effects, lexical repetition effects, and contextual disambiguation effects in healthy aged individuals and individuals with senile dementia of the Alzheimer type. *Brain & Language, 40,* 181-201.

Barco, P. P., Crosson, B., Bolesta, M. M., Werts, D., & Stout, R. (1991). Training awareness and compensation in post-acute head injury rehabilitation. In J. Kreutzer & P. Wehman (Eds.), *Cognitive rehabilitation for persons with traumatic brain injury: A functional approach* (pp. 129-146). Baltimore: Paul H. Brookes.

Baum, C. M., & Edwards, D. F. (1993). Cognitive performance in senile dementia of the Alzheimer's type: A kitchen task assessment. *American Journal of Occupational Therapy, 47,* 431-436.

Baum, C. M., Edwards, D. F., & Morrow-Howell, N. (1993). Identification and measurement of productive behaviors in senile dementia of the Alzheimer type. *The Gerontologist, 33,* 403-408.

Ben-Yishay, Y., & Diller, L. (1993). Cognitive remediation in traumatic brain injury: Update and issues. *Archives of Physical Medicine and Rehabilitation, 74,* 204-213.

Ben-Yishay, Y., Rattok J., & Diller, L. (1979). A clinical strategy for the systematic amelioration of attentional disturbances in severe head trauma patients. In Y. Ben-Yishay (Ed.), *Working approaches to remediation of cognitive deficits in brain damaged persons.* NYU Medical Center, Rehabilitation Monograph No. 60, pp. 1-27.

Benton, A. L. (1974). *The revised visual retention test* (4th ed.). New York: Psychological Corp.

Botwinick, J., Storandt, M., & Berg, L. (1986). A longitudinal, behavioral study of senile dementia of the Alzheimer's type. *Archives of Neurology, 43,* 1124-1127.

Bruer, J. T. (1993). *Schools for thought.* Cambridge, MA: MIT Press.

Burns, T. (1990). The cognitive performance test: A new tool for assessing Alzheimer's disease. *OT Week,* December 27. Rockville, MD: American Occupational Therapy Association.

Cermak, L. S., Verfaellie, M., & Chase, K. (1995). Implicit and explicit memory in amnesia: An analysis of data-driven and conceptually driven processes. *Neuropsychology, 9,* 281-290.

Clark, F. (1993). *Occupation imbedded in real life: Interweaving occupational science and occupational therapy.* Eleanor Slagle Lecture presented at the American Occupational Therapy Association 73rd Annual Conference & Exposition. Seattle, WA.

Cohen, J. D., & Servan-Schreiber, D. (1992). Context, cortex, and dopamine: A connectionist approach to behavior and biology of schizophrenia. *Psychological Review, 99,* 45-77.

Cohen, N. J., & Squire, L. R. (1980). Preserved learning and retention of pattern-analyzing skill in amnesia: Dissociation of knowing how and knowing that. *Science, 210,* 207-210.

Craik, F. I. M., & Jennings, J. M. (1992). Human memory. In F. I. M. Craik & T. A. Salthouse (Eds.), *The handbook of aging and cognition.* Hillsdale, NJ: Erlbaum Associates.

Crossen, J. R., & Wens, A. N. (1988). Residual neuropsychological deficits following head injury on the Wechsler Memory Scale—Revised. *Clinical Neuropsychologist, 2,* 393-399.

DeLuca, J. (1992). Rehabilitation of confabulation: The issue of unawareness of deficit. *NeuroRehabilitation, 2*(3), 23-30.

DePoy, E., & Burke, J. P. (1992). Viewing cognition through the lens of the Model of Human Occupation. In N. Katz (Ed.), *Cognitive rehabilitation: Models for intervention in occupational therapy.* Boston: Andover Medical Publishers.

D'Esposito, M., Onishi, K., Thompson, H., Robinson, K., Armstrong, C., & Grossman, M. (1996). Working memory impairments in multiple sclerosis: Evidence from a dual-task paradigm. *Neuropsychology, 10,* 51-56.

Duchek, J. M. (1991). Assessing cognition. In C. Christiansen & C. Baum (Eds.), *Occupational therapy: Overcoming human performance deficits.* Thorofare, NJ: SLACK Incorporated.

Duchek, J. M., Balota, D. A., Faust, M. E., & Ferraro, F. R. (1995). Inhibitory processes in young and older adults in a picture-word task. *Aging & Cognition, 2,* 156-167.

Duchek, J. M., Hunt, L., Ball, K., Buckles, V., & Morris, J. C. (in press). The role of selective attention in driving and dementia of the Alzheimer type. *Alzheimer's Disease and Associated Disorders.*

Dunn, W. (1993). The issue is: Measurement of function: Actions for the future. *American Journal of Occupational Therapy, 47,* 357-360.

Dunn, W., Brown, C., McClain, L. H., & Westman, K. (1994). In C. B. Royeen (Ed.), *AOTA self-study series: The ecology of human performance: A contextual perspective on human occupation.* Rockville, MD: American Occupational Therapy Association.

Dunn, W., Brown, C., & McGuigan, A. (1994). The ecology of human performance: A framework for considering the effect of context. *American Journal of Occupational Therapy, 48,* 595-607.

Earhart, C. A., & Allen, C. K. (1988). *Cognitive disabilities: Expanded activity analysis*. Colchester, CT: S & S Worldwide.

Evans, D. A., Funkenstein, H. H., Albert, M. S., Scherr, P. A., Cook, N. R., Chown, M. J., Hebert, L. E., Hennekens, C. H., & Taylor, J. O. (1989). Prevalence of Alzheimer's disease in a community population of older persons. *Journal of the American Medical Association, 262,* 2551-2556.

Ferraro, F. R., Balota, D. A., & Connor, L. T. (1993). Implicit memory and the formation of new associations in non-demented Parkinson's disease individuals and individuals with senile dementia of the Alzheimer type. *Brain & Cognition, 21,* 163-180.

Fisher, A. G. (1992). *Assessment of motor and process skills* (Res. ed. 6.1J). Unpublished test manual. Fort Collins, CO: Colorado State University, Department of Occupational Therapy.

Fisher, A. G., & Short-DeGraff, M. (1993). Nationally speaking— Improving functional assessment in occupational therapy: Recommendations and philosophy for change. *American Journal of Occupational Therapy, 47,* 199-202.

Gasquoine, P. G., & Gibbons, T. A. (1994). Lack of awareness of impairment in institutionalized, severely and chronically disabled survivors of traumatic brain injury: A preliminary investigation. *Journal of Head Trauma Rehabilitation, 9*(4), 16-24.

Gentile, A. M. (1987). Skill acquisition: Action, movement, and neuromotor processes. In J. H. Carr, R. B. Shepherd, J. Gordon, A. M. Gentile, & J. M. Held (Eds.), *Movement science foundations for physical therapy in rehabilitation* (pp. 93-154). Rockville, MD: Aspen Publishers, Inc.

Golden, C. J. (1981). A standardized version of Luria's neuropsychological tests: A quantitative and qualitative approach to neuropsychological evaluation. In S. B. Filskov & T. J. Boll (Eds.), *Handbook of clinical neuropsychology*. New York: Wiley.

Golden, C. J., Hammeke, T., & Purisch, A. (1978). Diagnostic validity of the Luria neuropsychological battery. *Journal of Consulting and Clinical Psychology, 46,* 1258-1265.

Goldstein, G. (1984). Comprehensive neuropsychological batteries. In G. Goldstein & M. Hersen (Eds.), *Handbook of psychological assessment*. New York: Pergamon Press.

Goldstein, G. (1987). Neuropsychological assessment for rehabilitation: Fixed batteries, automated systems, and non-psychometric methods. In M. J. Meier, A. L. Benton, & L. Diller (Eds.), *Neuropsychological rehabilitation*. New York: Guilford Press.

Graf, P., & Schacter, D. L. (1985). Implicit and explicit memory for new associations in normal and amnesic subjects. *Journal of Experimental Psychology: Learning, Memory, and Cognition, 11,* 501-518.

Grafman, J. (1984). Memory assessment and remediation in brain-injured patients: From theory to practice. In B. A. Edelstein & E. T. Couture (Eds.), *Behavioral assessment and rehabilitation of the traumatically brain-damaged*. New York: Plenum Press.

Grant, D. A., & Berg, E. A. (1948). A behavioral analysis of degree of reinforcement and ease of shifting to new responses in a Weigh-type card-sorting problem. *Journal of Experimental Psychology, 38,* 404-411.

Gronwall, D. M. A. (1977). Paced auditory serial addition task: A measure of recovery from concussion. *Perceptual and Motor Skills, 44,* 367-373.

Guilmette, T. J., & Rasile, D. (1995). Sensitivity, specificity, and diagnostic accuracy of three verbal memory measures in the assessment of mild brain injury. *Neuropsychology, 9,* 338-344.

Halstead, W. C. (1947). *Brain and intelligence: A quantitative study of the frontal lobes*. Chicago: The University of Chicago Press.

Hartley, A. A. (1992). Attention. In F. I. M. Craik & T. A. Salthouse (Eds.), *The handbook of aging and cognition*. Hillsdale, NJ: Erlbaum Associates.

Hartley, L. L. (1992). *Cognitive-communicative abilities following brain injury: A functional approach*. Los Angeles, CA: Singular Publishing Group.

Hasher, L., & Zachs, R. T. (1988). Working memory, comprehension, and aging: A review and a new view. In G. H. Bower (Ed.), *The psychology of learning and motivation* (Vol. 22, pp. 193-225). New York: Academic Press.

Kahneman, D. (1973). *Attention and effort*. Englewood Cliffs, NJ: Prentice-Hall.

Kandel, E. R. (1976). *Cellular basis of behavior: An introduction to behavioral neurobiology*. San Francisco: W. H. Freeman and Co.

Katz, N., Itzkovich, M., Averbuch, S., & Elazar, B. (1989). Lowenstein Occupational Therapy Cognitive Assessment (LOTCA) battery for brain-injured patients: Reliability and validity. *American Journal of Occupational Therapy, 43,* 184-191.

Kielhofner, G., & Henry, A. D. (1988). Development and investigation of the occupational performance history interview. *American Journal of Occupational Therapy, 42,* 489-498.

Kihlstrom, J. I., & Tobias, B. S. (1991). Anosognosia, consciousness, and the self. In G. P. Prigatano & D. L. Schacter (Eds.), *Awareness of deficit after brain injury: Clinical and theoretical issues* (pp. 198-222). New York: Oxford Press.

Knesevich, J. W., LaBarge, E., & Edwards, D. (1986). Predictive value of the Boston Naming Test in mild senile dementia of the Alzheimer type. *Psychiatric Research, 19,* 155-161.

Knopman, D. S., & Nissen, M. J. (1987). Implicit learning in patients with probable Alzheimer's disease. *Neurology, 37,* 784-788.

Kopelman, M. D. (1989). Remote and autobiographical memory, temporal context memory and frontal atrophy in Korsadoff and Alzheimer patients. *Neuropsychologia, 27,* 437-460.

Laver, A. J., & Powell, G. E. (1995). *The Structured Observational Test of Function (SOTOF)*. Windsor, England: NFER Nelson.

Lezak, M. D. (1978). Living with the characterologically altered brain-injured patient. *Journal of Clinical Psychiatry, 39,* 592-598.

Lezak, M. D. (1983). *Neuropsychological assessment*. New York: Oxford University Press.

MacLeod, C. M. (1991). Half a century of research on the stroop effect: An integrative review. *Psychological Review, 109,* 163-203.

Mangels, J. A., Gershberg, F. B., Shimamura, A. P., & Knight, R. T. (1996). Impaired retrieval from remote memory in patients with frontal lobe damage. *Neuropsychology, 10,* 32-41.

Moscovitch, M., Winocur, G., & McLachlan, D. (1986). Memory as assessed by recognition and reading time in normal and memory-impaired people with Alzheimer's disease and other neurological disorders. *Journal of Experimental Psychology: General, 115*, 331-347.

Nebes, R. D. (1992). Cognitive dysfunction in Alzheimer's disease. In F. I. M. Craik & T. A. Salthouse (Eds.), *The handbook of aging and cognition.* Hillsdale, NJ: Erlbaum Associates.

Neistadt, M. E. (1992). The Rabideau Kitchen Evaluation Revised: An assessment of meal preparation skills. *Occupational Therapy Journal of Research, 12*, 242-255.

Neistadt, M. E. (1993a). Perceptual retraining for adults with diffuse brain injury. *American Journal of Occupational Therapy, 48*, 225-233.

Neistadt, M. E. (1993b). A meal preparation treatment protocol for adults with brain injury. *American Journal of Occupational Therapy, 48*(5), 431-438.

Neistadt, M. E. (1993c). The neurobiology of learning: Implications for treatment of adults with brain injury. *American Journal of Occupational Therapy, 48*(5), 421-430.

Neistadt, M. E. (1994). Perceptual retraining for adults with diffuse brain injury. *American Journal of Occupational Therapy, 48*(3), 225-233.

Nygard, L., Bernspang, B., Fisher, A. G., & Winblad, B. (1994). Comparing motor and process ability of persons with suspected dementia in home and clinic settings. *American Journal of Occupational Therapy, 48*, 689-696.

Pan, A. W., & Fisher, A. G. (1994). The assessment of motor and process skills of persons with psychiatric disorders. *American Journal of Occupational Therapy, 48*, 775-780.

Parasuraman, R., & Nestor, P. G. (1991). Attention and driving skills in aging and Alzheimer's disease. *Human Factors, 33*(5), 539-557.

Park, S., Fisher, A. G., & Velazo, C. A. (1994). Using the Assessment of Motor and Process Skills to compare occupational performance between clinic and home settings. *American Journal of Occupational Therapy, 48*, 710-716.

Polkinghorne, D. E. (1988). *Narrative knowing and the human sciences.* Albany, NY: State University of New York Press.

Porn, I. (1984). An equilibrium model of health. In L. Nordenfelt & B. Lindahl (Eds.), *Health, disease, and casual explanation in medicine* (pp. 3-9). Dordrecht, Netherlands: D. Reidel Publishing Company.

Porn, I. (1993). Health and adaptedness. *Theoretical Medicine, 14*(4), 295-303.

Porteus, S. (1965). *Porteus Maze Test.* Palo Alto, CA: Pacific Books.

Posner, M. I. (1986). *Probing the mechanisms of selective attention.* Paper presented at the meeting of the Midwestern Psychological Association, Chicago, IL.

Posner, M. I., & Boies, S. W. (1971). Components of attention. *Psychological Review, 78*, 391-408.

Posner, M. I., & Rafal, R. D. (1987). Cognitive theories of attention and the rehabilitation of attentional deficits. In M. J. Meier, A. L. Benton, & L. Diller (Eds.), *Neuropsychological rehabilitation.* New York: Guilford Press.

Prigatano, G. P., Altman, I. M., & O'Brien, K. P. (1990). Behavioral limitations that traumatic-brain-injured patients tend to under-estimate. *The Clinical Neuropsychologist, 4*(2), 163-176.

Prigatano, G. P., & Schacter, D. L. (Eds.). (1991). *Awareness of deficit after brain injury: Clinical and theoretical issues.* New York: Oxford University Press.

Raven, J. C. (1960). *Guide to the standard progressive matrices.* New York: Psychological Corp.

Reid, D. B., & Kelly, M. P. (1993). Wechsler Memory Scale-Revised in closed head injury. *Journal of Clinical Psychology, 49*, 245-254.

Riessman, C. K. (1993). *Narrative analysis: Qualitative research methods* (Vol. 30). Newbury Park, CA: Sage Publications.

Schacter, D. L. (1994). Implicit memory: A new frontier for cognitive neuroscience. In M. S. Gazzaniga (Ed.), *The cognitive neurosciences.* Cambridge, MA: MIT Press.

Schmidt, R. A. (1988). *Motor control and learning: A behavioral emphasis* (2nd ed.). Champaign, IL: Human Kinetics.

Schmidt, R. A., & Bjork, R. A. (1992). New conceptualizations of practice. Common principles in three paradigms suggest new concept for training. *Psychological Science, 3*, 207-217.

Schwartz, R. K. (1985). *Therapy as learning.* Dubuque, IA: Kendall Publishing Company.

Seltzer, B., Vasterling, J. J., Hale, M. A., & Khurana, R. (1995). Unawareness of memory deficit in Alzheimer's disease: Relation to mood and other disease variables. *Neuropsychiatry, Neuropsychology and Behavioral Neurology, 8*(3), 176-181.

Simkins-Bullock, J., Brown, G. G., Greiffenstein, M., Malik, G. M., & McGillicuddy, J. (1994). Neuropsychological correlates of short-term memory distractor tasks among patients with surgical repair of anterior communicating artery aneurysms. *Neuropsychology, 8*, 246-254.

Spencer, J., Krefting, L., & Mattingly, C. (1993). Incorporation of ethnographic methods in occupational therapy assessment. *American Journal of Occupational Therapy, 47*, 303-310.

Statistical Package for Social Science. (1992). Chicago: SPSS, Inc.

Stroop, J. R. (1935). Studies of interference in serial verbal reaction. *Journal of Experimental Psychology, 18*, 643-662.

Tannock, R., Schachar, R. J., Carr, R. P., Chajczjk, D., & Logan, G. D. (1989). Effects of methylphenidate on inhibitory control in hyperactive children. *Journal of Abnormal Child Psychology, 17*, 473-491.

Toglia, J. P. (1989). Approaches to cognitive assessment of the brain injured adult: Traditional methods and dynamic investigation. *Occupational Therapy Practice, 1*, 36-55.

Toglia, J. P. (1991). Generalization of treatment—A multi-context approach to cognitive perceptual impairment in adults with brain injury. *American Journal of Occupational Therapy, 45*, 505-516.

Toglia, J. P. (1992). A dynamic interactional approach to cognitive rehabilitation. In N. Katz (Ed.), *Cognitive rehabilitation: Models for intervention in occupational therapy* (pp. 104-143). Andover, MA: Andover Medical Publishers.

Toglia, J. P. (1993). *The contextual memory test manual.* Tucson, AZ: Therapy Skill Builders.

Toglia, J. P. (1994a). Attention and memory. In C. B. Royeen (Ed.), *AOTA self-study series: Cognitive rehabilitation.* Rockville, MD: American Occupational Therapy Association.

Toglia, J. P. (1994b). *Dynamic assessment of categorization: TCA The Toglia Category Assessment.* Pequannock, NJ: Maddak, Inc.

Trombly, C. (1993). The issue is: Anticipating the future: Assessment of occupational function. *American Journal of Occupational Therapy, 47,* 253-257.

Tulving, E. (1972). Episodic and semantic memory. In E. Tulving & W. Donaldson (Eds.), *Organization of memory.* New York: Academic Press.

Vasterling, J. J., Seltzer, B., Foss, J. W., & Vanderbrook, V. (1995). Unawareness of deficit in Alzheimer's disease. *Neuropsychiatry, Neuropsychology and Behavioral Neurology, 8*(1), 26-32.

Vikki, J., Ahola, K., Holst, P., Ohman, J., Servo, A., & Heiskanen, O. (1994). Prediction of psychosocial recovery after head injury with cognitive tests and neurobehavioral ratings. *Journal of Clinical and Experimental Neuropsychology, 16,* 325-338.

Vygotsky, L. S. (1978). *Mind in society: The development of higher psychological processes.* Cambridge, MA: Harvard Press.

Wechsler, D. (1945a). *The measurement of adult intelligence.* Baltimore: Williams & Wilkins.

Wechsler, D. (1945b). A standardized memory scale for clinical use. *Journal of Psychology, 19,* 87-95.

Wechsler, D. (1981). *Wechsler Adult Intelligence Scale—Revised.* New York: Psychological Corp.

Weinstein, E. A., Friedland, R. P., & Wagner, E. E. (1994). Denial/unawareness of impairment and symbolic behavior in Alzheimer's disease. *Neuropsychiatry, Neuropsychology and Behavioral Neurology, 7*(3), 176-184.

Weitzman, E. A., & Miles, M. B. (1995). *Computer programs for qualitative data analysis.* Thousand Oaks, CA: Sage Publications, Inc.

Wertz, R. T. (1979). Word fluency measure. In F. L. Darley (Ed.), *Evaluation of appraisal techniques in speech and language pathology.* Reading, MA: Addison-Wesley.

Wilson, B., Cockburn, J., & Baddeley, A. (1985). *The Rivermead Behavioural Memory Test.* Thames, England: Thames Valley Test Company.

Wood, W., Abreu, B., Duval, M., & Gerber, D. (1994). Occupational performance and the functional approach. In C. B. Royeen (Ed.), *AOTA self-study series: Cognitive rehabilitation.* Rockville, MD: American Occupational Therapy Association.

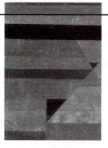

CHAPTER CONTENT OUTLINE

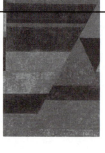

ABSTRACT

Psychological and emotional factors impact on occupational performance, health, and well-being in complex ways. To provide effective therapeutic intervention, these factors must be understood and addressed. In some cases, psychological difficulties can in and of themselves cause dysfunction; in other cases, psychological correlates of physical problems can reduce effectiveness of performance. Occupational therapists emphasize the relationship of self-identity to occupational performance, intervening through the use of therapeutic activities.

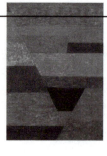

KEY TERMS

Self-concept

Self-esteem

Affect

Cultural values

Norms

Locus of control

Well-being

Motivation

Self-efficacy

Defense mechanisms

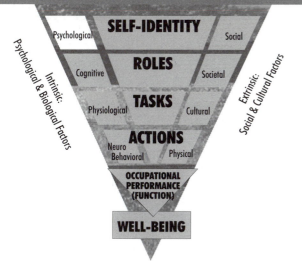

Coping with Psychological and Emotional Challenges

Bette R. Bonder, PhD, OTR/L, FAOTA

OBJECTIVES

The information in this chapter is intended to help the reader:

1. define the term psychological construct, and list and describe psychological constructs relevant to occupational performance

2. discuss the interaction of psychological factors with environmental factors as they contribute to occupational performance, well-being, and health

3. describe three psychological theories, and five occupational therapy theories relevant to psychological factors in occupational performance

4. describe major categories of psychological disorder

5. explain the relevance of psychological factors in occupational therapy intervention with individuals with physical disorders

6. discuss occupational therapy assessment and list instruments used to evaluate psychological factors in occupational performance

7. describe the settings in which occupational therapists provide mental health services

8. list and describe typical goals and modalities for occupational therapy intervention in mental health settings

9. discuss the literature evaluating effectiveness of occupational therapy in mental health settings, and the need for additional research.

"Employment is the chief cure for despair"
—Samuel Johnson

INTRODUCTION

Occupational therapy focuses on what people do: whether they can do what they need and want to do and whether their lives are meaningful and satisfying. A major assumption of occupational therapy is that activity is central to quality of life (Mattingly & Fleming, 1994). Further, it is assumed that quality of life, as reflected by activity, is an important and valuable therapeutic goal. People's decisions about what they want to do, how they assess their satisfaction with their activities, and even what they experience as essential undertakings are based on psychological factors that include individual needs, perceptions, and evaluations of the world in the context of personal experience. Thus, all performance is seen through a psychological/emotional screen. A homemaker who believes that an immaculate house is the most important measure of competence in that role will struggle with a psychological adjustment if she becomes the mother of toddlers, a role that makes an immaculate house difficult to achieve.

When a person is unable to accomplish desired or needed activities, regardless of the reason, psychological factors are central to his or her reaction to the situation. For example, spinal cord injury causes not only physical limitations, but also emotional consequences. Rehabilitation will be ineffective if it addresses either of these without consideration of the other; conversely, integration of all aspects of performance can yield more positive outcomes. By the same token, an individual with a diagnosed "psychiatric" condition may well have accompanying physical, cognitive, or sensory deficits that also require attention. An individual diagnosed with depression might also have arthritis that limits mobility and causes pain. Treatment of the depression without attention to the arthritis will be less successful than intervention that addresses both concerns, and the way in which they interact.

Occupational therapy considers all the reasons a person might be unable to perform needed or desired activities: sensorimotor, neuromuscular, motor, cognitive, and social as well as psychological (American Occupational Therapy Association [AOTA], 1994). In addition, occupational therapists recognize that performance occurs in the context of the person's environment. A supportive environment can facilitate performance in an individual with significant limitations in one or more performance components, while even the most functional of individuals might struggle in a hostile environment. Although it is complicated to do so, therapists must also address all components of the person's performance.

Bibliographic citation of this chapter: Bonder, B. (1997). Coping with psychological and emotional challenges. In C. Christiansen & C. Baum (Eds.), *Occupational therapy: Enabling function and well-being* (2nd ed.). Thorofare, NJ: SLACK Incorporated.

TABLE 12-1

Psychological Constructs

I. Intrinsic Factors

Self-Concept: Person's description of his or her attributes

Self-Esteem: Person's evaluation of his or her attributes

Affect: Person's internal experiences or feelings

II. Extrinsic Factors

Cultural Norms and Values: Beliefs and prescriptions for behavior shared by a group of individuals

Locus of Control: Belief about where control of individual actions rests

III. Outcomes of Interaction Between Intrinsic and Extrinsic Factors

Well-Being: Perceived sense of contentment or satisfaction

    Motivation: A drive toward action

    Self-Efficacy: Perceived performance capabilities

Occupational Performance: Effective accomplishment of roles, tasks and activities

Health: Perceived physical and psychological wellness

---

mance and the environment as well (Yerxa, 1988). The individual with a new spinal cord injury may be more highly motivated to engage in needed physical exercises if he or she is convinced that this will assist in accomplishment of valued life roles (Levine & Brayley, 1991), and if the environment is modified to ease the activity insofar as is possible. Other chapters address environmental factors and performance components. This chapter emphasizes psychological and emotional factors related to performance.

There have been numerous attempts to define psychological constructs (Bonder, 1993). In general, psychological constructs are internal factors related to the person's perceptions and feelings, demonstrated by the person's behavior. Psychological constructs are terms used to describe internal experience, personal reaction to the external environment, and psychological mechanisms by which the individual addresses relationships between environment and self. As reflected in the Person-Environment Occupational Performance Model (Christiansen & Baum, 1991; 1997), these constructs can be placed in three categories: intrinsic, extrinsic, and the outcomes of the interaction between intrinsic and extrinsic factors (Table 12-1). As neuroscience provides more information about the brain, we are beginning to get a clearer understanding of the mechanisms that support the psychological behaviors of the individual and why people with psychological deficits exhibit some of the behaviors they do. The neurological basis of motivation, cognition, and emotion are described in Chapter 8.

PSYCHOLOGICAL CONSTRUCTS

Intrinsic Psychological Factors

As reflected in the Person-Environment Occupational Performance Model described earlier in this text, contributions to self-identity are made by both intrinsic and extrinsic factors. Psychological factors intrinsic to the individual include self-concept, self-esteem, and affect.

Self-concept is the way in which individuals perceive themselves. It is reflected in their statements about who they are, both in terms of roles (mother, student, etc.) and attributes (smart, kind, etc.). Self-concept is descriptive, rather than evaluative, that is, it describes what one perceives as the self, but does not apply any value, either positive or negative, to that description. A person may have a self-concept that is not consistent with the way others see the individual. Such situations can lead to psychological difficulties, as the individual may be disappointed in interactions with others. For example, a person who perceives himself as having comedic talents might be disappointed and discouraged if his desired career as a stand-up comic never materializes.

Self-esteem refers to the relative value in which the individual holds the attributes that contribute to self-concept. An individual who describes him- or herself as "smart" might evaluate that either as positive or negative. Some adolescents whose self-concept includes a perception of self as intelligent might believe that this is not valued by peers and might therefore evaluate the attribute negatively, lowering self-esteem. An adult, however, might feel that intelligence is an admirable characteristic and experience heightened self-esteem because of a perception that he or she possesses the attribute. As with self-concept, self-esteem is largely internal to the person; however, inconsistency between the way others value the individual and ways the individual values him- or herself can be problematic.

Affect is the emotion or feeling that accompanies evaluation of self. The adolescent in the example above might feel unhappy about his or her perceived disadvantage, while the adult might find his or her intelligence a source of happiness. Affect or emotion can also contribute to psychological problems, as when it is inconsistent with the event or idea that caused it, or it is excessive or inadequate to the situation. For example, an individual who is sad frequently may be unpleasant to others, and as a result, have an impoverished social life.

These psychological factors all contribute to construction of self-identity, and to the roles, tasks, and occupations that express that self-identity.

Extrinsic Factors

The relationship of self to the environment is an equally important consideration. To a large extent, a person's self-identity is shaped by extrinsic factors in the environment. An individual will receive feedback or input from the environment responds to that behavior. The individual may experience dissonance if he or she is perceived by others in a way different from that in which he or she experiences him- or herself.

The environment provides many external cues to internal processes. Social and societal factors provide information that is processed through the screen of psyche. For example, among adolescents, social cues from peers and their interpretation by the individual have significant impact on self-esteem. Societal values, such as the importance of work, may affect the self-identity of an individual who finds him- or herself unemployed. Cultural values and norms provide direction to individuals about how to feel or how to perceive events. For example, an adolescent will feel bad about being smart to the extent that his or her adolescent culture indicates this to be an undesirable trait.

An important aspect of interaction of the individual with the environment relates to perception about where control over events rests, or *locus of control* (Rotter, 1966). Some individuals believe they can control in large extent what happens to them, that is, they have an *internal* locus of control; others believe the environment largely controls them, an *external* locus of control. Both behavior and assessment of events will be influenced by locus of control. For example, an individual with an internal locus of control may attribute success on the job to talent, while an individual with an external locus of control may attribute similar success to luck.

Obviously, these factors or constructs are not independent of each other. They interact in complicated ways that influence both behavior and feeling. For example, perceived personal attributes (self-concept) contribute to self-esteem based not only on the individual's affect about those characteristics, but the degree to which they are consistent with cultural values and norms and the feedback from others.

Outcomes of the Relationship between Self and the Environment

The desired outcomes of self-evaluation and of perceptions about personal relationship to the environment are effective occupational performance, health, and a sense of personal *well-being*. To the extent that the individual enjoys positive self-esteem because of good "fit" between personal perception and feedback from the environment, well-being will result. To the extent that the person does not experience

TABLE 12-2
Psychological Theories

Theory	Self	Self in Environment	Outcomes	Dysfunction
Analytic	id and ego	superego defense mechanisms	need satisfaction	inadequate ego formation
Behavioral	response to reinforcers	reinforcement punishment	adequate reinforcement	inadequate reinforcement
Cognitive	intellectual interpretation of experience	cognitive response	satisfaction as a result of effective interpretation of experience	depression or anxiety due to ineffective interpretation of experience

well-being, an expression of dissatisfaction will be evident. This might be an expression of negative affect or of defense mechanisms such as denial or projection. To resolve such a situation, the individual may undertake to change behavior, change the environment, or revise his or her perceptions. An inability to resolve these discrepancies may lead to psychological dysfunction.

Motivation describes the drive toward action. In general, motivation is related to the individual's wish for well-being. As described below, there is disagreement among theorists about whether motivation is largely an internal process or one that is mostly influenced by the environment. In either case, motivation leads the person to interact with the environment in ways that can produce well-being. Lack of motivation, or motivation to unproductive or ineffective action, can lead to dissatisfaction.

Perceived *self-efficacy* (Gage & Polatajko, 1994) is another result of effective interaction between the self and the environment. Self-efficacy is a "person's belief in his or her performance capabilities with respect to a specific task" (p. 783). To the extent that the individual is able to interact with the environment in ways that produce desired results, a sense of well-being and support of self-esteem, the individual will experience him- or herself as a capable, effective individual.

The interaction of these factors is demonstrated by the Person-Environment Occupational Performance Model (Christiansen & Baum, 1991; 1997). As it demonstrates, psychological factors alone will not ensure effective occupational performance, health and well-being. However, these factors are essential to these outcomes. Psychological factors alone cannot make a tone-deaf individual into a concert violinist; however, effective psychological coping mechanisms and a healthy self-identity can enable that individual to identify other strengths, acknowledge limitations, and find other means of expression.

Psychological Theories

Psychological theories are attempts to describe psychological constructs and their interaction in systematic ways that explain feelings and behaviors. Cognitive theorists (Beck, 1967; Ellis, 1973) emphasize primarily internal processes of the individual. They suggest that self-concept is largely determined by an intellectual or cognitive process of description, and that self-esteem rests on cognitive beliefs about that self-concept. External forces are relevant only insofar as they influence the individual's beliefs. Thus, cognitive theorists hold that locus of control is largely internal. Cultural norms and values contribute to the individual's intellectual understanding of events, but the individual has control over the degree to which those beliefs are incorporated into the self. Well-being is produced by consistency between self-concept and beliefs or interpretations about the attributes of the self.

Freudian analytic theorists (Freud, 1961) describe an interaction of internal forces and external forces as being mediated by a third force that integrates the demands of the other two. The internal force is called the id, and reflects the raw personal feelings, emotions, and evaluations that would occur in the absence of any input from the environment. These forces are largely driven toward pleasure. The external force is called the superego, and is in many ways consistent with the concept of conscience. The superego is the person's internal incorporation of cultural norms that may oppose the pure drive toward pleasure. The mediating structure is the ego. The ego is the factor that integrates the desires of the id and the restrictions placed by the superego; it is the reality principle that assists the individual to achieve pleasure in the context of a world filled with others whose needs must also be addressed. Thus, Freudian analysts see the person in the context of the environment, a view that reflects neither an entirely internal nor external locus of control.

A third group of theorists, the behaviorists (Skinner, 1971), focus primarily on the environment as the major force in the individual's actions. These theorists suggest that internal processes are largely unimportant. They suggest that individuals behave in ways that are reinforced by the environment, and that they avoid behaviors that are either not reinforced or are punished. Clearly behaviorists hold a view consistent with external locus of control. These theories are summarized in Table 12-2.

Psychological Constructs in Occupational Therapy

The essential element of psychological components, from the perspective of occupational therapy, is the focus on doing. The occupational therapist believes that "psychological variables address internal, unobservable processes that provide the person's drive toward activity" (Bonder, 1993, p. 212). Occupational therapists are not interested in the person's self-concept or affect as isolated factors, but rather, in the way that these factors contribute to effective performance of needed or desired activities. In addition, therapists are concerned about the reverse relationship; that is, the ways in which activities contribute to affect, self-concept, and self-esteem. For example, a therapist in a school setting would be concerned about how a student's self-concept affected academic performance, or, alternatively, how academic performance affected self-concept.

To explain these relationships, occupational therapy theories, unlike those of psychologists, focus on the components of performance and their relationships to each other. Chapter 4 discusses several occupational therapy models, each of which is relevant to a consideration of psychological and emotional issues in performance.

The Ecology of Human Performance Model (Dunn, Brown, & McGuigan, 1994) emphasizes the interaction of intrinsic and extrinsic factors in performance, with particular emphasis on context. As the match between circumstances and performance improves, self-identity will be increasingly accurate, occupational performance enhanced, and well-being increased.

The Person-Environment Occupational Performance Model (Christiansen & Baum, 1991; 1997) identifies a set of intrinsic (biological and psychological) factors as interacting with a set of intrinsic (social and cultural) factors, to produce a self-identity that guides role, task, and occupational selection and performance. As has already been discussed, psychological and emotional factors are central to the desired outcomes of effective occupational performance, health, and well-being.

The Model of Human Occupation (MOHO) (Kielhofner & Burke, 1980) conceptualizes the individual as an open system, with several subsystems that contribute to performance and evaluation of performance. The volition subsystem is an internal set of valued goals and beliefs. These valued goals are actualized through the habituation subsystem that reflects habits and roles. The performance subsystem includes the skills that enable the individual to accomplish the habits and roles to enact valued goals and beliefs.

The Person-Environment-Occupation Model (Law, Cooper, Strong, et al., 1997) posits a complex relationship between the person and the environment, with roles and activities expressing that relationship. Psychological factors are among those that influence and are influenced by the environment.

Occupational Adaptation (OA) (Schkade & Schultz, 1992; Schultz & Schkade, 1992) incorporates psychological variables with other factors contributing to performance as an integrated and complex schema directed at functional outcomes. OA suggests that the environment presents challenges to behavior and beliefs that must be met through the individual's ability to adapt or to acquire new skills. Because the environment changes frequently, the individual must become effective in adapting in order to achieve a sense of well-being. Developmental considerations are a component of this theory, as developmental stages present adaptational challenges to the self. Adaptation contributes to a sense of mastery, and mastery, in turn, to psychological well-being.

Some occupational therapy models focus at the impairment level, that is, they emphasize constituent components. Such models as the Cognitive Model (Allen, 1985) and Sensory Integration (Ayres, 1974) describe particular aspects of performance, rather than all constituents of ability. These theories have relevance in many situations, but are less comprehensive in describing deficit and remediation because they do not address issues of identity, self-esteem, and motivation. Further, when an individual has a performance deficit in another component area, or where the problem relates to poor person-environment fit (Lawton & Nahemow, 1973), these theories are less likely to be useful guides to practice. Psychological factors however, influence and are influenced by these other aspects of performance. A child who has a sensory integrative deficit may well experience alterations of self-concept that result in poor self-esteem. This contributes to even more problematic occupational performance, and has a negative impact on well-being.

VIEWS OF PSYCHOLOGICAL DYSFUNCTION

Psychological and occupational therapy theories describe not only what constitutes psychological well-being, but also how individuals become dysfunctional, and how that dysfunction manifests itself. Analysts describe psychological dysfunction in terms of formation of the ego and the relationship between id and superego. Someone who reports feeling

TABLE 12-3

Occupational Therapy Theories

Theory	Self	Self in Environment	Outcomes	Dysfunction
Model of Human Occupation	Subsystems: volition, performance, habituation	Behavior expressing values and skills	Well-integrated behaviors lead to well-being	Inadequate subsystem formation leads to inadequate performance and dissatisfaction
Occupational Adaptation	Adaptive capabilities	Changes in environment require adaptation	Effective adaptation leads to well-being	Ineffective adaptation leads to dissatisfaction
Ecology of Human Performance	Roles	Context for role performance	Effective performance	Poor match of roles/context causes poor performance
Person-Environment Occupational Performance	Psychological and other intrinsic factors	Social, societal, cultural factors	Occupational performance, well-being, health	Poor fit of intrinsic and extrinsic factors compromise function and well-being
Person-Environment-Occupation	Internal enabling or constraining factors	External enabling or constraining factors	Effective performance	Poor fit leads to compromised occupational performance

sad and withdrawn, symptoms of a disorder called depression, might be perceived by an analyst as having an excessively developed superego that prevents satisfaction of the needs of the id. To cope with the feelings that accompany difficulties around ego development or need satisfaction, analysts indicate that individuals develop psychological coping strategies known as *defense mechanisms*. These mechanisms include denial, the failure to acknowledge the problem; projection, the attribution of the problem to someone or something other than the self; and rationalization, the identification of intellectual explanations that minimize the problem. There are other defense mechanisms as well, and individuals may engage in one or several of them as their typical means of coping with problems. While everyone uses psychological defense mechanisms at times, their exaggerated or excessive use can contribute to psychological problems, according to analysts.

Behaviorists, on the other hand, believe dysfunction is the result of ineffective efforts to obtain reinforcement. Behaviorists would be reluctant to characterize internal emotions, and would focus instead on the person's behavior, so that in the case of someone who appeared depressed, the behaviorist would examine the individual's ability to receive adequate reinforcement from his or her environment, perhaps in the form of caring friends, for example. To cope with a lack of well-being, an individual might alter behaviors in an attempt to avoid negative consequences or encourage rein-

forcement. Such behavioral change might be positive, but might also lead to exacerbation of the problem, particularly if it occurs in a random fashion.

Cognitive theorists would suggest that individuals with psychological problems are ineffective or inaccurate in interpreting events and their own emotions. Someone who felt unpopular and therefore depressed might be viewed as misunderstanding the feelings of others.

Dysfunction, viewed by occupational therapy theorists, emphasizes the relationship of emotion to action. All five models described above attend to the important interaction of psychological factors with occupational performance. The Person-Environment Occupational Performance Model (Christiansen & Baum, 1991; 1997) identifies psychological factors as contributing to self-identity, and thereby to both well-being and occupational performance. The Model of Human Occupation (Kielhofner & Burke, 1980) would hold that someone who is depressed is lacking in valued goals and roles, or the skills to achieve those goals. The Occupational Adaptation model (Schkade & Schultz, 1992; Schultz & Schkade, 1992) theorizes that psychological dysfunction is the result of inability to adapt effectively during times of disequilibrium. Depression might be the result of inability to master a situation that called for change in performance. Table 19-3 summarizes the psychological constructs and beliefs about dysfunction of the theories described here.

Diagnosing Psychosocial Dysfunction

While various theories describe psychological dysfunction differently, it is necessary for professionals to communicate. To facilitate this, a diagnostic system has been developed to describe psychological, emotional, or social problems when these are a source of difficulty for the individual. The system provides a common language for all professionals, just as the *International Classification of Diseases* (ICD-10) (World Health Organization, 1990) does for professionals focusing on physical or biological disease. The diagnostic categorization for psychological disorders is found in the *Diagnostic and Statistical Manual* (DSM-IV) (American Psychiatric Association [APA], 1994), now in its fourth edition.

DSM-IV was developed through extensive discussion of task groups of experts (primarily psychiatrists, but with input from psychologists, social workers, and others), as well as clinical trials of various diagnostic categories to establish reliability and validity. The resulting list of diagnoses includes descriptions of specific factors that are considered in naming the individual's problem. These factors include type of onset, behaviors, duration, and typical course. DSM-IV purports to be atheoretical, to describe rather than to explain (Williams, 1988). This was important if all theorists were to accept it as the common diagnostic plan. An additional characteristic of DSM-IV is the inclusion of five axes, or dimensions. These include, in addition to the diagnosis on Axis I, the following: lifelong patterns of adaptation that contribute to dysfunction (Axis II); medical conditions that contribute to psychological problems (Axis III); level of stress experienced by the individual (Axis IV); and the patient or client's highest level of function (Axis V). This last axis is often not used by the psychiatrist or psychologist making the primary diagnosis, but is important to occupational therapists who focus on this aspect of the individual's life.

The development of DSM-IV and its characteristics have been described in detail elsewhere (Bonder, 1995). It is helpful here to briefly recount the main categories of psychiatric diagnosis, and to identify the ways in which occupational therapists might view them. The primary categories identified in the DSM-IV diagnostic listing include the following: 1) delirium and dementia; 2) schizophrenia and other psychotic disorders; 3) mood disorders; 4) substance-related disorders; 5) personality disorders; 6) anxiety disorders; 7) adjustment disorders; and 8) disorders of infancy, childhood, and adolescence.

Delirium and dementia are characterized by changes in cognition. Delirium usually accompanies some physical disorder, a high fever or a brain injury for example, and results in a change in consciousness, as well as disorientation. Dementia is a change in cognition without change in consciousness. Caused by a number of diseases, including Alzheimer's and Pick's diseases, as well as overmedication, dehydration, sensory deprivation, and substance abuse, dementia is most common among older individuals. Delirium and dementia alter both the self and the relationship between self and the environment as a result of difficulties perceiving, interpreting, and remembering events. In addition, impaired function is a significant characteristic from the perspective of occupational therapy.

Schizophrenia and other psychotic disorders are characterized by hallucinations, sensory experiences that are not in keeping with observable reality, such as hearing voices. Delusions, firmly held belief systems that are not consistent with observable reality, may also occur. Typical delusions include persecutory ideation, that the person is in danger of being harmed, and grandiosity, that the person is an extremely important figure. The hallucinations and delusions interfere with performance of life tasks.

Mood disorders include a number of forms of depression. Depression is characterized by lethargy and low energy, feelings of guilt and sadness, tearfulness, weight loss, and lack of ability to take pleasure in activities. At the other end of the spectrum are the manic disorders, characterized by extremely high energy, hyperactivity, irritability, and grandiosity. Some individuals fluctuate between depression and mania, a condition known as bipolar disorder. While these disorders are not specifically identified based on functional change, performance is most often affected. Individuals who are depressed tend to have poor self-esteem and little motivation. Individuals who are manic tend to have exaggeratedly positive self-esteem and to have difficulty carrying projects to completion.

Substance-related disorders refer to the constellation of disorders involving alcohol and drug abuse. Individuals with these disorders may abuse substances regularly or intermittently, and experience behavior changes as a result of intoxication. They are substantially unable or unwilling to avoid the substance. Substance-related disorders all contribute to functional problems, initially when the substance has been ingested recently, later, when the use becomes habitual, most of the time.

Personality disorders are related to long-standing personality characteristics that are patterns of behavior for the individual. Typically, personality disorders emerge in adolescence as patterns of adaptation, and persist thereafter. For example, individuals with histrionic personality disorder tend to be flamboyant, self-centered, and to have difficulties in interpersonal relationships. An individual may have an underlying personality disorder on which depression, an anxiety disorder, or other psychiatric disorder is superimposed. To date, no psychotropic medication has been found effective in dealing with these disorders, suggesting that they are, instead, learned patterns of behavior or adaptation. They may or may not lead to functional problems, depending to some extent on the degree to which the environment supports or accommodates the individual's behavior.

Anxiety disorders are characterized by either panic attacks or long-term generalized anxiety. Panic attacks are extreme anxiety reactions, with hyperventilation, sweatiness, shortness of breath, and profound feelings of fear. They may come upon the individual unexpectedly, or in reaction to a situation, as in the case of a fear of heights or enclosed spaces. More generalized anxiety is characterized by less severe but more constant feelings of fear or worry.

Adjustment disorders are short-term reactions to life changes, a divorce, move, or job change, for example. They are typically characterized by short-term depression and/or anxiety, and difficulty functioning in the new life situation.

Disorders of infancy, childhood, and adolescence include an array of disorders that have early onset. They include failure to thrive in infants, as well as developmental delay, pervasive developmental disorders like autism, and attention deficit hyperactivity disorder. In addition, children may experience depression or anxiety similar to older individuals. For example, children may experience school phobias, in which they become extremely anxious about leaving home for school. Children may also develop schizophrenia and other psychotic disorders, although these are rare.

A brief summary of the symptoms found in each category of disorder can be found in Table 12-4. In addition, the table summarizes the potential impact on performance of each category of disorder.

DSM-IV is relevant to occupational therapists because they must communicate with other professionals. Occupational therapists, however, formulate problems differently, and make a very different set of "diagnoses." As Rogers (1982) noted, it is quite possible for a medical diagnosis to be unaccompanied by functional deficits requiring occupational therapy. For example, when an individual has a cold, any functional problems will be short-lived and unlikely to require OT intervention. On the other hand, individuals may benefit from occupational therapy when they have no diagnosable medical condition. For example, an individual who has lost a job may need to learn job hunting skills in order to locate a new position. In this case, an occupational therapist might be able to intervene to prevent longer term dysfunction by assisting the individual to learn the new skills.

Emotional/Psychological Impact of Physical Dysfunction

Occupational therapists must address psychological factors in every setting. Individuals experiencing a "physical" illness may well experience accompanying psychological reactions, and intervention must be sensitive to these needs.

Many disorders considered to have primarily physical causes can also lead to emotional consequences. Cardiovascular accident (CVA) is an example. It may be difficult to assess the emotional consequences of CVA because of the accompanying cognitive or physical limitations that make standard instruments unreliable. However, clinical depression, with all its accompanying symptoms such as sadness, tearfulness, lethargy, and guilt, are frequently observed in people who have experienced CVA. Difficulty accomplishing meaningful life activities seems to be a major contributing factor, as is overprotection by caregivers (Thompson, Sobolew-Shubin, Graham, et al., 1989). In addition, however, clear biological changes related to post-CVA depression have been identified (Allman, 1991), contributing to better understanding of the likelihood that many so-called "psychological" disorders have biological causes.

Physical disability can lead to altered self-concept, lowered self-esteem, depression, and anxiety. These secondary consequences of newly acquired disability must be addressed to enhance motivation of the client to participate in all aspects of rehabilitation. For example, Mr. H. was a 65-year-old married male, recently retired from his job as a line worker in an auto factory when he suffered a cerebrovascular accident. The CVA left him with a right (dominant) side hemiplegia and balance problems. Mr. H. became quite sad, withdrawn, and lethargic. When questioned by the occupational therapist, he said tearfully that he had worked hard all his life, looking forward to retirement as a time to indulge his love of fishing, and that he was now unable to even hold a fishing rod. The occupational therapist, recognizing the importance of this leisure role to his self-concept and psychological well-being, worked with him to design a holder for the rod, and to teach him to reel in the line with a left-handed reel. As the project progressed, Mr. H. became increasingly optimistic and enthused, not only about fishing but also about other parts of his rehabilitation program. Several months later, the therapist received a note from Mr. H. with a picture of him, a smile on his face and a fish on his line.

In addition to psychological or emotional reactions to illness or disability, many individuals in medical settings have pre-existing or co-existing psychological problems. Among individuals admitted to general medical units, approximately 15% of patients have affective disorders such as depression and bipolar (manic-depressive) disorder (Mayou, Hawton, Feldman et al., 1991). Other psychological disorders are also common in medical settings, including anxiety disorders, adjustment disorders, and, less often, psychotic disorders such as schizophrenia.

TABLE 12-4

Classifications of Psychiatric Disorder

Category	Characteristics	Effect on Function

Delirium and dementia
    Alzheimer's Disease
    Pick's Disease
	Changes in cognition, especially memory	Negative impact on all areas of function

Schizophrenia
    Paranoid type
    Disorganized type
    Catatonic type
    Undifferentiated type
    Residual type
	Hallucinations, delusions	Negative impact on all areas of function

Mood disorders
    Major depression
    Dysthymia
    Manic disorder
    Bipolar Disorder
	Changes in affect, either depressed or excessively elated	Potential negative impact on performance, especially in social and work areas

Substance related disorders
    Dependence
    Abuse
    Intoxication
    Withdrawal
	Intoxication or withdrawal from mood or cognition altering substance	Potential negative impact on performance, especially social and work

Personality disorders
    Paranoid
    Schizoid
    Schizotypal
    Antisocial
    Borderline
    Histrionic
    Narcissistic
    Avoidant
    Dependent
    Obsessive-compulsive
	Difficulties in relating to others, adaptational problems	Negative impact on social performance, potential difficulties with work and leisure

Anxiety disorders
    Panic disorder
    Agoraphobia
    Phobia
    Obsessive-compulsive
    Post-traumatic stress
    Generalized anxiety
	Panic attacks or chronic anxiety	Potential negative impact on social, work, and leisure

Disorders of infancy, childhood, and adolescence
    Mental retardation
    Learning disorders
    Pervasive developmental disorders
    Attention deficit disorders
	Developmental delay in some or all areas; problematic behavior	Negative impact on some or all areas of performance. School performance tends to be affected in all these disorders.

Adjustment disorder	Difficulty adapting to new life situation	Negative impact on performance in sphere of life that is source of problem, possible generalizing of difficulty to other

The Occupational Therapy Perspective on Psychological Disorders

The division between psychological and physical disorders is increasingly recognized as arbitrary, and is now primarily based on symptoms, rather than on causes. Many psychiatric disorders are known to have biological etiologies, including schizophrenia (Szymanski, Kane, & Lieberman, 1991), dysthymia (Howland & Thase, 1991), and autism (Huebner, 1991). Further, many disorders respond to psychopharmacological intervention (Fischer, 1995), and the effectiveness of medical intervention to ameliorate symptoms is rapidly improving.

However, simply eliminating symptoms of psychiatric disorder does not assure avoidance of functional deficits. For example, the typical age range of onset for schizophrenia is late adolescence to early adulthood (APA, 1994). Individuals who develop schizophrenia at this time in their lives often fail to accomplish age-appropriate developmental tasks such as learning effective socialization skills with individuals of the opposite sex, or vocational skills that might lead to employment. Thus, even if the primary symptoms of schizophrenia such as hallucinations and delusions are controlled by medication, individuals with schizophrenia will need significant assistance, typically from an occupational therapist to achieve meaningful lives. For example, one client did quite well in a hospital setting when medication was administered to reduce her hallucinations. However, she was discharged home with no plan for how to spend the day, and quickly began to feel isolated and bored, stopped taking her medication, and began hallucinating again. During a second hospital stay, an occupational therapist helped her learn to identify interests, manage time, use public transportation to get to activities, and make friends. She remained on her medication and symptom-free for at least 2 years following that admission.

Occupational therapists focus on the functional deficits that are prominent features of many psychiatric disorders. Some psychiatric diagnoses are defined in part by deficits in self-care, work, or leisure performance (APA, 1994). These include schizophrenia, dementia, and developmental disorders. Other disorders may well result in, or derive from, performance deficits. Depression may result in poor work performance and poverty of social interaction due to the lethargy and anhedonia that characterize the disorder. Similarly, divorce or loss of a job may result in depression secondary to the stressful life event.

Consider the case of Mrs. B., a 40-year-old woman married to an attorney, mother to a 12-year-old girl and an 8-year-old boy, and employed until recently as a secretary at a large legal firm. A year previously, Mrs. B. was laid off from her job, as a result of corporate "right-sizing." She was quite hurt, because she felt she had been a good employee, and was expecting a promotion. She was also having difficulty at home with her daughter who had recently begun to behave in a "surly and uncooperative way" and her son, diagnosed as having an attention deficit disorder manifested by inattention, hyperactivity, and temper outbursts. Her husband worked long hours, and their traditional arrangement had been for her to take care of home-related matters; she felt a lack of support from him in this current, stressful period of her life.

Mrs. B. became lethargic, tearful, and unable to sleep. During the 8 months since losing her job, she lost weight, had difficulty getting out of bed in the morning, and described herself as hopeless and inept.

Mrs. B. had an affective disorder, major depression being the most likely diagnosis. A psychiatrist would prescribe an antidepressant medication that might well give Mrs. B. more energy and lift her mood. From the perspective of the occupational therapist, however, a good bit more would be required to return Mrs. B. to a fully satisfying life and to minimize the likelihood of further episodes of depression.

A therapist who subscribed to the Model of Human Occupation (Kielhofner & Burke, 1980) would be likely to formulate concerns around the volition subsystem, and the habituation subsystem. Mrs. B. had some valued roles, especially her work role, and was confronted with new situations for which she did not have a repertoire of skills, most notably those concerning her children. In addition, she appeared to lack either the necessary interpersonal skills or the emotional strength to deal with any resentment she felt toward a husband who provided inadequate support in home and family-related matters.

A therapist who subscribed to the Occupational Adaptation (Schkade & Schultz, 1992; Schultz & Schkade, 1992) model would, instead, consider the current challenges to Mrs. B.'s adaptation, and the adequacy of her adaptive skills. This therapist would consider Mrs. B.'s inability to demonstrate occupational mastery of the occupational challenges presented by her job loss and her family difficulties.

A therapist assessing the situation from the perspective of the Person-Environment Occupational Performance Model would examine the intrinsic factors, both psychological and biological, as well as the extrinsic factors (social and cultural) that have negatively affected self-identity, roles, tasks and activities, with the result of interfering with occupational performance and well-being.

THE TREATMENT PROCESS IN OCCUPATIONAL THERAPY IN MENTAL HEALTH

Assessment

Occupational therapy assessment considers all perform-ance components, regardless of the setting in which practice occurs. Psychological factors that affect performance must be carefully evaluated. While there are few standardized instruments that provide the specific information required by the occupational therapist, there are many mechanisms for obtaining data. Because so few instruments directly provide the necessary information, the goals of occupational therapy must be kept firmly in mind. For example, the therapist administering a standardized test of anxiety is not interested in anxiety, per se, but in "activity-related anxiety" (Bonder, 1993, p. 212-213).

Standard evaluations may be helpful, but those that elicit individual's experience are more helpful in some circum-stances (Vause-Earland, 1991). Thus, in addition to standard-ized assessments, therapists should plan to ask specific ques-tions. "Are you able to accomplish all your daily activities?" "Which are most difficult for you?" "What feelings do you experience prior to or while you are having difficulty?" "Does your anxiety interfere with your activities?"

A starting place for assessment is the *Global Assessment of Functioning Scale* (Endicott, Spitzer, Fleiss, & Cohen, 1976). This scale used as the basis of the DSM-IV (APA, 1994) Axis V diagnosis, and permits a rating between 1 and 100 as a gen-eral description of function. For example, someone who rates between 51 and 60 would have "moderate symptoms . . . *or* moderate difficulty in social, occupational, or school function-ing" (p. 32). This rating is quite imprecise, but conveys an overall impression of the individual's performance.

Role assessment inventories typically provide a broad perspective on the individual's activity constellation and sat-isfaction with those activities, and are a helpful starting place in assessing psychological components of function. A num-ber of structured interviews of this type have been developed in occupational therapy. These include the *Occupational History* (Moorhead, 1969; Florey & Michaelman, 1982; Kielhofner, et al., 1986), *Occupational Therapy Functional Screening Tool* (Kielhofner, 1985) *Occupational Role Screening Interview* (Florey & Michelman, 1982), and *Role Change Assessment* (Jackoway, Rogers, & Snow, 1987). The recently developed *Canadian Occupational Performance Measure* (COPM) (Pollack, 1993; Pollack, Baptiste, Law, et al, 1990) is particularly helpful in that it elicits information in a structured fashion that relates to the range of factors that the client perceives as interfering with performance.

Other instruments that can be used to provide a general perspective on performance are the *Activity Configuration* (Mosey, 1973), Role Checklist (Oakley, Kielhofner, Barris, & Reichler, 1986), *Comprehensive Occupational Therapy Evaluation* (COTE) (Brayman & Kirby, 1982), *Adolescent Role Assessment* (Black, 1976), and *Children's Self-Assessment of Occupational Functioning* (Curtin & Baron, 1986).

Assessing Performance Areas

Many standardized instruments have been designed specifically for use with individuals with individuals with psychiatric diagnoses. Some focus on performance areas. These include instruments that measure, for example, activi-ties of daily living (ADL). Among these is the *Milwaukee Evaluation of Daily Living Skills* (MEDLS) (Leonardelli, 1988), the *Scorable Self-Care Evaluation* (SCORE) (Clark & Peters, 1984), and the *Klein-Bell Activity of Daily Living Scale* (Klein & Bell, 1979). The *Bay Area Functional Performance Evaluation* (BaFPE) (Bloomer & Williams, 1986) assesses some ADL, some instrumental activities of daily living (IADL), and some components of performance, most notably cognitive abilities. Leisure interests, if not abil-ities, can be assessed with instruments like the *Interest Checklist* (Matsutsuyu, 1969), as well as the *Activity Configuration* (Mosey, 1973).

There are fewer examples of instruments specifically focused on occupational therapy considerations of work per-formance (Velozzo, 1991), although there are numerous instruments that provide various kinds of information that is useful in this area. The *Worker Role Interview* (Velozzo, Kielhofner, & Fisher, 1990) has potential to provide under-standing of the individual's work-related activities. Some vocational interest instruments like the *Strong-Campbell Interest Inventory* (Strong & Campbell, 1981) provide pro-files of client interests as compared with interests of success-ful individuals in an array of vocations. Other instruments provide information about performance components and skills (Mathiowetz, 1993), rather than about vocational per-formance as a whole. Jacobs (1991) has compiled a listing of work-related assessments, although these are not specific to psychological constructs.

Assessing Performance Components

Other instruments emphasize components of perform-ance. Many are not designed specifically for use with indi-viduals with psychological deficits (*Sensory Integration and Praxis Test* [Ayres, 1989]), while others have been designed with particular emphasis on this population.

Cognitive abilities, particularly those that describe the executive functions needed for task performance can be assessed with instruments like the *Allen Cognitive Level Test*

(ACL) (Allen, 1985; David & Riley, 1990) and the *Kitchen Task Assessment* (KTA) (Baum & Edwards, 1993). In addition, there is an array of neuropsychological instruments like the *Halstead-Reitan Neuropsychological Battery* (Boll, 1981) designed by psychologists, that provide invaluable information to occupational therapists. Caution must be exercised in using instruments developed by other professions for two reasons. First, they often require specialized training that is not part of typical entry level occupational therapy education. Second, they were standardized for different purposes, and interpretations for purposes of occupational therapy intervention must be made with this in mind.

Sensorimotor components are often measured in conjunction with cognitive ones. The *Halstead-Reitan* (Boll, 1981) looks at both, as do a number of other instruments. The *Sensory Integration and Praxis Test* (Ayres, 1989) is an example of an occupational therapy instrument that examines sensorimotor factors; it is standardized largely for use with children. The *Deuels Test of Motor Apraxia* (Edwards, Baum & Deuels, 1991) was developed to address apraxia in older adults and those with dementia. Numerous instruments assess motor performance, and are described in Chapter 8. A good resource for these instruments is the *Functional Tool Box* (Lewis & McNerney, 1995).

The *Assessment of Motor and Process Skills* (Baron, 1994; Pan & Fisher, 1994; Fisher, 1992) addresses two components of performance, cognitive and motor, through a performance-based observational method. Initially developed for use with adults with brain injuries, its use with individuals with Alzheimer's disease and other cognitive impairments has also been studied.

Perhaps the most difficult component to assess is the psychological component. This may be due in part to definitional problems. It is also difficult to evaluate phenomena that are primarily internal to the individual. A number of existing instruments in this area are what are called projective tests, i.e., they infer emotional state from observed performance. These include the *Azima Battery* (Azima & Azima, 1959), the *BH Battery* (Hemphill, 1982), and *Lerner's Magazine Picture Collage* (Lerner & Ross, 1977). These instruments require the patient to undertake an activity, for example making a collage, and then to talk about the process and product. The therapist observes emotional content (does the patient select images that are largely depressive in nature, for example), as well as the process, that may reflect motivation, ability to concentrate, hostility, locus of control, self-concept and self-esteem as well as other factors.

It is also possible to use projective instruments developed by other professions. The *House-Tree-Person* (Buck & Jolles, 1972) and *Draw-a-Person* (Machover, 1949) are examples of instruments developed initially by psychologists but used by some occupational therapists to provide information about body image, self-esteem, and perceptual abilities. Psychologists using these instruments usually complete at least one complete academic course devoted to their systematic administration and interpretation; occupational therapists without this training should not use them, and should be aware that unstandardized uses provide unstandardized information.

There is also a long list of instruments that measure various psychological constructs, including self-concept and self-esteem (*Multidimensional Self-Concept Scale* [Rotatori, 1994]), locus of control (*Rotter Locus of Control Inventory* [Rotter, 1966]), self-efficacy (Gage, Noh, Polatajko, et al., 1994), and personality characteristics generally (*Edwards Personal Preference Schedule* [Edwards, 1953]; *Sixteen Personality Factor* [16PF] [Cattell, Cattell, Cattell, Russell & Karol, 1994])

A number of instruments measure various forms of psychiatric disorder. A comprehensive screening instrument is the *Mental Status Examination* (Kaplan & Sadock, 1988), which is often administered in one of its many forms by a psychiatrist or psychologist as a way to decide which of the many more specific instruments would be helpful. Specific factors that can be evaluated by way of standardized instruments include depression (*Beck Depression Inventory* [Beck, 1967]; *Depression Adjective Check List* [Lubin, 1967]), anxiety (*Taylor Manifest Anxiety Scale* [Heineman, 1953]). Several of these measure a number of constructs on the same instrument (*Minnesota Multiphasic Personality Inventory* [MMPI] [Hathaway & McKinley, 1951]). The *Brief Psychiatric Rating Scale* (Overall & Gorham, 1962) measures somatic concern, anxiety, withdrawal, grandiosity, hallucinatory behavior, and other characteristics common in individuals with psychiatric disorders. All of these were developed for use by psychologists. Some require considerable training for effective use, others, like the *Beck Depression Inventory*, are relatively straightforward to administer and interpret. While a number of these can provide useful information, occupational therapists must keep in mind their purpose in assessing clients. As has already been noted, occupational therapists do not treat depression, but the activity-based consequences of depression. A summary of various instruments used in mental health settings by occupational therapists is can be found in Asher (1989).

An important consideration in the assessment process is the occupational therapist's role relative to psychotropic medication. As biological factors related to psychological disorders are better understood, medications to treat them effectively are becoming more available. However, treatment with these medications is still art as well as science (Fischer, 1995). Individuals react differently to varying kinds of medication and to different doses. For example, in treatment of depression, there are now three main types of medication (the tricyclic antidepressants, monoamine oxidase inhibitors, and selective serotonin reuptake inhibitors) with others also used occasionally. Each class of antidepressant has several drugs, with slightly different chemical compositions and effects. A particular individual may react better to one class of drug than another, or to different drugs within a class, or to different doses of a specific drug. To a large extent, effective medication must be determined through trial and effort. Because an important goal of these medical interventions is improved performance, the therapist must provide careful baseline information, and reassess as the medication reaches therapeutic blood levels. Further, the therapist must monitor side effects (e.g., tremor) that might negatively impact on function.

The instruments described here have varying mechanisms for administration. Some are interviews, others are observational measures, some are inventories or self-administered questionnaires. Advantages and disadvantages of each of these methods are discussed in Chapter 5. In general, the most effective assessment is one that uses several methods and covers a range of performance areas and components through screening, with careful attention to those areas identified through screening as presenting particular problems. A list of instruments and their uses is included in Table 12-5.

Returning to the case of Mrs. B., a set of assessment strategies can now be identified. Based on AOTA Uniform Terminology (AOTA, 1994), the therapist would consider both performance areas (activities of daily living; work and productive activities, and play or leisure), performance components (sensorimotor, cognitive integration and cognitive components, and psychosocial skills and psychological components), and performance contexts (temporal aspects and environment). The description of Mrs. B. above might emerge from a screening process, or be provided by the psychiatrist. The therapist would then pursue in detail those factors that seem most contributory to Mrs. B.'s performance difficulties. In this case, those would include psychosocial skills and psychological components. The factors listed in the Uniform Terminology Checklist (AOTA, 1994) are values, interests, self-concept, role performance, social conduct, interpersonal skills, self-expression, coping skills, time management, and self-control. The therapist would certainly consider performance contexts as well, those being temporal aspects and the physical, social, and cultural environment. In Mrs. B.'s case, the assessment of the social environment would include examination of the family constellation. The therapist could then consider what skills might be required in Mrs. B.'s situation, and an intervention could be structured to modify the environment, her skills, or both.

Uniform Terminology (AOTA, 1994) is a general guide of factors to consider. They must be placed in the context of a theory or frame of reference, however, to provide an explanation of how these factors interact to contribute to performance deficits.

The Ecology of Human Performance Model (Dunn et al., 1994) would encourage evaluation of performance in particular settings, through observation in relevant settings as well as standardized assessments. An *Occupational History* would provide a context for assessment and identify the settings in which assessment should occur.

Both the Person-Environment Performance (Law, et al., in press) and Person-Environment Occupational Performance (Christiansen & Baum, 1991; 1997) models would suggest a comprehensive assessment of the numerous intrinsic and extrinsic factors that contribute to performance, with particular attention to the interaction of these factors to produce effective occupational performance.

The Model of Human Occupation would suggest that Mrs. B. had lost valued roles. Administration of the *Occupational History* and *Occupational Role Screening Assessment* could clarify the specific nature of the loss. In addition, specific areas of performance might be assessed. If one of the valued roles lost related to work, an occupational inventory such as the *Strong-Campbell* might identify alternative interests.

The Occupational Adaptation frame of reference would suggest that Mrs. B. lacked the needed adaptive skills to cope with her changing circumstances. The *Multidimensional Self-Concept Scale* might provide information about Mrs. B.'s feelings of competence in her current situation, and her feelings about herself. The *Beck Depression Inventory* could reveal how much her current deficit in adaptation has impacted on her mood.

Intervention: Settings and Strategies

The environment in which primarily psychological problems are addressed is changing rapidly. This is a major factor in care. As in other kinds of health care, inpatient treatment is rapidly diminishing; where stays of several years were once common, inpatient care is now rare, and brief when it occurs (Bonder, 1995). It is not unusual to hear of stays as short as 24 hours. In place of inpatient care, some individuals are being seen in outpatient therapy, partial hospitalization situations and nursing homes. Increasingly, psychological interventions are provided in settings that are not identified exclusively with mental health. For example, therapists in schools often intervene with families to address psychological factors that impair school performance. The therapist may teach the family to work with their child to minimize anxiety that hampers learning. Therapists in work settings may need to help a client reduce fears of reinjury, as well as teach him or her how to stoop and lift.

As a result of these changes, as well as the fundamental principles of occupational therapy, therapists intervene to address psychological factors in many settings. These

TABLE 12-5

Occupational Therapy Assessments in Mental Health

Roles and Role Balance

Global Assessment Scale (Endicott et al., 1976)

Occupational History (Moorhead, 1969; Florey and Michaelman, 1982; Kielhofner et al., 1986)

Occupational Therapy Functional Screening Tool (Kielhofner, 1985)

Occupational Role Screening Interview (Florey & Michaelman, 1982)

Role Change Assessment (Jackoway, Rogers, & Snow, 1987)

Canadian Occupational Performance Measure (COPM) (Pollack, 1993; Pollack, Baptiste, & Law et al., 1990)

Activity Configuration (Mosey, 1973)

Role Checklist (Oakley et al., 1986)

Comprehensive Occupational Therapy Evaluation (COTE) (Brayman & Kirby, 1982)

Adolescent Role Assessment (Black, 1976)

Self-Assessment of Occupational Functioning (Curtin & Baron, 1986)

Functional Behavior Profile (Baum, Edwards & Morrow-Howell, 1993)

Performance Areas

ADL/IADL

Milwaukee Evaluation of Daily Living Skills (MEDLS) (Leonardelli, 1988)

Scorable Self-Care Evaluation (SCORE) (Clark & Peters, 1984)

Klein-Bell Activity of Daily Living Scale (Klein & Bell, 1979)

Bay Area Functional Performance Evaluation (BaFPE) (Bloomer & Williams, 1978)

Leisure

Interest Checklist (Matsutsuyu, 1969)

Activity Configuration (Mosey, 1973)

Knox Play Scale (1974)

Work

Strong-Campbell Interest Inventory (Strong & Campbell, 1981)

Worker Role Interview (Velozo, Kielhofner, & Fisher, 1990)

Performance Components

Cognitive

Allen Cognitive Level Test (ACL) (Allen, 1985; David & Riley, 1990).

Halstead-Reitan Neuropsychological Battery (Boll, 1981)

Kitchen Task Assessment (KTA) (Baum & Edwards, 1993)

Sensorymotor

Halstead-Reitan (Boll, 1981)

Sensory Integration and Praxis Tests (Ayres, 1989)

Assessment of Motor and Process Skills (AMPS) (Baron, 1994; Pan & Fisher, 1994; Fisher, 1992)

Deuel Test of Constructional Apraxia (Edwards, Baum & Deuel, 1991)

Motor

Assessment of Motor and Process Skills (Baron, 1994; Pan & Fisher, 1994; Fisher, 1992)

Psychological

Azima Battery (Azima & Azima, 1959)

BH Battery (Hemphill, 1982)

Lerner's Magazine Picture Collage (Lerner & Ross, 1977)

House-Tree-Person (Buck & Jolles, 1972)

Draw-a-Person (Machover, 1949)

Multidimensional Self-Concept Scale (Rotatori, 1994)

Rotter Locus of Control (Rotter, 1969)

Edwards Personal Preference Schedule (Edwards, 1953)

Self-Efficacy Scale (Gage, Noh, Polatajko, et al., 1994)

Beck Depression Inventory (Beck, 1967)

Depression Adjective Check List (Lubin, 1967)

Taylor Manifest Anxiety Scale (Heineman, 1953)

Minnesota Multiphasic Personality Inventory (Hathaway & McKinley, 1951)

Brief Psychiatric Rating Scale (Overall & Gorham, 1962)

Piers-Harris Children's Self-Concept Scale (1967)

Locus of Control Test for Children (Nowicki & Strickland, 1973)

Sixteen Personality Factor (16PF) (Cattell et al., 1994)

include not only traditional mental health inpatient settings, but also in sheltered workshops, schools, businesses, community health agencies, home health, nursing homes, homeless shelters, and prisons. A common set of goals and interventions may cross boundaries, but individuals in each setting there are unique factors to be considered, as well.

Prevention programs are becoming more common. These programs address both emotional and physical performance. For example, in industrial settings, an occupational therapist might be asked to structure work stations that minimize risk of repetitive motion syndrome, and at the same time, a work schedule that minimizes risk of excessive stress with its related problems. The Americans with Disabilities Act (ADA) requires that employers make reasonable accommodations for individuals with both emotional and physical disabilities. Christ and Stoffel (1992) note that such adaptations might include altering work schedules, structuring supervision appropriately, breaking tasks into manageable components, etc.

Habilitation programs are those that address specific skills of living. A sheltered workshop, for example, might provide vocational skills training for an individual with a developmental disability or chronic psychiatric disorder (Block, 1992). To be effective, it must also address issues of motivation, self-concept, self-esteem, and self-efficacy (Bolding & Llorens, 1991). Some individuals might need habilitation programs focused on self-care or social skills. This is particularly true of individuals who have had long-term, chronic disorders.

Inpatient programs are experiencing rapid transition. Most have greatly reduced length of stay, often by designing outpatient follow-up for clients. For example, therapeutic communities designed for individuals with substance abuse problems provide an environment in which an individual can withdraw safely from the substance and plan for a changed life (Carroll, 1992); Preparation for rapid transition to the community is an essential part of intervention in these settings. It has been noted that interdisciplinary teams work best in these settings. In addition, a particular role for OT in reducing substance abuse is providing alternative leisure interests (Mann & Talty, 1990).

Acute care inpatient facilities are now designed for careful evaluation (Robinson & Avallone, 1990) and for preparation for discharge (Atlas, 1992). In the now rare circumstances in which hospitalization is "long term," OT emphasizes daily living skills to facilitate deinstitutionalization (Hemphill & Werner, 1990).

Outpatient clinics and partial hospitalization (Gusich & Silverman, 1991) are increasingly substituting for in-patient care. These include halfway houses (Wilberding, 1991) that serve as a transition to the community or a temporary, partial shelter from the demands of community life. In partial hospital settings, clients might sleep and live in the facility while going to a job in the community. An occupational therapist in this kind of setting would focus on feelings and attitudes around competence and perceived competence in self-care and community living skills. Day hospitals, on the other hand, provide activities during the day, while clients return to their own homes in the evening. Occupational therapists might focus on vocational or leisure skills to enable clients to reintegrate into daily community life.

Community-based programs of various kinds provide support to individuals who may not be able to function comfortably without support (Learnard & Devereaux, 1992). One community mental health center had a weekly "hobby" group, during which the clients: 1) talked about their week, enabling the therapist to screen for emerging problems; 2) tried out various leisure activities to begin to establish interests; 3) practiced social skills; and 4) derived support and encouragement. Occupational therapists have an essential role in community mental health (Tricky & Kennedy, 1995) particularly as this is increasingly the site at which more individuals with more severe and chronic conditions are treated.

Home health is also increasingly a setting in which psychosocial intervention is provided. Although care is most often provided by a nurse whose main role is to administer medications, if issues of performance require attention the occupational therapist should undertake an environmental assessment to ensure that the person is capable of managing safely and independently in the home, complete an interest assessment to be certain the individual has a daily routine, and assist the individual in community integration. Environmental approaches are discussed in Chapter 11.

A less common site for occupational therapy is in crisis intervention (Miller & Robertson, 1991). This is a form of treatment in which the individual is seen during a period of emotional upheaval (e.g., divorce, death of a parent) for a very brief time. The focus of treatment is on resolution of the immediate situation. Occupational therapists can offer education and strategies for problem solving, particularly when the crisis is one related to role performance, for example, loss of a job.

Another less common but important site for occupational therapy services focused on psychosocial factors is in primary care (Devereaux & Walker, 1995). While most primary care emphasizes prevention of physical illness, screening for functional deficits can prevent secondary psychological disorder. For example, identifying an individual with an impoverished social life might facilitate intervention before isolation can lead to depression.

TABLE 12-6

Occupational Therapy Goals in Mental Health

Goal	Possible Modalities
Increased problem solving creativity interpersonal flexibility	Assertiveness training Expressive modalities (art, creative writing) Group discussion and activities Environmental modifications
Suicide prevention	Expressive modalities Support group interventions Participation in leisure activities
Improved family interaction	Group activities Discussion groups Assertiveness training
Reduction in problem behaviors	Sensory integration Behavioral programs with appropriate reinforcement and extinction Sensory input (listening to music, baking)
Vocational transition	Task analysis of work Assessment of interests Work skills training Practice
Time perspective and management	Education Practice
Activity balance and satisfaction	Interest assessment Group or individual discussion of interests Practice of new activities
Leisure interests	Interest assessment Experimentation with activities Discussion of resources
Self-esteem	All modalities above
Self-efficacy	Analysis of outcomes of activities
General health	Exercise Hobbies Social interaction Interests

Treatment Planning

Goals

Just as a frame of reference guides assessment, it also directs treatment. For example, for Mrs. B., goals based on MOHO might emphasize development of valued goals or reestablishing activities that allow expression of those valued goals. Goals based on OA might focus on learning adaptive strategies that permit Mrs. B. to adjust more easily as her circumstances change, teaching her problem-solving skills. Goals based on the Person-Environment Occupational Performance Model would emphasize not only Mrs. B's performance, but also the environment in which she must function. Education of the family regarding her needs would be an important strategy.

A number of goals can be identified as typical of occupational therapy intervention. These may be incorporated into treatment regardless of frame of reference. Some goals of occupational therapy, and modalities for implementing them are described in Table 12-6.

Problem-solving, creativity, interpersonal flexibility (Miller & Robertson, 1991; Nezu & Nezu, 1991) are important to individuals regardless of their psychiatric disorder. The world is an unpredictible place, and an array of strategies to meet daily challenges, as well as less frequent but more significant stresses is essential to effective performance. Therapists may enhance these abilities through teaching of problem-solving strategies, or through use of activities that require these characteristics and allow for practice.

Suicide prevention (Custer & Wassink, 1991) is an issue for many individuals who are depressed. Because guilt and anhedonia are so characteristic of people who are depressed, providing motivation or reasons for survival can be essential. Therapists must learn to watch clients who are suicidal to ensure that they do not harm themselves, but, equally important, must provide them with activities they can value and through which they can experience success, as a means to provide the will to survive.

Improved family interaction (Moyers, 1992) can be facilitated through use of groups as a practice arena for interpersonal skills. Many individuals who have psychiatric disorders also experience family problems, sometimes as a result of their disorder, sometimes as a contributing factor. The ability to identify feelings and needs clearly, often a difficulty in the context of the family, can be taught through assertiveness training. A client's ability to respond to the needs of others, sometimes equally problematic, can be taught through cooperative group activities. Also, families need to be give information to understand the deficits of their loved ones. They need to be aware that some behaviors are not willful on the part of the individual, and what strategies they can use to help the individual modulate behaviors. Further, they need to understand how their attitudes and behaviors may contribute to an environment that is not optimal to the individual's performance.

Reduction in problem behaviors (Reisman & Blakeney, 1991) that often accompany mental retardation, manic episodes, dementia and other psychiatric disorders, can be accomplished through engagement in activity. Sometimes patterned sensory input can be soothing to individuals who have mental retardation. Sensory integrative activities may also reduce some problem behaviors. For individuals with manic disorders, clear feedback and limit setting in the course of activity can be helpful.

Vocational transition (Richert, 1991) is particularly problematic for adolescents with psychiatric disorders and for individuals with chronic conditions. Simulating work environments in the clinic, providing work experience in a sheltered situation, discussing characteristics of effective workers, and instruction and practice of work-related skills such as using public transportation, interacting with a supervisor, and managing time, can be taught and practiced in the course of occupational therapy activities, particularly when the behavioral needs of the person can be matched to job demands.

Time perspective and time management (Suto & Frank, 1994) is a problem not only in work-related intervention, but in other areas of performance as well. Individuals who have mental retardation, brain injury, or who have chronic conditions may have difficulty understanding time. Practice in the occupational therapy environment, as well as discussion in group settings, can be helpful in adjusting to a time-focused external environment.

Activity balance and satisfaction (Larson, 1990) are issues for most individuals with psychiatric disorders, and are particular areas of emphasis for occupational therapy. It may be helpful to have the individual try out new activities, examine current activities, and map out plans for more satisfying involvement in the future. Assistance with resources for activities that are manageable financially, or that the individual can access can also support development of satisfying activity patterns. Working with families, the therapist can help everyone in the system understand the importance of activity in sustaining independence.

Leisure interests (Scaffa, 1991; Mann & Talty, 1990) are problematic for many individuals with psychiatric disorders. Such disorders as substance abuse are very likely to reemerge if the individual does not substitute satisfying leisure pursuits during the time previously spent using the substance. Exposure to an array of activities, planning for accomplishment of those activities, and practice can all assist the individual in developing leisure pursuits.

Self-esteem (Mayberry, 1990) is a goal addressed through all the strategies identified above. As the individual becomes more adept at managing feelings and situations, and develops more satisfying role balance and leisure activities, self-esteem is a likely outcome. However, the individual may also need assistance in interpreting what he or she is experiencing. Verbalization of abilities and identification of personal goals can assist in development of positive self-esteem.

An individual's ability to appropriately evaluate performance abilities (self-efficacy) is central to life satisfaction (Gage & Polatajko, 1994). Because psychosocial disorder is often associated with distorted perception, individuals may have unduly deflated or inflated views of their abilities. In such a situation, the goals for treatment would emphasize development of self-efficacy consistent with reality. One patient who was experiencing a manic episode told his therapist that he had "a perfect IQ." Such grandiosity is a typical sign of mania. This patient had both a distorted self-concept and an unrealistic sense of self-efficacy that appeared to contribute to an inappropriate sense of self-esteem. The therapist encouraged the patient to engage in activities he had never tried before. As he began to have difficulty completing them, his initial reaction was one of anger. Over time, however, he began to perceive the limitations of his perfection. At that point he was able to acknowledge to his therapist that being perfect was a weighty burden, and that he was relieved to know that he could make mistakes without causing catastrophe.

Modalities

Occupational therapists often use education, demonstration, discussion, and practice as methods to accomplish therapeutic goals. These interventions might be provided on a one-to-one basis, but are increasingly incorporated into groups. Groups are an efficient means of delivering care, and are especially effective in remediating some problems. For example, social competence is best addressed in group settings, since the group provides a natural practice arena (Donohue, Labovitz, & Miller, 1990; Dodge & Mallard, 1992). It is common to find that individuals with psychosocial disorders have problems in social settings because of distorted perceptions, lack of self-esteem, or lack of skills. Assertiveness can also be a problem, for example in individuals who, like Mrs. B., are depressed (Nezu & Nezu, 1991). Training a person to meet his or her interpersonal needs in effective and appropriate ways can lead to improved relationships, and groups provide a laboratory for feedback, modeling, and practice.

Occupational therapists emphasize the therapeutic value of doing. For example, a mime group might be helpful in enhancing body image and self-esteem (Probst & Howe, 1988). Similarly, storytelling might be an effective way to assist children to express emotion and deal with anxiety (Fazio, 1992). Crafts can provide experiences of competence, opportunities to evaluate skills and outcomes, and a mechanism for expression. For example, one client was severely depressed, and had a great deal of difficulty talking about her anger. She was able to use a woodworking project as a way to externalize the rage she had been controlling at great cost to her mental state. Table 12-6 provides a summary of typical occupational therapy goals and the types of interventions that might be considered.

OUTCOMES OF MENTAL HEALTH TREATMENT

Unfortunately, there are few systematic evaluations of outcomes of occupational therapy interventions directed toward psychological components of performance. There is evidence that groups do encourage cohesiveness, interpersonal learning, hope, universality (Falk-Kessler, Momich, & Perel, 1991). Another outcome study has validated the use of graded crafts in improving visuomotor integration in individuals with psychiatric disorders (Kleinman & Stalcup, 1991). Cognitive rehabilitation appears to improve attention in individuals with schizophrenia (Brown, Harwood, Hays, et al., 1993). This is a process by which, using computer games and

other cognitive practice mechanisms, individuals practice problem solving, reacting, recognizing information, and so on. It is unclear as yet whether the positive impact identified in these kinds of interventions are generalizable to everyday life situations. Sensory integration has been shown to reduce behavioral symptoms as measured on the *Nurses Observation Scale for Inpatient Evaluation* (Reisman & Blakeney, 1991). Many sensory-integrative methods useful with children are employed in mental health as well, including patterned proprioceptive input of various kinds. Some would argue that this is not SI as described by Ayres (1974) since spinning activities on suspended equipment are rarely included. However, rolling on large balls, play with a parachute, and other typical SI interventions have been described as a means to improve body-image and thereby self-concept, as well as to facilitate motor performance that may be impaired for individuals with some psychiatric disorders. There have been a number of descriptive studies in occupational therapy that describe programs in substance abuse, developmental delay, eating disorders, and others where individuals with primarily psychological problems are treated. An encouraging trend is the use of qualitative methods in research. Because the occupational therapy process is so complex, isolating effects on particular performance components is quite difficult. Qualitative methods encourage rich, thorough description of the therapeutic process and its outcomes, and are a promising method for examining therapeutic outcomes.

CONCLUSION

While this chapter has emphasized psychological factors influencing performance, it is essential to reiterate here the importance of recognizing that in real life, with real clients, there is no clear line among performance factors. Therapists must strive to identify all the factors that contribute to effective performance if they are to provide their clients with the best possible intervention, and achieve the best possible outcomes. No situation is without emotional correlates. However, emotional considerations alone are rarely adequate to explain or remediate difficulties. Effective therapists attend to psychological/emotional factors in every therapeutic encounter, recognizing the complexity of human experience and performance.

STUDY QUESTIONS

1. Psychological factors affect well-being for every individual. Why is this so? What psychological factors contribute to a positive sense of well-being?

2. How do the environment and an individual's psycho-

logical characteristics interact to support or impede performance and well-being?

3. Why is psychiatric diagnosis important to occupational therapists?

4. Why is it important to have a theoretical framework for understanding psychological functioning? Use one of the theories described in this chapter to support your answer.

5. What is the occupational therapist's role in pharmacological intervention for psychiatric disorder?

6. Assume you have a client who is extremely anxious about school performance. Based on at least one theory discussed in this chapter, describe how you would approach assessment. Identify instruments you might use, and what you would hope to learn.

7. For the client who is anxious about school, what might be some appropriate settings for intervention? What might be reasonable goals and modalities for treatment, and how might you know whether you are successful?

8. Can effectiveness of occupational therapy in mental health be determined based on existing studies of outcomes? What additional information is needed to document effectiveness?

RECOMMENDED READING

Asher, I. E. (1989). *An annotated index of occupational therapy evaluation tools.* Bethesda, MD: American Occupational Therapy Association.

Bonder, B. R. (1995). *Psychopathology and function* (2nd ed.). Thorofare, NJ: SLACK Incorporated.

Kielhofner, G. (1992). *Conceptual foundations of occupational therapy.* Philadelphia, PA: F.A. Davis.

Mattingly, C., & Fleming, M. H. (1994). *Clinical reasoning: Forms of inquiry in a therapeutic practice.* Philadelphia: F.A. Davis.

Schkade, J. K., & Schultz, S. (1992). Occupational adaptation: Toward a holistic approach for contemporary practice, part 1. *American Journal of Occupational Therapy, 46,* 829-838.

Schultz, S., & Schkade, J. K. (1992). Occupational adaptation: Toward a holistic approach for contemporary practice, part 2. *American Journal of Occupational Therapy, 46,* 917-926.

REFERENCES

Allen, C. (1985). *Occupational therapy for psychiatric diseases: Measurement and management of cognitive disabilities.* Boston: Little, Brown & Co.

Allman, P. (1991). Depressive disorders and emotionalism following stroke. *International Journal of Geriatric Psychiatry, 6,* 377-383.

American Occupational Therapy Association. (1994). *Uniform terminology for reporting occupational therapy services* (3rd ed.). Rockville, MD: Author.

American Psychiatric Association, Task Force on Nomenclature. (1994). *Diagnostic and statistical manual of mental disorders* (4th ed.). Washington, DC: Author.

Asher, I. E. (1989). *An annotated index of occupational therapy evaluation tools.* Rockville, MD: American Occupational Therapy Association.

Atlas, J. A. (1992). Brief treatment approaches to hospitalized adolescents. *Residential Treatment for Children & Youth, 9,* 5-13.

Ayres, J. (1974). *Sensory integration and learning disorders.* Los Angeles: Western Psychological Services.

Ayres, J. (1989). *Sensory integration and praxis tests.* Los Angeles: Western Psychological Services.

Azima, H., & Azima, F. (1959). Outline of a dynamic theory of occupational therapy. *American Journal of Occupational Therapy, 8,* 215.

Baron, K. B. (1994). Clinical interpretation of "The Assessment of Motor and Process Skills of Persons with Psychiatric Disorders." *American Journal of Occupational Therapy, 48,* 781-782.

Baum, C., Edwards, D. F., & Morrow-Howell, N. (1993). Identification and measurement of productive behaviors in senile dementia of the Alzheimer type. *Gerontologist, 33,* 403-408.

Beck, A. T. (1967). *Depression: Clinical, experimental and theoretical aspects.* New York: Harper & Row.

Black, M. (1976). The adolescent role assessment. *American Journal of Occupational Therapy, 30,* 73-79.

Block, L. (1992). The employment connection: The application of an individual supported employment program for persons with chronic mental health problems. *Canadian Journal of Community Mental Health, 11,* 79-89.

Bloomer, J., & Williams, S. C. (1986). *Bay Area Functional Performance Evaluation (BaFPE): Task oriented assessment and social interaction scale manual.* San Francisco: USCF.

Bolding, D. J., & Llorens, L. A. (1991). The effects of habilitative hospital admission on self-care, self-esteem, and frequency of physical care. *American Journal of Occupational Therapy, 45,* 796-800.

Boll, T. J. (1981). The Halstead-Reitan neuropsychological battery. In S. B. Filskov & T. J. Boll (Eds.), *Handbook of clinical neuropsychology.* New York: John Wiley & Sons.

Bonder, B. R. (1993). Issues in assessment of psychosocial components of function. *American Journal of Occupational Therapy, 47,* 211-216.

Bonder, B. R. (1995). *Psychopathology & function* (2nd ed.). Thorofare, NJ: SLACK Incorporated.

Brayman, S., & Kirby, T. (1982). The comprehensive occupational therapy evaluation. In B. Hemphill (Ed.), *The evaluation process in psychiatric occupational therapy.* Thorofare, NJ: SLACK Incorporated.

Brown, C., Harwood, K., Hays, C., Heckman, J., & Short, J. E. (1993). Effectiveness of cognitive rehabilitation for improving attention in patients with schizophrenia. *Occupational Therapy Journal of Research, 13,* 71-76.

Buck, J., & Jolles, I. (1972). *House-tree-person projective technique.* California: Western Psychological Services.

Carroll, J. F. X. (1992). The evolving American therapeutic community. *Alcoholism Treatment Quarterly, 9,* 175-181.

Cattell, R. B., Cattell, A. K. S., Cattell, H. E. P., Russell, M., & Karol, D. (1994). *Sixteen personality factor test.* Champaign, IL: Institute for Personality and Ability Testing.

Christ, P. A., & Stoffel, V. C. (1992). The Americans with Disabilities Act of 1990 and employees with mental impairments: Personal efficacy and the environment. *American Journal of Occupational Therapy, 46,* 434-443.

Christiansen, C., & Baum, C. (1991). *Occupational therapy: Overcoming human performance deficits.* Thorofare, NJ: SLACK, Incorporated.

Christiansen, C., & Baum, C. (1997). *Occupational therapy: Enabling function and well-being.* Thorofare, NJ: SLACK Incorporated.

Clark, E. N., & Peters, M. (1984). *The scoreable self-care evaluation.* Thorofare, NJ: SLACK Incorporated.

Curtin, C. & Baron, K. B. (1986). *The children's self-assessment of occupational functioning.* Chicago, IL: University of Illinois; 1986.

Custer, V. L., & Wassink, K. E. (1991). Occupational therapy intervention for an adult with depression and suicidal tendencies. *American Journal of Occupational Therapy, 45,* 845-825.

David, S. K., & Riley, W. T. (1990). The relationship of the Allen Cognitive Level Test to cognitive abilities and psychopathology. *American Journal of Occupational Therapy, 44,* 493-497.

Devereaux, E. B., & Walker, R. B. (1995). The role of occupational therapy in primary health care. *American Journal of Occupational Therapy, 49,* 391-396.

Dodge, E. P., & Mallard, A. R. (1992). Social skills training using a collaborative service delivery model. *Language, Speech, and Hearing Services in Schools, 23,* 130-135.

Donohue, M. V., Labovitz, D. R., & Miller, R. J. (1990). Social competence of female psychiatric patients: A study of sociability, social presence, socialization, diagnoses, and age of onset of psychosis. *Occupational Therapy Journal of Research, 10,* 163-176.

Dunn, W., Brown, C., & McGuigan, A. (1994). The ecology of human performance: A framework for considering the effect of context *American Journal of Occupational Therapy, 48,* 595-607.

Edwards, A. L. (1953). *Edwards Personal Preference Schedule.* New York: Psychological Corporation.

Edwards, D. F., Baum, C., & Deuel, R. K. (1991). Constructional apraxia in Alzheimer's disease: contributions to functional loss. *Physical & Occupational Therapy in Geriatrics, 9,* 53-68.

Ellis, A. (1973). *Humanistic psychology: A rational emotive approach.* New York: McGraw-Hill.

Endicott, J., Spitzer, R. L., Fleiss, J. L., & Cohen, J. (1976). The global assessment scale: A procedure for measuring overall severity of psychiatric disturbance. *Archives of General Psychiatry, 33,* 771.

Falk-Kessler, J., Momich, C., & Perel, S. (1991). Therapeutic factors in occupational therapy groups. *American Journal of Occupational Therapy, 45,* 59-66.

Fazio, L. S. (1992). Tell me a story: The therapeutic metaphor in the practice of pediatric occupational therapy. *American Journal of Occupational Therapy, 46,* 112-119.

Fischer, P. J. (1995). Psychopharmacology. In B. R. Bonder (Ed.), *Psychopathology and function* (2nd ed.). Thorofare, NJ: SLACK Incorporated, 183-219.

Fisher, A.G. (1992). *Assessment of motor and process skills* (Res. Ed. 6.1). Unpublished test manual, Department of Occupational Therapy, Fort Collins, CO: Colorado State University.

Florey, L. L., & Michaelman, S. M. (1982). Occupational role history: A screening tool for psychiatric occupational therapy. *American Journal of Occupational Therapy, 36,* 301-308.

Freud, S. (1961). The ego and the id. In *The complete psychological works of Sigmund Freud* (Vol. 9). London: Hogarth Press.

Gage, M., Noh, S., Polatajko, H. J., & Kaspar, V. (1994). Measuring perceived self-efficacy in occupational therapy. *American Journal of Occupational Therapy, 48,* 783-790.

Gage, M., & Polatajko, H. J. (1994). Enhancing occupational performance through an understanding of perceived self-efficacy. *American Journal of Occupational Therapy, 48,* 452-461.

Gusich, R. L., & Silverman, A. L. (1991). Basava Day Clinic: The model of human occupation as applied to psychiatric day hospitalization. *Occupational Therapy in Mental Health, 11,* 113-134.

Hathaway, S. R., & McKinley, J. C. (1951). *Minnesota Multiphasic Personality Inventory: Manual (Rev. ed.).* New York: The Psychological Corporation.

Heineman, C. E. (1953). A forced choice form of the Taylor Anxiety Scale. *Journal of Consulting Psychology, 17,* 447-454.

Hemphill, B. J. (Ed.). (1982). *The evaluative process in psychiatric occupational therapy.* Thorofare, NJ: SLACK Incorporated.

Hemphill, B. J., & Werner, P. C. (1990). Deinstitutionalization: A role for occupational therapy in the state hospital. *Occupational Therapy in Mental Health, 10,* 85-99.

Howland, R. H., & Thase, M. E. (1991). Biological studies of dysthymia. *Biological Psychiatry, 30,* 243-304.

Huebner, R. A. (1991). Autistic disorder: A neuropsychological enigma. *American Journal of Occupational Therapy, 46,* 487-501.

Jackoway, I. S., Rogers, J. C., & Snow, T. (1987). The role change assessment: An interview tool for evaluating older adults. *Occupational Therapy in Mental Health, 1,* 17-37.

Jacobs, K. (1991). *Occupational therapy: Work-related programs and assessments* (2nd ed.). Boston: Little, Brown.

Kaplan, H., & Sadock, B. (1988). *Modern synopsis of comprehensive psychiatry V* (5th ed.). Baltimore: Williams & Wilkins.

Kielhofner, G. (Ed.). (1985). *A model of human occupation: Theory and application.* Baltimore: Williams & Wilkins.

Kielhofner, G., & Burke, J. (1980). A model of human occupation, Part 1. Conceptual framework and content. *American Journal of Occupational Therapy, 34,* 572-581.

Kielhofner, G., Harlan, B., Bauer, D., & Maurer, P. (1986). The reliability of a historical interview with physically disabled respondents. *American Journal of Occupational Therapy, 40,* 551-556.

Klein, R. M. & Bell, B. (1979). *Klein-Bell activity of daily living scale: Manual.* Seattle: University of Washington, Division of Occupational Therapy.

Kleinman, B. L., & Stalcup, A. (1991). The effect of graded craft activities on visuomotor integration in an inpatient child psychiatry population. *American Journal of Occupational Therapy, 45,* 324-330.

Larson, K. B. (1990). Activity patterns and life changes in people with depression. *American Journal of Occupational Therapy, 44,* 902-906.

Law, M., Cooper, B. A., Strong, S., Stewart, D., Rigby, P., & Letts, L. (1997). A theoretical context for the practice of occupational therapy. In C. Christiansen & C. Baum (Eds.), *Occupational therapy: Enabling function and well-being.* Thorofare, NJ: SLACK Incorporated.

Lawton, M., & Nahemow, L. (1973). Ecology and the aging process. In C. Eisdorfer & M. P. Lawton (Eds.), *Psychology of adult development and aging.* Washington, DC: American Psychological Association.

Learnard, L. T., & Devereaux, E. (1992). A model for community practice. *Hospital and community psychiatry, 43,* 869-871.

Leonardelli, C. (1988). The Milwaukee Evaluation of Daily Living Skills (MEDLS). In B. Hemphill (Ed.), *Mental health assessment in occupational therapy.* Thorofare, NJ: SLACK Incorporated.

Lerner, C., & Ross, G. (1977). The magazine picture collage: The development of an objective scoring system. *American Journal of Occupational Therapy, 31,* 156-162.

Levine, R. E., & Brayley, C. R. (1991). Occupation as a therapeutic medium. In C. Christiansen & C. Baum (Eds.), *Occupational therapy: Overcoming human performance deficits* (pp. 591-631). Thorofare, NJ: SLACK Incorporated.

Lewis, C. B., & McNerney, T. (1995). *The functional tool box.* Washington, DC: Learn, Publ.

Lubin, B. (1967). *Manual for the depression adjective checklists.* San Diego: Educational and Industrial Testing Source.

Machover, K. (1949). *Personality projection in the drawing of the human figure.* Springfield, IL: Charles C. Thomas.

Mann, W. C., & Talty, P. (1990). Leisure activity profile measuring use of leisure time by persons with alcoholism. *American Journal of Occupational Therapy, 47,* 111-118.

Mathiowetz, V. (1993). Role of physical performance component evaluation in occupational therapy functional assessment. *American Journal of Occupational Therapy, 23,* 323-328.

Matsutsuyu, J. (1969). The interest checklist. *American Journal of Occupational Therapy, 23,* 323-328.

Mattingly, C., & Fleming, M. H. (1994). *Clinical reasoning: Forms of inquiry in a therapeutic practice.* Philadelphia: F.A. Davis.

Mayberry, W. (1990). Self-esteem in children: Considerations for measurement and intervention. *American Journal of Occupational Therapy, 44,* 729-734.

Mayou, R., Hawton, K., Feldman, E., & Ardern, M. (1991). Psychiatric problems among medical admissions. *Psychiatry in Medicine, 21,* 71-84.

Miller, V., & Robertson, S. (1991). A role for occupational therapy in crisis intervention and prevention. *Australian Occupational Therapy Journal, 38,* 143-146.

Moorhead, L. (1969). The occupational history. *American Journal of Occupational Therapy, 23,* 329-334.

Mosey, A. C. (1973). *Activities therapy.* New York: Raven Press Publishers.

Moyers, P. A. (1992). Occupational therapy intervention with the alcoholic's family. *American Journal of Occupational Therapy, 46,* 105-111.

Nezu, C. M., & Nezu, A. M. (1991). Assertiveness and problem-solving training for mildly mentally retarded personas with dual diagnoses. *Research in Developmental Disabilities, 12,* 371-386.

Nowicki, S., & Strickland, B. (1973). A locus of control scale for children. *Journal of Consulting and Clinical Psychology, 40,* 148-154.

Oakley, F., Kielhofner, G., Barris, R., & Reichler, R. K. (1986). The role checklist: Development and empirical assessment of reliability. *Occupational Therapy Journal of Research, 6,* 157-170.

Overall, J. E., & Gorham, D. R. (1962). The brief psychiatric rating scale. *Psychological Reports, 10,* 799-812.

Pan, A., & Fisher, A. G. (1994). The assessment of motor and process skills of persons with psychiatric disorders. *American Journal of Occupational Therapy, 48,* 775-780.

Piers, E. V., & Harris, D. B. (1967). *Piers-Harris children's self-concept scale.* Nashville, TN: Counselor Recordings and Tests.

Pollack, N. (1993). Client-centered assessment. *American Journal of Occupational Therapy, 47,* 298-301.

Pollack, N., Baptiste, S., Law, M., McColl, M. A., Opzoomer, A., & Polatajko, H. (1990). Occupational performance measure: A review based on guidelines for the client-centered practice of occupational therapy. *Canadian Journal of Occupational Therapy, 57,* 77-81.

Probst, D. L., & Howe, M. C. (1988). The effect of a mime group on chronic adult psychiatric clients' body-image, self-esteem, and movement-concept. *Occupational Therapy in Mental Health, 8,* 135-153.

Reisman, J. E., & Blakeney, A. B. (1991). Exploring sensory integrative treatment in chronic schizophrenia. *Occupational Therapy in Mental Health, 11,* 25-44.

Richert, G. Z. (1991). Vocational transition in acute care psychiatry. *Occupational Therapy in Mental Health, 10,* 43-62.

Robinson, A. M., & Avallone, J. (1992). Occupational therapy in acute inpatient psychiatry: An activities health approach. *American Journal of Occupational Therapy, 44,* 809-814.

Rogers, J. C. (1982). Order and disorder in medicine and occupational therapy. *American Journal of Occupational Therapy, 36,* 29-35.

Rotatori, A. F. (1994). Multidimensional self-concept scale. *Evaluation in Counseling and Development, 26,* 265-268.

Rotter, J. B. (1966). Generalised expectancies for internal versus external control of reinforcement. *Psychological Monographs, 80,* 1-28.

Scaffa, M. E. (1991). Alcoholism: An occupational behavior perspective. *Occupational Therapy in Mental Health,* 99-112.

Schkade, J. K., & Schultz, S. (1992). Occupational adaptation: Toward a holistic approach for contemporary practice, part 1. *American Journal of Occupational Therapy, 46,* 829-838.

Schultz, S., & Schkade, J. K. (1992). Occupational adaptation: Toward a holistic approach for contemporary practice, part 2. *American Journal of Occupational Therapy, 46,* 917-926.

Skinner, B. F. (1971). *Beyond freedom and dignity.* Toronto: Bantam.

Strong, E. K. Jr., & Campbell, D. P. (1981). *Strong-Campbell interest inventory* (Rev. ed.). Palo Alto, CA: Consulting Psychologists Press.

Suto, M., & Frank, G. (1994). Future time perspective and daily occupations of persons with chronic schizophrenia in a board and care home. *American Journal of Occupational Therapy, 48,* 7-18.

Szynanski, S., Kane, J. M., & Leiberman, J. A. (1991). A selective review of biological markers in schizophrenia. *Schizophrenia Bulletin, 17,* 99-111.

Thompson, S. C., Sobolew-Shubin, A., Graham, M.A., & Janigan, A. S. (1989). Psychosocial adjustment following a stroke. *Social Science in Medicine, 28,* 239-247.

Tricky, B. A., & Kennedy, D. B. (1995). Use of occupational therapists in mental health settings in South Carolina. *American Journal of Occupational Therapy, 49,* 452-455.

Vause-Earland, T. (1991). Perceptions of role assessment tools in the physical disability setting. *American Journal of Occupational Therapy, 45,* 26-31.

Velozzo, C. (1991). Development of the worker role interview. *National institute on disability and rehabilitative research final report.* Chicago, Ill: University of Illinois at Chicago.

Velozzo, C., Kielhofner, G., & Fisher, G. (1990). *A user's guide to the worker role interview.* Unpublished test manual. Chicago, Ill: University of Illinois at Chicago.

Wilberding, D. (1991). The quarterway house: More than an alternative of care. *Occupational Therapy in Mental Health, 11,* 65-92.

Williams, J. B. W. (1988). Psychiatric classification. In J. A. Talbott, R. E. Hales, & S. C. Yudofsky (Eds.), *The American psychiatric press textbook of psychiatry.* Washington, DC: American Psychiatric Press, 201-223.

World Health Organization. (1990). *International classification of diseases* (10th ed.). Geneva: Author.

Yerxa, E. (1988). Oversimplification: The hobgoblin of theory and practice in occupational therapy. *Canadian Journal of Occupational Therapy, 55,* 5-6.

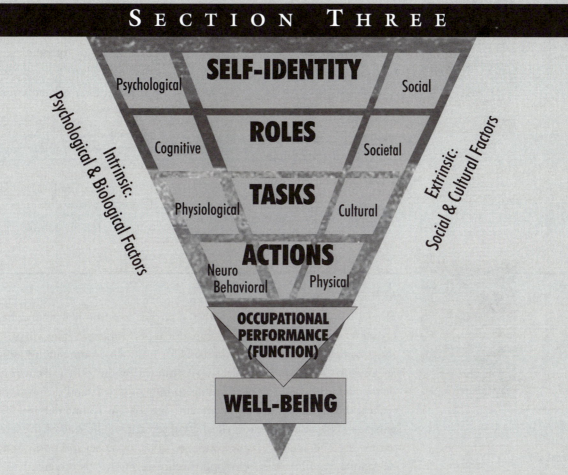

Psychological

SELF-IDENTITY

Social

Intrinsic:
Psychological & Biological Factors

Cognitive

ROLES

Societal

Extrinsic:
Social & Cultural Factors

Physiological

TASKS

Cultural

Neuro
Behavioral

ACTIONS

Physical

**OCCUPATIONAL
PERFORMANCE
(FUNCTION)**

WELL-BEING

Social and
Cultural Factors

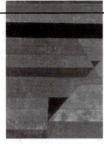

CHAPTER CONTENT OUTLINE

ABSTRACT

Human competencies interact with the physical environment in a dynamic, reciprocal relationship that shapes occupational performance. This chapter discusses these complex interactions as the basis for using environmental modifications as an effective therapeutic modality. Attributes of the physical environment are defined and described in relationship to human factors and occupational performance. Environmental assessment and use of environmental modification to enhance occupational performance are discussed. The role of the environment within six therapeutic frameworks (rehabilitation, sensorimotor, educational, behavioral, cognitive disability, and psychoeducational) is presented.

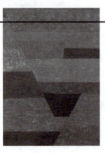

KEY TERMS

Physical environment

Object availability

Visual cues

Auditory cues

Safety

Press

Arousal

Tasks

Assistive devices

Alterations

Object modification

Task modification

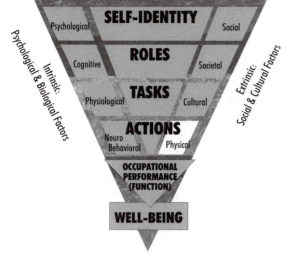

CHAPTER 13

The Role of the Physical Environment in Occupational Performance

Mary Corcoran, PhD, OTR/L, FAOTA, Laura Gitlin, PhD

OBJECTIVES

The information in this chapter is intended to help the reader:

1. define key attributes of the physical environment

2. describe the dynamic, reciprocal relationship among human competencies, the physical environment, and occupational performance

3. discuss several approaches to environmental assessment

4. identify strategies for enhancing occupational performance through environmental modifications

5. consider special issues in the introduction of environmental strategies, such as the personal meaning of objects and context-based instruction

6. discuss the use of environmental modifications in six therapeutic frameworks that typically structure occupational therapy services.

> "The physical settings occupied by people do not exist in isolation; rather, they are integral parts of a larger, complex system and must operate in concert with the social and organizational dimensions of this larger system."
>
> Cohen, U. and Weisman, G. (1991). *Holding onto home.* Baltimore, MD: Johns Hopkins University Press.

INTRODUCTION

This chapter emphasizes the important role of the physical environment in promoting human occupational performance. As discussed earlier, occupational performance is the result of complex interactions between human factors and attributes of the environment. Some environmental attributes interact with human capabilities to enable performance, while others present barriers to an individual's attempts at meaningful interactions with his or her surroundings. Moreover, the relationship between humans and their environment is a reciprocal one in that changes in either affect the other (Rogers, 1983; Christiansen, 1991). Because of this dynamic relationship, achieving and maintaining a just-right fit between abilities and environmental demands is a constant balancing process, much like walking a tightrope. When environmental demands are too low relative to an individual's abilities, he or she may reestablish balance by seeking a more challenging environment. When environmental challenges transcend an individual's abilities, skills and competencies are developed for more flexible and complex interactions with increasingly demanding environments.

Historically, occupational therapy literature has recognized the importance of creating opportunities for meaningful interactions with the environment as the basis for promoting health through occupation (Meyer, 1922; Reilly, 1962). Kiernat (1983) conceptualized the environment as an occupational therapy modality that is purposely manipulated to either challenge or support the client's competencies. In turn, the client's abilities expand in order to maintain a comfortable level of fit with the environment. This dynamic process of expanded abilities to maintain balanced integration is called adaptation (Ayres, 1979; Schultz and Schkade, 1992, Schkade and Schultz, 1992). It is a basic premise of occupational therapy that the ability to successfully adapt to evolving environmental challenges is essential to occupational performance.

In this chapter, we will explore the physical environment as one dimension of the context for occupational performance. We will discuss environmental assessment and modification as a way of enabling human performance and examine its implications for occupational therapy practice.

WHAT IS THE PHYSICAL ENVIRONMENT?

The physical environment is a complex, interacting array of built and natural objects. *Built objects* are created and con-

structed by humans and vary widely in terms of complexity, size, and purpose. Humans have had a longstanding fascination with building objects for practical reasons and as an outlet for creative urges. For instance, humans build objects to save labor (washing machines), for convenience (automatic teller banking machines), and as sources of comfort and beauty (paintings and sculptures). Use of technology has touched everyday life worldwide, shaping occupational performance through the use of machines to expand the limits of the human body.

As opposed to built objects, *natural objects* are those that occur as the result of forces of nature and also vary in regards to size, location, and composition. Natural objects in the physical environment include humans, although humans have also created a sociocultural environment, as is discussed in Chapter 15 of this book. Humans are important to this discussion of natural objects in the physical environment due to our innate tendency to shape and master other natural objects. Mastery over naturally occurring non-human objects is often attempted through the use of constructed objects, as is seen when a mountain is carved to build a new highway. Nature and humans are often in a dynamic state of tension in which constructed objects and the forces of nature are locked in a struggle for domination. An example of this tension was seen in the 1993 floods along the Mississippi River, which some experts say were exacerbated by an extensive system of flood control devices such as levies and dams.

Whether the physical environment is constructed of natural or built objects, or a combination, the effect on human performance is often profound. The concept of balanced interactions between people and the environment is central to the sensory integration frame of reference developed by Ayres (1978). Moreover, the philosophy of occupational therapy knowledge and practice reflects the importance of supporting occupational performance by enhancing the interaction of each client's characteristics with attributes of his or her environment.

ATTRIBUTES OF THE PHYSICAL ENVIRONMENT

The physical environment is filled with objects that support or impede occupational performance, depending on their interaction with our unique biopsychosocial makeup. For instance, a chair may be comfortable, but if we are feeling sleepy or bored with the reading material, that same chair may impede our ability to stay awake. Any change in either biopsychosocial status (e.g., a headache, anxiety about an upcoming event) or environment (e.g., distracting noises, an overly cluttered desktop) alters the interaction between us and our physical environment, thereby potentially affecting performance.

Attributes of the physical environment that are critical to

Bibliographic citation of this chapter: Corcoran, M., & Gitlin, L. (1997). The role of the physical environment in occupational performance. In C. Christiansen & C. Baum (Eds.), *Occupational therapy: Enabling function and well-being* (2nd ed.). Thorofare, NJ: SLACK Incorporated.

human performance have been grouped by the authors into three categories. The categories are object accessibility and availability, visual and auditory cues, and safety. Each is discussed in more detail in the following.

Object Availability and Accessibility

Objects must be both available and accessible if they are to support human performance of everyday tasks. Object availability refers to the presence or absence of an item (Barris et al., 1985). By comparison, object accessibility concerns the location of an object for convenient and efficient retrieval when needed. For example, think about situations where a needed object is available but not readily accessible, as in the case of infrequently-used serving dishes that are stored in difficult-to-reach places.

To improve the accessibility of available objects, most people create command control centers. These centers are designed to house most objects needed for a given task and are found commonly in homes and workplaces. Figure 13-1 shows one type of command control center, a medicine cabinet that holds items needed for personal grooming and self-medication. Other centers are usually established to address tasks such as handling finances and conducting telephone business. Command control centers may also be designed to allow an individual to remain in one space over time and perform all tasks needed without changing location. An example of this type of center includes the bedside table that usually holds items needed before sleep (reading materials), during the night (an illuminated dial), and upon awakening (an alarm clock). Command control centers are one typical way that individuals make needed items conveniently accessible.

For individuals with a disability, object availability and accessibility become critical. The importance of objects to occupational performance increases proportionally to limitations in motor and/or cognitive abilities. Individuals who have limited mobility are often provided with assistive devices (object availability), arranged to assure that they are within reach when needed (object accessibility). One example is a bathroom equipped with several assistive devices and conveniently located personal care products. In a similar manner, cognitive deficits related to dementia or schizophrenia are often treated by assembling all needed items for a certain task and placing those items together in a relevant and prominent location for easy accessibility. Clearly, adjusting the availability and accessibility of objects in the physical environment is potentially beneficial to address several types of performance deficits.

Visual and Auditory Cues

On any given day, most individuals are bombarded with sensory stimuli intended to shape their behavior. An entire

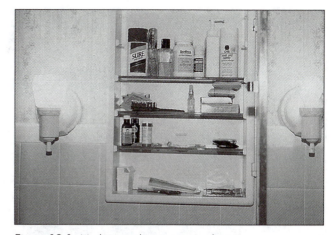

Figure 13-1. Medicine cabinet command center.

marketing industry has grown around the effort to create and deliver perfect messages that will result in the purchase of consumer goods. Some of these messages very subtly promote buying by bringing a thought to consciousness, such as placing candy at the grocery checkout to encourage impulse buying. Products are also promoted by appealing to an individual's personal image or by encouraging an emotional reaction to a product. For example, upbeat music or use of humor in an advertisement is often intended to establish a product, and its consumer, as fun. In this way, stimuli in the physical environment shapes behavior in myriad ways by establishing conscious or unconscious associations with specific objects.

Likewise, humans tend to surround themselves with sensory stimuli designed to shape their own behavior, including the use of conscious and unconscious messages. It is not uncommon for humans to make lists of things to do, post rules and responsibilities, and use music to establish a mood. These messages are known collectively as *cues*, defined as prompts or signals that promote a response. While any sensory system can be used to establish an environmental cue, the visual and auditory systems are the predominant pathways for this purpose.

While some cues are initiated by the individual whose behavior is targeted, other cues are established for that individual by others, such as supervisors, family members or caregivers. Parents often create a system of cues to shape their children's behavior (e.g., list of chores, visually appealing personal care products, a timer) and teach children to cue themselves (e.g., placing items needed for school next to the door). Individuals with newly acquired or chronic disabilities often use cues to assist themselves in the use of recommended techniques and procedures. Health care professionals understand the need for cues and promote their use through printed instructions regarding such procedures as home exercise programs or joint protection techniques. Cognitive disabilities may also give rise to environmental cues, as illus-

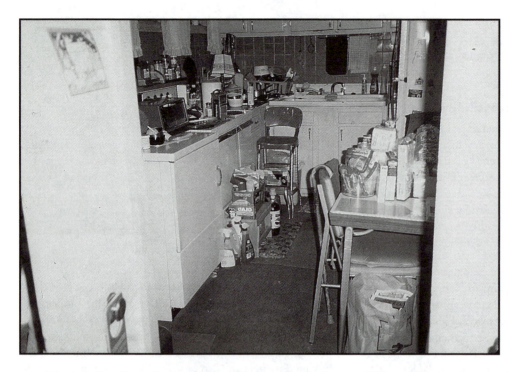

Figure 13-2. Home of a woman who is blind.

trated in use of reality orienting items (calendars or schedules) and written or pictorial instructions. Occupational therapists in particular have been labeled as "natural cuers" (Baum, 1995) in reference to their tendency to promote performance through carefully selected sensory stimuli.

Despite the fact that environmental cues can be powerful facilitators of performance, they are only effective if they are noticeable. Often, cues are masked by the presence of more powerful stimuli or lost in a barrage of multiple stimuli. The term *clutter* is used to describe physical environments where the presence of sensory stimuli exceeds the individual's capacity to process information (Mace, 1991). Figure 13-2 shows the home of an individual who lost her sight as a result of diabetes. In this illustration, the woman's home can be seen to contain many items, assembled in an effort to keep objects accessible. However, the woman was no longer able to efficiently gain tactile cues from her environment due to the excessive number of items. In addition, the excessive number of items created tripping hazards and her home had become unsafe. She required an occupational therapist to help her safely balance her need for object accessibility with her need to readily access tactile cues. One way of achieving this balance was to store objects that were not used on a daily basis in closed containers identified with Braille or embossed labels.

Safety

The ability of the physical environment to promote safe performance has received a great deal of attention in the dis-

ability and long-term care literature. This attention is warranted by high incidents of injury and death due to household and workplace accidents for any age group. Generally, issues of physical environmental safety can be divided into three categories including fall hazards, use of potentially dangerous items, and threat from fire or toxic substances.

Fall Hazards

Among the well elderly, falls are a major source of disability and mortality (Czaja, 1988). Many falls in the home can be attributed to extrinsic factors, such as unsafe use of objects, poor lighting, furniture in poor repair, tripping hazards, and lack of attention while using stairs (Studenski et al., 1994). A majority of falls occur on a stairway, and usually on the first step (Czaja, 1988). For the elderly requiring long-term care, falls occur with greater frequency and are accompanied by higher rates of morbidity and mortality (Studenski et al., 1994). Among nursing home clients, falls are estimated to occur at the rate of 1.5 per resident, and have been associated with attempts to transfer without help or exit the facility (Burnside, 1988). Fall hazards in institutions include emergency exit doors, typically required by building codes, that may promote unsafe exiting by nursing home residents who wander (Dickinson et al., 1995).

While older people are often the victims of falls, increasingly the public has become more aware of hazards to children presented by playgrounds and play equipment. Many areas have translated this awareness into legislation, mandating use of bicycle helmets for children under 12 and setting standards for the use of cushioning materials around playground equipment. However, these mandates are not found worldwide and childhood injuries from falls continue to rise.

Dangerous Items

The second category of environmental safety is related to the presence and safe use of potentially dangerous items. Much effort in public health is focused on identifying and removing household dangers, such as frayed electric cords. Uncontrolled access to medications, sharp kitchen implements, and electrical items pose a threat to children, as well as adults with impaired judgment.

There is increasing attention to the workplace and health threats imposed from the use of machinery, including injury due to accidents and repetitive trauma. While progress has been made in industrialized nations to regulate safety in industry, some third world countries have not yet addressed occupational hazards in the workplace. Regardless of level of industrialization, rural workers and farmers worldwide are particularly at risk of injury and death. In the United States, farm workers are estimated to be three times more likely to die on the job than the average American worker (Myers & Hard, 1995). Farming is an unregulated industry, usually involving isolated individuals working with dangerous items for long days to get the job done. In addition, children are often present and at risk of injury because many farms are family-run businesses.

Threat from Fire and Toxic Substances

The third safety area includes injury due to burns or exposure to toxic substances. Burns from fires or scalding claim the lives of thousands of victims yearly, usually the very young and very old. Exposure to toxic substances in the home, such as carbon monoxide and lead, is also a threat to the public health. While most fire and toxic substance exposures quickly result in death, others can result in chronic disability. Fortunately, most of these accidents are preventable with the use of protective devices (smoke and carbon dioxide detectors) and practices (removal of lead-based paints or products).

TRANSACTIONS BETWEEN HUMANS AND THE PHYSICAL ENVIRONMENT

Conceptualizing interactions with the physical environment transcends a simple comparison of environmental characteristics and human capacities. Influences between humans and the physical environment are dynamic and reciprocal in nature, so that each continually shapes the other (Christiansen, 1991). These interactions have been conceptualized in an emerging body of literature from several disciplines, including occupational therapy, psychology, engineering, urban design, and architecture. Exploration of these concepts as the basis for

understanding and enhancing the unique ways in which people interact with and within their environments is important.

Literature from the field of architecture has traditionally addressed how people interact with and within the environment, and in doing so, several descriptors have been developed in reference to spaces and the ways people use those spaces. One descriptor is that of *archetypal places* (Spivack, reported in Spencer, 1991), which focuses on the use of spaces for daily functions. Spencer (1991) concluded that the notion of archetypal places implies a "connection between space and activity patterns" (1991, p. 126) and joins other authors in urging occupational therapists to integrate the physical and sociocultural aspects of the physical environment (Gitlin & Burgh, 1995; Baum, 1991). Creation of archetypal places, such as establishing safe spaces for an impaired individual to wander freely, occurs naturally when people shape their own environments (Corcoran, 1992, 1994; Edwards, Baum, & Morrow-Howell, 1994; Olsen et al., 1993; Mann et al., 1994). Occupational therapists report application of this concept to many areas of practice, ranging from pediatrics (Richter & Oetter, 1990) to gerontology (Corcoran & Gitlin, 1992).

Human performance depends on the right mix of intrinsic and extrinsic factors (McEwen, 1990; David, 1990). Intrinsic factors are the unique biopsychosocial abilities that comprise each of us, labeled *performance components* in the American Occupational Therapy Association Uniform Terminology Document (1994) (see Appendix A). Extrinsic factors are harder to characterize because they exist in the perceptions of individuals about their physical and sociocultural environments. While environmental researchers suggest a number of schemes for conceptualizing extrinsic factors, most are based on Lawton and Nahmow's (1973) concepts of *press* and *arousal*. These concepts are applied here to the physical environment and its capacity to influence occupational performance.

Press

Environmental press is the degree to which the environment influences behavior (Mace, 1991). Characterized on a continuum of high to low, press represents a force that promotes human actions. For example, a playground full of enticing toys is labeled as high press because it will promote active play by children. Conversely, an environment with low press lacks challenges and opportunities for interactions.

Press must be considered in relation to an individual's level of competence in order to understand its effect on occupational performance. The high press of a playground full of toys promotes adaptation in the performance of a non-disabled child. However, for a child with motor problems, the press may be too high relative to competence because the child cannot physically access the toys. An imbalance exists

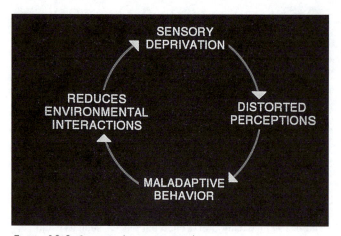

Figure 13-3. Sensory deprivation cycle.

between the disabled child's ability to interact with the environment and the press of the playground. For this child, adaptation of the child to his environment is not supported and the child's play performance is restricted.

For the elderly, adaptation is threatened as a consequence of normal aging processes, such as reduced vital capacity and changes in sensory acuity. Additionally, pathological conditions typically associated with aging, such as arthritis, can reduce an older person's adaptability even more. Therefore, the press of the environment is a crucial factor in the degree to which older people can live independently (Czaja, 1988). Struyk (1987) estimates that 46% of all elderly would enjoy enhanced performance in daily activities through the use of modified housing. However, he reports that, of a sample of 8,600 elderly-headed households with at least one member experiencing a health or mobility problem, only 10.3% had a modification. As proposed by Gitlin and Levine (1992), the meaning of assistive devices may be one factor in their underutilization by individuals with disabilities.

Arousal

Throughout the life span, the demands of the environment must arouse the human nervous system at a level that assures optimal interaction. If arousal is too high or too low, the individual may respond with frustration, leading to withdrawal, lethargy, or depression (McEwen, 1990; Barris et al., 1985). As with press, arousal must be considered in relation to an individual's initial state. A quiet, dark room has low arousal properties and may be useful for calming an anxious, stressed person. Likewise, any new parent knows that taking a cranky baby for a ride in the car often creates a perfect level of low arousal for the child to sleep. Gently rocked by the rhythm of the moving car, the child only experiences the uninteresting, unchanging stimuli of the car's interior.

Arousal that is too low relative to an individual's compe-

tence can contribute to sensory deprivation (Erber, 1979; Corcoran & Barrett, 1987). Sensory deprivation is defined as diminished ability to respond to the environment in the absence of an adequate stream of stimuli (Ayres, 1978; Corcoran & Barrett, 1987). In the elderly, sensory deprivation is characterized by symptoms such as disorientation, flexed posture, flattened affect, and poor concentration. As demonstrated in Figure 13-3, a cycle is established whereby lack of arousing stimuli leads to further deterioration of the individual's competence and leaves him or her less able to be aroused by the environment. Occupational performance declines as part of this downward spiral.

Fortunately, there is evidence to suggests that adjusting the arousal of the environment can, to some degree, reverse this cycle. Corcoran and Barrett (1987) designed and implemented an occupational therapy intervention for 16 long-term residents of a nursing home who exhibited symptoms of sensory deprivation. Before treatment was initiated, all 16 residents who participated in the study were totally dependent in self-care and severely limited in their basic task performance, such as decision making, attention span and initiation of activity. Randomly assigned to either a sensory stimulation group or a self-care group, these residents were treated twice weekly for a period of 16 weeks. The self-care group received an occupational therapy intervention that focused on reteaching feeding, dressing, and bathing skills. The sensory stimulation group received intervention designed to provide arousing sensory stimulation and promote adaptive interactions with the environment. For example, as shown in Figure 13-4, the sensory stimulation group relied heavily on firm touch to elicit an appropriate adaptive response. At the end of sixteen weeks, the self-care group showed no improvement in performance of ADL or basic task skills. The sensory stimulation group, however, demonstrated significant gains in some basic task skills, such as attention span, inappropriate attention-seeking, and cooperative behaviors. In addition, a few of the residents in the sensory stimulation group began feeding themselves finger foods, which represented an improvement in their occupational performance. Unfortunately, these positive changes were only sustained as long as a just-right fit existed between capabilities and environmental demands.

Tasks

Occupational therapists recognize the importance of performance in conceptualizing the area of interaction between individuals and the environment. Christiansen and Baum (1991) use a person-environment-occupational performance framework to organize knowledge about human and environmental factors that converge on performance. Likewise, a unique aspect of the environmental model by Barris and colleagues (1985), discussed earlier in this book, is its inclusion

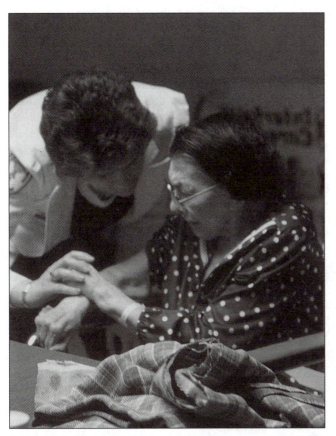

Figure 13-4. Firm touch in a sensory stimulation group.

TABLE 13-1

Environmental Principles for Intervention with Alzheimer Disease

1. Object availability may maintain or improve performance.
2. Surroundings should be simple.
3. Expectations about the use of objects should be static.
4. Presence of age-appropriate objects are important in maintaining ego integrity.
5. Task complexity may be mitigated through highly familiar gross motor activities with simple instructions.
6. Routines with rest breaks help reduce stress.
7. Criteria for success needs to be clear.
8. Tasks must lack negative consequences.
9. Family needs must be determined and addressed.
10. An atmosphere of collaboration must be facilitated with family caregivers.
11. One family member should be trained and supported as a care coordinator.
12. Unique family styles and norms must be understood and incorporated into the intervention.

Adapted from Corcoran, M. A. & Gitlin, L. N. (1992) Dementia management: An occupational therapy intervention for caregivers. *American Journal of Occupational Therapy, 46*(9), 801-808.

of the task layer as a point of interaction between people and the objects in their physical world. According to both these perspectives, individuals engage in tasks, usually involving the use of objects, to simultaneously meet a range of biological, social and/or cultural needs. For example, the task of grooming is highly variable, requires several objects chosen on the basis of personal preference and utility, and combines the purposes of health maintenance, social appropriateness, and self-expression. This variety in the simple task of grooming is due to the fact that tasks have several dimensions that may be intrinsic to the task itself, dependent on the physical attributes of the environment, or shaped by the performer (Christiansen, 1991). These task dimensions include the sequence of steps involved in the task, how the task is performed, when the task is conducted and with whom, and the symbolic meaning of engaging in the task (Barris et al., 1985). Environmental modifications aimed at the task level are often very effective in promoting occupational performance because they represent a functional reconciliation of environmental demands and individual capabilities. In addition, combining assistive devices with modifications at the task layer is important to the effective provision of assistive devices to older rehabilitation clients (Gitlin & Burgh, 1995).

Based on the Barris model, Corcoran and Gitlin (1991) established principles for environmental modifications which establish a "just-right fit" between an individual with Alzheimer disease and his or her surroundings (presented in Table 13-1). For example, Barris et al. (1985) theorized that objects can be thought of in terms of their complexity, and that a range of simple to complex objects contribute to the arousal and press of the environment. However, for adults with dementia, objects should be kept simple to match the adult's limited cognitive abilities and promote performance. Likewise, tasks must remain age- and gender-appropriate despite the need to reduce tasks to one or two steps. Corcoran and Gitlin's environmental principles for cognitively impaired adults differ from those that may be derived for a physically impaired but cognitively intact older person, whose need for novelty and arousal is high because access to the environment is restricted. In dementia management, "simplify surroundings" and "establish a routine" are examples of environmental principles stemming from broad conceptualization about humans and their interactions with the environment. These principles are presently being used as constructs in a study testing the effectiveness of an occupational therapy intervention that expands use of environmental modifications by caregivers in managing the effects of dementia (Corcoran & Gitlin, 1992; Gitlin & Corcoran, 1993, 1996).

Human factors engineers are also interested in the transactions among individuals, the environment, and performance, traditionally focusing on analysis of work-related tasks and systems for their degree of fit with human capabilities (Czaja, Weber, & Nair, 1993). Faletti (1984) suggested that the task analysis used by human factors engineers in industrial settings is relevant to studying performance problems in the elderly. Czaja and colleagues created a systematic analytical approach to task analysis, which they labeled a capability-demand approach. Using this approach, the physical demands (bending, reaching, lifting) of 25 daily tasks were compared with product information (height, weight, depth) and older adult capacities (strength, flexibility) to determine possible areas of mismatch between person and environment. They found that actions such as pushing/pulling, lifting, and carrying are common to many daily tasks but the physical demands of these actions exceeded the capability of many older people in the sample. For example, the authors reported that most middle kitchen cabinet shelves in their sample were 65 inches high and 12 inches deep. Because the average overhead reach of elderly females in their study was 68 inches, these women needed to stand on a stool to reach items placed back from the edge on the middle shelf. Installing shelving that is lower, narrower, or automatically adjustable can eliminate this potential source of accidental falls in the home. As this example demonstrates, capability-demand analysis is an exciting, systematic approach to evaluating and modifying objects and tasks to optimize human performance.

Interactions Between Sociocultural Factors and the Physical Environment

As we attempt to gain greater understanding of the reciprocal relationships among people, their surroundings, and performance, it becomes increasingly clear that sociocultural factors are an important part of that equation. On one hand, beliefs and values are critical to shaping our interactions with the environment, as illustrated in culturally-based patterns in architecture. On the other hand, the physical environment plays an important role in supporting people as they express themselves as members of a group or society. The dynamics between the physical and sociocultural dimensions of the environment can be harmonious or a source of tension, as is the case when people with disabilities are unable to create or access environments that support a cultural image. Although the sociocultural environment is discussed separately in this book, the following discussion is important to underscore specific ways in which belief and value systems shape and are supported by the physical environment.

Objects and other physical attributes of the environment are typically arranged to support culturally-derived daily routines and habit structures. The contents of command control centers mentioned earlier will differ depending on the user's everyday habits. For instance, if a woman is in the habit of applying her makeup in the bathroom, that command control center will contain her favorite makeup items, adequate lighting, and sufficient space to allow manipulation of several small objects. As in all human-environmental transactions, a dynamic process is present such that structural barriers shape habits and routines and vice versa. One woman with limited electrical outlets developed the habit of using her hair dryer in the dining room where fewer electrical demands existed. She modified the environment to support this habit by hanging an attractive mirror above the electrical outlet and clearing a nearby drawer to hold her supplies.

Natural and built objects often support the rituals and routines of everyday life. The routines of everyday life represent a variety of human dimensions, from cultural and religious to simple self-care. Reminding oneself to take a prescription medication often entails reminder notes or strategic placement of the medication itself in an area where the daily routine assures it will be seen. Items for religious or special occasion routines take on a symbolic meaning that intricately ties the object with the upcoming event. Holiday decorations and religious items are examples of objects necessary for enacting the routines and rituals of a family or cultural group. Many cultures use objects to assure good luck, such as a horseshoe. Objects are also central to the rituals of most of the world's religions. For example, Jewish traditions involve the use of many items, such as the Torah and prayer shawl.

The relationships between humans, their rituals, and the objects that support those rituals has been studied extensively by anthropologists. Turner (1986) proposed the importance of performing rituals to the evolution of the human brain, theorizing that the human cortex evolved to efficiently associate ritualistic use of objects and movements with emotional responses. This work is based on the premise that strong connections link human performance, human development, and the environment within the nervous system in ways that are not yet fully understood.

Not only does the physical environment potentially sustain routines and rituals, it is also an important factor in supporting a cultural group member's values, beliefs, and self-image. People everywhere design their surroundings to make a statement about themselves as individuals and as members of a cultural group. Decorations and artifacts in the home and workplace can provide an expressive outlet for its occupants, or the promotion of an image. Objects often serve as connections to family and friends (scrapbooks and photo albums) or symbols of status ("Dad's" chair in the living room) (Rubinstein, 1987). Promoting humility as a personal virtue, the buildings of some religious groups around the world feature short doorways that require bowing of the head to pass. Conversely, many cultures are associated with environments containing a lavish display of beautifully decorated items. The astute observer can learn much about an individual simply by noticing how he or she shapes the physical surroundings.

One of the best examples of the relationship between the physical environment and self-image is seen in clothing. Clothing choices usually reflect an individual's view of self, ranging from an image of oneself as traditional to unorthodox. The Amish reject modern styles, preferring unadorned clothing consistent with a "plain" image. More importantly, however, clothing represents an individual's roles in life, which change as he or she encounters developmental and social milestones. That little girl who wore nothing but pink party dresses may grow into a teenager wearing only jeans and T-shirts. After four years of college, she may be the owner of several business suits. At each stage, her clothing expresses who she is by representing the status, power, rights and responsibilities associated with her work and leisure roles.

As individuals experience decline in physical, social, or mental competence, their ability to express themselves through the physical environment is threatened. Although self-expression through the environment remains important, an individual with disabilities may not able to act on this urge. The surroundings may be filled with objects from roles that can no longer be enacted. Even worse, the environment may be filled with objects that represent a sick or disabled role, such as a hospital bed or other assistive devices. These objects may actually promote a view of the self as dependent (Gitlin, Luborsky, Schemm, & Burgh, in press). Through occupational therapy, disabled individuals can regain important, non-disabled life roles and the power to shape the environment in a way that reflects a positive self-image.

Interactions Between People with Disabling Conditions and the Physical Environment

To understand the role of the physical environment in promoting effective occupational performance by individuals with disabling conditions, we use a model of disability developed by the National Center for Medical Rehabilitation and Research (Badley, 1993). This model (Figure 13-5) demonstrates the progression of a disability from its pathology to its social consequences, as a basis for analyzing and modifying the effect of the environment on human performance.

In this model, a pathology involves an interruption or interference of normal physiological and developmental processes resulting in neurological or physiological deficits. The most basic consequence of a disease process is an impairment, or abnormality at the organ level that impacts either a cognitive process, motor ability, sensory process or psychological function. An impairment may then lead to functional limitations as represented by difficulty with basic components of performance such as sequencing, attending, sitting, rolling, or lifting. Functional limitations may lead to a disability in that an individual may experience difficulty with or an inability to perform daily self-care and instrumental activities of living. A disability, in turn, may impact the social roles that an individual assumes by limiting participation in leisure and work.

Using this schema, we can understand and adjust the specific impact of the environment for an individual with a disabling condition. An environmental strategy such as an assistive device for bathing (e.g., a tub seat, grab bars) directly targets the disability level. The strategy is designed to minimize the press imposed by the structure of the bathroom and the bathing activity. By offsetting an individual's loss of strength or balance with a technical aid, safe ADL performance in that environment is enhanced. The purpose of this type of environmental strategy is primarily restorative, that is, it is designed to compensate for losses and reestablish function. The strategy may also have a preventive effect at the impairment level of disablement in that it may reduce the risk of falling and the occurrence of other functional consequences. For example, individuals who are aging and beginning to experience age-related changes may benefit from grab bars in the bathroom and other strategies that address home safety. The role of environmental modifications as a prevention strategy has not been systematically evaluated by research but would appear to potentially prevent secondary conditions and excess disabilities that accompany a poor fit between human abilities and the environment.

Finally, an environmental strategy may ease the burden of care experienced by a family member by minimizing his or her physical effort and emotional strain involved in providing continued assistance with ADL. The potential benefit of an environmental strategy for a family caregiver is illustrated by the case of Mr. M, a 65-year-old male with a double lower limb amputation. Following discharge from rehabilitation and his return home, Mr. M was unable to ascend the stairs to sleep in his bedroom on the second floor. Mr. M and his wife initially modified a sleeping space on the first floor of their home. However, this arrangement required Mrs. M to use the stairs frequently to retrieve clothing and other daily necessities for Mr. M. This soon became a health hazard for Mrs. M, who had also recently been discharged from a hospital with coronary artery disease. To minimize the press of the environment, in this case, stair climbing and carrying articles, a stair glide was installed in the home. This enabled Mr. M to ascend and descend the stairs independently so that he could move back to his second-floor bedroom with his wife. In this case, the stair glide was a strategy that had a direct impact on the health and well-being of a caregiver.

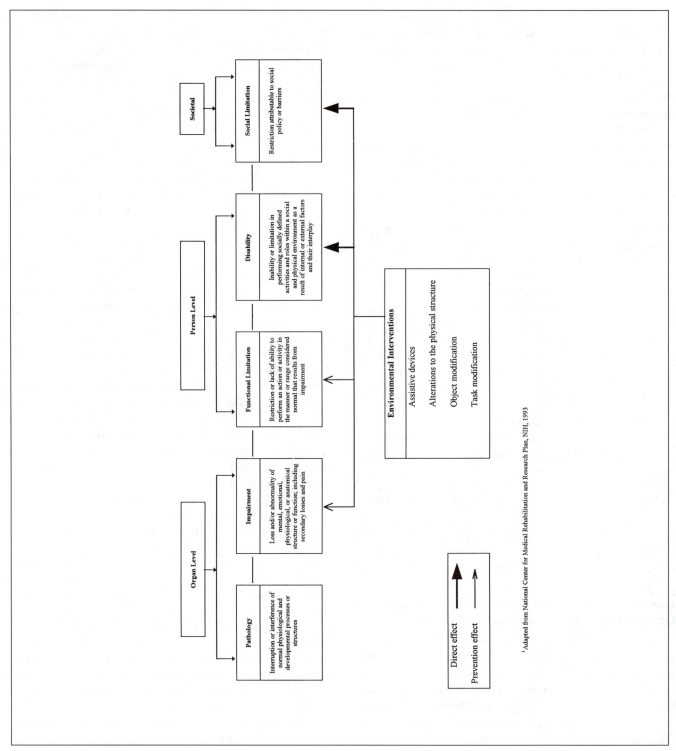

Figure 13-5. National Center for Medical Research and Rehabilitation Disablement Schema.

Predicting whether a suggested environmental modification will be accepted by an individual with a disabling condition may be difficult. When considering environmental modifications, occupational therapists must keep in mind that humans occasionally experience conflicting responses to a supportive environment. According to Parmelee and Lawton (1990) it is possible to enjoy the independence and security made possible by environmental supports, while at the same time resisting the restrictions to autonomy that accompany a low-risk environment. Labeled the autonomy-security dialectic (Parmelee and Lawton, 1990), this phenomenon is conceptualized as a tension between the wish to be safe and the need to be independent. As a result of this tension, the physical environment is constantly evaluated according to the balance between freedom to regulate oneself and absence of risk. The autonomy-security dialectic helps clarify why many individuals are ambivalent about assistive devices that allow the security of independent functioning but restrict choices about how the task is structured.

Thus far we have defined the physical environment and overviewed the complex relationships among human abilities, attributes of the physical environment, belief and value systems, and performance. The remainder of the chapter will focus on evaluating environmental influences on performance and explore broader practice issues introduced by an environmental approach in occupational therapy.

ENVIRONMENTAL ASSESSMENT

Occupational therapists work with clients in physical environments that are quite diverse. The rehabilitation center, home, adult day care center, work place, senior center or school present unique challenges to assessment and may require the development of tools that are designed to evaluate their specific dimensions.

Presently, occupational therapists tend to evaluate the physical dimensions of an environment by using self-made checklists or other self-generated forms. Using an assessment form in practice enables a therapist to assume a more comprehensive and consistent approach. However, there are a number of difficulties with existing self-made assessment tools. First, these tools, for the most part, have not been standardized nor tested for the consistency of measurement or reliability. The use of unstandardized forms, such as self-made checklists, makes it difficult to determine the reliability of a therapist's ratings, and whether all the relevant dimensions of the environment are consistently considered. Second, there tends to be an over-reliance on self-report by the client. Depending upon a client's self-report of his or her physical environment may be the only source of information available to a therapist. However, there is a tendency for clients and family members

tend to under-report barriers and issues in the environment. The third difficulty in environmental assessments is the use of observation without standardized procedures and definitions as to what to observe and how. Finally, there is a lack of consistency as to the domains of the environment that are assessed and a tendency to assess only one dimension of the environment, such as for its safety or accessibility. This unidimensional focus promotes a narrow view of the physical environment and limits our understanding of its multiple dimensions that impact occupational performance.

Although what needs to be evaluated and how is an unresolved issue, we can suggest some guiding principles to follow in assessing the physical dimensions of an environment in order to introduce an environmental change. There are four basic considerations in introducing an environmental strategy. These involve considering the:

1. nature of the environmental strategy such as the characteristics of an assistive device,
2. characteristics of the client, including his or her performance needs and desires,
3. characteristics of the family member or supportive network, including his or her own caregiving goals and personal needs and capabilities,
4. physical dimensions of the environment.

Other chapters of this book examine issues associated with assessing the person, whereas our purpose here is to consider the physical dimension of environments.

Assessing the Physical Attributes of an Environment

An assessment of the physical attributes of an environment is best achieved through a combination of strategies, including direct observation of the setting, an interview with the client, and an examination of the client's performance in that environment. It is most effective to walk through an environment accompanied by the client or caregiver, if at all possible. This allows the therapist to make observations and notations and clarify issues with the individual as they emerge. A comprehensive assessment would involve observing each room or environmental setting that is used by a client. For example, let's say you are working with a young adult with a spinal cord injury who is returning to school. It would be important to assess the entire physical dimensions of the school including entrances into and out of the school, as well as the accessibility of its corridors, bathrooms, and classrooms. Likewise, in assessing the physical environment of a client's home, a room-by-room assessment is necessary, as well as an examination of the physical dimensions of the entrances. Physical environments are not static and the placement of objects or the physical setup may vary or change throughout the day. It is important therefore to ascertain whether the observed conditions are

TABLE 13-2	
Typical Safety Considerations in the Physical Environment	
Dimension	**Example of Potential Hazards**
Tripping hazards	• throw rugs • slippery floors • raised thresholds
Lighting	• glare • inadequate
Stairways	• rise between steps too high
Electrical cords	• frayed • close to heat or oven
Furniture	• unstable • difficult to get out of

typical of that environment and how the setting may change throughout the day. This can be determined by asking the client or family member directly about the nature of the observation.

What then are the key dimensions of the physical environment that should be assessed in any type of setting? Here we discuss four dimensions: safety, object availability and accessibility, visual and auditory cues, and other dimensions.

Safety

In assessing an environment for its physical safety, the therapist is checking for conditions that may cause a fall or injury or that may place the individual at physical risk. Some of the factors that are routinely considered on a safety checklist are shown in Table 13-2. However, the specific conditions that are examined will obviously differ depending upon the environmental context. For example, the kitchen in the home may pose a different set of safety hazards than a bedroom and therefore specific features of the kitchen (e.g., oven, placement of electrical cords) need to be considered.

Object Availability and Accessibility

In assessing the environment for its availability and accessibility, the therapist considers a wide range of factors. With regard to availability, the therapist examines the environment to determine whether objects necessary to perform a given task can be easily obtained by the individual. For example, are objects for grooming available and/or labeled to facilitate use? Are there control centers in strategic locations in the environment (e.g., bedroom and living room) to enable an individual to use objects for a range of tasks?

With regard to accessibility, the therapist examines the environment to determine whether a client has access into and out of the environment. Once in the environment, does the client have access to other rooms, stairs, bathrooms? Is the furniture arranged to facilitate movement? When assessing object availability and accessibility in a specific space or room in the home, the following questions may be useful:

a. What activities are performed in this space/room?

b. For each activity performed, are essential items present?

c. Think about each activity in terms of sequence of actions and the motor and cognitive demands on the user. Can the user conveniently and safely access items at the time each is needed?

Visual and Auditory Cues

The physical arrangement of objects in a given setting provides cues for performance of tasks. For example, a place setting at the dining room table is a visual cue that a meal will be served. However, let's say that placed on the same table are newspapers, a pile of unpaid bills and a shopping list. Each object provides a cue for the performance of a different set of tasks. For individuals with a sensory deficit, multiple cues in a particular context may be confusing. Too many cues represent a form of environmental clutter that may be confusing to an individual. For example, children with sensory deficits may have difficulty concentrating if the classroom is too visually stimulating or cluttered with different environmental cues.

Clutter can only be assessed in reference to an individual's level of competence for processing information. For this reason, the effect of clutter is an issue for any individual whose occupational performance is at risk due to developmental delay or disabilities from motor or cognitive losses.

However, the effect of clutter is often difficult to recognize for individuals who are most severely compromised. To underscore the relationship between capacity and clutter, refer to the bathroom of a man with Alzheimer disease in Figure 13-6. Due to the presence of items for multiple grooming and cleaning tasks, this bathroom is considered cluttered in relation to the user's capacity to process stimuli. In fact, items for as few as two tasks are often impossible for an individual with Alzheimer disease to process correctly and therefore devastating to that person's occupational performance. Later in this chapter, environmental modifications will be presented that eliminate this subtle but disabling form of clutter.

Identifying visual and auditory cues requires careful observation and reasoning about the effect of the environment in relationship to the user's abilities. The following questions are designed to help develop observation and reasoning skills.

a. What are the predominant visual images in this space/room? Look for placement of items color, size, or emotional appeal to answer this question.

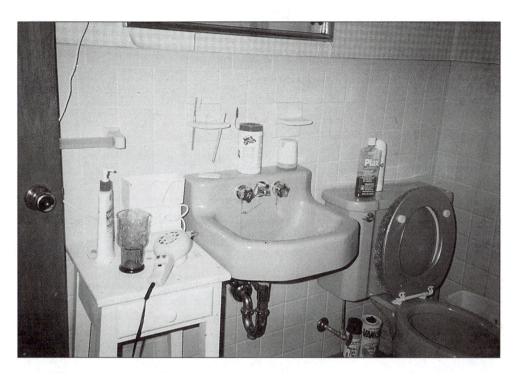

Figure 13-6. Bathroom of a person with Alzheimer disease.

b. What behavior or affective response is promoted by each of these visual cues? Do the cues promote responses that conflict (e.g. exercise equipment in an otherwise restful room) or converge in a powerful message? Given what you know about the abilities of the person who uses this room, how will he or she respond?

c. In relation to the user's abilities, does the room contain too many items, too few items, or just enough?

Other Dimensions

Other dimensions of the physical environment may be more difficult to assess. For example, is the physical environment comfortable? Is there adequate sensory stimulation? Is the physical environment aesthetically appealing to an individual? Assessment of these dimensions may affect the quality of life, sense of well-being, and occupational performance of an individual. Thus, these dimensions warrant careful evaluation by an occupational therapist.

Putting the Person Back in the Environment

Thus far we have discussed assessing dimensions of the physical environment without consideration of the person, his or her characteristics and interactions in that environment. Typically, assessments of the physical environment do not account for or include the "person" and his or her performance in that environment. However, it is this interaction that is critical to assess and which will lead to an effective treatment plan that includes an environmental strategy.

Let's say that in making a home visit you observe each room and note that the electrical outlets are exposed in the living room and kitchen and that tabletops and counters contain various items such as medicines, papers, scissors and other objects. Do these features represent safety hazards? They may put an individual at risk but this will depend upon the competence of that person within that environment. For example, exposed or opened outlets can pose a serious danger to curious toddlers. However, a household with older children need not be concerned about this aspect of the environment. Medications that are stored in open spaces or accessible locations can be a serious safety hazard for individuals with cognitive loss who may forget when to take medications and/or confuse these objects with food. Likewise, extreme clutter may present confusing cues to a person with a cognitive deficit and increase his or her disorientation. However, this may not necessarily be the case for an individual with a physical limitation. A person with a physical disability may function effectively in a cluttered environment. On the other hand, the lack of a ramp may present an environmental barrier for a client in a wheelchair or with an unsteady gait. The physical dimensions of the environment that need to be assessed may be different for individuals with a physical limitation than those with a cognitive deficit or for those who may experience both. There may be special considerations in assessing the environment based on the specific capabilities of the individual. Table 13-3 highlights some of these considerations. Characteristics other than impairment type may also influence an individual's performance in a given environment. Previous routines, personal habits and preferences and the meaning of a particular activity may also influence occupational performance.

TABLE 13-3

Special Considerations for Assessing the Environment

Environmental Dimension	Special Considerations	
	Physical Disability	Cognitive Disability
Safety	Are there tripping hazards?	Is medication accessible?
Accessibility	Are there ramps to entrance?	Are objects labeled?
Clutter	Are paths clear?	Are surfaces free of objects which offer different cues?

How can an occupational therapist assess the impact of the physical environment on a specific individual and assess, in turn, how that individual actively shapes and impacts the setting? Once again we lack well-developed assessment tools for this purpose and occupational therapists and researchers are trying to address this issue. The next generation of assessment tools must capture the interrelationships among different physical dimensions of the environment and the interplay between the person and environment.

Several assessments are currently available to therapists that attempt to assess persons in environments. One approach has been developed for use in rehabilitation to assist therapists in assessing how a client will interact with the home environment following discharge. This 10-minute test evaluates whether a client can recognize the danger inherent in an environment and is knowledgeable about the way to solve the problem (Robnett, 1995). This test involves arranging a kitchen unit in a rehabilitation setting with 10 hazards such as a sharp knife half off the counter, a spill on the floor, a cabinet door opened at head level. An OT would then accompany a client into the room and ask the client to describe potential dangers and solutions. This simple test can provide a great deal of information about how a client may handle the environment upon return home. This type of practical assessment however needs further testing and refinement to determine its reliability and the relationship of responses to cognitive and physical performance.

Another approach, developed by Margaret Christenson (1995), is the Enhancements Adapting Senior Environments (EASE) program. The EASE evaluation assists an occupational therapist to profile an older adult and his or her specific environmental barriers. Once a profile is established, EASE's database provides the therapist with possible solutions.

Another approach developed for use with older clients in the home has been developed by investigators from the Canada Mortgage and Housing Corporation (1995). In this approach, the therapist is guided to evaluate functional limitations as they are affected by or impact on different environmental features of the home. For example, for individuals who are experiencing difficulty with opening or closing doors, the therapist would assess grip, coordination, muscle weakness and mobility as well as the type of door handles throughout the home, the door or door spring width and operational force and the fit of the door frame. Based on this assessment, a number of recommendations are provided, which include changing the door handle, removing a nonessential door, or adjusting the door frame.

ENHANCING OCCUPATIONAL PERFORMANCE THROUGH ENVIRONMENTAL MODIFICATIONS

The goal of occupational therapy is to promote occupational performance by creating an opportunity for adaptation by an individual to the demands of the environment. Many therapists speak of a *just right fit* between abilities and environmental challenges that will facilitate adaptation. However, a just right fit is an elusive goal, depending on the client's competencies and the goals of treatment. For instance, if the goal of treatment is to help an anxious client feel comfortable with his or her occupational performance, Kiernat (1983) proposes modifying the demands of the environment to be slightly less than the individual's current level of skill. However, if the client requires challenge to maximize occupational performance, then the just right fit involves environmental demands that slightly exceed competence. Richter and Oetter (1990) illustrate these guidelines by applying Pearce's (1977) matrix of developmental progression to pediatric occupational therapy. In the first level of the matrix, the child requires a place of safety and security, similar to the environment of the womb. Environmental adaptations for children at this level involve use of close physical contact, such as small spaces and swaddling to promote the adaptive responses of calming and self-modulation. At the second level of developmental progression, the calmed child requires a safe, nurturing environment from which he can take risks. Environmental adaptations involve intermittent physical contact and can be achieved through use of therapeutic equipment such as swings and therapy balls. As the adaptive response of limited risk-taking is elicited, the occupational therapist adjusts the environment to provide greater challenges (toys for climbing and jumping), thus promoting further adaptation.

The next section of this chapter will broadly introduce environmental modifications to consider in relation to the client's competencies, his or her ability to promote adaptation, and the goals of treatment. This discussion is not intended to be an exhaustive review of all possible environmental modifications, but instead, an introduction to areas of consideration when using an environmental approach. We have identified four types of environmental modifications that directly address attributes of the physical environment described earlier. The introduction of a modification may have multiple purposes such as for function and safety and usually a combination of these strategies are implemented. The four types of modifications discussed here, examples of which are shown in Table 13-4, are assistive devices, alterations to the physical structure, object modifications, and task modifications.

Assistive Devices

Assistive devices are frequently prescribed for performance problems. In addition, assistive devices (such as closet organizers and extended shower hoses) are being marketed to the ablebodied population, advertised on the basis of their convenience, relaxation potential, and timesaving qualities.

Assistive devices are generally perceived by users to be an effective and important aids to their self-care and have been beneficial in reducing the need for help from another person (Gitlin, 1995b). Estimates of consistent use of prescribed assistive devices range from 50% to 85% (Gitlin, Schemm, Landsberg, & Burgh, in press; Gitlin, Levine, & Geiger, 1993; Bynum & Rogers, 1987; Geiger, 1990). The likelihood that an individual will use a device consistently is dependent in part on the occupational therapist's reasoning during a "complex series of interrelated decisions and clinical judgments" (Gitlin & Burgh, 1995, p. 996). Gitlin and Burgh (1995) used focus group methodology to identify six interdependent steps involved in decision making about which device to prescribe and how to best introduce use of the device. Those steps are: 1) selecting a device; 2) choosing an activity to practice use of the device; 3) determining the best time to introduce a device; 4) choosing an instructional site; 5) instructing in use of the device, and 6) reinforcing device use. These six steps act as a useful guideline for occupational therapists who incorporate assistive devices into their scheme for modifying the environment.

In the larger category of assistive devices is included modifications that are made for reasons of safety. While the physical environment can present many health and perfor-

---

TABLE 13-4
Four Major Types of Environmental Strategies

Strategy	Examples
Assistive devices	• grab bar • reacher • velcro clothing • canes • walkers • rocker knife
Devices for safety	• lighting • smoke detectors • sensing devices
Alterations to structures	• widening doors • stair glides • ramps
Modification of objects	• disabling stove • locks on doors • removal of throw rugs
Modification of tasks	• cuing (verbal, nonverbal, visual, auditory) • energy conservation

---

mance risks, occupational therapists must regard objects in terms of both cause and prevention. On one hand, items that are dangerous can be modified or removed to eliminate hazards, including those items used by clients in therapy and during everyday activities. Clients may also benefit, however, from information about assistive devices and modifications that are designed specifically to prevent injury.

Smoke and carbon dioxide detectors should be located on every level of the residence, especially the basement level. It is also important to have a detector installed in the client's bedroom that will contact the fire department automatically if not deactivated in a few minutes. Preferably, all smoke and carbon dioxide detectors should be wired directly into the electrical system of the home, eliminating the need for batteries. An emergency medical call device should be considered for the bathroom and the bedroom. Preferably, a voice-activated device should be purchased. Therapists should also consider modifications that improve function while preventing accidents and fires, such as a lightweight hair dryer that automatically activates when removed from the wall unit.

Newer appliances on the market, such as stoves and small appliances for heating water and food, have several useful safety features. Some stoves are equipped with sensing devices that shut the unit off automatically if an item begins to burn or is left unattended for a long period of time. Controls located in the front or on the side of the appliance are preferable, however a long reacher can be devised for use with older models. Counters placed next to the stove benefit the user by eliminating the need to carry hot heavy items. When possible, recommend cordless small appliances with rechargeable batteries. This reduces the need for reaching to unplug/plug in the appliance, and eliminates the danger of an electrical cord.

Visual input is an important safety modification as well as an object modification. Throughout the residence, all knobs should be labeled clearly with large print and colored to provide a visual contrast. Spigot knobs should be marked with blue (cold) and red (hot) paint, and the hot water temperature should never be set above 120 degrees.

Lighting can be modified to enhance visual input and safety. Some lighting is equipped with motion detectors, useful to prevent injuries when the client gets out of bed during the night. Also helpful is placing outside lights on an automatic timer. For the elderly, an increased need for light is accompanied by greater susceptibility to glare. Simply increasing the wattage of light bulbs in the area is likely to reflect more light and worsen the problem of glare. Use of high Color Rendering Index (CRI) full spectrum lamps will compensate increases in the level of illumination without increasing glare. Use of indirect lighting also helps to combat glare while improving visual clarity. Use of contrasting colors, preferably dark and light contrasts, are recommended for signs and stair risers. This also helps to reduce glare since the dark colors will not reflect light as readily as the lighter colors. Lighting should be installed in highly used passageways, such as halls and vestibules. It is also important to place light sources at the top and bottom of stairs, as these are the sites of most household falls (Studenski et al., 1994). To compensate for reduced depth perception on steps and in large rooms, lighting should be arranged to afford the most uniform illumination possible, thereby eliminating confusing pockets of light and shadow.

Safety modifications must always consider the overall level of clutter in the environment. As mentioned earlier, clutter can only be evaluated in relationship to the needs of the individual who is using the area. Clutter ranges from objects in a pathway to presence of items for more than one task. Occupational therapists may modify the environment by helping individuals to find safer storage places for items that present a tripping hazard and by suggesting furniture arrangements that increase the negotiable space in the home. Cordless telephones have been very useful in eliminating a source of falls due to cords in a pathway or hurrying to answer the telephone.

Alterations to the Physical Structure

Alterations to the physical structure include any adjustment to a permanent part of the building, including walls, floors, doorways, and staircases. Alterations are often made to enhance safe mobility, so installation of stair glides, ramps, and banisters are typical of modifications in this category. Alterations may also address safe mobility by repairing broken floor tiles, stair treads, replacing frayed carpets, and widening areas where a person with limited mobility must maneuver or make a transfer.

Doors are safety hazards in public areas and in the home. Any door requiring the side-by-side passage of two people should have a clear opening of no less than 48 inches. All glass doors, such as sliding doors and "full view" storm doors, should have a decal placed at chest height to avoid mistaking the glass for a clear opening. Color contrasts between the door and wall help those with low vision to locate the door.

On occasion, a door may be modified to disguise its presence instead of enhancing its visibility. Dickinson et al. (1995) explored the efficacy of several different types of window and door coverings for controlling dangerous exiting behavior by nursing home residents. They found that a cloth barrier, constructed of cotton material and attached at the sides with Velcro, reduced exiting behavior by 96%. A closed blind was much less effective, reducing the frequency of exiting by only 44%.

Be aware of body size and strength when designing environmental modifications. Avoid excessive reaching or bending by placing items strategically, and when possible, lowering cabinets and countertops. Little force should be needed to turn doorknobs and water spigots or these items should be replaced with L-shaped levers. In addition, while making modifications to the kitchen, bathroom, and work areas, always consider the need for a user to sit while performing tasks. Sitting to work usually requires lowered heights on work surfaces and room for accessible storage of a stool.

Privacy is another reason for alterations made to a physical structure, especially in the home. According to Barris et al (1985) personal preference for the use of space is determined by a group's culture. Therefore, it is not unusual for individuals with impaired mobility to resist converting a commonly-used room, such as the dining room, into a bedroom. Home alterations typically involve adding a separate, private, accessible bedroom and bathroom.

Information resources for ideas and specifications for physical alterations can be readily accessed through publications targeting specific populations, such as material published by the Alzheimer Association for caregivers of individuals with dementia.

Object Modification

Modifying objects typically involves making items available, easier to use, or more accessible. Within those broad parameters however, an extensive range of modifications exists.

Object availability entails choosing the items that most unobtrusively, but efficiently, address the targeted environmental deficiency. It has been suggested in the literature that individuals with chronic or slowly progressing disabilities are more likely to reject obvious adaptive devices (Faletti, 1984; Pynoos et al., 1987). Therefore, consider a non-medical item in preference to an assistive device in situations when both are able to support the individual in his or her occupational performance. For instance, consider the difference in appeal between a scoop dish and an ordinary bowl with very high sides.

Objects can be made easier to use by matching the requirements for their use to the sensorimotor and cognitive abilities of the individual. Use of built-up and extended handles are two examples of modifications that compensate for lack of muscle strength and/or range of motion. Cognitive problems may suggest the need for objects with instructions that are conveyed through pictures or highly simplified written instructions.

Maximizing the level of sensory input from an object is a typical modification that improves its usability. Object use by individuals with limited or undeveloped visual acuity (individuals below the age of 15 and above 50), and for individuals with a short attention span, should include enlarged print for greater visual impact. In addition, elderly people often are susceptible to glare, so using a dark background to absorb rather than reflect light may be beneficial. Along those same lines, glare can be controlled through the use of blinds and other coverings on brightly illuminated windows. While color coding helps to provide extra information, be aware of possible limitations in the client's ability to distinguish colors. For instance, the elderly typically have more difficulty distinguishing cool colors (blue and green) than hot colors (red, yellow, and orange).

In addition to visual input, auditory input from objects may be modified to make them more useful to individuals with hearing impairments. Because most congenital, acquired and age-related hearing problems involve deficits in the higher frequencies, smoke alarms and other auditory cues should be chosen based on their pitch in the middle to lower frequencies. Background noises should be kept to a minimum because they are often lower frequency sounds and can camouflage other auditory input.

When designing your own modifications or when modifying items used in therapy, make sure that all language and examples are standardized and universally familiar to the population. For example, the up position on a toggle switch is typically associated with "on," and a clockwise turn is expected to increase the volume or intensity.

Task Modification

Occupational therapists are specialists in analyzing and modifying tasks, and this topic has been discussed in greater detail in this book and other occupational therapy texts. We have included task modification in this chapter to draw attention to the importance of combining this therapeutic technique with the introduction of other types of environmental modifications. Just as with objects, tasks can be modified to manipulate the arousal and press potential of the environment. When using a combination of object and task modification, therapists should consider simplifying five dimensions of tasks, as developed by Barris et al (1985). They are: task complexity, temporal boundaries, rules, degree of seriousness/playfulness, and social implications. Task complexity refers to the skill level and sequence of actions related to a task. Manipulation of either or both are powerful tools which are available to occupational therapists as part of their entry-level training. Temporal boundaries include modification of the timing or scheduling of the task to make it simpler or more complex. An example of modifying the temporal boundaries includes creating a routine so information about the sequence and timing of tasks is predictable. Modifying tasks by changing the rules includes communication of the standards for performance in clear and unambiguous terms, as well as relaxing the rules when they cannot be observed due to reduced abilities. A task can be adjusted in terms of it seriousness or playfulness by emphasizing or de-emphasizing the consequences of the individual's actions. In modifying the social nature of the task, an occupational therapist can manipulate the level of cooperation and competitiveness of a task, as well as the opportunity to perform the task alone or in a group.

SPECIAL ISSUES IN INTRODUCING ENVIRONMENTAL MODIFICATIONS

Changing environments by introducing an assistive device or environmental alteration is a complex therapeutic intervention. There are a number of special considerations in using such an approach.

Clinical Reasoning

Mattingly and Fleming (1994) have documented that occupational therapists tend to reason in three ways, procedurally, interactively, and conditionally. In selecting and instructing in the use of an assistive device or environmental enhancement, occupational therapists also demonstrate a reasoning process that encompasses all three of these levels or

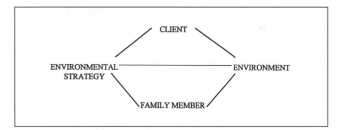

Figure 13-7. Four factors that guide clinical reasoning.

tracks (Gitlin & Burgh, 1995). When using procedural reasoning, the therapist asks "What does this person need?" On the procedural level, the therapist considers factors such as the patient's diagnosis, cognitive status and functional capacity. In reasoning at the interactive level, the therapist considers the personal goals and values of an individual and what he or she will accept as a strategy. When using conditional reasoning, the therapist evaluates multiple factors to seek a solution that optimizes the occupational performance of the individual.

As an occupational therapist reasons at each level to determine an appropriate environmental strategy, there are four basic factors that need to be considered during the assessment process (Figure 13-7). One factor involves the assistive device or environmental strategy itself such as its cost, level of difficulty of use, and its dimensions and fit with the physical environment. Another factor concerns the characteristics of the individual for which a strategy is sought. Factors such as the person's health, previous roles, values, current habits and personal goals are important considerations. A third factor that needs to be considered is the presence and roles of others in the environment. What is their role in caring for an individual as well as their own health and well-being and personal goals? The fourth consideration is that of the dimensions of the physical environment itself. Finally, the therapist must consider how all four factors interact and influence the desired outcome, occupational performance. That is, the therapist must consider the fit between the specific performance needs and desires of the person and his or her capabilities within a particular environment.

Personal Meaning of Objects

The physical environment, such as the home, is personal (Rubinstien, 1987). It is imbued with objects of personal significance and value and physical arrangements that have personal meanings. Changing the environment to accommodate functional loss can therefore be upsetting and difficult for an individual, even when these modifications may bring about improved performance or a better fit between the person and the environment. Introducing a modification may change a valued routine or deep-rooted preference for a way of organizing daily life (Frank, 1994; Gitlin, 1995a). Although the

goal of a modification is to enhance occupational performance, it may be difficult for an individual to accept such a strategy or require time for the change to be integrated into the person's environment and daily life. Recognizing the dilemma that functional loss and change may present is an important part of the therapeutic process involving environmental modifications.

Context-based Instruction

Most individuals need ample opportunity for practice, modification and refinement in using an environmental strategy. Short training periods with repeated opportunities for practice, experimentation, reevaluation and modification of the assistive device or environmental strategy is an effective approach. Demonstrating the use of an environmental strategy within the context in which it will be used enables the client to grasp its purpose and endorse its usefulness. The personal goals for occupational performance of individuals with chronic disability change over time with improvement or decline in health and functional status. Consequently, planning for the future or opportunities for reevaluation are important considerations in introducing an environmental strategy.

Family and Caregiver Involvement

Family members provide 90% of long-term care to individuals with functional dependence. Caregiver management of or direct participation in the daily routines of a family member appears to influence how and when assistive devices may be used in the home. Also, caregivers themselves may benefit greatly from the introduction of an environmental strategy. Nevertheless, caregivers receive very limited training in the use of devices when their family member is hospitalized and have limited knowledge as to the devices' potential benefit. Also, caregivers are rarely included in the decision-making process as to what types of devices would assist in the care of their family member (Gitlin, Corcoran, & Leinmiller-Eckhardt, 1995).

Markers of Success

We have said that changing the physical environment to enhance occupational performance involves rearranging personal and often treasured ways of being and doing. The use of environmental strategies must be integrated within the context of daily life and thus the success of the occupational therapist may need to be evaluated differently. What criteria can be used to judge whether an environmental strategy is being used successfully by a client?

There are four criteria of success that an occupational therapist can use. The first is whether the client integrates the strategy in daily routines. This can be assessed through direct observation and self-report. The second criteria of success involves observing whether the client modifies an environmental strategy to fit his or her particular environment. By modifying the strategy, an individual begins to shape it to fit his or her situation, personal preference and routine. A third criteria for success is whether the client is able to generalize a strategy to other problem areas. The fourth criteria that a therapist can use to judge success is whether the client's level of function or performance improves.

SPECIALIZED ENVIRONMENTS AND INTERVENTIONS

Most environmental modification occurs in the context of a larger intervention framework. Environmental modifications are a valuable aspect of several intervention schemes, including sensorimotor, behavioral, and educational frameworks. These frameworks and the role of environmental modifications to each will be discussed further in the next section of this chapter.

Some interventions are based exclusively on a person-environment-performance framework. Gallagher-Thompson (1994) referred to this type of intervention as "environmentally-oriented" (p. 103) and described it as focused more on what the individual has to accomplish to *improve* the situation as opposed to addressing how he or she *feels* about the situation. Interventions designed to modify the daily living environment are included. One example of an environmentally oriented intervention as described by Corcoran and Gitlin (1992), is designed to teach caregivers of elderly with dementia to use environmental modifications to manage problem behaviors in the home. This intervention is based on Barris and colleagues' conceptualization of the environment as consisting of four concentric layers encompassing the physical and sociocultural environment of the home. The majority of modifications recommended by Corcoran and Gitlin (1992) involve changes to the physical environment that are guided by information about the sociocultural environment.

While they cannot be considered an intervention protocol, the design of some physical spaces is based on environmental theory to address the needs of specified populations. Examples of such spaces include special classrooms for disabled children, dementia special care units in nursing homes, and sections of rehabilitation hospitals designed to simulate a street scene. The effectiveness of specially designed environments is only beginning to be tested, but initial results suggest their promise in terms of behavioral and functional outcomes (Dickinson et al., 1995; Sand et al., 1992).

ENVIRONMENTAL MODIFICATIONS IN COMBINATION WITH OTHER INTERVENTION FRAMEWORKS

Environmental modifications are a particularly powerful therapeutic aids when used in combination with other intervention frameworks. This sections examines the role of the environment in six therapeutic frameworks that typically structure occupational therapy services. They are: rehabilitation, sensorimotor, educational, psychoeducational, behavioral, and cognitive disability frameworks.

Rehabilitation Framework

In a rehabilitation framework, the primary focus is correcting the impairment in an effort to minimize or offset resultant disability. Treatment is typically concerned with enhancing the capabilities of the individual. Environmental modifications are occasionally used in the rehabilitation framework to maximize the therapeutic potential of activities. For instance, by placing an object toward the affected side of an individual with hemiplegia, weightshifting is promoted. Clients may even be taught to use these modifications on a long-term basis in order to sustain therapeutic gains.

When rehabilitation is not expected to result in further improvement of the individual's abilities, the rehabilitation approach also includes use of environmental modifications to compensate for permanent changes and reduce the level of disability. Traditionally, compensatory environmental changes within this framework include assistive devices and safety modifications.

Sensorimotor Framework

Treatment approaches that focus on use of selected sensory input to direct motor and affective responses are based on a sensorimotor framework. Many popular and effective treatment approaches are included the sensorimotor framework, such as sensory integration (SI), neurodevelopmental treatment (NDT), and proprioceptive neuromuscular facilitation (PNF). Manipulation of the physical environment lies at the heart of some sensorimotor approaches (e.g., SI) and is an important aspect of each.

The Ayres Clinic in Torrance, CA is a model for any clinic using an SI approach to promote a goal-directed adaptive response to an environmental demand (Slavik & Chew, 1990). Toward this end, objects in the environment are chosen for their therapeutic potential in helping a child to organize his or her own behavior. Such objects include equipment for vestibular, proprioceptive, and tactile input. The clinic is also designed with sliding doors to reduce sensory stimuli and safety features (thick mats) to lessen the poten-

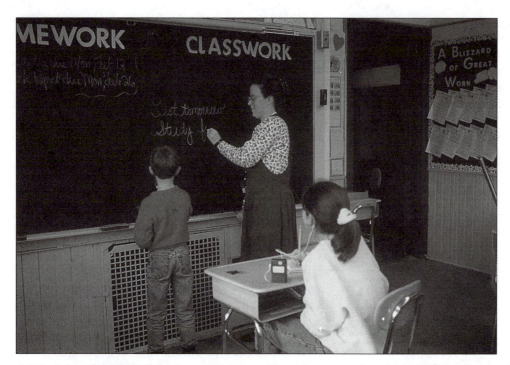

Figure 13-8. Hearing impaired child in the classroom.

tial for injury. Features of the Ayres Clinic have been adopted by many SI clinics around the world.

Neurodevelopmental Treatment (NDT), developed by Karl and Berta Bobath, involves the use of proprioceptive feedback to facilitate normal righting and equilibrium responses (Bobath and Bobath, 1972). Feedback is provided through positioning and the therapist's application of selected manual techniques. Environmental modifications are used primarily to promote optimal positioning (e.g., low stool, wooden chair) and to facilitate non-compensatory movements of the affected parts of the body (e.g., adjustable surfaces for weight-bearing). Non-compensatory use of the body is continued throughout the day, so clients' homes must be equipped with objects needed to perform bilateral and bimanual activities. Thus, it is important for a therapist using NDT to promote successful rehabilitation by adjusting both the clinic and home environments.

Educational Framework

In an educational framework the therapist often assumes a consultant role in relation to the teacher and parents. The efforts of the therapist must include training the teacher and parents to evaluate the environment from the perspective of the child being treated. That perspective may be unfamiliar at first, especially when the deficit is not easily understood, such as the effect of environmental noise on a hearing-impaired child. Occupational therapists may use equipment to allow the teacher to experience the disability, and recommend classroom techniques and assistive devices to adjust the environmental demands. Figure 13-8 shows a hearing-

impaired child and her teacher using several environmental modifications, including preferential seating to promote lip reading, an auditory trainer to amplify the teacher's voice, and visual cues written on the blackboard.

Occupational therapists working in the school system are faced with the challenges and rewards of treatment in the child's typical environment. It is common for occupational therapists in this setting to combine sensorimotor and educational frameworks in order to apply neurobehavioral concepts to the classroom. A school-based occupational therapist may not have access to equipment found in an SI clinic and must rely on a combination of portable assistive devices, environmental modifications to the classroom and techniques taught to the teacher and parents. For instance, treatment for tactile defensiveness may include use of a weighted vest, elimination of restrictive, irritating clothing, placement of the child at the end or beginning of line to avoid bumping, and firm pressure when touching (Koomar, 1990).

Psychoeducational Framework

A psychoeducational framework is typically used to provide support and information that enable individuals to manage long-term problems. Occupational therapists adopt a psychoeducational framework when they organize and conduct groups that address a variety of topics, ranging from assertiveness training to managing dementia-related problems in the home. Environmental modifications within this framework are organized into three categories, teaching supplies, experiential devices, and equipment recommendations for the client. Teaching supplies must be chosen carefully to promote the intended atmosphere for the group. Use of items typically associated with a classroom (e.g. blackboard, desks facing the "teacher) is appropriate for presentation of material, while more interaction and audience participation can be achieved with less formal items (e.g. chairs in a circle, flipchart). Teaching supplies also include reference materials distributed to participants for use outside the group. Experiential devices are chosen based on the topic. The psychoeducational model typically involves role play and the use of props can increase the realism and impact of these experiences. Additionally, groups which are focused on the management of chronic disability may include a discussion of recommended equipment. Often appropriate is demonstrating equipment options to the group and allowing the participants to try them before purchase.

Behavioral Framework

Based on a B.F. Skinner's concepts of stimulus-response, the behavioral framework modifies actions through the use of environmental influences. Typical applications of Skinner's concepts are behavior modification programs. Used in a variety of settings, behavior modification is a system of rewards for clearly identified positive behaviors. In school settings, students are rewarded with stickers or no-homework coupons for clean desks and outstanding academic performance. Mental health settings, day treatment centers, and sheltered workshops may rely heavily on behavior modification programs to adjust their clients' actions. The physical environment plays an important role in treatment based on the behavioral framework. Use of visual cues in the form of rewards or reminders about positive behaviors support the concepts of behavior modification. In addition, contracts signed by both client and staff are a powerful way to initiate the program.

Cognitive Disability Framework

Based on a cognitive disability framework, this neurobehavioral approach focuses on activity structure to promote occupational performance. Used widely in mental health, treatment based on the cognitive disability framework depends on provision of crucial environmental supports to cue the individual. The environmental modifications chosen are typically determined by the prognosis associated with the diagnosis. When the prognosis for independent functioning suggests improvement is possible, such as in depression or CVA, environmental modifications include grading tasks to challenge the individual. In dementia, however, improvements are not expected, so modifications focus on simplifying the objects and tasks in the environment (Corcoran & Gitlin, 1992; Levy, 1988). Figure 13-9 illustrates a highly simplified bathroom cabinet where objects are kept together in labeled containers, thereby providing access to needed

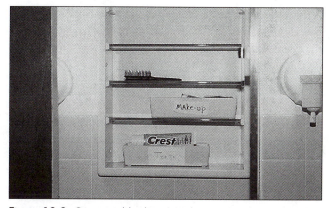

Figure 13-9. Organized bathroom cabinet.

objects while eliminating excessive visual cues (clutter). Caregivers must be included in decisions about environmental modifications for the management of cognitive disability in order to provide a consistent approach over time.

THE ENVIRONMENTALLY-MINDED OT ON A TEAM OF SERVICE PROVIDERS

Increasingly, occupational therapists will find themselves on an inter- or multidisciplinary team of health professionals. Despite the composition of the team, the occupational therapist is likely to possess the greatest expertise on the team for assessing and adjusting the fit between an individual's competencies and environmental demands. This suggests two directions for the occupational therapist's efforts as a team member, one in service to the client and the other as a resource for the team.

Occupational therapists have a primary responsibility to the client to create the best fit between abilities and environmental pressures. Much of this chapter has been focused on establishing and maintaining that fit. However, when other team members are involved, the role of the occupational therapist in relation to the client expands. The client who is being treated by a team of professionals will find it necessary to assimilate a considerable amount of information and accommodate several therapeutic regimes into the daily routine. An occupational therapist will be of service to the client in this effort by suggesting environmental modifications to manage information from other team members about exercises, recommendations, precautions, and procedures.

Occupational therapists can also serve as a resource to the team itself. Suggestions about environmental modifications during the conduct of therapeutic procedures can result in greater benefit and reduced frustration for both the team members and the client. The occupational therapist may also act as a resource for the timing of the introduction of therapeutic procedures based on an broad, comprehensive view of the client and environmental demands.

CHALLENGES FOR THE FUTURE

In response to demands for increased productivity and efficiency, it is sometimes tempting to take a simplistic approach to client issues, or to focus on one aspect of the individual (self-care) at the expense of other aspects (work and leisure). However, the relationship between people and their environments are so dynamic and complex that oversimplification is a disservice to the client and may confuse others about the value of occupational therapy. While it is important to assess each dimension of the person-environment-performance relationship comprehensively, it is equally important to recombine the individual with his or her environment to fully appreciate the therapeutic possibilities. Unfortunately, as stated earlier, current assessment tools and procedures have not advanced to the point where this can be easily accomplished. One challenge for the future is to monitor and study our clinical reasoning process as the basis for informing future assessment of person-environment fit. Mattingly and Fleming (1994) speak of conditional reasoning as the ability to create a mental image of an individual's performance given certain conditions. These conditions may include improved or refined abilities as well as environmental supports to occupational performance.

Another challenge for the future is the need to test the effectiveness of environmentally based services and environmental modifications. The benefits of such services have not traditionally been systematically examined using scientific methodology. Nonetheless, use of environmental modifications to remediate or prevent disability is widespread. As the managed care market evolves, pressure will increase to test the effectiveness of environmental modifications both in terms of cost and functional outcomes.

Finally, an emerging role for occupational therapists involves promoting environmental modifications as a primary prevention method. Just as seatbelts have become standard equipment on automobiles, it is also possible to educate consumers, developers, policymakers and planners as to the value of modifications to delay or prevent disability in specific populations, such as the well elderly.

This chapter has explored the physical environment as one dimension of the context for human performance. It has considered the transactional nature of the relationships among human capabilities, environmental attributes, and occupational performance as the basis for designing, introducing, and evaluating environmental modifications.

STUDY QUESTIONS

1. Name and describe three attributes of the physical environment.

2. Picture an individual with a specific disability in his or her home environment. Describe the press and arousal properties of the home and the ways in which the individual's culture is expressed.

3. Discuss the reasons why an individual may not accept an assistive device recommended to improve function.

4. Describe four major groupings of environmental modifications that may enhance occupational performance.

5. What role can/do environmental modifications play in your preferred intervention framework? How can that role be enhanced or expanded?

6. Explain the interactions among human abilities, environmental attributes, and occupational performance.

RECOMMENDED READINGS

Crabtree, J. L., & Crabtree, D. (1993). *Home caregiver's guide: Articles for adult daily living*. Tucson, AZ: Therapy Skill Builders.

Olsen, R. V., Ehrendrantz, E., & Hutchings, B. (1993). Creating supportive environments for people with dementia and their caregivers through home modifications. *Technology and Disability, 2*(4), 47-57.

Pynoos, J., Cohen, E., Davis, L., & Bernhardt, S. (1987). Home modifications: Improvements that extend independence. In V. Regnier & J. Pynoos (Eds.), *Housing the aged: Design directives and policy implications*. New York: Elsevier.

REFERENCES

American Occupational Therapy Association (1994). *Uniform terminology for occupational therapists* (3rd ed.). Bethesda, MD: Author.

Ayres, A. J. (1978). *Sensory integration and learning disorders*. Los Angeles: Western Psychological Services.

Ayres, A. J. (1979). *Sensory integration and the child*. Los Angeles: Western Psychological Services.

Badley, E. M. (1993). An introduction to the concepts and classifications of the international classification of impairments, disabilities, and handicaps. *Disability and Rehabilitation, 15*(4), 161-178.

Barris, R., Kielhofner, G., Levine, R. E., & Neville, A. M. (1985). Occupation as interaction with the environment. In G. Kielhofner (Ed.), *A model for human occupation*. Baltimore: Williams & Wilkins.

Baum, C. (1991). Addressing the needs of the cognitively impaired elderly from a family policy perspective. *American Journal of*

Occupational Therapy, 45, 595-606.

Baum, C. (1995). Practice and policy implications. Presentation at *Future directions in gerontology: Establishing therapeutic partnerships with elderly clients living in the community,* symposium, Philadelphia, PA.

Bobath, K., & Bobath, B. (1972). In P. H. Pearson & C. E. Williams (Eds.), *Physical therapy services in the developmental disabilities.* Springfield, IL: Charles C. Thomas.

Burnside, I. (1988). Nursing care. In L. R. Jarvik & C. H. Winograd (Eds.), *Treatment for the Alzheimer's patient: The long haul.* New York: Springer.

Bynum, H., & Rogers, J. C. (1987). The use and effectiveness of assistive devices possessed by patients seen in home care. *Occupational Therapy Journal of Research, 3,* 181-191.

Canada Mortgage and Housing Corporation. (1995). *Maintaining seniors' independence: A guide to home adaptations.* Author.

Christenson, M. A. (Spring, 1995). Assessing an elder's need for assistance: One technological tool. *Generations,* 54-55.

Christiansen, C. (1991). Occupational therapy: Intervention for life performance (pp. 3-44). In C. Christiansen & C. Baum (Eds.), *Occupational therapy: Overcoming human performance deficits.* Thorofare, NJ: SLACK Incorporated.

Corcoran, M. A. (1992). Gender differences in dementia management plans of spousal caregivers: Implications for occupational therapy. *American Journal of Occupational Therapy, 46*(11), 1006-1012.

Corcoran, M. A. (1994). Management decisions made by caregiver spouses of persons with Alzheimer's disease. *American Journal of Occupational Therapy, 48*(1), 38-45.

Corcoran, M. A., & Barrett, D. (1987). Utilizing sensory integration principles with regressed elderly patients (pp. 119-128). In Z. Mailloux (Ed.), *Sensory integrative approaches in occupational therapy.* New York: Haworth Press.

Corcoran, M. A., & Gitlin, L. N. (1991). Environmental influences on behavior of the elderly with dementia: Principles for intervention in the home. *Physical and Occupational Therapy in Geriatrics, 3-4,* S-22.

Corcoran, M. A., & Gitlin, L. N. (1992). Dementia management: An occupational therapy home-based intervention for caregivers. *American Journal of Occupational Therapy, 46*(9), 801-808.

Crabtree, J. L., & Crabtree, D. (1993). *Home caregivers guide: Articles for adult daily living.* Tucson, AR: Therapy Skill-Builders.

Czaja, S. J. (1988). Safety and security of the elderly: Implications for smart house design. *International Journal of Technology and Aging, 1*(1), 49-66.

Czaja, S. J., Weber, R. A., & Nair, S. N. (1993). A human factors analysis of ADL activities: A capability-demand approach. *The Journal of Gerontology, 48*(Special Issue), 44-48.

David, S. (1990). Environment: Implications for occupational therapy in mental health. In S. C. Merrill (Ed.), *Environment: Implications for occupational therapy practice.* Rockville, MD: American Occupational Therapy Association.

Dickinson, J. I., McLain-Kark, J., & Marshall-Baker, A. (1995). The effects of visual barriers on exiting behavior in a dementia care unit. *The Gerontologist, 35*(1), 127-130.

Edwards, D., Baum, C., & Morrow-Howell, N. (November, 1994). *Home environments of inner-city minority elderly with dementia: Do they facilitate or inhibit function?* Presentation at the Gerontological Society of America annual conference, Atlanta, GA.

Erber, J. T. (1979). The institutionalized geriatric patient considered in the framework of developmental deprivation. *Human Development, 22,* 165-179.

Faletti, M. V. (1984). Human factors research and functional environments for the aged. In I. Altman, M. P. Lawton, & J. F. Wohlwill (Eds.), *Elderly people and the environment.* New York: Plenum Press.

Frank, G. (1994). The personal meaning of self-care occupations. In C. Christiansen (Ed.), *Ways of living: Self-care strategies for special needs* (pp. 27-49). Rockville, MD: American Occupational Therapy Association.

Gallagher-Thompson, D. E. (1994). Direct services and interventions for caregivers: A review of extant programs and a look to the future. In M. Cantor (Ed.), *Family caregiving: Agenda for the future.* San Francisco: American Society on Aging.

Geiger, C. M. (1990). The utilization of assistive devices by patients discharged from an acute rehabilitation setting. *Physical and Occupational Therapy in Geriatrics, 9*(1), 3-25.

Gitlin, L. N. (1995a). Why older people accept or reject assistive technology. *Generations,* 41-45.

Gitlin, L. N. (1995b). Technology and self-care: What can social science research contribute to an understanding of technology use and aging. In press as proceedings of National Invitational Conference on Research Issues Related to Self-Care and Aging.

Gitlin, L. N., & Burgh, D. (1995). Issuing assistive devices to older patients in rehabilitation: An exploratory study. *American Occupational Therapy Association, 49*(10), 994-1001.

Gitlin, L. N., & Corcoran, M. (1993). Expanding caregiver ability to use environmental solutions for problems of bathing and incontinence in the elderly with dementia. *Technology and Disability, 2*(1), 12-21.

Gitlin, L. N., & Corcoran, M. (1996). Managing dementia at home: The role of home environmental modifications. *Topics in Geriatric Rehabilitation, 12*(2), 28-39.

Gitlin, L. N., Corcoran, M., & Eckhardt, S. (1995). Understanding the family perspective: A new framework for service provision. *American Journal of Occupational Therapy, 49*(8), 802-809.

Gitlin, L. N., & Levine, R. E. (1992). Prescribing adaptive devices to the elderly: Principles for treatment in the home. *International Journal of Technology and Aging, 5*(1), 107-120.

Gitlin, L. N., Levine, R. E., & Geiger, C. (1993). Adaptive device use in the home by older adults with mixed disabilities. *Archives of Physical Medicine and Rehabilitation, 74,* 149-152.

Gitlin, L. N., Schemm, R. L., Landsberg, L., & Burgh, D. Y. (In press). Factors predicting assistive device use in the home by older persons following rehabilitation. *Journal of Aging and Health.*

Kiemat, J. M. (1983). Environment: The hidden modality. *Physical and Occupational Therapy in Geriatrics, 2,* 3-12.

Koomar, J. (1990). Sensory integration treatment in the public schools. In S. C. Merrill (Ed.), *Environment: Implications for occupational therapy practice*. Rockville, MD: American Occupational Therapy Association.

Lawton, M. P., & Nahmow, L. (1973). Ecology and the aging process. In C. Eisendorfer & M. P. Lawton (Eds.), *Psychology of adult development and aging*. Washington, DC: American Psychological Association.

Levy, L. L. (1988). A practical guide to the care of the Alzheimer's disease victim: The cognitive disability perspective. *Topics in Geriatric Rehabilitation, 1*(2), 16-26.

Mace, N. L. (1991). The management of problem behaviors. In N. L. Mace (Ed.), *Dementia care: Patient, family, and community* (pp. 74-112). Baltimore: Johns Hopkins Press.

Mann, W. C., Hurren, D., Tomita, M., Bengali, M., & Steinfeld, E. (1994). Environmental problems in homes of elders with disabilities. *Occupational Therapy Journal of Research, 14*(3), 191-211.

Mattingly, C., & Fleming, M. H. (1994). *Clinical reasoning: Forms of inquiry in a therapeutic practice*. Philadelphia: F.A. Davis.

McEwen, M. (1990). The human-environment interface in occupational therapy: A theoretical and philosophical overview. In S. C. Merrill (Ed.), *Environment: Implications for occupational therapy practice*. Rockville, MD: American Occupational Therapy Association.

Meyer, A. (1922). The philosophy of occupational therapy. *The Archives of Occupational Therapy, 1*(1), 1-10.

Myers, J. R., & Hard, D. L. (1995). Work-related fatalities in the agricultural production and services sectors, 1980-1989. *American Journal of Industrial Medicine, 27*(1), 51-63.

Parmelee, P. A., & Lawton, M. P. (1990). The design of special environments for the aged. In J. E. Birren & K. Schaie (Eds.), *Handbook of the psychology of aging* (3rd ed.). New York: Academic Press, Inc.

Pearce, J. C. (1977). *The magical child*. New York: Bantam Books.

Reilly, M. (1962). Occupational therapy can be one of the great ideas of 20th century medicine. *American Journal of Occupational Therapy, 16*, 300-308.

Richter, E., & Oetter, P. (1990). Environmental matrices for sensory integrative treatment. In S. C. Merrill (Ed.), *Environment: Implications for occupational therapy practice*. Rockville, MD: American Occupational Therapy Association.

Robnett, R. (1995). Is your client safe at home? *OT Week, 9*(23), 22-23.

Rogers, J. C. (1983). Clinical reasoning: The ethics, science, and art. *American Journal of Occupational Therapy, 37*, 601-616.

Rubinstein, R. L. (1987). The significance of personal objects to older people. *Journal of Aging Studies, 1*(3), 225-238.

Sand, B. J., Yeaworth, R. C., & McCabe, B. W. (1992). Alzheimer's disease: Special care units in long-term care facilities. *Journal of Gerontological Nursing, 18*(10), 28-34.

Schkade, J. K., & Schultz, S. (1992). Occupational adaptation: Toward a holistic approach for contemporary practice, part 1. *American Journal of Occupational Therapy, 46*(9), 829-837.

Schultz, S., & Schkade, J. K. (1992). Occupational adaptation: Toward a holistic approach for contemporary practice, part 2. *American Journal of Occupational Therapy, 46*(10), 917-925.

Slavik, B. A., & Chew, T. (1990). The design of a sensory integration treatment facility. In S. C. Merrill (Ed.), *Environment: Implications for occupational therapy practice*. Rockville, MD: American Occupational Therapy Association.

Spencer, J. C. (1991). The physical environment and performance. In C. Christiansen & C. Baum (Eds.), *Occupational therapy: Overcoming human performance deficits* (pp. 125-142). Thorofare, NJ: SLACK Incorporated.

Struyk, R. (1987). Housing adaptations. In V. Regnier & J. Pynoos (Eds.), *Housing and the aged: Design directives and policy implications*. New York: Elsevier.

Studenski, S., Duncan, P. W., Chandler, J., Samsa, G., Prescott, B., Hogue, C., & Bearon, L. B. (1994). Predicting falls: The role of mobility and nonphysical factors. *Journal of the American Geriatrics Society, 42*, 297-302.

Turner, V. W. (1986). *The anthropology of performance*. New York: PAJ Publications.

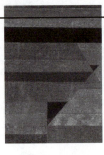

CHAPTER CONTENT OUTLINE

Introduction

The Search for Meaning

The Experience of Occupation

The Study of Meaning

Occupational Therapy and Meaning

Summary

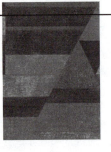

ABSTRACT

Daily occupations have two major dimensions: a visible dimension of performance and an invisible dimension of personal meaning. By attaching meaning to their occupations, individuals make sense out of their experiences and give coherence to their lives, a process that is strongly influenced by culture and ritual. The meaning of occupation is important to both occupational therapy theory and practice. Approaches to the study of meaning are described, followed by a discussion of meaning making in occupational therapy clinical practice. Therapists and clients together create therapeutic stories composed of meaningful experiences that fit into the larger context of clients' lives.

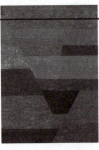

KEY TERMS

Client meanings

Culture

Flow

Meaningful

Meaningless

Narratives in practice

Occupational experience

Occupational task

Osgood's Semantic Differential

Qualitative research

Ritual

Social construction

Spirituality

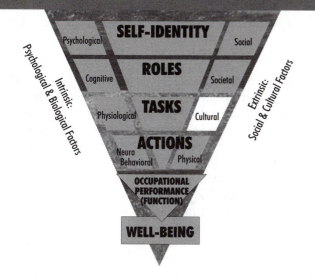

CHAPTER 14

SELF-IDENTITY
Psychological
Social
ROLES
Cognitive
Societal
TASKS
Physiological
Cultural
ACTIONS
Neuro Behavioral
Physical
OCCUPATIONAL PERFORMANCE (FUNCTION)
WELL-BEING
Intrinsic: Psychological & Biological Factors
Extrinsic: Social & Cultural Factors

Meaning and Occupation

Betty R. Hasselkus, PhD, OTR, FAOTA, Susan A. Rosa, MS, OTR

OBJECTIVES

The information in this chapter is intended to help the reader:

1. distinguish between the visible performance dimension of occupation and the invisible dimension of personal meaning

2. appreciate the importance of meaning in helping individuals make sense of and find coherence in their lives

3. recognize the influence of culture and ritual on the meanings people attach to their experiences and actions

4. discern the difference between the performance of an occupational task and the experience of engaging in an occupation

5. identify a variety of approaches to the study of meaning

6. recognize several reasons why it is important for occupational therapists to understand the meanings that their clients attach to the occupations in which they engage

7. identify at least two ways in which therapists can come to understand these meanings

8. become familiar with the concept of creating mutually meaningful therapeutic stories with clients.

> *"The activity of being a person is the activity of meaning-making."*
> Kegan, R. (1982). *The evolving self.* Cambridge, MA: Harvard University Press, p. 11.

INTRODUCTION

In the very early years of our profession, Meyer (1922) proposed that the daily occupations of human beings have two major dimensions: a dimension of performance and a dimension of personal meaning. We *perform* our ordinary and not-so-ordinary occupations every day and we attach *meaning* to these occupations in order to make sense out of our experiences. More than this, in occupational therapy, we hold to the belief that the meaning of our everyday activities is a major contributor to larger questions about the meaning of life; "Life is given meaning by what we do" (Fine & Kirkland, 1993, p. 20).

This chapter will focus on the meaning of occupations. Included will be: 1) a discussion of the concepts of meaningfulness and meaninglessness; 2) an exploration of meaning as it relates to the participation of individuals in everyday occupations; 3) a review of ways to study meaning; and 4) a discussion of the implications of meaning for carrying out occupational therapy. Narratives of therapists' and clients' experiences in practice will be used to illustrate key points and to enhance understandings of the importance of meaning in the therapeutic process. To understand the meaning of occupations is to better understand ourselves and the world in which we live. By doing so, we become more fully a part of that world.

THE SEARCH FOR MEANING

The search for meaning has been the object of philosophical discussion among ancient and contemporary thinkers. Frankl (1978) states that "the search for meaning is a distinctive characteristic of being human" (p. 29). People seek to make meaning out of their experiences in order to give coherence to their lives. It has also been said that the very act of being a person "is the activity of meaning-making" (Kegan, 1982, p. 11). To Yalom (1980), the lifelong tension between meaningfulness and meaninglessness is a fundamental feature of human life. He characterizes the search for meaning as one of four great themes of life, the others being the themes of isolation versus connectedness, death versus life, and restraint versus freedom.

Sources of personal meaning include our value orientation, i.e., the dimensions of life that seem good and important to us that we value. Examples are the valuing of individualism, patriotism, religiousity, altruism, dedication to a cause, and creativity. Frankl (1978) says that another source of meaning is being able to perceive a "possibility" embedded

in our reality (p. 38). In other words, we need to be able to see *potential* and *a future with possibilities* in order to experience meaningfulness. Reker and Wong (1988) propose that the greater the number and variety of sources for meaning that a person has, the greater will be the breadth of that person's sense of meaningfulness.

According to Frankl (1968), we can discover meaning in our lives in three ways: 1) through creativity, accomplishment, and doing; 2) by experiencing values; and 3) through pain and suffering. In being a therapist, we try to create meaning for ourselves and for our clients in the first and second ways by accomplishment and doing (carrying out therapy; enabling a client to carry out an activity) and by experiencing values (bringing about improvement, pleasure, independence).

Meaningfulness

We will begin with a quotation from an interview with an occupational therapist who participated in a study of the meaning of being a therapist (Hasselkus & Dickie, 1994). The intent of this quotation is to help us understand the nature of meaningfulness by focusing on the meaning of our own work, that of doing occupational therapy. This therapist was asked to think back over her practice and describe especially satisfying and dissatisfying experiences. The therapist quoted below describes a situation in which the patient, when first seen, was in a near-coma state, but as the story unfolds, it contains elements of order and purpose, possibilities, and a sense of great satisfaction. The therapist obviously found the experience to be personally meaningful and significant.

> *It was a woman in her 60s who was unresponsive and probably like [in a] coma, and was just beginning to eye track and nothing else, and was being NG [nasogastric]-tube fed. I was made aware of the patient by a dietitian. Through using some of the sensory stimulation with the patient and basic head trauma multi-sensory stim[ulation], we worked this lady to the point where she was sitting up and talking and remembering and feeding herself and doing ADL [activities of daily living], and was sent to a rehabilitation facility . . . [What was most satisfying was] the fact that the relationship she had with her family and how happy they all were to become a family and share again.*

Here is a story with a coherent beginning, middle, and end. Meaning for the therapist is created by the purposefulness and possibilities that are guiding the therapeutic process, the accomplishments that are realized, and the values of independent function and family happiness that are experienced. The therapist believes that, as a direct result of her work, the patient improved dramatically from a state of

Bibliographic citation of this chapter: Hasselkus, B. R., & Rosa, S. A. (1997). Meaning and occupation. In C. Christiansen & C. Baum (Eds.), *Occupational therapy: Enabling function and well-being* (2nd ed.). Thorofare, NJ: SLACK Incorporated.

"just beginning to eye track" to one of "sitting up" and "feeding herself." Deeds are done and values are experienced; meaningfulness is created. These therapeutic activities, devoted as they are to "leaving the world a better place to live in" (Yalom, 1980, p. 431), are typical sources of life meaning for occupational therapists.

Meaninglessness

In contrast, the following quotation is from a therapist's story of a very dissatisfying clinical experience that she had as a student. The dissatisfaction that the therapist expressed about this situation is strongly linked to the *meaninglessness* that the experience held for her. This story, like the one above, starts with a patient in a coma-like state:

> *The incident I found most dissatisfying occurred during my clinical work as a student.... A gentleman in his early 90s was referred for ADL in learning to feed himself. I do not even recall his diagnosis, but I never did understand why he was referred for OT. From the beginning it was evident that he was not able to respond. After several days of therapy, we were notified that the man had died.*

In this quote, the therapist describes a situation in therapy which made no sense to her ("I never did understand why he was referred for OT"). Although it is evident that the student continued to see the patient, the quotation infers that she did not perceive the situation to hold any promise for change. In large part, this quotation illustrates meaninglessness from the student's point of view, that is, she found herself in a situation in which she could see no useful role for herself and in which she could see no "possibilities" or goals to work for. (A word of caution: this is *not* meant to convey the message that occupational therapy with very old and dying patients is by its very nature meaningless, but rather that it appears to have been meaningless to this therapist as a student.)

Meaninglessness is, thus, associated with a lack of belief in the value, usefulness or importance of what we do (Yalom, 1980). The student therapist quoted above did not find the experience with the 90-year-old man to be personally meaningful to her. The experience seemed to have no sense of order, coherence, or purpose to her; she could not perceive the situation as holding any potential or future; she did not feel any sense of accomplishment.

These stories of practice given to us by therapists are stories of what therapists *do*. What we *do* in life is intimately connected to the meaning that we find in life. For occupational therapists, "what we do" may include such specialized occupational tasks as sensory stimulation or ADL as described in the interview above. But for everyone in the world, "what we do" is a phrase that refers more generally to

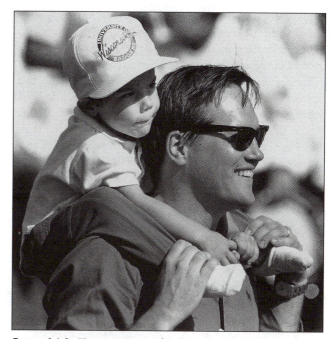

Figure 14-1. The experience of ordinary and familiar occupations. Courtesy of Jeff Miller, The University of Wisconsin—Madison.

the occupations of our everyday life. And it is from what we do, these deeds and the values they enable us to experience, that we find meaning in our lives.

The therapists' stories serve to illustrate the concepts of meaningfulness and meaninglessness in doing occupational therapy. The above examples relate to one thin slice of human occupation: certain people (occupational therapist, patient, dietitian, etc.) in a particular context (hospital, health care setting) doing particular things (ADL, dressing, feeding, sensory stimulation). We will proceed now to explore the nature of meaning more broadly in the context of everyday occupation, i.e., the meaning of "the ordinary and familiar things that people do every day" (American Occupational Therapy Association, 1995, p. 1015).

THE EXPERIENCE OF OCCUPATION

As stated in the first paragraph of this chapter, occupation has long been viewed as having both performance and meaning dimensions. This broad basic concept has been restated and redefined over the years in our professional literature. Fidler and Fidler (1978) speak of "doing and becoming"; their emphasis is on "doing" a purposeful action that enables the human being to "become," i.e., to develop in the psychological, social, and sensorimotor domains of life (Figure 14-1).

Fidler and Fidler, thus, recognize the reality of occupation per se but link it intimately with other invisible lifelong processes of human development. Nelson (1988) distinguishes between occupational form and occupational performance, with the former encompassing the physical and social context of the activity and the latter referring to the "doing" of the activity. Trombly (1995) proposes a model of occupational functioning in which the "doing" of the activity is organized by purposefulness and the motivation for occupation is derived from its meaning. Other descriptive terms have been introduced to enrich the multidimensional characterization of occupation (Christiansen, 1994a,b; Frank, 1994; Kielhofner, 1977, 1993; Rogers, 1982). Occupation, then, is human activity that has many aspects including the observable and the unobservable. Moreover, as Yerxa et al. (1990) have pointed out, the meaning aspects of occupation are of critical importance to fully understanding occupation as it relates to health and well-being.

To fully understand occupation, it is necessary to comprehend the experience of engagement...The same occupation may have a myriad of different meanings depending upon the goal of the individual, the environmental context, or mood...Eating may be done for survival, for social interaction as an important cultural ritual, as a symbol of a child's growing independence, or as a spiritual form of communion. (Yerxa et al., 1990, pp. 9-10)

The Experience and the Task

How do we come to have some understanding of this invisible *experience* of occupation? We can start by thinking about the distinction between the occupational task and the occupational experience. The occupational task encompasses the step-by-step mechanics of an activity, its observable characteristics and properties. The experience or meaning is derived from a person's characterization of the occupation in personally relevant terms. As an example, the task of getting dressed in the morning includes the mechanics of obtaining the clothes from the closet and drawers, taking nightclothes off, etc. The experience of getting dressed goes far beyond these mechanical procedures, and is embedded in one's age and gender, social status and social norms, and beliefs and values about attractiveness, neatness, and fashion. As Gelya Frank (1994) says, a self-care activity such as getting dressed is an activity that is both care of the self and an expression of the self.

The difference between the occupational task and the occupational experience can be further illustrated by quoting from another interview with an occupational therapist. This therapist described an experience of residential dining in a nursing home. Many of the nursing home residents were being fed by staff, and the therapist recognized that this approach accomplished the mechanics (task) of eating, but it certainly left much to be desired in terms of an eating experience. She wrote a proposal to change the dining room experience by incorporating important aspects of socialization and personal dignity.

There were quite a few folks that were not feeding themselves for one reason or another. Some were being fed just to expedite the different breakfast or lunch or dinner times. I saw a great need for these folks just to be, if they were able to feed themselves, to go ahead and do that...There were a lot of people who were aware and didn't want the food stuffed down them and wanted to be able to take their time eating...The lack of dignity that happened when they weren't able to feed themselves was really showing. So anyway, I wrote this all up and I recommended that they go ahead and let some of these people feed themselves and not separate [them from] a regular dining room and just to try to integrate them. And if some of the other people needed help, then some of the more able-bodied maybe could help, and so there was just more of a sense of community there.

The administrator of the facility did not approve of this therapist's proposal, and the emphasis continued to be on the task of people getting fed rather than on the equally important experience of eating. The therapist ultimately left this work situation to find another that better supported her concept of the importance of meaning in activities.

The Role of Culture

The meanings that activities have for us are the product of our culture. Cultures are shaped by human experience, and because individuals encounter differing experiences, even the simplest of activities can have many possible meanings. By understanding the role that culture plays in the shaping of meaning, we can become more aware of and sensitive to the inevitable differences that will exist between the meanings that activities will have for us as therapists and those they will have for our clients (Figure 14-2).

Defining Culture

Anthropologists define culture as all things that human beings learn as members of social groups. In our own literature, Barris, Kielhofner, Levine, and Neville (1985) defined culture as "the beliefs and perceptions, values and norms, and customs and behaviors that are shared by a group or society, and passed from one generation to the next through both formal and informal education" (p. 55). Simply stated, cultures are systems of shared meaning. These shared meanings underlie all our daily behaviors and occupations. Cultural traditions and conventions facilitate communication, prescribe behavior, and provide explanations of how the world works.

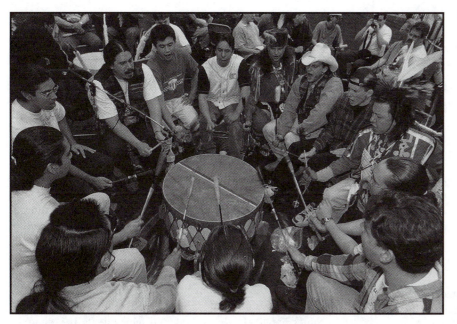

Figure 14-2. Cultural traditions prescribe behaviors. Courtesy of Jeff Miller, The University of Wisconsin—Madison.

Meaning is bestowed on things and events through language. Culture, therefore, is dependent on our biological capacity to think symbolically and use language. The intricate relationships between culture, language and meaning have been described by Bruner (1990):

> When we enter human life, it is as if we walk on stage into a play whose enactment is already in progress a play whose somewhat open plot determines what parts we may play and toward what denouements we may be heading. Others on stage already have a sense of what the play is about, enough of a sense to make negotiation with a newcomer possible...it is culture, not biology, that shapes human life and the human mind, that gives meaning to action by situating its underlying intentional states in an interpretive system. It does this by imposing the patterns inherent in the culture's symbolic systems its language and discourse modes, the forms of logical and narrative explication, and the patterns of mutually dependent communal life (p. 34).

The process through which shared meaning is created and maintained is frequently referred to as social construction (Berger & Luckman, 1966). The concept of "independence" is an example of a social construction; it is a concept that has been created and given a name in our culture and that is imbued with meanings that are shared by many in our society. The concept of independence in our culture includes such dimensions as individualism, initiative, self-reliance, and commitment to goals; such independence is valued and assumed to be desirable and good. Typically, occupational therapists value independence as it is defined in this way. Yet,

in some societies, independence is defined more as *inter*dependence, i.e., the concept of the rugged individual is discouraged and replaced by the reality and desirability of mutual dependencies among people as they live their daily lives. In this instance, the good of the group takes precedence over the good of the individual.

Multiple Levels of Culture

Culture exists on multiple levels. Neighborhoods, cities, and regions of a country may all represent subcultures within a larger culture. Even the small number of individuals who comprise families, with their shared opinions and ways of doing things, represent another level of subculture within their communities and neighborhoods (Sparring, 1991).

Similarly, professions can be viewed as cultures with a shared system of meanings, values and beliefs that are passed on from one generation to the next. Occupational therapists, for example, have a culture that reflects a blending of the values and expectations of white, middle-class North American society and the beliefs regarding the value of leisure and engagement in purposeful, functional activity (Krefting & Krefting, 1991). This culture represents our professional heritage (Figure 14-2).

Cultural differences are derived from the differences in the experiences of groups of people. These differences sometimes mean that concepts named in one culture may be absent in another. Differences among cultures means that, within all societies, some blending of cultures will occur; there will always be a range of meanings, even for those concepts that are strongly shared. Work, for instance, is an important concept across cultures, but even within our own society it can mean very different things. The meaning of

---

TABLE 14-1

Cultural Factors Influencing Performance

- Family structure
- Parental child-rearing styles or practices
- Economic status and history
- Educational background
- Age
- Marital status and history
- Vocational status and history
- Religion or spiritual orientation
- Political orientation
- Immediate environment
- Beliefs (about health, work, money, roles)
- Customs
- Values
- Health-related experiences

Different cultural factors influence human performance and can affect the perception of occupational therapy.

From Krefting L. H., & Krefting D. V. (1991). Cultural influences on performance. In C. Christiansen & C. Baum (Eds). Occupational Therapy: Overcoming human performance deficits. Thorofare, NJ: SLACK Incorporated.

---

work for women, for example, is different from the meaning for men. Culture dictates at what ages people work and do not work; retirement at age 65 is culturally expected in our society, while retirement at age 40 is a deviation from the age-related cultural norms of work activity.

Work is an example of a complex activity that has many levels of meaning. Yet even the simplest activities can have many possible meanings. An anthropologist, Clifford Geertz (1973), has used the example of quickly closing and opening one eye to illustrate the reality of many meanings. Our first thought might simply be, "That's a wink." But if we think further, we realize that this wink could be a flirting gesture, a deliberate signal meaning "I'm just kidding," an attempt to convey a sense of mutual conspiracy with someone, an imitation of someone else's wink with an intent to ridicule, etc. It is an action that, in our culture, can have many meanings. A personal anecdote illustrates this point further: While walking down a city street, a friend of ours, who was having eye trouble, was closing one eye to test out the vision in the other. A woman walking in the opposite direction suddenly "winked" back! In this case, the action of opening and closing the eye was not a wink at all, yet it was interpreted as a wink by another individual, based on what such an action had come to symbolize in this culture.

Frank's discussion about the meaning of self-care in people's lives gives vivid expression to the richness of the concept of multiple meanings as it relates to activities of daily living

(Frank, 1994). Her description of the social stigma that accompanies deviation from society's prescriptions for appropriate hygiene, dress, eating behavior, and methods of toileting also bears witness to the potential power that the meanings of even these ordinary occupations can have. Most of us are unaware of these commanding influences, a fact that is reflected in Hall's (1959) reference to culture as the "silent language." Only with conscious effort can we increase our awareness of the cultural influences in our own lives and the lives of others.

Individual cultural identities represent the integrated product of interactions with family members, peers, and others in the local community, in addition to the cultural influences of the region and country as a whole (Krefting & Krefting, 1991). In the United States, the blending of cultural traditions is widespread and longstanding, and the recent growth in the numbers of people with diverse ethnic backgrounds is producing a society that is ever richer and more heterogeneous. The range of possible meanings, belief systems, and values that occupational therapists in the United States are likely to encounter in their clients is potentially very great indeed (Table 14-1).

Culture and Health

Cultural influences are, of course, as prominent in activity related to health and disability as they are in any other daily occupations (see, for example, Payer, 1988; Kleinman, 1988). The way we define disability, the way we interact with health professionals, and our behaviors when ill or disabled are all strongly culturally grounded. Torres (1989), in her discussion of interactions with Hispanic patients in the hospital setting, described the well-developed system of folk medicine of these patients, their beliefs about illness as the will of God, and the traditional role of the Hispanic woman in caring for family members who are sick. Torres, who is a bilingual COTA of Hispanic heritage, felt the need to provide her services as a "culture broker" to both the patients and the medical staff. "I listen to their stories, let them know that their beliefs and customs are accepted, and then try to explain, in Spanish, what their problems are and how the medical staff plans to help solve them...It has also been my role to help the doctors understand the patients' beliefs when these matters are discussed in case conferences" (p. 3). This is just one example of cultural beliefs and customs that may affect health care practices.

In recent years, the concept of culture in health and health care has received increasing attention in our occupational therapy literature (Barney, 1991; Barris, Kielhofner, Levine, & Neville, 1985; Blakeney, 1987; Dyck, 1989; Jamieson, 1985; Krefting & Krefting, 1991; Krefting 1992; McCormack, Llorens, & Glogoski, 1991; McCree, 1989). Efforts to raise our awareness of the tremendous impact of culture on health occupations and the therapeutic process are extremely important to our efficacy as a profession. Barney

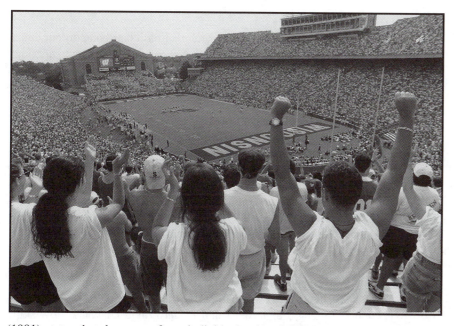

Figure 14-3. Rituals of a college football game. Courtesy of Jeff Miller, The University of Wisconsin—Madison.

(1991) states that, because of our individual cultural filters, "we may be ignorant of the customs, language, social relationship patterns, religion, and other practices of various ethnic and minority groups. In other words, we often do not know what we do not know" (p. 590). A "culturally holistic approach" (Barney, 1991, p. 592) in the health care we offer to clients will facilitate an optimal health care environment through cultural sensitivity and cultural continuity.

Rituals as Meaning

Rituals, or patterns of behavior that have strong elements of symbolism attached to them, are another expression of culture in our daily lives that are closely tied to occupation. The term "ritual" is often associated with religious ceremony. Organized religions provide opportunities for sacred rituals that involve the assembly of a group of people with a common focus of attention and a common emotional mood. Sacred symbols that hold meanings common to all members are present (Collins, 1988; Crepeau, 1995).

Secular rituals are also a part of our society. One has only to think of singing the national anthem at the beginning of a football game in a large athletic stadium 75,000 people focusing on the flag, patriotic symbol of our country to realize but one such ritual. Later in the game, when the team's mascot appears on the field, 75,000 people focus on this new symbol and shift en masse to a different emotional mood. Months later, when the spring commencement ceremony is held in that same stadium, several thousand people in the audience will focus on the school banners and emblems, the caps and gowns, and the potted ferns and dignitaries on the stage; all present are sharing yet a different emotional mood in a ritual with a different symbolic meaning. On a superfi-

cial level, what the people in the stadium are *doing* in all three circumstances looks very much the same; the *meaning* of the activity is, however, very different from one situation to the next (Figure 14-3).

Most of us do not think of our daily routines as rituals, but they can be just that. As defined by Driver (1991), rituals are "a known, richly symbolic pattern of behavior, the emphasis falling less upon the making and more upon the valued pattern and its panoply of associations" (p. 30). What differentiates rituals from simple routine activities, then, is their symbolism, i.e., their meaning (Crepeau, 1995).

Everyday rituals provide a rhythm to life. The action of rituals tends to soothe and calm, bringing a sense of order and stability to daily life (Moore & Myerhoff, 1977). The repetition of rituals "creates a sense of order because each aspect of the ritual can be anticipated from one event to the next" (Crepeau, 1995). At the age of about 8 years, the son of one of us (BH) had a grade school assignment to write a short paragraph about "home." The completed assignment contained the following sentence, poignantly revealing the meaning of "home" to a little boy: "At night I lie in bed and hear my mother sewing and my dad brushing his teeth." "Home" is the comfort and pleasure offered by familiar routines and ordinary activities. A mother's nightly routine of sitting at the sewing machine and a father's routine of brushing his teeth before going to bed were symbols of "home" to this child, strongly associated with a sense of place and comfort at the end of each day.

It can be seen, then, that rituals are one way that people both express meaning through occupation and create meaning from the occupation of others. Rituals may have a group focus or an individual focus. They are present in a wide variety of ways in our culture, ranging from the solemnity of a religious rite to the grandeur of the commencement ceremony to the ordinariness of everyday family activities. Routines and rituals make up very large parts of our daily behaviors and serve as important sources of meaning in our lives.

Spirituality as Meaning

Just as rituals are often narrowly understood only as they relate to religious ceremony, spirituality, too, is often associated only with religion. In an alternative view, spirituality has been defined recently as "the experience of meaning in everyday life activities" (Urbanowski & Vargo, 1994, p. 88). This definition places spirituality at the heart of occupation and the occupational therapy process.

Urbanowski and Vargo's (1994) conception of spirituality is an extension of the occupational performance model brought forward by the Canadian Association of Occupational Therapists (Law, Baptiste, Carswell, McColl, Polatajko, & Pollock, 1994). In this model of occupation, performance in everyday activities depends on capabilities of the individual in physical, mental, social and spiritual components. Thus spirituality emerges in this model as one of four key components that underlie occupation. Defined this way, spirituality becomes a dimension of occupation that can help individuals discover their meaningful connections to the rest of the world (Hettinger, 1996). Spirituality has been linked strongly to the inner transformation people experience after serious illness or injury, as they shift from a sense of being incomplete and victimized to a regained sense of agency and wholeness (Polkinghorne, 1996; Sullivan, 1993). Urbanowski and Vargo (1994) make the claim that every session that an occupational therapist has with a client has a spiritual dimension. It is important for therapists to seek understanding of the spiritual process that each client is experiencing by helping to identify the meaning of the client's future and the client's perception of future daily activities (Hettinger, 1996; Urbanowski & Vargo, 1994).

THE STUDY OF MEANING

We have characterized meaning as the invisible or hidden part of occupation, different from the form or performance of occupation which is behavioral and observable. The study of this invisible meaning of occupation is necessarily different from the study of its behavioral counterparts. For us, as occupational therapists, the study of the meaning of occupation is important to our theory and practice. We will describe three approaches to research on meaning that have contributed to our knowledge of occupation and to our occupational therapy practice.

Flow

One body of research that has contributed to our understanding of the meaning of occupation is the study of "flow" (Csikszentmihalyi, 1990; Csikszentmihalyi & Csikszentmihalyi, 1988). As Yerxa et al. (1990) stated, "To fully understand occupation, it is necessary to comprehend the experience of engagement in it" (p. 9). *Flow* is a term that describes the subjective quality of an experience during engagement in daily activities. A state of flow exists for people when their personal capabilities match the challenge of the tasks set before them. The flow experience includes such dimensions as a sense of control, clear goals, temporary loss of awareness of the self, enjoyment, an equilibrium of challenges and skills, and immediate feedback.

A person is in *optimal* flow when both the challenge of the task and the skill of the person are high; a person is in the opposite *apathy* when the challenge and the skill are both low. Two other modes of experience are *boredom* (low challenge, high skill) and *anxiety* (high challenge, low skill). When people are in flow, they feel strong, active, creative, and motivated; to be in optimal flow is to experience a "big personal high" (Larson, 1988, p. 166).

The Beeper Method

Flow is an elusive concept for research. Jacobs (1994) tried to study the optimal flow experience of occupational therapists at physical rehabilitation facilities in New England. Jacobs was only able to demonstrate that therapists are in flow "a small amount of the time" (p. 989), averaging once a day over a 5-day work week. Jacobs was attempting to investigate what factors contribute to flow in the work of occupational therapists and the relationship between flow and job satisfaction. She used M. Csikszentmihalyi's Experience Sampling Method (ESM) to systematically collect data on flow. The ESM is an ingenious method developed by M. Csikszentmihalyi to study the subjective experience of flow during people's ordinary everyday activities. Subjects wear a beeper or programmable wristwatch which is randomly activated seven times daily. When the signal sounds, the person stops whatever he or she is doing and fills out an Experience Sampling Form that contains questions about levels of concentration, sense of control, mood, level of challenge, importance of the activity, etc. This information is then compiled to help researchers understand the characteristics of the flow experience.

Have You Experienced Flow?

The theory of flow is grounded in psychological theories of the self and development (Csikszentmihalyi, 1988). According to Csikszentmihalyi, flow can only be sustained if both the challenges and the skills of a situation become ever more complex. This inner dynamic is what drives the self to higher and higher levels of complexity, i.e., it is what drives the human organism toward continual growth and development. We would invite you, the reader, to think back over your own recent life experiences and identify one in which you felt that you were in optimal flow. Were the purposes of the activity clear and did you have a sense of control during it? Did you lose your sense of time and place? Were you momentarily unaware of your own "self" and was your attention focused solely on the activity at hand? Csikszentmihalyi's research on the subjective experiences associated with occupations declares that this is the nature of the optimal flow experience.

Osgood's Scale

Another way to study meaning is to ask people to complete a standardized paper-and-pencil rating scale on meanings of activities. Osgood's Semantic Differential is a scale that has been used for this purpose (Osgood, Suci, & Tannenbaum, 1957). For example, a person may be asked to rate an activity somewhere on a seven-point scale between "good" and "bad" or between "excitable" and "calm." Osgood's original Semantic Differential had 50 of these bipolar adjectives. Further, Osgood found that these adjectives clustered into three large groupings: an evaluative group (such as good-bad), a potency group (such as rugged-delicate), and an activity group (such as active-passive) (Kerlinger, 1973). Ratings on this Differential may be summed and averaged to obtain a score; the score gives the researcher information on the meanings ascribed to the activity.

The use of Osgood's Semantic Differential is based on the assumption that activities have inherent characteristics that elicit certain responses from the people who engage in them. This is different from the assumption that people bring the meaning *to* the activity, or that meaning is created by the person in interaction with the activity.

Osgood's Semantic Differential has been used by a number of researchers in occupational therapy to study the meaning of activities. Katz and Cohen, for example, sought to study the meanings of four different craft activities—puppetry, woodworking, weaving, and ceramics—to occupational therapy students before and after training in each activity (1991). Their study combined the attempt to compare meanings of different activities with an experimental manipulation, i.e., before and after a workshop. Manipulations in other studies have included sharing and not sharing the materials for a project, creative and imitative activities, and keeping and not keeping the end product (Adelstein & Nelson, 1985; Carter, Nelson, & Duncombe, 1983; Rocker & Nelson, 1987). No differences were found in affective meaning in these studies except that creative activities were higher on power and eval-

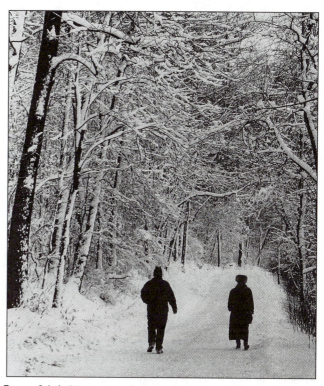

Figure 14-4. Discovering the meanings of everyday activities. Courtesy of Jeff Miller, The University of Wisconsin—Madison.

uative factors than imitative. As Katz and Cohen state, results from these studies are "inconsistent and limited to a few specific, short-term activities" (1991, p. 26). Nevertheless, research continues to be carried out using these instruments to study the meanings of purposeful activity.

Qualitative Research

A third way to study meaning is to use qualitative research approaches referred to as ethnography and phenomenology (Becker, 1992; Morse, 1994; VanManen, 1990). Using a qualitative approach, the researcher engages in observing, participating in the setting, in-depth interviewing, recording or videotaping ongoing activity, and eliciting subjects' stories to gain understanding of the subjective meaning of the phenomenon of interest. This approach to studying meaning is based on assumptions such as those expressed by Christiansen (1994b): "...we will never be able to accurately determine the meaning of an occupation by knowing or observing elements of its form and performance. The nature of this meaning can only be known to us if it is disclosed by the individual whom we are observing" (p. 8). In other words, to understand meanings, we need to do much more than merely observe people as they engage in occupation. We must *talk* to them (in-depth interviews, recording, eliciting their stories) to enable them to disclose the meaning to us. This process of facilitating disclosure in research is also used in occupational therapy practice to assist therapists as they seek to work together with their clients. The application of qualitative approaches to practice is discussed later in this chapter (Figure 14-4).

Qualitative information allows the interviewer to determine themes of meaning found in the detailed descriptions that have been collected. For example, Hasselkus (1989) conducted a series of in-depth ethnographic interviews with family caregivers who were caring for elderly family members in their homes in the community. The purpose of that ethnographic study was to understand the meaning of the family caregiving activities *from the perspective of the caregivers.* The interviews focused on the details of the caregiving day; a sense of "managing" was a prominent theme in the data. One family caregiver achieved a sense of managing through tightly scheduled daily routines of caregiving; another said, "I just got to take things as they come," suggesting his need for flexibility. Understanding individual meanings such as these can lead to better working relationships between therapists and family caregivers as they seek to carry out long-term care in community settings.

Other examples of qualitative research illustrate the array of possible topics and the rich potential for understandings offered by this approach to the study of meaning. Mattingly and Fleming (1993) used ethnographic interviews, participant observation, and videotaping to study the clinical reasoning processes of occupational therapists in practice; three major kinds of reasoning were interpreted from the data. Mulcahey (1992) studied the meaning of the experience of returning to high school after a spinal cord injury by carrying out intensive interviews with four adolescents who had sustained injuries within the previous 2 years; changes in the adolescents' self-images and coping patterns were described. Allen and Chin-Sang (1990) conducted in-depth interviews with 30 elderly African American women about their work histories and leisure experiences; the meaning of leisure for these women in old age was strongly related to their lifetimes of hard work. And finally, using occupational therapists' stories about satisfying and dissatisfying experiences in practice, Rosa and Hasselkus (1996) examined the patterns of helping between therapists and patients and found "working together" as a major theme of therapist satisfaction. These are but a few examples from many that are now in our literature (Figure 14-4).

Thus it can be seen that "meaning" is, indeed, a legitimate focus of research. The study of meaning takes many forms and offers us a rich resource for better understanding human occupation.

OCCUPATIONAL THERAPY AND MEANING

Placing an importance on the "meaning" of occupation influences the way we carry out our practice. Understanding a patient's perspective can mean the difference between success or failure in a therapy program. It is imperative that we learn how to gain understanding about the meanings attached to the occupations of the clients with whom we work. In the last section of this chapter, we will discuss the impact of meanings on the therapeutic relationship, the process of sharing meanings between therapist and client, and narrative theory as a source for meaning in practice.

Therapist and Client Meanings

We will start with an illustration of what can happen when a therapist does not place importance on the meaning of occupation to the client and consequently does not take the time to find out what that meaning is. This is a quotation from an interview with a therapist who described one of her "worst" experiences in practice.

> *[This patient] had a stroke and she refused treatment . . . When I would start on my way down the hallway she would start screaming as soon as she saw me coming. You know, I talked to her, I tried to explain to her that if we worked on her arm she might be able to use it . . . she had some movement so you could see that, you know, with therapy we could probably get some movement back. . . She just didn't really, you know, care. Those were not her goals and objectives. All she wanted to do was walk. . . Sometimes our expectations and the expectations of the people who we serve do not always meet eye to eye.*

This therapist and the patient she was trying to work with probably had not taken the time to try to understand the meaning of the situation to each other. The therapist believed strongly that what she had to offer this woman would lead to improvement in her function; the patient adamantly refused to have anything to do with the proposed therapy. If the therapist had started her therapy efforts by first seeking to understand the patient's feelings and perspective of the situation, and then sharing her own sense of the meaning of the situation, would this have made a difference? Possibly.

In fact, this therapist continued the interview with the following statement:

> *So, now my approach, from that experience, is different in that I explain the role of the occupational therapist and what we do and ask the resident, or anyone that I'm servicing, what is it that you want to*

do?...What is it that you find difficulty with? And let them, really, be more involved in determining goals and objectives if they are able to. That has worked better...and that's really important because a lot of times we'll do an evaluation or an assessment and we'll develop the goals, and not always have the involvement of the patient because we think that this is the best thing...And that's not always what the patient wants to do.

Asking a patient what he or she wants to do or feels is important is one way to understand the meaning of the situation to that person. When meaning is not considered, the therapist and patient may be unable to work together. Consideration of the patient's values and beliefs followed by a sincere effort to tailor the therapy to reflect those values and beliefs will maximize the potential for a full and satisfying therapeutic experience for both the patient and the therapist. A win-win situation is created out of a lose-lose situation. When personal meanings are not attended to, the therapist experiences one of her "worst" cases and the patient gets no therapy.

Meanings Shared in Practice

Kleinman (1988) was an early proponent of the concept of negotiation between professional and client. Kleinman urged that health care professionals be trained to seek out the perspectives of their clients and then to share their own perspectives, thus developing a relationship and a practice-based on mutual understandings and respect for each other's views. The process for doing such mutual sharing is very similar to the ethnographic interview process that is used in qualitative research.

The use of ethnographic methods in occupational therapy practice has been proposed by Hasselkus (1990) and Spencer, Krefting, and Mattingly (1993). Sometimes called "miniethnographies," the qualitative interview in therapy is a semi-structured exchange between the therapist and client. In this interaction, the therapist must discard the authoritative role and assume, instead, the role of a learner. Neither the therapist's nor the client's view should be overpowered by the other's already-constructed view of the situation (as occurred in the interview segment above where each was overpowered by the other). The purpose of the interview is for the therapist to understand the patient's point of view and for the patient to understand the therapist's view; ideally, a mutually agreed upon perspective will result. Table 14-2 lists techniques to be used in the first part of the interview, when the therapist is taking the time to learn from the patient. This approach lays the groundwork for the patient then being open to listening to the therapist's perspective.

TABLE 14-2

Ethnographic Interview Techniques

- The interviewer is the learner; the person being interviewed is the expert.
- The interview is semi-structured. Start with very global questions and then question further based on what the person starts talking about.
- Begin to incorporate the terms used by the client as he or she talks.
- Repeatedly express interest in what the person is saying.
- Be careful not to slip into the authority or expert role. Express ignorance appropriately.
- Build in opportunities for expansion and repetition.
- The interview should be asymmetrical, with the interviewee doing most of the talking.

From Hasselkus, B. R. (1990). Ethnographic interviewing: A tool for practice with family caregivers for the elderly. *Occupational Therapy Practice, 2*, 9-16. Copyright 1990 Aspen Publishers Inc.

A Home Care Example

Gitlin, Corcoran, and Leinmiller-Eckhardt (1995) discuss the impact of qualitative listening and sharing on the success of a home care program of occupational therapy. These authors state that, through the use of ethnographic techniques, the occupational therapist "is interested in the values, meanings, and viewpoints of persons and how persons make sense of or perceive their own context" (p. 803). Using a wonderful case example of two elderly sisters who lived in the community and cared for one sister's demented spouse, Gitlin et al describe the occupational therapist's initial recommendations intended to assist the caregivers with their difficult tasks. These recommendations included the use of home care services, major home modifications such as installing a stair glide, day care participation for the spouse, and preparation for possible nursing home placement. "These recommendations, which represent standard practice, were considered by the occupational therapist as critical for the well-being of both the care receiver and the caregivers" (p. 805). Nevertheless, in the next sentence, the authors state with chagrin, "Each suggestion, however, was rejected" (p. 805).

In their discussion of the case example, Gitlin et al noted that the therapist's recommendations represented a major change in the daily routines and image of the household as it was perceived by the family members. Further, these suggestions "reflected only the formal provider perspective that focused on the medical and dysfunctional aspects of the situation" (p. 805). The therapist did not yet understand what was meaningful in that household, and at that point she began to employ ethnographic techniques to reach a better understanding of the values and beliefs represented in the family. For example, the therapist carefully observed routines that were in place, objects that were present, and the language that was used by the family members to describe their situation.

New understandings emerged through this process. The therapist became aware of the sisters' primary concern for maintaining a sense of continuity and normality in the daily routines of the spouse as one way to preserve an image of what he used to do and the way he used to be. Informed by this new understanding, the therapist shifted her focus to more minor home modifications and teaching cuing techniques to the sisters to enhance the spouse's abilities in daily self-care activities. This shift in emphasis does not mean that the original recommendations were wrong; it simply means that they were not workable in this family context. As Gitlin et al conclude, a health care professional may be called on to modify or suspend his or her own beliefs about treatment in an effort to understand the meanings underlying a patient's or family's cultural context. The therapist must try to bring together the best of both worlds. This "bringing together" is what Krefting and Krefting (1991) refer to as the "negotiation of cultural filters in therapy" (p. 108).

Meaning-making Through Narratives

A school of thought exists that links the meaning of experiences in life with storytelling or narratives. Narrative theory proposes that individuals make meaning out of their experiences by creating stories or narratives about those experiences (Bruner, 1986, 1990; Coles, 1989; Polkinghorne, 1988; Mattingly, 1991, 1994). Stories have been described as the linguistic expression of our flow of experience (Polkinghorne, 1988); we construct stories out of our experiences in order to make sense of them. Manheimer (1989) calls this the "narrative quest"; he describes this quest as the individual's lifelong search for and creation of a personal life story as a way of defining the meaning of his or her life.

In therapy, eliciting patients' stories is one technique that can be used to gain understanding of patients' perspectives. Mattingly (1991) characterizes therapists' ways of thinking as narrative reasoning. "Therapists not only listen to the stories that their patients tell them, but also tell stories about their patients...an important part of this storytelling involves the therapist's understanding of the patient's way of dealing with disability" (p. 998). Thus, storytelling by patients, or the creation of narratives from patients' experiences, provides a window into the meaning of those experiences for occupational therapists. In our own research, we were eliciting stories from therapists when we asked them to describe very satisfying and very

dissatisfying experiences of practice. Through these narratives, we gained understanding about the meanings of those experiences (Hasselkus & Dickie, 1994). In therapy, when we start by asking a patient to describe for us their illness experience, we are, again, eliciting a story from that patient that will enable us to understand the meaning of the illness in his or her life.

Helfrich and Kielhofner (1994) further developed the concept of the patient's life story and its impact on the meaning of therapy. Both therapist and patient must share a view that the therapy makes sense and that it matters. The therapist creates, with the patient, a therapeutic story that fits the patient's own experience; the story unfolds through the shared experiences of therapy.

The sense of shared experiences of therapy contributing to a patient's larger life story is illustrated in an excerpt from another therapist's satisfying story of practice. This therapist worked in a nursing home. She described a horticulture therapy group that she "got involved with" and the subsequent party for group members that she held in her own home. The story offers a compelling example of shared experiences that build on the life narratives of both the therapist and residents of the nursing home.

> *I got involved with a horticulture therapy group and we entered a lot of the residents in the local flower show and they ended up winning The Best of Show! They were all pretty excited about that. These were people who had not experienced gardening or any real hobby or activity in quite a while.*
>
> *Then after the flower show was over, we decided to have a celebration. I have a house that's wheelchair accessible because I have a husband who is handicapped, so we had 33 residents from this nursing home to my house for a barbecue and a pool party. I think the most satisfying experience I've had as a therapist was seeing the benefit of my training and education. I had this house built, worked on the design and all that, and so it really truly was barrier free...Here we had 33 people, walkers, wheelchairs, you name it, and everybody was fine in their varying levels of independence, going to the bathroom. There were some people who were swimming in the pool for the first time in 25 years. It felt like a scene from the movie "Cocoon."*
>
> *I think for me, instead of seeing them, "Okay, well they've achieved functional level, they can be discharged from therapy," was seeing them in a naturalized environment or seeing them outside of their therapeutic setting and seeing them doing real things and hearing them give the feedback that they feel like real people and that what I had given them was hope back, and had given them something to really cherish. That's why I wanted to get into geriatrics in the first place.*

This is a therapist who, through the experience of doing, created brief therapeutic narratives that fit into each nursing home resident's larger life story. She and the residents created the narratives together, achieving what Mattingly calls narrative shaping of the therapeutic experience. Mattingly (1991) declares that this kind of therapy "is about much more than meeting specific treatment goals. It is about creating an experience that gives the participants a vision of themselves as actors in the world, that is, as more than just patients" (p. 1004). This is "doing real things" and feeling like "real people" and having "something to really cherish." For the therapist, this is why she "wanted to get into geriatrics in the first place." The story created in therapy fit into the larger life story of all of the participants—residents and therapist.

SUMMARY

Human occupation has two major dimensions: a visible dimension of performance and an invisible dimension of personal meaning. Performance refers to the doing of occupational tasks; meaning is revealed in the ways in which individuals characterize their occupations in personally relevant terms. Human life is meaningful to the extent that it makes sense and is perceived as having purpose and possible valued outcomes.

Meanings we attach to our actions are strongly influenced by the culture in which we live. Occupational therapists routinely interact with individuals whose life experiences are different or who have lived in different cultures and may assign different meanings to the same occupations. These meanings bring richness to the therapeutic interaction when acknowledged and integrated into the therapeutic process.

Because meaning represents an invisible dimension of occupation, we can only learn about the meanings that our clients attach to activities by asking them to tell us. By eliciting their stories, listening carefully and taking the time to understand their situations from their points of view, we are able to design therapeutic experiences that fit into the larger context of their lives.

The occupational therapy process thus incorporates the meanings of occupation as well as the observable performance components. We create therapeutic stories with our clients that nurture and sustain recovery and adaptation, and that provide the coherence and sense of possibility necessary to support a meaningful life. The discovery of meaning is central to that process.

STUDY QUESTIONS

1. What are the two dimensions of daily occupation?

2. How is culture defined? Give an example of the influence of culture on daily occupation.

3. What is the difference between ritual and habitual daily routine?

4. Occupational therapists try to create meaning for themselves and for their clients in what two ways?

5. Describe the difference between *performing* an occupational task and *experiencing* an occupational task.

6. What are four characteristics of "flow"?

7. Compare the following two methods of studying meaning: Osgood's Scale and qualitative in-depth interviews.

8. Name three characteristics of ethnographic interview techniques that can be used by therapists to gain understanding of clients' perspectives.

9. What is the meaning of narrative reasoning as described by Mattingly?

RECOMMENDED READINGS

Belenky, M. F., Clinchy, B. McV., Goldberger, N. R., & Tarule, J. M. (1986). *Women's ways of knowing*. New York: Basic Books.

Chinn, P. L. (Ed.). (1991). *Anthology of caring*. New York: National League for Nursing Press, #15-2392.

Christiansen, C. (1994). *Ways of living: Self-care strategies for special needs*. Rockville, MD: American Occupational Therapy Association.

Csikszentmihalyi, M., & Rochberg-Halton, E. (1981). *The meaning of things: Domestic symbols and the self*. New York: Cambridge University Press.

Dossey, L. (1991). *Meaning & medicine*. New York: Bantam Books.

Kaufman, S. R. (1986). *The ageless self: Sources of meaning in late life*. Madison, WI: University of Wisconsin Press.

Murphy, R. F. (1987). *The body silent*. New York: Henry Holt.

Plummer, K. (1983). *Documents of life*. Boston: George Allen & Unwin.

Sontag, S. (1990). *Illness as metaphor and AIDS and its metaphors*. New York: Anchor Books.

Spradley, J. P. (1979). *The ethnographic interview*. New York: Holt, Rinehart and Winston.

Swain, J., Finkelstein, V., French, S., & Oliver, M. (Eds.). (1993). *Disabling barriers—Enabling environments*. Newbury Park, CA: Sage Publications.

Tolstoy, L. *The death of Ivan Ilych and other stories*. (1960). New York: New American Library.

REFERENCES

Adelstein, L. A., & Nelson, D. L. (1985). Effects of sharing versus non-sharing on affective meaning in collage activities. *Occupational Therapy and Mental Health, 5*, 29-45.

Allen, K. R., & Chin-Sang, V. (1990). A lifetime of work: The context and meanings of leisure for aging black women. *Gerontologist, 30,* 734-740.

American Occupational Therapy Association. (1995). Position paper: Occupation. *American Journal of Occupational Therapy, 49,* 1015-1018.

Barney, K. (1991). From Ellis Island to assisted living: Meeting the needs of older adults from diverse cultures. *American Journal of Occupational Therapy, 45,* 586-593.

Barris, R., Kielhofner, G., Levine, R., & Neville, A. (1985). Occupation as interaction with the environment. In G. Kielhofner (Ed.), *A model of human occupation: Theory and application* (pp. 42-62). Baltimore: Williams & Wilkins.

Becker, C. S. (1992). *Living & relating: An introduction to phenomenology.* Newbury Park, CA: Sage.

Berger, P. L., & Luckman, T. (1966). *The social construction of reality.* New York: Doubleday.

Blakeney, A. B. (1987). Appalachian values: Implications for occupational therapists. *Occupational Therapy in Health Care, 4,* 57-72.

Bruner, J. (1986). *Actual minds, possible worlds.* Cambridge, MA: Harvard University Press.

Bruner, J. (1990). *Acts of meaning.* Cambridge, MA: Harvard University Press.

Carter, B. A., Nelson, D. L., & Duncombe, L. W. (1983). The effects of psychological type on the mood and meaning of two collage activities. *American Journal of Occupational Therapy, 37,* 688-693.

Christiansen, C. (1994a). A social framework for understanding self-care intervention. In C. Christiansen (Ed.), *Ways of living: Self-care strategies for special needs* (pp. 1-26). Rockville, MD: American Occupational Therapy Association.

Christiansen, C. (1994b). Classification and study in occupation: A review and discussion of taxonomies. *Journal of Occupational Science, 1,* 3-21.

Coles, R. (1989). *The call of stories.* Boston: Houghton Mifflin.

Collins, R. (1988). *Theoretical sociology.* San Diego, CA: Harcourt Brace Jovanovich.

Crepeau, E. B. (1995). Rituals (Module 6). In C. B. Royeen (Ed.), *The practice of the future: Putting occupation back into therapy.* Bethesda, MD: American Occupational Therapy Association.

Csikszentmihalyi, M. (1988). The flow experience and its significance for human psychology. In M. Csikszentmihalyi & I. Csikszentmihalyi (Eds.), *Optimal experience: Psychological studies of flow in consciousness* (pp. 15-35). Cambridge: Cambridge University Press.

Csikszentmihaly, M. (1990). *Flow: The psychology of optimal experience.* New York: Harper & Row.

Csikszentmihalyi, M., & Csikszentmihalyi, I. (1988). *Optimal experience: Psychological studies of flow in consciousness.* Cambridge: Cambridge University Press.

Driver, T. F. (1991). *The magic of ritual.* San Francisco: Harper.

Dyck, I. (1989). The immigrant client: Issues in developing culturally sensitive practice. *Canadian Journal of Occupational Therapy, 56,* 248-255.

Fidler, G. S., & Fidler J. W. (1978). Doing and becoming: Purposeful action and self-actualization. *American Journal of Occupational Therapy, 32,* 305-310.

Fine, S. B., & Kirkland, M. (1993). Vision of the American Occupational Therapy Foundation for occupational therapy in the 21st century. *OT Week, February 25,* 20-21.

Frank, G. (1994). The personal meaning of self-care occupations. In C. Christiansen (Ed.), *Ways of living: Self-care strategies for special needs* (pp. 27-49). Rockville, MD: American Occupational Therapy Association.

Frankl, V. E. (1968). *Man's search for meaning.* New York: Washington Square Press.

Frankl, V. E. (1978). *The unheard cry for meaning.* New York: Simon and Schuster.

Geertz, C. (1973). *The interpretation of culture: Selected essays.* New York: Basic Books.

Gitlin, L., Corcoran, M., & Leinmiller-Eckhardt, S. (1995). Understanding the family perspective: An ethnographic framework for providing occupational therapy in the home. *American Journal of Occupational Therapy, 49,* 802-809.

Hall, E. (1959). *The silent language.* New York: Doubleday.

Hasselkus, B. R. (1989). The meaning of daily activity in family caregiving for the elderly. *American Journal of Occupational Therapy, 43,* 649-656.

Hasselkus, B. R. (1990). Ethnographic interviewing: A tool for practice with family caregivers for the elderly. *Occupational Therapy Practice, 2,* 9-16.

Hasselkus, B. R., & Dickie, V. A. (1994). Doing occupational therapy: Dimensions of satisfaction and dissatisfaction. *American Journal of Occupational Therapy, 48,* 145-154.

Helfrich, C., & Kielhofner, G. (1994). Volitional narratives and the meaning of therapy. *American Journal of Occupational Therapy, 48,* 319-326.

Hettinger, J. (1996). Bringing spirituality into practice. *OT Week, June 13,* 16-18.

Jacobs, K. (1994). Flow and the occupational therapy practitioner. *American Journal of Occupational Therapy, 48,* 989-996.

Jamieson, M. (1985). The interaction of culture and learning: Implications for occupational therapy. *Canadian Journal of Occupational Therapy, 52,* 5-8.

Katz, N., & Cohen, E. (1991). Meanings ascribed to four craft activities before and after extensive learning. *Occupational Therapy Journal of Research, 11,* 24-39.

Kegan, R. (1982). *The evolving self.* Cambridge, MA: Harvard University Press.

Kerlinger, F. N. (1973). *Foundations of behavioral research* (2nd ed.). New York: Holt, Rinehart and Winston.

Kielhofner, G. (1977). Temporal adaptation: A conceptual framework for occupational therapy. *American Journal of Occupational Therapy, 31,* 235-242.

Kielhofner, G. (1993). *Conceptual foundations of occupational therapy.* Philadelphia: F.A. Davis.

Kleinman, A. (1988). *The illness narratives: Suffering, healing, and the human condition.* New York: Basic Books.

Krefting, L. H. (1992). Strategies for the development of occupational therapy in the third world. *American Journal of*

Occupational Therapy, 46, 758-761.

Krefting, L. H., & Krefting, D. V. (1991). Cultural influences on performance. In C. Christiansen & C. Baum (Eds.), *Occupational therapy: Overcoming human performance deficits* (pp. 100-122). Thorofare, NJ: SLACK Incorporated.

Larson, R. (1988). Flow in writing. In: M. Csikszentmihalyi & I. Csikszentmihalyi (Eds.), *Optimal experience: Psychological studies of flow in consciousness* (pp. 150-171). Cambridge: Cambridge University Press.

Law, M., Baptiste, S., Carswell, A., McColl, M. A., Polatajko, H., & Pollock, N. (1994). *Canadian Occupational Performance Measure*. Toronto: CAOT Publications.

Manheimer, R. J. (1989). The narrative quest in qualitative gerontology. *Journal of Aging Studies, 3*, 231-252.

Mattingly, C. (1991). The narrative nature of clinical reasoning. *American Journal of Occupational Therapy, 45*, 998-1005.

Mattingly, C. (1994). The concept of therapeutic employment. *Social Sciences Medicine, 38*, 811-822.

Mattingly, C., & Fleming, M. (Eds.). (1993). *Clinical reasoning: Forms of inquiry in therapeutic practice*. Philadelphia: F.A. Davis.

McCormack, G. L., Llorens, L. A., & Glogoski, C. (1991). Culturally diverse elders. In J. Kiernat (Ed.), *Occupational therapy and the older adult* (pp. 11-25). Gaithersburg, MD: Aspen.

McCree, S. (1989). Sensitivity to the black elderly client. *Gerontology SIS Newsletter, 12*, 1-2.

Meyer, A. (1922). The philosophy of occupational therapy. *Archives of Occupational Therapy, 1*, 1-10.

Moore, S. F., & Myerhoff, B. (1977). Introduction: Secular ritual: Forms and meanings. In S. F. Moore & B. Myerhoff (Eds.), *Secular ritual* (pp. 3-24). Assen/Amsterdam: VanGorcum.

Morse, J. M. (Ed.). (1994). *Critical issues in qualitative research methods*. Thousand Oaks, CA: Sage.

Mulcahey, M. J. (1992). Returning to school after a spinal cord injury: Perspectives from four adolescents. *American Journal of Occupational Therapy, 46*, 305-312.

Nelson, D. L. (1988). Occupation: Form and performance. *American Journal of Occupational Therapy, 42*, 633-641.

Osgood, C. E., Suci, G. J., & Tannenbaum, P. H. (1957). *The measurement of meaning*. Urbana, IL: University of Illinois Press.

Payer, L. (1988). *Medicine and culture*. New York: Penguin Books.

Polkinghorne, D. E. (1988). *Narrative knowing and the human sciences*. Albany, NY: State University of New York Press.

Polkinghorne, D. E. (1996). Transformative narratives: From victimic to agentic life plots. *American Journal of Occupational Therapy, 50*, 299-305.

Reker, G. T., & Wong, P. T. P. (1988). Aging as an individual process: Toward a theory of personal meaning. In J. E. Birren & V. L. Bengtson (Eds.), *Emergent theories of aging* (pp. 214-246). New York: Springer Publishing.

Rocker, J. D., & Nelson, D. L. (1987). Affective responses to keeping and not keeping an activity product. *American Journal of Occupational Therapy, 41*, 152-157.

Rogers, J. (1982). The spirit of independence: The evolution of a philosophy. *American Journal of Occupational Therapy, 36*, 709-715.

Rosa, S. A., & Hasselkus, B. R. (1996). Connecting with patients: The personal experience of professional helping. *Occupational Therapy Journal of Research, 16*, 245-260.

Sparling, J. W. (1991). The cultural definition of the family. *Physical and Occupational Therapy in Pediatrics, 11*, 17-29.

Spencer, J., Krefting, L., & Mattingly, C. (1993). Incorporation of ethnographic methods in occupational therapy assessment. *American Journal of Occupational Therapy, 47*, 303-309.

Sullivan, W. P. (1993). "It helps me to be a whole person": The role of spirituality among the mentally challenged. *Psychosocial Rehabilitation Journal, 16*, 125-134.

Torres, R. L. (1989). Contributions of a bilingual COTA to an occupational therapy program. *Gerontology SIS Newsletter, 12*, 3-4.

Trombly, C. A. (1995). Occupation: Purposefulness and meaningfulness as therapeutic mechanisms. *American Journal of Occupational Therapy, 49*, 960-972.

Urbanowski, R., & Vargo, J. (1994). Spirituality, daily practice, and the occupational performance model. *Canadian Journal of Occupational Therapy, 61*, 88-94.

VanManen, M. (1990). *Researching lived experience*. London, Ontario: State University of New York Press.

Yalom, I. D. (1980). *Existential psychotherapy*. New York: Basic Books.

Yerxa, E. J., Clark, F., Frank, G., et al. (1990). An introduction to occupational science: A foundation for occupational therapy in the 21st century. In J. A. Johnson & E. J. Yerxa (Eds.), *Occupational science: The foundation for new models of practice* (pp. 1-17). New York: Haworth Press.

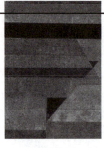

Chapter Content Outline

The Social-Cultural Normative Context: An Anthropological View

Societal Changes and Their Impact on Social Engagement

Social Policies Evolution

Issues in Environment-Centered Assessment

Environmental Factors

Macro, Meso, and Microsystemic analysis

Social Environment and Habitat Factors

Abstract

This chapter provides an overview of the role of the social environment as it influences the quality of social participation of people with disabilities. An anthropological view of normality and deviance is described, with physical and mental differences considered within this view. Societal developments which have influenced attitudes towards disability, including human rights, normalization, deinstitutionalization, and a broader definition of health are described. A new model of disability, oriented toward social change, political empowerment and social participation, is presented. Environmental determinants of social participation are proposed with definitions and elements of analysis.

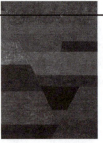

Key Terms

Sociocultural context

Normality

Impairment

Disability

Handicap situation

Deviance

Human rights

Inclusion

Stigma

Independent Living

Social exclusion

Social policies

Social change

Differences

Physical environment

Social environment

Barrier

Facilitator

Life habits

Social participation ICIDH

Environmental factors

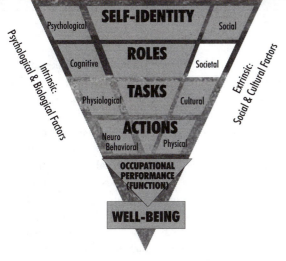

The Influence of the Social Environment on the Social Participation of People With Disabilities

Patrick Fougeyrollas, PhD

OBJECTIVES

The information in this chapter is intended to help the reader:

1. explain how the social environment creates barriers to the social participation of people with disabilities

2. understand perspectives on difference, deviance and normality from the field of social anthropology

3. identify environmental factors which limit potentially limit social participation and inclusion

4. discuss the evolution of social policies which affect the social participation of persons with disability

5. review issues in environment-centred assessment relevant to daily living and social participation

6. appreciate the importance of including social perspectives in assessment and intervention during the occupational therapy process.

> *"Disability is an issue that affects every individual, community, neighborhood, and family...It is more than a medical issue; it is a social, public health, and moral issue."*
>
> Pope and Tarlov, 1991, p.1.

THE SOCIOCULTURAL NORMATIVE CONTEXT: AN ANTHROPOLOGICAL VIEW

It is a universal rule, from the standpoint of anthropology, that each human being is unique and different from every other person. Each person develops within a particular cultural and ecological niche. A person's functional abilities, personal identity and daily routines are also a part of their uniqueness. This view of the individual provides a way of understanding how society contributes to handicapping conditions. This chapter proposes that the functional differences of the individual and conditions within the environment interact to create handicapping conditions. This occurs because the environment reflects social attitudes about what is expected and what is normal (Fougeyrollas, 1978; 1983; Jacquard, 1978).

The development of human beings is influenced profoundly by the cultures in which they learn social requirements. Societies ensure their continuation through the social learning process, which provides an understanding of the world and imparts values from a very early age. Newborns are immersed in a system of rules and expectations which shape their physical development and belief systems. The consequences of these social influences vary according to the constitutional differences of individuals.

An important part of societal influence relates to definitions of what is considered normal and expected. As children encounter these "boundaries", they are influenced to choose behaviors and adopt attitudes that conform to social expectations. In so choosing they acquire some possibilities but give up others. These are the consequences of any choice. The interaction between the person (before he or she notices that there is a difference) and the effect of the normative sociocultural context allows the individual to experience differences (or deviances) and be transformed by their effects.

The way in which the society recognizes and respects the differences in its members indicates its understanding of disability. Barriers imposed by society contribute to the consequences of disease and trauma for persons with disabilities. Even the act of identifying persons with disabilities as a separate category of people creates a label that results in social disadvantage or handicap.

Studies of persons with disabilities and the extent to which they are accepted by others in society traditionally have been studied within the category of social deviance. Social deviance refers to aspects of society considered outside the norm (Friedson, 1965). The study of deviance is most advanced in sociology, usually focusing on behaviors which are illegal or considered immoral. Crime, delinquency, or other practices (such as prostitution or drug use) judged unacceptable by mainstream society fall into this category (Durkheim, 1977; Merton, 1957). In general, these types of deviance imply some degree of individual responsibility for choosing the deviant behavior. Thus, most of the research on deviance has been aimed at finding an explanation for this process of choice. Over the last two decades, however, the focus of deviance research has shifted away from an analysis which examines the individual to approaches that emphasize how society contributes to such behaviors (Spitzer, 1975).

Persons with disabilities, because of their physical or mental impairments, experience situations where societal acceptance is comparable to that experienced by persons considered deviant in other ways. Unfortunately, people with disabilities have not chosen to be different and the idea of individual responsibility cannot be applied because their condition or state has been determined by pathology or injury, such as that which might result from a fall, a car accident or as the result of a genetic condition.

Theories on labeling and stigma (Goffman, 1963) have been proposed since the 1960's and have been further developed in more recent research on the social production of deviance or marginal status (Lemert, 1967; Ogien, 1995). These issues are addressed in Chapter 16.

Ironically, the reality of disability is that it does not involve a small segment of the population, but rather significant numbers at any given time (Bolduc, 1992). About 49 million Americans (one in seven) and 4 million Canadians (Statistics Canada, 1992) or about 15% of the population, have a physical or mental impairment that interferes with their daily activities. Yet only 25% of persons with disability are so severely disabled that they cannot work or participate in their communities (Pope & Tarlov, 1991). The medical, social and economic needs of an increasing segment of the population who have lost independent function because of irreversible pathology (or are at risk of losing independence because of the diseases or the consequences of aging) is of concern. These include seniors losing their independence because of factors related to aging, persons with mental disorders, persons with sensory, physical or intellectual impairments, persons traumatized by war, industrial, traffic or domestic accidents, and persons with chronic disease. Unfortunately, as a society we segregate these groups and do not have a coordinated effort to support their independence. There is, however, an increasing awareness of their needs because of the costs to the individual, to the family, and to society in terms of lost productivity and the cost of long term management.

Bibliographic citation of this chapter: Fougeyrollas, P. (1997). The influence of the social environment on the social participation of people with disabilities. In C. Christiansen & C. Baum (Eds.), *Occupational therapy: Enabling function and well-being* (2nd ed.). Thorofare, NJ: SLACK Incorporated.

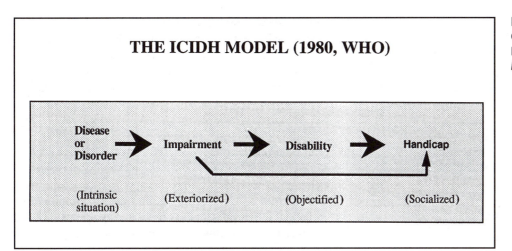

Figure 15-1. The International Classification of Impairments, Disabilities, and Handicaps Model.

SOCIETAL CHANGES AND THEIR IMPACT ON SOCIAL ENGAGEMENT

Over the past 25 years, societal changes have increased awareness of the issues surrounding disability and the social disadvantage often accompanying it. Policies relating to human rights, a recognition of the importance of promoting the inclusion of persons with disability in everyday society, deinstitutionalization, and a broadened concept of health as promoted by the World Health Organization (WHO), have contributed to these attitudinal changes.

The WHO redefined health to extend beyond the mere absence of disease. The WHO definition recognizes that a person without mental and social well-being cannot function optimally in his or her environment, and therefore cannot be considered healthy. At the same time, there has also been an evolution of comprehensive rehabilitation programs and social integration approaches in education, employment and transportation to reduce barriers and to support the full inclusion of persons with disability in society.

Additional efforts have built and strengthened communication among those involved in disability. In 1965, American sociologist Saad Nagi proposed definitions that differentiated between the acute disease process, anatomical or physiological impairment, functional limitation and disability (Nagi, 1965, 1991). His work identified rehabilitation as focusing primarily on functional limitations and disabilities. This contrasts with traditional medical intervention, which focuses on pathology. The Nagi concepts are still widely used in English-speaking North America.

The deviance and stigma theories developed by Freidson (1965) and Goffman (1963) introduced the ideas that physical limitations influence the attitudes of others because of values related to social expectations and cultural definitions of what constitutes a "normal" and acceptable range of performance. Their work contributed to our understanding of social obstacles that restrict the participation of individuals in

social roles. These ideas have helped change the views of disability from those focused on problems within the person, to those which recognize that disability is a societal problem with important social consequences (English, 1977; Groce and Scheer, 1990: Mottez, 1977; Phillips, 1990; Morvan & Paicheler, 1990).

In the 1970's a consumer movement emerged to defend the rights and facilitate the independent living of persons with disabilities. This movement pushed for a more adequate definition of equal opportunity and social participation. It also raised the need to have a mechanism to facilitate the development of policies and services to support the needs of individuals with the functional and social consequences of disease and trauma (Wolfensberger, 1972, 1992; Flynn & Nitsch, 1980; Bolduc, 1986, 1992; Fougeyrollas, 1983, 1988, 1990, 1995a; Granger, 1984: Minaire, 1992: Enns, 1989; and Barry, 1989). Groups representing persons with long term disabilities have pointed out that the curative medical model is not adequate to address the needs and experiences of their members, once the acute stage of the disease or injury has passed. Some groups in the International Disabled Persons Movement (Scandinavian and North American groups, Independent Living, Disabled People International) even argued that it was only necessary to struggle against environmental determinants of social exclusion, taking no interest in the person's physical limitations (DeJong, 1979; Enns, 1989; Hurst, 1993). This has prompted the need to have a mechanism to link information about the medical conditions, the rehabilitation process, and the environmental factors that either support or inhibit full societal participation.

In 1980, Dr. Philip Wood published (under sponsorship of the World Health Organization) an experimental classification related to organic, functional and social consequences of diseases. His system is the International Classification of Impairments, Disabilities and Handicaps (ICIDH), described elsewhere in this volume. Around this time, a number of other epidemiological and systemic models for classifying disability,

---

TABLE 15-1

Nomenclature of Life Habits

- Nutrition
- Physical condition
- Personal care
- Communication
- Housing
- Movement from place to place

- Responsibilities
- Family relations
- Interpersonal relations
- Community
- Education
- Employment
- Leisure and other custom ary activities

From Fougeyrollas, P., St-Michel, G., Blouin, M., 1989; Fougeyrollas, P., St-Michel, G., Bergeron, H., Cloutie, R., 1991)

---

chronic disease and injury were also developed (Duchvorth, 1983; Tremblay, 1982; Wan, 1974; Warren, 1977).

The ICIDH model (Figure 15-1) has fostered communication among scientists and has guided the development of assessments that have facilitated acquisition of knowledge about the person that will allow him or her to regain or acquire the skills necessary to carry out daily living requirements with the necessary support from the environment.

SOCIAL POLICIES EVOLUTION

In recent years, people with disabilities have exercised their civil rights. Their advocacy has given rise to new perspectives and has supported the development of a model of disability oriented toward social change, political empowerment and equalization of opportunity. These efforts have had an overall goal of full social participation (United Nations, 1983: Office des personnel handicapées, 1984; Enns, 1989; Barry, 1989; Fougeyrollas, 1983; 1995b; DeJong, 1979; Woodhill, 1992; Bickenbach, 1993; Oliver, 1990; Finkelstein, 1990; Flynn, 1993). This social change perspective implied the need for a comprehensive or holistic approach which considered individual physical or mental differences as well as environmental obstacles. Environmental obstacles create handicapping conditions unless they are removed. Thus, they are essential considerations in the process of facilitating social integration for persons with disability.

The Quebec and International Disabled Persons Movements' perspectives each define the concept of handicap as a consequence of the interaction between two important elements: the person with a disability and the environment. Handicap is a specific consequence of functional impairment, it occurs when the individual's performance of social activities is limited or impossible. Therefore, any definition of the con-

cept of handicap (or social disadvantage) must explicitly state the interactive relationship between the disabilities (which are individual characteristics) and environmental obstacles (physical and sociocultural factors in the environment).

A handicap affects a person's social participation, and can be defined as a disturbance in the performance of everyday living (in view of age, sex, and sociocultural identity) resulting from this interaction between capabilities and environmental characteristics (See Table 15-1). Using these criteria, the focus of occupational therapy should be to direct its efforts to help people avoid handicapping situations by supporting them in acquiring the skills and facilitating accommodations to carry out their customary daily occupations and social roles (Fougeyrollas et al, 1991).

Issues in Environment-Centred Assessment

Since the late 1980's, a consensus has evolved that views environmental variables as determinants of the social consequences of a person's impairments and disabilities (Badley, 1987; 1995; Chamie, 1989; Minaire, 1983, 1992; Soder, 1987; Verbrugge & Jette, 1994; Fougeyrollas, 1995; Christiansen, 1991). The environment includes the individual's usual surroundings such as home and work, interactions with people, and even more remote influences such as general economic conditions, the political climate and characteristics of the society or culture (Alexander & Fuhrer, 1984).

A paradigm change is allowing a movement away from the dominant biomedical conceptual models, which are centered on the individual, to the contemporary perspective of social change which centers on the environment. The goal is to reach a level of compatibility between people with disabilities and the characteristics of their social environments (Christiansen, 1991, Bolduc, 1995; Fougeyrollas, 1995a, 1995b; Swaim et al, 1993).

To identify and solve the problems outside the individual that create handicapping situations requires assessments that consider individual capabilities from the standpoint of environmental characteristics (which can include inaccessible facilities, poorly fitting tools or equipment, or discriminatory attitudes of employers). Measuring changes in handicapping situations over time is important if we are to determine which environmental modifications have the most beneficial effect in reducing social exclusion. These research results can be used to direct resource allocations.

The process of identifying handicapping situations requires a many faceted, multidisciplinary approach extending well beyond the health and social service fields. Such a process must even extend beyond the specific programs intended to compensate for the disabilities of people with mental and physical impairments. The approach must

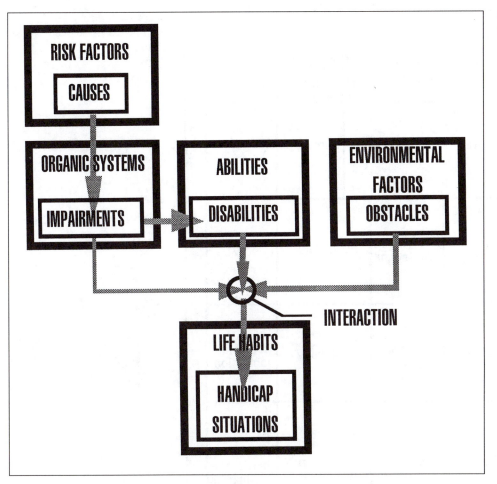

Figure 15-2. Handicap Creation Process.

involve an environment-centred analysis of the consequences of disabilities and their effects on socioeconomic organization, mentalities, sociocultural values and attitudes, legislation, and the physical environment. The approach is also relevant to town planners, engineers, architects, economic planners, lawyers, politicians, sociologists, anthropologists and the media, as well as the organizations representing people with disabilities which demand equality of opportunity. Figure 15-2 presents a conceptual model of the cultural process which results in handicapping conditions.

Currently, the evaluation tools used in rehabilitation combine functional limitations (actions such as grasp, stoop and reach) and the performance of complex activities (such as eating a meal, making one's bed or driving an automobile) and focus on the person and his or her problems (Alexander & Fuhrer, 1984). A problem exists in how functional assessment tools are developed. The functional evaluation of a person taking and holding an object, bringing it to his or her mouth and moving it left and right must ultimately relate to everyday situations, such as the movements required for eating Chinese noodle soup. Measures are needed that report the

ability of the person to perform tasks required in everyday living and how the environment supports the performance of those tasks. An example of environmental support would be human assistance (whether involving verbal instructions or physical assistance) or modification of the task (through using assistive technologies, task simplification, or modifications in the physical environment).

Environmental dimensions must be taken into consideration in assessment approaches which measure the consequences of impairment and disability. For example, performance scores should not be lower for persons who must use environmental support. Another factor that must be considered is the setting in which the assessment takes place. Assessments of daily living skills should be done (ideally) in the environment(s) in which they typically are performed. Performance in a clinical setting may be very different from that which occurs in an individuals usual surroundings (Alexander & Fuhrer, 1984). (Further information on these issues is provided in chapter five of this volume.)

The environmental barriers to social participation by persons with disabilities must be identified if they are to be

	Organic Structure	Internal functions	Functional aptitudes	Performance in social activities and social roles	Social and physical environment
O.M.S. Wood I.C.I.D.H. (1980)	Impairments		Disabilities	Handicaps	Ø
Nagi (1965)	Impairments		Functional Limitations	Disability	Ø
NCMRR (1993)	Impairments		Functional Limitations	Disability	Societal Limitation
CSICIDH (1991)	Impairments Organic systems		Abilities Disabilities	Life habits Handicap situations	Environmental barriers or facilitators

Figure 15-3. Attempt of correspondence between concepts.

overcome. To facilitate social change and to enable opportunities for full participation, it is important to focus on the interaction between an individual's characteristics (self-identity, abilities and limitations) and the characteristics of the environment which, in combination, result in handicapping situations (Figure 15-3).

ENVIRONMENTAL FACTORS

Environmental factors serve to inhibit or facilitate social participation depending on their interactions with personal characteristics. They determine whether or not a person can participate in common social activities, according to their age, sex and personal identity (as well as education, experience, and life history). The environment can be a barrier to anyone. Steps, heavy doors, poor lighting, or any number of variables can limit our ability to do what we need to do.

Five principle criteria must be included in any environ-

mental assessment scale: 1) accessibility; 2) accommodation; 3) resource availability; 4) social support; and 5) equality of opportunities (Whiteneck & Fougeyrollas, 1996; Figure 15-4).

Impairments, abilities and disabilities are linked to the person as are other internal personal identity variables, such as age, sex, life experience, education and cultural identity. Without an evaluation of environmental factors, there can be no ecological approach to avoid handicapping situations.

Bronfenbrenner (1979) describes three dimensions of analysis that make it possible to define the environmental setting. The choice of the dimension depends on the needs of the user. The three levels of environmental analysis are: macrosystemic (societal); mesosystemic (community), and microsystemic (personal).

Macrosystemic (societal) analysis considers the society as a whole. It provides basic reference documentation that is essential to study a target population. Without this level of

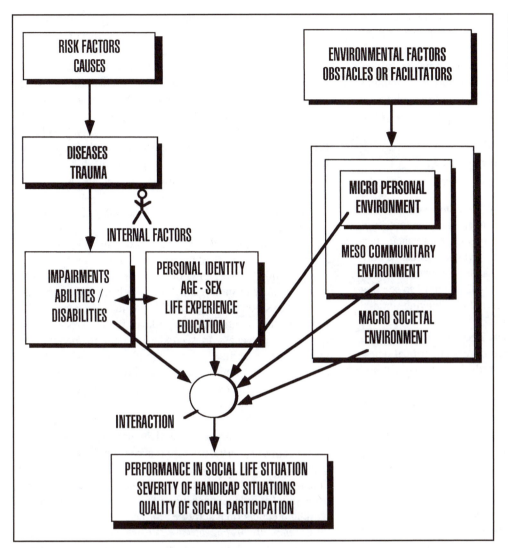

Figure 15-4. The Individual and Environment Determinants of Handicap Situations and Societal Participation. Adapted from Fougeyrollas, P. (1993).

analysis, interpretations of statistics on the severity of impairments, disabilities and handicapping situations cannot be made for use in planning programs and policies.

Mesosystemic (community) analysis is a more local analysis, assuming a community-wide focus. It allows officials of programs concerned with persons having impairments or disabilities to use the social environment to draw a picture of the immediate living conditions of the person or population being studied. The result of the analysis should be a description of the person's local environment or neighborhood, or the places he or she frequents in the course of carrying out social activities and fulfilling social roles. This type of analysis is vital for setting realistic and appropriate objectives for program planning in rehabilitation and assists in identifying community resources which can support social participation and involvement by people with disabilities.

Microsystemic (personal) analysis involves the immediate social environment of the person in the place where he or she lives. This level of analysis considers the individual's social activities and daily interactions with family and friends. Microsystemic (personal) analysis is the level of assessment used to determine eligibility for support programs, such as the number of hours required for personal assistant services, housekeeping, or the need for assistive technology. It is also the level of analysis that allows the clinician to form a relationship with the person to identify his or her goals, interests, self-perception of capabilities, extent of social participation, and access to resources. It is possible that when this personal level of analysis is not accomplished, the process of social disadvantage begins, because potentially handicapping conditions are not actively addressed at the critical early phases of rehabilitation.

Microsystemic analysis requires that rehabilitation professionals engage the problems faced by the individual where he or she lives, works or plays. For example, it is inadequate to provide a voice-activated computer to a client in a hospital or rehabilitation facility without a full understanding of how the person will work with the equipment, and whether or not the environment in which it will be used will facilitate or hinder its use. Additionally, it is important to know the habits, preferences, skills and interests of the person before any solutions are proposed that would affect how that person defines or wants to portray their self identity (McCuaig & Frank, 1994).

SOCIAL ENVIRONMENT OR HABITAT FACTORS

Social factors make up the systems and structures of organizations. Each of the following social factors contributes to the everyday lives of all citizens. These social factors can facilitate or inhibit everyday living and must be considered in the client-centred plans that are constructed to support person-environment fit. (Refer to Chapter 17 to see that many of these social factors are critical to achieving optimal levels of functional independence).

Social networks include: friends, peers, church congregations, and neighborhoods. These resources are critical determinants of social participation at the micropersonal and mesocommunity levels.

Family structure relates to the composition and operation of the family unit, including the extended family. The breakdown of traditional family units in contemporary, post-industrialized societies is a major factor of concern because it diminishes the resources available for personal assistance and maintenance of the home where families include persons with disabilities.

Organization of political systems and government refers to a macrosocietal dimension related to the organization of power in societies and institutions. It also relates to political authority, including political participation and representation in decision-making. This dimension is of crucial importance in the empowerment of people to make their own decisions and choices, and in getting access to information to help with decisions. At the collective level, it is linked to participation in planning, managing and evaluating services. Social policy orientations and contents belong to this macrosocietal domain.

Legal services include everything related to the access, use and quality of services linked to institutions with the power of jurisdiction, including courts of law and administrative tribunals. Exercising one's civil rights becomes highly problematic when legal services are not adapted to different ways of communication for people with intellectual or hearing disabilities.

Economic organizations relates to the production, distribution and use of wealth. It encompasses access to and organization of the labour market. This can be linked to the accommodation of a specific workstation on the microlevel

dimension, to the availability of jobs in the person's milieu at the mesocommunity level and to more macroeconomic constraints linked to the change in economic production (agriculture, technological revolutions, work-centred societies/ leisure-centred societies). This dimension includes the use of income from employment, social assistance programs, public or private insurance, and placements. This link to income security is frequently a high determinant of social exclusion (poverty). The quality of public and private disability insurance programs (e.g. veterans, work accident, road accident, disability pensions, care insurance) are at the heart of the evolution of social policies.

Health and social services include everything related to access, quality, or organization of health services, including prevention, hospital care, medical care, rehabilitation, social support, home care, shelters and residential resources.

Educational services include everything related to access, quality or the organization of private and public educational institutions. This environmental category can be linked to the situation of the child in the classroom, to the conditions of access to secondary school by people with intellectual disability, or behavioral problems, or to the equality of opportunity in a public educational system.

Public infrastructure services include everything related to access, quality and organization of commercial businesses, transportation (regular and adapted) communication, accommodation, and other services having to do with the local community infrastructure (energy supply, road maintenance and water supply, for example). This environmental dimension includes those mesosystemic (community) factors necessary for independent living and participation in leisure, work and educational activities for people with disabilities.

Community organizations is a category at the mesosocial environment level which includes access to and organization of groups such as religious, recreational, sports and mutual assistance activities (volunteers, self help and peer counseling). This category includes any group of citizens brought together by common interest such as the consumer movement, independent living centres and organizations relating to the promotion of rights for persons with disabilities.

Social rules includes ideologies, concepts, views, philosophies, and judgments specific to any sociocultural context.

Law refers to the category including legislation, bills of individual freedoms guaranteed by governments, regulations and official statutes. It includes laws, collective agreements, and regulations governing social assistance (for example, equality of opportunity programs).

Values and attitudes include mores, philosophies, customs and beliefs, social representations and the resulting behaviors of members of a specific group including citizens with disabilities themselves. This dimension is related to the labeling and stigma linked to visible differences or socially identified meaningful status.

Development covers activities related to the direct impact of human beings on their environment. Architecture is a developmental function as it includes all dimensions of universal design related to any kind of building. This dimension can apply to the microenvironment of home or the physical accessibility of any building in the community environment and is strongly related to norms developed by societies for universal architectural accessibility. These accessibility norms are a macrosystemic environmental dimension.

Land development includes urban and rural development shaping the physical dimension of geographical elements such as mountains, steep inclines, forests, plains, deserts, distances and waterways.

Technology includes other forms of development such as objects, furnishings, technical equipment and technology in general. This dimension includes assistive devices and other crucial social environmental determinants of independent living and social participation.

In addition, we must consider two dimensions linked to a physical environment having strong impact on social participation: 1) the climate, such as rain, snow, storms, heat and cold linked to a specific accommodation and 2) the amount of time for completing a task that is socioculturally defined and creates a social expectation for realizing a task in a specific social context, (e.g., preparing a meal, dressing, taking an examination, doing a work task).

It is not possible to understand the specific life habits (lifestyle) of a person from a simple evaluation of his or her abilities. A systematic analysis must be centered on the immediate physical and interrelated organizational context of the person's goals, the capabilities of the person (intrinsic factors supporting capacity) and the tasks and activities that will support goal achievement. Equally important is taking into account the lifestyle (life habits) and the community context where the person resides. This still is insufficient since the macrosystemic dimensions determine overall living conditions.

Often, handicapping situations are the result of negligence. Failure to address the facilitators and obstacles of social participation prevents understanding the complexity of the variables involved in producing or preventing handicapping situations. The unfolding of the individual and environmental determinants of the quality of social participation requires a team of individuals lead by the client. Some of these individuals are medically trained, some are policy officials, and some are family and friends. All are in the community and their actions construct the view of society.

Occupational therapists must use their knowledge to partner with clients and the community to remove barriers that limit the potential of those with conditions that require a modified environment. Only when health professionals and community leaders understand the impact their knowledge and attitudes can have, will the external determinants of social participation be focused on supporting autonomy and productivity of a total population, rather than compromising those who want to participate but are deterred by barriers that limit their potential.

A Case Example: Driving an Automobile

Mrs. X. Is 40 years old and living with a spinal cord impairment, the result of an accident involving the collapse of scaffolding used in the renovation of her house. She gets around through the use of a wheelchair. Driving an automobile was not one of Mrs. X's daily activities before the accident. She was living on a farm 15 kilometers out of town with her husband and could easily go into town by taking the bus. Some time after the accident her husband had to move to find work, confining Mrs. X to the farm. This resulted in a major handicapping situation for transportation, which consequently influenced her ability to live independently in her home.

This case study will demonstrate how environmental factors which influence automobile driving are more important to consider in this instance than the functional abilities required for driving. The case points out issues that must be addressed at all levels; that is, the person, the environment and the task performed each must be considered if a satisfactory level of occupational performance is to be achieved. We will now examine the influence that social environmental variables have on automobile driving in Mrs. X's situation.

Initially, under the microsystemic level, the analysis focuses on Mrs. X's abilities and disabilities and the requirements for diving a vehicle. Some modifications to her vehicle will be necessary in order to enable a match between her functional abilities and these driving requirements. For example, the installation of a manual brake and accelerator, as well as a steering aid will be necessary. Furthermore, the automobile must have an automatic transmission, and power brakes. It will not be possible for her to use her husband's old stick shift Camaro. At the microsystemic level, it is a question of eliminating the handicapping situation by modifying the vehicle in an adequate and practical way. It is equally important that the chosen vehicle must have door openings wide enough to allow easy access for Mrs. X's wheelchair, or in the case of a minivan, being adapted to include an electric lift.

At the mesosystemic level, conditions necessitate Mrs. X. to have enough capital to buy an adequate vehicle. Since the accident occurred in her home, Mrs. X is only eligible for a minimum amount of compensation by her personal insurance company. Her economic situation is now jeopardized and she must borrow enough money for the vehicle's down payment from her friend, who also guarantees a loan with the bank. We can see here the importance of her family and social network, as well as the economic level and the attitudes of those around her, as these will ultimately determine whether or not Mrs. X will be able to purchase a suitable vehicle.

For Mrs. X to get a temporary license, the automobile insurance company requires that she meet with a physician to obtain a medical certificate. Her chances of getting a temporary license and registering in a driving course now depend on the physician's knowledge of vehicle modifications which enable driving. Because Mrs. X is a high-school graduate, the driving course's written will not present any difficulties for her. However, the practical part of the course will present a handicap situation at the community or mesoenvironmental level.

The driving school in the nearest city does not have a modified vehicle, which obligate Mrs. X to provide the necessary vehicle in order to participate in the practical part of the course. She must then make an appointment in the nearest large city, 150 kilometres away where there is an occupational therapy clinic with a driving program that can determine the necessary vehicle modifications. Finding access to this kind of expertise can be considered a significant barrier to her goal of arranging transportation from her home to the neighboring town. Additionally, the driving school itself must be prepared to provide a suitable environment where Mrs. X can complete her training successfully.

At the macrosystemic level, the prohibitive cost of acquiring a suitable modified vehicle is influenced by the market availability of adapted driving devices, as well as the existence of a government program which provides compensation for the costs of vehicle modification.

It is essential to take into account Mrs. X's social life context, including her current projects, daily activities, family resources and social support, her access to health services and rehabilitation and assistive devices, amount of income, community resources such as the availability of adapted public transportation, and attitudes and knowledge of intervening or concerned persons. Also, the physical environment must be described, for example, distances to travel, the volume of traffic, the adequacy of roads and highways, parking, and technology, (i.e., an automatic minivan with assistive devices such as a lift and electric doors).

At the macrosystemic level, the presence and qualifying conditions of special needs compensation programs, the legislation and regulations surrounding the requirements for driver's licenses and the policies of insurance companies combine to form the social determinants of automobile driving.

It is now easy to understand why Mrs. X was bemused when her neighbor unexpectedly remarked, "I would have never believed someone in your state would be able to drive." We should all accept the challenge of making driving for Mrs. X a more normative experience.

STUDY QUESTIONS

1. Explain why one can say from an anthropological view that each human being is different, and is created as a social being.

2. Cite four dimensions of social policies influencing societal changes for people with disabilities over the past 25 years.

3. What is ICIDH?

4. Define a handicap situation.

5. Explain the differences between micro-, meso- and macrosystemic environmental analysis.

6. Give three examples in which societal barriers can be made into facilitators.

RECOMMENDED READINGS

Angelou, M. (1969). *I know why the caged bird sings*. New York: Random House.

Goffman, E. (1963). *Stigma: Notes on the management of spoiled identity*. Englewood Cliffs, NJ: Prentice-Hall.

Groce, N. E. (1985). *Everyone here spoke sign language: Hereditary deafness on Martha's Vineyard*. Cambridge, Mass: Harvard University Press.

Helander, B. (1995). Disability as incurable illness: Health, process and personhood in Southern Somalia. In B. Ingstad & S. Reynolds Whyte (Eds.), *Disability and culture*. Berkeley: University of California Press.

Murphy, R. F., Sheer, J., Murphy, Y., & Mack, R. (1988). Physical disability and social liminality: A study in the rituals of adversity. *Social Science and Medicine, 26*(2), 235-242.

Schussler, G. (1992). Coping strategies and individual meanings of illness. *Social Science and Medicine, 34*(4), 427-432.

REFERENCES

Alexander, J. L., & Fuhrer, M. J. (1984). Functional assessment of individuals with physical impairments. In A. S. Halpern & M. J. Fuhrer (Eds.), *Functional assessment in rehabilitation*. Baltimore, MD: Paul H. Brookes.

Badley, E. M. (1987). The ICIDH: Format, application in different settings and distinction between disability and handicap. *International Disabilities Studies, 9*, 122-125.

Badley, E. M. (1995). The genesis of handicap. Definition, models of disablement, and role of external factors. *Disability and Rehabilitation, 17*, 53-62.

Barry, M. (1989). The disability concept. *ICIDH International Network, 2*(2-3), 6-8.

Bickenbach, J. E. (1993). *Physical disability and social policy*. University of Toronto Press.

Bolduc, M. (1986). *Analyze de la cohérence de politiques québécoises à l'égard des personnel ayant des incapacités*. Québec, Ontario. Direction de l'évaluation des programmes. Ministère de la santé et des services sociaux.

Bolduc, M. (1995). *Une approche conceptuelle des conséquences des maladies et traumatisme qui tient mieux compte de ltenvironnement physique et social* (pp. 245-249). In: Actes du ème Congrès annuel de l'Association latine pour l'analyse des systèmes de santé. 25 au 27 mad. Montreal. Éditions Sciences des systèmes.

Bolduc, M. (1992). Making equal opportunity a reality: An insurance plan covering the additional costs associated with impairments, disabilities and handicap situations. *ICIDH International Network, 5*(1-2), 40-51.

Bronfenbrenner, U. (1979). *The ecology of human development, experiments by nature and design.* Cambridge, MA: Harvard University Press.

Chamie, M. (1989). Survey design strategies for the study of disability. *Bulletin World Health Statistics Quarterly, 42*, 122-140.

Christiansen, C. (1991). Occupational therapy: Intervention for life performance. In: C. Christiansen & C. Baum (Eds.), *Occupational therapy: Overcoming human performance deficits.* Thorofare, NJ: SLACK Incorporated.

Dejong, G. (1979). Independent living: From social movement to analytic paradigm. *Archives of Physical Medicine and Rehabilitation, 60*, 435-446.

Duchvorth, D. (1983). *The classification and measurement of disablement.* London, U.K.: Department of Health and Social Security. Social Research Branch, HMSO.

Durkheim, E. (1977). *Les règles de la méthode sociologique.* Paris, France: P.U.F.

English, W. R. (1977). *Combating stigma towards physically disabled persons.* New York, NY: Springer Publishing Co.

Enns, H. (1989). Disabled People International (DPI) statement on the WHO's ICIDH. January 1987. *International ICIDH Network*, 2(2-3), 28-30.

Finkelstein, V. (1989). Planning services together with disabled people: The importance of a common language. *World Health Statistics Quarterly, 42*, 177-179.

Flynn, R. J., & Nitsch, K. E. (1980). *Normalization, social integration and community services.* Baltimore, MD: University Park Press.

Flynn, R. J. (1993). Social integration between 1982 and 1992: Conceptual and operational definitions. *ICIDH International Network, 6*(2), 34-41.

Fougeyrollas, P. (1978). Normalité et corps, différents regards sur l'intégration sociale des handicapés physiques. *Anthropologie et Sociétés, 2*(2), 51:71.

Fougeyrollas, P. (1983). *Entre peaux: Logis de la différence. Du handicap à l'autonomie.* Thèse de maitrise. Département d'anthropologie. Quebec, Canada: Université Laval.

Fougeyrollas, P. (1988). *Prévenir, réduire et compenser les conséquences des maladies et traumatismes: Déficiences, incapacités et situations de handicaps.* Dossier thématique. Québec, Canada: Commission d'enquete sur la santé et les services sociaux.

Fougeyrollas, P. (1990). Les implications de la diffusion de la classification internationale des handicaps sur les politiques concernant les personnel handicapées. *Rapport trimestriel de statistiques sanitaires mondiales, 443*(4), 281-285.

Fougeyrollas, P. (1995). Documenting environmental factors for preventing the handicap creation process. *Disability and Rehabilitation, 17*, 145-153.

Fougeyrollas, P. (1995). *Le processus de production culturelle des handicaps.* Québec, Canada: CQCIDIH-SCCIDIH.

Fougeyrollas, P., St-Michel, G., Bergeron, N., & Cloutier, R. (1991). The handicap creation process: Analysis of the consultation. New full proposals. *ICIDH International Network, 4*(1-2), 8-37.

Fougeyrollas, P., St-Michel, G., & Blouin, M. (1989). Consultation: Proposal for revision of the third level of the ICIDH: The handicap. *International ICIDH Network, 2*(1), 8-32.

Freidson, E. (1995). Disability as social deviance. *Sociology and rehabilitation. A structural approach.* New York, NY: Dodd, Mead and Co.

Goffman, E. (1963). *Stigmate. Les usages sociaux des handicaps.* Paris, France: Les éditions de minuit.

Granger, C. V. (1984). A conceptual model for functional assessment. In: C. V. Granger & G. E.? (Eds.), *Functional assessment in rehabilitation medicine.* Baltimore, MD: Williams & Wilkins.

Groce N., & Scheer, J. (1990). Introduction. Cross cultural perspectives on disability. *Social Science and Medicine, 30*(8), V-VI.

Hurst, R. (1993). The definition of disability, our right to define ourselves. *ICIDH International Network, 6*(2), 7-8.

Jacquard, A. (1978). *Éloge de la différence. La génétique et les hommes.* Paris, France: Seuil.

Lemert, E. (1967). *Human deviance, social problems and social control.* Englewood Cliffs, NJ: Prentice Hall.

Merton, R. K. (1957). *Social theory and social structure.* New York, NY: Free Press of Glencoe.

Minaire, P. (1983). Le handicap en porte-à-faux. *Prospective et Santé, (26)*, 39-46.

Minaire, P. (1992). Disease, illness and health: Theoretical model of the disablement process. *Bulletin of the World Health Organization, 70*(3), 373-379.

Morvan, J. S., & Paicheler, H., et al. (1990). *Représentations et handicaps: Vers une clarification des concepts etdesméthodes.* Paris, France: CTNERHI-MIRE.

Mottez, B. (1977). A s'obstiner contre les déficiences on augmente souvent le handicap: ltexemple des sourds. *Sociologie et sociétés.* Québec, Canada: Les Presses de l'Université Laval.

Nagi, S. A. (1991). Disability concepts revisited: Implication for prevention in disability in America. *Toward a national agenda for prevention. Institute of medicine.* Washington DC: National Academy Press.

Office des personnel handicapées du Québec. (1984). On equal terms. *A policy for prevention and social integration of handicapped persons.* Québec, Canada: Les publications du Québec.

Ogien, A. (1995). *Sociologie de la déviance.* Paris, France: Armand Colin.

Oliver, M. (1990). *The politics of disablement.* London: Macmillan.

Phillips, M. (1990). Damaged goods: Oral narratives of the experience of disability in American culture. *Social Science and Medicine, 30*(8), 849-857.

Soder, M. (1987). Relative definition of handicap: Implications for research. *Upsala Journal Medical Science, 44*, 24-29.

Spitzer, S. (1975). Toward a Marcian theory of deviance. *Social Problems, 22*(5).

Statistics Canada. (1992). *Canadian health and activity limitation survey*. Ottawa, Canada: Author.

Swain, J., Finkelstein, V., French, S., & Oliver, M. (1993). *Disabling barriers—Enabling environments*. London, U.K.: Sage.

Tremblay, M. A. (1982). *Les nouveaux chemins de la guérison*. Non publié. Quebec, Canada: Miméo Université Laval.

United Nations. (1983). Decade of disabled persons 1983-1992. *World Program of Action Concerning Disabled Persons*. New York, NY: Author.

Verbrugge, L. M., & Jette, A. M. (1995). The disablement process. *Social Science and Medicine*.

Wan, T. T. H. (1974). Correlates and consequences of severe disabilities. *Journal of Occupational Medicine, 16,* 234-244.

Warren, M. D. (1977). *The need for rehabilitation*. Rehabilitation Today. London, U.K.: Update Publications.

Whiteneck, G., & Fougeyrollas, P. (1995, November). *Environmental Factors and ICIDH* (4th ed.). Task Force Position Paper. International Meeting on the Revision of ICIDH. Paris, France. Unpublished.

Wolfensberger, W. (1972). *The principle of normalization in human services*. Toronto, Ontario: National Institute of Mental Retardation.

Wolfensberger, W. (1992). *A brief introduction to Social Role Valorization as a high order concept for structuring human services* (2nd rev. ed.). Syracuse, NY: Training Institute for Human Service Planning, Leadership and Change Agentry. Syracuse University.

Woodhill, G. (1992). *Independent living and participation in research: A critical analysis*. Centre for Independent Living in Toronto.

World Health Organization. (1980-1993). *International classification of impairments, disabilities and handicaps. A manual related to the consequences of diseases*. Geneva, Switzerland.

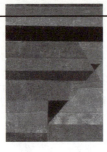

CHAPTER CONTENT OUTLINE

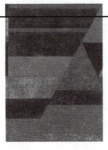

ABSTRACT

Stigma is a social phenomenon that separates people based on differences. This chapter provides an overview of stigma and the affect it has on the daily living and well-being of persons with disabilities. Stigma is compared and contrasted with other differences that exist among people in society. It is then considered in light of various models of disability, including the medical model, the economic model, the psychosocial model and the minority group model. The traditions and assumptions toward disability in each model are described and their consequences revealed. Sociopolitical changes that will foster environments and attitudes which enable positive self-identities for persons with disability are identified. The concept of equal environmental adaptations is proposed as an example of beneficial change which can counteract the negative consequences of stigma.

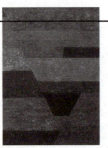

KEY TERMS

Stigma

Disability

Disability rights

ADA – Americans with Disability Act

Entitlement programs

Accessibility

Universal design

Equal environmental accommodations

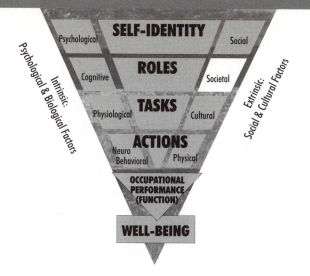

CHAPTER 16

Achieving Occupational Goals

The Social Effects of Stigma

David B. Gray, PhD, Harlan Hahn, PhD

OBJECTIVES

The information in this chapter is intended to help the reader:

1. acknowledge individuals with disabilities as persons with rights, skills and dignity

2. understand the negative influence of attributing undesirable attributes to persons with disability based on the distinguishing features of physical impairment

3. gain an understanding of the medical, economic, psychosocial, sociopolitical and minority group models of disability

4. provide a basis for establishing a mutually beneficial relationship with persons with disabilities

5. realize that disability has different meaning in different contexts at different ages

6. develop a concept that the environment can be modified to reduce excess disability through universal design, reasonable accommodations and accessible buildings

7. appreciate the influence occupational therapy can have on providing an enabling environment for people with disabilities.

> *"I also dislike people who try to talk down to my understanding. They are like people who when walking with you try to shorten their steps to suit yours; the hyposcrisy in both cases is equally exasperating."*
>
> Helen Keller (1880-1968), U.S. blind/deaf author, lecturer.

INTRODUCTION

One of the most important challenges facing students in occupational therapy today is the need to prepare for a career that allows them to work with clients as coequals. The ability to fulfill this personal opportunity and career responsibility will be fundamentally shaped and augmented by common perceptions of disability and chronic health conditions that have been acquired by occupational therapists during their training and by clients as they move from dependent patients to independent consumers. The interactive perceptions of the roles of the therapist and client develop from close interpersonal relationships that are influenced by prevalent social attitudes about disability. Thus, both the therapist and client need to understand how people with disabilities have been viewed historically and what new approaches are developing in response to the growing societal recognition of the civil rights and abilities of people with disabilities. This chapter seeks to examine various approaches to the study of disability, including medical, economic, and sociopolitical models, in an effort to promote a thorough understanding of the different means by which disability is interpreted. It is designed to permit occupational therapists to assess their own feelings about disability, their perceptions of client needs, their preparation for providing appropriate interventions, and their need to consider the client as an equal partner in the enablement process.

There is no single, invariable reaction to the impact of disability on a person's life—as a number of recent publications about life experiences by people with disability illustrate (Callahan, 1989; Price, 1993; Grealy, 1995; Hockenberry, 1995). Some people may be ashamed of their disabilities, some might express a sense of denial about the barriers that they confront, and others may define disability as a source of dignity and pride (Zola, 1982). Increasingly, however, the views of persons with disabilities have been affected by the growth of the disability rights movement and by studies which focus on the obstacles they encounter in the social and architectural environment (Batavia, 1992; Milam, 1993; Shapiro, 1993). From this perspective, disability can be regarded as the product of a disabling environment instead of personal defects or deficiencies (Hahn, 1985; Fougeyrollas, 1997). Ironically, this approach, which has contributed to a positive sense of identity for many persons with disabilities, may be less familiar to occupational therapists than traditional concepts of disability which have been constricted by focusing on overcoming impairments.

Bibliographic citation of this chapter: Gray, D. B., & Hahn, H. (1997). Achieving occupational goals: The social effects of stigma. In C. Christiansen & C. Baum (Eds.), *Occupational therapy: Enabling function and well-being* (2nd ed.). Thorofare, NJ: SLACK Incorporated.

By including environmental factors in the construct of the meaning of disability rather than attributing disability only to factors located within an individual, the focus of interventions can shift from the person's impairment to modifications to the physical and social environments where they live (Barker, 1948; Fine & Asch, 1988; Fougeyrollas & Gray, in press). This shift in locus of therapy has provided a reduction in physical and psychological stress to persons with disabilities. Perhaps most importantly, this emphasis on the social environment provides a firm foundation for cooperation between occupational therapists and their clients on a basis of genuine equality.

A Note on Language

Many people wonder about the kinds of words they should use in talking about people with disabilities. In view of the many negative terms about this matter that permeate the English language, these concerns are understandable. Yet perhaps the most important point to be made about this subject is that the struggle to eliminate bias on the basis of disability cannot be achieved simply by invoking socially acceptable terminology or by following prescribed rules of etiquette. Language is important because it shapes attitudes and behavior (Zola, 1993). The use of nondiscriminatory or inoffensive words, however, is only an initial approach rather than a final solution to the effort to gain full equality for citizens with disabilities (Bruce & Christiansen, 1988).

The most commonly accepted term at present is "people with disabilities." Words such as "crippled," "handicapped," and "invalid" have outdated and unfavorable connotations (Corcoran, 1977; Longmore, 1985; Bickenbach, 1993). Most writers also avoid the use of any of these words as a noun, i.e., "the disabled" or "the handicapped" are generally frowned upon. Many also insist on the formulation "persons with disabilities" to emphasize that disabilities do not significantly modify or alter personhood (Blaska, 1993). As the concept of a positive sense of identity based on disability gains increasing approval, some have begun to adopt "disabled" proudly as an adjective, e.g., a "disabled person." Others have even attempted to redefine discredited words such as "crippled" as a badge of honor or dignity. In the future, therefore, the vocabulary can be expected to reflect constant and growing changes. Perhaps the most predictable development is that people with disabilities, like other social groups, will continue to insist on the right to define themselves by labels of their own choosing.

THE DEFINITION OF STIGMA

Many of the conflicts in the interpretation of disability have revolved about the concept of stigma. Stigma is an undesirable difference that becomes a basis for separating an individual bearing such traits from the rest of society. The connotations of stigma include disgrace, disrepute, infamy, reproach, blemish, stain, perversion, and shame. The leading writer on this subject was Irving Goffman (1963), who believed that stigmatized individuals almost invariably incorporate these negative attributes into their own self-concepts. Another interpretation, however, is that stigma is imposed upon individuals by other people. Hence, stigma is not necessarily a reflection of low self-esteem. According to this view, stigma is much like prejudice based on race or ethnicity or gender (Fine & Asch, 1988). As a result, persons with disabilities are isolated or marginalized from the remainder of society, underemployed, undereducated, pitied, and prisoners of the misperceptions of others. Several Harris surveys of people with disabilities (National Council on the Handicapped, 1987; Harris, 1986, 1994) revealed that as a group, people with disabilities are the poorest, the least educated, and have the highest unemployment rates of any group in America.

INFLUENCE OF STIGMA

The life of Franklin D. Roosevelt illustrates the impact that stigma can exert at the highest levels of society (Figure 16-1). President Roosevelt led the allied countries to victory in a cataclysmic war, restored an economically devastated country to prosperity, and developed a system of social support for its citizens. Yet, he was so fearful of the stigma associated with his paraplegia that he spent much of his valuable energy hiding his inability to walk (Gallagher, 1985). In FDR's case, the stigma remains even after his death due to the refusal to erect a statue depicting FDR as he was, a man who used a wheelchair. Ability, achievement and adulation are rarely associated with people who cannot walk, hear or see. A statue of a great leader sitting in a wheelchair might be a realistic portrayal of FDR's life but would not reflect the public image that was created of him. The struggle between the reality and the image of physical disability continues at many levels. In *A Room With a View*, the main character Lucy and her fianceé Cecil engage in a discussion about the fences we build around ourselves to keep people out and the fences built by others to keep us out (Forster, 1908). FDR erected fences to keep people from entering into his life as a person with a disability and worked hard to avoid the fences built to keep him from participating in the activities he cherished. Recognizing that these challenges form an important aspect of the lives of people with disabilities may provide developing OTs with a valuable perspective on the problems they confront.

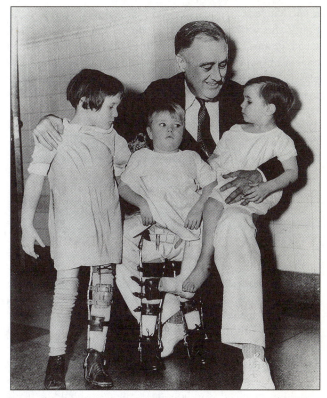

Figure 16-1. In this photo, President Franklin D. Roosevelt is shown in the early 1930s visiting some children at a treatment center for infantile paralysis (as poliomyelitis was commonly termed in that era). Photo courtesy of the National Archives and Records Administration, Franklin D. Roosevelt Library, Hyde Park, NY.

DILEMMA OF DIFFERENCE AND STIGMA

Research incorporating the concept of stigma has generally concluded that people with visible disabilities have been denied the opportunity to participate in society through systematic bias that is based on perceived difference. Efforts to redress these inequalities involve major contradictions. Irving Goffman (1963) noted that people facing stigmatizing conditions have two self-defeating options. First, demands for integration in "normal" settings require them to draw attention to their stigmatizing difference. These attempts to emphasize differences provide a basis for special services. However, these same criteria make the group visible as different from others in the culture (Wolfensberger, Nirje, Olshansky, Perske & Roos, 1972). The well-intentioned attempts at definition for the purpose of resource distribution seem to legitimize and reinforce the labels that created their unequal status in the first place. The more attention drawn to the differences, the stronger become the boundaries between stigmatized and nonstigmatized populations—the very situation the group set out to rectify! Yet, when groups de-emphasize their differences, they are in danger of incurring a reduction of the services they need. A classic example is the movement of people with developmental disabilities out of institutions into the community (Braddock, Hemp, Fujiura, Bachelder, and Mitchell, 1990). The dollars saved by closing institutions were rarely transferred to the creation of needed services in community settings. People with developmental disabilities have received decreased services, but the influence of social stigma has probably been somewhat reduced (Shapiro, 1993).

STIGMA AND MODELS OF DISABILITY

To engage in a meaningful discussion of phenomena associated with disabling conditions, a reality must be constructed that can be readily understood by most observers. The shared beliefs, assumptions and vocabulary of those concerned with disability can be used to explain why disability exists; who is categorized as disabled; what problems result from disability; when and where treatments should be provided; which, if any, social or physical environments should be changed; and how these changes should be made administratively and legally. The influence of models on the perception of the nature of disability is reviewed in this chapter. Decision-making behaviors may be influenced by our social constructions of reality, the kinds of questions we raise about our tasks, and the social arrangements, such as economic conditions, policies, and laws (Albrecht, 1992; Brooks, in press; Nagi, 1965, 1976, 1991).

The influence of models is so pervasive that we often describe problems and solutions as if we confine our thinking to only one model. One model can rarely, if ever, span the breadth of factors that may influence the issue we study. Thus, for those working in the field of occupational therapy, it is necessary to approach the analysis of problems faced by individuals with disabilities from several vantage points. Reliance on any single model is likely to miss important parts of the puzzle. In the United States and Sweden, surveys have been made to determine how many citizens have disabilities who may eventually use public housing. In the United States, a survey of housing needs in Houston, Texas, found that 10% of the residents needed special architectural modifications in their homes (Gilderbloom, Rosenthal & Bullard, 1987). The Swedish survey results were that over 40% of the population have mobility limitations that require planning for accessible housing (Brooks, in press). The difference in the survey results was in the inclusion and exclusion rules for who was considered to be a person with disability. In the U.S., disability was defined in the context of medical and economic mod-

els of chronic physical impairment. The population in need was described as low-income and elderly with disability. In 1972 Sweden, the definition of persons with mobility limitations included short-term physical conditions such as pregnancy or broken limbs. The results of the survey in Sweden was to require, by a specific law passed in 1984, that all public housing be accessible since it would be extremely expensive to remodel 40% of all public housing. In the U.S. the resolution to the problem was not based on survey numbers but on including housing access as civil rights of people with disabilities in the Americans with Disabilities Act (1990). In both countries, the concept of universal design of the built environment is providing architects and builders with the conceptual model for making the legal requirements for accessible housing come to fruition (Zola, 1989). An exploration of these models illustrates how occupational therapists can explore issues of stigma with their patients or clients. These efforts will assist the therapist in raising the issue of how stigma can influence their work as living environments for clients are developed. A recognition of stigma and its effects on people with disability can be used to educate citizens on issues and attitudes of importance to persons with disabilities.

MEDICAL MODEL

The medical model explains disability from the perspective that the cause of disability is the loss of, or reduction in, biological capacity to perform "normal" activities. Therefore, the treatment interventions for people with disabilities are biologically based. The goal is to cure the biological abnormality. The method becomes a reductionistic analysis of smaller and smaller components of the biological system. Distancing the unit of analysis from the person allows comparison of organs, tissues, cells and genes independent of the carrier, the unified whole individual. This approach also permits the study of the mechanisms of parts of the systems—what does what when? Thus, deviations from expected activity indicate a functional problem. These problems can be detected at a variety of levels—cellular products, images of structure/function anomalies, and physical sign (e.g., restricted motion, pain, temperature change). Accurate diagnosis of the biological factor(s) responsible for the conditions leads to effective treatments that can be administered in attempts to cure the abnormality in structure or function. To provide cures, the scientific approach is applied to the study of physical deficits and the mechanisms underlying these differences. This model has provided detailed descriptions of the biological factors leading to impairment and given rise to cures (e.g., polio). Search for the cure has formed the core belief system of the health care industry; receive services and we will "fix" you. Most of the

11 billion dollar annual budget of the National Institutes of Health is spent on research directed toward cure. A large portion of the national health care expenditures are spent on treating people with chronic conditions which presently are not curable (Rice & LaPlante, 1988; Pope & Tarlov, 1991).

Even when the medical community turns its attention to treating existing conditions, a fundamental flaw remains. The medical approach focuses almost exclusively on methods of altering the internal or biological characteristics of the individual. These interventions generally are not integrated with efforts to modify the external environment(s) where the person will live after medical treatments are completed. This makes it nearly impossible to explain outcome differences in the lives of people with similar and even identical impairments who were treated with the same medical intervention. The medical model provides a necessary but not sufficient answer to issues of disability. This is illustrated by the following study of children with cerebral palsy who were treated in 1948 during their childhood and then assessed when they were adults. A report in 1966 by Klapper and Birch states:

> ...however, the stigmatic remnants of childhood cerebral palsy appeared at each point to interfere with maximal social and economic achievement. Only the completely normal group of children who, as adults, were free from physical stigmata and awkwardness in gait or speech obtained full social profit from their physical progress. These had become the normal group in terms of sociability, and had the best economic prospects. The remainder, despite substantial progress in self-care and physical functioning, and substantial educational achievements were still stigmatized and socially isolated. Consequently, the progress made in the mechanics of functioning have not been reflected in any significant degree of independent living, social integration or interpersonal functioning. (p. 655)

One finding is especially interesting and should lead to further study. Individuals diagnosed with spastic cerebral palsy (CP) were the only group whose education went beyond high school. Is it possible that individuals with spastic CP may have a better prognosis for social integration? Reduction in spasticity through SDZ (selective dorsal rhizotomy) may augment this effect by decreasing the stigma associated with CP (Klapper & Birch, 1966).

Parsons (1961) proposed a concept of the "sick role" that required the individual to become exempt from ordinary social obligations provided that they devote their efforts to the ultimate goal of full recovery. The benefit for the persons with a disability is that at least they are held blameless for their condition. In addition, if these persons can convince

the medical gatekeeper that they are incapable of gainful employment, then they can qualify for financial support, health care when they are truly sick, housing credits, food stamps, assistive technologies and other benefits. The downside is that these benefits are contingent on staying "sick" which may never allow healthy persons with disabilities to get "well" (Wilkerson, Batavia, & DeJong, 1992); they are in lifelong rehabilitation and become wards of the medical industry (Albrecht, 1992; Oliver, 1996). The individuals may rely on meeting the medical community's categorization criteria to gain entry to very limited benefits which allow for a subsistence level of existence (Zola, 1982). Yet, people with disabilities are often blamed for using too much of the health care dollar and rationing may appear as managed care organizations take control of the health care industry (Albrecht, 1992; Orentlicher, 1994). These people are categorized so that they can never escape dependency, the very antithesis of goals of rehabilitation. Progress in one area may only change the emphasis in the treatment plan, not "heal" the impaired person. These are, from the medical perspective, bad patients (Bickenbach, 1993).

Setting Goals for Therapy

If persons with disabilities are not sick and cure is not possible, then is the goal to continue to focus on disablement, or might it be more appropriate to focus on enablement? Does one focus on impairments impervious to change or "solution" and waste resources analyzing how poorly people with these conditions perform, or does one expend energy to analyze how persons with similar impairments have adapted to environmental demands to meet the functional performance requirements and focus on what the person can do? Does understanding how a nonimpaired person solves a problem (moving from place to place in a home by walking) help a person with no or little lower limb function learn how to move within his or her environment (moving by pushing a wheelchair across rugs, around corners up and down slopes)? Would it not be better to compare performance on tasks for persons with similar physical impairments and use those who succeed as markers for possible growth and change in others in the same impairment group who are less successful in performing the task(s)?

This reliance on "normal" actions, activities and functions as therapeutic goals continues to be a dilemma for occupational therapy (Rogers & Holm, 1994). However, using within-group (e.g., people with spinal cord injury, head injury, affective disorders, amputations) comparisons to set realistic goals for improved performance may lead to two dilemmas. If one identifies the best performing members of a group as the ideal, then others who do not reach the performance levels of the "supercrip" may be labeled failures by themselves, their friends and therapists (Shear, 1986). For example, some persons with spinal cord injury may choose to focus their energy on learning to push a wheelchair and neglect their academic skills. Other persons with the same level of spinal cord injury may choose to operate an electric wheelchair rather than to use their energy pushing a manual wheelchair. They might choose to spend that time in developing skills that make their employment more likely. The definition of successful rehabilitation depends on the values of the persons doing the measures. For the therapist whose goal it is to teach the use of manual wheelchairs, the first person is a success and the second a failure (Bates, Spencer, Young, & Rintala, 1993). For the person, perhaps an occupational therapist, who is charged with returning the client to work, the first person is a failure and the second person a success. A success or failure only occurs if the therapist and client share the same goal (McCuaig & Frank, 1991).

Another danger of the within-group comparison approach is that the range of possible behaviors may be artificially restricted by the performance of group members if the entire group is expected to perform poorly. For example, for many years people with an extra 21st chromosome (Down syndrome) were described in terms of their very limited verbal and manual performance skills (Gray, 1975). In the decades of the 1950s and 1960s, parents, physicians and politicians (especially the Kennedy family) demanded that education, medical services and social activities be open to children with developmental disabilities (Boggs, 1987; Sloan & Stevens, 1976). This change in public attention resulted in social policies and programs to determine alternative forms of communication, specialized preparation for therapists and educators, early intervention with language acquisition training for the children and their parents (Kaiser & Gray, 1993), and work opportunities including sheltered, supported and competitive employment (Bellamy, Rhodes, Mank, & Albin, 1988; Kregel & Wehman, 1990). The stigma associated with developmental disabilities had limited the opportunities for individual growth for this entire population, thus creating unnecessary barriers that limited social participation.

Stigma and Therapy in the Medical Model

The medical approach to disability facilitated the identification of biological impairments. It also brought with it the stigma associated with inferiority, neediness, and dependence. Thus, the person becomes the exclusive target for change. Even today many health personnel are trained to view disability as residing within the person; and their treatments focus on changing the individual, instead of that person's environment. This approach to disability has led many soci-

eties to designate health care professionals as the gatekeepers to services for people with disabilities. Within the walls of the hospital and clinic facilities, this approach has some validity. However, when people with disabilities move from the hospital, they change their status from patients to citizens. As individuals re-integrate into home and community, they acquire other interests including the role of consumer of goods and services not related to impairments or health status (DeJong & Lifchez, 1983). The dilemma is created. Often, the only access to and funds for goods and services, unrelated or marginally related to the person's health needs, remains within the domain of health professionals who must write justifications for people with disabilities to qualify for food stamps, housing allowances, transportation (e.g., driver's permits, automobile adaptations, reduced fares on mass transit), assistive technology (e.g., wheelchairs, large print, auditory output of text, Braille devices, computer modifications), home modifications (e.g., ramps, elevators, bathrooms), personal assistance (e.g., help in getting out of bed, showering, cooking). The list of activities that require approval by medical personnel raises some questions (Batavia & Hammer, 1990). Is the cost of controlling access to these goods and services necessary? Do the costs of assessing entitlement, eligibility, insurance coverage exceed the provision of service costs? Do these life activities require medical supervision? Are health professionals trained to make these decisions? Should the control of decision-making in these areas reside with physician, therapist or client (Brooks, 1984)? These are questions that occupational therapists must struggle to address as they plan interventions.

Medical Control: Covington's Caveat

The intrusiveness of the medical interpretations of disabilities extends even beyond the grasp of competent physicians who are aware of its undue influence. The following episode in the life of an individual, George Covington, with very low vision (legally blind) shows how the medical system can influence stigma and fear (Covington, in press).

When George was in elementary school (Grim Elementary!) his teacher noticed that he was having trouble seeing the board and reading books. The principal of the school called George's mother and offered to take up a collection to buy him glasses. Despite numerous attempts by George, his mother and the family ophthalmologist to resist this futile but well-meaning gesture of charitable concern, the school insisted he have a pair of glasses. The physician complied by ordering George a pair of glasses with no correction. Not yet satisfied, the school made repeated suggestions that George attend the school for the blind like the "others" so he could be with his "kind." Not bowing to this socially acceptable method of treatment for the problems of the blind, George's mother kept him in public school because she believed he would have more choices later in life. He did. He has worked for the U.S. House Majority Leader James Wright and Vice President Dan Quayle, where he worked to reduce social barriers to people with disabilities to enable full participation in society. By avoiding the trap of expectations set by those who associate incompetence with physical impairments, George escaped the fate of many of his contemporaries.

ECONOMIC MODEL

If the medical model has been extended beyond its competencies and reaches too far into the lives of people with disabilities, then what framework can be used for understanding disability in the larger context of society? Some have suggested an economic analysis of disability costs. While it is beyond the scope of this chapter to fully develop an economic analysis of disability (Berkowitz, 1978; Berkowitz & Hill, 1986; Albrecht, 1992), some essentials of the argument that stigma influences employment practices and economic studies may be instructive. A fundamental premise of economic analysis is that the efficient production of goods and services represents a major societal priority. The assumption is that people with disabilities are less efficient human resources than people without disabilities (Bickenbach, 1993). Costly, large government-operated programs (e.g., Social Security) are based on the principle that if persons are not capable of substantial gainful employment due to disability, then they are entitled to certain benefits. But people with identical impairments vary greatly in their capacity to perform activities that have economic value. Here the economic model has relied on "medical determinations" of disability to categorize the likelihood of employment. This model requires persons with disabilities to submit to a series of medical examinations that either put them into an entitlement program or exclude them. In many cases, these decisions determine if a person lives, where the person lives, and the quality of life they can possibly achieve. The contingencies for admission to entitlement programs in the United States (e.g., Social Security Disability Income [SSDI], Social Security Supplemental Income [SSI], Medicaid, Medicare, Food Stamps, Meals on Wheels) include economic tests, "means tests." Virtually no accumulation of wealth is allowed and continued poverty maintains eligibility for these services. Like being caught in a spider's web, once captured by the system, it is nearly impossible to escape and return to a job that will provide monetary compensation at a level that will cover medical expenses and provide a minimal standard of living (Weaver, 1986).

Faulty Assumptions—Diagnosis Predicts Potential for Work

The economic approach to disability rests on several faulty assumptions. For many years, diagnostic categories have been used to determine work capacity but they do not necessarily predict functional capacity or performance on tasks that may have economic value (Berkowitz & Hill, 1986). Generalizations based on assignment to diagnostic categories paints the whole person with the brush of incompetence associated with a physical or mental impairment (Johnson, 1986). For example, paralysis due to spinal cord injury (diagnosis) often leads to no capacity for an action (walking) in one category of behaviors (mobility) that may be entirely unrelated to work tasks for which the person is fully qualified to perform (e.g., executive management, tax return preparation, medical management, occupational therapy). Functional capacity for work relies on a number of factors and resources (Frattali, 1993). The U.S. government is moving to develop tests of functional abilities to determine a person's capacity for substantial gainful employment (Committee on Childhood Disability, 1995). This approach provides an opportunity for health care professionals to use their skills to determine the strengths (abilities) of their clients in areas related to work performance. With this shift, people with disabilities will be allowed to focus on building skills for employment rather than stressing their limitations to qualify for benefits. To maximize the advantages of this change, the entitlement system will need to move to a distribution of benefits quite different than the current all-or-none approach. In fact, there have been some changes in the retention of benefits during trial employment periods. Gradual reduction of benefits as personal income and wealth increase would create incentives for many people with disabilities to leave the dependency status imposed by entitlement programs.

Occupational therapists and other health care professionals can provide invaluable assistance to people with disabilities by concentrating therapeutic interventions on building skills rather than focusing on the largely immutable aspects of impairment. Understanding the client's abilities and disabilities, desires and fears, and dreams and realities will advance the relevance of OT interventions. These efforts will make some, but clearly not all, people with disabilities, more efficient human resources; as a result, they will be more likely to fit into the competitive workplace. This approach to intervention planning and implementation may provide a solid justification for the role of occupational therapy in the future as services move from acute care facilities into the community and home and outcomes move from immediate reduction of costs to issues of well-being and sustained health.

Faulty Assumptions 2—Individual Employer and National Costs and Benefits

Another problem with economic analyses of the "cost" of disability stems from the use of segmented rather than holistic approaches. Such studies inevitably reach the conclusion that people with disabilities are not an efficient human resource. The argument is that it is always less costly to employ persons with no disability than to adapt the work site for those with disabilities (Bickenbach, 1993). Most economic studies include no measure of the training level of people with disability; type and cost of worksite modification; relative worker turnover rates; costs of keeping disabled people from work; employee benefits for which persons with a disability are not likely to participate (e.g., health clubs, vacation resorts, company cars); and workplace morale.

Equally important, focusing on the cost per person to each business leaves out an essential component of the analysis, namely a national economic assessment of the costs and benefits of different options for treating or employing people with disabilities. If one assumes that society will not terminate the lives of people with disabilities who are not efficient workers, then one must balance the cost of employment (training and access) with the costs of the maintenance of life for people with disabilities (e.g., personal assistance, institutions). The dependency-related alternatives add to the cost of products through increases in taxation. Do they equal or exceed the cost of making worksites accessible? The economic issue then becomes one of how to balance the costs of an individual component of the economy with the costs for the society as a whole. It raises the questions, "Who pays for training, accessibility, and reasonable accommodations?" And "How much financial resources should come from government, employers, insurance and personal savings or earnings?"

Stigma and Employment

Current employment practices assume that workers must adjust to the worksite conditions provided by employers. The employer's obligation is to provide the tools and materials for the worker to complete required tasks. Little attention has been paid to those aspects of employment that reduce the opportunities for people with disabilities resulting from stigma instead of functional restrictions. In fact, many economic models have postulated that stigma or discrimination toward impaired persons does not belong in economic analysis. That is, the reduction in earning potentials that result from stigma rather than functional limitations are not included in the economic analysis. In fact, civil rights legislation disrupts a pure economic analysis (Bickenbach, 1993).

If one wishes to understand the costs of stigma, one needs to go beyond the financial calculations of materials and labor to produce products. One needs to ask "What is the cost of correcting the conditions leading to stigma?" "What is cost of keeping people with disabilities out of the workplace compared to making the workplace accessible?" "What is the cost of making the workplace accessible verses the cost of providing employees without disabilities an adequate work site?"

An honest and even-handed approach to studying employment costs would include basic questions regarding expenditures that must be made for *all* employees. "What is the additional cost over and above provision of 'normal' office furniture for special furniture of people with disabilities?" From the perspective of persons with mobility disabilities, one might ask "What is cost of providing chairs for all employees in workplaces, auditoriums, lunch and dining rooms?" And "What is the cost of providing transportation for mobility disabled workers compared to providing company cars for non-mobility disabled employees?" Another approach to equity problems can be assessed from the position of people with visual impairments. They want to know why the employers are wasting money on lighting systems. Would it be fair to charge sighted people for light in their workplace? Is it fair to require blind people to pay for Braille machines, auditory tapes of meetings, building access technology, computer modifications to enhance images? Is it essential that the rugs and furniture be altered to meet the preferences of new executives? Do research laboratories transformed at great expense to attract cutting-edge scientists really improve efficiency? What about special dining facilities and housing for company executives compared to making reasonable accommodations for employees with disabilities? The point is that the provision of employment accommodations is not based solely on job requirements, even for people without impairments. Yet, changes made for workers with disabilities are scrutinized and debated for "fairness" to others in the workplace and often condemned as inefficient and as burdens to employers. The power of stigma is such that changes made for the benefit of nonimpaired workers are rarely subjected to cost analysis but modifications essential for persons with disabilities are hotly disputed.

The irony is that changes made to accommodate people with disabilities often benefit everyone (Mace, Hardie & Place, 1991). In fact, many changes made specifically to accommodate the needs of people with disabilities have been used more by people without disabilities than by those with disabilities (e.g., telephones, curb cuts, automatic doors, larger bathroom stalls, brighter lights, multimodal presentations). The use of curb cuts is undoubtedly higher for bikers, skate boarders, people pushing strollers with infant passengers, persons with leg muscle weakness, and small children than for people who use wheelchairs for mobility.

The economic approach is subject to criticism of limited scope of analysis just as the biomedical model has been. The economic model excludes the total costs to society of keeping people with disabilities out of work (e.g., income subsidies, housing, food stamps, health care, institutions, nursing homes, assistive technologies) and excludes the cost to relatives of people with disabilities who lose economic opportunities. It excludes the income generated by employed people with disabilities—taxes, unique products, cultural influence for the appreciation of humanity, the opportunity for giving others (those with and without disabilities) meaning to their lives. We are then left with the following questions: What is the proper unit of economic analysis for the cost of work site accommodations related to employing people with disabilities? Should these costs be adjusted for providing nonstigmatized worksite accommodations for nondisabled employees? Should these costs be weighed against the net costs of maintaining people with disabilities in the nonwork environment? Taking a broader view of the costs and benefits of employing people with disabilities may shed light on the merits of improving work opportunities for a large portion of the population of people with disabilities (Kemp, 1991). The outcomes of such studies may show that other populations of people with disabilities will fall outside the scope of this more encompassing economic analysis. Whatever the results of such broad-based economic studies, the picture of people with disabilities in or out the work force will be a more accurate depiction of the costs and benefits of social policies that both encourage employment (ADA) and those that reinforce dependency (Social Security and worker's compensation programs).

However inclusive, economic models usually do not embrace the concept of human values that go beyond economic efficiency. Some people with disability may choose not to participate in work that is paid. They may choose to remain unemployed, engage in volunteer activities or participate in compensated work on an intermittent basis in nontraditional settings. Occupational therapists will need to reflect on the type of economic opportunities available to their clients and work with them to reach a decision on interventions that develop the 'best' paths to self-satisfying occupations.

PSYCHOSOCIAL MODEL

Beatrice Wright (1960), Wolf Wolfensberger (1972), Constantina Safilios-Rothschild (1982) and others developed what has been called the deviance model of disability. "Deviance theory" concentrates on the analysis of social labels applied to behaviors that do not meet the norms of society (e.g., prostitution, drug use, depression, conduct disorders). As a result, the focus of deviance-based analyses shifts from the biology of the individual with a disability to the social environment in which he or she lives. The problem identified by this approach is that people with disabilities do not meet role expectations for people of their age, economic status, and similar characteristics. The solution is to make people with disabilities as much like normal people as possible in as normal a process as possible. To do this, one must assess just how different the person is. This led to studies of how severely depressed, frustrated, angry or unskilled people with disabilities "really" are. In short, how far from the mean or average of those assumed to be normally distributed characteristics are persons with disabilities? Treatments were aimed at reducing this gap.

The deviance model has been subjected to many criticisms, but defining normal roles is the paramount problem. Perceived relationships between body type and personalities, except in extreme conditions, are rarely instructive. The incidence of depression, anxiety, frustration, and lower self-esteem may be slightly higher for different populations of people with disabilities at various times of their lives, but the variability among those within the same impairment condition is large. The psychosocial model influenced classification schemes developed to gather data for planning services needed by people with disabilities to reduce the gap between their performance and normal activities. In 1980, Philip Wood and Elizabeth Badley working under the sponsorship of the World Health Organization (WHO), wrote the first version of the International Classification of Impairments, Disabilities and Handicaps (ICIDH). Fundamental to the concept of the handicap portion of this system is the idea that people with disabilities deviate from roles expected of them (WHO, 1980). That is, people with disabilities are judged in comparison to the performance of people without disabilities. The difference, in part, was attributed to social and environmental conditions; but in practice, assessments were based on a person's ability or inability to engage in activities within the standards of performance considered normal.

What is a Disability?

The description of what a disability is rests on the use of the word both in science and practical life issues—who is qualified for what depends on who calls whom what and when for how long. For scientific studies, people with disabilities are included or excluded from an experiment on the basis of their biological characteristics. In the context of economic benefits, disability is linked to work capacity. For civil rights legislation, disability has come to mean people who are or are perceived to be unable to perform major life activities (ADA, 1990). Irving Zola (1993) pointed out the importance and limitation of naming in all these contexts. There is a tension between using terms that describe differences apparent to the biological reality (i.e., impairment) of the disability (e.g., lame, cripple, deaf, blind) and words that associate the condition with a general trait of the person with the disability (e.g., suffering, confined to a wheelchair, burden, sick, invalid, defective). He advocated using language to connote that a person *has* a condition not that the person *is* one—a person with head injury rather than a head-injured person.

An example of the power of language was the creation of a "new" type of disability through legislation. The term *learning disability* was used as a categorical descriptor in the Education for All Handicapped Children Act (P.L. 94-142). This legislation allowed those children meeting the category criteria to receive special education funds and services. At the time the bill was passed into law (1975), less than 5% of federal special education funds were allotted to the education of children who fit the description of learning disability in 94-142. By the early 1990s over 50% of the Federal special education funds were spent on education for this group (U.S. Department of Education). Many national, state and local research projects have been funded to study "learning" disabilities. People with learning disabilities are included in civil rights legislation and litigation. The power of language to direct services, research and legislation is clearly demonstrated by the example of the term *learning disability*. With these benefits has come the realization that people with learning disabilities are and have been stigmatized as unintelligent, unemployable and asocial. The stigma associated with people with learning disability illustrates that negative attitudes toward people with disabilities are not confined to those with a physically visible impairment.

The reactions of people with disabilities to attempts to categorize them as impaired, disabled, handicapped, physically or mentally challenged, or children with special needs have not always been positive. Kemp (1981) objected to Jerry Lewis basing telethon pleas to raise money to support research for the cure of muscular dystrophy on his view of the horrible lives that children with MD have and the bleak future they all face. Pfieffer (1993) points out that the language used in the ICIDH to describe people with disability has a "... focus upon the disability and not the person. They lump together all of the stigmatized persons and dehumanize them" (p. 4). He points out that no one is normal for every physical or behavioral characteristic. Characterizing the whole person as deviant and in need based on one difference is bad biology, economics and politics (Hahn, 1993). Oliver (1996) maintains that disability is "the loss or limitation of opportunities to take part in the normal life of the community on an equal level with others due to physical and social barriers." Separating the causal link between impairments from the lack of social opportunities that people with impairments experience is at the core of the argument. The medical model supports the link and the social political model does not. The importance of the issue "what is disability?" lies in the control over the access to different types and levels of goods and services. No easy answers are apparent. However, awareness of the differing points of view is essential to understand the tensions between providers and recipients of services.

Stigma and Deviance

One valuable series of studies has considered the relationships between stigma and attitudes. This issue revolves around the nature of reactions by people without disabilities toward persons with disabilities and the source(s) of these responses. Jerome Siller (1986) posited that attitudes toward people with disabilities shape the social reception of visibly disabled people. He found that people without disabilities have difficulty knowing how to treat people with disabilities (interactional strain), tend to reject intimate interactions, and exclude persons with disabilities from social activities. Others adopt the attitude that people with disabilities should be treated with benevolence, often verging on authoritative and paternalistic interactions. Some observed interactions were actually based on hostile attitudes, especially when people with disabilities displayed emotions that were not a conventional part of social exchanges. Anxiety about the nondisabled persons' vulnerability to becoming disabled explained other actions. Generalizations of poor capabilities also were often made based on visible impairments. These studies helped to establish that attitudes provide the link between the concept of society-induced disadvantages (handicap) and observable and measurable empirical phenomena—reactions by nondisabled members of society. The lesson learned is that disadvantages experienced by people with disabilities are a result of systematic social processes based on stigma rather than functional limitations.

Fougeyrollas and Gray (in press) are studying the influences of stigma on the development of group homes for persons with severe mental or physical limitations in Quebec, Canada. Many prior attempts to locate group homes in residential neighborhoods have failed. An examination of the factors that led to failure showed that no efforts had been made to explain to the neighborhood inhabitants the nature of the people who would live in the group home; their strengths as well as weaknesses. No one had assessed the attitudes of the inhabitants of these neighborhoods about their willingness to accept people with severe physical or mental impairments. Information that has proven useful in reducing the anxiety of inhabitants of targeted neighborhoods includes knowing the number of people with disabilities who will live in the house, being assured that the new neighbors are not dangerous, discovering the number and quality of service providers, and having advance knowledge of structural modifications to neighborhood buildings and streets. Providing explanations about which changes might be made to the neighborhood to accommodate the new residence may have reduced the angry, hostile reactions of the residents who probably based their negative responses on stigmatized perceptions of people with severe physical and behavioral impairments. The importance of assessing social and environmental factors in developing programs for people with disabilities is but one example of how social stigma may be overcome through careful planning.

Just as societies stigmatize persons with disabilities, health professionals frequently have been criticized for paternalism, greed, overcontrol, insensitivity, and well-intentioned bungling (Rogers, 1992; Milam, 1993; Gallagher, 1995). Many persons with a disability tend to assume that all health professionals share the conceptual blinders of the medical model which prevent them from recognizing the importance of social and environmental barriers in everyday life. Thus the burden falls on these professionals to demonstrate their sensitivity to these concerns by considering the context of the whole person, by avoiding overgeneralizations, and by staying within their areas of competency. If not, they will have "noncompliant," "nonadhering," and uncooperative patients, clients or consumers who will pay the price of being both disabled and unhealthy (Corcoran, 1977).

People with disabilities have developed strategies to use these stigma-laden reactions by "normals." They try to pass as normal by displaying humor to show their positive attributes, becoming excessively self-effacing, speaking with sarcasm in describing their own stigmatized group (Hockenberry, 1995), demonstrating aggression to upset the normal (Price, 1993), and exaggerating accomplishments to show what a struggle it is to overcome the impairment. Many of these efforts represent an attempt to "pass," or to disguise their disabilities. But the shifting research paradigms have also produced a renewed search for a positive sense of identity based on disability (Hahn, 1988).

THE SOCIOPOLITICAL DEFINITION OF DISABILITY AND THE MINORITY GROUP MODEL

The major alternative to medical and economic models has been founded on a "sociopolitical" approach which defines disability as the product of interactions between individuals and the environment (Hahn, 1986). The emergence of this definition has presented a major challenge to the dominant viewpoints that have shaped the study of disability for many years. Traditionally, most concepts of disability had supported a "functional limitations" paradigm which identified decrements in individual performance as the basic cause of the difficulties of persons with disabilities and which sought to remedy these problems by improving

their personal capabilities and skills to the maximum extent possible (Hahn, 1985). By contrast, the sociopolitical perspective became the source of a "minority group" model which recognizes the environmental barriers confronting persons with disabilities as essentially similar to the obstacles faced by other disadvantaged groups in society. This model asserts that the effects of many disabling conditions can be alleviated primarily through the adoption of public laws and policies such as measures to combat attitudinal discrimination. The minority group model also shifts attention from a clinical orientation, which centers on the unique problems of each individual, to a collective approach, which seeks to solve such difficulties through government programs designed to improve the status of all people with disabilities (Hahn, 1994). The effort to reconcile these contrasting models and perspectives represents a crucial challenge to occupational therapy. The growing acceptance of the minority group model has produced major legislative accomplishments including the passage of the ADA of 1990.

The Minority Group Model

The major tenets of the minority group model are founded on the parallels between people with disabilities and other groups that have experienced discrimination based on race or ethnicity, gender, sexual orientation, and age. Historically, the social inequality of each of these groups was regarded as a result of innate biological characteristics. Women were perceived as inferior to men, African Americans were considered inferior to whites, gays and lesbians were viewed as the victims of an inherent biological predisposition to deviate from heterosexual norms, and older adults were treated as inferior to younger people. Gradually, advances in research based on different theoretical perspectives have provided increased support for the proposition that the status of these groups is socially and culturally determined. In other words, the disadvantages experienced by all of these groups can be traced to pervasive social and cultural influences rather than to personal or biological traits.

In the case of persons with disabilities, the assumption of biological inferiority often has been difficult to refute and replace with the concept fundamental to evolution, individual differences are essential to species survival. Darwin's theory of evolution holds that individual differences are passed on from generation to generation through natural selection by the environment. When environments change, the characteristics selected for continuation in the next generation change. In humans, selection factors for survival in our complex societies are largely culturally and politically determined. Those human characteristics that are highly valued at one time in one social system may differ from those human traits at another time in another society. The contrast was made all too clear by

German social policy in Adolph Hitler's era where diversity was exterminated rather than appreciated (Gallagher, 1995). The passage of ADA is a signal to the world that the United States is striving to make the physical, legal, employment and transportation aspects of the environment a level playing field for the wide diversity of American citizens with and without disabilities; racial majorities and minorities; men and women; and heterosexuals and homosexuals.

The minority group model is also based on the similarities between the social policy issues faced by people with disabilities and other disadvantaged groups. Like most minorities, persons with disabilities have been plagued by persistent discrimination in education, employment, housing, transportation, public accommodations, and communications. In fact, they have one of the highest rates of unemployment and welfare dependency in most societies. A substantial proportion subsist below the poverty line. Many have gone to separate schools, and most of them have confronted barriers in housing, transportation, communications, and public accommodations that exceed the rigid patterns of segregation imposed on other minorities (Harris, 1994). The numerous analogies between the policy issues confronted by citizens with disabilities and other disadvantaged segments of the population, therefore, indicated that the fundamental source of the problems of persons with disabilities could be attributed to attitudinal discrimination rather than to functional impairments.

The minority group model of disability has three major postulates. They are: a) the primary source of the difficulties encountered by people with disabilities can be traced to pervasive public attitudes; b) all aspects of the environment are fundamentally shaped or molded by public policy; and c) public policy is a reflection of prevalent social attitudes and values (Hahn, 1986). The implications of this reasoning indicate that discrimination against persons with disabilities cannot be ascribed merely to happenstance or coincidence; instead, these sentiments may reflect a subtle, though barely discernible, aversion that is buried deep within the human psyche. This question was addressed by a study that found that an unfavorable predisposition to persons with disabilities may be attributed to "existential" and "aesthetic" anxiety (Hahn, 1993). Existential anxiety refers to the fears of many people without disabilities individuals that they too could acquire a significant disability. Hence, they may tend to avoid, and to isolate, people with disabilities as a means of defending themselves against these worries. By contrast, aesthetic anxiety encompasses the uncertainties produced by relentless strivings in modern society to emulate idealized images of physical appearance that are promoted by the mass media. Almost by definition, the visible evidence of a significant bodily impairment or disability is often regarded as antithetical to these ideal standards; thus, unfavorable perceptions of persons with disabilities may reflect feelings of discomfort or

displeasure based primarily on aesthetic considerations. This study also asserted that, while existential anxiety might be especially compatible with the functional limitations paradigm, aesthetic anxiety may be most closely linked to the minority group model of disability. Consequently, this research has focused renewed attention on the significance of human, and especially physical differences in assessing the position of persons with disabilities in society. Although negative feelings and attitudes about people with disabilities may be suppressed by a posture of charitable benevolence or sympathy, unfavorable reactions to the perceptible characteristics of a disability and the patterns of avoidance that they tend to produce are a crucial component of the problems that must be addressed by any social support program, therapeutic intervention or service program designed to improve the status of persons with disabilities in society.

ATTITUDES ABOUT DISABILITY

The conceptualization of disability as difference has also spawned new classifications and measurements. Instead of equating disabilities with functional limitations, some researchers have proposed that disability can be defined by the concepts of visibility and labeling. Frequently, the most salient characteristics of an individual, and the ones that are most likely to evoke stigmatizing attitudes, are the obvious indications of an impairment. Some of these attributes such as the signs of mental retardation or amputations may be associated with the person, while other signifiers might be identified by necessary equipment or assistance including wheelchairs, white canes, and sign-language interpreters. For others with so-called hidden or invisible impairments, indications of a disability are apt to be revealed by notations in medical records, dossiers, or application forms. In either case, visual or recorded evidence of a disability often tends to elicit stereotypic perceptions that result in the exclusion of persons with disabilities from many social and economic activities. Hence, the mere presence of a disability, regardless of its functional implications, frequently spawns prejudiced reactions that restrict the opportunities available to the disabled minority.

The consequences of prejudicial or stigmatizing attitudes have been evident in many cases. In comparison to people without disabilities, persons with disabilities are less likely to engage in most forms of social participation. Evidence indicates, for example, that persons with disabilities have displayed lower involvement in everyday activities such as going to a supermarket or visiting restaurants, theaters, or concerts (Harris, 1986). Part of the explanation for these patterns can probably be attributed to inaccessible shops and buildings. Part of it might be ascribed to the fear of humiliation or ridicule that has long prevented people with disabilities from venturing into public activities. In any event, adverse attitudes often have a debilitating effect on individuals with disabilities. Many people with disabilities tend to absorb feelings of guilt and shame that produce a reduced sense of self-esteem.

A POSITIVE SENSE OF IDENTITY FOR PERSONS WITH DISABILITIES

The emergence of sociopolitical definition and disability rights movement, however, had a significant effect on the self-concepts of many individuals with disabilities. The realization that disability could be attributed to the effects of a disabling environment rather than to personal characteristics relieved them from a massive psychological burden. The struggle to eliminate stigma and prejudice provided them with an important sense of purpose. As a result, many persons with disabilities began to search for a positive sense of identity that would bolster their own efforts and enable them to recruit additional participants in the movement.

The effort to develop a positive sense of identity for persons with disabilities has tended to revolve about two major issues. Initially, many have argued that disability is an essential component of the diversity and heterogeneity of society. Instead of relying on medical cures to eradicate disabilities or on attempts to emulate idealized images of personal appearance, they have advocated that people must learn to appreciate the value of human differences, which contribute immeasurably to the richness of life experiences.

Perhaps the most significant advances toward the development of a positive sense of identity for persons with disabilities, however, have been made by explorations that focus on the everyday experience of living with a disability. In the immediate aftermath of a disabling event, people are usually compelled to ask two of the most difficult questions that can be posed to any human being, namely, "Why?" and "Why me?" There are no universal answers to such questions; but there is one response that appears to be almost invariable. After a disability, individuals tend to view their surroundings differently; their perceptions of the environment are not the same as they were before. More importantly, these different perspectives can be an important source of creativity. Persons with disabilities may gain a valuable source of insights and knowledge that is not readily available to people without disabilities. In addition, this creativity may become a crucial basis for empowerment. The capacity to discover innovative solutions to the numerous challenges that people with disabilities encounter in the environment can be an important means for improving their influence and status in the social structure. Finally, persons with disabilities have an unusual opportunity to become involved in a historic movement to extend and expand the definition of human and civil rights. All of these perspectives may contribute significantly to the effort to find meaning and purpose in life.

Occupational Therapy and the Disability Rights Movement

In a lecture on a college campus, an activist in the disability rights movement stated that his major problems stemmed from discriminatory attitudes instead of physical impairments. He believed that the principal solution to these difficulties was to gain equal rights rather than to reduce his functional limitations.

After his talk, he was questioned by an occupational therapist: "I'm surprised," she said, "because I've been working with disabled people for many years, and I've never heard any of them express these opinions before. How can you explain why your views are so different from theirs?"

In reply, he pointed out that the objectives of the disability rights movement have not yet achieved widespread recognition from the general public. "In addition," he said, "many of the people with whom occupational therapists work tend to be newly disabled. They have not gained the opportunity or the experience necessary to develop a different—or a positive—understanding of disability. Perhaps," he concluded, "occupational therapists might join the effort to promote this kind of understanding."

EQUAL ENVIRONMENTAL ADAPTATIONS

As a legal principle embodying respect for human differences, some advocates have proposed that judicial interpretations of laws prohibiting discrimination against persons with disabilities should be guided by the standard of Equal Environmental Adaptations (Hahn, 1993). Perhaps the clearest example of this concept is demonstrated by the presence of chairs as a ubiquitous feature of many environments. For most individuals without disabilities, chairs represent an essential and usually "taken for granted" facet of most habitats; but, for people who use wheelchairs, they may be superfluous. Rather than requiring persons with disabilities to achieve equivalent levels of functional competence, many contend that they should be provided with environmental adaptations that are at least commensurate with the advantages granted to the people without disabilities. As a concept designed to promote parity in the treatment of persons with disabilities and people without disabilities, the principle of Equal Environmental Adaptations represents an important attempt to fulfill the standard of equality within the context of an appreciation of human differences.

For occupational therapists, the word disability must designate more than a person's physical or mental impairment. The environmental conditions that proscribe the expression of that person's abilities are essential elements to understand the need for creating living conditions that foster his or her equal opportunity to participate in major life activities. Developing intervention programs that maximize access and minimize excess disability (cultural and physical barriers) to participation requires the therapist to understand and apply the principles of universal architectural design to create environments adapted to the needs of clients. Applying the fundamental universal design concept of maximal use for a widely diverse population of users should form the basis for advocating for and implementing policies, programs and interventions that increase access to social events (e.g., employment, recreation, education). Solutions to physical barrier removal in existing structures and in new construction seems to be within the reach of current technology (Welch & Ostroff, 1995). Even though it may not yet be grasped by the imagination, universal access to social activities stands as a challenge for the next generation of Americans. In a physical and social environment fully adapted to the needs and interests of people with disabilities, the effects of impairments on full participation in major life activities would be substantially reduced or even negligible.

CONCLUSION

In a fundamental sense, the foundation for the broad responsibilities confronting occupational therapists seemed to be established by a significant redefinition of disability or chronic health conditions that emerged during the 1980s. Unlike the almost exclusive reliance on a biomedical orientation stressing the loss or reduction of functional capacities that had dominated previous work, researchers and clinicians increasingly began to adopt a sociopolitical approach which defined disability as a product of the interaction between individuals and the environment. From this new perspective, disability is regarded primarily as the consequence of a disabling environment rather than personal defects or deficiencies. The principal difficulties encountered by persons with disabilities are located in surroundings outside the individual instead of internal or organic characteristics; and the search for solutions to these problems concentrated on efforts to reduce architectural, communication, and attitudinal barriers in the social environment. In many respects, this transition reflects a major shift of emphasis in the classic definition of disability (Nagi, 1991) as an "inability or limitation in performing socially defined roles and tasks expected of an individual within a sociocultural and physical environment." Whereas the medical approach focused primarily on inability or limitations and economic definitions centered on the performance of work or vocational roles and tasks, the sociopolitical perspective emphasizes the obstacles facing persons with disabilities in the social environment. This change encompasses extensive implications for the development of theory and practice in occupational therapy, especially as it moves beyond the institution to the community setting.

For persons with disabilities to fulfill their true potential, they must seek broader goals than the rehabilitation of their individual impairments. They may need to form coalitions and alliances that will enable them to become a powerful political constituency; promote equal rights for other disadvantaged groups; strive to enact policies that serve the interests of all people with disabilities; cooperate with occupational therapists and other professionals in the pursuit of common endeavors; and support research designed to reduce social, economic, and physical barriers to their full participation in society.

The implications of the minority group model also appear to indicate significant new roles for occupational therapy. Perhaps most importantly, occupational therapists can become valuable allies with persons with disabilities in the struggle to promote changes in the social environment. These activities might appropriately include the advocacy of new laws requiring that companies providing health service programs include people with disabilities in their plans, make provision for their acute and long-term needs, and furnish environmental modifications to reduce excess disability. Clearly, new legislation is needed to contribute funds for purchase of assistive technology. Finally, societal actions need to be monitored continuously to ensure that prior measures banning discrimination against people with disabilities are effectively implemented. Furthermore, occupational therapists may be an important source of support in the effort by persons with disabilities to develop a positive sense of identity. Both health professionals and people with disabilities must recognize that not all aspects of living with a disability are negative, and they may need to change their approach to these issues accordingly.

STUDY QUESTIONS

1. Define stigma and relate it to the lives of people with disabilities. How did it influence Franklin D. Roosevelt?

2. Can giving a group of people with disabilities special privileges lead to stigma? If so, give an example.

3. Review the strengths and weaknesses of the medical model of disability.

4. What are the costs and benefits of including people with disabilities in the U.S. workforce?

5. What is normal? How different does one have to be to

be abnormal, deviant and stigmatized?

6. Describe the minority group model of disability.

7. Review the concepts of disablement and enablement. give examples of each.

8. What is the ADA and how might it influence occupational therapy?

9. What is "equal environmental adaptation" and how does it relate to reasonable accommodation requirements of the ADA?

REFERENCES

Albrecht, G. L. (1992). *The disability business: Rehabilitation in America*. Newbury Park, CA: Sage Publications, Inc.

Americans with Disabilities Act of 1990, Public Law 101-336, 104 Stat. 327-378 (1990).

Barker, R. B. (1948). The social psychology of physical disability. *Journal of Social Issues, 4*(4), 28-37.

Batavia, A. I. (1992). Assessing the function of functional assessment: A consumer perspective. *Disability and Rehabilitation, 14*, 156-160.

Batavia, A., & Hammer, G. (1990). Toward the development of consumer-based criteria for the evaluation of assistive devices. *Journal of Rehabilitation Research, 27*, 425-436.

Bates, P. S., Spencer, J. C., Young, M. E., & Rintala, D. (1993). Assistive technology and the newly disabled adult: Adaptation to wheelchair use. *American Journal of Occupational Therapy, 47*, 1014-1021.

Bellamy, G. T., Rhodes, L. E., Mank, D. M., & Albin, J. M. (1988). *Supported employment: A community implementation guide*. Baltimore: Paul H. Brookes.

Berkowitz, M. (1978). *Work disincentives and rehabilitation*. Falls Church, VA: Institute for Information Studies.

Berkowitz, M., & Hill, M. A. (1986). Disability and the labor market: An overview. *Disability and the labor market: Economic problems, policies and programs*. Ithaca, NY: ILR Press [Cornell University].

Bickenbach, J. E. (1993). The question of language. *Physical disability and social policy*. Toronto: University of Toronto Press Inc.

Blaska, J. (1993). The power of language: Speak and write using "Person First" In M. Nagler (Ed.), *Perspectives on disability* (p. 27). Palo Alto, CA: Health Markets Research.

Boggs, E. M. (1987). Toward timely corrections of mental retardation/developmental disabilities policy. *American Journal of Mental Deficiency, 92*, 134-135.

Braddock, D., Hemp, R., Fujiura, G., Bachelder, L., & Mitchell, D. (1990). *The state of the states in developmental disabilities* (pp. 9-31). Baltimore: Paul H. Brookes.

Brooks, N. A. (1984). Opportunities for health promotion: Including the chronically ill and disabled. *Social Science in Medicine, 19*(4), 405-409.

Brooks, N. A. (1997, in review). Models for understanding reha-

bilitation and assistive technology. In D. B. Gray, L. A. Quatrano, & M. L. Lieberman (Eds.), *Using, designing and assessing assistive technology*. Baltimore: Paul H. Brookes.

Bruce, M. A., & Christiansen, C. H. (1988). Advocacy in word as well as deed. *American Journal of Occupational Therapy, 42*(3), 189-191.

Callahan, J. (1989). *He won't get far on foot: The autobiography of a dangerous man*. New York: Vintage.

Corcoran, P. J. (1977). Pejorative terms and attitudinal barriers. *Archives of Physical Medicine and Rehabilitation, 58*, 500.

Covington, G. (1997, in review). Why assistive technology doesn't work. In D. B. Gray, L. A. Quatrano, & M. L. Lieberman, (Eds.), *Using, designing and assessing assistive technology*. Baltimore: Paul H. Brookes.

DeJong, G., & Lifchez, R. (1983, June). Physical disability and public policy. *Scientific American*.

Fine, M., & Asch, A. (1988). Disability beyond stigma: Social interaction, discrimination, and activism. *Journal of Social Issues, 44*(1), 3-21.

Forster, E. M. (1908). *A room with a view*.

Fougeyrollas, P., & Gray, D. B. (1997, in review). ICIDH, handicap and environmental factors and social change: The importance of technology. In D. B. Gray, L. A. Quatrano, & M. L. Lieberman (Eds.), *Using, designing and assessing assistive technology*. Baltimore: Paul H. Brookes.

Frattali, C. M. (1993). Perspectives on functional assessment: Its use for policy making. *Disability and Rehabilitation, 15*(1), 1-9.

Gallagher, H. G. (1985). *FDR's splendid deception*. Arlington, VA: Vandamere Press.

Gallagher, H. G. (1995). *By trust betrayed patients. Physicians and the license to kill in the Third Reich*. Arlington, VA: Vandamere Press.

Gilderbloom, J., Rosenthal, M., & Bullard, D. (1987). *Designing, locating and financing housing and transportation services for low-income, elderly, and disabled persons*. Houston, TX: University of Houston Center for Public Policy.

Goffman, I. (1963). *Stigma: Notes on the management of spoiled identity*. Englewood Cliffs, NJ: Prentice-Hall.

Gray, D. B. (1975). The effects of etiology, drug and visual stimuli on fixed-interval panel pushing in a population of Downs and non-Downs syndrome retarded males. *Dissertation Abstracts International, XXXV*(12).

Grealy, L. (1994). *Autobiography of a face*. New York: Houghton Mifflin Co.

Hahn, H. (1985). Changing perceptions of disability and the future of rehabilitation. In L. G. Perlman & G. F. Austin (Eds.), *Societal influences in rehabilitation planning: A blueprint for the 21st century. A report of the Ninth Mary E. Switzer Seminar* (pp. 53-64). Alexandria, VA: National Rehabilitation Association.

Hahn, H. (1986). Disability and the urban environment: A perspective on Los Angeles. *Society and Space, 4*, 273-288.

Hahn, H. (1988). The politics of physical differences: Disability and discrimination. *Journal of Social Issues, 44*(1), 39-48.

Hahn, H. (1993). Can disability be beautiful? In M. Nagler (Ed.),

Perspectives on disability (pp. 217-226). Palo Alto, CA: Health Markets Research.

Hahn, H. (1993, August). Equality and the environment: The interpretation of reasonable accommodation in the Americans with Disabilities Act. *Journal of Rehabilitation Administration, 17,* 101-106.

Hahn, H. (1993). The political implications of disability definitions and data. *Journal of Disability Policy Studies, 4*(2), 41-52.

Hahn, H. (1994). The minority group model of disability: Implications for medical sociology. In R. Weitz & J. Jacobs Kronenfeld (Eds.), *Research in the sociology of health care* (pp. 3-24). Greenwich, CT: JAI Press.

Harris, L., & Associates. (1986). *The ICD survey I: Disabled Americans' self perceptions: Bringing disabled Americans into the mainstream.* New York: International Center for the Disabled.

Harris, L., & Associates. (1994). N.O.D. survey of Americans with disabilities. *Business Week,* May 30.

Hockenberry, J. (1995). *Moving violations: War zones, wheelchairs, and declarations of independence.* Hyperion.

Johnson, W. G. (1986). The Rehabilitation Act and discrimination against handicapped workers: Does the cure fit the disease. In M. Berkowitz & M. A. Hill (Eds.), *Disability and the labor market: Economic problems, policies and programs* (pp. 242-260). Ithaca, NY: ILR Press.

Kaiser, A. P., & Gray, D. B. (Eds.). (1993). *Enhancing children's communication: Research foundations for intervention.* Baltimore: Paul H. Brookes.

Kemp, E. J. (1981). Aiding the disabled: No pity please. *The New York Times,* September 4.

Kemp, E. J. (1991). A labor lawyer's guide to the Americans with Disabilities Act. *NOVA Law Review, 15*(1), 31-65.

Klapper, Z. S., & Birch, H. G. (1966). The relation of childhood characteristics to outcome in young adults with cerebral palsy. *Developmental Medicine and Child Neurology, 8,* 645-656.

Kregel, J., & Wehman, P. (1990). Supported employment: Promises deferred for persons with severe handicaps. In J. Kregel, P. Wehman, & M. S. Shater (Eds.), *Supported employment for persons with severe disabilities: From research to practice* (Vol. III, p. 33).

Longmore, P. K. (1985). A note on language and the social identity of disabled people. *Am Behav Scient, 28*(3),419-423.

Mace, R., Hardie, G., & Place, J. (1991). Accessible environments: Toward universal design. In W. F. E. Preisler, J. Vischer, and E. T. White (Eds.), *Design intervention: Toward a more humane architecture.* New York: Van Norstrand Reinhold.

McCuaig, M., & Frank, G. (1991). The able self: Adaptive patterns and choices in independent living for a person with cerebral palsy. *American Journal of Occupational Therapy, 45,* 224-234.

Milam, L. W. (1993). *CripZen: A manual for survival.* San Diego, CA: Mho & Mho Works.

Nagi, S. Z. (1965). Some conceptual issues in disability and rehabilitation. In M. B. Sussman (Ed.), *Sociology and rehabilitation.* Washington, DC: American Sociological Association.

Nagi, S. Z. (1976). An epidemiology of disability among adults in the United States. *Milbank Mem Fund Q Health & Society, 54*(4), 439-468.

Nagi, S. Z. (1991). In A. M. Pope & A. R. Tarlov (Eds.), *Disability in America: Toward a national agenda for prevention.* Washington, DC: National Academy Press, Institute of America, National Academy of Sciences.

National Council on the Handicapped. (1987). Harris poll on employment: Disabled employees rated excellent. *Focus,* 3.

Oliver, M. (1996). *Defining impairment and disability: Issues at stake.* Unpublished manuscript.

Orentlicher, D. (1994). Rationing and the Americans with Disabilities Act. *Journal of the American Medical Association, 271*(24).

Parsons, T. (1961). *The social system.* Glencoe, IL: Free Press.

Pfieffer, D. (1993). Disabling definitions: Is the World Health Organization normal? *Perspectives, 11*(3), 4-9.

Pope, A. M., & Tarlov, A. R. (Eds.). (1991). *Disability in America: Toward a national agenda for prevention.* Washington, DC: National Academy Press, Institute of America, National Academy of Sciences.

Price, R. (1993). *A whole new life.* New York: Atheneum Macmillan.

Restructuring the SSI Disability Program for children and adolescents. (1995, May). Report from the Committee on Childhood Disability to the Disability Policy Panel of the National Academy of Social Insurance (pp. 1-55). Washington, DC.

Rice, D. P., & LaPlante, M. P. (1988). *Cost of chronic comorbidity.* In American Public Health Association Annual Meeting Program. Washington, DC.

Rogers, J., & Matsumura, M. (1991). *Mother to be: A guide to pregnancy and birth for women with disabilities.* New York: Demos Publications.

Rogers, J. C., & Holm, M. B. (1994). Accepting the challenge of outcome research: Examining the effectiveness of occupational therapy practice. *American Journal of Occupational Therapy, 48*(10), 871-876.

Safilios-Rothschild, C. (1982). Social and psychological parameters of friendship and intimacy for disabled people. In M. Eisenberg, C. Griggs, & R. Duval (Eds.), *Disabled people as second-class citizens* (pp. 40-52). New York: Springer.

Shapiro, J. P. (1993). *No pity: People with disabilities forging a new civil rights movement.* New York: Times Books, Random House, Inc.

Shear, M. (1986, November-December). No more supercrip. *New Directions for Women,* 10.

Siller, J. (1986). The measurement of attitudes towards physically disabled persons. In C. P. Herman, M. P. Zana, & E. T. Higgins (Eds.), *Physical appearance, stigma, and social behavior.* Hillsdale, NJ: Lawrence Erlbaum.

Sloan, W., & Stevens, H. A. (1976). *A century of concern: A history of the American Association on Mental Deficiency 1876-1976.* Washington, DC: American Association on Mental Deficiency, Inc.

U. S. Department of Education, Office of Special Education. Annual reports to Congress on the implementation of the Education and Handicapped Act from 1977 through 1994.

Weaver, C. L. (1986). Social security disability policy in the 1980s and beyond. In M. Berkowitz & M. A. Hill (Eds.), *Disability and the labor market: Economic problems, policies and programs* (pp. 29-63). Ithaca, NY: ILR Press.

Welch, P., & Ostroff, E. (1995). *The Universal Design Education Project in strategies for teaching Universal Design* (pp. 19-30). Berkeley, CA: Adaptive Environments Center, Boston and MIG Communications.

Wilkerson, D. L., Batavia, A. I., & DeJong, G. (1992). The use of functional status measures for payment of medical rehabilitation services. *Archives of Physical Medicine and Rehabilitation, 73*, 11-120.

Wolfensberger, W., Nirje, B., Olshansky, S., Perske R., & Roos, P. (1972). *The principle of normalization in human services.* Toronto: National Institute of Mental Retardation, Leonard Crainford.

World Health Organization. (1980). *International classification of impairments, disabilities, and handicaps.* Geneva, Switzerland: Author.

Wright, B. A. (1960). *Physical disability: A psycho-social approach.* New York: Harper & Row.

Zola, I. K. (1982a). Disincentives to independent living. *Archives of Physical Medicine and Rehabilitation, 63,* 396.

Zola, I. K. (1982b). *Missing pieces: Chronicle of living with a disability.* Philadelphia: Temple University Press.

Zola, I. K. (1989). Toward the necessary universalizing of a disability policy. *Milbank Quarterly, 67*(Suppl. 2, Pt. 2), 401-430.

Zola, I. K. (1993). Self, identity and the naming question: Reflections on the language of disability. In M. Nagler (Ed.), *Perspectives on disability* (pp. 15-24). Ontario, Canada.

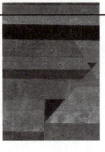

CHAPTER CONTENT OUTLINE

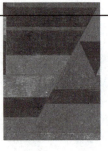

ABSTRACT

Occupational therapists have been aware for most of this century of a relationship between social support and occupation. While other professionals may also have much to offer in the area of social support, occupational therapists have a unique role in promoting occupational performance through the involvement of the social network, in marshaling support from the network for occupational performance achievements, and in enhancing the capacity of occupational therapy clients for giving and receiving support. This chapter reviews the concept of social support, particularly as is pertains to occupational therapists and others working with people with disabilities. The chapter summarizes the existing literature on network characteristics, sources, types, and evaluation of social support by people with disabilities. It then explores principles for therapeutic intervention in the area of social support. Measures of social support are reviewed with recommendations for use in occupational therapy. Principles for intervention are summarized, and intervention at different levels, including individual, couple, family and community, are explored. Finally, professional attitudes toward the support system are challenged, relative to research findings.

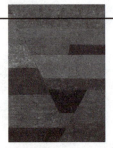

KEY TERMS

Social support

Social network

Instrumental support

Informational support

Index individual

CHAPTER 17

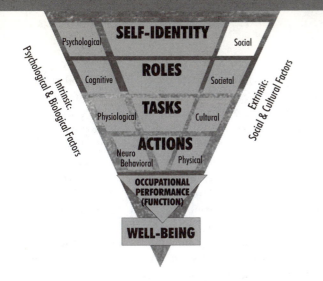

Social Support and Occupational Therapy

Mary Ann McColl, PhD, OT(C)

OBJECTIVES

The information in this chapter is intended to help the reader:

1. understand the concept of social support and its relationship to occupation and well-being
2. review current knowledge about social support among people with disability
3. identify options for assessing a client's degree of social support
4. identify principles, levels and alternatives for social support intervention
5. view social support from the perspective of persons with a disability.

"The secret of continuing development...
is the discovery through a variety of relationships
that social expectations can be changed and that
difference can be a source of strength."
Mary Catherine Bateson

Social Support

The experience of being cared for and loved, valued and esteemed, and able to count on others should the need arise.

Figure 17-1. Definition of social support. From Cobb, 1974; McColl & Friedland, 1989.

INTRODUCTION

Occupational therapists have been aware for most of this century of a relationship between social support and occupation (Kelleher, 1925; Kindwall & McLean, 1941). Both clinical practice and research provide evidence that social support affects occupation, as well as other outcomes, from well-being to mortality (Berkman & Syme, 1979; Bruhn, 1991; Gottlieb & Selby, 1989; Nicaise, Jonckers, Smits, Provost & Asiel, 1993; Oxman, Berkman, Kasl, Freeman, & Barrett, 1992). In fact, its effect may exceed that of well-established risk factors, like smoking (Orth-Gomer, Rosengren, & Wilhelmsen, 1993).

The model guiding our thinking about occupation in this book shows occupation as being influenced by both intrinsic and extrinsic factors (Christiansen & Baum, 1997). Social support affects occupation, health and well-being through both avenues: intrinsic factors such as one's disposition toward social relationships and ability to participate in relationships; and extrinsic factors such as the availability of supportive others and the accessibility of support venues. Thus social support is a legitimate concern of occupational therapists, and not something to be simply delegated to other professionals. While other professionals may also have much to offer in the area of social support, occupational therapists have a unique role in promoting occupational performance through the involvement of the social network, in marshalling support from the network for occupational performance achievements and in enhancing the capacity of occupational therapy clients for giving and receiving support.

Most of what we know about social support comes from work with able-bodied populations, often the elderly

(Bowling, 1991). However, the experience of disability offers a particular context for social support (Dimatteo and Hays, 1981). This context includes both intrinsic and extrinsic factors that people with disabilities share with the population as a whole, such as age, gender and social situation (Krahn, 1993). It also includes a number of unique contextual factors related to the disability and its effects on everyday life (Weinberger, Tierney, Booher, & Hiner, 1990). The disability-related context of social support has been explored by a number of authors, all of whom agree that intrinsic factors such as pain and activity limitations, and extrinsic factors such as accessibility and stigma, all contribute to a unique context for the development and functioning of social relationships (Dunkel-Schetter & Bennett, 1990; Johnson & Troll, 1994; Lanza & Revenson, 1993; O'Brien, 1993; Schulz, Tompkins, & Wood, 1987; Tilden & Weinert, 1987; Wortman & Conway, 1985).

The purpose of this chapter is to review the concept of social support, particularly as it pertains to occupational therapists and others working with people with disabilities. The chapter addresses the following questions:
1. What do we currently know about the social support systems of people with disabilities?
2. How can occupational therapists work with people with disabilities to enhance occupation through social support (Figure 17-1)?

DEFINITION

A definition of social support will serve as the basis for the following discussion. As a general statement, social support is defined as: the experience of being cared for and loved, valued and esteemed, and able to count on others should the need arise (Cobb, 1974; McColl & Friedland, 1989).

This definition describes social support as an experienced rather than an observed phenomenon (Dunkell-Schetter & Bennett, 1990). That is, support is viewed as experienced or subjective, rather than behavioural or objective. There is now sufficient evidence to confirm that the subjective dimension is most influential for health (Orth-Gomer, et al., 1993; Sarason, Pierce, & Sarason, 1990). In other words, as House (1981) very eloquently puts it, social support has to be perceived to be effective.

Social support is a multidimensional construct. Several decades ago, researchers strove to determine a single definition for social support that would encapsulate its true essence. They attempted to isolate which of many known dimensions of social support was most influential, and therefore most essential (see McColl & Skinner, 1988). More recently, researchers have recognized the need to expand the topic. Thus instead of working toward agreement on a single

Bibliographic citation of this chapter: McColl, M. A. (1997). Social support and occupational therapy. In C. Christiansen & C. Baum (Eds.), *Occupational therapy: Enabling function and well-being* (2nd ed.). Thorofare, NJ: SLACK Incorporated.

definition of social support, researchers now recognize the plurality of the construct, and attempt to capture the many different aspects of support. In fact, some would say that social support is no longer considered a single concept at all, but rather a category of concepts, all related to the beneficial effects of social relationships (Dimatteo & Hays, 1981; Kobasa et al., 1991; Norris, Stephens & Kinney, 1990). Thus the term "social support" may be thought of as an umbrella term, covering a variety of more specific dimensions of social relationships.

Of the many dimensions along which social support can be described, four are examined in the chapter: network structure, types of support, sources of support, and evaluation of support. Structural aspects of support systems, such as availability, size, density and dispersion, may be helpful in attempting to understand the composition of the network. Functional types of support are also instructive in describing support systems. One of the most popular taxonomies for types of support is that used by Cohen and colleagues (Cohen & Wills, 1985; Cohen & Syme, 1985; Cohen, Mermelstein, Kamarck, & Hoberman, 1985) referring to instrumental support (tangibly assisting the individual), belonging support (making the individual feel securely attached), informational support (furnishing information, advice or guidance), and esteem support (enhancing self-esteem through reflected esteem).

Source represents another dimension of social support that may be helpful in understanding its effects. Sources are divided primarily into formal and informal sources, with formal sources of support being those to which everyone should have access (e.g., groups, institutions, organizations and professionals) and informal sources being those to which individuals uniquely have access because of who they are (such as spouse, family and friends) (McColl & Friedland, 1994). These two categories of support can be further specified; for example, informal sources can be rated on the degree of intimacy, obligation and reciprocity in the relationship. Relationships within both categories are governed by rules, conventions and social norms that define the type and extent of support that can be provided (Antonucci & Jackson, 1990).

Evaluation of support is the fourth dimension that may be used to characterize support. This concept is similar to what some authors refer to as adequacy of support or satisfaction with support (Henderson, Duncan-Jones, Byrne, & Scott, 1980). Underlying this notion of evaluation is an internal assessment of the extent to which social support fulfills needs, complements individual coping or meets expectations. This is perhaps the most purely subjective aspect of social support, because the criteria used for evaluation are usually not explicit.

SOCIAL SUPPORT AMONG PEOPLE WITH DISABILITIES

These four dimensions will be used to organize information about social support. The following section summarizes what we know about social support among people with disabilities.

Network Characteristics

One of the most notable observations about the social networks of people with disabilities is their size. Most authors describe the networks of people with disabilities as being smaller, less dense and less complex than those of able-bodied contemporaries (Antonucci & Jackson, 1990; Knox & Parmenter, 1993; Krahn, 1993). While most adults in the general population have networks of 8 to 15 individuals (Schulz & Rau, 1985), estimates for those with disabilities vary widely. Schulz and Decker (1985) found that the mean network size for 100 people with spinal cord injuries was 2.3 persons. Wineman (1990) described the social networks of people with multiple sclerosis as comprised of nine individuals for men and 10 for women. She also found that those with the progressive type of MS had larger networks than those with the episodic type. Norris and colleagues (1990), in a study of 48 stroke survivors, found network size to be, on average, four. Perhaps the most dramatic finding about network size in several studies was that the modal network size was 1, suggesting that a large proportion of the population derived all of their support from a single individual (Schultz & Decker, 1985; Knox & Parmenter, 1993; Kinsella, Ford, & Moran, 1989; Norris et al., 1990). This concentration of support in one supporter leaves these individuals extremely vulnerable to the loss of that supporter and places a great deal of stress on the supporter, thus increasing the risk of loss.

Numerous authors have suggested reasons for the contraction of the social networks of individuals with disabilities. Fitzpatrick and colleagues (1991) studied individuals with rheumatoid arthritis, and found that the more disability and pain individuals experienced, the less likely they were to have diffuse relationships, or relationships that are not characterized by intimacy and/or obligation. While close relationships, such as family, were not significantly affected by pain and disability, the difficulties of maintaining diffuse relationships in the presence of disability seem, in some cases, to be overwhelming.

Wortman and Conway (1985) note that the disability itself imposes constraints on interactions with the support system. For example, a mobility impairment may decrease the accessibility of some locations where support could be obtained. Wortman (1984) notes that communication problems may also inhibit the ability of individuals with some

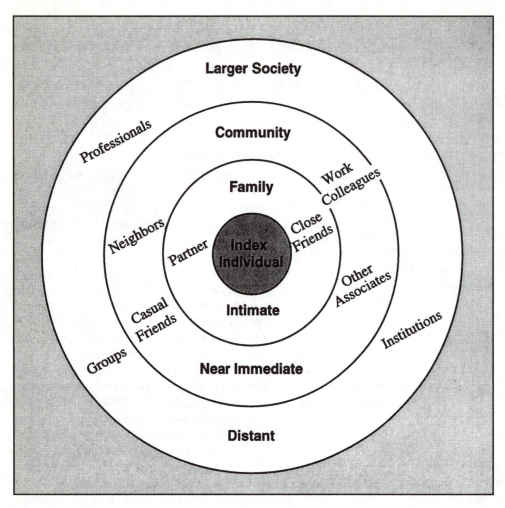

Figure 17-2. Levels of the social environment. Adapted from Davidson, 1991.

kinds of disability to maintain diffuse relationships. In addition, social barriers, such as inability to easily maintain normative social behaviours (such as eye contact) may further limit the ability of someone with a disability to sustain a social network. Wortman (1984) also notes that social stigma, ignorance and fear may adversely affect the social support systems of individuals with disabilities. In particular, there may be a concern among possible supporters about the extent of support needs of the disabled individual, and the possible obligations that may be associated with a relationship with him or her.

Silver, Wortman and Crofton (1990) found that the perceptions of how well an individual was coping already influenced whether or not support was offered. Those who appeared to be coping best received the most offers of support. McNett (1987) suggests the opposite: that social support is most likely to be offered when it becomes apparent that personal coping is inadequate. Thus while we might like to believe the latter — that supporters respond in an altruistic way to those who appear to need support — there is some

evidence that in fact the reverse is true. Support accrues to those who appear to need it least, and to those who may be the easiest to support. Also, the presence of a disability may serve to enlarge the network, by including family helpers who might not otherwise be involved, service providers and disabled peers (Krol et al., 1993; Stoller & Pugliesi, 1988).

Schulz and Rau (1985) note the importance of the time of onset of disability for network size over the lifespan. They refer to statistically and temporally normative and non-normative events as having different effects on the social network. Whereas a stroke in an older person would be considered a statistically and temporally normative event, a spinal cord injury in a young person would be considered both statistically and temporally non-normative. The non-normative event, such as the early onset or traumatic disability, requires greater adjustment on the part of both the index individual and the members of his or her social network, and is therefore expected to have a negative effect on network size (Figure 17-2).

Sources of Support

Sources of support may be thought of as concentric circles around an index individual, that is, the person receiving support (McColl & Friedland, 1989; Grady, 1995; Davidson, 1991). Nearest the centre are family and close friends, then casual friends and associates, then the community at large, including professionals, groups and institutions. The importance of individuals at each of these levels seems notably different for people with disabilities than for members of the general population. Researchers point to the fact that networks of people with disabilities are dominated by family members to a far greater extent than the networks of able-bodied people (Knox & Parmenter, 1993; Norris et al., 1990). Several authors talk about an implicit ordering of support provision by various sources. An interesting observation about these hierarchies of support is that family consistently occupies the top spots (Brillhart, 1988; Croog, Lipson, & Levine, 1972; O'Brien, 1993; Schultz & Decker, 1985). Family relationships seem to be relatively robust in the face of stressors like a disability. A number of authors have noted that while family relationships are present in disabled samples at approximately the same rate as in able-bodied samples, diffuse relationships are not (Fitzpatrick, Newman, Lamb, & Shipley, 1988; Kinsella et al., 1989). Depending on the age of the index person, the most involved sources of support are reported to be parents, spouses or siblings.

Family or kin ties have a number of characteristics that may make them particularly meaningful in the lives of people with disabilities. Family ties are characterized by different constraints, obligations and types of interaction than non-kin ties (Dakof & Taylor, 1990; Gonzalez, Goeppinger, & Lorig, 1990). Antonucci and Jackson (1990) refer to the different sets of rules that apply to different relationships; in particular to different norms for reciprocity. They use the analogy of a "support bank," where an index individual may take out a long-term loans of help and support from a family member with flexible repayment terms. In non-kin relationships, however, individuals may usually only make only short-term loans, and are expected to reciprocate in a direct and tangible manner. The flexibility of kin relationships serves people with disabilities well, since the nature and manner of reciprocity is not always obvious, and the experience of indebtedness in relationships can be intensely negative (Antonucci & Jackson, 1990). In addition, kin often have a longitudinal view of the person and his or her disability. In the case of a noncongenital onset, they may remember the person before the onset of disability, and therefore may be perceived as knowing the essential person, both with and without the disability.

It may oversimplify to say that family relationships are more supportive than other types of relationships. Research has shown that while family are preferred for some support functions, particularly the more intimate or longstanding functions, friends and other associates are preferred for other kinds of support. In the post-stroke period, Norris and colleagues (1990) found that family members performed 92% of all functional assistance and 83% of all errands. Croog and colleagues (1972) interviewed men who had experienced their first myocardial infarction, and found that kin were perceived as most helpful when they offered financial or practical functions, while friends and community associates were associated most often with moral or emotional support. Further, friends were most responsive in times of crisis, whereas family offered a more stable level of background support.

Several authors have also pointed to the importance of diffuse or community relationships (Anson, Stanwyck, & Krause, 1993; Fitzpatrick et al., 1988, 1991). Research with people who had experienced strokes showed that community contacts, such as neighbours and work colleagues, were most influential in terms of adjustment to community living (Friedland & McColl, 1987). Fitzpatrick and colleagues (1991) suggested that diffuse relationships were more onerous to maintain, thus to the extent that these were present, the individual probably had a generally well-developed support system. Current research with people with acquired brain injuries (McColl, Carlson, Johnston, Minnes, Shue & Willer, 1996) underlines the importance of friendships, particularly making new friends in the process of community integration.

Fischer and colleagues (1989) point to the underutilization of support groups for people with disabilities. Cluff and Cluff (1983) suggest that community groups may fulfill functions that neither professionals nor close relationships can, such as social comparison, socialization and information-sharing. Furthermore, group supports have been shown to result in fewer negative interactions, and to persist even when individuals come and go from the network (Felton & Berry, 1992).

Knox and Parmenter (1993) mention the importance of support from others with the same disability. Besides the obvious benefits associated with sharing similar experiences, the support of others with the same disability can fulfill a number of other functions. It can provide an environment where the individual does not need to compete with able-bodied others, feel conspicuous because of the disability, and has some status or position other than that afforded by the disability. In effect, these relationships based on the shared experience of disability allow for a focus on issues associated with the disability while neutralizing the importance of the disability in the relationship.

Finally, a number of authors have commented on relationships with professionals, and have confirmed that beyond the acute stage, people with disabilities tend to have no more contact with professionals and other formal sources of support than people in the general population (Croog et al., 1972). Decker and Schultz (1985), in a sample of 100 spinal

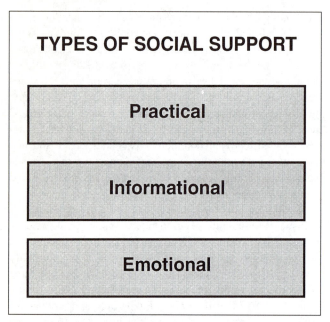

TYPES OF SOCIAL SUPPORT

Practical

Informational

Emotional

Figure 17-3. Types of social support.

cord injured individuals, found that 85% never used formal sources of support, and only 6% used formal supports regularly. These findings assist in dispelling the myth that people with disabilities are high-volume users in the service sector, and that they use formal sources to substitute for informal sources of support. Dakof and Taylor (1990) suggest that the main function that people with disabilities seek from formal sources is informational support consistent with the professional role.

Types of Support

Most taxonomies of types of support include a practical type (instrumental, aid, tangible), an informational type (advice, guidance) and an emotional type (esteem, belonging, moral support). Types of support are generally differentiated in an effort to assess the fit between a stressful situation and the support received. Jacobson (1986) suggests that the type of support needed may be anticipated to some extent, based on the unfolding response to a stressful event. He uses the classical stage theory of adjustment to loss (Bowlby, 1980) to predict the support needs of people in a variety of stressful situations, including the onset of disability or chronic illness. In the crisis phase accompanying onset, he suggests that emotional support will be most meaningful; in the transition phase, informational support and, in the long-term deficit phase, tangible support. Broadhead and Kaplan (1991) develop this idea more fully, looking at the specific supportive functions that are required at each stage following cancer onset. Their analysis shows

an ebb and flow of the various types of support over the period from diagnosis to the terminal stages, in response to predictable stressful events.

Different types of support have also been shown to have different relationships with outcomes, like adjustment, quality of life and occupational function. While emotional support has consistently been shown to have a positive relationship to outcomes (McColl & Rosenthal, 1994; Weinberger et al., 1990), other types of support are not so uniformly perceived as supportive. For example, several studies have shown a negative relationship between instrumental support and both occupational and adjustment outcomes. Norris and colleagues (1990), in a sample of stroke survivors, found that tangible support was related to ADL dependency, but were uncertain as to the direction of this relationship. Taal and colleagues (1993) found a similar relationship in people with rheumatoid arthritis, however, Weinberger and colleagues (1990) found the opposite in a sample with osteoarthritis. People with spinal cord injuries showed a negative relationship between tangible support and psychosocial outcomes (McColl, Lei, & Skinner, 1994). However, this finding can be interpreted in two ways: it could mean that dependency on others generally leads to negative psychosocial consequences, or it could simply mean that those with the most problems receive the most tangible support. Either way, it seems that the need for tangible support is experienced as somewhat of a double-edged sword; while helpful on the one hand, it reinforces dependency on the other.

Informational support seems to be perceived as helpful only when delivered by sources with established credibility, such as professionals or others who have undergone a similar experience (Dakof & Taylor, 1990; Lehmann, Ellard, & Wortman, 1986), making a strong statement for a client-centred approach. Advice from close informal supporters was perceived aversively in several studies (Manne & Zautra, 1989). This may present difficulties for families in the initial stages of adjustment to the disability of a family member (Figure 17-3).

Evaluation of Support

The evaluation of support is defined as the extent to which support is perceived as positive, supportive, helpful and satisfactory. Research with people with strokes and spinal cord injuries (Friedland & McColl, 1989; McColl & Skinner, 1995) suggests that the support they receive is generally perceived positively. Schulz and Decker (1985) also, in their sample with spinal cord injuries, found that subjects were generally satisfied with their support system. Little is known about predictors of satisfaction with support, but two studies offer some insight. In a study of 38 individuals with acquired brain injuries, none of the many variables considered significantly predicted perceived adequacy of support (Kinsella et al., 1989). Even when the availability of support was rated as low, the adequacy of support continued to be rated highly. Kinsella and associates (1989) acknowledge that cognitive impairment may be a factor in this finding, however, they allow for the fact that satisfaction with support may be unrelated to quantitative parameters like availability. O'Brien (1993), in studying people with multiple sclerosis, found that as both severity and duration of disability increased, satisfaction with support decreased, suggesting that the support system may "wear down" over the course of a lifelong disability, particularly a progressive one. Alternately, as people with progressive disabilities become more disabled, their needs and expectations may be less frequently met by their supporters, leading to dissatisfaction and a sense of social isolation.

Support is remarkably consistent across source and type. In a sample of men post-myocardial infarction, the most consistent predictor of the evaluation of one type of support was the evaluation of other types of support (Croog et al., 1972). Thus people with positive relationships in one sphere of their lives tend to view relationships in other spheres positively as well. This finding has been interpreted as an overall disposition to perceive support, and perhaps other aspects of life as well, either positively or negatively as a general rule.

ENHANCING SOCIAL SUPPORT AMONG PEOPLE WITH DISABILITIES

As we agree that social support is good for people with disabilities, and there can be little doubt that it is, then how can occupational therapists in institutions and in the community enhance the availability and adequacy of support to ultimately enhance occupation? The logical synthesis of the foregoing discussion is a compilation of the research as it applies to assessment and intervention; that is, to our ability to assess and enhance social support and occupation for people with disabilities, both during rehabilitation and within the community.

Assessment

A number of authors have made recommendations about assessing social support. Most prevalent among these are recommendations for conceptual clarity (Thoits, 1985), psychometrically sound assessments (Cohen & Wills, 1985) and sensitivity to issues of people with disabilities (Wortman, 1984).

At the root of all assessment issues in social support is the need for conceptual clarity and definition. Each of us knows what it feels like to have support in certain situations and none in others. As a theoretical construct, social support is readily accessible to us at an intuitive level. Because of its

intuitive nature, much of the early work on measuring social support was done from an atheoretical standpoint (Aldwin & Revenson, 1987; Antonucci & Israel, 1986). Definitions of social support were often based on intuitive conceptualizations rather than explicit theoretical or empirical ones. The result was that assessments of social support proliferated, each based on a different definition of support, and each representing an apparent improvement over previously published assessments (McColl & Skinner, 1988).

Assessment is an essential first step in intervention. What is assessed and how it is assessed are dictated by the definition underlying the assessment. Theoretical specificity about definition becomes especially important when considering a concept like social support, which is multi-dimensional and theoretically complex. Remembering the definition of social support used earlier in this chapter, assessments have been classified according to the four dimensions of support: structure, type, source and evaluation. Nine of the more popular assessments were classified to assist occupational therapists in choosing assessments for social support.

Structure

Perhaps the most widely used structural measure of social support is the Social Network Index (Berkman & Syme, 1979). This measure was used for longitudinal epidemiological studies showing the relationship between the availability of social support and mortality over a 12-year period (Berkman & Syme, 1979; Berkman & Breslow, 1983). It is a brief measure that assesses the availability of a spouse, family and close friends, and church and other community organizations.

The Social Relationships Scale (McFarlane et al., 1980) takes another approach to assessing availability. It asks respondents whether or not they have support in stressful situations related to six areas of life: home/family, work, money, personal, health and social. It also provides some information on the evaluation dimension in that it asks individuals to rate the helpfulness and reciprocity in relationships associated with each of these six areas.

The Social Support Questionnaire (Sarason et al., 1983) has an availability component as well as an evaluation component. The SSQ is made up of two subscales: one giving the number of supporters available in each of 27 situations and the other giving the satisfaction with support received. The availability score represents the average number of supporters the index person has in any given situation.

Finally, the Interview Schedule for Social Interaction (Henderson et al., 1980) also assesses the availability (as well as the adequacy or evaluation) of two types of support: attachments or close relationships and integration or diffuse relationships. Scores are computed for the availability of attachments (AVAT) and the availability of social integration (AVSI).

Types

Perhaps the most widely used assessment of types of social support is the Interpersonal Support Evaluation List (Cohen et al., 1985). The ISEL consists of 40 questions about the availability of someone to provide tangible support, emotional support, informational support and esteem support. In research with people with spinal cord injuries and acquired brain injuries, an adapted version of the ISEL was developed to provide more specific information about disability-related situations (McColl & Skinner, 1995).

The Social Support Questionnaire by Schaeffer and colleagues (1981) also gives information about types of support. It asks respondents about nine different situations and the extent to which they had tangible support, emotional support and informational support. The three scores for the SSQ represent the number of people available to provide each type of support.

Finally, the Norbeck Social Support Questionnaire (Norbeck et al., 1981, 1983) assesses the availability of three types of support consistent with Kahn's (1979) conceptualization of social support: aid, affirmation and affect. Scores for each type include items on the frequency and duration of contact with supporters in each area.

Sources

Two measures focus on sources of social support. The Perceived Social Support Measure (Procidano & Heller, 1983) is composed of two sections: one for family and one for friends. Each section results in a score based on 20 analogous items asking about support, information and feedback provided by each source.

The other assessment focusing on source is the Social Support Inventory for People with Disabilities (McColl & Friedland, 1989). The SSIPD is made up of five sections corresponding to five sources: intimate/confidante, family and close friends, acquaintances and associates, community groups and professionals. Five scores may be calculated on quantitative and qualitative aspects of relationships with these sources.

Evaluation

A number of the assessments mentioned offer the evaluation perspective on social support: the Social Relationships Scale (McFarlane et al., 1980); the Social Support Questionnaire (Sarason et al., 1983); the Interview Schedule for Social Interaction (Henderson et al., 1980); and the Social Support Inventory for People with Disabilities (McColl & Friedland, 1989).

Besides conceptual clarity, the second issue in the assessment of social support is the reliability and validity of social support measures. For each of the measures discussed, information about psychometric properties is available in the orig-

inal citations, as well as in several reviews of measurement in social support (McColl & Skinner, 1988; Cohen & Wills, 1985; Donald & Ware, 1984; Turner, Frankel & Levin, 1983). One particular issue in the validity of assessments of social support is the validity of self-report versus observed approaches. If perceived support is of interest, then self-report is inevitable, with no opportunity for objective corroboration. On the other hand, if observed support is assessed, then no information is available about the extent to which the index individual is experiencing the support. Antonucci and Israel (1986) described a phenomenon called veridicality, referring to the agreement about support exchanged between a recipient and a provider. They found that veridicality was only moderate; only about 79% of the time recipients and providers agreed as to the fact that a supportive exchange had occurred. In the case of an unsubstantiated report, the inevitable question arises as to who to believe: the index person reporting on whether or not support was received or another person reporting on whether or not support was given. Perhaps the resolution to this dilemma lies in House's (1981) comment, referred to earlier, that support must be perceived in order to exert any beneficial effect on the occupation, health or well-being of an individual.

A final problem of assessing social support is the need for instruments to address the unique needs and problems of people with a disability. Wortman and Conway (1985) emphasize the importance of assessing support specifically for people with disabilities and tailoring support measures to capture those dimensions that are most meaningful. Wortman (1984) outlines three factors that impinge on the assessment of support for people with disabilities. First, information on social support in the general population is inadequate as a normative standard for support for people with disabilities. Because of differences in the need for support to overcome fears and concerns, reinforce self-concept and assist in meeting role responsibilities, independent norms are necessary that have been generated on samples of people with similar disabilities, and therefore, similar contexts for support. Second, assessments of social support among people with disabilities must take account of the logistical problems of developing and maintaining social ties when one is ill or physically limited. In other words, the ideal assessment of social support for someone with a disability would take account of the environment in which he or she exists, and the opportunities available for social interaction. Third, it is important to recognize that some of the issues faced by people with disabilities in social relationships are very subtle problems associated with other peoples' fears, ignorance and stigmatization of disability. This adds a dimension to social relationships that is difficult to quantify or isolate, but is nonetheless a factor in the support systems of people with disabilities. Manne and Zautra (1989) discuss some of the subtle negative messages transmitted by network members to individuals with disabilities. Silver, Wortman and Crofton (1990) report that the presence of a disability elicited a certain amount of avoidance from network members, despite the apparent need for support.

Principles for Intervention

In the same way that assessment approaches must be based on an explicit theoretical approach, intervention efforts must also be carefully and consistently based on theoretical principles that explain how the intervention is expected to affect outcomes. The choice of theoretical view, based on research of people with similar disabilities to those of the population concerned, then guides a number of other decisions about how intervention should be structured. For a review of theoretical approaches to social support, see McColl (1996).

To date, interventions to improve social support have not met with unqualified success. The question remains as to whether or not this impressive resource is amenable to therapeutic manipulation. The mixed success of intervention studies leaves some doubt as to whether it is (Bowers, Clark-Mahoney, Forshee, Reiner, Schilling, & Snyder, 1987; Cwikel & Israel, 1989; Fischer et al., 1989; Friedland & McColl, 1992; Moser, Clements, Brecht & Weiner, 1993). Further, the research to date leaves many questions unanswered as to which elements of support can be used in intervention.

Besides the use of an explicit theoretical approach, a number of specific principles for remediation may be extrapolated from the research findings. First, while it appears that formal sources of support are more amenable to change than informal sources, informal sources are clearly the most influential for health outcomes (Antonucci & Jackson, 1990). The challenge, therefore, is to enhance the support-giving potential of informal sources without institutionalizing or formalizing them (Gottlieb, 1985; Lanza & Revenson, 1993). The informal nature of close supports is such that they are highly idiosyncratic and individualized. Therefore individualized intervention approaches may be necessary, such as individual, couple and family counseling, that are respectful of the unique parameters of the support relationships involved.

Second, the timing of supportive inputs has repeatedly been shown to be important. Antonucci and Jackson (1990) refer to a developmental perspective on social support, and Krahn (1993) develops the idea further, stating that individual and family development, as well as the development of a specific stressful event, all affect the perceived availability and adequacy of social support. Jacobson (1986) and Broadhead and Kaplan (1991) expand the idea of a developmental sequence for the specific stressful event. Relying on loss theory, they suggest that a stressful event has a temporal sequence of its own, and that social support must coincide with this sequence in order to be perceived as helpful. Thus the balance of emotional, instrumental and informational support must change over time to be optimally supportive and to correspond with the timetable for adjustment. Research with people with spinal cord injuries over their first year post-rehabilitation (McColl et al., 1994) shows that while coping stays remarkably constant over the year, the composition of the support system changes. The initial system is dominated by informational support, presumably from professionals, whereas the support system at one year contains more than twice as much emotional support as either of the other two types (instrumental or informational).

A number of authors have noted a further temporal phenomenon regarding social support following a stressful event, particularly a disability. At the onset, there is often an influx of support, however, as time goes on, support "wears down" (Kutner, 1987; Lanza & Revenson, 1993), or its effects "wear off" (Burton, Kline, Lindsay, & Heidenheim, 1988). Either way, support does not continue to be the same potent resource for health over the long term. The challenge for intervention then is to monitor the temporal fluctuations in the support system in such a way as to capture these changes as they begin. To do so, service providers would need to assess sources, types, structure and satisfaction with support from the perspectives of both the index individual and the key supporters. The sustainability of support may depend on the extent to which supporters' needs are assessed (Hobfoll & Stephens, 1991) and support for supporters is considered in intervention planning (Coyne, Ellard, & Smith, 1990).

A final issue of the timing of social support involves recognizing that its effects are exerted both contemporaneously and longitudinally (Antonucci & Jackson, 1990). Thus while some support has a relatively immediate effect on the recipient, other supports may have effects over a long period or at some future time. Therefore, the support offered to help with a current problem may in fact be perceived as irrelevant to the present situation, but may have an effect on some future stressor. Similarly, support exchanged in the past may exert its effect in a current stressful situation. The idea of a "support bank," as expressed by Antonucci and Jackson (1990) and described earlier, captures this idea. Supports developed as part of an intervention today thus may be believed to have both short- and long-term effects (Table 17-1).

A third important concept in the development of social support interventions is reciprocity. Reciprocity in relationships is important for everyone; several studies show the importance for outcomes not only of getting, but also of giving, social support (Anson et al., 1993; Heller et al., 1991). But as Antonucci and Jackson (1990) point out, reciprocity may be doubly important in relationships with people with disabilities. While everyone perceives an imbalance or inequity in a relationship as uncomfortable, Antonucci and

TABLE 17-1

Summary of Principles for Social Support Intervention

1. Intervention must be based on theoretical principles.
2. The need for social support has a temporal sequence.
   - Different types of support are needed at different times.
   - Support has both immediate and long-lasting effects.
   - The potency of support sometimes diminishes over time.
3. Reciprocity and balance in social relationships are important.
4. The amount of social support needed depends on the individual.

Jackson (1990) suggest that it can be downright aversive for someone with a disability. This may be a function partly of the emphasis in rehabilitation on independence. In a qualitative study of aging men with spinal cord injuries (McColl & Rosenthal, 1994), participants expressed the ultimate importance attached to independence and their abhorrence of the prospect of any increase in the need for help. Corbet (1993) too talks about the independence ethic, and its origins in the values underlying traditional rehabilitation. Schultz and associates (1987) discuss the ultimate failure of reciprocity in a relationship, when one member comes to be perceived as a burden. They found the perception that one was burdensome to others to be significantly related to depression. This fact, combined with real constraints on the ability to reciprocate in some situations, creates a potential problem of equity in relationships. The challenge to providers is to facilitate the negotiation of reciprocal relationships that are manageable and satisfying for all concerned. This may involve making the nature of reciprocity more explicit, increasing the value attached to supportive functions offered by the disabled member, or redefining relationships and roles to change the balance of reciprocity. Buunk and Hoorens (1992) refer to "support book-keeping," meaning the accounting process all of us do implicitly on who does what for whom. This process may need to become more explicit in relationships where reciprocity is a potential problem. All of these measures may be inevitably easier in family relationships, where the norms of reciprocity are usually more flexible than in friend or colleague relationships (Buunk & Hoorens, 1992; Norris et al., 1990; Antonucci & Jackson, 1990; Dakof & Taylor, 1990).

A final principle for intervention involves the quantitative parameter of support. How much new support should be fostered? The literature offers no real answers to this question, except to suggest that social support is highly variable, and that while some people with objectively vast support systems are unhappy and feel unsupported, others with only one or two contacts are highly satisfied (Cutrona, 1986). Further the literature shows us that not all relationships are supportive, some relationships can be experienced as intrinsically negative (Buunk & Hoorens, 1992; Manne & Zautra, 1989), intentionally supportive acts can sometimes be misdirected or miscarried (Coyne et al., 1990), and too much support can be stifling and undermining (Bruhn, 1991). Thus, the only apparent answer to the question of "How much?" is "However much a person wants." One solution to the ambiguity around quantity seems to be to adopt a client-centred approach to the development of support, and to attempt to achieve a perceived balance of support, as experienced by the individual.

Levels of Intervention

The principles discussed so far refer to intervention in social support at the level of specific relationships. This is probably a function of the fact that the literature on social support focusses on support exchanged in dyads. However, as Bruhn (1991) points out, intervention for social support can be conducted on a number of levels. Perhaps most often overlooked is social support intervention at the individual level. Much of the evidence discussed has not involved the objective parameters of relationships at all, but rather it has referred to an individual's perceptions of the adequacy or availability of supports. It may not be necessary for any objective changes to take place in relationships for this construct, perceived support, to be altered. Individual psychotherapy may offer individuals the opportunity to explore the nature of their relationships and their expectations and beliefs about support. Further it may offer them tactics for the development of more positive, constructive, and ultimately health-promoting perspectives on the supports given and received.

Intervention at the level of specific dyads has been discussed briefly. It usually involves efforts to renegotiate existing relationships or to broker desired relationships. A program designed for stroke survivors and their networks is an example (Friedland & McColl, 1989). However, several other interesting approaches to the development of support in dyads are described in the literature. Based on models with other populations where a common stressor is shared (e.g., AIDS, alcoholism), peer support or buddy support may have some interesting applications. Wilson and Thompson (1983) describe a program where individuals leaving rehabilitation after a spinal cord injury were paired with long-term survivors, who provided informational support, advice, and in some cases, emotional support. Despite disagreements in the literature, telephone dyads may also be worth exploring

(Heller et al., 1991). Hassett and colleagues (1993) describe a computer bulletin board for people with disabilities as a source of support for about 15% of subscribers.

Perhaps the most common intervention approach found in the literature on social support is the group approach. Groups may have a number of different functions, from mutual aid and information-sharing, such as the group described by Glennon and Smith (1990), to sharing feelings and experiences, as in the typical psychotherapy group, to teaching new skills, like assertiveness or stress management (Lanza & Revenson, 1993). Although several authors observed compelling benefits from group participation in rehabilitation (Bowers et al., 1987; Fischer et al., 1989), Lanza and Revenson (1993) counsel against assuming that the informal benefits of social support can be conveyed through a formal group process. Gottlieb (1985) notes that groups can seldom offer the intensity needed in relationships for beneficial effects to accrue. Joice, Thompson and Glynn (1990) found that support group participants were less enthusiastic about group effectiveness than the staff thought they were, and in fact, the most positive effect of the group was on staff morale.

Finally, Gonzalez and coauthors (1990) point out that social support intervention can also be offered on the community level. Through strategies like outreach, community development and other public health approaches, community resources can potentially be mobilized to foster a community that is more supportive to its members with disabilities. Grady (1995) offers strategies and challenges to occupational therapists for developing communities that are more inclusive of members with disabilities. One example of the process through which occupational therapists might become involved in capacity-building in communities is community-based rehabilitation (CBR) (Peat & Boyce, 1993). Community-based rehabilitation is defined as "a strategy within community development for rehabilitation, equalization of opportunities and social integration of people with disabilities. CBR is implemented by people with disabilities themselves, their families, communities and appropriate health, education and social services" (International Labour Organization/United Nations Educational, Scientific and Cultural Organization/World Health Organization, 1994). Although originally conceived for applications in the developing world, where traditional institutional and professional rehabilitation resources were often not readily available, the idea of CBR has captured the attention of western rehabilitators as well (Peat & Boyce, 1993; McColl & Paterson, in press). As we come to better understand the importance of community in our society (Condelucci, 1991; McKnight, 1988), the community development approach for social support may be increasingly accessible.

CONCLUSION

Although the rhetoric of rehabilitation over the past few decades has acknowledged the importance of families and support systems for rehabilitation outcomes, the reality may not match. A disturbing study by Watson (1987) showed that while rehabilitation professionals expressed a belief in the value of family participation in rehabilitation, a majority of them also held a number of notably less constructive views: families get in the way of rehabilitation, families are generally difficult to work with, families really don't understand the problems being dealt with in rehabilitation, the decision-making hierarchy should continue to favour professionals and families are expected to cooperate quietly with professionals. In other words, participation of the family and other members of the support system was valued, as long as it did not affect how rehabilitation professionals functioned. Family members and other supporters were seen strictly as reinforcers of the professional's initiatives, and whenever they departed from that role, they risked being marginalized in the rehabilitation process. This same attitude toward the support systems of consumers was recently illustrated in a letter to the editor of the *American Journal of Occupational Therapy* from a woman who is both the mother of a disabled child and an occupational therapist herself:

...when I have participated at team meetings as an occupational therapist, my opinion has been sought after and respected, yet when I have attended team meetings for my son, I have been treated as if I could not possibly understand what is best for him and should just do as I am told (Minshull, 1994).

The powerful and voluminous evidence in the literature suggests that professionals may have it backwards. Rather than being the principal agents of change in rehabilitation, professionals may be just one of an array of supporters who help people with disabilities through difficult times, at the onset of their disability and throughout their lives. To the extent that the entire support system, formal and informal, can be mobilized to provide support for people with disabilities and function in an integrated and coordinated fashion, the outcomes of occupational therapy—occupation, health and well-being—are sure to improve.

STUDY QUESTIONS

1. Define social support and identify two or three issues associated with the definition.

2. Suggest a structure for analyzing: a) an individual's support system, and b) a community's support system.

3. Compare two or three measures of social support according to the underlying aspects of support that they measure.

4. Identify the knowledge, skills, and attitudes required for an occupational therapist to assist someone to make changes in his or her support system.

5. Explain how social support relates to the model of occupational performance outlined in Chapter 3.

ACKNOWLEDGMENT

I gratefully acknowledge my three principal collaborators in research on social support: Judith Friedland, Harvey Skinner and Carolyn Rosenthal. Further, I acknowledge the financial support of National Health Research and Development Program, Health Canada; Ontario Mental Health Foundation; and Ontario Ministry of Community and Social Services.

REFERENCES

Aldwin, C. M., & Revenson, T. A. (1987). Does coping help? *Journal of Personality and Social Psychology, 53,* 337-348.

Anson, C. A., Stanwyck, D. J. & Krause, J. S. (1993). Social support and health status in spinal cord injury. *Paraplegia, 31,* 632-638.

Antonucci, T. C., & Israel, B. A. (1986). Veridicality of social support: A comparison of principal and network members' responses. *Journal of Consulting and Clinical Psychology, 54,* 432-437.

Antonucci, T. C., & Jackson, S. S. (1990). The role of reciprocity in social support. In B. R. Sarason, I. G. Sarason, & G. R. Pierce (Eds.), *Social support: An interactional view.* New York: John Wiley & Sons.

Bateson, M. C. (1990). *Composing a life.* New York: Plume.

Berkman, L. F., & Breslow, L. (1983). *Health and ways of living: Findings of the Alameda County study.* New York: Oxford University Press.

Berkman, L. F., & Syme, L. (1979). Social networks, host resistance and mortality: A follow-up study of Alameda County residents. *American Journal of Epidemiology, 109,* 186-207.

Bowers, J. E., Clark-Mahoney, J. P., Forshee, T., Reiner, A., Schilling, J. E., & Snyder, B. S. (1987). Analysis of a support group for young spinal cord-injured males. *Rehabilitation Nursing, 12,* 313-315.

Bowlby, J. (1980). *Attachment and loss* (Vol. III). *Loss: Sadness and depression.* New York: Basic Books.

Bowlby, J. (1988). Developmental psychiatry comes of age. *American Journal of Psychiatry, 145,* 1-10.

Bowling, A. (1991). Social support and social networks: Their relationship to the successful and unsuccessful survival of elderly people in the community. An analysis of concepts and a review of the evidence. *Family Practice, 8,* 68-83.

Brilihart, B. (1988). Family support for the disabled. *Rehabilitation Nursing, 13,* 316-319.

Broadhead, W. E., & Kaplan, B. H. (1991). Social support and the cancer patient: Implications for future research and clinical care. *Cancer, 67,* 794-799.

Bruhn, J. G. (1991). People need people: Perspectives on the meaning and measurement of social support. *Integrative Physiological and Behavioral Science, 26,* 325-329.

Burton, H. J., Kline, S. A., Lindsay, R. M., & Heidenheim, M. A. (1988). The role of support in influencing outcome of end-stage renal disease. *General Hospital Psychiatry, 10,* 260-266.

Buunk, B. P., & Hoorens, V. (1992). Social support and stress: The role of social comparison and social exchange processes. *British Journal of Clinical Psychology, 31,* 445-457.

Christiansen, C., & Baum, C. (1997). *Occupational therapy: Enabling function and well-being* (2nd ed.). Thorofare, NJ: SLACK Incorporated.

Cluff, C. B., & Cluff, L. E. (1983). Informal support for disabled persons: A role for religious and community organizations. *Journal of Chronic Disability, 36,* 815-820.

Cobb, S. (1974). A model for life events and their consequences. In B. S. Dohrenwend & B. P. Dohrenwend (Eds.), *Stressful life events: Their nature and consequences.* New York: John Wiley and Sons.

Cohen, S., Mermelstein, R., Kamarck, T., & Hoberman, H. M. (1985). Measuring the functional components of social support. In I. G. Sarason & B. R. Sarason (Eds.), *Social support: Theory, research and applications.* (pp. 7-94). Boston: Martinus Nijhoff.

Cohen, S., & Syme, S. C. (1985). Issues in the study and application of social support. In S. Cohen & S. C. Syme (Eds.), *Social support and health.* Orlando: Academic Press.

Cohen, S., & Wills, T. A. (1985). Stress, social support and the buffering hypothesis. *Psychological Bulletin, 98,* 310-357.

Condelucci, A. (1991). *Interdependence: The road to community.* Winter Park, FL: PMD Publishers Gr.

Corbet, B. (1993). What price independence? In G. G. Whiteneck, S. W. Charlifue, K. Gerhart, D. P. Lammertse, S. Manley, R. Menter, & R. Seedroff (Eds.), *Aging with spinal cord injury.* New York: Demos Publ.

Coyne, J. C., Ellard, J. H., & Smith, D. A. F. (1990). Social support, interdependence and the dilemmas of helping. In B. R. Sarason, I. G. Sarason, & G. R. Pierce (Eds.), *Social support: An interactional view.* New York: John Wiley & Sons.

Croog, S. H., Lipson, A., & Levine, S. (1972). Help patterns in severe illness: The roles of kin network, non-family resources, and institutions. *Journal of Marriage and the Family, 34,* 32-41.

Cutrona, C. (1986). Objective determinants of perceived social support. *Journal of Personality and Social Psychology, 50,* 349-355.

Cwikel, J. M., & Israel, B. A. (1989). Examining mechanisms of social networks: A review of health related intervention studies. *Public Health Reviews, 15,* 159-193.

Dakof, G., & Taylor, S. E. (1990). Victims' perceptions of social support: What is helpful from whom? *Journal of Personality and Social Psychology, 58,* 80-89.

Davidson, H. (1991). Performance and the social environment. In C. Christiansen & C. Baum (Eds.), *Occupational therapy: Overcoming human performance deficits.* Thorofare, NJ:

SLACK Incorporated.

Decker, S. D., & Schulz, R. (1985). Correlates of life satisfaction and depression in middle-aged and elderly spinal cord-injured persons. *American Journal of Occupational Therapy, 39,* 740-745.

DiMatteo, M. R., & Hays, R. (1981). Social support and serious illness. In B. H. Gottlieb (Ed.), *Social networks and social support* (pp. 117-148). Beverly Hills, CA: Sage.

Donald, C. A., & Ware, J. E. (1984). The measurement of social support. *Research in Community Mental Health, 4,* 325-370.

Dunkel-Schetter, C., & Bennett, T. L. (1990). Differentiating the cognitive and behavioural aspects of social support. In B. R. Sarason, I. G. Sarason, & G. R. Pierce (Eds.), *Social support: An interactional view.* New York: John Wiley & Sons.

Felton, B. J., & Berry, C. (1992). Groups as social network members: Overlooked sources of social support. *American Journal of Community Psychology, 20,* 253-261.

Fischer, S., Pallapothu, S., & Cummings, V. (1989). Over fifty support groups for patients in a rehabilitation hospital. *American Journal of Physical Medicine and Rehabilitation, 68*(1), 24-25.

Fitzpatrick, R., Newman, S., Archer, R., & Shipley, M. (1991). Social support, disability and depression: A longitudinal study of rheumatoid arthritis. *Social Science and Medicine, 33,* 605-611.

Fitzpatrick, R., Newman, S., Lamb, R., & Shipley, M. (1988). Social relationships and psychological well-being in rheumatoid arthritis. *Social Science and Medicine, 27,* 399-403.

Friedland, J., & McColl, M. A. (1987). Social support and psychosocial dysfunction after stroke: Buffering effects in a community sample. *Archives of Physical Medicine and Rehabilitation, 68,* 475-480.

Friedland, J., & McColl, M. A. (1989). Social support for stroke survivors: Development and evaluation of an intervention program. *Physical and Occupational Therapy in Geriatrics, 7*(3), 55-69.

Friedland, J,. & McColl, M. A. (1992). Social support intervention after stroke: Results of a randomized trial. *Archives of Physical Medicine and Rehabilitation, 73,* 573-581.

Glennon, T. P., & Smith, B. S. (1990). Questions asked by patients and their support groups during family conferences on inpatient rehabilitation units. *Archives of Physical Medicine and Rehabilitation, 71,* 699-702.

Gonzalez, V. M., Goeppinger, J., & Lorig, K. (1990). Four psychosocial theories and their application to patient education and clinical practice. *Arthritis Care and Research, 3*(2), 132-143.

Gottlieb, B. H. (1985). Social networks and social support: An overview of research, practice and policy implications. *Health Education Quarterly, 12,* 5-22.

Gottlieb, B. H., & Selby, P. M. (1989). *Social support and mental health: A review of the literature.* University of Guelph, Ontario, Canada.

Grady, A. (1995). Building inclusive community: A challenge for occupational therapists. *American Journal of Occupational Therapy, 49,* 300-310.

Hassett, M., Lowder, C., & Rutan, D. (1993). Use of computer network bulletin board systems by disabled persons.

Heller, L., Thompson, M. G., Trueba, P. E., Hogg, J. R., & Vlachos-Weber, I. (1991). Peer support telephone dyads for elderly women: Was this the wrong intervention? *American Journal of Community Psychology, 19,* 53-74.

Henderson, S., Duncan-Jones, P., Byrne, D. G., & Scott, R. (1980). Measuring social relationships: The interview schedule for Social Interaction. *Psychological Medicine, 10,* 723-734.

House, J. S. (1981). *Work stress and social support.* Reading, MA: Addison-Wesley.

International Labour Organization/United Nations Educational, Scientific and Cultural Organization/World Health Organization. (1994). *Community-based rehabilitation for and with people with disabilities: Joint position paper.* Geneva, Switzerland: World Health Organization.

Jacobson, D. E. (1986). Types and timing of social support. *Journal of Health and Social Behavior, 27,* 250-264.

Johnson, C. L., & Troll, L. E. (1994). Constraints and facilitators to friendships in late late life. *The Gerontologist, 34,* 79-87.

Joice, A., Thomson, M., & Glynn, A. (1990). Carers support groups: Meeting the needs of carers and staff. *British Journal of Occupational Therapy, 53,* 136-138.

Kahn, R. (1979). Aging and social support. In M. W. Riley (Ed.), *Aging from birth to death* (p. 7791). Boulder, CO: Westview Press.

Kelleher, J. P. (1925). Motivation of social interest. *Archives of Occupational Therapy, 4,* 365-371.

Kindwall, J. A., & McLean, J. (1941). One hand for the ship. *Occupational Therapy and Rehabilitation, 20,* 223-229.

Kinsella, G., Ford, B., & Moran, C. (1989). Survival of social relationships following head injury. *International Disability Studies, 11,* 9-14.

Knox, M., & Parmenter, T. R. (1993). Social networks and support mechanisms for people with mild intellectual disability in competitive employment. *International Journal of Rehabilitation, 16,* 1-12.

Kobasa, S. C. O., Spinetta, J. J., Cohen, J., Crano, W. D., Hatchett, S., Kaplan, B. H., Lansky, S. B., Prout, M. N., Ruckdeschel, J. C., Siegal, K., & Wellisch, D. K. (1991). Social environment and social support. *Cancer, 67,* 788-793.

Krahn, G. (1993). Conceptualizing social support in families of children with special health needs. *Family Process, 32,* 235-248.

Krol, B., Sanderman, R., & Suurmeijer, T. P. B. M. (1993). Social support, rheumatoid arthritis and quality of life: Concepts, measurement and research. *Patient Education and Counseling, 20,* 101-120.

Kutner, N. G. (1987). Social ties, social support, and perceived health status among chronically ill people. *Social Science and Medicine, 25,* 29-34.

Lanza, A. F., & Revenson, T. A. (1993). Social support interventions for rheumatoid arthritis patients: The cart before the horse? *Health Education Quarterly, 20*(1), 97-117.

Lehmann, D. R., Ellard, J. H., & Wortman, C. B. (1986). Social support for the bereaved: Recipients' and providers' perspectives on what is helpful. *Journal of Consulting and Clinical Psychology, 54,* 438-446.

Manne, S. L., & Zautra, A. J. (1989). Spouse criticism and support:

Their association with coping and psychological adjustment among women with rheumatoid arthritis. *Journal of Personality and Social Psychology, 56,* 608-617.

McColl, M. A. (1996). Social support, disability and rehabilitation. *Critical Reviews in Physical and Rehabilitation Medicine, 7*(4), 315-333.

McColl, M. A., Carlson, P., Johnston, J., Minnes, P., Shue, K., & Willer, B. (1996). Consumer perspectives on the definition of community integration. Paper presented at New Beginnings Conference, Canadian Head Injury Coalition, Halifax, NS.

McColl, M. A., & Friedland, J. (1989). Development of a multidimensional index for assessing social support in rehabilitation. *Occupational Therapy Journal of Research, 9,* 218-234.

McColl, M. A., & Friedland, J. (1994). Social support, aging and disability. *Topics in Geriatric Rehabilitation, 9,* 54-71.

McColl, M. A., Lei, H. & Skinner, H. A. (1994) Structural relationships between social support and coping. *Social Science and Medicine, 41,* 395-407.

McColl, M. A., & Paterson, J. (1997). Critical dimensions of community based rehabilitation. *Canadian Journal of Rehabilitation* (in press).

McColl, M. A., & Rosenthal, C. (1994) A model of resource needs of aging spinal cord injured men. *Paraplegia, 32,* 261-270.

McColl, M. A., & Skinner, H. A. (1988). Concepts and measurement of social support in a rehabilitation setting. *Canadian Journal of Rehabilitation, 2*(2), 93-107.

McColl, M. A., & Skinner, H. A. (1995). Assessing inter- and intrapersonal resources for community living. *Disability and Rehabilitation, 17,* 24-34.

McFarlane, A. H., Norman, G. R., Streiner, D. L., Roy, R., & Scott, D. J. (1980). A longitudinal study of the influence of the social environment on health status: A preliminary report. *Journal of Health and Social Behaviour, 21,* 124-133.

McKnight, J. (1988). *Beyond community service.* Evanston IL: Centre for Urban Affairs and Policy Research.

McNett, S. C. (1987). Social support, threat and coping responses and effectiveness in the functionally disabled. *Nursing Research, 36,* 98-103.

Minschull, H. (1994). Treat parents of child with special needs as members of the team (letter). *American Journal of Occupational Therapy, 48,* 951.

Moser, D. K., Clements, P. J., Brecht, M. L., & Weiner, S. R. (1993). Predictors of psychosocial adjustment in systemic sclerosis. *Arthritis and Rheumatism, 36,* 1398-1405.

Nicaise, J., Jonckers, J., Smets, P., Provost, J., & Asiel, M. (1993). Social rehabilitation of the elderly after surgical intervention. *Acta Chirurgica Belgica, 93,* 122-125.

Norbeck, J. S., Lindsey, A. M., & Carrieri, V. L. (1981). The development of an instrument to measure social support. *Nursing Research, 30,* 264-269.

Norbeck, J. S., Lindsey, A. M., & Carrieri, V. L. (1983). Further development of the Norbeck social support questionnaire: Normative data and validity testing. *Nursing Research, 32,* 49.

Norris, V. K., Stephens, M. A., & Kinney, J. K. (1990). The impact of family interactions on recovery from stroke: Help or hindrance? *The Gerontologist, 30*(4), 535-542.

O'Brien, M. T. (1993). Multiple sclerosis: The role of social support and disability. *Clinical Nursing Research, 2*(1), 67-85.

Orth-Gomer, K., Rosengren, A., & Wilhelmsen, L. (1993). Lack of social support and incidence of coronary heart disease in middle-aged Swedish men. *Psychosomatic Medicine, 55,* 3743.

Oxman, T. E., Berkman, L. F., Kasl, S., Freeman, D. H., & Barrett, J. (1992). Social support and depressive symptoms in the elderly. *American Journal of Epidemiology, 135,* 356-368.

Peat, M., & Boyce, W. (1993) Canadian community rehabilitation services: Challenges for the future. *Canadian Journal of Rehabilitation, 6,* 2819.

Procidano, M. E., & Heller, I. (1983). Measures of perceived social support from friends and from family: Three validation studies. *American Journal of Community Psychology, 11,* 124.

Sarason, I. G., Levine, H. M., Basham, R. B., & Sarason, B. R. (1983). Assessing social support: The Social Support Questionnaire. *Journal of Personality and Social Psychology, 44,* 127-139.

Sarason, B. R., Pierce, G. R., & Sarason, I. G. (1990). Social support: The sense of acceptance and the role of relationships. In I. B. Sarason, B. R. Sarason, & G. R. Pierce (Eds.), *Social support: An interactional view.* New York: Wiley.

Sarason, B. R., Pierce, G. R., & Sarason, I. G. (1990). Traditional views of social support and their impact on assessment. In I. B. Sarason, B. R. Sarason, & G. R. Pierce (Eds.), *Social support: An interactional view.* New York: Wiley.

Schaefer, C., Coyne, J. C., & Lazarus, R. S. (1981). The health-related functions of social support. *Journal of Behavioural Medicine, 4,* 381-405.

Schulz, R., & Decker, S. (1985). Long-term adjustment to physical disability: The role of social support, perceived control, and self-blame. *Journal of Personality and Social Psychology, 48,* 1162-1172.

Schulz, R., & Rau, M. T. (1985). Social support through the life course. In S. Cohen & S. L. Syme (Eds.), *Social support and health.* New York: Academic Press.

Schulz R., Tompkins, C. A., & Wood, D. (1987). The social psychology of caregiving: Physical and psychological costs of providing support to the disabled. *Journal of Applied Social Psychology, 17,* 401-428.

Silver, R. C., Wortman, C. B., & Crofton, C. (1990). The role of coping in support provision: The self-presentational dilemma of victims of life crises. In I. B. Sarason, B. R. Sarason, & G. R. Pierce (Eds.), *Social support: An interactional view.* New York: Wiley.

Stoller, E. P., & Pugliesi, K. L. (1988) Informal networks of community-based elderly. *Research on Aging, 10,* 499-516.

Taal, E., Rasker, J. J., Seydel, E. R., & Wiegman, O. (1993). Health status, adherence with health recommendations, self-efficacy and social support in patients with rheumatoid arthritis. *Patient Education and Counseling, 20,* 63-76.

Thoits, P. A. (1985). Social support and psychological well-being: Theoretical possibilities. In B. R. Sarason & I. G. Sarason (Eds.), *Social support: Theory, research and applications.* Boston: Martinus Nijhoff.

Tilden, V. P., & Weinert, C. (1987). Social support and the chronically ill individual. *Nursing Clinics of North America, 22,* 613-620.

Turner, R. J., Frankel, B. G., & Levin, D. M. (1983). Social support: Conceptualization, measurement and implications for mental health. *Research in Community Mental Health, 3,* 67-111.

Watson, P. G. (1987). Family participation in the rehabilitation process: The rehabilitators' perspective. *Rehabilitation Nursing, 12*(2), 70-73.

Weinberger, M., Tierney, W. M., Booher, P., & Hiner, S. L. (1990). Social support, stress and functional status in patients with osteoarthritis. *Social Science and Medicine, 30,* 503-508.

Wilson, W. C., & Thompson, D. D. (1983). The Virginia communi-ty cadre: Community reintegration of persons with spinal cord injuries. *Rehabilitation Literature, 44,* 19-23.

Wineman, N. M. (1990). Adaptation to multiple sclerosis: The role of social support, functional disability, and perceived uncertain-ty. *Nursing Research, 39,* 294-299.

Wortman, C. B. (1984). Social support and the cancer patient: Conceptual and methodological issues. *Cancer, 53,* 239-260.

Wortman, C. B., & Conway, T. L. (1985). The role of social support in adaptation and recovery from physical illness. In S. Cohen & S. L. Syme (Eds.), *Social support and health.* New York: Academic Press.

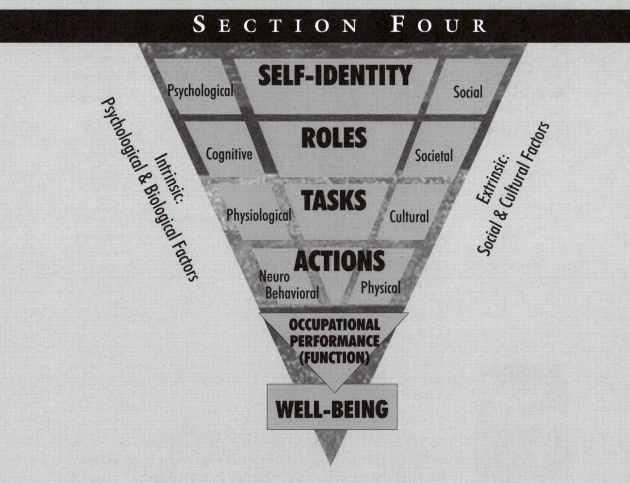

Interventions:
Achieving Function and
Well-Being Through
Occupation

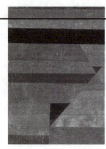

Chapter Content Outline

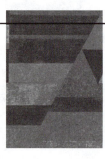

Abstract

Why and how do we choose our occupations? There is a process of human development in which the societal values learned by the child are expressed in occupational participation. The mechanism of this process is described in this chapter. The fit of this process within models of occupation which have been developed by theorists in occupational therapy is proposed. The underpinnings of this process in terms of major theories of psychological development and action are described.

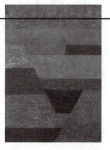

Key Terms

Occupational competence

Affordance

Effectancy

Ability

Self-efficacy

Self-actualization

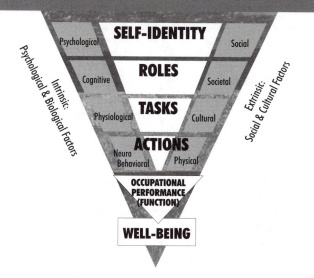

Occupational Competence Across the Life Span

Leonard N. Matheson, PhD, Paula C. Bohr, PhD, OTR, FAOTA

OBJECTIVES

The information in this chapter is intended to help the reader:

1. understand the interacting effect of the individual's abilities, the role's demands, and the environment's affordances and limitations on the development of occupational competence

2. understand the mechanism of the development of occupational competence

3. appreciate the importance of societal values in shaping the occupational development of the individual

4. identify major developmental theorists and aspects of their theories which pertain to the development of occupational competence

5. apply the concepts of occupational competence to the study of the disability experience and ways in which therapists can provide appropriate intervention.

"As long as the environment remains safe and adaptation enables him or her to ignore it, the person's purpose will continue to compete with bodily demands for change and variation."

Paul Branton, 1972

INTRODUCTION

Philosophically, occupational therapists have conceived of humans as social beings who define themselves in terms of our occupations, "the use that we make of ourselves" (Meyer, 1922 p. 5). In recent years, theorists in this discipline have constructed models which describe systems of occupational behavior and performance which are multifaceted, ecological and dynamic (e.g.. Kielhofner, 1985; Dunn, et al, 1994; Law, et al, 1996; Christiansen & Baum, 1997). In recent years, other models of change and development in occupational behavior and occupational performance across the life span (e.g.. Coster, 1995a & 1995b; Llorens, 1991) have been proposed. Thus far, however, no unifying theory or model which focuses on the mechanisms of the life span development of occupational behavior or performance has been proposed. In this chapter a new model of development which is based on the earlier work of many theorists and researchers from diverse fields will be presented. The "occupational competence model of human development" describes a mechanism of life span occupational development which addresses the question: "At any particular point in life, why do people participate in certain occupational activities?" This is a corollary to the unanswered question posed by Birren and Birren (1990, p. 15): "How does behavior become organized over time?" Scientists describe such a basic question as involving a "first principle" (Reilly, 1962), something that is fundamental and irreducible. In this chapter, the authors present a first principle of occupational therapy: People do occupational activity in order to develop role competence. This extends the perspective of developmental psychology which considers "the environmental context of the individual as well as the individual's historical background and adaptive strategies" (Birren & Birren, 1990, p. 16) to include occupational role as an organizing focus in people's lives. Further, the occupational competence model of human development describes the need people feel to develop role competence as the fundamental reason people look for and accept the challenges that are part of their roles; why the person with a poorly defined role is uncomfortable; and why people feel sad, frightened and angry when they lose their ability to fulfill their roles as a consequence of injury or illness.

Another question which the occupational competence model can address is: "Why does a person become an occupational therapist?" There are many important reasons to become an occupational therapist that have to do with values, goals and dreams which are unique to each of us. The occupational competence model suggests that becoming an occupational therapist provides you with what you believe is the best opportunity to meet the need that you have to develop and maintain competence as an adult in society. This hypothesis is based on what Robert W. White (1971) describes as the "urge towards competence," a basic part of human nature which is applicable to us all. White's concept holds that the motivation to acquire the substantial number of skills required to competently perform a societal role cannot be explained through motivational theories that are based on drive reduction or the resolution of childhood conflicts. That is, you are not developing competence as an occupational therapist simply to reduce hunger or fear or to prove something to your parents, but to have a sense of yourself as a competent person. Christiansen (1991, p. 20) reports that "there is considerable agreement that the single characteristic of the individual which has the greatest influence on performance is one's sense of competence."

White proposes that competence should be considered an intrinsic need. He describes competence as having to do with "an organism's capacity to interact effectively with its environment" (1959, p. 297). He defines competence as being "sufficient or adequate to meet the demands of a situation or task" (1971, p. 273). White points out that all infant animals naturally explore their environments. Describing infant behavior once his or her basic needs have been met as being primarily exploratory, White argues that the opportunity to experience novelty and the obvious challenge that such an experience entails is so strongly sought by the infant that it suggests a primary drive. The healthy and content infant who is not asleep is most satisfied when she is engaged in exploring her environment through play activity. Exploratory behavior is strongly motivated and is both self-reinforcing and necessary for survival. There seems to be a need for engagement in activity.

White (1974) describes the basic drives for exploration, activity and manipulation as being a response to a primary motivation for competence. He argues that humans do more than simply maintain themselves, but exhibit growth behavior in terms of an increase of autonomy and what Angyal described as "a characteristic tendency toward self-determination" (in White, 1959, p. 324). Others have described this as a "need for competence" (Harter, 1978), "personal causation" (De Charms, 1968, Bandura & Schunk, 1981, and Oakley, et al, 1985, Kielhofner, et al, 1995), "emergent interactive agency" (Bandura, 1989) or "self-determination" (Deci and Ryan, 1985). In the occupational therapy literature, Clark, et al (1991, p. 303) also recognize the motivational importance of competence such that "occupation is fired by the human system's drive for efficacy and competence."

A key precept of the field of occupational therapy is that the development of competence is based on "the experience of

Bibliographic citation of this chapter: Matheson, L. & Bohr, P. (1997). Occupational competence across the life span. In C. Christiansen & C. Baum (Eds.), *Occupational therapy: Enabling function and well-being* (2nd ed.). Thorofare, NJ: SLACK Incorporated.

occupation or doing...by learning skills and strategies necessary for coping with problems and adapting to limitations" (Christiansen, 1991, p. 9) in the interplay between the person, his or her roles and the environment (Baum & Christiansen, 1996; Law, et al, 1996). As noted by Dunn, Brown and McGuigan (1994, p. 595), "Occupational therapy is interested in the interrelationship of humans and their contexts and the effect of these contexts on performance." The occupational competence model emphasizes a person-centered ecological approach to rehabilitation. In this model, adaptation is based on the person's striving toward acceptable compromise with the environment (White, 1974) to optimize occupational role function (Baum, 1991). It is important to recognize that the occupational competence model represents a continuous dynamical system, a concept from Chaos Theory in which there is an ongoing interaction between the person, his or her roles, and the environment. The person has values and goals, the roles have demands, and the environment has threats and affordances. In this model, the individual's role functions as an "attractor state" (Peak & Frame, 1994, p. 131) which describes a factor tending to impose structure on a continuous dynamical system. The person orchestrates an "adaptive compromise" (White, 1974, p. 54) with environmental and role demands. The term we propose to describe this constant process is "negotiation." Just as the person in the role of the long-distance runner negotiates with symptoms experienced early in a race by adjusting her stride length, pace or breathing pattern, so must all individuals adapt by negotiating with their environments in order to be optimally competent in their roles. The runner neither ignores nor capitulates to her symptoms, because to do either would result in performance that is less than optimally competent. To the degree that her ongoing and dynamic negotiation is successful, she will fully utilize her capacity to perform as a runner. In many ways, her ability to adapt in this negotiative manner determines her ultimate display of capacity.

This first principle (that people do occupational activity in order to develop role competence) is important because it helps to explain not only our behavior but the behavior of the people we want to help. Further, studying this as a developmental theory is important because it helps to explain the patterns of development which people display as they adapt to diminutional changes with advanced age, a process which may mimic the response to impairment of persons at all ages. Finally, rather than describe a developmental system which has discrete stages, the patterns of development in the occupational competence model are dynamic, described as "triadic reciprocal causation" (Bandura, 1989, p. 1175), based on interaction between the person, his or her role demands and the environment.

This chapter addresses the ethology of persons as occupational beings, which goes beyond description and attempts to explain *why* and *how* occupational behavior develops across the life span. Ethology, which is the systematic study of the formation of character, is fundamental to the study of the development of occupational behavior because it deals with the core characteristics of being human. One of our most important core characteristics is that we are social animals. We exist in societies, which are cohesive groups of people who share common goals, values, purposes and ways of looking at the world. In society we occupy at least one role, to do something which contributes to our society's survival. Society rewards us for fulfilling our role. In fact, society guided us to that role because society had a need to have someone fulfill our role. Societal roles are the media through which society channels our urge toward competence. Thus, our development occurs, guided by societal needs. As we begin a new role, the demands of the role present challenges which we seek because of our urge towards competence. If we are successful in meeting that challenge, we grow; we experience occupational development. To the degree that we are acculturated or fully included in our society, we are in tune with our society's needs. We are in a position to optimally fulfill this role and will be rewarded by society. Conversely, to the degree that we are alienated from our society, we are unable to meet our society's needs and will struggle to fulfill our role. Society will not only not reward us, but may punish us for attempting to maintain competence for a role that either is irrelevant or is threatening to society. Nevertheless, we continue to develop our abilities to perform our role because we have a need to maintain role competence because doing is fundamental to being.

The focus of this chapter will be on the adaptations of the person in response to the press of both the social role and the environment. This chapter will not study the development of the role and environment, although it must be recognized that both role and environment also change over time and are worthy of study. The rapidity of change in the person is on a scale to which humans can easily relate. The pace of change in roles and environment is much slower and requires a longer historical perspective and is beyond this chapter's scope.

This chapter explores what happens when our occupational involvement is disrupted by illness or injury. White (1974, p. 52) regards the human as a system. He points out that a living system tends to do more than merely maintain itself as intact as possible and display "extensive re-balancing processes when injured or deformed." The person who is injured wants to not only recover but wants to continue to grow. The person who has become occupationally disabled usually experiences a sense of loss because the roles which provided an opportunity to develop competence and meet valued goals cannot be fulfilled. The experience of loss focuses on diminished ability to meet the person's perception of the role performance expectations from society, including family, friends, employers and caregivers. This concern is expressed, often with much anguish, as "What will I do?!" When this occurs, there is a strong urge to develop new means to reassert role competence, although this will have to be accomplished with less capacity than before the disability occurred. If an existing role is not able to be resumed, attempts will be made to adapt the role. If adaptation is not possible or is not adequate to allow the person to maintain competence, the urge toward competence will lead the person to begin a new role that he or she believes to be feasible. Some people are overwhelmed by this challenge and become helpless and depressed, while others assume the patient role (Mechanic, 1962; Pilowski, 1987; Matheson, 1991). Some people respond by developing vigorous and exciting new roles to meet society's needs in creative ways. This chapter examines the reasons why people develop these various responses. An understanding of these dynamics will set the stage for our attempts as therapists to provide effective and valued assistance.

OCCUPATIONAL COMPETENCE

The occupational competence model of human development describes how individuals adapt to changing capacities and assimilate new roles across the life span and how that development influences behavior. The model uses some terms which may be familiar, but are formally defined in Table 18-1.

In this chapter, "occupation" is the term used to denote the activities in which people are engaged to support their roles. "Competence" is the term used to denote the ability to interact effectively with the environment while maintaining individuality and growth (White, 1960), performing the occupational tasks which are essential to these roles. Occupational competence is based on the individual's successful performance of tasks which support the type and level of activity that is necessary to meet socioculturally defined role demands. The occupational competence of the individual is achieved by occupational performance, which is, in turn, a consequence of occupational behavior. Thus, the purpose of occupational behavior is to maintain occupational competence in response to role demands.

A corollary to the occupational competence model is that occupational behavior develops over the life span in the service of occupational performance in order to maintain role competence. An occupational behavior which produces a particular outcome at a young age may not produce the same outcome at a later age because time-linked changes in the person or in the environment may have improved or diminished the individual's ability to perform that task or the degree to which the environment is supportive of task per-

formance. The research literature indicates that, with advancing age, adults are generally able to maintain productivity (Salthouse & Maurer, 1996). The worker who is performing a demanding job will do this work in different ways as his or her physical abilities (Nygård et al., 1991) and cognitive abilities (Schaie, 1996) change with age. In order to achieve the same occupational performance at a later age, the individual copes with these changes by constantly adjusting his or her behavior (Lazarus & Folkman, 1984). In this way, occupational behavior is dynamically linked to development of the biological, psychological and sociocultural aspects of the individual across the life span, when these are taken within the context of his or her role demands.

The occupational competence model of human development emphasizes the ecological nature of occupational performance which inextricably links the person and the environment, specifically through the role challenges that the environment provides (Oborne et al., 1993). This developmental perspective considers the person in terms of goals, abilities, effectancies and environmental affordances. The occupational competence model hypothesizes that development occurs in response to societally mediated role challenges presented to the individual. Occupational competence does not develop automatically as a consequence of the development of capacity, but is developed within the context of the individual's capacity as a consequence of motivation to maintain his or her role. Instrumentally, occupational competence is developed in response to the stimulus of task challenges posed by role demands and anticipated role demands (Branton, 1987). The adaptive response to the task challenge is characterized by gaining knowledge about environmental affordances, acquiring skills, and developing of effectancies which are pertinent to each.

Occupational competence is tied to individual roles and varies as the demands of the role vary, usually in a gradual and dependable developmental progression. As the individual matures and ages, various roles are undertaken, each composed of numerous demands which pose varying levels and types of challenge to the person. To the degree that the individual is able to meet the role demands, he or she becomes occupationally competent. The development of occupational competence follows a progression across the life span and is influenced by factors which are common across the species without regard to culture or society, such as changes in physical and cognitive capacity. Occupational development occurs in the individual's quest to establish and maintain occupational competence in systematic patterns of behavioral response to culturally determined role-based challenges which typically are referred to as "growth and development" in the early years and as "aging" in the later years.

Conceptual Basis of Occupational Competence

Occupational competence is based on five related concepts which must be explicated: capacity; effectance; affordance; competence; and self-efficacy.

Capacity

Capacity refers to the current potential of the individual to perform tasks. In childhood, capacity is based on the infant's physiological development. Individuals can be thought of as "open systems" (Von Bertalanfy, 1968) composed of numerous physiological, psychological and sociocultural subsystems which support occupational performance. While each subsystem has its own capacity, occupational competence is a consequence of their complementary effect. This calculus of occupational competence can be described as occurring in time so that the combined effects of these system changes allow patterned changes in what people do. As the individual matures, his or her capacities change in a manner which is unique to each subsystem and which has similarity across individuals. This age-based linkage of the various systems has been described as a "clock shop" (Schroots & Birren, 1990) in that the systems seem to age independently but have a finite life span. In old age, the systems begin to "run down" at a rate which has some modest degree of correlation within the individual. Similarity across individuals is guaranteed by the common genetic pool which members of the species share. Similarity is substantially affected by cultural differences, roughly in correspondence to the degree that the natural development of the subsystem depends on cultural influences. Capacity puts a ceiling on the range and magnitude of abilities people can develop. As people age, some abilities diminish as a consequence of changes in capacity and by changes in the availability of opportunities to develop abilities based on the acquisition of skills and knowledge. This process of adaptation is driven by the urge to be competent in life roles. Thus, withdrawal or retirement from life roles with advancing age may not merely reflect, but may presage, diminished ability.

Effectance

Effectance refers to the individual's extent and focus of capacity which is pertinent to the task challenges posed by role demands. Effectancy is differentiated from capacity as the child develops skills; skill to reach, skill to walk, skill to communicate. Effectance can be developed up to the individual's capacity given sufficient effort, motivation and skill development. Competence is task-based. Competence is differentiated from effectance through the application of effort. As the child is faced with a task for which she has the necessary effectancy, she can demonstrate competence to achieve

---

TABLE 18-1
Definitions

Accommodation: The process whereby the organization of information within a schema must be revised or altered due to the inability to fit new information into any existing mental category.

Adaptation: The satisfactory adjustment of individuals within their environment over time. Successful adaptation equates with quality of life.

Affordance: Anything which the environment can offer the individual which is pertinent to the role challenge and can facilitate role competence.

Assimilation: The expansion of data within a given category or sub-category of a schema by incorporation of new information within the existing representational structure without requiring any reorganization or modification of prior knowledge.

Capacity: The immediate potential of the individual to perform tasks which support occupational performance.

Competence: The ability to interact effectively with the environment while maintaining individuality and growth (White, 1960).

Effectance: The sub-set of the individual's abilities pertinent to the task challenges posed by role demands.

Ethology: The systematic study of the formation of the core characteristics of being human.

Mastery: The achievement of skill to a criterion level of success.

Occupation: Engagement in activities, tasks, and roles for the purpose of productive pursuit, maintaining oneself in the environment, and for purposes of relaxation, entertainment, creativity, and celebration; activities in which people are engaged to support their roles.

Occupational behavior: The set of responses which allow the individual to maintain role competence.

Occupational development: The systematic progression of change which occurs across the life span in response to an individual's role-based challenges.

Role competence. Achievement of the behaviors which have some socially agreed-upon function and for which there is an accepted code of norms.

Self-efficacy: The feelings that people have about their ability to be successful in using a particular coping strategy or problem-solving approach.

---

mastery if she chooses to expend effort. Without the effort, effectance can be inherent, but competence cannot be demonstrated. Effectance and ability are similar, but not identical.

Effectance is the subset of the individual's abilities which are relevant to role demands. For example, the individual in the student role develops effectancies for that role which are not pertinent to some of the student's other roles as sister, aunt or daughter. After graduation, if the role which replaces the student role does not require these "student" effectancies, they continue to exist as abilities, but, because the are not necessary to meet a role challenge (to maintain occupational competence as a student), they lie fallow and may degrade. Effectancies develop as a consequence of successful participation in meaningful activities which challenge the individual's perception of competence. White argues that the motivational aspect of competence is a consequence of an "effectance urge" which begins in childhood. He reports that "the effectance urge represents what the neuromuscular system wants to do when it is otherwise unoccupied or is gently stimulated by the environment...effectance motivation is persistent in the sense that it regularly occupies the spare waking time between episodes of homeostatic crisis" (1959, p. 321).

Affordance

Affordances are based on what the environment can offer the individual which is pertinent to the role challenge. Environmental affordances are intertwined with the individual's effectancies. Effectancies can be considered innate in the individual and have a genetic basis, while environmental affordances can be considered innate in the environment and have a psychological basis. In fact, environmental affordances do not exist outside of the relationship between the person and the environment, based on the person's psychological appraisal of the environment. Gibson's (1979) concept of ecological physics held that affordances are properties of the environment that can only be identified with reference to the observer. They reflect the functional link between the environment and the individual. For example, a pencil can exist physically, but will not become an affordance until it has psychological reality in the service of an individual's application of effectancies to meet role demands. A sharp pencil can provide environmental affordances which may be limited to spearing small fish for the non-literate native hunter. Alternately, it may be used to create an artistic masterpiece in the hands of an individual who has the effectancies to fulfill the role of artist, such as Shakespeare or Mozart. These masters would not perceive the sharp pencil as an effective hunting instrument, just as the hunter would not perceive it as an implement for communication. Gibson coined the term "direct perception" to signify how an affordance enters awareness. Direct perception is immediate and sensory dependent, without cognitive interpretation. This is a necessary characteristic of affordance in that competence often is demonstrated as rapidly emitted habit-based behavior which would be critically slowed by cognitive interpretation. People learn about affordances by using them. Once learned, they can be used by the person without the need for cognitive interpretation. Put another way, the direct perception of an affordance depends on the individual's experience of doing in which the affordance was found to be useful. As Flach, et al (1995) report, "A direct perceptual system resolves ambiguities through acting on the environment by looking, touching, and manipulating ..." (p. 9).

Affordances and effectancies work in a supplemental manner to support the individual's effort to perform tasks competently. A two-dimensional model of effectance and affordance will illustrate this concept. In Figure 18-1, the supplementary relationship between effectance and affordance is described. This graphic describes the necessity for the individual to supplement one for the other in order to develop competence. The occupational competence model holds that each person configures the match of effectancies and affordances to perform role tasks with optimal self-perceived efficiency. Conceptually, the urge toward competence provides the motivation to facilitate growth out of the experience of overwhelm by explorational activities in both effectancies and affordances. Given successful exploration that is sustained, competence develops. As task competence aggregates, role competence occurs. Because role demands are variable, at any given time the individual is likely to have areas in which there is more than adequate task competence. This leads to the opportunity for occupational actualization of the individual and expansion of the role. Throughout life, the healthy individual constantly mixes personal and environmental resources to achieve role competence. In order to maintain role competence, the individual develops excess resources which are not implemented unless called upon but are perceived by the individual to be available to go beyond insuring role maintenance to further role development in a manner that reflects his or her personal goals and values.

Growth occurs when the combined effects of affordance and effectance are inadequate to the role demands and the individual's self-efficacy beliefs allow the urge toward competence to be expressed. The experience of overwhelm occurs when the individual's self-efficacy beliefs are poor. One means of responding to overwhelm is to become depressed and emotionally insulated from the role challenge. Another means of responding to overwhelm is to become alienated from the society which has posed the role demand. Alternately, the individual can be moved out of overwhelm by therapeutic intervention through independent increases in either affordance or effectance or through a combination of both. From overwhelm, improvement in affordance leads to environmental dependence. In contrast, improvement in effectance leads to self-adaptive survival in which the individual often is isolated and fragile. Movement to self-efficacy sustaining growth occurs when both affordance and effectance are improved and exploration occurs.

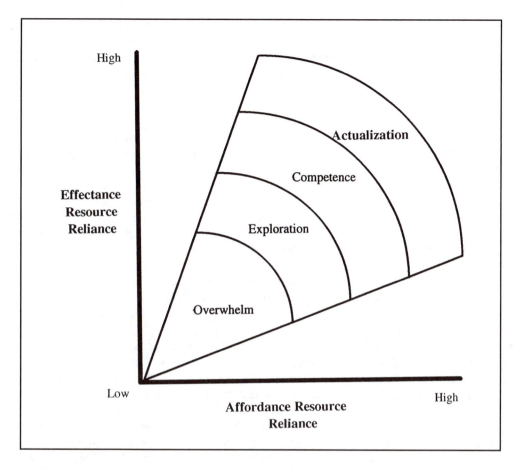

Figure 18-1. Occupational competence results from the supplemental integration of effectancies and affordances, stimulated by the urge towards competence.

Competence

Competence is a process of mind (Bateson, 1979) in which effectancies and affordances constantly must be marshaled to manage changing role demands. Faced with a role which is challenging and valued, the individual exhibits exploratory behavior in order to begin to develop task competence. Task competence is based on the adaptation of existing abilities and the development of new effectancies, applied in concert with pertinent affordances. As task competence is achieved, additional role-tasks are accepted as challenges. The individual's successful application of effectancies, displayed in occupational behavior, using the environmental affordances, results in task competence. As task competencies are aggregated, occupational role competence develops. This process begins in early childhood. It is seen in play behavior as the child pretends to undertake a role task for which he or she does not yet have the capacity. The mimicry of adult occupational role behavior is an expression of the urge toward competence and provides a valuable opportunity for the culture to direct the child's growth.

In response to a challenging role, if the occupational outcome of the behavior is judged by the individual to be successful, awareness of competence results. Awareness of occupational competence is a cognitive phenomenon, measured in terms of a standard of performance held by the individual. This prototype is role-specific so that performance in the role is compared to some standard of performance held by the individual for that role. For example, the piano student who begins study with a master soon integrates the master's standards as his own. He strives to achieve this new personal prototype. At some point in the student's development, it will become apparent that the student's capacity is greater or lesser than the master's. At this point, the student may begin to shift his prototype to conform to actual capacity. If the shift does not occur, a mismatch will leave the student stunted or frustrated because the urge toward competence cannot be fully expressed.

The competence prototype is also important in the preservation of competence in the face of diminishing capacity (Frey & Ruble, 1990). This can be seen clearly in aging athletes. Some aging athletes adapt to diminution of effectancies by shifting their field of play to "seniors" or "masters" events and continue to experience success as they are able to express competence in this new context. Other aging athletes continue to compete in their usual and customary roles and experience frustration as their effectancies are mismatched to these role demands. The occupational competence model of development predicts that the former athletes would be more satisfied and better adjusted than the latter.

Self-Efficacy

Self-efficacy is a cornerstone of healthy adulthood. Albert Bandura (1977) points out that self-efficacy is based on the person's perception of competence and that these self-perceptions affect psychosocial function. Individuals' perceptions of their abilities affect how they behave, their level of motivation, thought processes, and emotional reactions to challenging circumstances. Bandura argues that self-efficacy assists in the development of competence through its effect on the individual's appraisal of specific task challenges as: 1) being within the individual's ability so that mastery may be attempted, and 2) through its effect on perseverance to meet the challenge and overcome obstacles to the initial application of effectancies.

Self-efficacy affects the degree to which the individual perceives that he or she has the effectance to successfully address a challenge. Self-efficacy is concerned with judgments about how well one can organize effectancies and affordances to meet task role challenges which present risk. Without adequate self-efficacy, the individual will not attempt to meet the challenge or may capitulate without having persevered to the extent required to overcome the challenge. Self-efficacy beliefs make it more likely that the individual will attempt to overcome a particular task or role challenge and will increase perseverance in the face of initial performance failure, so that competence can be achieved. In addition, self-efficacy beliefs facilitate exploration in new areas of task role performance. In this way, task competence becomes generalized to the role.

For example, Tanya, a gymnast who, at age 14, experienced a below-the-elbow amputation returned to her sport to attempt floor exercise routines with a prosthesis because she had the self-efficacy to perceive that she had the combination of effectancies and affordances to be successful in that event. She refrains from attempting the balance beam because her self-efficacy does not extend to that task. Without regard to whether or not she is able to perform in the floor exercises or on the balance beam, her self-efficacy guided her to attempt one and to forego the other. Given success in the floor exercises, Tanya may eventually attempt the balance beam.

Self-efficacy is an important consequence of the individual's demonstrated competence in the performance of tasks that are meaningful. The value of the task and the individual's appreciation of the adequacy of his or her response are necessary for self-efficacy to occur. In Tanya's situation, her ability to value her success in the floor exercises was crucial. If she demonstrated the ability to perform the floor exercises at a level which she did not value, there would have been no improvement in her self-efficacy.

Dynamic Interaction of Resources

Effectancies, affordances, competence and self-efficacy are unique to the interface of the individual, his or her environment and his role challenges. Actor Christopher Reeve experienced a C3-4 spinal cord injury in 1995 and became quadriplegic. In addition to having access to all of the necessary medical care and rehabilitation, he received excellent support from his family, friends and colleagues. Most needs that were identified were met. As a consequence, Mr. Reeve quickly re-established himself as a public figure and resumed his career as an actor within his functional capacity, relying on his vocal and intellectual capacities. This is a good example of an environment which was responsive. It had affordances which could be perceived by Mr. Reeve which he used to develop new effectancies based on his residual capacities which were, in turn, pertinent to the tasks which comprised his new role as a voice actor. Mr. Reeve demonstrated what Bandura (1990) describes as "reciprocal causation...when people believe the environment is controllable on matters of import to them, they are strongly motivated to exercise fully their personal efficacy, which enhances the likelihood of success" (p. 338).

In contrast to a responsive environment, an environment which is non-responsive to the person's goals can lead to "learned helplessness" (Peterson, Maier and Seligman, 1993) which can cause depression. Peter Jones (a real person with a fictitious name) was 15 years old when he suffered a C5-6 spinal cord injury during a high school football game and became quadriplegic. Although Peter had all of the necessary medical care and rehabilitation, and received excellent support from his family and friends, he became depressed, withdrawn and suicidal. From his point of view, the assistance he was offered was not pertinent to his goals of being a football player and high school student once again and he had no other goals to pursue. Even though the resources were virtually the same as those offered to Mr. Reeve, because Peter could not identify a role in which he might be able to demonstrate competence, he did not utilize the resources. An important difference between the experience of these two people was that Mr. Reeve perceived that he had occupational roles which he could resume, given the utility of the affordances to catalyze and make useful his residual effectancies. Peter did not perceive that he had such roles to which he could return. After a few years of emotional turmoil, Peter was introduced to a mouth-stick artist who suggested to him that he try to express himself in that medium. Although quite reluctant, he made the attempt and found it to be a meaningful challenge which he was capable of addressing. At that point in time, he began to make use of many of the environmental affordances he previously had ignored. As he developed skill as an artist, he developed self-efficacy which extended beyond his skills with a mouth stick. He became actively involved with his family once again and returned to school, taking classes in art at a community college. He gradually resumed roles which were typical of other young men, including that of husband and father. None of the roles which Peter attempted were easy for him. All were so challenging that he could not have been successful without the availability of significant environmental affordances which were implemented by his effectancies, orchestrated by his self-efficacy and driven by his urge to regain sociocultural role competence. The occupational competence model predicts that this dynamic person-centered catalysis will be similar for all people who take on new and challenging roles after experiencing a disability; it was only the types of effectancies, affordances and roles which were different for Mr. Reeve and for Peter.

Human Nature, Motivation and Societal Structure

As noted above, occupational competence does not develop haphazardly, but in response to challenges based on role demands. The occupational competence model hypothesizes that the urge toward the competent fulfillment of role demands is a primary human motive. Competence is based on the application of effectancies in successful transactions with the environment, using the environmental affordances and overcoming the challenges presented by the individual's sociocultural role. Figure 18-2 describes the dynamic nature of these relationships.

The occupational competence model describes the growth of competence as occurring in response to role demands based on three dynamically interacting components: person, role and environment. This growth is compelling and urgent, demanded of the person by the person's valuation of the role. If the demand is too great, overwhelm can occur and lead to decompensation and death. If the demand is not sufficient or the role not highly valued, a lower level of effort will be expended, increasing the likelihood that competence will not result. In terms of dynamical systems theory, growth of competence is equivalent to "hunting at the edge of chaos" which Hancock and Chignell (1995, p. 41) argue "allows the most thorough exploration of the possibilities that the landscape presents and represents the epitome of adaptability." Occupational competence occurs at the interface between the individual, his or her role demands and the pertinent environment. Ability reflects the individual's capacity to take advantage of environmental affordances. Effectance is based on the individual's physical and psychological capacities as they relate to role demands. Environmental affordances are a subset of the capacity of the environment to provide support for the individual. The subset is delimited by the individual's effectancies as he or she strives to meet role demands. The individual is challenged by

role demands and applies effectancies to environmental affordances in order to meet these demands. Thus, one aspect of the individual's effectance is his or her ability to perceive and acknowledge environmental affordances. The person who is optimally occupationally competent achieves that level of performance through a mix of effectance that is pertinent to the task roles and affordances that are useful in support of his or her effectance.

Occupational competence will be sustained when the demands that have been successfully met are perceived as part of the role, the abilities, effectancies and affordances are perceived as adequate, and the role is meaningful and valued. For example, the single African American mother of three who is living in low-income housing learns computer skills which she hopes will allow her to transition from her present living situation. If her culture does not value her skills or will not acknowledge her attempt to improve herself, she may begin to devalue her achievement and competence in her new work role. The individual's valuing of role competence is greatly influenced by sociocultural factors. Such devaluing has been demonstrated in studies of competence development in school children. Veroff (1969) reports that children begin with standards of competence that are dependent on their own performance in manipulating their environments early in life but, during school years, begin to shift to social standards. Phillips and Zimmerman (1990) studied perceived competence in children grades three through nine who were identified as being above average in academic achievement. Proportionally more girls than boys had high perceived competence in the third grade; this was balanced in the fifth grade and offset in favor of boys in the ninth grade. For the children who perceived themselves as having low competence, the age shift was much more stark. The third grade and fifth grade found an equal number of boys and girls in this group. In the ninth grade, all of the children with low perceived competence were girls. This is all the more striking when we recall that all of these children were above average in academic achievement. Perhaps the most suggestive finding in this study focused on sex-role identity, in which children with feminine sex-role identities more often had low perceived competence than children with masculine or androgynous identities.

The development of occupational competence is guided by self-efficacy beliefs. The successful performance of occupational tasks results in increased self-efficacy to the extent that the task is meaningful to, and valued by, the person. Valuing is a process that is dependent on society and cultural learning that occurs as society provides approbation or disgust in response to the individual's occupational role performance.

Links between behavior, society and the evolution of species have been widely discussed (e.g., Bronfenbrenner, 1977 and Wilson, 1978). In human society, because of the dependence of self-efficacy beliefs on values, they are crucial

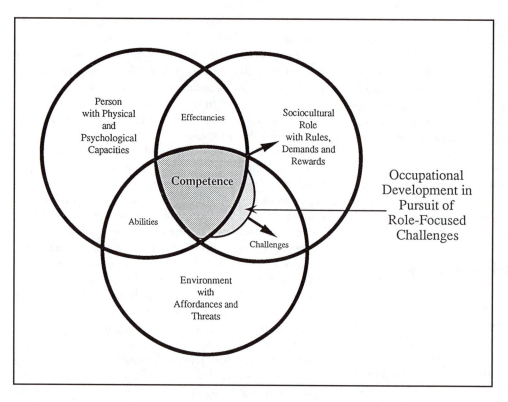

to the community's ability to guide the individual's competence striving to tasks which are important to the community. Thus, altruism and self-sacrifice, both types of behavior which threaten the individual but are important to preserve the community, are found among other occupational behaviors that preserve the individual. Although these behaviors are threatening to the individual's survival, if they are necessary to the community's survival, they must be displayed by members of the community in appropriate roles. The degree to which the individual species member is acculturated will determine the extent to which the individual will adopt the societal value of sacrifice to sustain the species. Examples abound, such as the parent working late to provide for his or her family, the fireman entering a burning building to save a child, or the soldier who risks injury to contribute to society's defense. Acculturation leads to a repertoire of behaviors which includes sacrifice and altruism. In contrast, cultural alienation leads to decreased sacrifice and to selfishness. Occupational competence is the medium through which the individual's behaviors are channeled by social conventions to meet the needs of the community. For the species, the ability of the individual to sacrifice ensures its survival. That such altruistic behavior is more highly valued than individual survival points to the ideal of cultural competence. Healthy cultures value and reward "heroic" behavior which supports the ability of the culture to compete and survive. Altruistic behavior is one expression of occupational competence. Society often requires individual sacrifice for the greater good of

other members and for the good of society as a whole. This was evident just before Christmas, 1995, when United States soldiers shipped out to Bosnia Herzegovina to participate in the NATO peacekeeping effort. Within the context of their occupational competence, these soldiers and their families made sacrifices that were very painful and frightening and completely at odds with survival. Successful self-sacrificial behavior occurs when the individual applies effectance in combination with environmental affordances to achieve or maintain role competence as part of being a parent, policeman or soldier. Altruism is required to fulfill these roles because society requires the consequence. This helps to explain the apparently contradictory behaviors of individual survival and sacrifice. The intertwining ideals of human competence and cultural competence are transmitted throughout the culture as values that the society embraces and celebrates. Although Bandura maintains that self-efficacy beliefs are task-specific, the inclusion of self-sacrificial tasks in a role's prototype suggests that it may be more appropriate to consider self-efficacy beliefs to be role-specific. This is a useful area for research.

Society's imposition of role demands is guided by its valuing of the person as a contributor to the maintenance and growth of society. Society imposes roles which are consistent with its recognition of the potential of the individual. Society can facilitate the development of the individual by posing demands that are integral components of valued roles which exceed the individual's current level of occupational competence. To the degree that the individual is acculturated and participating in the society, the role demand will be accepted and integrated by the individual, providing a spur to growth. The individual will experience growth when the role demands are consistent with his or her capacity and the person is given an opportunity to respond. Role acquisition presents the challenge which triggers the development of occupational competence.

Occupational competence is pertinent to each role and drives the growth of the person. It also drives the development of society, although over a much greater time scale. This can be illustrated by examining the roles of women in the United States during World War II. In response to the demands of the war, American women became employed in jobs in the industrial sector which previously had been dominated by men. Some women became riveters and bomb makers while others became pilots or draftspersons. These women faced role demands to which they responded by developing occupational competence which changed dramatically and permanently the way that they and the American culture considered "women's roles." Thus, the opportunities in the culture for demonstration of occupational competence broadened quickly and permanently. Occupational competence was so highly valued on an individual basis that, at war's end, many women resisted resumption of their prior roles and either remained in new roles or returned to their old roles while retaining their new roles.

Emergence of Occupational Competence

Occupational competence is motivated by what White (1959) described as an "effectance motive" that begins in childhood. White does not discount the effect of physiologic maturation, but emphasizes that competence in learning to adapt to these changes is the source of a substantial portion of the difference between individuals. White (1959, p. 324) relies on Angyal's thesis that "the general dynamic trend of the organism is toward an increase of autonomy...the human being has a characteristic tendency towards self-determination...a tendency to resist external influences and to subordinate the heteronomous forces of the physical and social environment to its own sphere of influence." Development of competence during childhood and adolescence reflects rapid increases in the individual's underlying capacity and ability to use that capacity at the same time that the individual is exposed to increasing levels of demand. The challenges that these demands place on the individual lead to a response. The competent response occurs under certain circumstances and can lead to an increase in self-efficacy which, in turn, increases the likelihood that competence will be developed in response to additional challenges.

The individual's urge to preserve occupational competence provides motivation to emit behavior intended to achieve successful performance in tasks which are challenges to his or her competence. If the outcome of the behavior is successful in meeting the challenge, competence results. If the response is inadequate, self-efficacy beliefs can lead to perseverance which may lead to success. For the person with a functional limitation which interferes with valued role performance, the urge to maintain competence is of paramount importance (Bandura, 1982). When it is present, it provides motivation to overcome or adapt to the functional limitation so that competence in role performance is regained. Its absence signals depression or may lead to adaptation for death.

In summary, the development of occupational competence requires the successful completion of a series of steps. Occupational competence emerges when the following circumstances occur:

1. The individual perceives a challenge to his or her role competence;
2. The individual knows what must be done to meet the challenge;
3. The individual perceives that he or she has the effectancies in combination with environmental affordances which are adequate to meet the challenge;
4. The individual is willing to address the challenge;
5. The individual has a relevant self-efficacy belief and believes that he or she can succeed;
6. The individual has the effectancies in combination with the environmental affordances that will allow success;
7. The individual applies effort to take on the challenge;
8. The response or outcome is as expected or approximates the response or outcome that was expected;
9. The response or outcome is both apprehended and appreciated by the individual.

The occupational competence model of human development is deterministic only to the extent that it posits that behavior has its basis in the genetic endowment of the individual (Bronfenbrenner, 1977; Wilson, 1978). Beyond physiologic maturation, the individual's development occurs in response to role demands and environmental affordances. The model allows for free will which exists for the person in the valuing of the roles that he or she assumes. In turn, task competence for these occupational roles leads to increased self-efficacy for role tasks and further development of the individual's unique effectancies. The developing values of the individual determines which roles are pursued.

Occupational Competence in Response to Age-Linked Changes

The concept of maturation reflects the observation that members of species progress through patterned stages of behavioral and biological development. Arnold Gesell argued that maturation of the human was primarily influenced by innate and endogenous factors but acknowledged the possible influence of environment on development. He described development in terms of five major fields of behavior: adaptive behavior, gross motor behavior, fine motor behavior, language behavior and personal social behavior (Knoblock & Pasamanick, 1974). He viewed each of the fields as following a rigid sequence and hierarchy of development which were the result of a "natural biologic unfolding" of the individual. Based on his descriptions, Gesell produced age-related standards for motor, language and social skills. The parameters Gesell defined have been used to detect developmental delay. Since Gesell's ages or stages of development were predictable sequences and cycles of development, they are often used as a basis for developmental assessments and as a basis for planning therapeutic intervention. Unfortunately, viewing development from such a rigid perspective allows the importance of individuality and the importance of the whole person to be overlooked (Bing, 1968). Additionally, the normative data which Gesell reported were based on observations of a specific population of children at a specific time in history. The standards of development Gesell identified are not entirely applicable across cultures or with specific populations. Like Gesell, the occupational competence model recognizes age-related changes of the individual. However, it acknowledges the strong influence of both the environment and roles on the development of the individual over the lifespan. Occupational competence inextricably links the person to the environment through valued role demands. Through this linkage, the occupational competence model assumes that performance is not modal to the stage of development but to the demands of the role. Early in life, role demands may be relatively uniform across a culture. However, as people reach adulthood, roles become so diverse that a biologic basis for occupational performance provides only broad parameters within which unique competencies are able to be developed.

Changes in capacity with age have appreciable effects on occupational competence. A wide variety of changes occur that appear to be age linked. Some of these changes are important for occupational therapists to understand. Since 1884, when Sir Francis Galton gathered behavioral data on men and women age 5 to 80 at the International Health Exposition in London, England, age differences in performance have been noted. Galton found age-linked differences in strength, reaction time, and auditory perception of high-pitched tones. Since this pioneering work, life span developmental psychologists have studied age-linked differences in human performance with cross-sectional models which compare people of different ages. Actual age changes have been studied with longitudinal models that compare people at different points in time. These researchers have begun to con-

sider the human life span as being characterized in terms of changes in the person's capacity for biological, social, and psychological self-regulation (Birren, 1988). Depending on the domain of function, self-regulation develops from childhood, through adolescence and into early and middle adulthood. The rate of development varies across domains and the developmental peaks are different, depending on the domain. Life span scientists study the degree to which the various domains are independent or "entrained." They point out that an ecological balance of capacities is a characteristic of human health and well-being, and that compensation for degrading capacity occurs within the person and within the person's environment in order to maintain self-regulation. These changes in capacity can be studied from various perspectives, including:

1. *Biological Age* (Birren, 1959): An estimate of the individual's present position with respect to his or her potential life span; how much longer the person will live. Related to the rate of biologic aging is "functional age," an index of an individual's ability to adapt to the environment (Birren & Renner, 1977).

2. *Psychological Age*: This has to do with "age-related adaptive capacities of the individual" (Birren, 1959, p. 18) such as perception, learning and memory.

3. *Social Age*: Social age has to do with the individual's societal roles within the context of his or her culture (Birren, 1959) and the "expectations of his group and society" (Birren, 1964, p. 10). Neugarten and Datan (1973) describe society as having an age-status structure with a "social time clock."

Table 18-2 summarizes some of the important developments which occur with age, organized in terms of subsystems. There are considerable inter-individual differences with "across-the-board" degradation rarely found, even at age 80 (Schaie, 1990). In addition, degradation in task performance can be mediated by intervention and practice can minimize age changes. For example, degradation in psychomotor speed with age is worsened by the complexity of the task. Older individuals have disproportionately slower response times as complexity increases. Practice can eliminate most of the effect due to complexity but not the effect due to psychomotor slowing (Salthouse, 1988; Stones & Kozma 1989). Spirduso and MacRae (1990, p. 194) report that "as individuals age, with practice a multitude of compensatory mechanisms can be developed that result in little observable difference in some types of skilled performance of older and younger individuals." Individuals develop compensatory mechanisms for coping with the decrements in cognitive processing with age. In addition, several researchers (Schooler, 1990; Hoyer, 1987) have reported that the individual's occupational involvement may mediate age decrements.

As an example, Schooler found that job conditions which promote occupational self-direction increase intellectual flexibility, whereas jobs which limit occupational self-direction decrease intellectual flexibility. Miller et al. (1985) found that the degree to which complex work can increase intellectual flexibility remains the same across the life span, but the complexity of the individual's occupational demands does not, especially as workers near retirement. Thus, part of the intellectual decrement reported in the elderly may result from the reduced complexity of their work environments producing lower levels of demand, which, in turn, allows age-related biologic decrements to be more powerfully expressed.

Clearly, that development can occur in response to challenge and may even require challenge. Development and restoration after an injury can occur apace with physiologic change and tissue repair without challenge but even physiologic change can be guided or shaped by challenge (Mooney, 1992). Challenges are presented by the social context through one's roles and are role driven or timed in that the role determines most of the challenges the person will receive. The ability to meet the challenge determines whether the role is appropriate for that point in the person's development. Growth can be characterized as the development of ability to respond to a challenge. Senescing occurs when challenges are not met, either because they are not presented to the individual, as in retirement, or because they overwhelm the individual. When challenges are not able to be met adequately, either adaptation or degradation can occur. Decompensation, or in the extreme, death, occurs when challenges so overwhelm the individual that he or she is not able to respond. It is not clear how to differentially predict the difference in response.

Age-related changes will influence the individual's occupational competence unless the individual adapts to those changes. At the point of an organism's development when capacity ceases to increase or begins to decrease, it becomes necessary to compensate by increasing skills, knowledge and effort to improve effectancy or by seeking environmental resources. In this way occupational competence is preserved.

The occupational competence model acknowledges that each of the human systems matures based on the combined effects of the individual's genetic makeup and environmental influences. Because of this, it is important to distinguish age changes from age differences. Age differences take into account both changes with age and differences that are related to individuals' respective age cohorts. For example, changes that take place in the development of self-concept during adolescence are likely to be substantially different for U.S. citizens who were born in 1920 compared with people who were born in 1960. Whatever difference is found would also be likely to be distinct from the difference that would

be found over the same time span in the !Kung! people of the Kalahari Desert. To the degree that the aspects of the individual are more biologically based and less psychologically based, age changes will be resistant to epochal differences. Conversely, age changes which are primarily psychological or social are quite likely to be affected by epochal differences in society and in the broader culture. Age differences typically are studied through the use of cross-sectional models which look at people of different ages at one point in time. Age changes, on the other hand, typically are studied through the use of longitudinal models which consider individuals or groups of individuals across at least two points in time. Each model has important limitations and presents challenges to the scientist in terms of confounding effects which obscure the effect that the scientist is attempting to study (Schaie, 1977).

Distinguishing description of age changes from the explanations for the cause of those changes is important. Much more research has described the differences which appear to be related to age and the changes which are a consequence of age than to explain the causes for these differences and changes. As growth proceeds from infancy through childhood and into adolescence, causal models of development become increasingly complex. Although scientists have spent decades searching for causal models of development which are generally applicable across cultures, across generations and across the life span, relatively few have been identified.

Although tempting, it is not correct to think of aging as occurring over predictable stages or having discrete strata which can be identified and labeled. These are convenient but can be misleading if we are not careful. The usual changes with age occur gradually, over months or years, with noteworthy developmental markers which are shared across individuals. For example, gradual changes in sexual maturity occur in human females over a period of several years in adolescence, with menarche being the developmental marker often used as a reference of physiological sexual maturity. Menarche is a marker which is useful in organizing our thinking about this particular issue, but it can lead to confusion if we use it to describe age changes in all of her systems, including those which are as diverse as the endocrine and social systems. Sexual maturity can be described as a stage of development which is uniquely pertinent to each system. For example, human females in diverse cultures achieve physiologic sexual maturity at roughly the same chronological age, with minimal inter-cultural differences. However, sexual maturity in terms of females' social development varies tremendously across cultures. Although there is consistency within a culture, there are vast differences among cultures. To the degree that the system under study is not closely linked to the individual's physiological development, cultural influence will be more profound.

TABLE 18-2

Sub-system Developments Which Occur with Age

Cardiovascular System	Musculoskeletal System	Brain and Nervous System	Sensory System	Endocrine System	Female Reproductive System	Male Reproductive System
Thickness of the left ventricle increases and arteries become thicker and less flexible with age.	Loss of bone density begins for both sexes in the fifties and accelerates for women at menopause.	Brain weight increases until age 20 and decreases thereafter.	Eye lens becomes thicker and heavier, resulting in increased prevalence of presbyopia.	Level of thyroid hormone declines with age.	Number of eggs in ovaries decreases with age, with increasing prevalence of chromosomal defects.	The prostate gland increases with age, usually as a consequence of benign cell growth.
Maximum heart rate decreases 1 beat per year, even in well-trained athletes.	Intervertebral spinal discs decrease in size. Changes in posture result in loss of height.	Energy metabolism in the brain declines with age.	Hearing higher sound frequencies declines with age, greater in men than women.	Level of growth hormone declines with age.	The weight and size of the uterus decreases to 50% in size in menopause.	Testosterone levels decrease with age.
Pumping capacity is stable in persons free of heart disease.	Body weight increases through middle age and decreases after age 65.	Prevalence of dementias increases with age.	Decline in ability to smell begins earlier in life than other sensory losses and is widespread.	Level of insulin declines with age while blood sugar increases slightly.	The vagina becomes smaller after menopause.	Penile erectile ability decreases with age.
VO₂ max declines .5% to 1% per from age 25, depending on fitness.	Strength declines after age 30. Upper limb decline is less pronounced than back or lower limb decline.	Short term memory declines with age. Intelligence.	Touch sensitivity decreases with age.	Hormone receptors decline in numbers and efficiency with age.	Vaginal tissues become more fragile and local glandular secretions decrease.	Prevalence of primary impotence increases with age.
Peak systolic blood pressure increases with age.	Endurance declines with age less than strength. Diminished fitness explains much of the loss.	Response speed slows with age disproportionately with increased task complexity.	Pain sensitivity decreases with age.	Ability to maintain normal levels of blood glucose declines with age.	Breast tissue undergoes involution and decreases in size after menopause for most women.	Sexual capacity and drive decreases with age.

The occupational competence model of human development suggests a perspective on the study of aging which is in contrast to models of aging which meet the criteria proposed by Strehler (1977) as deleterious, progressive and unavoidable. The occupational competence model may be more in line with Schroots' (1988) characterization of human development in terms of increasingly complex and enriched behavioral repertoires of behaviors from which the individual can strategically select to adapt to changing demands and capacities. It also seems to be consistent with an "integrative" theory of human development posited by Birren and Birren (1990, p. 16) which focuses on compensation. They note that "the older organism is presumed to maintain performance by compensating for deleterious changes in component processes." In commenting on the development of research on aging, they describe "an evolving ecological perspective in the psychology of aging that looks at the environmental context of the individual as well as the individual's historical background and adaptive strategies." (1991, p. 16). The occupational competence model uses occupational role competence as a factor which integrates the changes occurring in the individual and his environment over time. As an integrative factor, it also suggests that occupational role competence may offer an organizational strategy with which to approach the study of human aging. Figure 18-3 gives an example of the development of a typical person's occupational competence across the life span in terms of societal phases which are organized around occupational roles.

In this model, occupational development is composed of the life span changes in occupational performance which are exhibited by the individual in a societal role within an environment in response to the urge to develop and maintain occupational role competence. The dynamism occurs among the three components as well as over time in that role acquisition is age-linked.

Life Span Development of Occupational Competence

Occupational competence is role-directed. Because age-graded changes in societal demands decrease in adulthood (Baltes et al., 1980), patterns of occupational development become more diverse and difficult to characterize. However, the dynamics of the interplay among the person, roles and the environment continues. One example is presented in Figure 18-3. Beginning at preschool age, when the child begins to take on role responsibilities at home and in the immediate community under the direct supervision of older family members, the environment predominates. Competence is primarily a consequence of environmental affordances which are attuned to the unique abilities of the child as he or she develops physically. Role behaviors

emerge to meet the parents' role-based demands for self-care and communication. As the child moves into primary grades, role demands greatly increase in concert with the evolving physical, psychological, and sociocultural capacity of the child. Role challenges are much greater and are equivalent to environmental affordances. For the secondary student, personal capacities have greatly increased and are the focus of attention. Although environmental affordances and role demands continue to be high, the secondary student has become centered on the self and is self-directed. Environmental affordances and role demands are minimized and may even be rejected. The young careerist maintains the level of personal capacity found in the secondary student and continues to develop it gradually. In addition, integration of environmental affordances and role demands accelerates. The individual selects roles consistent with perception of abilities and cultural values. The vocational role begins to be established. The individual becomes adept in using environmental affordances and in recognizing and minimizing threats before they impact competence. The mature careerist finds a balance among personal effectancies, environmental affordances, and role demands. The first diminution of personal effectancies is noted and is offset by development of new effectancies that are not limited by the diminishing subsystem, coupled with more active use of environmental affordances so that role demands are able to be met. The active retired person begins to experience accelerated diminution of personal effectancy as a result of subsystem degradation with age. Role demands are changed and lessened with increased reliance on environmental affordances. The frail retired individual experiences accelerated diminution of personal capacities along with constriction of role demands. Greater reliance on environmental affordances is necessary and is sought to maintain competence in the individual's few remaining roles.

Occupational Competence and Development of Personality

The occupational competence model attempts to integrate existing theories of personality and human development to provide therapeutic intervention to individuals who have experienced a loss of occupational involvement and, as a result, are in a crisis. The occupational competence model conceptualizes basic human nature as organized around the organism's maintenance of competence as the person develops. Personality has to do with the appreciation, marshaling, and use of the resources necessary to maintain competence. The uniqueness of the individual is expressed in personality. Maddi (1989, p. 8) defines personality as a "stable set of tendencies and characteristics that determine those commonalties and differences in people's psychological behavior that

SOCIETY PHASE	PERSON, ROLE, ENVIRONMENT INTERACTION	CONTRIBUTIONS TO COMPETENCE
Pre-school		**Person** - Physical capacities, especially gross motor skills, evolve. Self begins to be expressed as individuality. Assertiveness and communication style are reflected in personality. **Role** - Behaviors emerge to meet parents rule-based demands for self-care & communication. **Environment** - Threats are minimized as the individual learns to manipulate the environment to maximize affordances.
Primary student		**Person** - Physical, psychological and sociocultural capacities expand. Competence develops in response to environmental and role challenges. **Role** - Role demands, rules and rewards are prescribed by other individuals and society. **Environment** - Impact of threats are minimized by the individual. Individual integrates the ability to control & use environmental affordances.
Secondary student		**Person** - Physical capacities evolve as a result of biological & physical maturation. Individuality & self-efficacy result from self-evaluation of role demands & use of environmental affordances. **Role** - Individual rejects roles prescribed by adults and society & begins to experiment with role behaviors. **Environment** - Individual minimizes environmental affordances to exert "self".
Young careerist		**Person** - Physical capacities reach their maximum. Individual conforms to cultural and social demands while maintaining a sense of identity and individuality. Individual structures time and environment to maximize competence. **Role** - Individual selects roles consistent with their perception of their abilities & cultural values. Vocational role begins to be established. **Environment** - Individual becomes more adept in utilizing environmental affordances & recognizing or minimizing threats before they impact competence.
Mature careerist		**Person** - Abilities, diminished as a result of maturation, are optimized through structuring of the environment. Personhood is established within the context of current society and culture. **Role** - Firmly established roles allow individual to gain control over financial, physical and personal environments. **Environment** - Individual minimizes environmental treats to abilities by restructuring or adapting the environment. Individual efficiently and effectively uses environmental affordances to meet role demands.
Active retired		**Person** - Abilities continue to diminish as a result of maturation. Personhood established within a culture of retirement. **Role** - Primary work role is abandoned. Leisure and other life roles fill time once dominated by work. Individual may continue in a modified work role. **Environment** - Major environmental treats to abilities are handled by restructuring or adapting the environment. Individual becomes less efficient and effective use of environmental affordances to meet role demands.
Frail retired		**Person** - Physical capacities are diminishing with biological and physiological maturation. Personal identify is diminished as the roles which defined the individual are removed. **Role** - Primary life roles are abandoned or are being minimized by society. Individual becomes dependent on others as capacities limit the individuals ability to utilize environmental affordances. **Environment** - Diminished capacities impact the individual's ability to respond to the environment.

Figure 18-3. Occupational competence is role-organized, based on the person's values within the contexts of the environment. As roles change, personal and environmental resources change.

have continuity in time and that may not be easily understood as the sole result of the social and biological pressures of the moment." Among other things, personality reflects the unique acculturation of the individual, which affects valuing of roles, the tasks associated with those roles, and, thereby, occupational role competence.

Personality develops as the individual encounters the familial and social environments. These environments impose demands on the individual through tasks which are usually age-appropriate given the morés of that family or societal unit. The need for survival within the familial or social environment requires that age-appropriate task demands be placed on the individual. The age appropriateness is determined by the competencies level of the individual, which are, in turn, cultivated and monitored by the family and societal unit.

Various theorists have described personality as developing across some or all of the life span (Maddi, 1989). Depending on the perspective of the personality theorist, the individual's personality develops in response to various challenges within the context of changes in competence. The development of self-worth also appears to be linked to success in developing competencies in areas which are important to the person (James, 1892). More recently, Harter (1985, 1990) has emphasized the interdependence between self-worth and competence. Other theorists who have developed theories of personality without a focus on the importance of competence have, nevertheless, provided important contributions to the occupational competence model of human development. Those theorists whose models are most relevant are presented here.

Freud and Instincts

The Psychoanalytic school, founded by Sigmund Freud, characterized development of personality as determined by the struggle between the developing individual's natural instincts within the constraints imposed by society. All behavior is caused and, thus, can be explained. The individual's earlier experiences are understood within the developmental context of his instinctual human nature. Freud held that personality was well-established by adulthood and that human development occurs in five "psychosexual stages" which are presented in Table 18-3. Physical capacity develops as the child shifts the primary focus of pleasure from one area of the body to another. Freud's structural model of personality (composed of the Id, Ego and Superego) ascribes motivation to the "life instinct" found in the Id, which produces libidinal energy. The life instinct supports the individual's preservation and competes with the "death instinct" which threatens the individual with destruction. Personality development occurs as the child matures and receives an optimal level of gratification at each stage so that he can pass through to the next stage without fixation. Freud's

model of motivation is based on tension-reduction, in which the frustration of basic needs produce tension that leads to the Id's primary process, which is to achieve gratification and reduce the tension. Freud's determinism, which emphasized tension reduction as the primary motivator of behavior, leaves little room for free will or choice. Freud's notion of the importance of the unconscious is a significant contribution to the occupational competence model in that it is the repository of the individual's values, which influence role selection.

Erikson and Psychosocial Development

Erik Erikson was a student of Freud's who believed that personality was based on more than instinct. He argued that the development of the Ego was influenced by the social and cultural environment. He developed eight stages of psychosocial development, presented in terms of successive crises which must be resolved (Table 18-4). Erikson described the development of the "autonomous will" of the child, which he has labeled the "sense of industry" (Erikson, 1985). He described mastery as an important component of development throughout childhood and adolescence. The model which Erikson described begins with exploration leading to activity and manipulation, and finally, to mastery. In the occupational competence model, mastery reflects successful task performance and provides one basis of occupational competence.

Rogers and Personal Development

Carl Rogers was the founder and leading proponent of humanistic phenomenology. Rogers' view of human nature was that we are inherently growth-oriented and predisposed to activities which enhance and provide value to the organism. Rogers argued that humans have a natural tendency toward actualization and stressed the importance of the individual's self-perception. Humans behave in accord with their subjective experience of themselves and their environments. The description of human character posited by Rogers (1980) is consistent with White (1971) who argued that neither behaviorism nor psychoanalysis provide an adequate explanation of the development of the human being as a system which is "alive, growing, self-expanding, and is itself a source of influence, as well as one shaped by outside influences" (p. 272). For Rogers, effective action on the external environment is reinforcing simply because of its effectiveness. He notes that there is inherent satisfaction in influencing the environment from what he calls a "feeling of efficacy." He did not describe a mechanism for the development of competence, but noted that learning about efficacy develops a "sense of competence" which is an aggregation of experiences concerning the individual's ability to affect the environment.

Rogers described "the actualizing tendency" as the basic human motive (Maddi, 1989, p. 98). He argued that the human

TABLE 18-3

Developmental Theories of Childhood and Adolescence

Age	Jean Piaget **Cognitive Development Periods**	Sigmund Freud **Psychosexual Development Stages**	Lawrence Kohlberg **Moral Development Levels**
Birth	**Sensorimotor period**	**Oral Stage**	
6 mos	Development focuses on the experience of the self and self in the environment. The child senses and reacts. The first learned social behaviors, crying to communicate needs, is noted at 8 to 12 months.	Mouth is the primary area of gratification of impulses. Id is dominant.	
12 mos			
18 mos		**Anal Stage**	
24 mos		Gratification results from elimination. Conflict between the Id and reality, in the form of parents' demands for control of behavior, begins the development of the Ego.	
	Preoperational Thinking Period		
3 yrs	The use of symbols and formal language begins to appear. Logic is not yet present.		
4 yrs		**Phallic Stage**	
5 yrs		Genitals are the primary area of gratification. Superego develops, signaling a conscience.	**Preconventional Morality**
6 yrs		**Latency Stage**	The child relies on external controls and the standards of others. Avoiding punishment and receiving reward is characteristic of hedonistic behavior.
7 yrs		Calm before the storm of puberty. Diminution of interest in sexual gratification. Identification with parent of the same gender occurs.	
8 yrs	**Concrete Operations Period** Children begin to develop concepts and to apply logic to problem solving.		
9 yrs			
10 yrs			**Conventional Morality**
11 yrs			Sociocultural awareness and desire to be accepted in the community directs behavior. Concern for law and order is demonstrated.
12 yrs	**Formal Operations Period** The ability to perform abstract thinking and to apply logic to novel experiences develops.	**Genital Stage** Hormonal changes signal the onset of sexual maturity. Focus is on adult modes of sexual expression. Satisfying intimate relationships outside of the family of origin are developed.	
13 yrs			**Postconventional**
14 yrs			Morality is based on the prevailing "social contract." Standards of the community are internalized and judgment to compare oneself to these standards is demonstrated.
15 yrs			
18 yrs			
21 yrs +			

TABLE 18-4

Life Span Developmental Theories

Age	Havighurst **Developmental Tasks**	Erik Erikson **Psychosocial** **Development Crises**	Daniel J. Levinson **Biopsychosicial Eras**
Birth	**Infancy and Early Childhood**	**Basic Trust vs. Mistrust**	**Childhood**
	Individual learns to walk, talk, eat, and control elimination.	Learns to trust caretakers.	Rapid growth and development occur. Individuation of the child
2 yrs		**Autonomy vs. Shame and Doubt**	begins with gradually increasing
	Sex differences are learned. The individual is involved cognitively with language, physical reality	Discovery of sense of autonomy.	biological and psychological separation from the mother.
4 yrs		**Initiative vs. Guilt**	
	and forming concepts, and begins to develop a conscience.	Conscious control of environment.	
6 yrs	**Middle Childhood**	**Industry vs. Inferiority**	
8 yrs	The individual learns physical skills to achieve competence in	Determination to achieve mastery develops.	
10 yrs	play, and is learning to get along with peers in appropriate social and sexual roles. Personal independence begins to be achieved.		
12 yrs	**Adolescence**	**Identity vs. Role Confusion**	
14 yrs	The individual begins to have mature relationships with peers of	Childhood crises are mastered. Identity is linked to mastery.	
16 yrs	both sexes and learns social and gender roles. Emotional independence from parents		
18 yrs	begins to be achieved.		**Early Adult Transition**
	Early Adulthood	**Intimacy vs. Isolation**	Relationships with family of origin are modified as childhood
20 yrs	The individual is selecting and learning to live with a mate and	Differentiation in role development. Development of	dependence is replaced with independence and adult identity.
25 yrs	deciding to begin or not begin a family. The individual establishes a home and begins employment.	intimate relationships.	**Entering the Adult World**
30 yrs	**Middle Age**	**Generativity vs. Stagnation**	**Age 30 Transition**
40 yrs	The individual achieves social responsibility and satisfactory	Contributions to society overcome self-absorption.	**Settling down**
	career performance. Commitment to an intimate relationship occurs.		**Mid-Life Transition**
50 yrs	The individual begins to adjust to gradual physiologic changes.		**Middle Adulthood**
60 yrs	**Later Maturity**	**Ego Integrity vs. Despair**	**Late Adult Transition**
70 yrs	Adjusting to deteriorating health, reduced income, and death of	Acceptance and integration of oneself and inevitable death.	**Late Adulthood**
80 yrs	spouse. Focus is on establishing satisfactory living arrangements.		

organism tends to maintain itself and to strive for enhancement. He offered a concept which he termed the "organismic valuing process" by which the individual evaluates experiences in self-referent terms. This is a primary feature of human nature. As a secondary feature, the individual has the capacity and tendency to symbolize experiences. Rogers stressed the need for the individual to have a sense of free will and believed in the self as the primary determinant of behavior. Rogers' emphasis on the individual's valuing of experience makes an important contribution to the occupational competence model. Valuing is based on the individual's degree and type of societal acculturation. Like White, Rogers does not describe stages of development, but describes how personality development can occur within a therapeutic context.

Maslow and Self-Actualization

The notion that humans seek stimulation from their environments and roles has been studied extensively. Early contributions by Goldstein (1963) and Maslow (1968), who described the motive of self-actualization in terms of the individual's need to be challenged and stimulated by tasks and roles. Maslow argues that development occurs across a hierarchy of needs. Maslow describes human potential as being able to be "actualized" under certain conditions and that each person has the potential to experience such actualization. He describes humans as "choosing, deciding, seeking animals" who have "come to the point in biological history where we now are responsible for our own evolution. We have become self-evolvers. Evolution means selecting and therefore choosing and deciding and this means valuing" (Maslow, 1971, p. 10). He argues that development can be facilitated by assisting the individual to become aware of his or her identity. He describes people who are self-actualizing as making their work part of the self. He notes that these people are dedicated to work tasks that are selected based on intrinsic values. Maslow's contribution to the occupational competence model stems from his emphasis on the valuing of occupational roles and the need for challenge imposed by the environment. The occupational competence model posits that the combined effects of the environment and the individual's valued roles challenge the individual. In response, the urge toward competence leads to growth directed at that challenge.

Havighurst and Society

Robert J. Havighurst focused on developmental tasks which are based on individual needs mediated by societal demands. Havighurst's theory emphasizes an individual's learning of specific tasks at each stage of development (see Table 18-4) to meet social expectations. Developmental behaviors result from the reconciliation of societal requirements and individual needs. Havighurst (1979) believed in the ability of the individual to learn rather than just respond

to situations. Learning of developmental behaviors occurs during "sensitive periods." These sensitive periods are the times when the individual is most likely to integrate previous learning and social guidance to achieve new task skills. When the individual is able to learn particular skills, that individual is able to achieve competence in meeting age-appropriate role demands. According to Havighurst, biological, sociological and psychological influences allow the individual to learn age-appropriate skills. The skills which Havighurst identified for each of the six developmental stages reflect not only these influences but the implications for learning at each of the stages. As with Havighurst, the occupational competence model recognizes the societal control of role acquisition.

Levinson and Biopsychosocial Eras

Daniel J. Levinson (1996) performed biographical studies through in-depth structured interviews of small groups of men and women who were selected to be representative of modal roles in American society. He has developed an age-linked view of adult development which recognizes the importance of interaction of the biological, psychological and social aspects of the person over time. The life cycle is hypothesized to have three eras, early adulthood, middle adulthood, and late adulthood, each with its own set of developmental periods (see Table 18-4). Levinson argues that the individual's life structure is primarily composed of relationships with other people. He uses life structure in a manner that is analogous to personality structure, arguing that there are patterns of development and dynamics in each that can be discovered. Although his work has attracted much popular attention, the scientific value of this approach is not yet widely accepted. Perhaps Levinson's most important contribution to the occupational competence development model is the breadth of human experience that he has studied, suggesting that a inclusive, dynamic and non-linear model is appropriate.

Behaviorism and Occupational Competence

The occupational competence model of human development assumes that the person's abilities are learned, as are the application of abilities to become effectancies and the perception of affordances in the pursuit of role competence. The following section will describe models of learning which are pertinent to the development and maintenance of occupational competence.

Watson and Skinner

John B. Watson argued that individuals developed entirely in response to environmental influences. Watson emphasized respondent learning or classical conditioning and identified the phenomena of stimulus generalization and extinction. Years later, B.F. Skinner (1974) stressed the importance of the "functional relationship" between environmental conditions and behavior. He argued that environment affects our emotional lives as well. Like Freud, both Watson and Skinner were deterministic in their views of human behavior and development, although they certainly held competing views of the primary determining factors and their scope of study. The environment for Watson and Skinner was the primary determinant of behavior and of the individual's development. In contrast to Watson's emphasis on respondent learning, Skinner focused on reinforcement of "operant behavior." Operant behavior is that which has an effect on the environment and is controlled by an environmental consequence of the effect. The consequence of the behavior provides reinforcement so that it is increasingly likely to be emitted by the individual. Skinner argued that the development of the infant is guided by behaviors which are reinforced selectively by the environment. Many behaviors are emitted by the infant. Those which are reinforced are more likely to be emitted again, given similar environmental circumstances. Both respondent and operant behaviors can be identified in the individual's repertoire. Skinner argued that the operant behaviors identified the person as unique and was akin to personality, although he would prefer to describe this as a consequence of his "personal history of reinforcement."

Skinner's emphasis on the genetic basis of a capacity for operant behavior and the emphasis on the environmental reinforcement of behavior places the locus of behavioral control in the environment. However, it does not rule out individuals' configuration of the environment so that individual agency is not able to be achieved. Skinner's view of human nature was that we can be individuals who are unique, based entirely on a combination of our genetic endowment and our unique collection of reinforcing experiences. The occupational competence model relies on operant conditioning to learn skills so that capacity is transformed to ability. Ability focused by values and applied to societal roles becomes effectance. Effectance combined with affordance leads to competence. The operant model hinges on the valuing of the effect of the consequence of behavior.

Competence and Cognitive Development

In response to a task challenge posed by a situational demand, the individual applies effectance and affordances which are pertinent. A competent response that is apprehended and appreciated by the individual leads to self-efficacy if the task is a component of a valued role. Competence has a perceptual underpinning in that the individual must apprehend his or her adequacy. Competence has an emotional component in that the individual must appreciate his or her adequacy. Competence has an evaluative component in that

the individual must judge the response to be adequate. Thus, the cognitive development of the person or the cognitive deficits acquired by disease or injury places limits on the development of occupational competence.

Piaget and Cognitive Development

The notion that cognitive development progresses through stages was first put forth by J.M. Baldwin, a prominent American psychologist (1895). Jean Piaget was a Swiss biologist who became an adherent to Baldwin's pioneering work. Piaget came to believe that development occurs as the result of maturation of the person's intellectual capacity, shaped by environmental challenges to which the person must adapt. Piaget (1954) defined adaptation as the organism's ability to adjust to change in order to fit into its environment. The individual uses assimilation and accommodation to adapt. Assimilation is defined as the processing of information in a manner which is compatible with the individual's perception of reality. Assimilation fits information into a schema, a predetermined framework held in the mind. Accommodation is defined as changes in the cognitive structures which are required to integrate aspects of experience which cannot be assimilated. Both Piaget's model of human cognitive development and the occupational competence model describe development as a consequence of environmental challenges (see Table 18-3). While the occupational competence model focuses on development of the individual's multi-system negotiation with the environment in order to meet role demands, Piaget emphasizes cognitive adaptation.

Vygotsky and Social Cognitive Development

Lev Vygotsky described development in terms of a social cognitive theory. He described the development of cognitive function as shaped by cultural influence, especially through language. For Vygotsky, language is necessary for thinking to occur and is the individual's primary tool for interacting with parents and important others in the "zone of proximal development" (1978, p. 84-91). Early in life, crying is oral communication on a family-centered basis. As the child's circle of social contact widens and his cognitive abilities, motor abilities, and cultural abilities develop, speech becomes necessary. The culture shapes the child's cognitive development and literally how he views the world. Both Vygotsky and Piaget understood communicative behavior to be central to development. Even at a preverbal age, crying behavior is learned in interaction with the environment. Its function is to help the infant establish control over the environment. The occupational competence model views extensions of this behavior into adulthood. During periods of life when occupational competence is not sufficient to maintain the person's role, variants of crying behavior serve to control the environment (Matheson, 1991).

Kohlberg and Moral Development

Lawrence Kohlberg has built on the ideas of Piaget and Vygotsky with reference to the acculturation of the child in terms of morality. Given the assumption that cognitive function both directs and reflects behavior, Kohlberg presented to subjects of various ages vignettes which pose moral dilemmas. The justification for resolution of the dilemma was found by Kohlberg to be patterned, sequential, and somewhat age-linked. Three different and sequential levels of moral judgment, each with two stages were able to be identified. Research on Kohlberg's stage model has resulted in only inconsistent support, with differences found between genders and much more variability among people in general. A modification of the original model to exclude the sixth stage (because it is rarely found) and to sharpen the stage descriptors has led to greater support for the developmental nature of the model.

Bandura and Personal Agency

The social cognitive approach is based on what Albert Bandura (1989) describes as a "microanalysis of perceived coping capabilities" rather than on global personality traits. In social cognitive theory, personal agency (being the cause of one's behavior) is based on the notion that human behavior is regulated in terms of cognitive processes. For Bandura, self-generated messages which are self-efficacy beliefs lie at the very heart of the causal process, functioning as "proximal determinants" of motivation and action. Self-efficacy develops from the experience of success which the individual has with challenging and meaningful tasks. For Bandura (1990), motivation requires discrepancy production through the acceptance of a meaningful challenge to produce disequilibrium. Action is directed toward reduction of this discrepancy. Bandura's work has provided important underpinnings to model of occupational competence, especially his research with self-efficacy development.

Seligman and Learned Helplessness

Seligman (1975) and Peterson, Maier and Seligman (1993) have described a situation in which repeated exposure to uncontrollable situations leads to a generalized sense of inefficacy so that the individual becomes passive and apathetic and the ability to distinguish controllable from uncontrollable situations is diminished. This phenomenon is based on three essential components:

1. The fact that there is a random relationship between one's behavior and the outcome of a situation. No matter what one does, the outcome is not changed.
2. The cognitive appraisal which an individual makes of the situation. The first step is to perceive as uncontrollable an event that is uncontrollable or to misperceive as uncontrollable an event that is controllable. The second step is to explain to oneself why the event is uncontrollable. Was the lack of control due to my own action or was it just bad luck? The third step is to develop an expectation about the likelihood of this occurring again in the future.
3. Change of behavior so that the individual becomes more passive in other situations that are different from the one in which the individual experienced uncontrollability.

The learned helplessness phenomenon is important to the occupational competence model in that it describes the consequences both of a nonresponsive environment and the central importance of the individual's direct perception of affordances based on experience. People become helpless in response to environments which are perceived to be nonresponsive; this quality of the environment does not exist independent of the individual's perception.

OCCUPATIONAL COMPETENCE AND DISABILITY

Physical, mental or emotional impairments which are sufficient to create functional limitations and disrupt the individual's occupational competence are said to cause the person to become "disabled." This categorization of a person as being disabled is problematic since competence is a graduated phenomenon for which there is no predictable delineation between competence and incompetence. Competence is personally relevant and cannot be entirely defined by anyone other than that individual. Although each of us pays attention to the opinions of those who are important to us, we each make the determination of our competence for ourselves. Our definition of our own competence allows each of us to recognize our abilities while acknowledging that a certain degree of incompetence is necessary for growth to occur.

The labeling of disability is a sociobehavioral phenomenon which poses challenges for individuals identified by their societies as having disabilities and for the rehabilitation professionals with whom they interact. Disability must continue to be recognized as a social, political, and cultural convention at least as much as it is a part of the human experience. Although the social relativity of disability renders it somewhat murky as a concept, the occupational competence model of human development posits a reciprocal relationship between competence and disability. This is certainly a simplistic and artificial convention. However, it is one that has value in that it emphasizes the ecological nature of the relationship of the person within the society which has created the disability.

Disruption of occupational roles by the onset of a disability is tempered by many factors unique to the newly-disabled individual, many of which we do not understand. Neugarten (1968) reported that persons who experience expected negative life events are more likely to take them in stride than persons for whom the events are completely unexpected. For example, a myocardial infarction for a man at age 50 is likely to be less disruptive if his father had a myocardial infarction at that age than for a man whose father had no such experience. Others (Brim and Ryff, 1980) have studied this issue and have generally found that a person's ability to anticipate negative life events prepares that person to handle them if they arise. White (1974) describes the person's ability to transcend immediate experience through anticipation of the future as an important expansion of the human's environment which requires much broader strategies of adaptation. In White's view, the anticipation presents challenges to the person which require the development of greater competence. Thus, when the event occurs, the individual's competence is more likely to be adequate. White cites work by Hamburg and Adams (1967) in which people who suffered severe injuries which threatened to restrict future activity were able to search for information while keeping distress within manageable limits and maintaining personal worth and relationships. He notes that the ability to develop strategies of adaptation in anticipation of potential future problems is a peculiarly human attribute. Further, he notes that role rehearsal is an effective means to develop competence and self-esteem. White concludes that "strategies of adaptation lead not just to equilibrium, but to development" (1974, p. 64).

After the onset of an impairment, the newly-disabled person must begin explorational activity which will lead to adaptation and re-establishment of functional self-efficacy and resumption of occupational competence. The focus of this exploration will be affected greatly by the person's culture and its value system (Coster, 1995a). Thus, the person must be considered within the context of his or her environment (Dunn, Brown, McGuigan, 1994) in a "collaboration among the person, the family, and the occupational therapist" (p. 603). Early in the adaptation process, the person experiences a self-evaluative appraisal process in which role demands are inventoried and matched to perceived functional abilities. The collection of information about both demands and abilities is most accurate if it occurs experientially. Often, this is facilitated through a functional capacity evaluation and visits to the environments in which the person's roles are to be performed. The experience-based information about task competence obtained from such evaluations may facilitate a more rational self-perception.

The primary difficulties encountered during early adaptation to a serious impairment have to do with the individual's questioning of self-worth-related role competence and both social and familial acceptability. Although occupational competence may be lost, the loss is anticipated to be temporary if the person will either be able to re-establish competence in the original roles or move on to new roles in which competence can be established.

The self-evaluative appraisal process often is problematic for the person with a disability, although the perception of competence in the tasks which comprise one's roles is believed by Bandura (1990) generally to be optimistic. That is, "when people err in their self-appraisal, they tend to overestimate their capabilities..." (p. 343). However, the individual's perception of ability may be negatively colored by the ongoing experience of disability (Matheson et al., 1993). Older people and persons with disabilities may have an opposite tendency. This is illustrated by the fact that elderly people often develop an "illusion of incompetence" (Langer, 1979) in response to the relinquishment of control after retirement and with the advent of health problems associated with age. Similarly, people with disabilities may have a tendency to view their competencies in an unnecessarily negative light.

The disabled person's perception of competence arises from experience. Christiansen (1991) reports that "the extent to which individuals are able to develop a positive sense of self and belief in their autonomy is largely based on their successes in dealing with environmental challenges..." (pp. 19-20). Christiansen argues that competence is based on environmental mastery which is achieved through occupational activity, occupation being defined broadly as "purposeful involvement." This is the primary way in which people's self-efficacy beliefs can be enhanced (Bandura, 1990). Ancillary methods include modeling of effective behavior, persuasion of the person that he will be effective if he makes an adequate attempt, and positive alteration of the feedback that the person experiences after an attempt has failed. These methods are components of effective rehabilitation strategies such as work hardening, an intervention that has its roots in occupational therapy (Matheson et al., 1985). In such an approach, the person with a disability performs functional goal setting and exploration in valued tasks which become progressively more demanding. Various activities which are valued by the person are attempted in a real or well-simulated work environment. If this explorational activity is successful, the behavior is reinforced and additional exploration at a higher level of challenge is undertaken. This is consistent with Bandura and Schunk's (1981) notion of "proximal self-motivation", it also is consistent with Gage's (1992) and Gage and Polatajko's (1994) arguments concerning the limited utility of demonstrations of competence in the occupational therapy clinic, and with Dunn, Brown and McGuigan's (1994) emphasis on the "ecology of human performance." Success in "real world" tasks shapes subsequent behavior through mastery and the development of expectancies about ability to perform. Thus, it is important that goal setting be calibrated to the patient's capacity. If the patient's functional exploration is unsuccessful, explorational behavior will be negatively reinforced. The immediate effect of this negative reinforcement is that exploration becomes less frequent. A more enduring effect of unsuccessful exploration is the self-referent belief that this experience has helped to develop; a belief about functional inefficacy. This will negatively affect the person's self-perception and self-referent reports to others.

Rehabilitation programs can be composed of elements of restoration, education and adaptation. The occupational competence model indicates that each provides value in assisting the person to re-establish role competence. Since the interaction between a person with a disability and a rehabilitation professional often draws attention to an absence of abilities and may actually induce a feeling of incompetence (Langer & Chanowitz, 1987), it is important that restoration focuses on the capacities of the person which have been diminished by the impairment. Maximizing the capacities which are critical to the maintenance of the valued roles should be the focus for intervention. To the degree that restoration of lost capacity is able to occur, the need for adaptation will be minimized. It is important to remember that the expression of capacity in the person's abilities is dependent on the development of skill. Thus, when capacity is diminished, some offset can be gained by improving skill to more efficiently use the person's residual capacity. At the same time, providing opportunities for the person to experience his or her value by using adaptive mechanisms and environmental resources such as described by Law (1991) and Baum (1991) can lead to development through actualization of his or her capacity.

Education of the individual contributes to the development of occupational competence which is separate from skill development based on the capacity of the person. Occupational competence is partially reliant on the individual's perception of environmental affordances. In many ways, the perceptual ability and perceptual style of the individual place primary limitations on the use of environmental affordances. The individual must be able to perceive the available resources and appreciate how they can be helpful. Without this perception and subsequent valuation, the resource may as well not exist. Valuation of the pertinence of the affordance is based, in part, on the individual's self-efficacy beliefs. In turn, perception of the value of the affordance is based on the meaning of the task and its importance to the goals of the individual. Thus, apprehension of the meaning of the task within the context of the individual's goals will affect how the resource will be valued. Finally, appreciation of the adequacy of the individual's response given the application of effectancies and the use of the affordances to respond to the environmental demands will set the stage for subsequent encounters with this environment. If use of an affordance has led to successful completion of a meaningful task, the individual will be more likely to perceive and value the affordance, and make use of it again. In other words, the individual learns to use both internal and external resources more effectively.

As the benefits of restoration and education are being experienced, adaptation is necessary. Adaptation is based on three groups of factors, including the person's perception of abilities and effectancies, environmental affordances and threats, and role demands and rewards. In the occupational competence model, adaptation is spurred by the urge to develop and maintain role competence, and is based on the perceived adequacy of the dynamic adjustment of each of the three groups. In rehabilitation, adaptation begins in a surrogate environment which provides structured affordances and minimizes threat along with simulated role demands. The skill of the care provider is to assist the recipient to use this surrogate environment to rehearse resumption of the role. Because the person needs to perform the role demands in real life, the therapeutic process must merge the experience of the structured environment into the actual living environment. The surrogate environment provides a temporary transition in which the clinician becomes an adaptive consultant. As it was so eloquently described by Zola (in Baum, 1991), adaptation is a life-long process which extends far beyond the formal rehabilitation experience and focuses on potential quality of life.

Perhaps the most effective way to understand how the occupational competence model is expressed in rehabilitation is to observe a person who experiences a disability as it unfolds. Let us meet our guide, Larry, as we continue to explore the relationship between *doing* and *being*. Larry is a 46-year-old plumber. He is married, the father of four children aged 6 to 17 years. His wife Linda works part-time at a preschool day care center. Larry is a journeyman plumber, having entered the Union apprenticeship program after graduation from high school. Aside from the apprenticeship program, he has no other training or education beyond high school. Larry and his family live in the suburbs of a large city in a home in a family neighborhood. Larry has been active in Little League, Youth Soccer, the Boy Scouts, and has been actively involved with his children. Larry is a big man, approximately 30 pounds overweight and a one-pack-a-day smoker. Aside from his activities with his children and at work, he leads a sedentary life and does no regular exercise. On the day after Christmas, Larry suffered a stroke. We meet him 3 days after the stroke as he is being discharged from the local hospital. His impairment is described as "left hemiplegia without facial paralysis or visual field involvement." After introducing ourselves and establishing rapport, the following dialogue occurs:

O.T.: *Larry, what type of work do you do?*

Larry: *I'm a plumber. Been a plumber for 25 years.*

O.T.: *How will this stroke affect your work?*

Larry: *I don't know...My wife's worried about that, but I think I'll be OK. The doctors are going to let me know tomorrow. That's all I know.*

In the early phase of medical recovery, adaptation begins with Larry denying the most troubling consequences of his stroke. Denial is a universal defense mechanism that protects Larry from the emotional pain of his loss. He continues to perceive his capacities as they were before his stroke. This helps him maintain a personal prototype of competence which is acceptable for his roles of husband and father.

Let's look in on Larry several days later, when the denial has begun to break down, leading to disbelief and despair:

O.T.: *Hi, Larry! How's it going?*

Larry: *Not too well.*

O.T.: *Why? What's up?*

Larry: *They say I won't work as a plumber again. It's all I know. I just can't believe it! How am I going to take care of my family? What kind of father or husband can I be? I gotta get outta the house, give it a try. I could get a helper. My boy is 17, he could help me. I know I can do it!*

Larry's emotions combine sadness with anxiety and fear. The denial is no longer effective in shielding him from some of the worst aspects of his new circumstance. He now vacillates between disbelief and despair. He has begun to realize that his effectancies are inadequate to support the task demands of his previous role and he is attempting to find affordances which can adequately compensate. What can we do, as therapists? We could have anticipated his current state when we first met him. We could have introduced ourselves like this:

O.T.: *Larry, I'm an occupational therapist, which means that I help people get back to doing things they want to do after something like this. When you need help, I'll be available.*

Such an introduction would not have helped Larry avoid moving into despair and disbelief, but it might help him move through these experiences faster. It would have signaled Larry that, at some point in the future, he would need assistance to "get back to doing things" that are important to him. In addition, by placing him in control of the relationship, we respect and support his interpersonal competence, which often gets disregarded in medical relationships. Some time later, Larry contacts us by telephone and asks us to come by the house for a talk:

Larry: *You said last week that you help people get back to what they want to do. That's what I want. Can you help me?*

O.T.: *Sure. We can be very effective. I've helped lots of people get back to work. What do you want to do?*

Larry: *I want to be a plumber, but I don't think I can. I don't know anything else.*

It is apparent that Larry has defined his occupational competence quite narrowly. Let us explore this to see if we can get him to think more broadly.

O.T.: *How good a plumber were you?*

Larry: *I was great! I was always being requested. On big jobs, I was foreman because I knew how to get people to do the job right.*

O.T.: *So, you weren't just a plumber, you were a manager or leader?*

Larry: *I guess so, yeah.*

O.T.: *Why were you good at getting people to do the job right?*

Larry: *I knew plumbing. I knew how to motivate people.*

(It is evident that Larry has begun to "let go" of his occupational roles. He is speaking of them in the past tense. Because we want to help Larry expand his awareness of his effectancies, we gently challenge him with this observation followed by a question.)

O.T.: *Sounds like you don't know plumbing or how to motivate people any more. How can that be?*

Larry: *You're right. I'm figuring I can't be a plumber since I don't have two good hands and have trouble walking. I'm all washed up.*

O.T.: *That's a mistake a lot of people make.*

At this point we have begun to remind Larry of his residual task competence. We can see his mood brighten and his confidence start to return. We have tapped into his urge toward competence and his self-efficacy beliefs. We might want to finish off this session by talking with Larry about his goals.

O.T.: *Larry, what do you want to do with the rest of your life?*

Larry: *I told you. I want to be a plumber, but I can't!*

O.T.: *I'm going to write that down here, because if it's something you still want, it's important. What else do you want?*

Larry: *Gosh, I don't know. To take care of my kids and be a good husband again.*

O.T.: *Great. Let's break those down into bite-size chunks. First, to take care of your kids. How do you do that?*

Larry: *I provide for them, do things with them, protect them, give them guidance and discipline.*

O.T.: *All right! Let me list those separately. To provide what?*

Larry: *A home, clothes, money to do things they want to do. Take vacations together. At least one decent car.*

O.T.: *I'll list those separately.*

After listing 12 to 15 goal statements, we helped Larry prioritize them, beginning with the goal that's least important and working backwards to the goal that's most important. We are assisting Larry to become clear about his role responsibilities and demands. We closed this session by asking him to review the goal list with his wife and make changes before we type it up. We tell him that we'd like him to give this to people who are important to him, like his doctor, brothers, sisters, older children, spouse, and so forth.

The next topics we can address have to do with Larry's perceptions of his effectancies and environmental affordances. In the next session, we ask him about his functional abilities in several basic areas, such as sitting, standing, walking, climbing stairs, lifting and carrying. We also ask him about his ability to perform activities of daily living and his perception of the needs which will need to be met to allow him to begin to address his goals.

We are helping Larry to differentiate the consequences of his impairment. His functional limitations offset his competencies differentially. For Larry, his competencies which are tied to his physical capacity have been more severely impacted than his competencies which are tied to his interpersonal capacity or his intellectual capacity. To the degree that we can help Larry reestablish his self-efficacy beliefs, he can be expected to pursue re-establishment of task competence in these areas which are still available to him. To the degree that task competence can be reestablished, role competence will follow. Because such intervention can be expected to help Larry maintain a high level of motivation and focus his attention and the attention of the treatment team, rehabilitation can be expected to progress well and the specific interventions that are intended to restore, educate and help Larry to adapt to life after the stroke can be expected to be optimally effective.

SUMMARY

Occupational competence is role-directed. It develops because humans, as social beings, feel the need to look for and accept challenges that are a part of their social roles. It is sustained when the role is meaningful and valued by the individual, the individual's abilities and environmental supports are perceived as adequate, effort is expended, and the role challenges are met successfully. Occupational competence is pertinent to each role the individual undertakes and actually drives the growth of the individual. The occupational competence model of human development describes how individuals accommodate to, and select new roles across the life span in concert with changes in capacities. As a new valued role is begun, the demands of the role present challenges which the individual seeks to meet because of an urge toward competence. The issue of value of the role challenges is important in that this is the way in which society directs individuals to take on necessary roles. The valuation of the role by society is accepted by an acculturated member of the society who, in turn, values his or her occupational competence and develops self-efficacy beliefs.

The development of occupational competence is a dynamic process with ongoing negotiation between the person, his or her roles and the environment. Growth occurs when the combination of the individual's extent or focus of capacity pertinent to task challenges posed by valued role demands (effectancies) and perception of what the environment can offer pertinent to the role challenges (affordances) is inadequate. Under certain circumstances, the innate urge toward competence will be expressed by the individual who

addresses the challenge and overcomes the inadequacy. However, this process does not occur unless the individual has self-efficacy beliefs which lead to exploration and an attempt to address the challenge. Self-efficacy beliefs affect how the individual behaves in response to such a challenge, especially his or her level of motivation and perseverance. In this way self-efficacy is crucial to sustain the growth of the individual as he or she pursues new and challenging roles.

Disruption of occupational roles by the onset of a disability results in questioning of self-worth and, often, denigration of occupational role competence. The person who becomes occupationally disabled may experience a sense of loss because of a perceived inability to fulfill the roles which provided an opportunity to maintain competence. When self-efficacy beliefs are poor, the experience of overwhelm can occur in which the individual will not attempt to meet the role challenges or may capitulate without having persevered to the extent required to overcome the challenges. The result may be that the individual becomes depressed, emotionally insulated from the role challenges, or alienated from society. Therapeutic intervention can move the individual out of this state of overwhelm.

Initially, the therapeutic process provides the individual a surrogate environment in which structured affordances are provided and threats are minimized so that the individual can be successful in rehearsing the tasks necessary to resume a meaningful role. It is important that the individual experiences successful exploration of tasks which will allow the generalization of competence necessary to undertake higher levels of role challenge. Ensuring this incremental task-based success is the reason that treatment goals should be person-centered and calibrated to the individual's capacity. If the explorational activity is unsuccessful, the frequency with which the individual attempts exploration will decrease.

Success is most likely by focusing on improving the individual's effectancies in concert with the pertinent environmental affordances so that task competency can occur and adequate self-efficacy beliefs emerge. This approach to intervention allows the individual to develop new means to assert role competence despite decreased capacity. Education is an important component of treatment at this stage. It facilitates awareness of environmental affordances and appreciation of how they can be helpful in performing tasks which are meaningful. Reinforcement of the value of the affordances through successful completion of the meaningful task makes it more likely that the affordance will be accessed again.

When restoration of lost capacity is not possible and the previous role cannot be resumed, the therapist must assist the individual in adapting the role. Adaptation must consider the individual's goals and values, perception of abilities and effectancies, the environmental affordances and threats and the role demands and rewards. The effectiveness of the dynamic adjustment of these factors is facilitated by the urge to develop and maintain role competence. The therapist works as an adaptive consultant to allow the individual to rehearse adaptations in the structured environment of the clinic prior to merging the experience of the structured environment into the actual living situation.

STUDY QUESTIONS

1. Draw a flow chart describing the development of occupational competence. What are the key elements which provide positive and negative control of the person's development?

2. What is the importance of self-efficacy in sustaining the development of a person with a newly-acquired disability?

3. Must the development of occupational competence be client-centered? If so, why? If not, why not?

4. Who is more likely to be successful? A person with a history of occupational competence who has become severely disabled, or a person who is able-bodied who has a poor history of occupational competence?

5. How does effectance differ from ability? How is it dependent on ability?

6. Why aren't affordances able to be universally recognized and identified?

7. Why is facilitating the development of occupational competence almost as important as saving a person's life?

8. What effectancies of you as an occupational therapist will be most important in developing another person's occupational competence?

REFERENCES

Baldwin, J. M. (1895). *Mental development in the child and race: Methods and processes.* New York: Macmillan.

Baltes, P. B., Reese, H. W., Lipsitt, L. P. (1980). Life span developmental psychology. *Annual Review of Psychology, 31*, 65-110.

Bandura, A. (1989) Human agency in social cognitive theory. *American Psychologist, 44*(9), 1175-1184.

Bandura, A. (1982) Self-efficacy mechanism in human agency. *American Psychologist, 7*(2), 122-147.

Bandura, A. (1977). Self-efficacy: toward a unifying theory of behavioral change. *Psychological Review, 84*, 191-215.

Bandura, A. (1990). Conclusion: Reflections on non-ability determinants of competence. In R. Sternberg & J. Kolligian (Eds.), *Competence considered.* (pp. 315-362). New Haven: Yale University Press.

Bandura, A., Schunk D. H. (1981). Cultivating competence, self-efficacy, and intrinsic interest through proximal self-motivation. *Journal of Personality and Social Psychology, 41*(3), 586-598.

Bateson, G. (1979). *Mind and nature: A necessary unity.* New York, E. P. Dutton.

Baum, C. (1991). Identification and use of environmental resources. In C. Christiansen & C. Baum (Eds.), *Occupational therapy: Overcoming human performance deficits* (pp. 789-802) Thorofare, NJ: SLACK Incorporated.

Baum, C. & Christiansen, C. (1997). Doing and health. In C. Christiansen & C. Baum (Eds.), *Occupational therapy: Enabling function and well-being.* (2nd ed.). Thorofare, NJ: SLACK Incorporated.

Bing, R. K. (1968). Discussion of Mosey's recapitulation of ontogenesis. *American Journal of Occupational Therapy, 22*, 433-435.

Birren, J. E. (1959). Principles of research on aging. In J. E. Birren (Ed.), *Handbook of aging and the individual* (pp. 3-42). Chicago: University of Chicago Press.

Birren, J. E. (1964). *The psychology of aging.* Englewood Cliffs, NJ: Prentice-Hall.

Birren, J. E. (1988). A contribution to the theory of aging: As a counterpart to development. In J. E. Birren & V. L. Bengston (Eds.), *Emergent theories of aging* (pp. 153-176). New York: Springer.

Birren, J. E., Birren, B. A. (1990). The concepts, models, and history of the psychology of aging. In J. E. Birren & K. W. Schaie (Eds.), *Handbook of the psychology of aging* (pp. 1-20). San Diego: Academic Press.

Birren, J. E., & Renner, V. J. (1977). Research on the psychology of aging: Principles and Experimentation. In J. E. Birren & K. W. Schaie (Eds.), *Handbook of the psychology of aging* (pp. 3-38). New York: Van Nostrand Reinhold.

Branton, P. (1993). In praise of ergonomics: A personal perspective. International Review of Ergonomics, 1, 1-20. In D. Oborne, R. Branton, F. Leal, P. Shipley, & T. Stewart (Eds.), *Person-centered ergonomics: A Brantonian view of human factors.* London: Taylor and Francis.

Brim, O. G., & Ryff, C. D. (1980). On the properties of life events. In P. B. Baltes & O. G. Brim (Eds.), *Life span development and behavior.* New York: Academic Press.

Bronfenbrenner, U. (1977). Towards an experimental ecology of human development. *American Psychologist, 32*, 513-531.

Christiansen, C. (1991). Occupational therapy: Intervention for life performance. In C. Christiansen & C. Baum (Eds.), *Occupational therapy: Overcoming human performance deficits* (pp. 3-44). Thorofare, NJ: SLACK Incorporated.

Clark, F., Parham, D., Carlson, M., Frank, G., Jackson, J., Pierce., D., Wolfe, R., & Zemke, R. (1991). Occupational science: Academic innovation in the service of occupational therapy's future. *American Journal of Occupational Therapy, 45*, 300-310.

Coster, W. (1995a). Developmental aspects of occupation. *The study of the future: Putting occupation back into therapy.* Bethesda, MD: American Occupational Therapy Association.

Coster, W. (1995b). Development. In C. A. Trombly (Ed.),

Occupational therapy for physical dysfunction, fourth edition. Baltimore: Williams and Wilkins.

DeCharms, R. (1968). *Personal causation.* New York: Academic Press.

Deci, E. L., & Ryan, R. M. (1985). *Intrinsic motivation and self-determination in human behavior.* New York: Plenum Press.

Dunn, W., Brown, C., & McGuigan, A. (1994). The ecology of human performance: A framework for considering the effect of context. *American Journal of Occupational Therapy, 48*(7), 595-607.

Erikson, E. (1985). *Childhood and society.* New York: W.W. Norton.

Flach, J., Hancock, P., Caird, J., & Vicente, K. (1995). *Global perspectives on the ecology of human machine systems.* Hillsdale, NJ: Lawrence Erlbaum Associates.

Frey, K. S., & Ruble, D. N. (1990). Strategies for comparative evaluation: Maintaining a sense of competence across the life span. In R. Sternberg & J. Kolligian (Eds.), *Competence considered* (pp. 167-189). New Haven: Yale University Press.

Gage, M. (1992). The appraisal method of coping: An assessment and intervention model for occupational therapy. *American Journal of Occupational Therapy, 46*, 353-362.

Gage, M., & Polatajko, H. (1994). Enhancing occupational performance through an understanding of perceived self-efficacy. *American Journal of Occupational Therapy, 48*, 452-461.

Gibson, J. J. (1979). *The ecological approach to visual perception.* Boston: Houghton Mifflin.

Goldstein, K. (1963). *The organism.* Boston: Beacon Press.

Hamburg, D. A., & Adams, J. E., (1967). A perspective on coping behavior: Seeking and utilizing information in major transitions. *Archives of General Psychiatry, 17*, 277-284.

Hancock, P. A., Chignell, M. H. (1995). In J. Flach, P. Hancock, J. Caird, & K. Vicente. (1995). *Global perspectives on the ecology of human machine systems.* Hillsdale, NJ: Lawrence Erlbaum Associates.

Harter, S. (1978). Effectance motivation reconsidered: Toward a developmental model. *Human Development, 21*, 34-64.

Harter, S. (1985). Competence as a dimension of self-evaluation: Toward a comprehensive model of self-worth. In R. Leahy (Ed.), *The development of the self* (pp. 55-118). New York: Academic Press.

Harter, S. (1990). Causes, correlates, and the functional role of global self-worth: A life span perspective. In R. Sternberg & J. Kolligian (Eds.), *Competence considered* (pp. 67-97). New Haven: Yale University Press.

Havighurst, R. J. (1979). *Developmental tasks and education.* New York: David McKay.

Hoyer, W. (1987). Acquisition of knowledge and the decentralization of *g* in adult intellectual development. In C. Schooler & K. W. Schaie (Eds.), *Cognitive functioning and social structure over the life course* (pp. 120-141). Trenton, NJ: Ablex.

James, W. (1892). *Psychology: The briefer courses.* New York: Henry Holt & Company.

Kielhofner, G. (1985). *A model of human occupation: Theory and application.* Baltimore: Williams & Wilkins.

Kielhofner, G., Borell, L., Burk, J., Helfrich, C., & Nygard, L.

(1995). Volition subsystem. In G. Kielhofner (Ed.), *A model of human occupation: Theory and application* (pp. 39-62). Baltimore: Williams & Wilkins.

Knoblock, H. & Pasamanick, B. (1974). *Gesell and Armatruda's developmental diagnosis.* New York: Harper & Row.

Langer, E. J. & Chanowitz, B. (1987). A new perspective for the study of disability. In H. E. Yuker (Ed.), *Attitudes towards persons with disabilities.* New York: Springer.

Langer, E. J., Rodin, J., Beck, P., Spitzer, L., & Weinman, C. (1979). Environmental determinants of memory improvement in late adulthood. *Journal of Personality and Social Psychology, 37*, 2014-2025.

Law, M. (1991). The environment: A focus for occupational therapy. *Canadian Journal of Occupational Therapy, 58*(4), 171-179.

Law, M., Cooper, B., Strong, S., Stewart, D., Rigby, P, & Leits, L. (1996). The person-environment-occupational model: A transactive approach to occupational performance. *Canadian Journal of Occupational Therapy, 63*(1), 9-23.

Lazarus, R. S., & Folkman, S. (1984). *Stress, appraisal and coping.* New York: Springer.

Levinson, D. J. (1996). *The seasons of a woman's life.* New York: Alfred A. Knopf.

Llorens, L. A. (1991). Performance tasks and roles throughout the life span. In C. Christiansen & C. Baum (Eds.), *Occupational therapy: Overcoming human performance deficits* (pp. 45-68). Thorofare, NJ: SLACK Incorporated.

Maddi, S. R. (1989). *Personality theories: A comparative analysis.* Pacific Grove: Brooks/Cole.

Maslow, A. H. (1968). *Toward a psychology of being.* Princeton: Van Nostrand.

Maslow, A. H. (1971). *The farther reaches of human nature.* New York: Viking.

Matheson, L. N. (1991). Symptom magnification syndrome structured interview: Rationale and procedure. *Journal of Occupational Rehabilitation, 1*(1), 43-56.

Matheson, L. N., Matheson, M. L., & Grant, J. (1993). Development of a measure of perceived functional ability. *Journal of Occupational Rehabilitation, 3*(1), 15-30.

Matheson, L. N., Ogden, L. D., Violette, K., & Schultz, K. (1985). Work hardening: Occupational therapy in industrial rehabilitation. *American Journal of Occupational Therapy, 39*(5), 314-321.

Mechanic, D. (1962). The concept of illness behaviour. *Journal of Chronic Diseases, 15*, 189-194.

Meyer, A. (1922). The philosophy of occupation therapy. *Archives of Occupational Therapy, 1*(1), 1-10.

Miller, J., Slomcyznski, K. M., & Kohn, M. L. (1985). Continuity of learning generalization throughout the life span: The impact of job on intellectual processes in the United States. *American Journal of Sociology, 91*, 993-615.

Mooney V. (1992). Function and the industrial back pain patient. *Journal of Occupational Rehabilitation, 2*(3), 95-102.

Neugarten, B. L. (1968). *Middle age and aging: A reader in social psychology.* Chicago: University of Chicago Press.

Neugarten, B. L., & Datan, N. (1973). Sociological perspectives on the life cycle. In P. B. Baltes & K. W. Schaie (Eds.), *Lifespan developmental psychology: Personality and socialization* (pp. 53-69). New York: Academic Press.

Nygård, C. H., Eskelinen, L., Suvanto, S., Tuomi, K., & Ilmarinen, J. (1991). Associations between functional capacity and work ability among elderly municipal employees. *Scandinavian Journal of Work and Environmental Health, 17*(suppl 1):122-127.

Oakley, F., Kielhofner, G., & Barris, R. (1985). An occupational therapy approach to assessing psychiatric patients' adaptive functioning. *American Journal of Occupational Therapy, 39,* 147-154.

Oborne, D., Branton, R., Leal, F., Shipley, P., & Stewart, T. (Eds.), (1993). *Person-centered ergonomics: A Brantonian view of human factors.* London: Taylor and Francis.

Peak, D. & Frame, M. (1994). *Chaos under control: The art and science of complexity.* New York: W.H. Freeman and Company.

Peterson, C., Maier S. F., & Seligman M. E. P. (1993). *Learned helplessness.* New York, Oxford University Press.

Phillips, D. A., & Zimmerman, M. (1990). The developmental course of perceived competence and incompetence among competent children. In R. Sternberg & J. Kolligian (Eds.), *Competence considered* (pp. 41-66). New Haven: Yale University Press.

Piaget, J. (1954). *The construction of reality in the child.* New York: Basic Books.

Pilowsky I. (1987). Abnormal illness behaviour. *Psychiatric Medicine, 5*(2):85-91.

Reilly, M. (1962). Occupational therapy can be one of the great ideas of 20th century medicine. *American Journal of Occupational Therapy; 16*(1), 87-105.

Rogers, C. R. (1980). *A way of being.* Boston: Houghton Mifflin.

Salthouse, T. A. (1988). Cognitive aspects of motor functioning. In J. A. Joseph (Ed.), *Central determinants of age-related declines in motor function* (pp. 33-41). New York: New York Academy of Sciences.

Salthouse, T. A., & Maurer, T. J. (1996). Aging, job performance and career development. In J. E. Birren & K. W. Schaie (Eds.), *Handbook of the psychology of aging* (pp. 353-364). San Diego: Academic Press.

Schaie, K. W. (1977). Quasi-experimental research designs in the psychology of aging. In J. E. Birren & K. W. Schaie (Eds.), *Handbook of the psychology of aging* (pp. 39-69). San Diego: Academic Press.

Schaie, K. W. (1990). The optimization of cognitive function in old age: Predictions based on cohort sequential and longitudinal data. In P. B. Baltes & M. M. Baltes (Eds.), *Successful aging: perspectives from the behavioral sciences* (pp. 94-117). Cambridge: Cambridge University Press.

Schaie, K. W. (1996). Intellectual development in adulthood. In J.

E. Birren and K. W. Schaie (Eds.), *Handbook of the psychology of aging* (pp. 266-286). San Diego: Academic Press.

Schooler, C. (1990). Psychosocial factors and effective cognitive functioning in adulthood. In J. Birren, & K. W. Schaie (Eds.), *Handbook of the psychology of aging* (pp. 347-358). San Diego: Academic Press.

Schroots, J. J. F. (1988). On growing, formative change and age. In J. E. Birren & V. L. Bengston (Eds.), *Emergent theories of aging* (pp. 299-329). New York: Springer.

Schroots, J. F., & Birren, J. E. (1990). Concepts of time and aging in science. In J. E. Birren & K. W. Schaie (Eds.), *Handbook of the psychology of aging* (pp. 45-67). San Diego, Academic Press.

Seligman M. E. P. (1975). *Helplessness: On depression, development and death.* New York: WH Freeman.

Skinner, B. F. (1974). *About behaviorism.* New York: Albert A. Knopf.

Spirduso, W. W. & MacRae, P. G. (1990). In J. E. Birren & K. W. Schaie (Eds.), *Handbook of the psychology of aging* (pp. 183-200). San Diego, Academic Press.

Stones, M. J. & Kozma, A. (1989). Physical activity, age and cognitive motor performance. In M. L. Howe & C. J. Brainerd (Eds.), *Cognitive development in adulthood: Progress in cognitive development research.* New York: Springer.

Strehler, B. (1977). *Time, cells and aging.* New York: Academic Press.

Veroff, J., (1969). Social comparison and the development of achievement motivation. In C. P. Smith (Ed.), *Achievement-related motives in children* (pp. 46-101). New York: Basic Books.

Von Bertalanfy, L. (1968). *General systems theory.* New York, Braziller.

Vygotsky, L. S. (1978). Mind in society: The development of higher mental processes. In M. Cole, V. John-Steiner, S. Scribner & E. Souberman (Eds.), *Mind in society.* Cambridge, MA: Harvard University Press.

White, R. W. (1959). Motivation reconsidered: the concept of competence. *Psychiatric Review, 66,* 197-333.

White, R. W. (1960). Competence and the psychosexual stages of development. Nebraska Symposium on Motivation, pp. 1-12.

White R. W. (1974). Strategies of adaptation: an attempt at systematic description. In G. V. Coliho, D. A. Hamburg, & J. E. Adams (Eds.), *Coping and adaptation.* New York: Basic Books.

White R. W. (1971). The urge toward competence. *American Journal of Occupational Therapy, 25,* 271-274.

Wilson, E. O. (1978). *On human nature.* Cambridge, MA: Harvard University Press.

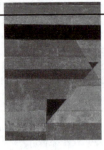

Chapter Content Outline

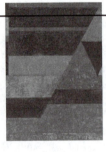

Abstract

Adaptation is central to the practice of occupational therapy and appears as a continuous thread in the occupational therapy literature from 1922 to 1990. A review of this literature reveals the major concepts embedded in the occupational therapy perspective on adaptation. From a study of those concepts, a paradigm of adaptation through and for occupation emerges. This paradigm of adaptation suggests that the role of occupational therapy is to facilitate the internal adaptation process of clients with an approach that is holistic and client-centered in order to enhance occupational performance. It is through engagement in the tasks and occupations which make up an occupational role, that internal adaptation is most readily facilitated and the outcome of intervention most effective. A discussion of one such approach, Occupational Adaptation, demonstrates the adaptation paradigm.

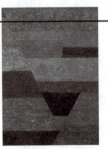

Key Terms

Occupations	Person Systems
Adaptation	Relative Mastery
Occupational Adaptation (the process)	Internal Adaptation Process
Occupational Adaptation (the state)	Adaptation Gestalt
Occupational Environment	Adaptive Response Mechanism

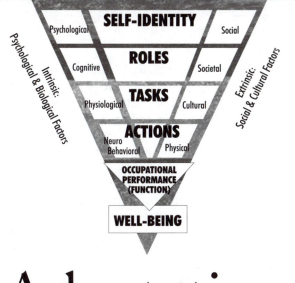

Adaptation

Sally Schultz, PhD, OTR, Janette Schkade, PhD, OTR

OBJECTIVES

The information in this chapter is intended to help the reader:

1. gain an understanding of the historical significance of adaptation within the profession

2. be able to trace the strand of adaptation through some of the profession's most noteworthy literature

3. be able to articulate the relationship between occupation and adaptation

4. have a rudimentary knowledge of the Occupational Adaptation Frame of Reference and its connection with the Paradigm of Adaptation

5. articulate the means and methods to promote internal adaptation within the context of therapeutic intervention.

"Go to the people, work with them, learn from them, respect them, start with what they know, build with what they have. And when the work is done, the task accomplished, the people will say, 'we have done this ourselves'."

Lao Tsu, China, 700 BC

INTRODUCTION

Occupational therapists often experience an interesting phenomenon in their daily practice. They observe that patients or clients with similar deficits or the same disability have remarkably different results from therapy. Some appear to respond quite well to treatment, adapt readily to changes in their lifestyle, and experience favorable outcomes. Others have a more difficult time and seem to encounter many problems in adjusting to their conditions. Clearly, factors other than the nature or the severity of the condition, or even the type of intervention, account for these differences (Christiansen, 1991, p. 70).

This chapter proposes that individual adaptation is a significant factor affecting the response to physical and psychosocial problems. While, the occupational therapy literature has historically championed the role of therapy in helping the individual adapt, direction as to how to accomplish this has been minimal. There are numerous references to the need for therapists to "elicit an adaptive response" (e.g., Ayres, 1972a; King, 1978; Kleinman and Bulkley, 1982). However, there is little explanation of how an individual generates an adaptive response, and equally as important, how a therapist affects the quality of the adaptive response. This chapter provides an explanation of individual adaptation, the underlying adaptive process and its relationship to occupational performance, as well as a therapeutic approach that may be used to influence individual adaptation.

Other disciplines have addressed adaptation in human growth and development (e.g., Cohen & Lazarus, 1979; Erickson, 1985; Piaget & Inhelder, 1969; White, 1974) Much of this work emphasizes the relationship between stress and coping. While the two terms coping and adaptation are often used interchangeably, Cohen and Lazarus (1979) cautioned that the terms should be viewed in a hierarchy with adaptation as the more encompassing. Coping implies specific reactions to specific situations, whereas adaptation is a broader conceptualization of the fit between the individual's capacities and the demands for performance (Christiansen, 1991).

ADAPTATION—SIGNIFICANCE TO OCCUPATIONAL PERFORMANCE

The Person Environment Performance Framework (see Chapter 3) provides a generic explanation of transactions which occur between the individual and the environment

Bibliographic citation of this chapter: Schultz, S., & Schkade, J. (1997). Adaptation. In C. Christiansen & C. Baum (Eds.), *Occupational therapy: Enabling function and well-being* (2nd ed.). Thorofare, NJ: SLACK Incorporated.

through occupation. In this framework, health and well-being are dependent upon the individual's ability to successfully perform relevant activities, tasks, and roles. Occupation is the means by which performance is actualized. The process, however, is much more complicated than it appears. Each person's occupational perfomance is affected by intrinsic factors, such as abilities, skills, personality values and motivation, and extrinsic factors, such as the built environment, social networks, cultural traditions, and societal rules and expectations. The individual must engage in a complex transaction between these factors and the relevant occupations. This transaction may be best understood as a process of individual adaptation. Occupational performance is a product of the individual's ability to reconcile these factors. The way in which the factors become organized represents the individual's adaptation. Sometimes the transactions are routine and predictable; sometimes unusual and unexpected. Some adaptations will yield positive results; while others are negative. A gap in meeting performance expectations may be more a function of poor adaptation than one of functional skills or environmental demands.

If adaptation is the mechanism by which person-environment transactions are negotiated, then it is the individual's internal adaptation which therapists must facilitate to have the greatest impact on occupational performance. As many others in the profession have stated, the therapist's task is to help "close the gap" between adaptive capacity and environmental demands (e.g., King, 1978; Llorens, 1970; Reilly, 1962). Therapists may incorrectly assume that as the patient acquires more functional skills, or begins using assistive devices, adaptation is occurring. The individual's internal adaptation may remain unchanged. In fact, unless the individual's process of adaptation is facilitated by the therapist, adaptation may not begin until therapy is either discontinued or the therapist is not around.

ADAPTATION—UNIVERSAL CONCEPT

A close look at the occupational therapy literature confirms that adaptation is a concept so fundamental to the field that it is recognized as a universally accepted treatment goal. Adaptation is not only viewed as an important goal, but also as a measure of therapeutic effectiveness. However, like so many values that exist as "givens" within a specific culture, the profession's understanding of adaptation is varied, and perhaps elusive. The profession may have embraced adaptation without fully understanding its multiple dimensions. Universal concepts such as adaptation, or for example "the therapeutic relationship," often suffer from being so pervasive that the need for definition, comparison, and guidelines for implementation is overlooked. Although most therapists would be quick to assert that they promote their client's adaptation, there may be considerable variance among those therapists as to what constitutes adaptation, and how it is accomplished. This chapter begins with an historical overview of some of occupational therapy's most widely recognized literature on adaptation. This is followed by a synthesis of the literature which delineates the relationship between adaptation and occupational therapy. The last section provides a description of one theoretical perspective which illustrates the relationship and its practical application with clients.

VARIOUS DEFINITIONS WITHIN PRACTICE

Occupational therapists use the term adaptation to communicate a number of different meanings. For example, adaptation is the term used to describe changes made in the client's home environment as well as to describe assistive devices the client uses to complete self-care activities. Both of these uses are directed at changes made, usually by the therapist, in the client's physical surroundings. While some practitioners use adaptation to characterize a compensation the client has been taught in order to cope with an underlying impairment, others may use adaptation to discuss a client's level of adjustment or acceptance of a loss in functional skills. Other practitioners may use adaptation to describe the client's internal response to a significant challenge in performing occupational roles. Regardless of such variance, since the origin of the profession there has been a consistent strand of thought which is identifiable within the body of knowledge, i.e., the phenomenological process of human adaptation and its relevance to occupational therapy.

The occupational therapy literature contains a number of terms that may seem to have the same meaning, e.g. adaptive process, adaptive mode, adaptive patterns, adaptive behavior, adaptive functioning, occupational adaptation, adaptive response, adaptive strategy, etc. Although these terms may appear to be interchangeable, the reader is cautioned against making this assumption, as these terms have distinct definitions when associated with specific theoretical models.

THE CONCEPTUAL EVOLUTION OF ADAPTATION

This section provides an overview of adaptation as presented in the profession's early literature from 1922 to 1979. Familiarity with the underpinnings of adaptation is necessary to understand the evolution of the adaptation concept from 1980 to 1990 (the second half of this section). The references

included in these two discussions are generally accepted as among those most frequently cited in the profession's body of knowledge.

Understanding of Adaptation

Perhaps the earliest and most recognized publication to state the significance of the adaptation phenomenon was Adolph Meyer's 1922 landmark article. In this work (which became accepted as the profession's original statement of philosophy), Meyer urged health care providers to divert their focus from diagnosing and prescribing treatment to conquer disease, and attend to what he proposed was the more important issue: that successful treatment extends far beyond the underlying disease. He stated that in his opinion, "... many formidable diseases are largely problems of adaptation and not some mysterious devil in disguise" (p. 1).

Meyer asserted that psychiatry was among the first medical specialties to "recognize the need of adaptation and the value of work as a sovereign help in the problems of adaptation" (p. 1). He identified occupation as the most effective tool to positively influence what he identified as the patient's primary problem: adaptation. The role of therapy was defined as giving opportunities for the patient to engage in meaningful occupations (rather than prescriptions). According to Meyer, engaging the patient in activity that incorporated the patient's "hands and muscles, and a happy appreciation of time" (p. 2) was the preferred treatment modality to affect problems of adaptation.

The First Principle and Its Related Hypothesis

Reilly's (1962) often-cited lecture reclaimed elements of the profession's founding beliefs that had become essentially dormant for many years due to the profession's tendency to seek an identity through emulating others. Reilly's lecture provided what is probably the most frequently cited quotation in the profession's literature. The words, "That man, through the use of his hands as they are energized by mind and will, can influence the state of his own health" (p. 2) emerged as a fundamental hypothesis and have resounded through the profession. This quotation is consistent with Meyer's emphasis on work and its relationship to adaptation.

Reilly asserted that her hypothesis represented the profession's fundamental belief that had been "passed on for proof by the early founders" (p. 2). In the latter part of her lecture, Reilly identified what she called the profession's First Principle. She stated, "The logic of occupational therapy rests upon the principle that man has a need to master his environment, to alter and improve it...Severe dysfunction and unhappiness occurs when this need is blocked" (p. 6).

According to Reilly, the function of such a first principle is to provide a basis for the profession's body of knowledge, treatment process, and application techniques. She concluded that although content on sensorimotor, cognitive and psychosocial systems would always be relevant, the profession's body of knowledge should focus on work. She described the capacity to work as a developmental process in which the individual adapts by learning how to integrate motor and cognitive functions to experience control over the environment and satisfaction in performance. She concluded that the treatment process should, therefore, be focused on work satisfaction. With this orientation, the therapist acts to facilitate the client's active, creative problem-solving within tasks directly associated with the individual's life roles. The therapist's method is to create the setting necessary for the above-described treatment process to occur. Reilly defined remedial procedures, directed at the client's underlying functional deficits, as techniques.

The Relationship Between Theories of Motivation and Adaptation

Reilly's (1962) assertion that all individuals have an innate need to master, alter and improve the environment spurred efforts within the profession to better understand the nature of such motivation, how it is triggered, and how it can be harnessed by the occupational therapist to promote individual adaptation. Explanations for motivation are either explicitly or implicitly stated throughout the remainder of the literature discussed.

Motivation, Meaning and Adaptation

White (1959), a psychologist, offered a perspective on motivation (known as the urge toward competency) which, for the time, was a significant departure from the two prevailing theories on motivation: psychoanalysis and behaviorism. White countered that the human being is as much a creator of experiences as a passive recipient. He asserted that although the urge toward competency reflects the desire to master the environment, he believed that the "urge" actually stems from the pleasure or "joy in being a cause" (Groos, 1901). White described this form of satisfaction as "intrinsic" (p. 272) to communicate that there was no need for extrinsic (or external) sources of affirmation.

Yerxa's (1967) Eleanor Clarke Slagle Lecture emphasized the significance of personal meaning as a motivation for adaptation. She claimed that choice and self-initiated activity may be the primary source of motivation in human adaptation. She also proposed that adaptive changes are as much a consequence of internal desire as external demand. Her comments on the acquisition of movement skills being internally created as well as externally stimulated, illustrate her congruence with White's (1959) theory on motivation.

Florey's (1969) seminal article directly incorporated White's (1959) theory. She proposed that the concept of intrinsic motivation had the potential to serve as a frame of reference to guide practice. Florey asserted that intrinsic motivation (i.e., internal, self-directed influence and self-reward) is, in fact, the preferred explanation of motivation for occupational therapy. Florey concluded that "it is the self-reward of independent action that underlies competent behavior" (p. 320).

Relationship Between Human Development, Adaptation and Occupational Therapy

The 1969 Eleanor Clarke Slagle Lecture (Llorens, 1970) provided what may have been the first organized framework for occupational therapy practice with an overarching emphasis on human adaptation. Llorens' 10 premises present the occupational therapist as an "enculturation agent" (p. 93), e.g., one who helps the client achieve the highest level of performance within a cultural context.

Llorens stated that dysfunction occurs when trauma or disease creates a "gap" between expectations from the culture and the client's ability to perform. Thus, the task of therapy is to help the client close the gap, further described as "a disparity between expected coping behavior and the client's adaptive facility" (p. 94). The therapist improves adaptive facility (a combination of necessary skills and abilities) by engaging the client in selected activities and relationships. Llorens emphasized that the client's experience of mastery and satisfaction is necessary for adaptation (or change in adaptive facility) to occur. Llorens concluded that such interventions are valuable in that they serve to "prevent potential maladaptation." A logical inference is that perhaps the greater value of such interventions is their potential to promote the client's adaptation and enculturation.

Emphasis on the Client as the Agent of Change

Smith (1972), another psychologist frequently cited in literature on adaptation, proposed a perspective on the therapeutic ends and means of occupational therapy. His perspectives were consistent with those of White (1959), Yerxa (1967), and Florey (1969). In summary, Smith suggested that occupational therapy replaces the concept of helping the client adjust, to one of helping the client become competent, i.e., an agent rather than a patient. Smith urged occupational therapists to focus on the client's spark of intrinsic motivation. As he stated, the problem of occupational therapy is to "...nurture and fan the spark of intrinsic motivation, not quench it" (p. 11) and "...give the client practice in thinking how to control the world, not adjust to it" (p. 15).

Smith observed that most individuals perceive themselves as patients when referred to occupational therapy. Such role orientation (with its implied dependency) places even greater demand on therapists to reposition the patient into the role of agent, wherein the patient is proactive and functions as a consumer of health care. With patient agency as the focus, the client has the potential to use personal resources to self-direct adaptation in a way that the client can function as an "origin" i.e., a doer, or an actor who does not adjust to life, but actively lives it. DeCharms (1968) contrasted his description of the "origin" as one who creates life experiences, with the "pawn," who views life as determined by external forces with little opportunity to change those forces. Smith expanded upon White's (1959) explanation of the motivational core underlying competency. Smith proposed that the motivation leading to competency is a cyclical cluster of attitudes toward the self and the world. He identified self-respect (attitude toward self as a significant and effective person) and hopefulness (attitude regarding potential to be effective in the world) as characteristic of the two crucial attitudes which develop competency. Smith also asserted that individuals use the same two categories of attitudes (toward self and potential in the world) to produce the motivation that leads to incompetence. Helplessness and hopelessness were identified as the two attitudes which produce cyclical incompetence.

As with the preceding discussion on Reilly, White, Yerxa, and Florey, Smith emphasized not only the environment's demand for adaptation, but the individual's potential as a generator of adaptation demands which result from the individual's actions. While the environment presents demands for adaptation, the individual emerges as the primary actor in creating those environments and respective demands.

Adaptation as a Key Concept within Additional Practice Frameworks

Work that was done on motivation theory and its effect on occupation and adaptation led to the development of practice frameworks designed to provide a theoretical explanation of the therapy process. Adaptation became one of the most consistent elements within these frameworks. In 1972, Shannon proposed the Work-Play Frame of Reference. His work was based on the theory of occupational behavior generated by Reilly and her protégés. Shannon's stated intent was to provide an alternative to the current focus on illness or injury and redirect therapy toward emphasis on the behaviors or skills of the individual. The skills he stressed were those he described as being directly related to what he described as successful adaptation, i.e., resumption of the individual's life plan and life tasks. He called for a shift from adapting activities for the purpose of treating pathology, to promoting the individual's adaptation to life. In addition, Shannon proposed that the client's adaptation process may be the primary interest of the profession.

A few years later, Shannon (1977) made an impassioned plea for occupational therapists to return to those beliefs that originally legitimized the profession. He espoused that occu-

pational therapy had abandoned "substantive" rationality for "functional" rationality. This shift resulted in treatment that stressed efficiency to achieve ends with disregard for the relative desirability of the ends. According to Shannon, occupational therapy had become "derailed." The original understanding of adaptation as a competency phenomenon was in danger of being replaced by more simplistic explanations that focused on stimulus-response, instincts, drives, or neuromuscular patterning. He warned that Reilly's (1962) hypothesis was being subverted by a technique hypothesis that promoted "the laying on of hands" by therapists, and a rejection of the client as a "creative being capable of directing his own future" (p. 233). Shannon concluded that such framing of the treatment focus would increase the client's dependency and reduce potential for adaptation. Shannon's comments reflect his concern that the profession was in danger of losing its concern with adaptation, that is influenced by the individual, and at risk for reframing therapy into a process controlled by the therapist and other external influences.

Shannon asserted that the profession has a primary practice domain consisting of two elements that should guide intervention: 1) temporal adaptation—how one occupies time as demanded by activities in work, play, rest and sleep; and 2) behavioral competencies—those performance skills required for successful temporal adaptation. He completed this two-part proposal by overlaying Matsutsuyu's (1971) perspectives on role and its relationship to occupation. Matsutsuyu offered that the individual should not be viewed in the context of presenting disease or disability, but within the context of the roles occupied by that person, such as: pre-schooler, homemaker, or retiree. Therefore, the individual's occupational roles emerge as the framework for understanding the individual's unique performance demands and tailoring treatment to promote successful adaptation within those roles. Shannon's perspectives are consistent with the profession's evolving theory on adaptation and motivation theory. He juxtaposed these ideas with another key concept that has historical significance within the profession's developing body of knowledge: the occupational role.

Kielhofner (1977) elaborated upon the concept of temporal adaptation and Reilly's theory of occupational behavior in a preliminary framework for practice. In contrast to Matsutsuyu (1971), Kielhofner proposed that the individual's adaptation should be viewed within the broader context of time. He asserted that the way in which the individual used and organized time (daily habits) was the best measure of adaptiveness. He contrasted this with the concept of activities of daily living, asserting that temporal adaptation is much more than a checklist of self-care skills. Kielhofner defined temporal adaptation as a "descriptive term for integration of an entire spectrum of activities, the organization of which supports health on an ongoing daily life basis" (p. 236). He suggested the term temporal dysfunction to describe problems within the individual's organization. Kielhofner stated that it is the experience of actions in time, i.e., "that he or she has acted, is acting, and will continue to act" (p. 237) that transforms the nature of the individual's adaptation. He proposed that within the individual there is an inner process in which the past and future serve as reference points for human adaptation. The process of adaptation is thus fueled by the individual's awareness of agenthood and respective placement in time. Kielhofner concluded that temporal adaptation is unique to the individual and is a culmination of socialization processes experienced throughout the life span. As with others cited in this review of literature, he recognized the importance of roles, commenting that "adaptation requires individuals to use their time in a manner that supports their roles" (p. 239).

Fidler and Fidler (1978) also emphasized the use of time and its significance to adaptation within their conceptual framework of "doing." They defined doing as a process of testing capacities through feedback from interaction with human and nonhuman objects. They stated that it is through such doing that the individual acquires the ability to adapt and fulfill life roles. The greater the individual's repertoire of doing experiences, the greater the range of action alternatives or adaptive behavior. Their ideas are consistent with White's (1959) premise that there is an innate drive to master and explore the environment. Fidler and Fidler espoused that there is no greater sense of satisfaction than that which comes from successful doing, as long as the individual has accomplished it from one's own resources. They cautioned practitioners against the tendency to misinterpret doing as simply random activity. Doing must be directly linked to the individual's present life roles, as well as age, biology and culture. They stressed the necessity to understand the relationship between the concept of doing and human adaptation for interventions to be therapeutic.

The Fidlers' understanding of doing may be viewed as analogous to the phenomenon of adaptation. As they stated, doing is the means by which the individual adapts. A logical extension of their work is to propose that doing (or occupation that is personally meaningful), can be best understood as the action component of the adaptation process. The Fidlers' emphasis on satisfaction, self-initiation, and the relationship between doing and individual roles, adds additional support for viewing doing as behavior or action that exists within the more comprehensive dimension of adaptation.

Proposal for the Science of Adaptive Responses

The 1978 Eleanor Clarke Slagle Lecture solidified adaptation as a core concept within the profession. In her lecture, King (1978) asserted that the profession was in dire need of synthesis and unification, and that the concept of adaptation had the potential to fulfill this need. She reported that this idea stemmed from being reminded of Ayres' (1972a) phrase "eliciting a related adaptive response" (p. 114). King stated that "eliciting an adaptive response" was probably the one thing that every therapist does. She also noted that (within the literature of that time) adaptation was mentioned in almost every article. King concluded that, although adaptation was an ever-present concept in almost all of the profession's arenas, its significance had not been articulated beyond being an implicit assumption. She stated, "I have not found that we have rigorously analyzed the concept or used it consciously to explain our function in any broad sense...it is time that some of our implicit assumptions about adaptation be made explicit" (p. 431).

King's lecture identified four normative characteristics of the adaptive process. Her first assertion was that adaptation is dependent upon the individual having a positive or active role. She emphasized that an "adaptive response cannot be imposed, it must be actively created" (p. 432) by the adapting person. Second, she asserted that adaptation occurs only when it is called forth by demands embedded within the activity/environment. For example, the individual's adaptive process is activated when the desire to perform an activity is blocked by personal or environmental limitations. Thus, a naturalistic condition demands that the individual generate an alternate approach to the activity (i.e., an adaptive response). King described the therapist's task as providing the environmental experiences/demands which trigger the individual's adaptive process. She emphasized the necessity of employing the client's real-life environment. Therapists were cautioned to realize that an adaptive response does not actually occur until the client incorporates the adaptation into routine actions. The third characteristic proposed by King was that personal adaptation does not occur at the conscious or cognitive level. She urged therapists to avoid focusing the client's cognitive attention on the adaptive response being elicited. She asserted that doing so would actually interfere with adaptation. Instead, the therapist should provide experiences that naturally activate the client's potential for an adaptive response. King offered her belief that in occupational therapy always there are always two sources of motivation within the client: "...the most distinguishing characteristic of occupational therapy, derived from a simple truth about adaptation, is that there is always a double motivation..." (p. 433).

The client's first motivation is direct and refers to the activity itself, e.g., the individual's motivation to catch a ball or make a vase. The client's second motivation is indirect, it is, however, a constant. The second motivation is the urge that all human beings have to adapt. King espoused that it is the second source of motivation, the client's urge for personal adaptation, that occupational therapy should promote. She stated that even though personal adaptation is the more subtle of the two motivations, and not as easily recognized by the client or others, it is the therapist's duty to ensure its understanding. King asserted that *"the use of purposeful activity to elicit an adaptive response is the realm of occupational therapy and that which most accurately distinguishes the profession from all others"* [italics added by authors].

"The fourth characteristic of the adaptive response is that it is self-reinforcing" (p. 433). King described the personal experience of mastering the environment's demands as a stimulus that motivates the individual to accept even greater challenge. She espoused that while performance of the activity may be a desirable outcome, the more important product is the experience of mastery that follows a successful adaptive response and the effect which that experience has on adaptation.

Adoption of a Statement of Philosophy

The profession's formal Statement of Philosophy (American Occupational Therapy Association [AOTA], 1979) reflects the significance of the concept of adaptation and its evolution as an essential element within the profession's body of knowledge. In the first two paragraphs of the Statement, the term purposeful activity is used five times; while the term adaptation appears six times in fewer than ten sentences. The Statement begins by providing a definition of adaptation and its significance. Adaptation is presented as a normative process that is continually present across the life span. Adaptation is defined as a change in function that supports survival and self-actualization. Dysfunction occurs as a consequence of disruption in the adaptation process caused by biological, psychological, or environmental factors. Purposeful activity is viewed as a facilitator of the adaptive process. The Statement posits that "occupational therapy is based on the belief that purposeful activity (occupation) may be used to ameliorate dysfunction as well as elicit maximum adaptation" (p. 785).

In many ways, the Statement of Philosophy is an amalgamation of the profession's current understanding of adaptation. The Statement proposes the normative process of adaptation as a framework for occupational therapists to understand human development, function, and dysfunction. The significance of occupation is presented as the preferred medium to tap into what may be conceptualized as the target for therapy; the individual's adaptation process.

Contemporary Thought on Adaptation

With the formal adoption of the 1979 Statement of Philosophy by the Representative Assembly, adaptation became indisputable as one of the profession's fundamental concepts. The need to clarify the profession's understanding of intervention and its effect on adaptation was heightened. In response, the years between 1980 and 1990 were a period of heightened scholarly activity. Rapid expansion of the profession's general body of knowledge and further elaboration on the phenomenon of adaptation occurred. The works of several authors are recognized as major contributions. The following discussion introduces perspectives from some of the most widely known.

Emergence of a Model of Human Occupation

This model was introduced in a four-part series, Part I by Kielhofner and Burke (1980). The stated intent of the model was to provide a framework for the profession's core concepts as well as a tool to organize a broader science of human occupation. Kielhofner and Burke combined the concepts of general systems theory with a systemic explanation of human occupation. The model consisted of four elements: *input* (information from the environment), *throughput* (organization of information flow through three subsystems: volition, habituation, and performance), *output* (occupational behavior), and *feedback* (information on results of output). Each of the three subsystems was conceptualized as having a specific effect on output.

In this model, the volition subsystem is the source of the individual's motivation to explore and master. The habituation subsystem functions to organize the individual's patterns of behavior in a way that will satisfy both the individual's urge to explore and the environment's demands. The performance subsystem is the source of skills the individual needs to act on the environment. In Part II, Kielhofner (1980a) elaborated the concept of temporal adaptation to describe the "unfolding of occupational behavior over the life span" (p. 663). The third article, Part III, (Kielhofner, 1980b) provided a discussion on adaptation. Kielhofner defined adaptation "as a process requiring both internal satisfaction to the system and fulfillment of the environment's demands" (p. 737). He stated that change is the central theme of the open system and discussed that change occurs through two cycles in the system: the benign cycle and the vicious cycle. The benign cycle is adaptive and satisfies the need for mastery and external demands. The vicious cycle is maladaptive and perpetuates feelings of incompetence and fails to meet external demands. In Part IV, Kielhofner, Burke, and Igi (1980) proposed that change in the system is primarily guided by the volitional subsystem. Occupational therapy is provided to reorganize the system. The therapist elicits a response that will help the client make the adaptation necessary to replace the vicious cycle with a benign cycle.

The model of human occupation marked a turning point in the method used to articulate future conceptual relationships. Although the majority of the concepts within this model had been discussed by previous occupational therapy authors, the model provided further clarity through the use of a conceptual diagram. Future models began to routinely incorporate such visual representations.

Examination of Old Values and Suggestions for New Directions

In 1981, Jerry Johnson was asked to give a national conference presentation in which she would introduce the theme of general sessions by Gail Fidler, A. Joy Huss, and Virginia Scardina, three renowned authorities in their practice areas. The purpose of the four presentations was to examine the profession's old values, and to suggest new concepts to replace the old treatment symbols. The four speakers intimated that, in fact, the proposed "new" concepts may be a more accurate reflection of the underlying meaning of the old values. These four presentations were then published as a set. Johnson (1981) revealed that when asked to present, she viewed the task as relatively simple since she had given considerable thought to the profession's values throughout her career. However, when she began to write, "the process was slow and arduous" (p. 589). She found the relationship between competency, adaptation, and integration (three of the profession's core concepts) to be ambiguous and tenuous. She concluded that these three concepts were explained more by anecdote than definition. Johnson responded with an articulation of the following relationship between these three concepts: competence (having capacities equal to expectations); adaptation (changing to meet shifts in circumstances); and integration (reconstituting a renewed whole). She summarized the purpose of occupational therapy by stating that we assess the individual's functioning within occupational performance in order to provide therapy that will result in adaptation and subsequent integration.

Fidler's (1981) comments professed the need to examine "symbols of the past such as crafts, kinesiology, and peg boards," and replace them with the concepts: "competence, adaptation, and integration" (p. 567). She stressed that replacement of old symbols with concepts does not mean that the profession's old values are being discarded. She asserted that the concepts would more accurately represent the actual meaning of the old values. Fidler reiterated Yerxa's (1967) concern for the lack of specificity in the profession's core concepts. She argued that competency is what enables the individual to adapt and, therefore, competency should be the primary focus of the profession. Her review of the literature revealed that, even though purposeful activity was accepted as the primary means to develop competency, except for Reilly and associates, there was an "impressive lack of information relative to the meaning and uses of activities" (p. 569).

In the second publication, Huss (1981), called for an increased emphasis on teaching occupational therapy students how to use occupations to elicit an adaptive response that will help clients reach their maximum adaptive potential. She criticized the use of non-occupation-based therapies in that they have no potential to demand adaptation from the client. The last speaker (Scardina, 1981) traced the evolution of sensory integration theory and its application. In this work, Scardina stressed that neither activities nor the use of specialized equipment are therapeutic. She asserted that therapy is the guided use of activities that will, first and foremost, elicit an adaptive response that provides improved integration of sensation. Scardina issued the caveat, that regardless of what the therapist does, the therapist cannot reorganize the individual's brain, only the individual can.

Additional Models Proposed

Kleinman and Bulkley (1982) elaborated upon King's (1978) proposal that "individual adaptation" be recognized as the primary domain of practice. They introduced the "adaptation continuum" (p. 16) to provide a broader conceptualization of human adaptation. The adaptation continuum consists of four types of adaptation occurring in the following sequence: homeostatic reactions; adaptive responses; adaptive skills, and adaptive patterns. Homeostatic reactions are mechanical and physiological responses, reflecting the capacity to perform. Adaptive responses (the integration of sensorimotor, cognitive, social, emotional, cultural components) develop into adaptive skills due to repetition or combination of adaptive responses. Adaptive patterns are combinations of skills that reflect more complex patterns of performance over time. Kleinman and Bulkley affirmed that the function of occupational therapy is to elicit adaptive responses. They described neuromuscular facilitation, relaxation exercises, work simplification, assistive devices, and so forth, as "subordinate activity designed to prepare for performance" (p. 18). They concluded that the focus in all settings is to elicit adaptive responses that meet the therapy goal of building adaptive skills. In their opinion, this is what distinguishes occupational therapy from other helping professions. Several provocative questions complete their discussion. What is the specific benefit of the adaptive response? What is the mechanism by which it occurs? Are there states of the individual (e.g., relaxation, happiness, disappointment) which are more conducive to adaptive responses? What are maladaptive responses?

Howe and Briggs (1982) suggested an ecological system model. They described states of both illness and health as "ecological adaptation" (p. 322). The goal in this model is to help individuals cope with the environment, adapt, change it, and to master life tasks relative to themselves and their environment. As with the model of human occupation, the ecological system model incorporated the general systems theory framework of input, throughput, output, and feedback. Howe and Briggs combined the systems framework with an explanation of the environment as a series of embedded layers ranging from the inner life space (where cognitive, psychological, and physiological operations process input) to three layers of extended life spaces (immediate, social, and ideological). Life tasks and roles are performed within the extended life spaces. The nature of these behaviors becomes increasingly complex over time. The match between role performance and internal/external expectations is processed as feedback that either the individual or society may use to alter the system by influencing expectations and performances. Howe and Briggs identified two forms of motivation for the development of performance skills: 1) the drive to survive, and 2) the drive to develop competency or feelings of efficacy. They determined whether a behavior is functional or dysfunctional by evaluating its appropriateness to life tasks and effectiveness in meeting expectations. The approach to treatment is centered on adaptation. Howe and Briggs asserted that therapists should use purposeful activity presented in a way that complies with the characteristics necessary (King, 1978) to elicit an adaptive response. They supported their perspective with the statement that, "The adaptive process has been at the center of occupational therapy's theory and practice since its origin as a profession." (p. 326).

The concept of internal adaptation was proposed by Reed and Sanderson (1983) as representing a generic model that existed intuitively within the profession. They defined a generic model as a set of beliefs which are focused on a specific outcome. According to Reed and Sanderson, such models provide an explanation of why occupational therapy is valuable, but do little for directing day-to-day practice. In the generic Internal Adaptation model, the concept of adaptation is defined as the changes or adjustments made by a person in order to meet the demands of the environment. Reed and Sanderson commented that the model's conceptualization of adaptation is congruent with the core values of occupational therapy. The model fosters the individual being in control of self; the use of purposeful occupation as the primary therapy modality; and an appreciation of internal adaptation as a lifelong normative process. King's (1978) work, on the characteristics of an adaptive response, was discussed as an example of the generic, albeit intuitive, model. While Reed and Sanderson recognized that internal adaptation was an attractive model, they cautioned that therapists must be well disciplined to use the generic model. For example, they stated that a focus on internal adaptation requires adherence to a specific definition of purposeful. Reed and Sanderson emphasized that within the generic model, "purposeful" (1983, p. 46) should only be used in reference to what the individual finds purposeful, not the therapist or society. Furthermore, since it is much more difficult to provide client-driven therapy than therapist-driven, the therapist must develop an in-depth understanding of appropriate methods and techniques that are consistent with the theoretical principles.

Reed and Sanderson (1983) and Reed (1984) proposed a frame of reference entitled "Adaptation Through Occupation" (1984, p. 491). In the first work (1983), the authors provided 11 assumptions to explain the nature of the interactive relationship between adaptation, occupation, and the environment. In the first assumption, occupation is defined as that which enables individuals to either adapt to the environment or adapt the environment to themselves. The second assumption proposes that occupational competency affects the individual's potential to adapt. Third, all occupations require some combination of "abilities, knowledge and attitudes" (1983, p. 74). Two of the 11 assumptions stress the influence that environmental changes (including changes within the individual) have on the individual's occupations. Several other assumptions refer to the potential that the individual has to affect the environment, as well as therapeutic management of the environment to promote the individual's adaptation within occupation. The remaining assumptions address the importance of a healthful balance of occupations, the individual's need to guide therapy, and skills that are relevant to the individual.

The proposed frame of reference defines "adaptation as an interaction process between the physical, psychobiological and sociocultural environments" (1983, p. 78). In the 1984 version of the proposed framework, Reed stated that occupation is the tool to achieve adaptation through "that which engages a person's time, energy and attention" (p. 491). This work provides additional clarification of "purposeful," stating that the term should be limited to defining those activities which society values. Reed incorporated the term "meaningful occupation" (1984, p. 502) into the framework to define those activities which the individual finds personally rewarding. Reed and Sanderson (1983) professed that their focus on individual satisfaction was not incidental, but vital. They espoused that the "best adaptation occurs" (1983, p. 79) when the individual's "ultimate satisfaction" serves as the primary therapeutic objective.

Definition of Occupation and its Relation to Adaptation

Nelson (1988) asserted that the profession was in need of a definition for occupation that reflects how it is used in practice. For example, some therapists use the term occupation to identify the actual activity. Others use occupation to describe the doing of the activity. Nelson responded to this dilemma by developing a model of occupation that has two dimensions: form and performance. He used the term, occupational form, to describe the activity, e.g., the steps, structure, parameters. He used occupational performance to characterize the individual's doing of the activity. Nelson defined occupation as a "dynamic relationship between occupational form and occupational performance" (p. 633). The following is a brief overview of this dynamic relationship and its impact on human adaptation.

Nelson asserted that activities contain both form and performance elements. Some aspects of an activity's occupational form are fixed, and consequently, shape performance. However other aspects of the occupational form are flexible, and are shaped by such factors as the individual's developmental level, sense of purpose, and experience of meaning in the activity. Occupational form is also influenced by occupational performance. This occurs in not only current occupational forms but in future occupational forms as well. The nature of future forms is shaped by the individual's success at combining present performance skills with adaptations in the developmental structure (abilities, skills, processes) that are necessary for future occupations. Such adaptations occur when occupational performance is inadequate to satisfy the individual's sense of purpose.

Nelson's work offered further comment on the relationship between occupation and adaptation. He cited Fidler and Fidler (1978); King (1978); and Meyer (1922) to support his suggestion that adaptation is the term which best describes the change process facilitated by occupational therapy. He concluded that adaptation (which can be either positive or negative) occurs within two domains: the individual's sense of purpose, and the individual's developmental structure. In summary, while Nelson focused on defining occupation, he also provided an explanation of the reciprocal relationship between occupation and human adaptation.

Proposal to Develop a Discipline of Occupational Science

A group of faculty and students at the University of Southern California began the development of a basic science for occupational therapy (Yerxa, Clark, Frank, Jackson, Parham, Pierce, Stein, and Zemke, 1990). The authors were quick to point out that applications were to be developed by practitioners, leaving the basic science free to focus on universal concepts that would ultimately enable therapists to do a better job with their patients. The USC group lamented that therapists are faced with the demand to reduce incapacity without having sufficient knowledge of capacity, i.e., "how humans develop and sustain independence, adapt to environmental challenges, and learn competency" (p. 4). Thus occupational science is described as the study of three primary areas: the need for occupation; the capacity to engage in occupation; and the orchestration of daily occupations within the environment over the life span.

The roots of occupational science are attributed to Meyer (1922), Slagle (1922), Reilly (1962, 1966, 1969), and Ayres (1972a, 1979). The authors acknowledged that perspectives on occupation from other disciplines will help shape the developing science. The following provides a summary of the initial conceptualization of occupational science and its relationship to adaptation as discussed in this chapter.

Occupation is the core concept of occupational science. The USC group defined occupation as "chunks of activity within the on-going stream of human behavior" (p. 5). These chunks can be either playful or productive, however in either case, they are typically self-initiated; goal-directed and socially sanctioned. Individuals carry out occupation by using adaptive skills that they find satisfying. Although not directly stated, occupational science appears to be based on an *a priori* assumption; that is, the belief that there is an innate human drive to act on the environment toward the experience of competency (White, 1974). This assumption explains the theory of motivation for occupation.

Occupational behavior is an additional key concept, describing the actions that are part of "willful planning and organizing of resources, which the individual experiences as engaging." The "building blocks" of occupational behaviors are rules, habits and skills. The individual's occupational roles (Reilly, 1969) determine which rules, habits and skills are relevant to occupational therapy. The USC group added their perspective on time to their discussion on occupational behavior. They asserted that perception of "time use" (as a source of satisfaction and support for values and goals) affects which occupations and related behaviors the individual selects to include in patterns of daily living.

The environment (made up of social, cultural, physical and spiritual factors) is another key concept. It's significance lies in a second basic assumption of occupational science: occupation occurs as an action on the environment or as a response to challenges from the environment. Therefore, the environment forms the context for occupation (Dunn, Brown & McGuigan, 1994).

Yerxa et al. (1990) asserted that two other concepts, meaning and challenge, determine whether a particular occupation is health promoting. What is meaningful to one may not be to another. The challenge to one may be too complex, due to inadequate skills, whereas for another, it is too simple. Consequently, occupation must be individualized to provide the right match between individual skills and values as well as the therapeutic goal.

In summary, occupational science intends to provide basic research on occupation that goes beyond the practice of occupational therapy toward the interdisciplinary body of knowledge on humankind. Yerxa et al. proposed that the study of occupation will produce an understanding of human behavior that will benefit society at large, as well as the practice of occupational therapy.

The initial articulation of occupational science makes only one direct comment on adaptation, "the blend of daily occupation...and perception of quality of life...mediates adaptation" (p. 5,6). However, one can deduce that adaptation is an underlying, albeit even intuitive, theme throughout the discussion. The significance of the adaptation phenomenon is undeniable given the theories cited as the foundation for the proposed science. (See previous analysis of Meyer's,

Reilly's and Ayres' perspectives on adaptation and its relevance to occupational therapy.)

The Phenomenon of Adaptation: Focus of 1990 Slagle Lecture

The 1980s ended with Fine's 1990 Eleanor Clarke Slagle Lecture (Fine, 1991) on the "experience of adversity and the drive to rise above it" (p. 493). She stated that these "two themes characterize the human condition." Fine reviewed literature from numerous disciplines to articulate her explanation of resilience and human adaptability. She found that even contradictory theories affirmed a human capacity to withstand traumatic disruption, create adaptive responses, and reintegrate. While challenges develop adaptive skills, challenge can also exceed capacity, promoting disintegration. Fine asked the core question: "Who rises above adversity?" (p. 493). What enables some individuals to withstand life-threatening conditions? The remainder of her lecture responds. She cautioned therapists that limiting outcome measures to behavioral skills is an incomplete assessment of adaptation. Resilience is both a response to the situation, and a response to feelings about the situation. She provided numerous examples showing the necessity of hope, will, meaning, and the ability to ignore things beyond one's control. Fine identified four tasks that the therapist does that promote the client's reintegration. The occupational therapist helps the client: find meaning; handle feelings about the situation; understand the reality of the situation; and develop the performance skills needed. Fine suggested therapists examine their role, and perhaps reframe practice models. She lamented that the profession may have left behind a fundamental value (i.e., clients' perceptions of themselves and their situation). She concluded, "evidence suggests that we may have reframed rehabilitation to fit the economy more than the client" (p. 501).

SIGNIFICANCE OF ADAPTATION WITHIN OCCUPATIONAL THERAPY

The profession's body of knowledge contains overwhelming evidence of a consistent strand of thought on adaptation. However, the strand has not been clearly identified and systematically organized. The literature argues that although adaptation has been an ever-present concept, it is recognized more as an implicit, tacit aspect of the profession's art, than a primary element of practice. The profession assumes that occupational therapists have a natural understanding of adaptation and how it is accomplished. Although there has been considerable debate in recent years on the definition of occupation, the process of promoting the client's adaptation has received little direct scrutiny. Such oversight continues even though almost every professional writing

makes reference to helping the client adapt, adapting the environment, or promoting adaptation. The remainder of this section responds to the need for a formal articulation of the underlying strand on adaptation and its significance to occupational therapy.

Identification of the Strand on Adaptation

The strand, an interwoven set of perspectives on individual adaptation, was identified by a review of the literature discussed in the first section of this chapter. Recurring themes, concepts, and assumptions regarding adaptation and its relationship to the value, purpose, and goal of occupation therapy were systematically recorded. Forty frequent "statements on the phenomenon of adaptation" were identified. The statements were then analyzed to determine their similarity and interrelationship. The following set of 10 beliefs emerged as elements of the strand on adaptation:

1. There is an innate urge to affect the environment.
2. Adaptive facility and environmental expectations are predictive of the person-environment transaction.
3. There is a need to experience mastery in person-environment transactions.
4. Person-environment transactions occur in the form of occupations.
5. Perception of mastery results from goodness of fit between adaptive facility and expectation.
6. Demand for adaptation appears when the "fit" is inadequate.
7. Adaptation is a form of change that occurs in:
   - sensorimotor, cognitive, or psychosocial skills
   - adaptive responses
   - physical, social, or cultural expectations/demands
8. Mastery over expectations yields satisfaction.
9. The experience of joy resulting from being a successful agent of change fuels the urge to affect the environment.
10. Maladaptation is an unsuccessful attempt to meet expectations.

These 10 elements provide the core for the strand on adaptation. The relationship between the strand and occupational therapy was based on the literature reviewed, and is proposed as follows: Occupational therapy develops the individual's ability to adapt so that person-environment transactions produce occupational performance with mastery and satisfaction.

Table 19-1 connects each of these 10 elements with the authors reviewed in this chapter. This table is intended to provide a general relationship between these readings and the identified elements of adaptation; it should not be viewed as an exhaustive explanation of the authors' perspectives on adaptation and occupational performance. The reader is encouraged to read the original works for a more comprehensive understanding.

.TABLE 19-1

Strand on Adaptation—Core Elements

Elements of Strand on Adaptation	Authors Emphasizing the Element	Significance Within the Evolving Strand
Innate urge to affect the environment	Meyer, 1922; White, 1959; Reilly, 1962; Shannon, 1972; 1977; Kielhofner & Burke, 1980; Howe & Briggs, 1982; Yerxa et al., 1990	Identifies core motivation that leads to adaptation.
The adaptive facility/environmental expectations predict person-environment transactions.	DeCharms, 1968; Llorens, 1970; Smith, 1972	Clarifies the interactive relationship between innate qualities and what individuals choose to do in life.
Need to experience mastery in person-environment transactions.	Meyer, 1922; White, 1959; Reilly, l962; Yerxa, 1967; Kielhofner, 1977; Yerxa, et al., 1990	Emphasizes the importance that mastery has in the progression of person-environment transactions.
Person-environment transactions occur in the form of occupations.	Meyer, 1922; Reilly, 1962; Llorens, 1970; Shannon, 1972 & 1977; Fidler & Fidler 1978; King, 1978; Johnson, 1981; Huss, 1981; Howe & Briggs, 1982; Nelson, 1988; Yerxa et al., 1990	Clarifies that occupations are the vehicle for affecting adaptation within person-environment transactions.
A perception of mastery results from the fit between adaptive facility and expectation of occupation.	Llorens, 1970; Kielhofner, 1977; King, 1978; Kleinman & Bulkley, 1982	Articulates that mastery is an individual perception.
Demand for adaptation appears when the fit is inadequate.	Reilly, 1962; Llorens, 1970; King, 1978; Scardina, 1981; Reed & Sanderson, 1983; Nelson, 1988	States that the perception of mastery activates the adaptation process.
Adaptation is change which occurs in sensorimotor, cognitive, or psychosocial skills; adaptive responses; physical, social or cultural expectations/demands.	Reilly, 1962; Yerxa, 1967; Llorens, 1970; Shannon, 1977; King, 1978; AOTA, 1979; Kielhofner, 1980a; Reed & Sanderson, 1983	Confirms that adaptation is a holistic, cyclical process.
Mastery over expectations yields satisfaction.	Meyer, 1922; Yerxa, 1967; Florey, 1969; Llorens, 1978; Fidler & Fidler, 1978; Smith, 1972; Shannon, 1977	Articulates the importance of satisfaction as an outcome of adaptive responses.
The experience or joy resulting from being a successful agent of change fuels the urge to affect the environment.	Meyer, 1922; White, 1959; Reilly, 1962; DeCharms, 1968; Florey, 1969; Llorens, 1970; Smith, 1972; Fidler & Fidler, 1978; Reed & Sanderson, 1983	Provides an explanation of how successful adaptation promotes increasing ability in occupational performance.
Maladaptation is an unsuccessful attempt to meet expectations.	Meyer, 1922; Reilly, 1962; Llorens, 1970; Kielhofner, 1980a; Kleinman & Bulkley, 1982; Fine, 1991	Communicates that adaptation can result in either a positive or negative transaction between the person and the environment.

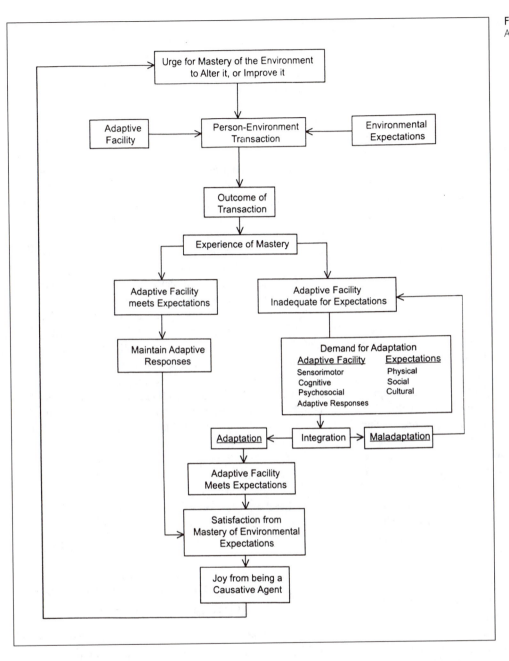

Figure 19-1. Paradigm of Adaptation.

The second step in clarifying the strand on adaptation was to examine the conceptual relationship between the elements. Figure 19-1, the Paradigm of Adaptation, represents both the identified elements and their organization. This figure is our explanation of adaptation as it is understood within the profession's body of knowledge. The figure organizes the 10 elements into a configuration that represents the flow of events in adaptation. Although the Paradigm of Adaptation is an addition to the profession's body of knowledge, the elements that make up the structure are in no way novel. We propose that these elements have been ever-present within the art of practice. As with many concepts, often associated with what is often called "common sense," the profession's beliefs on the process of internal adaptation, have been given little direct attention, sometimes all but ignored. The result has been that some therapists incorporate isolated elements of the strand (e.g., adaptation limited to physical changes such as assistive devices and environmental modifications). A comprehensive perspective on adaptation offers the therapist multiple avenues for potential effect on the individual's occupational performance.

ADAPTATION AS A PARADIGM OF THE PROFESSION

We assert that promoting internal adaptation has been and will always be an integral part of occupational therapy. The success of person-environment transactions depends upon the quality and nature of the individual's adaptive processes. When individuals experience physical or psychosocial trauma the frequency and complexity of person-environment transactions is magnified. Since adaptation is a normative process, the patient or client will attempt to adapt whether the therapist facilitates it or not. The outcome may be positive or negative. Therapists who facilitate person-environment transactions by promoting internal adaptation will affect the client's overall occupational performance as well as those specific skills addressed in therapy.

The range of treatment methods may lead to the erroneous conclusion that adaptation is essentially a technique. Therapists will use various elements of the strand on adaptation at different times, and in different contexts. The authors suggest that adaptation is far more than a technique. It is proposed that adaptation embodies a dimension of practice that reflects the essence of the profession's purpose and uniqueness. The promotion of internal adaptation is a highly sophisticated process of therapy that has remained at the tacit level of understanding. It is a universal component of practice. For the majority of therapists, elements of the strand on adaptation are a day-to-day consideration. The prominence of the elements of adaptation within practice suggests that adaptation is more to the profession than a collected set of interventions.

We propose that adaptation is of such significance that it functions as a paradigm within occupational therapy. The literature cited in the previous discussion offers substantive testimony. The continuum of adaptation techniques, approaches, and methods speaks to the universality of adaptation. The perpetuation of adaptation principles (as tacit knowledge passed on from generation to generation) demonstrates the power that adaptation holds within the profession. Adaptation is a concept with such multiple facets that it is more than an aspect of practice. Identification of adaptation as one of the profession's paradigms appears to be appropriate and timely. While paradigms may exist without formal recognition, they are less resistant to external threat, and their utility is usually compromised. If the paradigm of adaptation remains tacit, the concept of adaptation as a medium to enhance occupational performance will lose its potential to differentiate occupational therapy from other professions. As health care continues to evolve, adherence to core paradigms may be essential to occupational therapy assuming a role that is consistent with its legacy.

Figure 19-1 presents an initial structure for studying the proposed Paradigm of Adaptation. The literature reviewed in the beginning of this chapter provides the rationale for the identification of the elements and their sequence.

In summary, noted authorities have consistently promoted personal adaptation as the primary motive of occupational therapy. Numerous leaders have asserted that adaptation is at the core of all interventions. Within these perspectives, health is understood more as a relative state of adaptation than as freedom from disease or disability. Thus, the purpose of occupational therapy is to help the client produce adaptive responses that will yield satisfaction in the performance of life roles. Dysfunction is defined as a disruption in the individual's normative cycle of adaptation, rather than a problem in functional skills, independence, or activities of daily living. The role of the therapist is to help the client become more adaptive. The effect is observable in the quality of the client's transactions between the intrinsic and extrinsic factors of occupational performance. Many therapists have intuitively incorporated an emphasis on individual adaptation into their therapy program. The paradigm of adaptation may bridge some of the fragmentation caused by specialization, as well as provide new perspectives on the contribution of occupational therapy in health and wellness programming.

The profession's literature contains a rich and complex discussion on humanity and the purpose that occupational therapy serves. We believe that there is a continuous strand of thought in the literature that can be articulated as a prevailing theme within the profession. That is, the literature consistently alludes to the vital importance of what is best described as an inextricable link between occupation and adaptation. This relationship is understood not as a cause and effect, but as an interaction that is in a continuous process of ebb and flow. We assert that the profession's understanding of the link between these two concepts reflects its origin and its future.

OCCUPATIONAL ADAPTATION—A THEORETICAL FRAME OF REFERENCE FOR A PARADIGM OF ADAPTATION

The proposal for a paradigm of adaptation was based on a chronological review of occupational therapy literature through 1990. Differing views of the role of adaptation and its nature within occupational functioning exist. While the strand of adaptation is clearly present in this diverse body of work, only a few perspectives were elaborated into a fully articulated theoretical system whose central theme is on the individual's internal adaptation through person-environment transactions. Only two theories existing within this time frame met this criterion: *Sensory Integration*, first articulated by Ayres (1972a, 1972b), and *Spatiotemporal Adaptation* by Gilfoyle, Grady and Moore (1981, 1990), which was based on the work of Piaget (Flavell, 1963; Piaget & Inhelder, 1969). These two theories should be further examined for their potential to represent a paradigm of adaptation because of the extent to which they have been developed and the extent to which the individual's internal adaptation is paramount.

Sensory integration addresses the internal adaptive response in children whose central nervous systems are unable to receive, interpret and organize sensory information which can then be used to promote competence in the usual developmental tasks of childhood. Ayres' view was that the nervous system's ability to modify dysfunctional integration of sensory information tapered off at about age 10. In a later elaboration of sensory integration, Koomar and Bundy (1991) allude to the possibility that the theory could apply to older children and adults but did not develop this application. Therefore, sensory integration is limited in its scope to function as an overarching theoretical system illustrating a paradigm of adaptation because of its relatively narrow focus, both in terms of problems addressed and age of clients. *Spatiotemporal adaptation* is focused on developmental sensorimotor adaptation in the child from 0 to 5 years of age and thus is limited in its utility as a generic, overarching system for the study and practice of occupational therapy based on a paradigm of adaptation. Both sensory integration and spatiotemporal adaptation are beautifully articulated and organized theoretical systems. The occupational therapist whose client population of concern is young children should be strongly encouraged to study these two perspectives in depth.

In 1992, another theoretical perspective with the potential to reflect a paradigm of adaption emerged. Occupational adaptation (Schkade & Schultz, 1992; Schultz & Schkade, 1992) describes an internal adaptation process which begins developing at birth and continues to be refined over the life span. It provides an expansive umbrella under which a broad scope of study and practice, consistent with a paradigm of adaptation, is possible. The remainder of this chapter focuses on the perspective within occupational adaptation, a theoretical frame of reference. (Schkade & Schultz, 1992; Schultz & Schkade, 1992; Schkade & Schultz, 1993; Schultz & Schkade, 1994; Garrett & Schkade, 1995; Pasek & Schkade, 1996). Occupational adaptation is seen as a normative process for developing competence in occupational performance through a process of internal adaptation. Disruption in this normative process, as a result of illness, trauma, congenital conditions, etc., is the focus of intervention provided by the therapist who practices from this perspective. Therapists practice tacitly within a similar set of ideas which guides their thinking.

Schön (1983) discussed the importance of practice which appears tacit or intuitive. In his book, *The Reflective Practitioner*, Schon described how professionals from many disciplines can articulate their tacit practice by analyzing the manner in which they decide what problems to address. He proposed that the manner of "setting the problem" reflects the central function of practice. Schon deliberately distinguished "problem setting" from "technical problem solving." Schon stated:

*When we set the problem, we select what we will treat as the "things" of the situation, we set the boundaries of our attention to it, and we impose upon it a coherence which allows us to say what is wrong and in what directions the situation needs to be changed. Problem setting is a process in which, interactively, we **name** the things to which we will attend and **frame** the context in which we will attend to them (p. 40).*

Occupational adaptation is a way to "name" the things to which occupational therapists pay attention and "frame" the intervention context (the questions asked and the approaches employed) when the occupational therapist practices within a paradigm of adaptation which serves occupational performance.

The Occupational Adaptation Process

Occupational Adaptation assumes that individuals are occupational beings who develop competence in occupational performance through the activities of an internal adaptation process. (See Chapter 18 by Matheson and Bohr for an elaboration of the development of occupational performance competence.) Key terms for occupational adaptation appear in Table 19-2. This internal adaptation process exists to enable the individual to respond to challenges over a lifetime. These are challenges which require some form of change in the individual's response approach if movement toward competence will occur. Occupational adaptation assumes that engagement in occupations that are personally meaningful to the individual will be most beneficial in promoting the healthy action of the internal adaptation process and therefore most likely to enhance occupational performance. Thus occupation is our most powerful therapeutic medium and competent occupational performance is our intervention goal.

Occupational Adaptation views the person as consisting of sensorimotor, cognitive and psychosocial systems. This conceptualization was chosen because these are terms with which occupational therapists are familiar through their appearance in Uniform Terminology (AOTA, 1994) as "Occupational Performance Components." These person systems are seen in a particular individual to be the influence of genetic/familial, environmental and experiential/phenomenological subsystems which feed into the person systems to make them what they are. As described earlier in this book, the occupational person is similarly represented as operating through physiological, psychological, neuro-behavioral and cognitive factors or intrinsic factors (see Chapter 3).

Occupational performance takes place within a context consisting of work/school, leisure/play and self-care envi-

---

TABLE 19-2

Key Terms

Occupations are activities that are characterized by three essential properties. These properties form the necessary and sufficient conditions for occupations.

- Active participation by the individual
- Meaning to the individual
- A process that ends in a product, whether the product is tangible or intangible (e.g., a piece of furniture or a sense of accomplishment).

Adaptation is a change the person makes in his or her response approach when that person encounters an occupational challenge. This change is implemented when the individual's customary response approaches are found inadequate for producing some degree of mastery over the challenge.

Occupational adaptation (the process) is a series of actions, internal to the individual, which unfold as the individual is faced with an occupational challenge. The individual engages this process with the intention to produce a response that will result in an experience of relative mastery over the challenge.

Occupational adaptation (the state) is a state of competency toward which human beings aspire. The existence and strength of this state in an individual is a function of the extent to which occupational responses have been effective in producing relative mastery over occupational challenges and the extent to which such responses have successfully generalized to a variety of occupational challenges.

---

ronments. This conceptualization came from Uniform Terminology (AOTA, 1994) which classifies these as "Occupational Performance Areas." Just as the person systems are particular to an individual because of subsystems that influence them, occupational environments are what they are because of physical, social and cultural subsystems that influence them. These subsystems are reflected in Uniform Terminology (AOTA, 1994) by the category of "Context." In Chapter 3, Christiansen and Baum discuss these influences as extrinsic factors, which they label societal, cultural, social and physical. Dunn, Brown and McGuigan (1994) also provide an elaboration of context and its importance in intervention.

Occupational performance then is the individual engaging in transactions with occupational environments. Performance is embedded in occupational roles. Christiansen and Baum reflect these roles as consisting of multiple occupations which are formed into various tasks inherent in these roles. These roles carry performance expectations which come from the individual (internal expectations) and from the physical, social and cultural factors in the occupational environment (external expectations). These are similar to the intrinsic and extrinsic factors in Christiansen and Baum terminology. These role expectations guide the individual's quest for responding masterfully and adaptively.

As the person responds to the occupational challenge, the internal adaptation process is engaged. This internal process exists to create a response that is masterful and adaptive. When the process is functioning well, masterful and adaptive responses are likely to be the result. If, however, the process is dysfunctional, the response will be lacking in mastery and dysadaptive. Three subprocesses reflect the functions of the adaptive process. A response must be:
- generated (adaptive response generation subprocess)
- evaluated (adaptive response evaluation subprocess)
- integrated (adaptive response integration subprocess)

Occupational Adaptation proposes that the adaptive response generation subprocess consists of an adaptive response mechanism which selects a level of adaptation energy, an adaptive response mode and an adaptive response behavior (Table 19-3). The output of the mechanism is then configured into an adaptation gestalt (or a plan for the response) which includes participation of all three person systems: sensorimotor, cognitive, and psychosocial. Thus, the adaptive response in occupational performance is always a holistic one. See Figure 19-2 for examples.

Following expression of the occupational response, the individual then evaluates the effect of that response in terms of *relative mastery*. Relative mastery consists of:
- efficiency (use of time, energy and resources)
- effectiveness (extent to which the desired result occurred)
- satisfaction to self/society (extent to which the response outcome was personally gratifying and socially well regarded).

Relative mastery is phenomenological and nonstandardized because it is assessed against the particular set of intrinsic and extrinsic expectations peculiar to the occupational role and the context within which it is expressed.

The third subprocess, adaptive response integration, takes the output of the generation and evaluation activity, synthesizes the occupational event and integrates it into the person for future use. If the individual experienced positive relative mastery, then the state of occupational adaptation will be strengthened. If, however, the individual experienced no rela-

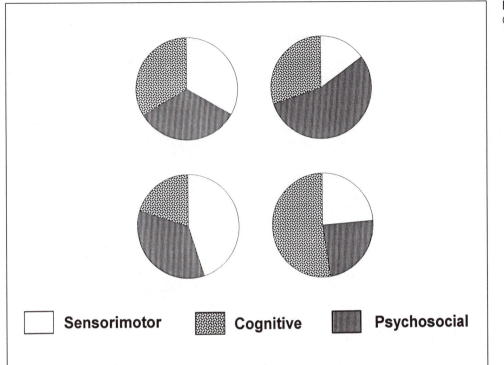

Figure 19-2. Adaptation Gestalt Configurations.

☐ **Sensorimotor**   ▨ **Cognitive**   ▥ **Psychosocial**

tive mastery or if the event was so aversive as to be experienced as negative relative mastery two integration possibilities exist. Should the individual learn from the aversive experience that a different approach will be necessary to prevent repetition of dysfunctional responses, the state of occupational adaptation will be reinforced even though the event was experienced as negative. When the individual does not recognize the need for a different approach under similar circumstances, the dysfunctional behavior will likely be repeated and the state of occupational dysadaptation will be reinforced.

The occupational environment will also assess the individual's response and information fed back into the physical, social and cultural subsystems. This feedback to the environment provides the potential for the individual to impact occupational role expectations. The environmental expectations may change as a result of this information or they may remain the same, even intensified.

The Occupational Adaptation Schematic

The Occupational adaptation process is represented as a schematic seen in Figure 19-3. This figure reflects a kind of cross-section of the process, which has just been described, stopped in time so that a picture of the process flow emerges. In real time, the person will be dealing with multiple occupational challenges. Some of these challenges will be of brief duration during very temporary events, such as when parking a car in a tight space. Others will be of extended duration, such as when dealing with major life transitions, whether

those transitions involve positive events such as birth of a new child or aversive ones brought on by disease or trauma with protracted loss. In other words, persons may cycle very rapidly through a single event, such as the car parking example which quickly resolves. Persons dealing with chronic and disabling conditions will be repeatedly cycling through multiple events related to the disabling condition. These events call for the adaptation process to be functioning well if positive relative mastery is to be experienced. For example a person affected by severe rheumatoid arthritis will persistently encounter the need for adaptation with respect to frequently occurring occupational challenges if occupational functioning is to be minimally disrupted. Occupational adaptation is seen at its most profound during challenges that involve major life transitions. During these times, the process is most at risk for disruption and dysfunction.

The three elements in occupational adaptation are seen in the schematic as the person, the occupational environment and the interaction of the first two to form the third element. Arrows connecting the elements in both directions indicate the communicative and mutually influencing nature of these elements. The respective constants in the three elements are the desire for mastery, the demand for mastery and the press for mastery. These constants provide motivational influences which are enduringly present. A particular occupational challenge is the result of the interplay between these forces; it signals the beginning of a particular occupational event. The remainder of the occupational adaptation process, as previ-

---

TABLE 19-3
Adaptive Response Mechanism

Adaptation Energy*	Adaptive Response Modes	Adaptive Response Behaviors**
Primary: Focused attention; high energy usage at intense activity, more structured. *Secondary:* More creative, sophisticated; low energy usage; disregards structure in favor of alternative approaches	*Existing:* Response patterns in adaptive repertoire from previous successful uses. *Modified:* Changes in existing mode when existing mode fails to achieve success. *New:* Uniquely different mode developed as existing and modified fail to achieve success.	*Primitive:* Hyperstabilized in all person systems. "Frozen" or stereotypic. No adaptive movement (no variety in behavior that can lead to adaptation). *Transitional:* Hypermobile in all person systems. High activity level; random; unmodulated; variable. Variability can result in behavior more likely to produce response that can lead to adaptation. *Mature:* Blended mobility and stability in all person systems. Goal directed; modulated. Most likely to produce adaptive and masterful response to challenge.

*See influence of Selye, H. (1956). *Stress of Life*. New York: McGraw-Hill.

---

ously described, occurs in the adaptive response subprocesses, as well as the evaluation and incorporation by the occupational environment.

Guiding Principles for Intervention

The overarching principle of intervention from an occupational adaptation perspective is that the focus of intervention is to positively impact occupational performance through the internal adaptation process. When the therapist successfully engages this internal process, the client begins to act as his or her own agent of change. The following principles guide the approach of the therapist practicing from this perspective.

1) Occupational adaptation is not a collection of techniques but a way of directing the therapist's thinking about intervention in the individual's internal adaptation process.
2) Intervention is guided, not by concerns about general skill development, but by the requirements of an *occupational role* that is identified by the client as meaningful. This role takes place within an environmental context about which the client or family must educate the therapist. Evaluation of strengths and deficits in *sensorimotor, cognitive and psychosocial systems* is measured against what promotes or inhibits the client's ability to carry out the meaningful role.
3) A personally meaningful intervention focused on the internal adaptation process will be more efficient and the outcomes more likely to generalize to other contexts than

intervention focused on general skill development.
4) Intervention is a combination of method
- Occupational readiness is designed to address deficits in the sensorimotor, cognitive and/or psychosocial systems. These interventions prepare or ready these systems to engage in occupation.
- Occupational activities simulate or replicate tasks of the meaningful occupational role that will guide intervention and that will direct the focus on the client's internal adaptation process. These activities must meet the three required properties for occupations: active participation by the client; meaning to the client; process ending in a tangible or intangible product.
5) The client evaluates his or her progress in terms of relative mastery:
- use of time, energy and resources (efficiency);
- extent to which the desired goal was achieved (effectiveness);
- degree to which the personal actions producing the outcome were personally and socially well regarded (satisfaction to self and society).
6) The therapist assesses client progress with standard assessment tools and with indications that the client's internal adaptation process has been affected:
- spontaneous generalization to other activities;
- initiation of new approaches in novel situations;
- increase in relative mastery.

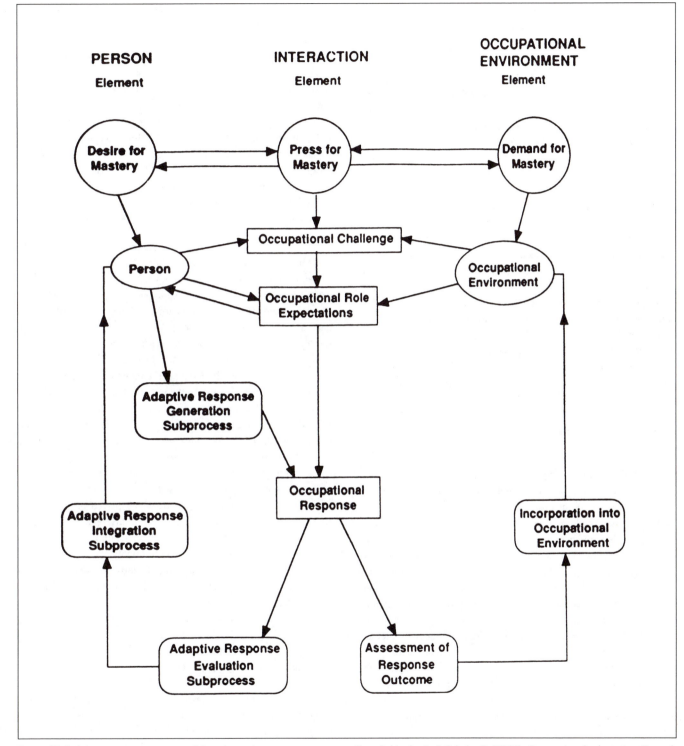

Figure 19-3. Schematic representation of the relationships among constructs. From Schkade, J., & Schultz, S. (1992). Occupational adaptation: Toward a holistic approach to contemporary practice. Part I. *American Journal of Occupational Therapy, 46,* 9. Copyright 1992 by the American Occupational Therapy Association, Inc. Reprinted with permission.

Case Studies

Two cases demonstrate the therapeutic power of focus on the client's internal adaptation process. "The Preacher" illustrates how use of a meaningful activity within a preferred role facilitates occupational performance. This case describes what occurred when the client was asked to perform in a familiar and meaningful activity (preaching) as opposed to an unfamiliar and non-meaningful activity (standard clinic protocol). The sensorimotor deficits which had been the focus of intervention had not been responsive to efforts of a multidisciplinary team of therapists. The creation of an environment associated with the ministry (occupational role) capitalized on familiar role-related activities and tasks. Literally overnight, the client surprised and delighted the therapeutic team with the true capability of his sensorimotor system. He directed his own performance without prompts or assistance from the therapists.

"The Water Skier" is an example of how the therapist uses an occupational role selected by the client to drive the intervention process. This therapist leads the client to identify the role of most importance to him, in this case a leisure role. The client then educates the therapist in the physical, social and cultural expectations of the role. These expectations direct the therapist to assess the ability of the client's person systems to engage in the role. With knowledge of his abilities and limitations and the role expectations the therapist, collaborating with the client, develops an intervention program designed to facilitate his internal adaptation process. She sets the stage for the client to function as his own agent of change and enhance occupational performance in his chosen role.

The Preacher

Mr. Jones was a 68-year-old retired minister who had suffered a stroke. He presented with the characteristic neurologic damage which left him with problems in movement and speech. He had been in rehabilitation for almost 4 months with therapeutic intervention of the multidisciplinary team focused on intervention in the sensorimotor system, i.e., emphasis on standing tolerance, shifting his weight while in standing, being able to reach across his body in diagonal patterns, speech articulation disorders. After a considerable time and effort, the team had concluded that the patient was not a good candidate for walking. His documented standing tolerance was a maximum of 5 minutes and his difficulty in weight shifting was extreme. At this point, the therapist was introduced to occupational adaptation and the importance of personally meaningful activity associated with an occupational role as a therapeutic medium. In a conversation with Mr. Jones, the therapist discovered that he was a minister who most desired to return to the task of preaching in that occupational role. She told him that the next day she would bring a podium into the room where the bible study group, of which Mr. Jones was a member, would meet and she wanted him to preach. Mr. Jones expressed fear and apprehension that he would not be able to preach. The next day, a Friday, the therapist brought a podium into the room and put it in place. As soon as Mr. Jones saw this symbol of the physical subsystem from the occupational environment of preaching, he began to articulate a list of things he could talk about. Despite his apprehensions about standing and talking, Mr. Jones was assisted into standing and he began to preach. For 20 minutes, Mr. Jones stood and preached. As he preached, he weight shifted. He gestured, crossing midline, to the full extent of his range of motion. He spoke in the most powerful voice he could summon. At the end of the 20 minutes when Mr. Jones sat down, he burst into a song. Then he cried. The following Monday, Mr. Jones began to walk. Engagement in an occupational activity meaningful to Mr. Jones set the stage for him to maximize remaining capabilities and act as his own agent of therapeutic change. The sensorimotor and speech performance requirements were thus allowed to emerge in a more automatic fashion under Mr. Jones' self-direction.

Case reported by Jessica Dolecheck, MA, L/OTR.

The Water Skier

Mr. Moore was a 27-year-old single male who had sustained a flexor tendon laceration of the left wrist. After surgery, splinting and exercises he returned to work as a computer programmer using only his right hand. He was referred for continued rehabilitation to a hand clinic. Intervention was originally planned with the assumption that return to work should be the focus. As this plan was followed, it became apparent that Mr. Moore was disinterested in the therapy and performed in a very perfunctory way. Because of Mr. Moore's lackluster response to the treatment approach, the occupational therapist decided to use an occupational adaptation approach with Mr. Moore. He chose to focus on his leisure role as a competitive water skier. The therapist learned about the environmental demands of Mr. Moore's chosen role:

- *Physical*—Static and dynamic handling of equipment with speed and accuracy, maximum resistance to the upper extremities, good overall body condition, all of which placed him at risk of re-injury; components of task relative to injury related to grasping and manipulating a ski rope handle: 1) maintaining a stable grasp with moderate to maximum force comfortably. 2) rapidly manipulating the handle between right and left hands, 3) dynamic and static upper extremity strength and endurance to resist force of water/rope.

- *Social*—Interaction with competitors, team members, and officials;

- *Cultural*—Performance per competition regulations (speed, time, and number of tricks performed).

Person systems assessment revealed:

- *Sensorimotor*—Appearance. Incision closed at wrist, scar red and tender, skin dry; Range of Motion. Normal passive finger flexion, full finger extension within limits of splint (0 degrees at IP's and 60 degrees at MP's), wrist held in flexion at 60 degrees; Shoulder/elbow range of motion. Normal; Strength. Not assessed at this time; Edema. Moderate at left wrist, especially over scar, mild in digits; Sensation. Impaired one point localization over thenar eminence, normal sensation throughout rest of hand; Pain. Dull pain over dorsal and volar aspects of wrist.

• *Cognitive*—very attentive to instruction; very verbal about his injury and previous lifestyle; able to comprehend instructions; no difficulty with memory.

• *Psychosocial*—very anxious about his hand and very protective of it; expressed increased confidence with therapist input on treatment; important social support system is through water skiing activities.

This assessment of *occupational role* performance demands resulted in an intervention plan consisting of tissue-healing goals with standard splinting, exercise, heat, compression methods, etc. (*occupational readiness*) and occupational role goals with engagement in water ski-related activities (*occupational activity*). Water ski-related activities began at the *social* level, then progressive involvement in *physical* aspects, beginning with driving the boat for other skiers. Mr. Moore helped plan a fitness program to maintain general body strength and endurance for skiing. Graded functional activities to improve object manipulation progressed to simulation of ski rope handle manipulation with progressive resistance. Mr. Moore also rated himself periodically on efficiency, effectiveness and satisfaction to self/others (relative mastery) of rehab progress toward participation in water skiing. Mr. Moore completed his course of therapy with active involvement in and adherence to his intervention plan. When discharged from therapy, he commented to the O.T. that he planned to use the evaluation of relative mastery in other areas of his life.

Case reported by Kimberly Norton, MA, OTR, CHT

CONCLUSION

Internal adaptation is critical to the integrity of healthy occupational functioning and thus has significant implications for both prevention and remediation efforts led by occupational therapists. This chapter has focused on the importance of the client's internal adaptation process as a central theme for occupational therapy intervention. Adaptation as an integral force is supported by a body of literature which spans the profession's history. The appearance and reappearance of the strand of adaptation has been persistent and pervasive. It has been spun by our most influential thinkers and woven with passion into the fabric of occupational therapy thought and theory.

The client's internal adaptation can be used by therapists to direct the selection of the things to which we will pay attention when helping the client address his or own occupational dysfunction, or in Schon's (1983) words cited earlier, "setting the problems" we will address. This is strong medicine for occupational therapists who are notorious for claiming that what we do is tacit and intuitive and cannot be articulated. Internal adaptation provides a way to "name" our focus. Theoretical perspectives on adaptation, both now and in the future, assist us to "frame" the context in which those

problems are challenged. We submit that facilitation of the client's internal adaptation process leads to competence in occupational functioning that endures long after the therapeutic relationship has been forgotten.

The work of validating, through application and research, the power of a client's internal adaptation is underway by therapists who are using this concept in intervention. The cases reported in this chapter provide examples. Each therapist who employs internal adaptation as a means to enhance occupational functioning can make significant contributions to this body of work. The continuation and intensification of this effort will be important for the advancement of our profession. Realization of our most potent tool for influencing the health and well-being of our clients depends on it.

REFERENCES

American Occupational Therapy Association. (1979). Statement of philosophy. *American Journal of Occupational Therapy, 33,* 781-813.

American Occupational Therapy Association. (1994). Uniform terminology for occupational therapy (3rd ed.). *American Journal of Occupational Therapy, 48,* 1047-1054.

Ayres, A. J. (1972a). *Sensory integration and learning disorders.* Los Angeles: Western Psychological Services.

Ayres, A. J. (1972b). *Southern California sensory integration tests manual.* Los Angeles: Western Psychological Services.

Ayres, J. (1979). *Sensorimotor integration and the child.* Los Angeles: Western Psychological Serivces.

Baum, C., & Christiansen C. (1997). Person-environment occupational performance: A conceptual model for practice. In C. Christiansen & C. Baum, (Eds.), *Occupational therapy: Enabling function and well-being* (2nd ed.). Thorofare, NJ: SLACK Incorporated.

Christiansen, C. (1991). Performance deficits as sources of stress: Coping theory and occupational therapy. In C. Christiansen & C. Baum, (Eds.), *Occupational therapy: Overcoming human performance deficits.* Thorofare, NJ: SLACK Incorporated.

Christiansen, C., & Baum, C. (1997). Occupational therapy: Philosophy/principles/practice. In C. Christiansen & C. Baum, (Eds.), *Occupational therapy: Achieving human performance needs in daily living* (2nd ed.). Thorofare, NJ: SLACK Incorporated.

Cohen, F., & Lazarus, R., (1979). Coping with the stress of illness. In G. C. Stone, F. Cohen, N. E. Adler, et al. (Eds.), *Health psychology: A handbook* (pp. 217-254). San Francisco: Jossey Bass.

DeCharms, R. (1968). *Personal causation: The internal affective determinant of behavior.* New York: Academic Press.

Dunn, W., Brown, C., & McGuigan, A. (1994). Ecology of human performance: A framework for considering the effect of context. *American Journal of Occupational Therapy, 48*(7), 595-607.

Erickson, E. (1985). *Childhood and society.* New York: W.W. Norton.

Fidler, G. (1981). From crafts to competence. *American Journal of Occupational Therapy, 35*(9), 567-573.

Fidler, G., & Fidler, J. (1978). Doing and becoming: Purposeful action and self-actualization. *American Journal of Occupational Therapy, 32*(5), 305-310.

Fine, S. (1991). Resilience and human adaptability: Who rises above adversity? *American Journal of Occupational Therapy, 45*(6), 493-503.

Flavell, J. (1963). *The developmental psychology of Jean Piaget.* Princeton, NJ: Van Nostrand.

Florey, L. (1969). Intrinsic motivation: the dynamics of occupational therapy theory. *American Journal of Occupational Therapy, 23*(4), 319.

Garrett, S., & Schkade, J. K. (1995). The occupational adaptation model of professional development as applied to level II fieldwork in occupational therapy. *American Journal of Occupational Therapy, 49,* 119-126.

Gilfoyle, E., Grady, A., & Moore, J. (1981). *Children adapt.* Thorofare, NJ: SLACK Incorporated.

Gilfoyle, E., Grady, A., & Moore, J. (1990). *Children adapt* (2nd ed.). Thorofare, NJ: SLACK Incorporated.

Groos, K. (1901). *The play of men.* New York: Appleton.

Howe, M., & Briggs, A. (1982). Ecological systems model for occupational therapy. *American Journal of Occupational Therapy, 36*(5), 322-327.

Huss, A. (1981). From kinesiology to adaptation. *American Journal of Occupational Therapy 35*(9), 574-580.

Johnson, J. (1981). Old values—new directions: Competence, adaptation, integration. *American Journal of Occupational Therapy, 35,* 589-598.

Kielhofner, G. (1977). Temporal adaptation: A conceptual framework for occupational therapy. *American Journal of Occupational Therapy, 31,* 235-242.

Kielhofner, G. (1980a). A model of human occupation, part two: Ontogenesis from the perspective of temporal adaptation. *American Journal of Occupational Therapy, 34,* 657-663.

Kielhofner, G. (1980b). A model of human occupation, part three: Benign and vicious cycles. *American Journal of Occupational Therapy, 34,* 731-737.

Kielhofner, G., & Burke, J. (1980). A model of human occupation, part one: Conceptual framework and content. *American Journal of Occupational Therapy, 34,* 572-581.

Kielhofner, G., Burke, J., & Igi, C. (1980). A model of human occupation, part four: Assessment and intervention. *American Journal of Occupational Therapy, 34,* 777-788.

King, L. (1978). Toward a science of adaptive responses—1978 Eleanor Clarke Slagle lecture. *American Journal of Occupational Therapy, 32*(7), 429-437.

Kleinman, B., & Bulkley, B. (1982). Some implications of a science of adaptive responses. *American Journal of Occupational Therapy, 36,* 16-19.

Koomar, J. A., & Bundy, A. C. (1991). The art and science of creating direct intervention from theory. In A. Fisher, E. Murray, & A. Bundy (Eds.), *Sensory integration theory and practice.* Philadelphia: F.A. Davis.

Llorens, L. (1970). Facilitating growth and development: The

promise of occupational therapy. *American Journal of Occupational Therapy, 24,* 93-101.

Matheson, L., & Bohr, P. (in press). Identity and growth: Self and development across the lifespan. In C. Christiansen & C. Baum (Eds.), *Occupational therapy: Enabling function and wel-being* (2nd ed.). Thorofare, NJ: SLACK Incorporated.

Matsutsuyu, J. (1971). Occupational behavior—A perspective on work and play. *American Journal of Occupational Therapy, 25,* 291-292.

Meyer, A. (1922). The philosophy of occupational therapy. *The Archives of Occupational Therapy, 1,* 1-10.

Nelson, D. (1988). Occupation: Form and performance. *American Journal of Occupational Therapy, 42,* 633-641.

Pasek, P. B., & Schkade, J. K. (1996). Effects of a skiing experience on adolescents with limb deficiencies: an occupational adaptation perspective. *American Journal of Occupational Therapy, 50,* 24-31.

Piaget, J., & Inhelder, B. (1969). *The psychology of the child.* New York: Basic Books.

Reed, K. (1984). *Models of practice in occupational therapy.* Baltimore: Williams & Wilkins.

Reed, K., & Sanderson, S. (1983). *Concepts of occupational therapy* (2nd ed.). Baltimore: Williams & Wilkins.

Reilly, M. (1966). A psychiatric occupational therapy program as a teaching model. *American Journal of Occupational Therapy, 20,* 60-67.

Reilly, M. (1969). The educational process. *American Journal of Occupational Therapy, 23,* 299-307.

Reilly, M. (1962). Occupational therapy can be one of the great ideas of 20th century medicine. *American Journal of Occupational Therapy, 16*(1), 1-9.

Scardina, V. (1981). From pegboards to integration. *American Journal of Occupational Therapy, 35*(9), 581-588.

Schkade, J. K., & Schultz, S. (1992). Occupational adaptation: Toward a holistic approach to contemporary practice. Part I. *American Journal of Occupational Therapy, 46,* 829-837.

Schkade, J. K., & Schultz, S. (1993). Occupational adaptation—an integrative frame of reference. In H. Hopkins & H. Smith (Eds.), *Willard and Spackman's Occupational Therapy* (8th ed.). Philadelphia: J.B. Lippincott Company.

Schon, D. A. (1983). *The reflective practitioner.* New York: Basic Books.

Schultz, S., & Schkade, J. K. (1992). Occupational adaptation: Toward a holistic approach to contemporary practice. Part 2. *American Journal of Occupational Therapy, 46,* 917-926.

Schultz, S. & Schkade, J. K. (1994). Home health care: a window of opportunity to synthesize practice. Home & Community Health, *Special interest Section Newsletter, American Occupational Therapy Association, 1,* 1-4.

Shannon, P. (1972). Work-play theory and the occupational therapy process. *American Journal of Occupational Therapy, 26*(4), 169-172.

Shannon, P. (1977). The derailment of occupational therapy. *American Journal of Occupational Therapy, 31*(4), 229-234.

Slagle, E. (1922). Training aids for mental patients. *Occupational Therapy and Rehabilitation, 1,* 11-14.

Smith, M. (1974). A perspective on therapeutic ends and means. Competence and adaptation. *American Journal of Occupational Therapy, 28*(1), 11-15.

White, R. (1959). Motivation reconsidered: The concept of competence. *Psychological Review, 66,* 297-333.

White, R. (1974). Strategies of adaptation: An attempt at systematic description. In G. V. Coehlo, D. A. Hamburg, & J. E. Adams (Eds.), *Coping and adaptation.* New York: Basic Books.

Yerxa, E., Clark, F., Frank, G., Jackson, J., Parham, D., Pierce, D., Stein, C., & Zemke, R. (1990). An introduction to occupational science, a foundation for occupational therapy in the 21st century. *Occupational Therapy in Health Care, 6*(4), 1-17.

Yerxa, E. (1967). Authentic occupational therapy. *American Journal of Occupational Therapy, 21,* 1-9.

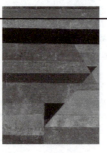

CHAPTER CONTENT OUTLINE

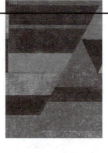

ABSTRACT

This chapter gives a historical perspective of the field of assistive technology. Current terminology is reviewed and legislation that governs access to information and technology by consumers is described. Two conceptual models are presented to provide the context for assistive technology application. In the context of consumer responsive practice in assistive technology, environments of practice as well as the service delivery process are presented.

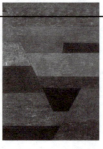

KEY TERMS

Consumer Responsive Practice

The Rehabilitation Engineering and Assistive Technology Society of North America (RESNA)

Mobility Technologies

Seating/Positioning Technologies

Augmentative and Alternative Communication (AAC)

Access (man/machine interface)

Society for Automotive Engineers (SAE)

Universal Access Design

Human-Environment/Technology Interface Model (HETI)

Human Activity Assistive Technology Model (HAAT)

Rehabilitation Engineering Research Centers (RERC)

National Institute on Disability Related Research (NIDRR)

Office of Vocational Rehabilitation (OVR)

National Registry of Rehabilitation Technology Suppliers (NRRTS)

Rehabilitation Technology Supplier (RTS)

Assistive Technology Supplier (ATS)

Assistive Technology Practitioner (ATP)

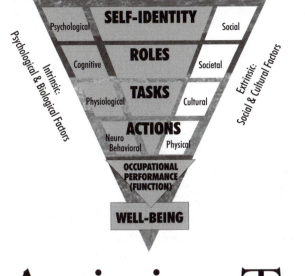

CHAPTER 20

Assistive Technology

Elaine Trefler, MEd, OTR, FAOTA, Douglas Hobson, PhD

OBJECTIVES

The information in this chapter is intended to help the reader:

1. define key terms used in the field of assistive technology

2. describe the possible roles for occupational therapists related to assistive technology application

3. list possible settings for occupational therapists to practice in assistive technology

4. discuss two models of assistive technology application

5. list and explain the components of a service delivery program for assistive technology.

> *"If opportunity is the distance between what is and what could be"*
> *(Crimmins, 1995, p. 129) then assistive technology*
> *provides the opportunity for persons with physical disabilities that*
> *have things to do and places to go."*
>
> C. Baum (in press)

INTRODUCTION

Consumer Responsive Practice

The scope and focus of occupational therapy practice is changing. At one time, most of the people who received occupational therapy intervention were patients in hospitals or rehabilitation facilities. For some years, therapists did home, school or worksite visits as a component of their delivery of services. However, in the last 10 years, more and more therapists are practicing in the community, and instead of therapy services being part of the medical model of "we know best," they are providing a more consumer responsive model of intervention.

In a consumer responsive model, therapists assist people with disabilities to define their own goals and decide, based on the advice and information provided by professionals, the course of action to follow. In the field of assistive technology (AT), the occupational therapist would advise clients by assisting them in stating and prioritizing their goals, determining what assistive technology to choose based on their personal goals and technology options, and helping them integrate the assistive technology into their daily routine through training and follow-up services. Evaluations for assistive technology should ideally take place in the environment in which the consumer will use the technology. In other words, if a wheelchair is the assistive technology under consideration because the client needs to be independent in mobility on a university campus, then the evaluation should include a visit to the campus to determine terrain, building accessibility, distances traveled and transportation issues related to getting to and from the campus. A person's posture and function could be measured in a clinic, but to be truly client responsive, seating needs at home, work, school and in the community must also be considered. This client-centered process is used to develop partnerships between therapists and consumers to ensure appropriate selection and use of assistive technology.

In the United States, an assistive technology device is defined in Public Law 100-407 as "any item, piece of equipment or product system whether acquired commercially off the shelf, modified, or customized that is used to increase or improve functional capabilities of individuals with disabilities." This definition encompasses the technology itself, not the application or process involved in ensuring that people with disabilities receive the product they need and learn how to use it. It is the total scope of the evaluation, application, follow-up, information gathering and sharing, ensuring quality of products and personnel that is changing the meaning of the words "assistive technology" from the individual product into a field of practice. The knowledge base is evolving. The state of practice is evolving. In this chapter, we will discuss the *field* of assistive technology in its evolving state, not assistive technology *products*. We can be sure of this: the field of assistive technology is here to stay, and occupational therapists have a primary role in the development of the field of assistive technology, and will recommend assistive technology to clients who wish to live independently. As a result, all aspects of the field are subject to change, at times rapidly, in the years to come.

History of Assistive Technology and Occupational Therapy

Occupational therapists have been employing assistive technology in professional practice for years. Perhaps the most famous piece of technology in our profession is the buttonhook that launched the commercial enterprise Be OK®, begun by Fred Sammons in 1958. From buttonhooks to computers, seating systems to robotics, the technology available which can enable persons with disabilities to function to their maximum potential has been part of the occupational therapist's tools of practice. The 1990s have brought a proliferation of opportunities for occupational therapists to be involved in the design and development of technologies, the application of technologies in many environments, the participation as members of a team in many formats, and as advocates and information resources for consumers and colleagues.

Occupational therapists are well-suited for the role of assistive technology practitioners (ATP). Defined by RESNA, the Rehabilitation Engineering and Assistive Technology Society of North America, an ATP is a person with professional credentials in a recognized field of practice such as Occupational Therapy, Physical Therapy, Speech and Language Pathology, Special Education or Rehabilitation Counseling, who has chosen to practice in the field of Assistive Technology. Many occupational therapists are practical problem-solvers, are adaptive, and work well as members of a team. With a strong medical background, therapists thrive in the community workplace, including applications in the homes, schools and workplaces of persons with disabilities. Skills in problem-solving, counseling and planning enable therapists to assist people with disabilities to define and solve their functional challenges and to apply assistive technology when appropriate.

Bibliographic citation of this chapter: Trefler, E. & Hobson, D. (1997). Assistive technology. In C. Christiansen & C. Baum (Eds.), *Occupational therapy: Enabling function and well-being* (2nd Ed.). Thorofare, NJ: SLACK Incorporated.

Definitions of Technology

Technology means different things to different people, therefore it helps to understand the varied perspectives from which technology is defined. Some definitions are based on the composition of the hardware; others are based on what it does; and still others focus on the newness or innovation of the technique or device. Many definitions are best described as dichotomies, as reflected in the following section.

High Technology versus Low Technology

Low technology usually refers to assistive devices such as button hooks, dressing sticks, long-handled sponges, rocker knives, forks, Dycem^{TM}, Velcro^{TM}, and wash mitts. Many others round out an entire menagerie of low technological devices. Special devices for writing, splints, mouth-wands, head sticks, special seating systems, and even more common devices such as eyeglasses fall within this category.

High technology usually is differentiated from low technology by the use of electronics. Any device which requires electricity is considered to be high technology, particularly those devices which use integrated microchips for electronic processing. The definitions of low and high technology change over time. The more familiar and common a technological device becomes, the more likely it is to be termed low technology. For example, the telephone was once considered high technology but today would be considered low technology. Calculators, radios, televisions, bank teller machines, and dishwashers have been perceived as less "high tech" as they have become more prolific in everyday use. One way of viewing this distinction would be to consider low technology as commonplace and high technology as having exotic features or devices.

Custom versus Commercial Technology

An important distinction among the types of technology is how they are made and whether they are available commercially. In the past, most devices were custom-made since few devices were available commercially. But within the last decade, this situation has changed drastically, and therapists now use commercial products which cost much less.

Cost-effectiveness is a very important issue in the current health care and educational environment. A product made on an assembly line is much less expensive than a product which takes one to six hours to individually fabricate in the occupational therapy clinic. Commercial devices such as splints have become more available in a variety of sizes and styles which can be fitted quickly and modified to the client, thus avoiding the high cost of custom-made splints. The use of custom-made technologies is greatly shrinking as more commercially-available technologies are used.

From Smith, R. (1991). Technological approaches to performance enhancement. In C. Christiansen & C. Baum (Eds.), *Occupational therapy: Enabling function and well-being* (2nd Ed.). Thorofare, NJ: SLACK Incorporated.

This trend has critical implications for occupational therapy practice. Occupational therapists are doing less of this custom fabrication and more selection of the appropriate commercial products. Because of this, one of the new skills required by occupational therapists is the ability to review, analyze, and evaluate countless product descriptions in the extensive technology literature and databases to determine the best commercial product for their patient/client.

Minimal versus Maximal Technology

Technological applications to enhance human performance are used across a wide range of human ability levels. Technological devices once were implemented primarily to assist and support human performance deficits; today they are being used to substitute for performance deficits. For example, in the past, technology intervention was limited to using a wash mitt or a long-handled sponge to assist individuals with washing and bathing activities. These devices provided some minimal assistance to improve an individual's independence. Although this minimal technology continues to be used, there are maximal technologies available for the person with severe motor deficits (e.g., high level quadriplegia) such as robots that can grab a sponge, dip the sponge into water, and wash the face.

Appliance versus Tool

Technology can be applied as an appliance or as a tool (Rodgers, 1985). The distinction between tools and appliances is crucial for proper technology application. An appliance operates independently; for example, a refrigerator serves its technological function by operating by itself once it is plugged in. Other appliance technologies include hearing aids, eyeglasses, and certain splints. They do not require the development of particular skills in order to be used.

In contrast, a tool requires certain skills and/or manipulation to serve a useful function. People think of some tools or higher technologies as appliances that require very little effort. This misunderstanding can have serious consequences. For example, communication aids are often thought to be a simple type of technology that helps an individual speak or write. However, communication aids cannot operate on their own and require many hours of both the user's time to learn their operation and the therapist's time to teach the user. Such tools of higher technology should not be perceived as an easy answer, but rather as implements that require skill and time in order to help individuals improve their performance and become more independent. When potentially valuable tools are treated as appliances and training is not provided, the devices frequently end up being discarded or not used because the client does not know how to use them correctly. Just as a cook must learn to use a stove to make savory meals, one who wears a flexor hinge (tenodesis) splint must learn to manipulate the splint for grasp and pinch, and those who use a communication aid must develop the language skills and mechanical operations of the device to be able to functionally converse. Without user training, these tools may only exhibit a fraction of their potential.

DEFINITIONS IN ASSISTIVE TECHNOLOGY

Definitions in the field have been well presented by Smith (1991) (see box).

Definitions are still evolving. For example, some use the term *low technology* while others use *light technology* to describe a device that is simple to use and does not contain electronic components. However, even more interesting is the interpretation of what a low/light technology device is. Is the telephone a low/light technology device or a high technology device? It is certainly simple to use, but in itself it is quite a complex piece of hard technology. Sometimes technology can be so well-designed that the consumer considers it low/light technology. The complexity of the design of the technology is often transparent. As well, some technologies may seem high technology when first introduced, but as time passes, constant exposure makes it seem lighter. This has been true for telephones, VCRs and, for some, computers.

Assistive technology enables or enhances a person's ability to be independent. During the evaluation, the consumer and therapist focus on the abilities of the consumer and whether assistive technology can assist in the task of independent living. Some devices take the place of a missing function, such as an augmentative communication device with speech output which enables persons without spoken communication to speak. A wheelchair may enable a person who cannot walk to move independently in his or her environment. Other devices, such as seating systems, enhance a person's ability to sit by providing greater comfort, function and stability.

OVERVIEW OF ASSISTIVE TECHNOLOGIES

Major areas of assistive technologies will be introduced and references to acquire specific information will be presented.

Mobility

Mobility technologies include wheelchairs, walkers, canes, orthotic devices, FES (functional electrical stimulation), laser canes and any other assistive device that would assist a person with a mobility disability, be it motor or sensory, to move about in his or her environment. There are very few people who have a working knowledge of all the possible commercial options. Therefore, people usually acquire expertise in certain areas, such as wheelchairs. There are hundreds of varieties of wheelchairs, each offering a different array of electro-mechanical characteristics that need to be understood as part of the selection process. Fortunately, there are now several ways that the practitioner and the consumer can obtain useful information. A classification system has been developed which sets a conceptual framework for understanding the different types of wheelchairs that are produced commercially (Hobson, 1990). Magazines such as *Paraplegic News* and *Sports and Spokes* annually publish the specifications on most of the manual and powered wheelchairs commonly found in the North American marketplace. These reviews are based on standardized testing that is carried out by manufacturers following the ANSI/RESNA wheelchair standards (Axelson, Minkel & Chesney, 1994). Since the testing and measurements are done and reported in a standard way, it is now possible to make accurate comparisons between products, a tremendous advancement for wheelchair specialists and the consumers they serve.

Seating/Positioning

Many people cannot use wheelchairs as they come from the manufacturer. Specialized seating is required to help persons attain a comfortable and functional seated posture for activities that enable them to access work, attend educational programs, and participate in recreational activities. Orthotic supports, seating systems in wheelchairs, chairs that promote dynamic posture in the workplace, and chairs for the elderly that fit properly, are safe and encourage movement, all fit into the broad category of sitting technology. There are a number of pulished resources to help therapists with issues of seating needs based on diagnosis and physical/functional status (Trefler, Hobson, Johnson Taylor, Monahan & Shaw, 1993), evaluation practices (Bergen, Presperin & Tallman, 1990; Trefler et al., 1993; Zollars, 1996), and terminology (Medhat & Hobson, 1992). These references also discuss the selection process, evaluation tools, biomechanics of supported sitting and materials properties of weight relieving technologies. A classification system of specialized seating has been developed which provides a conceptual framework for understanding the features of the various technologies and their potential applications (Trefler et al., 1993).

Sensation

People with limited or no sensation are prone to skin injury; special seating technology can assist in the prevention of tissue breakdown. Specially designed cushions and backs for wheelchairs and mattresses that have pressure distributing characteristics achieve this objective. Technology has also been developed to remind people to relieve pressure at determined intervals or to do it for them mechanically.

Access/Interface (Human/machine Interface)

In order to use assistive technology, people with disabilities need to be able to operate the technology. With limitations in motor and/or sensory systems, persons often require the assembly or design of individualized systems. This could be as simple as several switches or a miniaturized keyboard, or as complex as an integrated control system that allows a person to drive a wheelchair and operate a computer and a communication device using only one switch.

Communication (Augmentative and Alternative)

Because of motor or sensory limitations, some individuals cannot communicate with spoken or written words. There are communication systems that enable people to communicate using synthesized voice or printed output. Systems for people who are deaf allow them to communicate over the phone or through computer interfaces. Laptop computers with appropriate software can enable persons to communicate faster and with less effort than previously possible. Some basic guidelines for selecting an augmentative communication system, including strategies for securing funding, have been proposed (Jones & Jones, 1990; Angelo, 1997; Cook & Hussey, 1995).

Transportation

Modified vans and cars enable persons with disabilities to independently drive a vehicle. Wheelchair tie downs and occupant restraints in personal vehicles and in public transportation vehicles are allowing people to be safely transported to their chosen destination. Fortunately, voluntary performance standards for restraint and tie down technologies are currently being developed by a task group within the Society for Automotive Engineers (SAE). Standards for hand controls have just been revised for another 5 years. Other standards relate to van body modifications and wheelchair lifts. These standards provide the rehabilitation engineer with a set of tools that can be used to confirm safety compliance of modified transportation equipment. Currently in development are transport wheelchair and vehicle powered controls standards.

Universal Access Design

Universal access design is a concept that supports the design of environments and their contained products so people with disabilities, or those who are aging and/or acquire a disability, can use or readily adapt their environments or products. Paul Grayson, among others, has published extensively regarding the need to rethink how we design our living environments (Grayson, 1991). Vanderheiden and the Denno

lead group of the Honeywell SSD Center, have prepared excellent human factors guidelines for product designers. These guidelines provide invaluable information on access characteristics to allow use by the elderly and persons with disabilities (Denno et al., 1992; Vanderheiden & Vanderheiden, 1991).

Activities of Daily Living (ADL)

ADL technology enables a person to live independently as much as possible. Devices such as environmental control units, bathroom aids, dressing assists, automatic door openers and alarms are all considered aids to daily living. Many are inexpensive and can be purchased through careful selection in stores or through catalogues. Others are quite expensive and must be ordered through vendors who specialize in technology for independent living, or must be modified or built to address the specific needs of a person.

School and Work

Technology that supports people in the workplace or in an educational environment can cover applications such as computer work stations, modified bathrooms, and transportation to and from work or school. Students need the ability to take notes and do assignments. Working people have myriad special tasks that may need to be analyzed and modified to enable independence and productivity. An extensive overview of rehabilitation engineering in the workplace, which includes a review of different types of workplaces, and the process of accommodation (including case examples), has been prepared (Weisman, 1990), as well as a workbook to assist in the design of workplace modifications (Mueller, 1990).

Recreation

A component of living that is often overlooked by the professional community is the desire and in fact the need, of people with disabilities to participate in recreational activities. Many of the adaptive recreational technologies have been developed by persons with disabilities themselves in their effort to participate and be competitive in sports. Competitive wheelchair racing, archery, skiing, and bicycling, and technology that enables people to bowl, play pool, and fly their own airplanes are just a few areas in which equipment has been adapted for specific recreational purposes (Enders & Hall, 1990).

Community and Workplace Access

There is probably no other single legislation that has had a more profound impact on the lives of people with disabilities in the U.S. than the Americans with Disabilities Act, signed into law by President Bush in August, 1990. The civil rights

---

TABLE 20-1

Technology Related Conferences

RESNA - the Rehabilitation Engineering and Assistive
Technology Association of North America
1700 Moore St.
Arlington, VA 22209-1903
http://www.resna.org/resna/reshome.htm

American Occupational Therapy Association (AOTA)
4720 Montgomery Lane
P.O. Box 31220
Bethesda, MD 20824-1220
301/652-2682
http://www.infl.com.aota

International Society of Augmentative and Alternative
Communication
428 East Preston Street
Baltimore, MD 21202-3993

Human Factors and Ergonomics Society
P.O. Box 1369
Santa Monica, CA 90406
310/394-1811

United States Society of Augmentative and Alternative
Communication
P.O. Box 5271
Evanston, IL 60204-5271
847/869-2122

Closing the Gap
(computer applications and AAC)
P.O. Box 68
Henderson, MN 56044
507/248-3294
http://www.closingthegap.com

Technology and Persons with Disabilities
Center on Disabilities (CSUN)
(computer applications and AAC)
California State University, Northridge
18111 Nordhoff St.
Northridge, CA 91330-8340

International Seating Symposium
University of Pittsburgh, SHRS
Forbes Tower, Suite 5044
Pittsburgh, PA 15260
412/647-1270
http://www.pft5xx36.ft90.upmc.edu/RTP/RERCHP.html

---

legislation mandates that all people with disabilities have access to public facilities, and that reasonable accommodations be made by employers to allow persons with disabilities to access employment opportunities. The impact of this legislation is now sweeping America and leading to changes in the way people view the rights of persons with disabilities.

Consumer independence is the optimal goal of occupational therapy. If a person is unable to perform a task such as writing a term paper, a number of choices become available, depending on the needs and available resources of the person. Many issues impact on the choices, including cost, time frame in which a solution is needed, ease of operation, product availability, and availability of maintenance and repair.

The field of assistive technology is rapidly changing. Clinicians working in this area need a vehicle for staying in touch with the latest advances. Table 20-1 lists organizations or groups that hold technology-related conferences. RESNA is the primary interdisciplinary professional association that addresses a full range of rehabilitation technology. Table 20-2 lists the special interest groups of RESNA.

In providing assistive technology, it is important to keep the solution as simple and cost-effective as possible. Figure 20-1 illustrates the preferred hierarchy of possible intervention strategies.

- The first choice would be to modify the task. If the person wants to have the paper typed, he or she could find someone to type it.
- If the person wants to type it using a computer, he or she would need to be able to access the keyboard of a commercially available computer system. If this person has a motor impairment that prevents him or her from using a standard keyboard, the therapist may investigate positioning the keyboard and the person to provide a more ergonomically designed work station. Simple placement of the keyboard in an alternate location or the use of an alternate posture might be all that is necessary.
- If the client is still unable to operate the keyboard, an alternate commercial product may be sought. There are ergonomic keyboards with alternate designs and sizes that might enable the person to use his or her fine motor skills more effectively for keyboard operation.
- The next option may be to modify a commercially available device to fit the consumer's needs. If the placement of a commercial keyboard needs modification, an easel or ramp might be used. If the client cannot execute a two key function, software could be loaded into the computer that would enable the person to perform two key functions using only one key at a time. In some cases, this option resides in the operating system of the computer, such as Sticky Keys in the Macintosh.
- The final choice, because of cost, time and availability, would be to custom design a product. In the case of a

computer application, custom software could be written or a custom access method could be developed. In the past few years, alternate sized keyboards have become commercially available for persons with disabilities. These large or small keyboards have reduced the need for customization even further.

THE CONCEPTUAL FRAMEWORK FOR INTERFACING PEOPLE WITH ASSISTIVE TECHNOLOGY

Introduction

One of the major contributions and challenges for the occupational therapist is to identify the abilities, needs and life goals of a person with disabilities and then guide him or her on a self-directed course that incrementally progresses towards the person's identified goals. The occupational therapist, who is also an assistive technology practitioner (ATP), will be specifically skilled at assessing needs and introducing the potential of assistive technology as a means of supplementing a person's abilities. The prime purpose of the assistive technology intervention is to minimize the mismatch between the person's abilities and the demands of environments in which they endeavor to carry out activities of self-care, work, education or recreation. Since this conceptual framework is the fundamental "raison d'être" for assistive technology, the following presents a brief overview of the conceptual models that have been developed to help explain the relationship between people, technology and the environment. Furthermore, an understanding of these models, as they are applied to assistive technology, further defines the role of the occupational therapist, because many of the professional activities involved in the implementation of the model(s) are to a large extent those of the therapist.

One of the exciting aspects of the assistive technology field is that it is still undergoing rapid development and change. The three interrelated conceptual frameworks that are presented build on preceding models, and others will follow. The basis of the models is founded on the human-machine interaction models developed by human factors researchers, beginning in the early 1970s.

The Human-Environment/Technology Model (HETI)

The first model was developed by Roger Smith (Smith, 1991), and is termed the human-environment/technology model (HETI). Conceptually, there are six primary functions technology can serve; three of them address human deficits and the other three address the technological environment.

TABLE 20-2
Special Interest Groups of RESNA

SIG-01	Service Delivery & Public Policy
SIG-02	Personal Transportation
SIG-03	Augmentative & Alternative Communication
SIG-04	Dysphagia: Feeding, Swallowing & Saliva Control
SIG-05	Quantitative Functional Assessment
SIG-06	Special Education
SIG-07	Technology Transfer
SIG-08	Sensory Loss & Technology
SIG-09	Wheeled Mobility & Seating
SIG-10	Electrical Stimulation
SIG-11	Computer Applications
SIG-12	Rural Rehabilitation
SIG-13	Assistive Robotics & Mechatronics
SIG-14	Job Accommodation
SIG-15	Information Networking
SIG-16	Gerontology
SIG-17	International Appropriate Technology
SIG-18	Tech Art
SIG-19	Universal Access
SIG-20	Cognitive Disabilities and Technologies

HETI is the framework for understanding these functional relationships, as shown schematically in Figure 20-2. HETI proposes that a person must first receive information in order to interact with the environment. The person must then process the information to make meaningful judgments and proper decisions. Finally, the person must respond motorically to the information. This is consistent with sensory input, cognitive throughput, and motor output, which is the base of much occupational therapy theory and practice. In this conceptual model, these three functional capacities are labeled human input (HI), human processing (HP), and human output (HO). All *sensory* dimensions fall under human input, including perceptions that are tactile, proprioceptive, visual, vestibular, auditory, olfactory, and gustatory. Human processing is made up of all *cognitive* dimensions, including memory, orientation, attention span, recognition, thought processing, problem-solving, generalization, sequencing, concept formation, categorization, and other intellectual operations. Human output includes the *neuromo-*

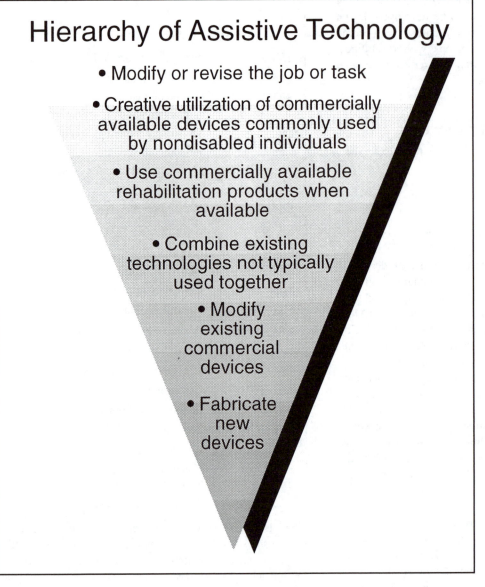

Hierarchy of Assistive Technology

- Modify or revise the job or task
- Creative utilization of commercially available devices commonly used by nondisabled individuals
- Use commercially available rehabilitation products when available
- Combine existing technologies not typically used together
- Modify existing commercial devices
- Fabricate new devices

Figure 20-1. Hierarchy of Assistive Technology. From Symms, J. & Ross, D. (1991). Presented at Pacific Regional RESNA Conference, Long Beach, CA.

tor dimensions, such as fine motor coordination, gross motor coordination, muscle tone, reflexes, range of motion, strength, endurance, soft tissue integrity, skeletal integrity, postural control, and activity tolerance.

In the Smith approach, adequate sensation, cognitive skills, and motor skills are generic in their interaction with the environment and not specific to a given activity. For example, visual sensation allows an individual to visually perceive all of the environment. Deficits in visual perception do not affect one specific activity, but tend to encompass many activities. Therefore, both visual skills and visual deficits tend to be fundamental.

The second half of the HETI Model is the machine or technology environment. The components mirror the human side of the model. Any type of dynamic and functional machine has some type of method to sense or receive information, hence the environment/technology input (EI). These types of technologies also have a specific function and purpose which are termed environment/technology applications (EA). Functional machines and technology are useless unless there is a way to demonstrate their capabilities through some motor or display presentation, which is the environment/technology output (EO). The technology half of the model tends to be fairly specific to one or a few activities, such as computers or electronically controlled wheelchairs; thus, they are more limited in application, as opposed to the more generic capabilities and functions of the human half of the model.

To illustrate this model, consider the example of a person

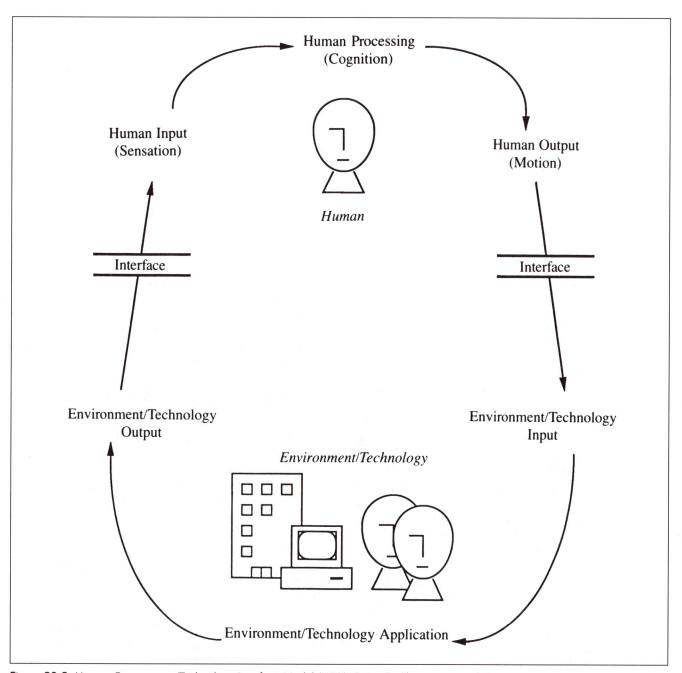

Figure 20-2. Human-Environment/Technology Interface Model (HETI). From C. Christiansen and C. Baum. (1991). *Occupational therapy: Overcoming human performance deficits.* Thorofare, NJ: SLACK Incorporated. Used with permission.

interacting with a computer. When people first encounter a computer, they must see the computer, the keyboard or mouse, and visually perceive the display on the computer monitor (HI). As they use the computer, they must integrate information (words, pictures) that they read or see from the monitor and convert that information into appropriate motor responses. When the computer beeps to indicate an error, they must decide what the beep signifies (HP). Motor output is then

aimed back to the computer (HO). This human-machine interaction, however, would be absolutely useless if the computer did not have some method of acknowledging and acting on the person's motor output. The person presses a key or moves a mouse to tell the computer what to do next (EI). But the computer must have a program which reads, interprets, and analyzes what the key and mouse movements mean. The particular computer program becomes the computer's processing side

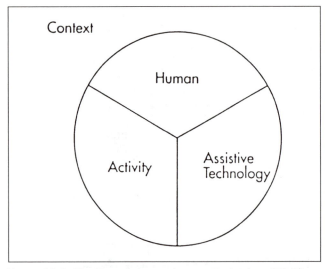

Figure 20-3. The Human Activity Assistive Technology (HAAT) Model.

of the human's cognitive processing (EA). The computer then must convert the new information it has calculated into a presentation which is perceivable by a human being. It takes its imperceptible (below human threshold) electronic impulses and converts them into auditory signals and visual displays (EO). This completes the human-machine cycle.

Smith claims these six components are essential for the functioning of the human-technology model. If an individual needed to use a computer, but had any disability in sensory perception, cognitive processing, or motor output, the person would have difficulty using the computer. Likewise, this would be a non-functional interaction if the computer had a disability. A non-functioning computer would either fail to accept information the way the person was providing it, fail to process information in appropriate applications, or fail to output information so the person could perceive it. This model operates in a cycle and, as in most chains, is only as strong as its weakest link. Consequently, if an individual were blind, the cycle would be broken and the person could not use a computer (or powered wheelchair) unless one of two things were to occur: 1) either the person's input system (blindness) was somehow remediated, or 2) the computer expressed some additional type of output which could be perceived by somebody who could not see the monitor.

Another example can be seen in a person driving a power wheelchair, in which the person needs to see where he or she is going (HI), decide where to go (HP), and control the joystick (HO). The wheelchair requires a method of control, which is the joystick (EA), which can actually move the chair in that direction (EO). The model assists the therapist by identifying potential breakdown sites in therapeutic interventions and provides a framework for discussing the human potential and limitations of technology.

The HETI model illustrates the interrelatedness between the person and technology and how we should think in terms of recognizing the essential contributions of both the person and technology, if one is have a unified interactive system. The analogy between the human (sensation, cognition, motion) and technology components (input, application, output) really seems to work well for computer-based technology in which the computer carries out an activity analogous to the human processing or cognition. In many assistive technology applications, especially low tech applications, this analogy has less meaning. Furthermore, the Smith model fails to emphasize the goals and activities of the individual, or the influence of the contexts in which the person will be carrying out the activities.

More recently, Cook and Hussey extended the conceptual models to place more emphasis on identifying life roles and related activities, and the influence of the environment or context in which the person performs the activity using an assistive technology device. They also suggest that the expanded perspective provides a systematic means of differentiating and measuring human versus system performance (Cook and Hussey, 1995).

The Human Activity Assistive Technology (HAAT) Model

The HAAT model also draws from more recent human factors research. Similarly, the purpose is to provide a framework for studying human performance in a wide range of tasks involving technology, including computers, telecommunications equipment, industrial processes, and vocational tasks (Bailey, 1989). The HAAT model is an adaptation of the Bailey human factors model, expanding the context to include social and cultural factors, as well as environments and physical conditions such as temperature, noise and lighting level. Assistive technologies are specifically shown, and their relationship to the other three components (human, context and activity) is illustrated. The four component adapted model is shown in Figure 20-3. The four components and their interrelationships as developed by Cook and Hussey will be briefly discussed.

The Cook and Hussey model is composed of four fundamental components: the human, an activity (or occupation) the human wishes to perform, the context or environment in which the person wishes to perform the activity, and the assistive technology which enables the person to successfully carry out the activity. Each of the components shown in Figure 20-3 plays a unique part in the total system. The specification of a system begins with a need or desire by the person to perform an activity. The activity (e.g., cooking, writing, playing tennis) defines the goal of the assistive technology system. This activity is accomplished by completing a set of tasks. Each activity is carried out within a context. The combination of activity and context allows specification of the human skills required for attainment of the goal. If the person lacks the necessary skills to accomplish the activity, then assistive technologies may be used. This use still requires skills. However, they are adapted to the individual capabilities of the person and then matched to an assistive technology system, the function of which is to accomplish the desired activity.

The interaction among the components of the HAAT model can be illustrated by an example. Tony needs to write reports. Thus, writing is his activity. He is required to accomplish this as part of his work, and this specifies part of the context. Because of a spinal cord injury, Tony is unable to use his hands, but he is able to speak clearly. A voice recognition system (the assistive technology) is obtained for him. This system allows Tony to use his skills (speaking) to accomplish the activity (writing) by translating what Tony says into computer-recognizable characters. As Tony speaks, the assistive technology recognizes what he says and sends it to the computer as if it had been typed. Since there are other workers in the office, Tony uses a noise canceling microphone to avoid errors in voice recognition, and he works in a cubicle to avoid bothering other workers. These further define the context of this system. Tony's assistive technology system consists of the activity (writing), the context (at work in a noisy office), the human skills (speaking), and the assistive technology (voice recognition). For any other individual, one or more parts of this system may be different. For example, another person may be able to type, but only with an enlarged keyboard. A third person may need to write at home, rather than at work.

Thus, each assistive technology system is unique. It is therefore the role of the occupational therapist to assess the skills and abilities of the individual, determine his or her functional goals and the activities necessary to realize them, understand the influences of the context(s) in which the activity will be carried out, and assist the individual to make appropriate selections of assistive technologies that will enhance his or her ability to achieve the desired activities of daily life. Let us now examine a little further the two differentiating aspects (activity and context) of the HAAT model.

Activity

The activity (or occupation) is the fundamental element of the HAAT model and defines the overall goal of the assistive technology system. In *Uniform Terminology for Occupational Therapy, Second Edition* (American Occupational Therapy Association, 1989) occupations are categorized within three basic performance areas: self-care, work and school, play and leisure. Self-care activities include dressing, hygiene, grooming, bathing, eating, communica-

tion, taking medications, sexual expression, and mobility. Included in work/school are home management activities, educational activities, vocational activities, and care of others. The play and leisure area includes activities related to self-expression, enjoyment, or relaxation.

The occupations that an individual performs are determined by the life roles that individual fulfills. Christiansen (1991) defines roles as "distinctive positions in society, each having a defined status and specific expectations for behavior." He goes on to say that, "although roles are occupied by persons, they define performance expectations and are viewed as attributes of performance and not of individuals" (p. 28). A person can have multiple roles simultaneously, and roles change throughout the person's lifespan. Examples of roles we hold during our lifetime include student, parent, son or daughter, sibling, employee, friend, and homemaker. The life role of the individual influences the activities performed by the individual.

Occupations can be broken down into smaller tasks and actions. For example, the task of paying bills typically includes a series of actions such as opening the envelope, reading the amount, writing a check for the appropriate amount, putting the check in the envelope with the bill, recording the check in the check register, sealing the envelope, placing a stamp on the envelope, and putting the envelope in the mail box. The skills and abilities intrinsic to the human allow the individual to complete a series of tasks to produce the functional outcome of the occupation or activity. It is important that the occupational therapist be aware of these different components of the activity. By identifying the life roles an individual has, activities carried out by that individual can be determined. Viewing the task in terms of the underlying actions allows us to see whether the individual has the required intrinsic skills and abilities or whether alternative approaches are necessary.

Contexts

The HAAT model also introduces the concept of contexts, i.e., where the activity is being performed. The context includes four major considerations. These are: 1) setting (e.g., at home, at work in the community), 2) social context (with peers, with strangers), 3) cultural context, and 4) physical context, measured by temperature, moisture, light, etc. The contexts in which the human carries out the activity are frequently forgotten when assistive technology application is considered. However, the context is often the determining factor in the success or failure of the assistive technology system.

Setting. The type of setting dictates the characteristics of the assistive technology system, and a system that is successful in one environment may not be in another. For example, a manual wheelchair that has solid hard rubber tiers may work well around the house but not on rough outdoor terrain. In some cases, the number of settings in which the system is to be used is limited to one or two. But in many cases, the system will need to function across all of these settings, and flexibility in the system to do this is absolutely necessary.

Social and Cultural Contexts. For assistive technology use, the social aspects of the context can be the most important. Since we are concerned with aiding human performance in communication, mobility, and manipulation, we must be concerned with the social context in which this performance takes place. Social context is closely related to and influenced by culture. Krefting and Krefting (1991) define culture based on three concepts: 1) "culture is a system of learned patterns of behavior"; 2) it is "shared by members of the group rather than being the property of an individual," and 3) it includes effective mechanisms for interacting with others and with the environment (p. 102). Thus, these three elements of culture clearly couple it to the HAAT model and emphasize the importance of cultural considerations in the design and implementation of assistive technology systems. This cultural screen differs for each of us, and it biases the way we interact with others and the ways in which we perceive various actions, tasks, and life roles. For example, in some cultures leisure is recognized as a desirable and socially acceptable pursuit. However, in other cultures, pursuit of leisure time is thought to indicate laziness and lack of productivity. If the occupational therapist and the consumer have differing cultural screens, then they may have difficulty establishing and achieving mutual goals. For example, if the occupational therapist views leisure as a desirable and satisfying occupation, he or she may recommend assistive technology systems that enable leisure activities to take place. This could include modified computer or video games, an adapted wheelchair for tennis or other sports, or adaptations of board games. However, if the consumer is from a culture in which leisure is viewed as being nonproductive, he or she may reject these assistive technology systems as frivolous.

Physical Context. The environmental conditions that exist where the system is being used are called the *physical context*. Three commonly measured parameters—heat (related to temperature), sound, and light—most directly affect the performance of assistive technologies. Many materials are sensitive to temperature and affected by excessive heat or cold. For example, the properties of foams and gels used in seat cushions can change under conditions of very high or very low temperatures. Liquid crystal displays are affected by temperature as well as by ambient (existing) light. Taken together, these three parameters describe the physical context in which assistive technologies are used. When recommending specific technologies, an understanding of the assistive technology and how it performs in specific environmental conditions is important in order to avoid malfunction of the technology and disappointment for the user.

A natural outcome of the HAAT model is the ability to identify where in the process a difficulty may reside, as well as document outcomes of the intervention.

THE ENVIRONMENTAL MISMATCH MODEL

Persons with disabilities no longer wish to be viewed by others as a group distinct from the remainder of society. The vast majority are no longer in acute rehabilitation phases, or they have matured with a stable congenital disability and simply wish to pursue their life's goals the same as all other people. For the most part they do not view themselves as being medical patients and therefore resent the notion of having to return to the medical system to have their needs met, including their assistive technology services. This view of persons with disabilities is a departure from the traditional view, and one which occupational therapists must be cognizant of if they are to be responsive to desires and needs of people who spend the majority of their lives in community environments. This paradigm shift suggests an additional conceptual building block that needs to be added to the above described models.

If we examine our built environment, i.e., the places where people live, work, become educated and recreate, we find that these environments, and the products found in them, are to a large extent made for so-called "normal" adults. That is, people who have normal strength, good vision, good coordination, are of average size, average weight, etc. If you are a child, a mother with a child, a person of short or tall stature, or elderly and feeble, chances are the environment or tools or appliances within the environment may not match your needs, depending on how far you vary from the norm. However subtle, there is a mismatch between you and the built environment in which you must function in order to carry out your daily activities. Examples of this mismatch abound. Standard seat sizes and controls in cars do not accommodate people of tall or short stature, the average print size in most publications or electronic controls assumes vision within normal ranges, access to many buildings and public vehicles still assumes normal agility to negotiate steps, most homes are built on multiple levels, most room lighting and sound systems assume normal sight and hearing. The fact is that many people, young and old, who are not seen as disabled are not adequately accommodated by our built environment.

If we now see persons with disabilities within the same context, it provides a conceptual framework for responding to needs and providing services that is a departure from current practices, and more closely aligned with how persons with disabilities view themselves. That is, society should view disability as nothing more than another variation of the norm for which the built environment is incapable of meeting the person's needs. Within this context, and in keeping with the models discussed above, the primary purpose of assistive technol-

TABLE 20-3

Recent Major U.S. Federal Legislation that has Impacted Assistive Technologies

Legislation	Major assistive technology impact
Rehabilitation Act of 1973	Mandated reasonable accommodation, LRE in federally funded employment and higher education; requires both assistive technology device and services
Education for All Handicapped Children Act of 1975 (PL 94-142)	Extended reasonable accommodation and LRE to age 5-21 education; mandated IEP for each child; assistive technology plays major role in gaining access to educational programs
Handicapped Infants and Toddlers Act (PL 99-457)	Extended PL 94-142 to infants and to ages 3-5 years; expanded emphasis on educationally related assistive technologies
1986 Amendments to The Rehabilitation Act of 1973 (PL 99-506)	Required all states to include provision for assistive technology services in both state plan and IWRP for each client; Section 508 mandated equal access to electronic office equipment for all Federal employees
Technology-Related Assistance for Individuals with Disabilities Act of 1988 (PL 100-407)	First legislation specifically related to assistive technologies; extends Section 508 to all funded states, mandates consumer-driven assistive technology services and statewide system change
Americans with Disabilities Act (ADA) of 1990 (PL 101-336)	Civil rights act for disabled; extends Sections 503, 504, 508, and other provisions to all citizens in terms of public accommodation, private employment, transportation, and telecommunications
Individuals with Disabilities Education Act (IDEA)	Reauthorization of PL 92-102. Extends assistive technology device and service definitions to education
Reauthorization of the Rehabilitation Act of 1973	Brings rehabilitation act language and mandate in line with ADA; defines rehabilitation technology as rehabilitation engineering and assistive technology devices and services; mandates rehabilitation technology as primary benefit to be included in IWRP

ogy is to bridge the gap between the functional abilities of persons and the limitations of their environment and its products to meet their needs. However, this paradigm shift places the burden on society to accommodate the needs to all people rather than to view those that vary from the norm as being distinct and different with special needs.

This concept of creating environments and contained products that accommodate an ever-broadening definition of normal has been termed *universal design*. By definition, universal design has as its goal to minimize the need for assistive technology. However, it should be clear that built environments and products, however accommodating, will never meet the needs of all persons with disabilities, and therefore assistive technologies will be needed to supplement the remaining deficiencies in the environment.

LEGISLATION

Beginning with the Rehabilitation Act of 1973, various pieces of legislation have worked toward providing people with disabilities access to education, work and the community (Fillippo, Inge & Barcus, 1995; Cook & Hussey, 1995) (Table 20-3).

However, there remains a gap between legislation and implementation. Perhaps the Americans with Disabilities Act (ADA) has come closest to a piece of civil rights legislation for people with disabilities. Through reasonable accommodation, people in the United States are gaining access to public buildings, many places of employment, public transportation and recreational facilities. It is against the law to deny employment solely based on a person's disability.

As with any legislation, there are some who choose to ignore it or simply deny that it applies to them. The result is litigation, an often costly and lengthy process. But persons with disabilities, for the first time, have the law on their side. Progress, though never rapid or complete, is at least moving in the direction of providing fair access to the community, education and work.

Occupational therapists provide information in the area of legislation and consumer rights. Working in school systems with children ages 3 to 21, occupational therapists in the United States are involved in the development of the Individualized Education Plan (IEP), or in preschool settings for children birth to 2, with the Individualized Family Service Plan (IFSP), which is more family-oriented. AT may be required to enable the child to participate in the educational program. A child might need a page turner in order to read the assignment or an enlarged computer keyboard in order to write the homework assignment. In the workplace, we may work with the client and his or her vocational rehabilitation counselor to write the Individualized Written Rehabilitation Plan (IWRP), in which assistive technology services may enable a person to return to work or be retrained. A custom file folder separator might enable a person to access files he or she would need in a day, or a Braille reader would enable a person who is blind to review necessary documents.

Occupational therapists should have information that could lead consumers to Centers for Independent Living (CILs) where they would find peer counselors, information specialists or advocacy services. Although some occupational therapists actually can provide advocacy information, generally they act as referral sources to persons who are experts in legal and advocacy issues.

EDUCATION

Assistive Technology is just beginning to enter into the curriculum in occupational therapy preservice education programs. Kanny, Anson & Smith (1992) completed a survey of 59 occupational therapy education programs at the undergraduate and graduate levels. Approximately 50% indicated that less than 20 hours of training in assistive technology was being offered. Another 25% provided between 20 and 50 hours of training, and the rest provided more than 50 hours of training. As the skills and knowledge base in assistive technology are clearly defined and competencies for occupational therapists are formalized, all OTs will need to have at least an entry level competence. All preservice programs will need to include assistive technology so that their students can succeed in incorporating it into their repertoire of practice skills, which are tested in credentialing examinations.

In the interim, either for programs that do not have faculty who are experienced in assistive technology or for therapists who are already in practice and wish to upgrade their skills, there are a number of models of assistive technology education that provide the training. Many professional associations in occupational therapy include assistive technology courses in their pre-conference program at their annual conferences, and there is often a technology tract that attendees can choose. RESNA always has 2 days of instructional courses preceding the annual conference, with a series of

morning seminars and special sessions supplementing the full conference program. A number of university programs sponsor assistive technology continuing education programs to augment or actually serve as coursework for their own students and others. Other meetings, such as the International Seating Symposium (ISS), Closing the Gap, the National Medical Trade Show, and Technology and Persons with Disabilities (CSUN), provide a variety of educational experiences.

Another approach is to include a full course in assistive technology for preservice occupational therapists. Specialized electives are possible at several universities such as the Tech Spec. at the University of Wisconsin-Madison. Also, there is now a masters program in assistive technology at the University of Pittsburgh in the Department of Rehabilitation Science and Technology. Students who are occupational therapists, engineers, speech and language pathologists, and others who hold undergraduate degrees can enroll in a multidisciplinary masters program. Students take a program of study that prepares them to specialize in service delivery or research in the area of AT.

Finally, the AOTA has produced a home study program in assistive technology. Edited by J. Hammel, PhD, the program includes study modules in various assistive technology application areas. Home study materials are provided, as well as the opportunity to discuss issues on-line.

RESEARCH

Occupational therapists can become involved in either basic or applied/clinical research projects related to assistive technology. In the applied research area, therapists are involved with consumers and engineers in the evaluation and comparison of existing products, outcomes intervention, the development of new service delivery mechanisms, present use patterns of technologies, design of new technologies, the surveying of consumers satisfaction with products or the process of delivery of assistive technology, and the development of new methods of assessment, documentation and prescription. In the basic research area, therapists are part of research teams investigating the effects of functional electrical stimulation on the upper extremity, types of grasp used by children with cerebral palsy when using tools/toys, and the effectiveness of seating intervention on posture, respiration and function and so forth. In a very general sense, the difference between these two types of research is that applied research looks at issues of current practice, while basic research is adding to the knowledge base of the field.

Preservice and postgraduate programs are now providing didactic and practical experiences for therapists to learn the research skills. Clinical practice in assistive technology will

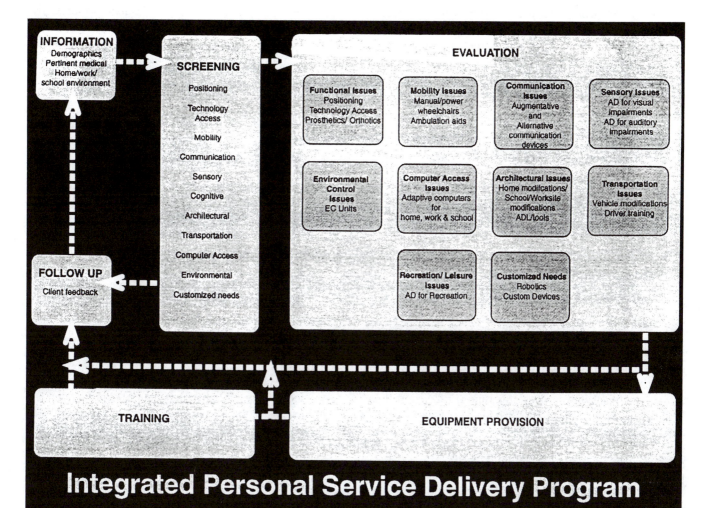

Figure 20-4. Integrated Personal Service Delivery Program.

provide the basis for excellent research projects.

ACTIVITIES FOR OCCUPATIONAL THERAPISTS IN ASSISTIVE TECHNOLOGY

Service Delivery

An assistive technology program should augment traditional therapy programs. The model described is being implemented by the University of Pittsburgh Medical Center. The program, called the Center for Assistive Technology (CAT), can represent any comprehensive technology service delivery program in either a state agency, a rehabilitation center, or a university based program. Proposed steps in a service delivery process are seen in Figure 20-4. The components of the program will be described.

Referral/Information

As assistive technology programs expand beyond the medical model to a community-based practice, referrals can be accepted from a wide variety of sources. Physician referrals are most common, but therapists, persons with disabilities, their families, community advocates, teachers, and vocational rehabilitation counselors are beginning to broaden the referral base. It is important to keep the client's primary physician informed of the referral and recommendations. This is particularly important if a letter of medical necessity or a prescription is necessary, but it also serves to keep the physician a part of the person's core team and is a way to educate the physician in the benefits of assistive technology. Seating and mobility technologies still require a physician's prescription for funding. Other technologies, such as environmental control units (ECUs) and computer technologies, can be purchased by some third party payers such as vocational rehabilitation, without physician involvement.

Information Gathering

The information gathered in an AT assessment must come from both traditional and non-traditional sources. Traditional sources include the physician and hospital records, school or work histories, and a personal interview which would focus on the client's needs, expectations and interests. It is important to know the person's age, diagnosis, rehabilitation history, grade in school, work history and how he or she spends leisure time.

A review of scales of activities of daily living which are used to assist therapists in selecting appropriate functional measures (Law & Letts, 1989) did not include AT in the measure of independence. *OT Fact* includes the use of AT to some extent, but there is no test in which the use of AT would raise the person's scale to independent when he or she uses AT to achieve performance. Therapists who use such scales as the Functional Independence Measure (FIM) report that their clients are more functional than the score indicates. It is anticipated that a revised version of the FIM will enable clients to use AT to perform tasks without having an adverse effect on their score. New measures of client satisfaction are being introduced (Demers, Weiss-Lambrou & Ska, 1996).

Additional information is helpful. For example, it has been shown that some people have a predisposition to the use of technology (Scherer, 1991). One could administer the Assistive Technology, the Educational Technology, the Workplace or Health Care Technology Predisposition's Assessment components of Scherer's series of assessments for selecting and evaluating technologies. The series includes a test entitled The Assistive Technology Device Predisposition Assessment, which enables the occupational therapist and consumer to determine the likelihood of the consumer being a candidate for assistive technology intervention. As well, consumer goals, desires and needs need to be documented, with the consumer giving priority to his or her own life goals. Because technology abandonment is a real concern (Batavia & Hammer, 1990), it is essential that therapists know a person's past history with AT use, his or her present attitudes, needs and goals, so that mistakes, which are often costly, can be avoided. Therapy evaluations are most often performed to establish functional goals for treatment. The therapist in the technology team must be able to interpret the functional abilities of the consumer and his or her goals to determine if assistive technology would be ben-

eficial. For example, if a consumer is able to operate a joystick but not a keyboard, and he or she wants to operate a computer, the therapist must recommend a computer access system that is operated with a joystick.

Screening

Not all referrals to an AT clinic are appropriate. Consumers might receive services more quickly and more cost-effectively by pursuing another route. For example, if a person needs a simple feeding adaptation, it would be much more efficient if the treatment therapist worked with the client in the context of his or her rehabilitation to provide an adapted spoon or plate. If, however, all low technology devices had been considered and there was still a problem, then the AT team might be consulted to see if a custom designed device would be appropriate. If a person used a wheelchair that required maintenance, the consumer would be encouraged to contact the shop where the wheelchair was purchased for the needed service. However, if the disrepair is at the point where a new prescription is necessary, the AT referral is appropriate.

Screening assists the AT team to determine those technologies from which the consumer might benefit. Technology categories to consider would be positioning, access technology, mobility, architecture, transportation and environmental access, as previously described in this chapter. Also, technologies for people with sensory, cognitive and communication impairments would become part of the screening. Questions might alert the consumer to possibilities he or she had not considered. For example, a parent might bring a child to the clinic for a bath aid because that is the one activity that is causing the most stress at home. While at the clinic, the therapist might share information with the family about other appropriate technology such as a powered wheelchair or an AAC device. Information gathered during the screening will also assist the technology team to be better prepared in terms of time allocation for the assessment. They could also assemble any equipment that might be useful to have during the evaluation.

Once the client has identified the technology areas of concern, a full evaluation is scheduled. Therapists, in conjunction with engineers and others, provide a full evaluation of physical, functional and sensory needs, as well as environmental issues. Evaluations can run for an hour, days or even longer when needs are complex. Often the evaluation enables the client to try several AT devices to determine which he or she can most easily operate, which he or she likes the best, and which is most compatible with the client's environment and lifestyle. Care must be taken not to extend the evaluation beyond a reasonable time. At some point, the consumer must commit to a course of action and begin to implement the plan to acquire the technology. This is difficult in an area of practice where each day brings technical advances. Just as the general public must choose a car or computer which will be less than ideal in a year, the user of assistive technology must acquire his or her own solution and begin to use it as soon as is feasible.

Equipment Acquisition/Provision

In general, assistive technology is expensive. Most consumers do not purchase the technology they need but rely on assistance of third party payers. Insurance carriers, government sponsored programs such as Medicaid and Medicare, school systems, the Office of Vocational Rehabilitation (OVR), and non-profit agencies such as United Cerebral Palsy provide funds for some technologies for some people in some locations. Some families pay for the needed technology themselves. The funding process is complex with complete documentation required, including at times a physician signature. Most states have a Tech Act Project that has a complete resource of funding opportunities in that state. These projects are funded under Public Law 100-407 and their locations can be found by contacting RESNA, which provides technical assistance to all projects. Rehabilitation Technology Suppliers, AT clinics and Centers for Independent Living (CIL's) are all knowledgeable resources. Whatever the source, funding must be found before the equipment is ordered.

Once the equipment has been procured, the client usually returns to the clinic for fitting and training. There are many stories of equipment being delivered directly to consumers that is never used because no one could assemble the pieces. In other situations, the consumer forgot how to use the technology, and rather than ask for help, just placed the equipment out of sight. A session in the clinic and at the home, work or school is highly recommended to avoid this problem.

Training

Occupational therapists are often involved in either direct training or training of a trainer such as a teacher or parent. The therapist in the AT clinic can train school system therapists, teachers, parents, nursing home personnel, community based therapists or nurses, the consumers themselves or their caregivers to be the actual trainers. It is always better to have the training occur in the environment in which the consumer will be using the technology. If a child is receiving a powered wheelchair, the initial checkout of ability and skill level can be done at the clinic. Once the occupational therapist is confident that the equipment and its operation are clear to the child and are working to expectation, the rest of the training should occur in the environments in which the child will be using the chair on a daily basis. That means the parents and school therapist or teacher must understand the operation of

the equipment and the functional expectations. They can then be the trainers in the school, home and community in which the child spends his or her day. If problems occur, the therapist must remain a resource, especially if problems are related to equipment performance.

Follow-up

Follow-up can take many forms. For simple technologies, a phone call may be all that is required. For more complex systems, follow-up clinic visits, calls to teachers or family members, home visits or visits to the worksite may be indicated. In all cases, follow-up provides valuable information. First, the effectiveness of the technology intervention can be monitored and/or measured. Second, if the intervention is not working smoothly, assistance can be provided before abandonment occurs, and finally, timing for changes in technology can be anticipated. Following an appropriate schedule, clients can be contacted and information obtained can be used as a screening to determine if further evaluation as warranted. At that point, the consumer might enter the service delivery flow for the second time.

THE OCCUPATIONAL THERAPIST AND ASSISTIVE TECHNOLOGY PRACTICE

Occupational therapists are involved in many aspects of AT, from providing the evaluations, recommendations and training in a service delivery program to being involved in product development and research. In all phases, the therapist ensures that the physical, social and functional needs of consumers are addressed (Figure 20-5).

Service Delivery

Many occupational therapists practicing today employ AT as a modality for their consumers. If the AT used is low technology and part of a overall intervention plan, the therapist would be expected to have a general knowledge base and would be considered a generalist. If the AT used is high technology and is provided as part of a comprehensive AT program, the therapist in that program would be expected to have a much higher level of expertise and would be considered a specialist. As a generalist, therapists would be competent in recommending low technology assistive technology and would refer consumers to an assistive technology team if either the technology needed was high technology or if the technology required was multifaceted and integration of several technologies was required. As a generalist, therapists can be employed in any of the traditional occupational therapy settings and have the expertise to incorporate AT

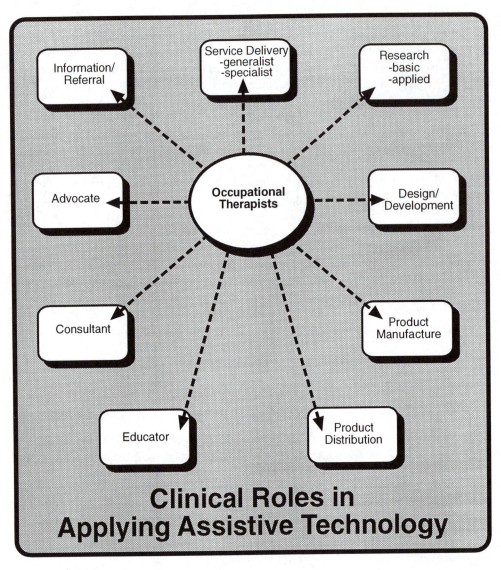

Figure 20-5. Clinical Roles in Applying Assistive Technology.

into their evaluation process. They would know where to find information on AT and know when the expertise of a specialist was required.

Therapists who desire to be specialists in AT would pursue advanced training either formally or through on-the-job experience. Because the field of AT is so broad, it is likely that specialization in one of the areas of AT would occur. Therapists might specialize in the delivery of ECU's or seating and wheeled mobility or AAC.

Research

Therapists who become specialists in AT often work as part of research teams. Because of occupational therapists' strong background in clinical service, they are often well-suited to present excellent questions for research. Generalist therapists in school systems may be asked to participate in

research. For example, if the research team was interested in knowing if a child was more independent in mobility using a manual or powered wheelchair, the therapist in the school system might be involved in selecting possible subjects, monitoring counters on the wheelchairs that recorded miles traveled, or even teaching the child to use the powered chair. Practicing therapists also develop excellent research questions based on their daily practice and their observations.

Design/Development

A component of any service delivery program is the custom designing of individual solutions when there is not a commercially available solution. On a one-on-one basis, this is the custom design of a product. When the solution meets the needs of a number of consumers, then a product becomes more viable for mass production. Seating systems of the standardized modular variety came about when individual designs showed the potential of meeting a broader market. The MPI (Trefler & Hobson, 1975) was such a system because it met the needs of about 60% of the moderately involved children with cerebral palsy that were seen in a seating clinic. Occupational therapists were involved with the determination of the component shapes, sizes and their integration. In addition to defining product parameters, therapists are often responsible for field testing products and providing much needed clinical feedback to designers and manufacturers.

Product Manufacture

Once products are designed and field tested, therapists are not often involved in taking the product through the manufacturing phase. They might evaluate the final product in field trials or assist with determining some of the materials to be used. In this case, therapists in a sheltered workshop might be asked to evaluate whether a newly developed tool is effective and to give feedback to the developers. In very few cases would a therapist actually fabricate devices for mass market sales.

Product Distribution/Sales

Products must be distributed widely so that consumers can have access to them. Occupational therapists are now entering the assistive technology sales force. Therapists must be cautious of a conflict of interest in this field of employment. Most who sell only one line of products refrain from doing consumer evaluations unless it has already been determined that the product they represent is being recommended by an independent technology team.

Education

In order for consumers to have the AT they need, therapists must know of its availability. They must also be trained to incorporate AT into treatment plans. It is anticipated that all university based programs in occupational therapy will provide training in assistive technology. Strategies for inclusion of assistive technology material into occupational therapy curriculum are available. As well, books, journals, and magazines that focus on AT all provide resources for students of occupational therapy to acquire a knowledge base in assistive technology.

Consultants

Therapists can be consultants in assistive technology in several capacities. They may work as part of a specialty team and consult with therapists who are generalists. Consultants generally present their recommendations to the primary care group in a format that can be easily used by the contracting party. For example, a specialist providing technology recom-

mendations to a vocational rehabilitation counselor should attempt to justify the technology in terms of work related functions. Options of optimal and compromise solutions, complete with costs, sources of purchase, service and training, should be included. If providing consultation directly to a consumer, options, costs and sources are also important. In addition, a component of the recommendation should be educational in nature so the consumer has all the information necessary to make a wise decision. Consultation services should also recommend a course of implementation that would include training and recommended timing of follow-up.

Occupational therapists are traditional sources of information for consumers and their families. Relationships built during evaluation and treatment often put consumers at ease. Consumers are traditionally referred to colleagues with specific expertise. Occupational therapists refer people for medical follow-up such as eye exams, for physical therapy, and for driving evaluations if the facility does not have the expertise or equipment. In the United States, with the funding of Public Law 100-407, information and referral has become more organized and comprehensive in the area of assistive technology. Information specialists provide consumers with information about services in their area, technologies, funding possibilities and perhaps legal services related to acquisition of services.

Traditionally, occupational therapists have been advocates for consumers. Our primary goal is to enable clients to be as functional and independent as possible. This is done through treatment, individual recommendations about equipment, and perhaps most important, helping them to be well informed.

THE APPLICATION OF ASSISTIVE TECHNOLOGY IN FACILITY AND COMMUNITY SETTINGS

Changing trends in health care are causing the systems of financing to change. Traditional environments in which AT has been provided are changing. Large multidisciplinary clinics, under managed care, are being scrutinized. As well, the commercial market is becoming more competitive with traditional health care facilities. Occupational therapists are involved in the application of AT in many traditional and nontraditional environments. They must be able to address issues of effectiveness and efficiency as well as outcomes such as the impact of AT on function and well-being (Figure 20-6).

Assistive Technology Program in a Rehabilitation Facility

Almost every comprehensive hospital or rehabilitation facility has at least one occupational therapist on staff. Many commercially available technologies can be provided

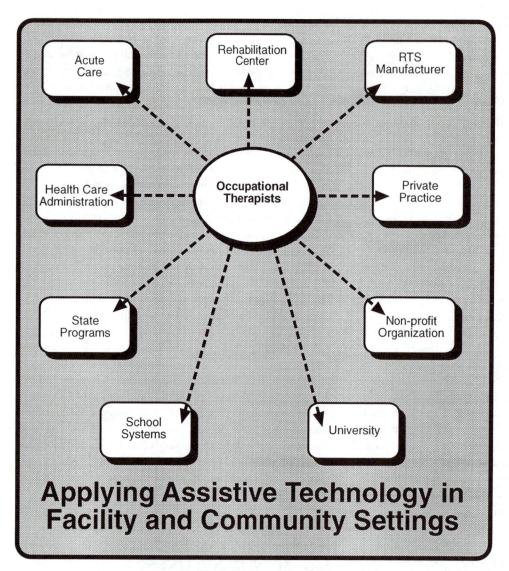

Figure 20-6. Applying Assistive Technology in Facility and Community Settings.

Acute Care

Rehabilitation Center

RTS Manufacturer

Health Care Administration

Occupational Therapists

Private Practice

State Programs

Non-profit Organization

School Systems

University

Applying Assistive Technology in Facility and Community Settings

through the occupational therapy department. However, with customized products or the products requiring complex modification or design, the assistance of a technical staff is advised. There are a variety of different models that the administration can choose, several of which can involve the occupational therapist directly.

Occupational therapy departments might choose to hire a carpenter or technician to work under the direction of the therapists. Larger facilities that deal with clients with complex problems, such as head and spinal cord injuries, might choose to set up an assistive technology service. In some situations, this AT service would employ occupational therapists directly in the specialty service, while others would choose to have the primary occupational therapist work with the engineer in problem-solving and provision. Either model works well as long as mutual professionals respect each other, and open communication precedes the application of technology.

If the therapist is employed in the assistive technology or rehabilitation engineering department, most often he or she acts as a consultant to the primary treatment therapist and helps to interpret the client's needs to the technical team. The primary therapist can help with problem definition, the initial fitting and training, and bring back to the technical team any problems or success stories. Programs in which the primary therapist works directly with the engineer pose a greater potential for communication problems. Each therapist will have different vocabularies and expectations with which to communicate with the technical team members. The engineers or technicians will have design ideas of their own, which they will want to employ in the problem solving process. If the process is to work positively to solve the real problems of the client, then all professionals involved must adopt a similar vocabulary, and effort must be spent assuring that communications have been appropriately processed. Otherwise, with the best for the client in mind, the therapist will state a functional need and perhaps a solution which will be misinterpreted by the technical team, and the end product may not be appropriate. We must make every effort to put the responsibility on the professional team to solve the real problem as stated by the client, and not on the client to make the wrong solution work.

Assistive Technology Program in an Acute Care Facility

There are not many assistive technology programs located directly in acute care facilities as hospital stays are so short that implementation of AT services is unlikely. In acute care it is often advisable to monitor progression of a rehabilitation program before implementing AT services and the numbers of clients requiring AT services during their acute phase would not warrant the personnel required for an in-house AT service. More likely, occupational therapists would have the resources of community-based rehabilitation technology professionals as consultants. Depending on the scope of work, there may be biomedical engineers available for consultation. Therapists have been involved in positioning premature infants, persons with head injuries and stroke as well as others. Consultants can assist with the implementation of ECU units in the hospital rooms, simple augmentative communication devices and temporary mobility devices. It is common for intervention in the acute care facility to be temporary, and to use only the technology available in the occupational therapy department.

The Technology Service Delivery Program in a University

Throughout the United States, there are a number of service delivery programs located in universities. Often, but not always, they are part of a larger, federally supported Rehabilitation Engineering Research Center (RERC), funded by the National Institute on Disability Related Research (NIDRR). Service delivery programs in AT are usually administered by a technical director and have a physician as part of the team. They are supported by fee for service, although they may have some grant funds to underwrite service or the fitting of prototype devices. Universities would also have an education component, and often a research component funded by local, state and/or national grants. Occupational therapists can play an active role in all three aspects of university-based programs.

A service program can be coordinated by an OT. Clients can be of all ages and disabilities, and the most frequently recommended and provided technical services include seating and mobility systems, augmentative communication devices, ADL devices and computer access and worksite and home modifications. This type of clinic was described previously in this chapter as the Center for Assistive Technology

at the University of Pittsburgh.

School Systems

Many children with special needs receive their educational technology within their education program. Occupational therapists, in conjunction with speech pathologists and teachers, work with families to enable children to fully participate in their education program. In the larger school systems in the 1960s and 1970s many school districts had specially designated schools for children with disabilities. AT expertise was supported by the State Department of Education, which provided evaluation and training expertise from a central program. Individual school districts had access to AT services and some had an AT program on site. However, there has been a shift in philosophy and now most children are mainstreamed into their local area school system. There are many educational and social advantages of this shift. However, the challenge of getting technology to the children has become more complex. There is greater need to teach all educators of the value of AT and when children using specific pieces of equipment are in their classrooms, teachers must be provided assistance in incorporating the technology into the classroom activities.

Each school system and state Education Department can choose to provide training programs for teachers, parents and support staff, funds to hire AT specialists within the state system, equipment, loaner equipment, funds to the schools directly or none of the above. Occupational therapists must understand the school system mandate in their area and determine if positions are available as employees of the education system or as consultants to it.

State Agency Based Program

State agencies can include the Office of Vocational Rehabilitation (OVR), state schools for the blind or state homes/schools for people with developmental disabilities. With the 1986 amendments to the Rehabilitation Act, all clients eligible for vocational rehabilitation with OVR must have AT services considered in their Individualized Written Rehabilitation Plan. With that in mind, some states are employing rehabilitation engineers to provide AT service to clients within the state agency. Occupational therapists can be involved in the evaluation, problem-solving, and provision process. This is a new arena for occupational therapists and some of the state agencies must be convinced that it is cost-effective for therapists to be part of the technology team for the state.

The Rehabilitation Technology Sales Industry

The role of the rehabilitation technology supplier (RTS) is changing. From a commercial establishment with few trained personnel selling only commercially available health care products, many facilities are now providing custom equipment and specializing as rehabilitation specialists. They are being required to combine commercially available equipment choices and to develop custom solutions. Companies are beginning to hire or train an informed sales force to become resource people for the ever increasing number of complex and expensive technical aids. Large dealership networks are providing their own training programs. Out of concern for quality assurance, a number of RTSs have formed the National Registry of Rehabilitation Technology Suppliers (NRRTS). NRRTS supports continuing education programs, as well as a credentialing program for their members. The concern is to provide consumers, therapists, funders, and others some indication as to who in the RTS field is qualified to provide custom fitting and problem-solving as a member of a team of experts. As with any evolving field, terminology is changing. A supplier who successfully completes the RESNA credentialling exam is referred to as an assistive technology supplier (ATS). If this person is a member of NRRTS, and provides consumers with product choices, he or she can use the designation of rehabilitation technology supplier-certified (RTS-C). A person with the RTS-C credential is likely to provide the highest quality of service to consumers in the seating/wheelchair field.

The involvement of the therapist is increasing nationally in the RTS network. Companies that deal with custom seating and mobility systems, complex environmental control (ECU) applications, and other areas of high technology that require customization, are hiring occupational therapists as staff members or as consultants. The RTS relies heavily on the medical prescription which is formulated by the technology team, of which the occupational therapist is a key member.

Occupational therapists can consult with product manufacturers. They can train dealers in product application, provide ideas and feedback on new products, develop training literature and run education programs. This is not the RTS network in which the dealer carries a variety of products by different manufacturers. It is the product manufacturer itself.

An ethical challenge faces the therapist who takes a position within the industry side of assistive technology. If the therapist is involved in the education program of the company with materials that are not product specific, then there is no obvious conflict of interest. However, if the therapist is part of the product development, part of the marketing of product even in the provision of education, then a conflict of interest is possible if this same therapist is employed by a facility which requires therapists to be involved in the prescription process. There is always the question of whether the product is being recommended because it is the most appropriate for the client, or because the therapist knows that product best or is employed by the product manufacturer. If this is the case, then the therapist might consider working full-time with the manufacturer and offering consultation services with the prescribing therapist. Involvement with the commercial sector can be stimulating, stressful and financially rewarding, but therapists who have been educated to work in the medical model must be open to the new and often competitive nature of private industry.

Private Practice in Assistive Technology

Private practice AT programs can either be owned by the therapist who hires technical support, which may be a technician or a rehabilitation engineer, or owned by the rehabilitation engineer who employees the therapist. The focus of the practice will vary with the interest of the owner, the needs of the local clients and the available of funding. For example, many are providing services for vocational rehabilitation clients because OVR will pay for the services offered. Private companies are being formed by therapists with the intent of providing specialty consultant services to existing programs nationwide. These companies sell expertise related to service delivery, management, funding, education, or quality management, to list just a few.

Local Affiliate of a National Nonprofit Disability Organization

Spread across the nation are programs which are motivated by a nonprofit disability-oriented focus. The Muscular Dystrophy Association, United Cerebral Palsy, and National Easter Seals Programs are in almost every large metropolitan area or at least represented state by state. If the client population represented by the agency has needs for AT, the agency may choose to fund AT devices for eligible persons, provide low cost loans, information or advocacy services. In most cases, the local affiliate has the option of how to meet these needs. Occupational therapists could evaluate requests for AT, or they could work directly in either AT or direct care services of the local affiliate. Therapists, for example, provide services in many Easter Seals early intervention programs. They could be involved in the evaluation, recommendation and training in the use of appropriate AT.

Miscellaneous Programs Including Information/Resource Centers and Volunteers

Occupational therapists are finding a new role as information managers. The availability of technology is changing so rapidly that information brokers are becoming sought after in many states and localities. With their knowledge of disability and of equipment, occupational therapists are uniquely suited to organize and operate information services. These types of services can and do include written materials such as catalogues, books, personal files, and electronic media such as databases, which can be both local or remote.

Treatment therapists, clients and other community and health care workers can use the information specialist in locating the most appropriate technical solution for a functional need. In some situations, actual loan or trial equipment use can be arranged at a resource center. Each state is required to establish a statewide information and referral network in response to Public Law 100-407. Within many Tech Act projects, occupational therapists might organize and provide information, facilitate services for people with disabilities, and in management of the projects themselves, organization and operation of such resource centers.

Volunteer Networks

Volunteer networks are mentioned with caution. Individuals or companies, especially those in the high technology sphere, would like to perform community service. Also, university faculty are looking for meaningful projects for students. Although well-meaning, the caution comes from several directions. Often volunteers are working in isolation and do not know what products are already on the market. The time frame might not meet with the needs of the client, who usually needs the solution immediately, not before graduation. And who is to provide the follow-up and maintenance of the equipment once the employee has left the company or the student has graduated? Often the occupational therapist is the one to contact the volunteer group in trying to locate an affordable solution to a client's problem. The therapist works with the volunteer in problem definition and has a responsibility to the client to educate both the volunteer and the client as to available products. This is not to say that this process never works. It is only to caution therapists to look carefully and not to create a long-term problem for the client.

FUTURE (EVOLVING ISSUES)

Consumers of any service or product are entitled to an assurance of quality. If one purchases a new automobile, assurance that the product is of an acceptable performance standard and comes with a warrantee is desired. If there is need for maintenance or repair, the consumer assumes that the person performing the repairs has had sufficient training and/or experience to do the job correctly. Persons with disabilities are entitled to the same quality in products they purchase and in the personnel who recommend them. Clients must be able to assume that the personnel recommending product options, teaching them how to use them and providing the maintenance and repair, are well trained.

Under the auspices of the AOTA, special interest section on assistive technology, Hammel and Smith(1993) have proposed three levels of occupational therapist competence.

These competencies are in review at the moment and are not mandatory in terms of practice.

- Foundation level therapists would have received an orientation to assistive technology in their professional training. These therapists should consider assistive technology as a possible modality for their clients regardless of diagnosis and stage of their rehabilitation. It includes an "awareness of and knowledge of the types of assistive technology, their uses, and their applicability to the individual clients within occupational therapy frameworks." Occupational therapists at the foundation level should also be aware of resources of information and referral for their clients' particular needs, and be willing to refer them to technology specialists as appropriate.

- Technology Specialist Level 1 therapists would have taken some form of specialized training in assistive technology, such as a dedicated course, electives and perhaps an additional clerkship in an assistive technology service delivery program (Pirtizlaff & Smith, 1991). At this level, therapists could provide initial troubleshooting related to assistive technology and apply low technology solutions in their practice. They may also take on the role of coordinating assistive technology services.

- Technology Specialist Level 2 therapists would have completed intensive training in assistive technology through internships, apprenticeships, continuing education and/or formal education programs. These therapists would be qualified to apply assistive technology either as team members or independently, depending on the service delivery model they are working within.

Quality products, qualified professionals and informed consumers form the AT team that ensures that consumers have and use appropriate assistive technology. In occupational therapy practice we have the obligation to provide AT as part of intervention. Whether therapists provide AT in their own practices or refer the client to a specialist will vary widely according to the qualifications and experience of the therapist, the complexity of the consumer's needs and the resources available in the community.

REFERENCES

Angelo, J. (1996). *Assistive technology for rehabilitation therapists.* Philadelphia: F. A. Davis.

Axelson, P., Minkel, J., & Chesney, D. (1994). *A guide to wheelchair selection: How to use the ANSI/RESNA wheelchair standards to buy a wheelchair.* Washington, DC: PVA.

Bailey, R. W. (1989). *Human performance engineering* (2nd ed.). Englewood Cliffs, NJ: Prentice Hall.

Batavia, A. E., & Hammer, G. S. (1990). Toward the development of consumer-based criteria for evaluation of assistive devices. *Journal of Rehabilitation Research and Development, 27*(4),

425-436.

Baum, C. M. (in press). Achieving effectiveness with a client-centered approach: A person-environment interaction. In Gray, Quatrano & Liberman (Eds.), *Designing and using assistive technology: The human perspective.* Baltimore: Paul H. Brookes.

Bergen, A. F., Presperin, J., & Tallman, T. (1990). *Positioning for function, wheelchairs and other assistive technologies.* Valhalla, NY: Valhalla Rehabilitation Publications, Ltd.

Cook, A., & Hussey, S. (1995). A framework for assistive technologies. In A. Cook & S. Hussey (Eds.), *Assistive technology: Principles and practices* (p. 45-76). St. Louis: Mosby Year Book.

Crimmins, J. C. (1995). *The American promise: Adventures in grass-roots democracy.* Companion to the PBS Series. San Francisco: KQED Books.

Demers, L., Weiss-Lambrou, R., & Ska, B. (1996). Development of the Quebec User Evaluation of Satisfaction with Assistive Technology (Quest). *Assistive Technology, 8.1,* 3-11.

Deno, J. H., et al. (1992). *Human factors design guidelines for the elderly and people with disabilities.* Minneapolis: Honeywell, Incorporated.

Enders, A., & Hall, M. (1990). *Assistive technology sourcebook.* Arlington, VA: RESNA Press.

Flippo, K. F., Inge, J., & Barcus, J. M. (1995). *Assistive technology: A resource for school, work, and community.* Baltimore: Paul Brookes Co.

Gradel, K. (1990). Open the customer service window NOW!! *Smart Exchanges, 3,* 1.

Gradel, K. (1991). Customer service: What is its place in assistive technology and employment services? *Journal of Vocational Rehabilitation,* Spring.

Kanny, E., Anson, D., & Smith, R. O. (1992). Technology training for occupational therapists: A survey of entry-level curricula. *Occupational Therapy Journal of Research, 11,* 311-319.

Little, J. (1991). Rethinking rehab: Are you a quarterback coach? *TeamRehab Report,* Mar/April, 23-26.

Mace, R. (1991). *Designs for special needs.* Raleigh, NC: Institute for Barrier Free Environments.

Manne, W. C., & Kathleen, A. B. (1995). Assessment services: Person, device, family, and environment. In W. C. Manne & A. B. Kathleen (Eds.), *Assistive technology for persons with disabilities* (p. 299-317). Bethesda, MD: American Occupational Therapy Association.

McAlees, D. C. (1995). *Operationalizing consumer decision making and choice in the VR process.* Stout, WI: University of Wisconsin-Stout.

Medhat, M., & Hobson, D. (1992). *Standardization of terminology and descriptive methods for specialized seating.* Arlington, VA: RESNA Press.

Mueller, J. (1990). *The workplace workbook: An illustrated guide to job accommodation and assistive technology.* Wichita, KS: The Dole Foundation.

RESNA. (1987). *Rehabilitation technology service delivery: A practical guide.* Arlington, VA: Author.

RESNA Technical Assistance Project. (1992). *Assistive technology and the individualized education program.* Arlington, VA: RESNA Press.

Scherer, M. J. (1994). *Living in the state of stuck.* Cambridge, MA: Brookline Books.

Smith, R. (1991) Technological approaches to performance enhancement. In C. Christiansen & C. Baum (Eds.), *Occupational therapy: Overcoming human performance deficits* (pp. 747-788). Thorofare, NJ: SLACK Incorporated.

Smith, R. O. (1992). Technology and disability. *American Journal of Occupational Therapy, 1*(3), 22-30.

Trefler, E. T., Hobson, D. A., Johnson Taylor, S., Monahan, L. C., & Shaw, C. G. (1993). *Seating and mobility for persons with physical disabilities.* Tucson, AZ: Therapy Skill Builders.

Trefler, E. T., Tooms, R. E., & Hobson, D. A. (1978). Seating for Cerebral-Palsied Children. *Inter Clinic Information Bulletin, Vol XVII.* (1), 1-8.

Vanderheiden, C. G. (1987). Service delivery mechanism in rehabilitation technology. *American Journal of Occupational Therapy, 41*(11), 703-771.

Vanderheiden G., & Vanderheiden K. (199). *Accessibility design guidelines for the design of consumer products to increase their accessibility to people with disabilities or who are aging.* Trace R & D Center, Madison, WI: University of Wisconsin-Madison.

Weisman, G. (1991). Rehabilitation engineering in the workplace. In R. V. Smith & J. Leslie (Eds.), *Rehabilitation engineering.* Boca Ratan, FL: CRC Press Inc.

Zollars, J. A. (1996). *Special seating: An illustrated guide.* Minneapolis, MN: Otto Book Rehabilitation.

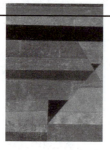

CHAPTER CONTENT OUTLINE

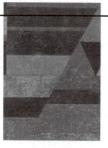

ABSTRACT

The challenge of working with people with disabilities is a multidimensional one that practicing therapists face every day. Perhaps the most fundamental aspect of this challenge is the determination of the best and most effective way for a therapist to get along with the people she or he serves. This chapter explores four models of the relationship between occupational therapists and the people they serve (biomedical rehabilitation, client-centered rehabilitation, a community-based rehabilitation and independent living). It outlines the basic tenets of each of these four models, and the circumstances under which each is most applicable. Finally, the chapter follows two consumers of occupational therapy services, through the process of rehabilitation and reintegration. These examples demonstrate how person, environment, and occupational performance can be addressed within each model, and how different models are more or less applicable under different circumstances and at different times.

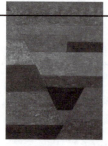

KEY TERMS

Disability

Models of service

Independent living

Client-centred

Community-based rehabilitation

Biomedical rehabilitation

Client-centred rehabilitation

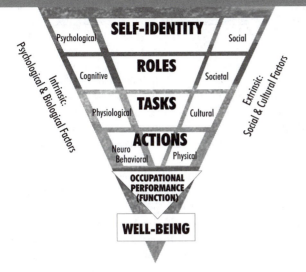

CHAPTER 21

SELF-IDENTITY

Psychological

Social

ROLES

Cognitive

Societal

TASKS

Physiological

Cultural

ACTIONS

Neuro Behavioral

Physical

Intrinsic: Psychological & Biological Factors

Extrinsic: Social & Cultural Factors

OCCUPATIONAL PERFORMANCE (FUNCTION)

WELL-BEING

Meeting the Challenges of Disability

Models for Enabling Function and Well-Being

Mary Ann McColl, PhD, OT(C), Nancy Gerein, PhD, Fraser Valentine, MA

OBJECTIVES

The information in this chapter is intended to help the reader:

1. understand the history and assumptions underlying four models for providing service to persons with disabling conditions: biomedical, client-centred, community-based, and independent living

2. compare and contrast each service model in terms of its advantages and disadvantages

3. identify circumstances where each service model may be most appropriate

4. identify, using case examples, how factors related to the person, his or her environment and occupational performance influence intervention at four different stages.

"The real challenge comes from the realization of multiple alternatives and the invention of new models. Aspiration ceases to be a one-way street...and instead becomes open in all directions, claiming the possibility of inclusion and setting an individual course among the many ways of being human...

Mary Catherin Bateson , p. 62.

Introduction

The challenge of working with people with disabilities is a multidimensional one that practicing therapists face every day. Perhaps the most fundamental aspect of this challenge is the determination of the best and most effective way for a therapist to get along with the people he or she serves. What is the best model of service for each person at each stage in their rehabilitation and their pursuit of integrated independent living? What are the factors and assumptions that are associated with different models of service?

This chapter explores four models of the relationship between occupational therapists and the people they serve (biomedical rehabilitation, client-centred rehabilitation, community-based rehabilitation and independent living). It outlines the basic tenets of each of these four models, and the circumstances under which each is most applicable. Finally, the chapter follows two consumers of occupational therapy services, through the process of rehabilitation and reintegration. These examples demonstrates how person, environment and occupational performance can be addressed within each model, and how different models are more or less applicable under different circumstances and at different times.

Biomedical Rehabilitation

Traditionally, occupational therapists have functioned within a biomedical rehabilitation model of service delivery. *Biomedical rehabilitation* is described in the United Nation's (1983) definition of rehabilitation as "a goal-oriented and time-limited process aimed at enabling an impaired person to reach an optimum mental, physical and/or social functional level." This view of rehabilitation arose in the early part of this century, as waves of veterans returned from the First World War, many with permanent disabilities (McColl, Law & Stewart, 1993; Symington, 1994). It existed virtually unchallenged for the first 50 or 60 years of the profession's existence. Its dominance over the thinking of occupational therapists was strengthened in the 1950s and 1960s, as the status of professionals became enhanced by the scientific revolution (McColl, Law & Stewart, 1993).

In its modern iteration, biomedical rehabilitation is usually undertaken by a team of rehabilitation professionals, often headed by a physician (preferably a specialist in rehabilitation medicine). This team collaborates to assess and diagnose functional problems related to an impairment or

Bibliographic citation of this chapter: McColl, M. A., Gerein, N. & Valentine, F. (1997). Meeting the challenges of disability: Models for enabling function and well-being. In C. Christiansen & C. Baum (Eds.), *Occupational therapy: Enabling function and well-being* (2nd ed.). Thorofare, NJ: SLACK Incorporated.

disability, set goals and priorities, implement interventions to promote optimum functioning, assess progress and discontinue services when an optimal level has been reached (Bakheit, 1995). The recipient of services is usually referred to as a patient, denoting that he or she has limited responsibility in the therapeutic process, other than to simply be the object or recipient of service.

A number of assumptions underlie the biomedical approach to occupational therapy. First, it is assumed that the patient, or recipient of services, has an objective impairment that causes the disability (Schlaff, 1993). Thus the need for service arises because the patient has some normative deviation in everyday functioning (Bickenbach, 1992). The root of his or her difficulties lies within him- or herself, and can be objectively detected and measured using biomedical technology.

A second assumption of the biomedical approach is that professionals have information and skills that give them an advantage over patients in terms of understanding the nature of the problems and knowing what to do about them. A corollary to this is that patients themselves are ill-equipped to make decisions about the nature and course of rehabilitation, because they lack this specialized expertise.

A third assumption of the biomedical model is that the problems associated with disability can be understood by reducing them to a series of subproblems associated with different body systems. These subproblems are best solved by a team of professionals, each working on a carefully defined area about which he or she has special expertise. The combination of efforts by an appropriately constituted team will result in the best possible outcomes for the patient.

Finally, the biomedical model assumes that the patient and members of his or her support system will cooperate with the therapeutic team, primarily because of the recognized expertise of the team, and the implicit good sense of its recommendations. This cooperator role for the patient and family is reminiscent of what Parsons (1975) described as the sick role. Within the sick role, the patient has two freedoms and two responsibilities. The two freedoms are freedom from responsibility for the impairment, and freedom from normal social roles for the duration of the impairment. The two responsibilities are to pursue optimal functioning and to cooperate with service providers.

Although the traditional biomedical approach to rehabilitation has lost favour in some circles in recent years, it must have some advantages, or it would surely not have prevailed for more than half a century. Although it is often portrayed in the literature of the last decade or so as draconian and authoritarian, one principal advantage of the biomedical approach is that it is primarily benevolent. Consistent with the Hippocratic Oath and other expressions of benevolent intent, the intent is to do good toward others. Beange (1987) refers to health professionals within a biomedical approach as "benevolent dictators," recognizing their authority, but also acknowledging their benevolent intent.

Another advantage of the biomedical approach is the inherent willingness of professionals to shoulder responsibility for others in situations where they may truly not be able to assume decision-making authority. For example, some people, in the wake of the onset of a disability, would be incapable of planning or decision making because of the magnitude of the medical and psychological issues. In such instances, professionals who function according to a biomedical model assume responsibility for determining the course of therapy that they believe will be most advantageous for the individual. In this way, precious weeks are not lost and further complications incurred while waiting for the medical, psychological and social situation to stabilize.

There are also, however, several possible disadvantages to the use of the biomedical model. This very willingness of professionals to assume responsibility for decision making in therapy can be experienced as disempowering and alienating to individuals with disabilities who are capable of making their own decisions. At its extreme, this disempowerment is manifested as institutionalization, where individuals are rendered literally incapable of functioning outside of an institution, because of their inability to make even the smallest of decisions.

Another disadvantage of the biomedical model is that its relevance is time limited. The freedoms and responsibilities associated with the patient role cannot become lifelong patterns, although the impairments or disabilities which initially invoked them may be lifelong. For example, individuals cannot be expected to make a career out of pursuing recovery, nor can they be allowed the freedom from social role obligations indefinitely. Thus, at some point, another model of service will be necessary for providers who have long-term relationships with people with disabilities, as many occupational therapists do.

The final, and perhaps most damning disadvantage of the biomedical model, is that it denies an essential area of expertise in its professional decision-making process. This expertise lies within the patient, and it pertains to the experience of living with a disability. To the extent that the disability is not merely an objective occurrence, as this model assumes, but also an experienced phenomenon, this phenomenological expertise is essential to good service.

In response to some of these disadvantages, occupational therapists have sought other models of service delivery to guide their interactions with consumers. One of these is the client-centred approach.

CLIENT-CENTRED REHABILITATION

Client-centred rehabilitation is a therapeutic orientation whereby clients engage the assistance and support of a therapist to facilitate their problem solving and the achievement of their own goals. According to this model, clients seek a therapist, explain their problems, and in an environment of understanding, trust and acceptance, pursue change toward their goals (Burnard & Morrison, 1991). By its very name, it differentiates itself from the biomedical model by calling the recipients of service *clients*. Unlike a patient, who is simply the object of service, a client seeks the advice of a professional in managing some aspect of his or her life (Herzberg, 1990; Patterson & Marks, 1992). Thus the language implies that in a client-centred model, the client is in charge, and is seeking from the relationship with the professional what he or she needs, and discarding that which he or she does not feel is necessary at this time.

The exact origin of client-centred practice, as referred to by occupational therapists, is somewhat ambiguous (Canadian Association of Occupational Therapists, 1991). One's first thought is that it must be an extension of client-centred therapy, as defined by Carl Rogers (1942). Rogers described a nondirective approach to therapy, where the therapist's role is to create an environment of trust and support, furnishing clients with the opportunity to use their own problem-solving capacities to realize their therapeutic goals. However, other definitions of client-centred practice in the recent literature suggest other origins of the client-centred ideology (Preston, 1994). For example, Baradell (1990) talks about client-centred consultation as a model of professional consulting, using individual case histories as a basis for discussion. Braddy and Gray (1987) discuss client-centred practice as self-instruction and mutual aid.

SUMMARY: BIOMEDICAL REHABILITATION

Assumptions:
1. There is an objective impairment that is causing the disability;
2. Professionals have the knowledge and skill necessary to solve the problems of individual with disabilities;
3. Problems can be analyzed into their component parts and solved systematically.

Advantages:
1. Benevolence;
2. Professionals willing to assume responsibility.

Disadvantages:
1. Disempowering;
2. Time-limited in its relevance;
3. Lacks expertise about living with a disability.

Robinson (1991) equates case management and managed care approaches with client-centred practice. These latter definitions seem to emerge from recent social influences on health care delivery systems, like demedicalization and consumerism (Holyoke & Elkan, 1995; Pollock, 1993).

For the purposes of this discussion, our definition of client-centred therapy is closest to Rogers' original conception of it. There are a number of assumptions to the client-centred approach that may assist in differentiating it from other models. The first assumption of client-centred therapy is that clients know what they want from therapy and what they need to reach their optimum level of functional performance. Thus the agenda for therapy is established by the client. This assumption is the ultimate extension of one of the most basic values of occupational therapists: the belief in the uniqueness and worth of every individual (Clarke, Scott & Krupa, 1993).

A second assumption of the client-centred approach is that the only relevant frame of reference or vantage point for therapy is that of the client. While the therapist may have knowledge and expertise about certain aspects of disability and therapy, he or she can never fully understand the values, beliefs and experiences of the client, and must therefore accept the client's reports as the most relevant source of information about the progress of therapy.

A third assumption of the client-centred approach is that the dominance of professionals in the process of therapy is in fact counter-therapeutic (Goodall, 1992). Professional dominance creates dependency, disempowerment, and ultimately institutionalization.

The fourth and final assumption of the client-centred approach is that the therapist cannot actually promote change; he or she can only create an environment that facilitates change. This concept was first introduced to the occupational therapy literature by Meyer (1922) when occupational therapy first began. Change or new learning takes place only when an individual identifies it as necessary for the maintenance or development of the self (Rogers, 1965). Thus any contention by the therapist that he or she is the agent of change is misguided, since the only agent of change can be the individual him- or herself, and the most potentially valuable role for the therapist is to support the client through the change with information, ideas, suggestions, resources, and the communication of trust and belief in the ability of the client to succeed.

The client-centred approach has achieved considerable prominence in the past several years, yet the rhetoric associated with it often violates some of these assumptions. For example, we often hear about therapists "allowing clients to make decisions" or "involving clients in the process of therapy" within a client-centred approach. Kerfoot and LeClair (1991) suggest that therapists may even use client-centred rhetoric as a means of guiding or manipulating the therapeutic agenda. Client-centred practice is not simply a more

respectful way to deliver a professionally dominated or biomedical rehabilitation. Rather it is a different model of service delivery altogether, where the therapist is engaged by the individual to assist with the achievement of personal goals in occupational performance.

This approach, like the others, has a number of advantages and disadvantages. Its main advantage is its tendency to enhance self-esteem, mastery, independence, resourcefulness and empowerment among clients (Emener, 1991; Goodall, 1992). Because of this, service delivered according to a client-centred model is perceived by clients as excellent service (Kerfoot & LeClair, 1991).

A second advantage to the client-centred approach is the extent to which it supports a truly individualized or "tailored" approach to therapy (Brown, 1992). Because clients identify therapeutic goals and activities that are pertinent to their unique circumstances and context, no two occupational therapy programs can look exactly alike. Thus therapists are constantly challenged to use all three forms of clinical reasoning to understand the client's context (interactional), understand the details of the disability (procedural) and understand the effect of the disability on the client's life (conditional) (Mattingly & Fleming, 1994).

The third advantage of the client-centred approach is the opportunity that it presents for the therapist's own personal and professional growth and development. Unlike the traditional model, where the therapist is the expert and people are learning from him or her, in the client-centred model, the client is the expert. There is thus an opportunity for the therapist to learn more about disability and its manifestations in peoples' lives, more about the multidimensional nature of human occupational performance, and more about him- or herself, both within the therapeutic role and more generally in human relationships.

There are also a number of disadvantages to working from a client-centred perspective. Because the approach is essentially nondirective, some clients perceive the therapist operating from this perspective as less skilled and less effective (Schroeder & Bloom, 1979; Jaffe & Kipper, 1982; Wanigaratne & Barker, 1995). The conventional perception of a health care practitioner is that of a person who will take charge and make things better. Thus for those who hold to this view, there must be a certain amount of disappointment in a therapist who asks how he or she can be of service.

A second disadvantage of the client-centred approach is the ambiguity around the nature of the therapeutic relationship. A number of authors in the occupational therapy literature have described it as a "partnership." While this definition is intuitively pleasing, in that it invokes the image of two people working closely together toward a common purpose, the partnership idea falls down when we look more closely at the definition. Webster's dictionary describes a partnership as a contractual arrangement whereby two or more individuals share in the liability for any losses and the benefits of any gains. This is clearly not the case in the relationship between a therapist and a client; the losses and gains are both primarily incurred by the client. The consequences of this ambiguity may be a level of discomfort on the part of the therapist and the client as to who is responsible for what, and what each might expect from the other.

A third disadvantage of the client-centred approach is the need for fairly significant technical and structural change in health care systems to accommodate this change in ideology from the biomedical approach. As an example, a number of reviews of the literature show that there are few (if any) occupational therapy assessments that are suitable for application in a client-centred practice (Pollock et al., 1990; Pollock, 1993; Trombly, 1993). Structural changes also will be required to allow systems to accommodate the needs and conveniences of clients, rather than of therapists (Holyoke & Elkan, 1995; Robinson, 1991; Carlisle, 1992; Brider, 1992). For example, outpatient service outside of regular business hours is uncommon in current systems, yet for many people, therapy would be considerably more accessible if it were available evenings and weekends.

Finally, a disadvantage of the client-centred approach is that it may not be acceptable to all therapists. Rogers (1965) himself admits that the success or failure of client-centred therapy is often a function of the therapist's personality, and his or her respect for others and belief in their resourcefulness and adaptiveness. To determine your own orientation toward client-centredness, ask yourself whose interests, opinions and goals prevail when client and therapist disagree as to the appropriate course of action.

COMMUNITY-BASED REHABILITATION

Community-based rehabilitation (CBR) is a third model for the delivery of rehabilitation services to people with disabilities. CBR is defined as "a strategy within community development for the rehabilitation, equalization of opportunities and social integration of all people with disabilities. CBR is implemented through the combined efforts of people with disabilities themselves, their families and communities, and the appropriate health, education, vocational and social services" (International Labour Organization, United Nations, Educational Scientific and Cultural Organization, World Health Organization, 1994).

CBR emerged in developing countries, where traditional rehabilitation services, which rely on highly trained professionals and well-equipped facilities, could not adequately serve the needs of people with disabilities. In developed countries, interest in CBR was sparked by its apparent applicability to underserved populations, such as rural communities and minority groups, and by its emphasis on community participation, particularly of people with disabilities. CBR in the developed world includes home-based services, outreach services and community development programs for issues related to disability. The definition of community in CBR may be geographical, referring to a particular area or locality, or it may be relational, referring to a group with shared interests and values, mutual obligations, a common history, or other affinity (Miles, 1994).

The essential difference between CBR and the two approaches to rehabilitation just discussed lies in CBR's emphasis on the social origins of issues relating to disability. CBR aims for a redistribution of community resources in favor of community members with disabilities. The whole community is the target of CBR programs, although people with disabilities themselves are the primary beneficiaries (Lysack & Kaufert, 1994).

CBR programs vary widely throughout the world, due to the differences among communities in which they operate. However most CBR programs have a number of features in common. Through community participation in social action, CBR programs assist communities to develop a greater awareness and understanding of community members who have disabilities. They also help communities to work together to identify and overcome barriers which prevent people with disabilities from participating in the life of the community. Human and financial resources of the community are used, and simple rehabilitation techniques are

---

SUMMARY: CLIENT-CENTRED REHABILITATION

Assumptions:
1. Clients know what they want and need from therapy;
2. Ultimate relevance of the client's perspective on problems;
3. Professional dominance is counter-therapeutic;
4. Therapist cannot be the instrument of change, only the facilitator.

Advantages:
1. Empowering;
2. Highly individualized;
3. Opportunity for personal growth for therapist.

Disadvantages:
1. Perception of less skilled, active role for therapist;
2. Ambiguity about client-therapist relationship;
3. Need for structural change to support client-centred practice;
4. Based on therapist personality and beliefs.

taught by professionals to families and community members, who carry them out with people with disabilities. Vocational skill development and income-generating activities are often included in CBR programs (O'Toole, 1991; Peat & Boyce, 1993).

A number of assumptions underlie CBR. First, people with disabilities are assumed not to exist in isolation; rather, they are seen as embedded in a web of family, kin and community. The community both supports people with disabilities and benefits from their contributions to the economic and social environment. Rather than viewing disability as an individual matter, CBR views the issues of people with disabilities as the issues of the whole community. It builds on the family units and the norms of communal support to improve the lives of individuals and the community (Lysack & Kaufert, 1994). CBR programs are thus founded on principles of community development. Community development is defined as a process by which people work collectively to define common problems, discuss strategies for change, make decisions, act on and evaluate their decisions. Implicit in the term is strong participation and ownership of the process by the community (Compton, 1971).

A second assumption of CBR is that individuals and communities have at their disposal the resources to influence their own health. This assumption is shared by another popular movement in health care, the health promotion movement. Health promotion is defined as "the process of enabling people to increase control over the determinants of health" (Wallerstein, 1992). It includes both individual and collective learning, to empower people to assume mastery over aspects of the environment that affect their health. To this end, empowerment education is a health promotion strategy within CBR, aimed at developing in people with disabilities and their communities the capacity to identify the fundamental causes of disadvantage and to develop social and personal action plans to change the situation (Wallerstein, 1992).

Lastly, CBR assumes that it is more important (and more possible) to make small improvements to the quality of life of all people with disabilities in a community than to provide the highest standard of care for a privileged few (O'Toole, 1991). The lives of all people with disabilities are improved when communities view them as integral members, and engage collaboratively in a process of community problem-solving. This can be achieved by providing information and training to community members, providing basic aids and adaptations, and making simple, inexpensive accommodations, all of which benefit the majority of people with disabilities.

Thus the roots of CBR lie jointly in the philosophies of community development and health promotion. The principle of individual and community self-determination is the common thread between health promotion and community development which underlies CBR when applied to the issues of people with disabilities.

There are a number of inherent advantages to the community-based rehabilitation approach to delivering services to people with disabilities. An important advantage is that CBR makes service accessible to a much larger number of people with disabilities and their families than traditional service models. Furthermore, this model of service delivery is not dependent on the availability of highly trained professionals and resource-intensive institutions. Thus it is an extremely cost-effective approach to providing a basic level of service to a large number of individuals.

A second advantage of the CBR approach is that many community members, both disabled and able-bodied, increase their knowledge, skill and understanding about disability. Through exchanges between people with disabilities and professionals, and through participation in social action, individuals develop skills and competencies which are useful in many situations besides CBR. People with disabilities are seen as contributors to community life, while other community members learn to value the contributions that they can make when afforded the opportunity.

The third and perhaps most compelling advantage of CBR is the increase in competency that occurs in the community in which a CBR program resides. Through the process of community development, communities learn to listen to disadvantaged or marginalized groups, engage in collective problem-solving, and marshal resources which were often previously unknown or underused. Reliance on the community's own people and resources reduces its dependence on external resources and helps to ensure that programs continue over the long term.

The final advantage of CBR is its inherent sensitivity to the social, economic and cultural issues of the community. Because CBR is planned by the community to meet needs it defines, with professionals providing support where requested, programs tend to be technically, socially and financially acceptable, and may engender more commitment from the community. People with disabilities are also fully involved in the program, therefore the systems developed by the community to encourage the integration of people with disabilities may be more holistic and comprehensive than those developed by professionals (Banerjee, 1992).

On the other hand, there are also disadvantages to CBR. First, because CBR is delivered in the community, its applicability is restricted to issues of people living in the community. Thus it is of limited utility to people with newly acquired disabilities. Those individuals usually require one of the more resource-intensive models of service at least at the initial phase. Also for individuals living in the community with complex multiple disabilities, CBR may not be able to respond completely to their needs. For example, CBR is ill-equipped to provide highly technical or specialized service.

Another disadvantage of this approach is that it may take a long time to develop individual and community abilities to respond to the issues of community members with disabilities. Because the progress of the program may depend on changing community structures, the time frame may be longer than that for individual rehabilitation. This can be discouraging for people with disabilities, and can ultimately endanger the program's credibility and success. Further, success may be difficult to demonstrate; indicators of community development and community competence are not well developed since research in this area is relatively young (Bichmann, Rifkin & Shrestha, 1989; Hawe, 1994).

A third disadvantage of CBR is that the continuity of the program can be threatened by changes in the community, such as turnover in CBR volunteers, changes in the interests of the community, and changes to the resources available for the program. Perhaps the most threatening of these is a change in the priority that a community assigns to issues of its members with disabilities. In a fiscal environment of scarce resources, CBR programs are vulnerable to shifting priorities away from issues of a minority disadvantaged group, such as people with disabilities.

The fourth and final disadvantage of the CBR approach is

SUMMARY: COMMUNITY-BASED REHABILITATION

Assumptions:
1. People with disabilities must be seen in the context of their communities;
2. Individuals and communities can influence their own health;
3. Small improvements to the quality of life of all people in a community is preferable to maximum improvements for a few.

Advantages:
1. Increases accessibility of service;
2. All community members increase their understanding of issues of disability;
3. Communities develop their ability to solve problems collectively;
4. Services are inherently sensitive to the context and culture.

Disadvantages:
1. Applicable only to people living in the community;
2. May take longer to achieve specific benefits;
3. Vulnerable to changes in resources and attitudes of community;
4. Rehabilitation professionals unprepared for community development/health promotion roles.

---

lack of preparedness of most rehabilitation professionals for community development and health promotion roles. While individual practitioners may be interested in this approach, they may not be certain how to intervene at the level of a community, instead of at the level of the individual. Since CBR programs are by definition "owned" by the community, the role of the professional is defined by the community. That role is usually not to implement programs, but to enhance the ability of people with disabilities and communities to achieve their own goals (Boyce & Peat, 1995). Professionals may find the roles that communities and people with disabilities wish them to take on in conflict with their own ideas. For example, professionals may want to control clinical aspects of programs, be involved in organizational aspects and bow out of fund-raising. People with disabilities, on the other hand, may want to share in control of clinical aspects, fully control organizational aspects, and delegate fund-raising to influential professionals (O'Toole, 1991).

INDEPENDENT LIVING

Finally, *independent living* (IL) is a fourth model for the delivery of services to persons with disabilities. This model differs significantly from biomedical, client-centred and community-based rehabilitation models in that it developed out of a collective political movement of persons with disabilities (DeJong, 1979; Driedger, 1989; Oliver, 1990). No longer willing to accept lifelong dependent relationships with professionals, people with disabilities asserted a political strategy in the 1960s and 1970s to promote a view of disability as a socially constructed phenomenon (Oliver, 1990). Independent living represents a new attitude, a new set of organizing principles, and a new approach to service delivery, aimed to ensure people with disabilities access to housing, health care, transportation, employment, education, and mobility. These aims were achieved through self-help and peer support, research and service development, and referral and advocacy (Canadian Association of Independent Living Centres [CAILC], 1989; DeJong, 1979; DeLoach et al., 1983).

The primary goal of IL is to ensure access to resources and full participation for people with disabilities in society (Cole, 1979; CAILC, 1989). Although this goal may seem similar in many ways to that of traditional rehabilitation, IL's central distinction can be found in the way in which the goal is addressed. Unlike previously outlined models, in IL the initiative for control of service rests with consumers/individuals themselves, rather than with programs, institutions or professionals (Cole, 1979; DeLoach et. al., 1983). Perhaps the greatest strength of the independent living approach is its commitment to placing in the hands of people with disabilities themselves control of the resources which affect their daily lives (Ben-Sira, 1983; DeJong, 1979). The IL approach, first developed by persons with disabilities themselves, has received considerable attention in medical and rehabilitation circles in North America and indeed around the world.

A number of assumptions inform the IL model. First, the model understands people with disabilities as consumers of services, rather than as patients or clients. Consumers are seen as being in control of the resources that affect their lives, and able to make informed choices about the disposition of those resources to meet needs (Gadacz, 1994). This assumption requires a different view of people with disabilities and a different type of relationship between consumers and providers. Hierarchical relationships with professionals are incompatible with the view of consumers as autonomous and rationally driven (Oliver, 1990; DeJong, 1979).

A second assumption of the IL approach is that disablement stems not from the individual him- or herself, but rather from the environment in which the individual lives (Driedger, 1989). This approach does not understand disabilities as deficits, but rather as conditions of life. IL advocates that individuals are disabled by inaccessible buildings, lack of access to education, unemployment, and hostile attitudes. Disablement lies not in the physical condition of the individual, but in the construction of society (Brisenden, 1986). Therefore, the means to overcome disablement lies also in the environment and in greater access to resources, such as education, living arrangements and mobility.

A third assumption of the IL approach is that the management of a medically stable disability is a personal matter first, and a medical matter second (DeJong, 1979). While acknowledging the need for rehabilitation in acute disabling episodes, the independent living approach sees this need as a strictly time-limited one. Once the medical condition stabilizes, proponents of the IL approach believe that people with disabilities are competent to assume responsibility over the resources that affect their lives, and to make informed choices over their setting, context and circumstances, whether medical or nonmedical (Gadacz, 1994).

As in all previously outlined approaches, the IL model has a number of advantages and disadvantages. Its most important advantage is its commitment to providing people with disabilities with control over the resources which affect their daily lives, thereby enhancing their ability to act autonomously and achieve mastery and self-respect. For example, within an IL approach, people who require a personal attendant to assist with daily self-care would be provided with resources to directly hire, supervise and fire personal attendants (whereas in traditional models, they would be referred by professionals to a program which would dictate to them the terms and conditions of attendant care that they were entitled to receive). The inherent increase in self-determination and participation associated with this approach represents increased independence and self-respect

for people with disabilities (Boland & Alonso, 1982).

The second advantage of the IL approach is its focus on self-help, and its recognition of the significant contributions that persons with disabilities can make to the lives of others and to society as a whole. Similar to the personal and professional growth of the therapist under the client-centred approach, independent living offers growth potential for individuals with disabilities themselves as well as for communities. Persons with disabilities are assisted, often by others with disabilities, to live independent lives in the community, and make significant and meaningful contributions. One example of self-help within the IL approach has been the development of Independent Living Resource Centres. These centres are community-based, consumer-controlled response centres, aimed at addressing the needs of persons with disabilities in the community, and ensuring that these needs can be met in a non-institutional setting (CAILC, 1994).

The third advantage of the independent living approach is its focus on citizenship, equality, and participation in society for people with disabilities. This holistic, nonmedical approach offers expression to the sociopolitical nature of people with disabilities, both individually and collectively (CAILC, 1994). It diverts the focus of service away from the impairment and disability, and onto the real issues of day-to-

---

SUMMARY: INDEPENDENT LIVING

Assumptions:
1. People with disabilities are rational, informed consumers of service;
2. Disablement stems from the environment, not the individual;
3. Disability is a life-long personal issue, and a time-limited medical issue;

Advantages:
1. Promotes self-determination, mastery and self-respect among people with disabilities;
2. Focuses on contributions that people with disabilities make;
3. Focuses on equal participation of people with disabilities in all aspects of daily life.

Disadvantages:
1. Many of basic tenets unfamiliar to professionals;
2. Not applicable for some disabled people, especially those who find IL unsuitable for their personal circumstances;
3. Difficulty in evaluating long-term outcomes of independent living.

TABLE 21-1
Comparison of Four Models of Service to People with Disabilities

	Biomedical rehabilitation	Client-centred rehabilitation	Community-based rehabilitation	Independent living
Decision-making	professional to patient	client to professional	community	consumer
Role of professional	assess; make treatment recommendations; provide treatment	consultant to fulfill goals of client	assist community to solve problems involving disabled community members	limited consultation
Role of consumer	sick-role (Parsons, 1966)	digest information; communicate decision; participate in therapy	stimulus to community action; participate in community problem-solving	self-help; mutual aid; advocacy
Relevant expertise	professional	both professional and consumer	community and consumer	consumers and peers

day life, like employment, access, housing and transportation. It offers a sociopolitical context for these issues, and focuses on promoting change in social structures to enhance equity and participation of people with disabilities in all aspects of society (Oliver, 1990).

Some disadvantages of the IL approach must also be outlined. First, this approach is relatively new (emerging first in the United States in the 1970s, and later in Canada). As a result, there is still some ambiguity surrounding the tenets of the movement itself and the meaning of some of its central concepts. For example, the concept of "independence" means different things to different people. Within an IL approach, the term "independence" is often replaced with the term "autonomy," meaning freedom from domination by social structures, institutions and professionals; control over the resources necessary for daily life; and, expression of the sociopolitical nature of the individual (Brisenden, 1986; DeJong, 1979; Oliver, 1990). This definition of independence differs in many ways from the traditional definition of independence, meaning that an individual is capable of living alone in the community. Research is underway that attempts to close this conceptual gap (Boland & Alonso, 1982; Walton et. al., 1980; Berrol, 1979).

A second disadvantage is that some of the strategies commonly used in the IL approach may not be for everybody (Cole, 1979). For instance, for most people with newly acquired or exacerbated disabilities, the IL approach does not deal with the basic issues that arise at this time. Furthermore, the IL approach, like the community-based approach, is incompatible with inpatient or institutional service delivery. However, even

in these instances, some of the principles of independent living may be applied. For example, the use of peer counselling can be implemented even within an institutional setting, and by doing so, one acknowledges the autonomy and expertise that lies within the community of people with disabilities.

The third and final disadvantage is the difficulty in determining long-term outcomes of the IL approach. Because the goals of rehabilitation from an IL perspective are dramatically different from the goals of traditional rehabilitation models, research approaches used previously to evaluate traditional rehabilitation do not apply (Crewe & Zola, 1983; Williams, 1983). Again, like community-based rehabilitation, there is consensus in the literature that IL evaluation must occur at two levels: the individual and the community (DeLoach et al., 1983). DeJong and Hughes (1982) suggest measures for evaluating the growth and development of individuals with disabilities within the community. More research is needed which involves people with disabilities in all aspects of design, implementation and analysis, and which leads to a better understanding of the impact of the ILmodel on both persons with disabilities and on communities as a whole.

APPLICATIONS OF THE FOUR MODELS OF SERVICE

Using the model of occupation presented in Chapter 3, two applications are described of the four models of service discussed (Table 21-1). In each, an effort has been made to

---

TABLE 21-2

Person, Environment, and Occupational Performance for Steven at Acute Stage

Intrinsic Factors	**Extrinsic Factors**	**Occupational Performance**
Acute Care:		
Physiological: Immediately following his surgery, Steven was able to make only gross movements of his arms and shoulders, and was unable to use his hands for a functional grasp. He had no sensation or movement below the level of his mid-chest, and no control over his bowel or bladder.	*Physical*: In the acute hospital following his surgery, Steven's environment consisted of his semi-private hospital room.	*Self-care*: Soon after his surgery, Steven was assisted to sit up in bed, and to begin to resume responsibility for basic self-care activities, such as feeding. Where necessary, he was furnished with adaptive devices to do so. Otherwise, he was dependent on the unit staff for virtually all his needs.
Psychological: Steven was frightened and overwhelmed, and often appeared barely aware of what was going on around him. He experienced periods of anxiety and agitation, but otherwise was cooperative.	*Social*: His social environment consisted of his roommate, a 72-year-old man who had had a stroke, the unit staff at the hospital, his mother who stayed with him most of the day and the early evening, and his other family members and friends who came to visit regularly. Occasionally, Steven's girlfriend also visited, but this was difficult for everybody.	*Productivity*: The productive part of Steven's day was occupied with therapy, tests, and other hospital procedures.
Neurobehavioural: The level of neurological damage was identified as C6-7, meaning he was unlikely to resume walking or to regain normal use of his arms and hands.	*Cultural*: Steven's cultural environment at this stage was the culture of the hospital and the health care system. This culture imposes many rules and constraints on the behaviour and freedom of patients. These rules are not always well explained to patients, and are often misunderstood.	*Leisure*: Steven's leisure activities consisted of visiting with family and friends, making phone calls, and watching television in his room. He required assistance to use the phone or the TV. He shared a hospital room with an older gentleman, so he had some companionship, but little privacy.
Cognitive: Steven did not lose consciousness at the time of the accident, and is not expected to have sustained any cognitive impairment, therefore, no cognitive assessment was planned.	*Societal*: Within the hospital, Steven was largely sheltered from societal influences. He has had almost no experience with anyone with a disability before now, but he was aware that society generally treats people with disabilities differently.	

---

identify several models of service for each individual. Further, we have tried to show how different models may be more or less applicable at different points along the continuum of rehabilitation and life with a disability.

The first example follows Steven over a 3-year period following his accident, and tracks the models of occupational therapy services used at each of four intervals or stages: the acute care stage; the inpatient rehabilitation stage; the outpatient rehabilitation phase; the postrehabilitation phase.

Case Example 1: Steven

Steven is a 17-year-old young man who lives with his parents and two younger siblings. The family owns and operates a dairy farm, and have lived in the same rural community for several generations. Steven was ready to enter his last year of high school when he was injured in a motor vehicle accident near his home last summer. He sustained a C6-7 spinal fracture. At the time of his accident,

Steven was taken by ambulance to the trauma centre 40 minutes away. His fracture was surgically stabilized, and he was placed in a halo-traction vest until his spine was stable.

Acute Care

Steven's first encounter with an occupational therapist was with Janet at the trauma centre. Steven's occupational performance at that time is described in Table 21-2. The prevailing model of service in the trauma centre was the biomedical model. Based on the assumption that Steven was not in a position to direct his own care at the acute stage, and given the knowledge and skill of the therapists and doctors about the neurological condition, decisions about therapy were made by the team, in consultation with Steven's parents, and communicated to Steven in a manner that was sensitive to the psychological and social issues at play. Treatments focused on the intrinsic factors underlying

TABLE 21-3

Person, Environment, and Occupational Performance for Steven at Transfer to Rehabilitation

Intrinsic Factors	**Extrinsic Factors**	**Occupational Performance**
Inpatient Rehabilitation:	*Physical*: Steven's physical environment was the rehabilitation centre, which was ideally accessible to someone in a wheelchair. There he shared a room with three other men.	*Self-care*: Steven had begun to perform some of his own rudimentary self-care, but was still dependent on the unit staff for many of his needs.
Physiological: At the time of transfer to the rehabilitation centre, Steven was able to sit up for several hours at a time, but needed maximum assistance to transfer to the wheelchair. He was beginning to develop spasticity in his legs, and still had little strength in his arms.	*Social*: His social environment still consisted largely of the unit staff, his three roommates, his family, and friends. His mother has moved back home and visited with other family members several evenings per week. Weekends home were planned, as soon as the house could be made ready for him. Steven's girlfriend had stopped visiting by this time, but several high school friends remained in touch.	*Productivity*: The productive part of Steven's day continued to be occupied with therapy. Some discussions had begun about future productivity, and the skills and abilities that Steven has that might lead to future productivity.
Psychological: Steven was beginning to understand the implications of what had happened to him. He began to ask staff tentative questions about what lay ahead of him.		*Leisure*: Steven's leisure activities continue to be dominated by visits with family and friends, phone calls and television. However, peer relationships with roommates and other residents of the rehabilitation centre had become important to him.
Neurobehavioral: The neurological status was clear by this point, and little further change or recovery was expected.	*Cultural*: Steven's cultural environment at this stage was the culture of the rehabilitation centre, and was somewhat less restrictive than the culture of the trauma centre. Its emphasis was on independence and self-care.	
Cognitive: Cognitive functioning was not assessed, since day-to-day functioning did not suggest cognitive problems.	*Societal*: Steven remained largely sheltered from societal influences.	

Steven's disability, including his physical, psychological and neurological condition.

Initially, Janet came by daily to ensure that Steven was positioned appropriately in his bed to prevent contractures, that he was as comfortable as possible, that his skin was not breaking down at any of the pressure points and that he was able to communicate with nursing staff, family and friends. In order to meet these goals, she provided Steven with foot drop splints to maintain his ankle position, and resting splints to protect his wrists. Janet performed several basic assessments of Steven's physical, psychological and neurological functioning, including manual muscle testing, range of motion, sensation, tone, hand function and functional independence, using the Functional Independence Measure (FIM) (Keith, Granger, Hamilton & Sherwin, 1987). Janet also provided Steven with an adapted call bell that he could operate independently if he needed assistance from nursing or support staff, and adaptive equipment for self-care and feeding. Finally, she organized with the evening staff to provide assistance to Steven in making telephone calls.

By the end of 4 weeks, Steven was able to sit up in a high back wheelchair for several hours at a time. At this point, the team conferred and determined that Steven's condition was medically stable, and it was appropriate that he be transferred to the rehabilitation hospital across the street.

Inpatient Rehabilitation

Still wearing his halo-traction device, Steven was transferred to the rehabilitation centre. His status, environment and occupation at that time are described in Table 21-3.

On his second day at the centre, Steven met Lloyd, his new occupational therapist. Lloyd, like many of his colleagues in the rehabilitation centre, functioned from a client-centred model of service. Therefore, on his first meeting with Steven, Lloyd's first priority was to get to know Steven, and begin to develop an understanding of the meaning of this injury in Steven's life. Given that Steven's injury was still fairly recent and he was feeling overwhelmed, this meeting required a great deal of skill on Lloyd's part. Lloyd's primary objective was to communicate to Steven his desire to understand the situation from Steven's perspective, and his commitment to help him solve his problems. Lloyd used a number of techniques and activities to learn more about Steven's life before his injury, his home and family, his plans and hopes for the future. For example, Steven and Lloyd completed a detailed occupational history and a time use diary for a typical day. With Lloyd's help, Steven developed a social network diagram to describe his home and family, and discussed the elements of the diagram with Lloyd as they went along. Lloyd also began to introduce the idea of the future by asking Steven to project the diagram forward in time. Steven realized that he was virtually unable to do this, and began to tentatively explore various scenarios that might shed some light on the future. Lloyd and Steven made several attempts to use a narrative approach to raise issues about Steven's rehabilitation plans. They wrote a story about the accident, the rehabilitation process and the next few chapters in Steven's life. Through the narrative, they began to set long- and short-term goals for rehabilitation. Using the Canadian Occupational Performance Measure (Law et al., 1990), Steven identified a number of specific problems of occupational performance that he was concerned about: his inability to get around, the fact that he was missing school and falling behind, and the strained relationship with his girlfriend.

Steven's long-term goals were to walk again, to patch things up with his girlfriend and to finish high school and to begin learning from his father about the operation of the farm. In the short term, he was quite amenable to the physical aspects of therapy, but resistant to learning daily living skills involving the wheelchair or other adaptive devices. Therefore short term goals were developed that focused strictly on developing strength, balance and physical capabilities, getting around in the hospital and looking after himself on the ward.

Steven participated actively in rehabilitation for 4 months, during which time, he developed strength, tone and balance, as well as a functional tenodesis grasp. He became independent in the basic elements of self-care and able to propel the wheelchair independently. From time to time, assistive devices were introduced for the sake of expediency, and accepted as short-term solutions. However, Steven would not agree to order a wheelchair of his own, and he became angry when it was repeatedly suggested by team members and by family. He continued to use one of the centre's chairs on a loan basis.

About 2 months into his rehabilitation, discussions began about the possibility that Steven might go home for a weekend. Reactions of family varied from fear and apprehension to excitement and anticipation. Steven himself experienced the same range of mixed feelings. To begin the process of adjusting to the idea of going home, and making the home environment ready for Steven, Lloyd and Steven did a number of visualization exercises, including detailed visualization of driving up to the farm, entering the house, eating Thanksgiving dinner and helping with the farm chores. Steven began to identify the feelings associated with going home, most prominent of which was his fear of failure and his embarrassment at being seen in the wheelchair. He also began to identify some of the barriers to accessibility, and some of the adjustment issues that he might face on weekends home. Steven accompanied Lloyd on a home visit to assess for structural modifications, but did not actually bring the wheelchair or get out of the car. Plans were developed for an exterior ramp, a downstairs bedroom and an adapted main floor bathroom. Also, Steven's mother was taught to manage his bowel and bladder routine.

Steven's first weekend home at month 3 pointed out some of the limitations of the loaner wheelchair — its width, lack of reclining back, inadequate footrests and general heaviness, making future discussions possible about the selection of a more attractive and suitable wheelchair. Otherwise the weekend was quite low-key, with no visitors, and was generally agreed by everyone to be a success. Subsequent weekends were used to identify problems in various aspects of home life, and to begin the process of connecting with friends, neighbours and community members. During the week, Lloyd and Steven sought solutions to each new issue as it arose.

Steven's visits home also raised issues in his mind about his ability to follow his original career path of taking over the farm, however in the short term, everyone agreed that his first priority must be to complete high school. Steven was discharged home after 4 months of rehabilitation to his parents' partially renovated farmhouse, with plans to resume high school after Christmas.

Outpatient Rehabilitation

Just before Christmas, Steven returned home and was visited by a community occupational therapist named Sylvie. Sylvie was hired by Steven's insurance company to assess Steven's needs for community living, and to make recommendations about what was necessary to ensure Steven's return to school and preparation for gainful employment in the future. Using a traditional approach, Sylvie began by assessing Steven's ability to fulfill his self-care roles at home and to pursue his education. As a result, she uncovered the occupational profile described in Table 21-4. At the end of a long visit, reassured that Steven and his family felt confident of their ability to manage over the Christmas holidays, Sylvie arranged to come back immediately after the New Year.

TABLE 21-4

Person, Environment, and Occupational Performance for Steven Upon Returning Home

Intrinsic Factors	Extrinsic Factors	Occupational Performance
Outpatient Rehabilitation:		
Physiological: At the time of discharge home, about six months after his injury, Steven's physical condition was excellent for someone with quadriplegia. He had developed good strength in his remaining active muscles, but still had no sensation below the level of his lesion, and no voluntary bowel or bladder function. He was able to transfer independently, propel his wheelchair and use a functional grasp for a wide range of objects.	*Physical*: Steven moved home with his family. The home was adapted, with a ramp leading up to the back door and a modified main floor bedroom and bathroom. It still had many of the architectural barriers of an older home, such as narrow hallways and small rooms.	*Self-care*: Currently, Steven performs almost all of his self-care independently, but receives assistance from his mother with his bowel and bladder program. His morning routine takes about 90 minutes.
Psychological: Psychologically, Steven had been having a difficult time. He was resentful about his situation, fearful about resuming community living, and depressed about his prospects for the future.	*Social*: Steven's social environment consisted primarily of his family and a few close friends, one from before the accident and two from the rehab centre. Steven's girlfriend came by the house a couple of times, but conversation was strained and uncomfortable.	*Productivity*: Steven is willing to return to school to complete his high school diploma, but otherwise has little enthusiasm for the topic of future productivity.
Neurobehavioural: No change.	*Cultural*: Steven's cultural environment at this stage was that of a small rural farming community. Beliefs about work and family run deep, and the dominant attitude among neighbours and family friends is one of support, but also of pity.	*Leisure*: Steven's leisure activities include spending time with his younger siblings, listening to music, playing computer games, and watching TV. He has not resumed community social activities, except for visiting with one male friend.
Cognitive: No change.	*Societal*: Steven was aware that at 17 years of age, he is expected to focus on preparing for future productive employment by completing his education and training for a job. There was previously an expectation that he would farm alongside his father, and take over responsibility for the farm as his father prepared to retire.	

On her second visit, about 3 weeks later, Sylvie discovered that Steven and his family had managed very successfully over the holidays, and that they had effectively problem-solved most of the issues that had arisen. Steven however had not left the house, he was expressing some reluctance about returning to school, and family relationships were severely strained. Steven's mother revealed to Sylvie that a local service club was planning a fund-raising event in the community hall 3 weeks hence, to raise money to help pay for an adapted van. Steven was expected to attend and was flatly stating that he would not.

Recognizing that the issues faced by Steven and his family involved the whole community to some extent, Sylvie reconsidered her approach, and began the process of community development that is central to community-based rehabilitation. She began by asking Steven and his family to identify the individuals and structures that comprised their community. They identified neighbours, Steven's friends, the church, the store, the school, and the service club, of which Steven's father was a member. Sylvie sought the family's and Steven's permission to talk to each of these people about how the community might participate in the process of facilitating Steven's re-engagement with the community, return to school and plan for future productivity. Sylvie thus acted as a catalyst to a process whereby the community assumed ownership of some of the issues that Steven faced, assessed its resources to deal with these issues, and developed a sustainable plan to make changes.

She and Steven met first with the school principal, Steven's teacher, the student council president and the school bus driver. They collectively problem-solved about adapting the bus with a lift and wheelchair tie-down, altering the pick-up schedule to allow Steven time for his morning routine, making one entrance to the school fully accessible, ensuring that the entrance was kept clear of snow, bicycles and other obstacles, altering the timetable and room allocations to accommodate Steven's schedule and developing a rotation schedule for fellow students to provide peer assistance to Steven throughout the school day. Steven was furnished with a beeper in case of emergencies, and three students were taught to assist with emptying Steven's leg bag when necessary.

Steven, however, continued to refuse to go to school, out of fear and embarrassment at the reactions of the other students. Thus when school resumed after the holidays, members of Steven's homeroom took turns bringing notes and assignments to Steven at home. After 3 weeks, he had a visit from virtually everyone, and had overcome his fear of the "first day." By the end of January, he was attending school on a part-time basis, with plans to graduate the following year.

The visits of his classmates and other community members also assisted with Steven's willingness to attend the community fund-raiser. He discovered at that time also that the store in the village had been rearranged to allow passage of his wheelchair and the single step at the front entrance had been ramped. The store had been a place where Steven and his friends had always convened informally. From time to time in the past, the storekeeper had shooed them away, however this action sent a clear message that the teenagers were welcome patrons.

Post-rehabilitation

Steven finished high school in the spring, almost 2 years after his injury. He was 19 years old and anxious to be more independent of his family. He found the necessity of his mothers' help with personal care increasingly degrading. He recognized the growth that had taken place in his community to afford him the kinds of opportunities it had, but he still felt like a "charity case" and could not shake the feeling that deep down, people felt sorry for him and always would. They remembered him as an ablebodied teenager, and he saw the reflection of that image in their eyes. He felt he couldn't continue to live with reminders of the past in all his social relationships. Even his part-time job in the store offered little to his sense of self-sufficiency and self-respect (Table 21-5).

Steven's family was horrified at the thought of his moving out. They had not a clue how to begin to assemble the resources needed for Steven to live alone. They called Sylvie for some advice. Sylvie was able to obtain authorization for two visits to help Steven secure appropriate housing and to assess the need for ongoing supports. Recognizing the limits of her ability to help Steven with the challenges he faced, and his need for self-determination and autonomy, Sylvie

referred Steven to the Independent Living Resource Centre (ILRC) in town, and also encouraged him to contact his friend from the rehabilitation centre who now lived independently in town. Sylvie advised that she would become more involved if requested, but that other services were more appropriate to help Steven with the issues he faced now.

Steven called his buddy Raymond, whom he had been in touch with by phone over the intervening year since leaving rehab, but had not seen for some time. Raymond's disability was slightly less severe than Steven's, but they shared an understanding that was largely unspoken, and recognized by both to be unique to that relationship. Steven told Raymond of his plans, and Raymond invited him in to town to see his place. Steven arranged with his mother to take him into town, leave him alone for the day, and pick him up again about supper time. Steven also arranged a visit to the ILRC for the same day.

Steven returned home that evening exuberant at the possibilities for independent living. He had put his name on a waiting list for an accessible apartment, knowing that he might wait up to a year for a suitable place. In the meantime, his experience with Raymond had shown him that he had some work to do to be ready when his name came up. First and foremost, he needed to learn to drive. The ILRC recommended a driving instructor who specialized in teaching car transfers and hand-controlled driving. Steven was surprised to discover at his first lesson that the instructor also had a disability. Using his own van, that had been purchased jointly by his insurance company and the community, Steven got his driver's license before the end of the summer.

By fall, he was driving into town to attend community college, training to be a data systems analyst. On one of his free afternoons each week, he volunteered at the ILRC, answering phones, doing office work, and developing a computerized catalogue for the centre's resource library. By the following spring, a suitable apartment had become available, and Steven prepared to move into town.

He contacted Sylvie again to make the first of her two authorized visits. Together they assessed the apartment and identified the need for several minor adaptations. More importantly however, they began to discuss the need for attendant care. Sylvie recommended to the insurance company that Steven be provided with 4 hours of attendant care a day, 2 hours each morning and evening. She further recommended that the resources to support this assistance be placed in a trust fund to be managed by Steven, and accounted for on an annual basis.

The insurance company agreed to all of Sylvie's recommendations, except the last one, that Steven take responsibility for the management of his personal assistance. They insisted that Steven acquire attendant services through a program run by the rehabilitation centre. In his haste to begin his new life, Steven accepted these conditions and moved into his

---

TABLE 21-5

Long-term Person, Environment, and Occupational Performance for Steven

Intrinsic Factors	Extrinsic Factors	Occupational Performance
Post-Rehabilitation:	*Physical*: Steven's physical environment continued to be his parents' home and surrounding community, but Steven had begun to discuss moving into his own apartment in town, about 40 minutes drive away.	*Self-care*: Steven has developed a stable and consistent self-care program, that can be maintained with some assistance from his mother during the morning and evening.
Physiological: No change.		
Psychological: A year and a half after his injury, Steven became anxious to begin to pursue living on his own and becoming independent in a number of ways.	*Social*: Steven's social environment was still dominated by family, but also included students and staff at school, friends and neighbours.	*Productivity*: Steven has returned to high school and has completed his diploma. He hopes to train for a job as a police or taxi dispatcher, but sees little opportunity for himself in their own small community. Although he assists wherever possible with the daily and seasonal chores of the farm, he has no ambitions to farm himself.
Neurobehavioral: No change.	*Cultural*: Steven's cultural environment now has several layers, because he participates in various aspects of the community. The school has its own culture, oriented around achievement; the community has a culture, which values work and family, and the family has a culture aimed at protecting Steven from harm.	
Cognitive: No change.		
	Societal: Steven has begun to be acutely aware of the larger society, and of the constraints and opportunities it affords him.	*Leisure*: Steven's leisure activities include socializing with friends, hanging out at the store in the village, fishing with adapted equipment, and riding his ATV.

---

apartment. However, after several months, Steven became dissatisfied with his attendant. He did not really like having a woman do his personal care, and she was often late in the mornings, causing him to miss classes. When he complained to the program manager at the rehab centre, he was told that there was no one else they could send. Therefore, he sought the support of the ILRC to advocate on his behalf with the insurance company to allow him to hire and manage his own personal assistance. Using information about the models used by other people to manage their own attendants, and the corporate assurance of accountability from the ILRC, the insurance company agreed to a pilot project whereby Steven would have sole authority over the resources to purchase his personal assistance. The ILRC would annually audit the accounts. Steven sought advice and information from the ILRC about how to advertise for, interview, hire and train an attendant, how to supervise and give feedback to an attendant, and how to terminate a work relationship if necessary. Steven's first attendant was an occupational therapy student, who worked with Steven throughout the duration of his degree, and upon graduation, moved away but remained a close friend.

Case Example 2: Sandy

Sandy is a 35-year-old woman who has lived alone in a subsidized housing complex for much of her adult life, and has little contact with her family or other members of her community. As a young woman, she was a good student, and was enrolled in an engineering program at university. However, at the age of 19, she experienced her first episode of schizophrenia, and was forced to drop out of school. Since then, she has made several attempts to take additional courses toward her degree, but has never been able to complete them. Sandy has been in and out of the hospital many times over the past 16 years. She has recently been hospitalized for another acute episode, where she discontinued her medication and quickly became delusional and paranoid.

Acute Care

Sandy was admitted by ambulance to the emergency unit of the hospital in her area about 10:00 one night, because voices were telling her that she was "a blight on society and didn't deserve to live." This had apparently been going on for 2 or 3 days, with increasing intensity, to the point where Sandy was

---

TABLE 21-6

Person, Environment, and Occupational Performance for Sandy at Admission

Intrinsic Factors	**Extrinsic Factors**	**Occupational Performance**
Inpatient Rehabilitation:		

Intrinsic Factors

Inpatient Rehabilitation:

Physiological: Sandy was admitted to hospital in a condition that could only be described as deteriorated and fragile. She was malnourished, sleep-deprived, and unclean. Her posture was somewhat stooped and her movements appeared to require a great deal of effort.

Psychological: Sandy was fearful and confused at the time of admission. She spent any unstructured time in her room alone, and expressed doubts about her ability to interact with other patients and staff, to say nothing of members of the outside community. She was compliant with institutional routines, and sought frequent reassurance from staff.

Neurobehavioral: Not assessed on this admission.

Cognitive: Mental status evaluation indicated that Sandy was oriented, although somewhat suspicious and fearful.

Extrinsic Factors

Physical: At this stage, Sandy's physical environment is the rehabilitation unit of a large psychiatric hospital.

Social: Sandy's social environment consists almost entirely of the unit staff. She is not in touch with her family or anyone else from the community.

Cultural: Sandy's cultural environment is institutional at this point. The culture of the rehabilitation unit is oriented toward independence in the community.

Societal: Sandy's societal environment is composed of her memories of the feelings he had of not fitting in society.

Occupational Performance

Self-care: Sandy's self-care has deteriorated significantly, to the point where health and hygeine are issues. Her appearance is described by staff as "frightening."

Productivity: Sandy's productivity roles while in rehabilitation involve participating in therapy, so that it becomes possible to resume independent living.

Leisure: Sandy has little in the way of leisure or recreational interests, but is willing to take part in most of the activities of the unit. She does not socialize easily, but participates in a solitary way.

---

afraid to leave her apartment, and afraid to go to sleep. She phoned a crisis help line, and agreed to meet the counselor at the emergency department of the hospital (Table 21-6).

As an inpatient on a short-stay mental health unit, Sandy was initially stabilized on medication, and attention was directed at her general health and physical state. After a couple of days, she met Janice, the occupational therapist. Janice practices occupational therapy from a client-centred perspective, and therefore her first meeting with Sandy was spent finding out about her in her own words. Janice makes it a practice never to read a client's chart until after she has met him or her, and heard about problems in the client's own words. For the sake of safety, she asks nursing staff about any special instructions prior to this first meeting.

Sandy told Janice about the night she came into hospital, and characterized it as the logical culmination of her general inability to "make something of herself." She expressed profound disappointment in her life to date, and pointed to normative social milestones that she had failed to achieve, such as career, marriage and children. Janice guided the interview to find out more about specific problems that Sandy might experience in the areas of self-care, productivity and leisure.

Sandy specified her most pressing problems as having nothing to do all day, being lonely and being afraid of another episode like the one that brought her here. Further, Sandy made clear that she did not wish to return to her apartment.

Over the course of a 10-day admission, Janice and Sandy explored a number of different long-term living options. With the cooperation of the psychiatrist and social worker, Sandy was assisted in securing a place in a community boarding home for people with mental illnesses.

Janice and Sandy also explored her use of time and the need for a balance in her daily activities. They did detailed time and occupation diaries, and identified temporal structures and patterns that could help Sandy to add meaning to her day-to-day life. Part of this process involved the identification of resources in Sandy's new community that might become part of her routine, such as a community clubhouse. However, in order to comfortably access these, Janice and Sandy had to work together to develop and rehearse strategies for making contact, attending initially and sustaining participation. At the end of 10 days, Sandy was discharged to the boarding home, and Janice was authorized to provide outreach follow-up to Sandy for a transitional 6-week period (Table 21-7).

TABLE 21-7

Long-Term Person, Environment, and Occupational Performance of Sandy

Intrinsic Factors	Extrinsic Factors	Occupational Performance
Post-Rehabilitation:		

Intrinsic Factors

Post-Rehabilitation:

Physiological: Sandy left the hospital considerably more physically healthy than when she arrived. She continues to appear physically somewhat fragile.

Psychological: Sandy was psychologically stabilized when she moved to the boarding home, but remains extremely shy and unsure of herself. She has little confidence in her ability to make real changes in her life. In addition, she is nervous and apprehensive about her ability to fit into her new environment. She is somewhat overwhelmed by the many changes facing her, and worried about sliding back into illness.

Neurobehavioral: No change.

Cognitive: No more paranoid or explicit suicidal ideation.

Extrinsic Factors

Physical: Sandy's physical environment is a three-storey mental health boarding home in the heart of a large city. She lives with 8 other residents in a partially supported setting.

Social: Sandys's social environment consists mainly of boarding home staff (manager, cook, and night supervisor) and fellow residents.

Cultural: The cultural environment of the boarding home is somewhat bereft initially. One does not have the sense that there is much interaction among residents, and the culture is clearly defined by the manager, with little input from residents. The boarding home itself is somewhat marginalized in the larger community, as are its members.

Societal: Sandy is aware that she is somewhat out of step with the mainstream of society, and that people regard her differently because of her disability. Her societal environment is therefore perceived as alienating and unfriendly.

Occupational Performance

Self-care: Sandy has resumed maintaining a good standard of personal care and hygeine. At the boarding home, she has her meals and housekeeping mostly done for her.

Productivity: Sandy is at a loss as to how she will fill the productive part of her day in this new environment. She has identified some possible community resources, but has not yet had the opportunity to explore them.

Leisure: Sandy has little in the way of leisure activities. Her hope that her new collective living arrangement would help her to make friends and use her time in more fulfilling ways seem destined to be disappointed.

Outpatient Rehabilitation

Janice made her first visit to the boarding home the day after Sandy moved in. She found Sandy sitting on the bed in her room, with the door open a crack. She reported having her meals at the appointed times, but having met none of her neighbours. Mealtimes were brief and mostly silent. Sandy was very disappointed at how this was turning out.

Janice saw in the boarding home a community with the capacity to provide a better quality of life for its members, through collective problem-solving. Using a community-based rehabilitation approach, she began to identify stakeholders in this community, including the residents themselves, the boarding home owner, manager and staff, several neighbours, the owner of a local coffee shop where residents commonly convened, staff of a day program Sandy was planning to attend, and the organizers of a community clubhouse run by former psychiatric patients. In her initial contact, she asked each of these people to identify problems or issues they might have, especially as they applied to the boarding home and its residents. Not surprisingly, issues diverged widely, and included everything from residents wandering the streets to inadequate finances. All were invited to an evening meeting to address these issues, held in the coffee shop.

Janice facilitated the meeting, attempting to ensure that everyone had an opportunity to raise their issues. By the end of the meeting, the group had tentatively and, in some cases, reluctantly agreed to several initiatives. The boarding home staff would review aspects of daily operation that could be assumed by residents; the boarding home operator and manager agreed to explore ways in which the residents could have more say in how the home ran, its rules and regulations; Janice agreed to provide several informal information sessions to neighbours and local business people about mental illness and its consequences for individuals; residents agreed to form a planning council to plan at least one community social outing per week. Finally, the group had identified several resources and supports within the community that they could call on for help if they needed it.

Janice visited the home once or twice a week for the 6-week follow-up period. During that time, Sandy began to take a more active role in several kitchen and laundry duties in the home, she participated tentatively in a couple of outings with other residents, she began volunteer work with a community newspaper, and began to trust her next-door neighbour enough to tell her something about herself. Janice also witnessed the beginning of a process of development whereby individuals recognized their links and responsibilities to one another, and their capacity to solve problems collaboratively with the resources available in the community.

Despite her improved relationship with her roommate, Sandy continued to feel that there were many issues about which she wished to talk to someone. She recognized that she needed to talk to someone who had experienced some of the things that she had experienced with her illness, but did not wish to sacrifice her privacy within the boarding home. She had heard about a support group for people with mental illness, and decided to make some inquiries. In so doing, she discovered that the support group was part of a centre, called the Survivors' Centre, that embraced an independent living philosophy, with individuals with mental illness helping and supporting others in similar circumstances. In addition to the weekly support group, the centre offered peer support through telephone dyads, resource information and referral to other services within the community, a weekly movie night, a monthly supper club, a public education committee, an emergency hotline, and a volunteer and vocational training program. In addition, the Centre ran several commercial enterprises, including a cafe, a dry-cleaning business, a car wash and a recycling centre. After much thought, Sandy called and went down to the Centre for an orientation. Initially, she took the name of another woman whose circumstances were similar to her own, but who had just been discharged from hospital, and agreed to call her and see how she was doing. Bit by bit over the next few months, Sandy tried out more of the Centre's activities. Now, 2 years later, she is the manager of the recycling centre. Her involvement with the Centre has resulted in her gaining confidence in her ability to contribute to her community, finding others with whom she shares important experiences relating to her illness, and broadening the scope of her daily life to include a more meaningful balance of activities.

CONCLUSION

The challenge of working with people with disabilities can be met in a variety of different ways. In this chapter, we have outlined four different approaches to addressing issues of disability and occupational dysfunction. Each of these approaches assists in the development of occupational functioning, but each requires different assumptions about the person, the environment and the nature of occupation. Further, each has advantages and disadvantages that makes it more or less applicable in different settings, at different times in the process of rehabilitation and community integration, and for different individuals.

For many years, occupational therapists have functioned primarily from only one model of service: the biomedical model. While this model of service has served some consumers of occupational therapy services well, it has apparently been counter-therapeutic for others. But occupational therapists need not be restricted to a single model of service delivery. The chapter describes three alternatives to the biomedical model, each based on a different belief system about the nature and origins of disability. As occupational therapists become more skilled in areas like phenomenology, community development and sociopolitical analysis, the potential utility of other models of services increases. The occupational therapist who has in his or her therapeutic repertoire the ability to assess a situation and choose between models will undoubtedly be better prepared to meet the challenge of working with people with disabilities. He or she will be able to choose an approach to service that is based not simply on his or her own preferences, but on a multidimensional assessment of the person, environment and occupational needs of people like Steven or Sandy.

STUDY QUESTIONS

1. Define each of the four models of service covered in the chapter.

2. Compare and contrast any two of the four models in terms of:

   - their view of disability;
   - their applicability to occupational therapy;
   - the role of the therapist;
   - the skills required by practitioners;
   - other attitudes and aptitudes needed to function from each perspective.

3. Identify your own readiness to practice from each of the four perspectives. What would you like to learn to allow you to expand your repertoire to include all four models of practice?

ACKNOWLEDGMENT

The authors gratefully acknowledge the assistance of the following people in conceptualizing and preparing the case studies: Terry Krupa, Tanya Packer, Lynda Rankin, Kirby Rowe and Beth tenHove.

REFERENCES

Bakheit, A. M. O. (1995). Delivery of rehabilitation services: An integrated hospital-community approach. *Clinical Rehabilitation, 9*, 142-149.

Banerjee, R. (1992). CBR—Is it an appropriate alternative? *Sharing strengths—A workshop on community-based rehabilitation.* Seva-in-Action, Bangalore, India.

Baradell, J. V. (1990). Client-centred case consultation and single case research design: Application to case management. *Archives of Psychiatric Nursing, 4,* 12-17.

Bateson, M. C. (1990). *Composing a life.* New York: Plume.

Beange, H. (1987). Our clients' health: Their responsibility or ours? *Australia and New Zealand Journal of Developmental Disabilities, 13*, 175-177.

Ben-Sira, Z. (1983). Societal integration of the disabled: Power struggle or enhancement of individual coping capacities. *Social Science and Medicine, 17*, 1011-1014.

Berrol, S. (1979). Independent living programs: The role of the able-bodied professional. *Archives of Physical Medicine and Rehabilitation, 60*, 456-457.

Bichmann, W., Rifkin, S., & Shrestha, M. (1989). Toward the measurement of community participation. *World Health Forum, 10*, 467-472.

Bickenbach, J. (1992) *Physical disability and social policy.* Toronto: University of Toronto Press.

Boland, J. M., & Alonso, G. (1982). A comparison: Independent living rehabilitation and vocational rehabilitation. *Journal of Rehabilitation, 48*, 56-59.

Boyce, W., & Peat, M. (1995). A comprehensive approach to research in Community Based Rehabilitation. *NU News on Health Care in Developing Countries, 2*(95), 15-18.

Braddy, B. A., & Gray, D. O. (1987). Employment services for older job seekers: A comparison of two client-centred approaches. *The Gerontologist, 27*, 565-568.

Brider, P. (1992). Patient-focused care. *American Journal of Nursing, 9*, 27-33.

Brisenden, S. (1986). Independent living and the medical model of disability. *Disability, Handicap & Society, 1*, 173-179.

Brown, S. J. (1992). Tailoring nursing care to the individual client: Empirical challenge of a theoretical concept. *Research in Nursing and Health, 15*, 39-46.

Burnard, P., & Morrison, P. (1991). Client-centred counselling: A study of nurses' attitudes. *Nurse Education Today, 11*, 104-109.

Canadian Association of Independent Living Centres. (1989). *Independent living promotion kit.* Ottawa: Author.

Canadian Association of Independent Living Centres. (1994). *A time for change, the time for choices.* Ottawa: Author.

Canadian Association of Occupational Therapists. (1991). *Occupational therapy guidelines for client-centred practice.* Toronto: Author.

Carlisle, D. (1992). Patients first. *Nursing Times, 88*(12), 16-17.

Clarke, C., Scott, E., & Krupa, T. (1993). Involving clients in program evaluation and research. *Canadian Journal of Occupational Therapy, 60*, 192-199.

Cole, J. A. (1979). What's new about independent living. *Archives of Physical Medicine and Rehabilitation, 60*, 458-461.

Compton, F. (1972). Community development theory and practice. In J. A. Draper (Ed.), *Citizen participation: Canada. A book of readings.* Toronto: New Press.

Crewe, N. M., & Zola, I. K. (1983). *Independent living for physically disabled people: Developing, implementing and evaluating self-help rehabilitation programs.* Washington: Jossey-Bass Publishers.

DeJong, G. (1979). Independent living: From social movement to analytic paradigm. *Archives of Physical Medicine and Rehabilitation, 60*, 435-446.

DeJong, G., & Hughes, J. (1982). Independent living: Methodology for measuring long-term outcomes. *Archives of Physical Medicine and Rehabilitation, 63*, 68-73.

DeLoach, C. P., Wilkins, R. D., & Walker, G. W. (1983). *Independent living: Philosophy, process and services.* Baltimore: University Park Press.

Driedger, D. (1989). *The last civil rights movement: Disabled peoples' international.* New York: St. Martin's Press.

Emener, W. G. (1991). Empowerment in rehabilitation: An empowerment philosophy for rehabilitation in the 20th century. *Journal of Rehabilitation, 57*(4), 7-12.

Gadacz, R. (1994). *Rethinking disability: New structures, new relationships.* Edmonton: University of Alberta Press.

Goodall, C. (1992). Preserving dignity for disabled people. *Nursing Standard, 6*(35), 25-27.

Hawe, P. (1994). Capturing the meaning of "community" in community intervention evaluation: Some contributions from community psychology. *Health Promotion International, 9*(3), 199-210.

Herzberg, S. R. (1990). Client or patient: Which term is more appropriate for use in occupational therapy? *American Journal of Occupational Therapy, 44*, 561-565.

Holyoke, P., & Elkan, L. (1995). *Rehabilitation services inventory and quality.* Toronto: Institute for Work and Health.

International Labour Organization, United Nations Educational, Scientific and Cultural Organization, World Health Organization. (1994). *Community-based rehabilitation for and with people with disabilities.* Geneva: WHO.

Jaffe, Y., & Kipper, D. A. (1982). Appeal of rational-emotive and client-centred therapies to first-year psychology and non-psychology students. *Psychological Reports, 50*, 781-782.

Keith, R. A., Granger, C. V., Hamilton, B. B., & Sherwin, F. S. (1987). The Functional Independence Measure: A new tool for rehabilitation. *Advances in Clinical Rehabilitation, 1*, 6-8.

Kerfoot, K. M., & LeClair, C. (1991). Building a patient-focused unit: The nurse manager's challenge. *Nursing Economics, 9*, 441-443.

Law, M., Baptiste, S., McColl, M. A., Opzoomer, A., Polatajko, H.,

& Pollock, N. (1990). The Canadian Occupational Performance Measure: An outcome measurement protocol for occupational therapy. *Canadian Journal of Occupational Therapy, 57,* 82-87.

Lysack, C., & Kaufert, J. (1994). Comparing the origins and ideologies of the independent living movement and community based rehabilitation. *International Journal of Rehabilitation Research, 17,* 231-240.

Mattingly, C., & Fleming, M. (1994) *Clinical reasoning: Forms of inquiry in a therapeutic practice.* Philadelphia: F.A. Davis Co.

McColl, M. A., Law, M., & Stewart, D. (1993). *Theoretical basis of occupational therapy: An annotated bibliography.* Thorofare, NJ: SLACK Incorporated.

Meyer, A. (1922). The philosophy of occupational therapy. *Archives of Occupational Therapy, 1,* 1-10.

Miles, M. (1994). *Information based rehabilitation and research.* CBR Symposium. Bangalore, India.

Oliver, M. (1990). *The politics of disablement.* London: MacMillan.

O'Toole, B. J. (1991). *Guide to community-based rehabilitation services. Guides for special education.* Paris: UNESCO.

Parsons, T. (1975). The sick role and the role of the physician reconsidered. *Health and Society, 25,* 258-278.

Patterson, J. B., & Marks, C. (1992). The client as customer: Achieving service quality and customer satisfaction in rehabilitation. *Journal of Rehabilitation, 58*(4), 16-20.

Peat, M., & Boyce, W. (1993). Canadian community rehabilitation services: Challenges for the future. *Canadian Journal of Rehabilitation, 6,* 281-289.

Pollock, N. (1993). Client-centred assessment. *American Journal of Occupational Therapy, 47,* 298-301.

Pollock, N., Baptiste, S., Law, M., McColl, M. A., Opzoomer, A., & Polatajko, H. (1990). Occupational performance measures: A review based on the Guidelines for Client-centred Practice. *Canadian Journal of Occupational Therapy, 57*(2), 82-87.

Preston, K. (1994). Rehabilitation nursing: A client-centred philosophy. *American Journal of Nursing, 94*(2), 66-70.

Robinson, N. C. (1991). A patient-centred framework for restructuring care. *Journal of Organizational Nursing and Administration, 21*(9), 29-34.

Rogers, C. (1942). *Counselling and psychotherapy: Newer concepts in practice.* Boston: Houghton-Mifflin Co.

Rogers, C. (1965). *Client-centred therapy: Its current practice, implications and theory.* Boston: Houghton-Mifflin Co.

Schlaff, C. (1993). From dependency to self-advocacy: Redefining disability. *American Journal of Occupational Therapy, 47,* 943-948.

Schroeder, D. H., & Bloom, L. J. (1979). Attraction to therapy and therapist credibility as a function of therapy orientation. *Journal of Clinical Psychology, 35,* 683-686.

Symington, D. (1994). Megatrends in rehabilitation: A Canadian perspective. *International Journal of Rehabilitation Research, 17,* 1-14.

Trombly, C. (1993). Anticipating the future: Assessment of occupational function. *American Journal of Occupational Therapy, 47,* 253-257.

United Nations (1983). *World program of action concerning disabled persons.* New York: Author.

Wallerstein, N. (1992). Powerlessness, empowerment, and health: Implications for health promotion programs. *American Journal of Health Promotion, 6*(3), 197-205.

Walton, K. M., Schwab, L. O., Cassatt-Dunn, M. A., & Wright, V. K. (1980). Techniques and concepts: Independent living. Perceptions by professionals in rehabilitation. *Journal of Rehabilitation, 46*(3), 57-63.

Wanigaratne, S., & Barker, C. (1995). Clients' preferences for styles of therapy. *British Journal of Clinical Psychology, 34,* 215-222.

Williams, G. H. (1983). The movement for independent living: An evaluation and critique. *Social Science and Medicine, 1,* 1003-1010.

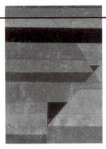

Chapter Content Outline

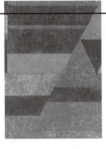

Abstract

Occupational therapy, with its focus on enabling and improving occupational performance, has been implicitly oriented toward well-being since its inception. Its core values and practices endorse prevention and health maintenance, and these issues need to be addressed explicitly over the entire lifespan. Changes in health care delivery demand more focus on prevention throughout the continuum of care, beginning in the acute care setting and focusing increasingly on community settings. This chapter discusses resources, trends, and public health functions that provide a foundation for strengthening a prevention and health maintenance approach to occupational therapy. Information is provided about resources, theories and applications that examine health as a community and social issue, not just a medical care concern. Theoretical approaches to behavior change are described for possible application by occupational therapists. Therapist roles are discussed, followed by examples of programs that address health promotion and prevention across the lifespan to illustrate the concepts and techniques from this chapter.

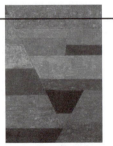

Key Terms

Prevention: Primary, secondary and tertiary

Health promotion

Secondary conditions

Agent-host-environment framework

Incidence & prevalence

Needs assessment approaches

Key informant approach

Community forum

Rates under treatment

Social indicator approach

Social Learning Theory

Self-efficacy

Health Belief Model

Community empowerment

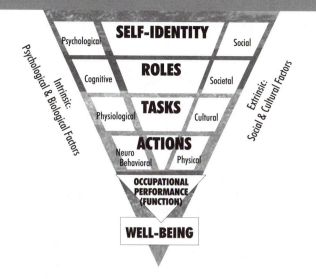

CHAPTER 22

Prevention of Disability and Maintenance of Health

Kathy Kniepmann, EdM, MPH, CHES, OTR/C

OBJECTIVES

The information in this chapter is intended to help the reader:

1. describe the three levels of prevention and explain health promotion, health education, and secondary conditions

2. identify key national resources and describe their implications for occupational therapy's efforts to address health promotion and prevention

3. describe needs assessment techniques that could be used by an occupational therapist for program planning

4. explain Social Learning Theory, the Health Belief Model, and community empowerment as approaches to behavior change for health promotion or prevention

5. relate the public health/community framework to the practice of occupational therapy

6. identify ways that occupational therapists can address prevention and health promotion throughout the lifespan and across the continuum of care.

> *"We are a profession possessing knowledge that is particularly necessary to maintain the health of people. To move from therapist to health agent demands us to change but to change in a forward, positive way...we must be willing to know more."*
>
> Finn, 1972

Introduction

Several decades ago there was growing concern about safety in a city on a mountaintop accessible only by dangerous, winding roads. This community had an increasing number of accidents and injuries, especially at night. The hospital built a larger emergency room and a modern trauma unit. They expanded emergency services and organized a patrol to call for help immediately with accidents, and later expanded their rehabilitation services. The hospital modernized the ambulance system, and improved their service coordination in exemplary ways. Several doctors gave conference presentations about their model services for trauma care and wrote articles in important journals. They won several awards and had national acclaim for this work. A therapist however, suggested that the community look at changing the bigger picture. She recommended better lighting for roads, more guardrails, improved driver's education, and wider roads with less hairpin turns. She also suggested developing a public transportation system which could decrease the number of accidents by inexperienced or inebriated drivers and provide options for people who had difficulty with vision or decreased reaction time. The health providers rejected these suggestions, retorting that they needed to address health issues, not road design, education, or transportation systems.

This tale from public health mythology dramatizes problems of the twentieth-century U.S. health care system. Financing mechanisms have supported a remedial approach to medical and health care. Services have been designed reactively, responding to problems rather than addressing causes or contributory factors. Medical knowledge and skill in remedial care has expanded dramatically, with extensive resources for managing infectious diseases, trauma, and acute care. This expansion has had definite benefits, but many drawbacks as well. As a physician from the Institute of Medicine wrote, "the success of curative and corrective medical strategies has proved a necessary but not sufficient component of enhanced health care" (Thier, 1990, p. S136). This tide has been shifting, as health management trends and national initiatives are pushing for prevention, health promotion, and a community focus for the health care system. Factors such as the aging of the population, increased rates of chronic diseases, soaring health care costs, and increased rates of survival from spinal cord injury, head injury, and other trauma have mandated a shift to prevention in response to a changing society (Caserta, 1995; Daltroy & Liang, 1993; DeJong, 1995; McLeroy, Bibeau, Steckler & Glanz, 1988;

Bibliographic citation of this chapter: Kniepmann, K. (1997). Prevention of disability and maintenance of health. In C. Christiansen & C. Baum (Eds.), *Occupational therapy: Enabling function and well-being* (2nd ed.). Thorofare, NJ: SLACK Incorporated.

Marge, 1988; Rothman & Levine, 1992; Tarlov & Pope, 1991; US Department of Health and Human Services, 1990; Yang, Fink, Mirsch, Robbins & Rubenstein, 1995).

The philosophy, history, knowledge, and skills of occupational therapy places the profession in an ideal position to serve as primary care providers and community health agents. Occupational therapists can play key roles in the design of data collection and surveillance systems, in planning and implementing community needs assessment, and in advocacy—both for specific clients or constituencies and for society, by influencing policy formation, program design, implementation, and evaluation. As community activists, occupational therapists can educate people who are at risk, or those who have health problems, to help them maximize their occupational performance and quality of life. As essential members of interdisciplinary service delivery teams, occupational therapists can provide innovative, effective leadership for the design and management of programs for health promotion and prevention. By basing these programs on current knowledge and designing them soundly to test new questions, they formulate ways to improve the health of individuals, communities, and society.

This chapter will define key terminology in health promotion and prevention and describe essential resource documents. Core functions of public health will be explained, followed by a description of selected theoretical approaches to health promotion and prevention. Roles will be identified for occupational therapists to enhance health and prevent problems that interfere with success in daily living. Descriptions of selected programs will be provided to illustrate prevention and health promotion potential for occupational therapy.

Terminology

The terms prevention, health promotion and wellness are used many ways. This chapter will use the following definitions.

Prevention, in a narrow sense, means averting the development of disease. In more common use, it consists of measures that limit the progression of disease at any point along its course (Rothman & Levine, 1992). Prevention can be differentiated into three levels—primary, secondary, and tertiary (Figure 22-1).

Primary prevention is geared to supporting or protecting the health and well being of society at large. Efforts are designed to avoid "onset of pathologic processes by reducing susceptibility, controlling exposure to disease-causing agents, and eliminating or at least minimizing behaviors and environmental factors that increase the risk of disease or injury that can cause disabling conditions" (Tarlov & Pope, 1991). *Secondary prevention* directs efforts to populations who are considered "at risk." This involves the early detection of a

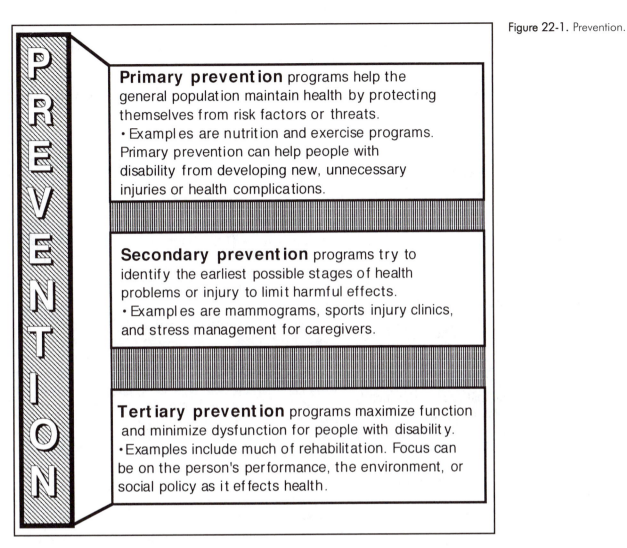

Figure 22-1. Prevention.

potential health problem, followed by the implementation of interventions that are designed to halt, reverse, or at least slow the progression of that condition (Tarlov & Pope, 1991). Examples are immunization of at risk populations (such as flu shots for seniors and health care workers) and screening for hypertension. Secondary prevention can also include programs designed to help build skills for people at risk, such as with parenting classes for teens who may be at high risk for stress and parenting difficulties. *Tertiary prevention* strives to maximize function and minimize the detrimental effects of illness or injury. This could be done by focusing on the person's function, the environment as it effects the person's behavior, or social policy as it effects individual and group health. *Disability in America* urges a more active integration of rehabilitation with public health to address tertiary prevention for people with disabilities, explaining that:

...modifying or eliminating social and physical obstacles to personal autonomy and societal partici-

pation present opportunities for prevention strategies that are not often enough accepted into the traditional province of public health. Measures designed to foster independent living and help ensure a reasonable quality of life should clearly be major elements of disability prevention policies and strategies. (Tarlov & Pope, 1991, p. 107)

Health is defined holistically by the World Health Organization as "the extent to which an individual or group is able, on the one hand, to realize aspirations and satisfy needs, and, on the other hand, to change or cope with the environment. Health is, therefore, seen as a resource for everyday life ... a positive concept emphasizing social and personal resources, as well as physical capacities" (World Health Organization, 1986a, p. 74). This parallels the perspectives of many leaders in occupational therapy, particularly Wilcock, an international leader based in Australia, who states that occupation helps people "adapt to environmental changes and to flourish as individuals" (Wilcock, 1993, p.17) and views the balanced use of capacities as essential for health and survival.

Health education is any combination of educational, organizational, economic, and environmental supports for behavior conducive to health (Green & Johnson, 1983). The health education process is that continuum of learning which enables people, as individuals and as members of social structures, to voluntarily make decisions, modify behaviors, and change social conditions in health-enhancing ways (Joint Committee on Health Education Terminology, 1991).

Health promotion relates individual lifestyle to health status, with a focus on individual behavior that can influence one's health in a broad sense.

Disability in America explains health promotion as a means of health maintenance and enhancement (Tarlov & Pope, 1991). Occupational therapy literature includes an expanded perspective, describing it as "the practice of informing, educating, facilitating behavioral change, and using cultural support so people can assume responsibility for living a lifestyle that is centered on optimal well-being" (American Occupational Therapy Association, 1989, p. 806). Jaffe identifies health promotion as a core philosophical orientation of the profession and urges occupational therapists to "use their many skills to develop techniques and programs that enhance health, prevent disease, and improve the social climate that fosters and promotes a healthy society" (Jaffe, 1985, p. 502).

The Ottawa Charter, developed from the first international conference on health promotion in 1986, emphasizes a much broader approach to health than through medical care by the health sector (World Health Organization [WHO], 1986b). Conference participants concurred that health promotion needs to include efforts in five arenas: 1) building of healthy public policy; 2) creation of supportive environments; 3) strengthening of community development; 4) educating for enhanced life skills — particularly to help people "cope with chronic illness and injuries" so they can "make choices conducive to health" (WHO, 1986b, p. iv); and 5) reorienting health services beyond clinical and curative services to focus on the needs of the whole person.

Health promotion and *disease prevention* are defined together as "the aggregate of all purposeful activities designed to improve personal and public health through a combination of strategies, including the competent implementation of behavioral change strategies, health education, health protection measures, risk factor detection, health enhancement and health maintenance" (Joint Committee on Health Education Terminology, 1991, p. 99).

Secondary conditions, sometimes called secondary disabilities, can include pathology, impairments, or functional limitations. They are physical or mental health problems that derive from the primary disabling condition. The Institute of Medicine report states that individuals with disabling conditions have a 'narrow margin of health' which requires attention to prevent secondary conditions that unnecessarily increase the severity of the disability (Tarlov & Pope, 1991).

CURRENT MANDATES FOR A SHIFT OF SERVICES

Occupational therapists have made major contributions to the design and delivery of rehabilitation services or tertiary prevention. They can make even a more dramatic contribution to the formulation of research questions and implementation of studies to improve tertiary prevention (Baum, 1991). Effective emergency and acute care can prevent death, but rehabilitation determines the quality of life and can prevent secondary disabilities (Snell, 1993). With decreasing lengths of stay, attention to secondary and primary prevention in the community is essential for the future of occupational therapy. The profession has a knowledge and skill base, as well as a philosophy, that is ideal for addressing primary and secondary prevention as well as health promotion (AOTA, 1979; Finn, 1972; Grossman, 1991; Jaffe, 1985; Johnson, 1986; Learnard & Devereaux, 1992; Letts, Fraser, Finlayson & Walls, 1993; Reitz, 1992; Rothman & Levine, 1992; Townsend, 1991; Wiemer, 1972).

Statistics and economics press health professionals to address prevention and health promotion. Approximately 34 to 43 million U.S. citizens have some kind of disability that affects their ability to function (Tarlov & Pope, 1991). For an unmeasured number of those people, ability may be limited much more by external factors such as attitudes, policies, and environmental barriers. Disability costs the nation almost $200 billion annually in medical care and lost productivity (Tarlov & Pope, 1991). Having an activity limitation more than doubles the average number of physician visits per year (National Center for Health Statistics, 1981). The toll from costs of lost productivity, lost taxes, increased spending on expensive remediation and especially human suffering is enormous and much may be avoidable (Tarlov & Pope, 1991; U.S. Department of Health and Human Services, 1990). Health education and public health experts bemoan the lack of empirical evidence about the effectiveness of prevention, especially in the community (Tarlov & Pope, 1991; Clark & McLeroy, 1995). A major challenge for all health professions is to determine what kinds of programs make a difference, for whom, and which professions or teams are best qualified to develop and implement such services.

KEY NATIONAL INITIATIVES AND RESOURCES

Over the past decade, major national initiatives have focused efforts in the prevention and health promotion arena. The most important documents have come from the Office of the Surgeon General, the U.S. Department of Health and Human Services—Public Health Service, the Institute of Medicine, the Pew Commission, WHO's Healthy Communities and Healthy Toronto 2000, and the Centers for Disease Control and Prevention. These documents will be highlighted, with discussion of their implications for occupational therapy.

Healthy People 2000

Healthy People 2000 National Health Promotion and Disease Prevention Objectives offer a major guiding force for the development of health promotion and prevention efforts. This breakthrough document grew from *Healthy People*, the 1979 U.S. Surgeon General's Report, which was followed by an agenda for the 1980's: *Promoting Health/Preventing Disease: Objectives for the Nation.* Follow up has shown some improvement, but underlined the need for more defined objectives with surveillance and data systems. Healthy People 2000 is the culmination of over three years of effort with all 50 state health departments, a consortium of over 300 national organizations, and 7 regional hearings for testimony from hundreds of individuals and organizations. Over 10,000 people contributed to the total process. Healthy People lists specific targets to improve the health of the nation for each objective. Occupational therapists should be familiar with these objectives and identify ways they can make essential contributions to improving their community and the nation's health (Figure 22-2).

Three major goals guide the 22 objective areas of Healthy People 2000 (p. 43):

1. Increase the span of healthy life for all Americans;
2. reduce health disparities among Americans and
3. achieve access to preventive services for all Americans.

This document identifies people with disabilities as a special population, emphasizing the need to "prevent the longer-term consequences of functional impairments that can severely affect the quality of one's life" (U.S. Department of Health and Human Services, 1990, p. 39). The health promotion needs for this population are accentuated by the risk for future problems from secondary conditions that could increase functional limitations and decrease occupational performance. The report cites the lack of adequate rehabilitation or maintenance therapy as significant factors contributing to secondary health problems, providing a strong plea for occupational therapy involvement.

Healthy People 2000
priority areas

Health Promotion
Physical Activity and Fitness
Nutrition
Tobacco
Alcohol and Other Drugs
Family Planning
Mental Health and Mental Disorders
Violent and Abusive Behavior
Educational and Community Based Programs

Health Protection
Unintentional Injuries
Occupational Safety and Health
Environmental Health
Food and Drug Safety
Oral Health

Preventive Services
Maternal and Infant Health
Heart Disease
Cancer
Diabetes and Chronic Disabling Conditions
HIV Infection
Sexually Transmitted Diseases
Immunization and Infectious Diseases
Clinical Preventive Services

Figure 22-2. Healthy People 2000 priority areas. From U.S. Department of Health & Human Services, Public Health Services (1990). Healthy People 2000 - National Health Promotion and Disease Prevention Objectives. Washington DC: U.S. Government Printing Office.

Many of the objectives include specific targets for people with disabilities. The following objectives challenge the occupational therapist to action as the effort fits well within their expertise and skills. Other objectives could foster interdisciplinary activities.

- Reduce to no more than 20% the proportion of people with disabilities who engage in no leisure-time physical activity.
- Reduce to less than 40% the proportion of people with disabilities aged 18 and older who experienced adverse health effects from stress within the past year.
- Reduce the incidence of secondary disabilities associated with injuries of the head and spinal cord to no more than 16 and 2.6 per 100,000 people, respectively.
- Increase to at least 40% the proportion of people with chronic and disabling conditions who receive formal

patient education including information about community and self-help resources as an integral part of the management of their condition.

Healthy Cities/Healthy Communities

Healthy Cities/Healthy Communities is an ecological approach that addresses health by examining the interrelationship of social policy as it shapes the human-made environment, which in turn affects individual persons within the community (Hancock, 1993a). This model has been utilized in many locales throughout Europe, North America, Australia, Asia, and Africa since its inception in 1986. The focus is more on social and political change to meet the needs of communities than on trying to change individual behaviors related to specific diagnostic related health risks. Although both person and environment are addressed, the emphasis is on community action to build environments that are more conducive to health of all community members. Hancock explains that:

> ...a healthy city is not necessarily one that has high health status, though that is important; rather, it is one that is conscious of health, striving continually to be more healthy and to take health into account in all decisions- in other words, healthy public policy at the local level (Hancock, 1993b).

Local government, with high level participation by its citizens, can develop policies that set the stage by assuring social, political, environmental, and economic factors that are conducive to health. Other community factors to address include a stable and sustainable ecosystem, community empowerment and participation, and urban planning (Hancock, 1993b).

Occupational therapists have valuable knowledge and skills to contribute to the healthy communities movement as role model participants in planning, as consultants, and through encouragement of self-advocacy among citizens who may feel disenfranchised due to disability or risk for disability. Enactment of healthy cities principles could include community gardening to improve nutrition through citizen involvement as well as development of shelters for homeless persons and literacy programs (Hancock, 1988).

Disability in America

Disability in America: Toward a National Agenda for Prevention (Tarlov & Pope, 1991) proposes a comprehensive national program of disability prevention that "goes beyond the medical model to consider and address the needs of people with disabling conditions after those conditions exist and after they have been 'treated' and 'rehabilitated'." (p. v). Throughout the publication, the authors emphasize a view of

disability that is not limited to the person but is "a social issue and not just a physical condition ... a person is not always disabled by paralysis but more commonly by the way he or she is treated by others and restricted from performing normal social roles" (p. vi). Such a perspective on disability prevention directs occupational therapists to go beyond performance components to address environmental factors; to help clients develop self-advocacy and other coping skills; and to educate society in ways that will decrease social barriers.

Disability in America recommends a comprehensive approach for prevention of secondary conditions in people with disabilities that addresses: 1) the organization and delivery of services (including independent living centers); 2) availability of appropriate assistive technology, as well as adequate training in the use of these technologies; 3) adoption of health-promoting behavior; 4) education (of the public, health care professionals and of people with disability); and 5) consideration of environmental factors (social and physical).

Several of these recommendations would benefit from the expertise of knowledgeable and skilled occupational therapists (Table 22-1).

Practitioners for 2005

Healthy America: Practitioners for 2005, an agenda for action for U.S. health professional schools (Shugars, O'Neil & Bader, 1991), defines an exciting, innovative vision of health professionals trained to address the changing needs of society. They compellingly predict a need for professionals with expanded abilities and new attitudes by the year 2005. The competencies they suggest are particularly relevant to health promotion and prevention endeavors and address issues basic to occupational therapy. Selected competencies are:

- Care for the community's health
- Practice prevention —primary and secondary, for all people.
- Involve patients and families in the decision-making process
- Promote healthy lifestyles
- Assess and use technology appropriately
- Understand the role of the physical environment
- Emphasize primary care

Healthy America declares that the health care system or its many microsystems in the United States has paid minimal attention to prevention or to social and emotional factors, with too much distance between health professionals and patients or families. It urges containing incurable diseases or conditions in ways that facilitate maximal quality of life. The Pew report is geared toward the education of health professionals, but its outline of competencies and issues should guide ongoing professional development to address health promotion and prevention in community settings.

Centers for Disease Control and Prevention

A central mission of the Centers for Disease Control and Prevention (CDC) is to promote healthy lifestyles and prevent unnecessary disease, disability, and injury. The CDC has a variety of resources for research and program development, including extensive information on the Internet. It initiated an Injury Control Program in 1985 with research focus on prevention, acute care and rehabilitation. Soon after, they created the Disabilities Prevention Program to reduce the incidence and severity of primary and secondary disabilities and to promote independence, productivity, and community integration for people with disabilities. This program, in the National Center for Environmental Health, establishes surveillance systems and identifies risk factors. It is also involved in developing interventions to prevent secondary conditions and funding of state capacity building projects. CDC is federally funded and its resources are publicly available.

CONDITIONS LEADING TO ACTIVITY LIMITATIONS

As life expectancy increases in the United States, the number of people with disabilities is growing. People are living longer and medical services are dramatically improving the survival rates from trauma. National Health Interview Survey data from 1988 showed that these percentages of people with activity limitations listed the following categories as the main causes of their disability (Figure 22-3):

- Mobility limitations: 38%
- Chronic diseases (diabetes, cancer, respiratory, or circulatory): 8%
- Sensory limitations: 8%

The prevalence of the main causes of disability varies according to age grouping (Tarlov & Pope, 1991, p. 59) (Figure 22-4).

Occupational therapists are well qualified to help people address each of these conditions in ways that maximize occupational performance and thereby prevent or minimize difficulties with the client's goals for a meaningful life. By utilizing health promotion, prevention, and public health principles and knowledge, occupational therapists can help develop important strategies and resources to support maximal function, individual or family choices for improved quality of life, and a healthier society.

A FRAMEWORK FOR PREVENTION AND HEALTH PROMOTION

Wilcock (1993), along with many other occupational therapists, emphasizes the importance of balancing work,

---

TABLE 22-1

List of Recommendations from National Agenda for the Prevention of Disability

Organization and Coordination

Develop leadership of National Disability Prevention Program at CDC

Develop an enhanced role for the private sector

Establish a national advisory committee

Establish a federal interagency council

Critically assess progress periodically

Surveillance

Develop a conceptual framework and standard measures of disability

Develop a national disability surveillance system

Revise the National Health Interview Survey

Conduct a comprehensive longitudinal survey of disability

Develop disability indices

Research

Develop a comprehensive research program

Emphasize longitudinal research

Conduct research on socioeconomic and psychosocial disadvantage

Expand research on preventive and therapeutic interventions

Upgrade training for research on disability prevention

Access to Care and Preventive Services

Provide comprehensive health services to all mothers and children

Provide effective family planning and prenatal services

Develop new health service delivery strategies for people with disabilities

Develop new health promotion models for people with disabilities

Foster local capacity building and demonstration projects

Continue effective prevention programs

Provide comprehensive vocational services

Professional and Public Education

Upgrade medical education and training of physicians

Upgrade the training of allied professionals

Establish a program of grants for education and training

Provide more public education on the prevention of disability

Provide more training opportunities for family members and personal attendants of people with disabling conditions

Reprinted with permission from *Disability in America.* Copyright 1991 by the National Academy of Sciences. Courtesy of the National Academy Press, Washington, D.C.

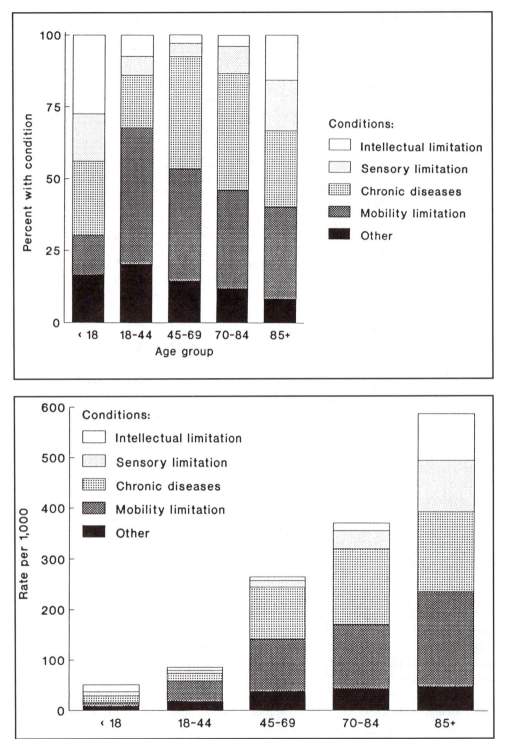

Figure 22-3. Prevalence of main causes of activity limitation, by age, 1983-1985. Calculated from LaPlante, 1988. Reprinted with permission from *Disability in America*. Copyright 1991 by the National Academy of Sciences. Courtesy of the National Academy Press, Washington DC.

Figure 22-4. Percentage distribution of main causes of activity limitation, by age, 1983-1985. Calculated from LaPlante, 1988. Reprinted with permission from *Disability in America*. Copyright 1991 by the National Academy of Sciences. Courtesy of the National Academy Press, Washington, D.C.

self care, and leisure for a productive, happy life. Occupational therapists must accept the challenge to focus on prevention. The Community Practice Team at the Program in Occupational Therapy of Washington University School of Medicine emphasizes that obstacles in the home or community can interfere with occupational performance and quality of life, proposing that such "difficulties are often persistent and complex, requiring solutions at the community level... which can address both personal and environmental factors affecting the performance of meaningful activities"

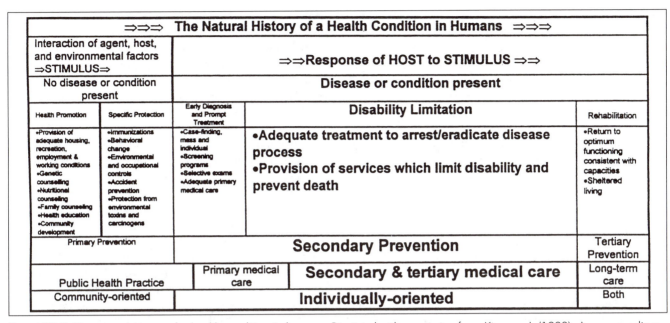

Figure 22-5. The natural history of a health condition in humans. Reprinted with permission from Kimmey, J. (1993). A new paradigm for health reform. Unpublished manuscript.

(Community Practice Team, 1996). The team includes experienced occupational therapists working in partnership with community agencies, professionals from a variety of backgrounds, and lay people to develop model programs that promote maximal health of individuals with disability or who are at risk.

Recent attempts at prevention have occurred primarily in settings such as hospitals, doctor's offices, or clinics. However, health is defined by performance in many other settings. Occupational therapists must identify ways to move into the day-to-day settings where health habits, illness, and injury occur. Community-based practice was outlined by Leavell and Clark in their 1965 publication of *Preventive Medicine for the Doctor in His Community: An Epidemiological Approach* (Leavell & Clark, 1965). Understanding the natural history of diseases or health problems in populations was emphasized as paramount to prevention and health promotion. They formulated a model for levels of prevention based on agent-host-environment interaction. That model, updated by Kimmey in the early 1990s, provides a paradigm that can be used to define important roles and intervention opportunities for occupational therapy (Figure 22-5).

The agent-host-environment framework from the field of public health examines the interrelationship of constructs that influence health status. The *host* can be the individual person, a group, or a community. Host factors include genetics, nutrition, health habits, general physical condition, occupation, and socioeconomic status. *Agent factors* or vectors

are the causes of illness or injury. Examples of agent factors include viruses or fungi, noise, hazardous equipment, poor lighting, and psychological stressors. *Environment*, in this framework, refers to the general surroundings such as living conditions or work settings that can shape host-agent interaction (Kimmey, 1993). Changes in any of those three arenas —agent, host, or environment—can create an imbalance that interferes with health and therefore is likely to create problems for performance.

Health promotion supports host or person factors (behavior, knowledge, attitudes, of individuals or groups) as well as environmental factors that enhance health. Health protection increases host resistance; such measures would include immunization programs, use of bike helmets, and passenger restraints. Leavell and Clark (1965) proposed that an imbalance or changed relationship between agent, host, and environment creates a stimulus that may interfere with health. Based on this model, an evolving mandate for the community occupational therapy practitioner is to assure provision of programs that support development of skills in coping, self-care, activity, and self-advocacy that will maximize the quality of life and minimize suffering in a cost-effective fashion. Access to primary care, as well as screening, is important to prevent problems that can cause disabilities. This can also prevent secondary conditions from developing in people with disabilities or minimize the effects of secondary conditions through secondary prevention efforts such as screening.

When changes of individuals' health status cause illness or injury, rehabilitation can help achieve function that is compatible with their capacities and interests. In this context, rehabilitation serves as tertiary prevention by limiting suffering and maximizing occupational performance in ways that are meaningful to individuals, families, or groups. Tertiary prevention is a proven expertise of occupational therapists. A major challenge for occupational therapists is to find innovative, effective, and economical ways to "move upstream" by transferring the knowledge and skill base of occupational therapy to address all levels of prevention. This is most efficiently and effectively done with a shift from a purely individual service orientation to a community-oriented approach that addresses personal, interpersonal, and collective health issues.

PRACTICING IN THE COMMUNITY

Community means more than a geographic location for practice, but includes an orientation to collective health, social priorities, and different modes for service provision. In her 1971 Eleanor Clarke Slagle lecture, Finn (1972) emphasized the need for community-based prevention programs, explaining that occupational therapists need to increase their knowledge about primary institutions such as schools, families, the law, businesses, and the church so they can "understand more fully their functions, their goals, their policies, and their methods of operation" (p. 62). Such knowledge will enable them to facilitate communication and collaboration with community resources for meaningful and effective programs.

An understanding of community resources is essential to ensure a partnership in program planning and implementation. As the Pew Commission emphasizes, "(p)ractitioners should have a broad understanding of the determinants of health...and be able to work with others in the community to integrate a range of services and activities that promote, protect and improve health" (Shugars et al., 1991, p. 18).

CORE PUBLIC HEALTH FUNCTIONS

Occupational therapists are based primarily in rehabilitation facilities, hospitals, or school settings according to the AOTA (Member Data Survey, 1990). The multidisciplinary field of public health is population based and addresses communities with responsibility for the core functions of *assessment, policy development*, and *assurance*. In public health, assurance includes health protection, community health promotion, health service quality assurance, targeted outreach, and service coordination. Health professionals from many disciplines are involved with public health. Occupational therapists can contribute to its core functions and be active partici-

pants in public health efforts to improve community health. The following definitions introduce public health foundations.

Community assessment involves gathering information about the health status of a community, its risks or hazards, needs, and available resources as well as utilization patterns. It has similarities to the occupational therapy process of patient/client evaluation— gathering information about problems, resources, priorities, and activity patterns. The "community" could be a geographic entity (town or city) or it could be a housing project, a neighborhood, a school and its surrounding resources for children, or a workplace.

Determining the extent of various health problems in a community involves epidemiological study of patterns of illness or injury. Two important epidemiological measures are incidence and prevalence. *Incidence* is the number of newly developed cases or events of a given illness/injury in a population during a designated time period. It is expressed as the number of new "cases" divided by the total number at risk (Hennekens & Buring, 1987). For example, the incidence of hip fractures or Colles' fractures may rise in icy winter months. *Prevalence* is the proportion of people who currently have a given condition, calculated as the number of existing cases of a disease divided by the total population at a given point in time (Hennekens & Buring, 1987).

Data on the incidence and prevalence of functional limitations, disabilities, and occupational performance problems in a community could help to identify possible needs for resources to address health promotion and prevention goals.

Prevalence does not necessarily indicate need, but it can help define populations who merit further attention for potential benefit from preventive services (Patrick, 1994). Discussion with community members would help determine whether further action should be pursued. Monitoring incidence and prevalence over time could help determine the effects of programs. Incidence and prevalence data may be available from local health departments, managed care plans, or other agencies.

Community needs assessment should not be done only by outside experts. Community members should take active responsibility for planning and implementing programs that influence their health (DeMars, 1992; Simmons, Nelson, Roberts, Salisbury, Kane-Williams, & Benson, 1989; Twible, 1992; Institute for Alternative Futures, 1992; U.S. Department of Health and Human Services, 1991; Steckler, Allegrante, Altman, Brown, Burdine, Goodman, & Jorgensen, 1995; Mullen, Evans, Forster, Gottlieb, Kreuter, Moon, O'Rourke, & Strecher 1995; Simmons-Morton, Greene & Gottlieb, 1995). Needs assessment and resource development should engage members of the target audience to increase investment and to assure that programs are designed to meet their needs. The target audience could be the community at large or it could be a designated group such as people with similar risks or conditions. Occupational therapists can serve as consultants and catalysts for needs assessment and planning, involving community members in the process.

Needs assessment can also be done to gather information about a specific health issue or a population of interest. For example, an occupational therapist working with toddlers who have disabilities may become concerned about developing community resources for support and education of the toddlers' parents. *Needs assessment approaches* (Table 22-2) that would be valuable for an occupational therapist working in the community include key informant approach, community forum, social indicators, rates under treatment, and surveys (Warheit, Bell & Schwab, 1977; Moore, 1987; McKillip, 1987) as well as review of relevant literature to utilize and build on the existing body of knowledge. Using a combination of techniques for information gathering from a variety of sources is important. This helps construct a clearer and broader picture of the nature and extent of needs in the population of interest. Occupational therapists, with their understanding of person-environment-occupation fit, could help formulate questions and select appropriate assessment techniques to determine what kinds of services, resources, or activities should be developed to maximize a community's health. Community strengths and resources should also be noted. Such information drives planning of programs to meet the needs of a given community while utilizing state-of-the-art principles and the existing occupational therapy body of knowledge.

The *key informant approach* to needs assessment asks information of individuals who are selected for their assumed familiarity with the needs of the community as a whole or with the target population for a potential program. Although this process may be less time-consuming than other approaches, the informants do not necessarily represent the community adequately and may bias the findings. Exclusion of certain individuals or representatives from some groups in the community could cause subsequent alienation. Subgroups of the community may be overlooked.

Community forums invite any residents to discuss their concerns at open "town hall" type meetings. This demonstrates an attempted partnership with the entire community and can increase general investment, although disadvantages include possible skewed attendance or participation.

Rates under treatment examines data from service delivery sites such as clinics, hospitals, schools, and mental health centers to ascertain who (sociodemographically) is using what kinds of services. Confidentiality policies may limit access to information, and this data does not indicate who might be getting care elsewhere. The *social indicators approach* examines data from public records—census, county health department, police records, housing offices. An advantage is not needing to reinvent the wheel with new sur-

veys or collection techniques; a disadvantage is that the measures are less direct and the reliability or validity may be questionable (Warheit, Bell, & Schwab, 1977). *Surveys* can be done to collect information on specific questions from a sample or an entire population. Written questionnaires or phone interviews can be used. Directness and control of questions are advantages, but expense and possibility of low response are disadvantages. Other techniques such as focus groups, nominal group process, delphi method and interpretive structural modeling also can be used for needs assessment. They are described well by Moore (1987).

After gathering information about community health concerns and needs, the next step in needs assessment is identifying existing resources that are available to meet the population's identified needs. What kinds of services are currently available, in what settings? Are people aware of the services/programs that exist to meet the needs of the community? Are there barriers to access (price, hours, stigma)? How much are they used? Can they be expanded, or are new services needed?

For *policy development*, another core function of public health, occupational therapists' input could help assure social policy that supports maximal occupational performance of all citizens. Occupational therapists need to monitor legislation, attentive to its implications for environments that are conducive to performance and responsive to diverse human needs. Input to the political process is essential.

THEORETICAL APPROACHES TO BEHAVIOR CHANGE

Health education and psychology provide several theories that can guide the design of community health interventions. Social learning theory addresses individual health behavior change, particularly through group interactions, and the health belief model proposes a framework for understanding decisions about preventive or protective actions. An additional approach, community empowerment, examines health as a social resource, with health improvements involving active participation of the entire community.

Social Learning Theory and Self-Efficacy

Social learning theory (Figure 22-6) includes concepts and strategies that have been used to guide the development of programs for skill development related to a wide range of health behaviors including chronic disease management (Simmons et al, 1989; Lorig & Holman, 1993; Mahowald, Steveken, Young, & Ytterberg, 1988; Robertson & Keller, 1992) and has been used specifically to support the development of health-promoting behaviors in persons with disabil-

TABLE 22-2

Sample Needs Assessment

Scenario: An occupational therapist has been contacted by the director of a retirement community to determine what kinds of programs would help the residents maintain or improve their health as they are getting older, developing more symptoms, and "aging in place." The director would like recommendations about the needs of the community and what kinds of new programs should be developed.

Needs assessment helps to find out:
- What is the nature and extent of the problem or issue?
- What resources and strengths exist in this population or community?
- How well are current resources serving the needs of the population?
- What else should be done?
- How can the problems/issues best be addressed in this community?
- Who should be involved in further planning and implementation?

Note: Involving members of the "target population" in the needs assessment process can increase their investment in the program and their sense of ownership. This also makes the program development more responsive to them.

Target Population: Seniors living in the retirement community

Needs Assessment–Approaches and Techniques

Approach or technique	Source	Kinds of information
Literature review	Journals, Books, Internet	What kinds of programs have been developed for similar settings/ populations? Examine theory, techniques, effectiveness. What worked/ failed and why? Information will be tailored to address needs of this specific population
Surveys	Residents	What kinds of services programs would they like? Explore concerns, needs, values, interests, past experience with health or wellness programs. Ask about culture, health status, function, socialization, leisure activities
Surveys	Family/caregivers	What do they think would help the seniors maintain or improve quality of life? What are the seniors' main problems and what are their strengths? What would make it easier for these caregivers to manage? (Possibilities: respite, household assistance, self-care training, adaptations of the environment for safety and accessibility)
Community forum	People at open meeting	Responses to open-ended questions about existent services and needs. What would help residents stay healthy, get healthier, or lead a more satisfying life? Gather ideas for programs
Rates under treatment	Local clinics, mental health center	Confidentiality may limit access, but try to obtain statistics on rates of various diagnoses and functional problems—falls, insomnia, depression, nutritional problems, chronic diseases
Social Indicators	Census bureau Housing office — residency data Police records for area	Age structure and gender of the population; percent living alone, average duration of residency, rate of turnover, average household size/ composition; crime rates and times of risk, accident rates, data on elder abuse or domestic violence, possibly number of calls for lost persons

TABLE 22-2 (continued)

Sample Needs Assessment

| Key informants | People who know these folks: apartment managers, senior club officers, beauticians, barbers, activity leaders, dining hall staff, facility and maintenance crew | Behavior and personality of these seniors. What are they like? How do they like to learn, how do they express concerns, attitudes to change, help seeking behavior? What kinds of services and activities have been popular here and which have failed – any ideas why? What comments have you heard about services or health concerns? What kind of sub-groups are there here? Do they associate with each other during activities or do you think they would prefer separate activities by gender or religion for instance? How do these residents respond to outsiders? Are there opinion leaders in this community – who are they? |

Note: Health care professionals can also serve as key informants. For this scenario, possible questions would be: Do these seniors follow through on recommendations for health promotion and wellness? Who do they turn to for advice about symptom management?

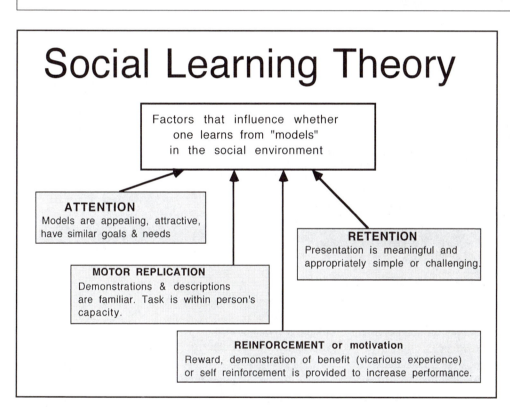

Figure 22-6. Social Learning Theory.

ities (Stuifbergen & Becker, 1994). Bandura developed social learning theory, sometimes called social cognitive theory, as a means of explaining the acquisition of new behaviors, particularly from observational learning. He identified four factors that influence how people learn from watching others in their environments: Attention, retention, motor replication, and motivation or reinforcement. Each of these influences will be discussed. *Attention* is based on factors such as the model's attractiveness or similarity to one's self and one's needs or goals. *Retention* is essential for future use

of the information. The manner of presentation, including coherence, meaningfulness and appropriate level of simplicity or challenge all contribute to retention. *Motor replication* is important for behavioral learning. Mental images can more easily be translated into actions if the model and the instructor in the model utilize familiar actions or describe them in familiar ways. *Reinforcement* or *motivation* influences the likelihood of initially attempting and continually performing the modeled behavior. Reinforcement can be direct (in the form of a reward), vicarious (when the model demonstrates

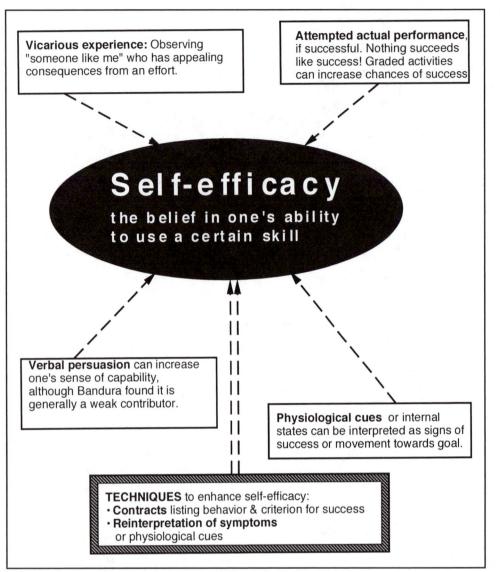

Figure 22-7. Self-efficacy.

Vicarious experience: Observing "someone like me" who has appealing consequences from an effort.

Attempted actual performance, if successful. Nothing succeeds like success! Graded activities can increase chances of success

Self-efficacy
the belief in one's ability to use a certain skill

Verbal persuasion can increase one's sense of capability, although Bandura found it is generally a weak contributor.

Physiological cues or internal states can be interpreted as signs of success or movement towards goal.

TECHNIQUES to enhance self-efficacy:
• **Contracts** listing behavior & criterion for success
• **Reinterpretation of symptoms** or physiological cues

experiencing benefits of the action), or self reinforcing (based on internal evaluation of the experience).

These four factors influence the likelihood that one will attempt to replicate new behaviors. Occupational therapists can include these factors in planning programs with clients to maximize their observational learning of skills for promoting their health and preventing secondary conditions.

Successful skill performance in therapy or an instructional setting is not necessarily linked to use of that skill in daily life. Unpredictable complications or barriers may deter the individual from using newly learned skills. Bandura found that actual day-to-day performance is influenced by a construct he named self-efficacy (Bandura, 1977;1986).

Self-efficacy is defined as a belief in one's ability to perform a given task successfully (Figure 22-7). It predicts the

likelihood that someone will attempt a given behavior and especially whether that person will continue working at it, despite possible difficulties. An understanding of self-efficacy can enable occupational therapists to enhance occupational performance of their clients (Gage & Polatajko, 1993). Unlike self-esteem, which is a more global construct, self-efficacy can be high for some skills and much lower for others, depending on a number of factors. Self-efficacy is based on four sources of information: vicarious experience, verbal persuasion, actual performance, and physiological cues.

Vicarious experience involves observation of someone else performing a task effectively. Particularly if it is someone who shares similar attributes ("someone like me"), vicarious experience can increase persons' beliefs in their own ability to perform a given task. Convincing communication, or *verbal per-*

suasion, can influence someone to feel more capable to perform a given skill. Bandura found that, although it can make some difference, it is the weakest contributor to perceived self-efficacy. Attempted *actual performance*, if successful, contributes significantly to one's sense of self-efficacy. As the adage goes, "nothing succeeds like success." An occupational therapist can evaluate the individual's performance components to determine strengths and capacities, then grade activities the client has chosen. This can set the stage for individuals or group members to try to perform familiar activities in new ways with success, thus contributing to self-efficacy. Interpretations of *physiological cues* or internal states can additionally influence one's perception of self-efficacy. If mild fatigue is interpreted as a sign of successful efforts, one's self-efficacy is likely to increase (i.e., "I did it right; I can do it again!"). That same state of fatigue could be interpreted by another person as a sign of strain and impending severe pain, thus decreasing one's perceived self-efficacy ("I blew it"; "This is going to kill me yet"; "I'll just never get it right").

Two techniques to enhance self-efficacy, contracting and reinterpretation of physiological cues, can be particularly useful to occupational therapists. *Contracting* can support goals that involve acquisition of new skills or change of behavior patterns (see Chapter 6). The Canadian Occupational Performance Measure provides such a tool as the client's goals become the focus of intervention. Contracts specify behaviors to be performed and a measurable criterion for success such as frequency and duration. This should involve a manageable challenge—something that will expand one's repertoire of behavior, but is realistic. In the Stanford Arthritis Self-Management Program (Lorig & Holman, 1993), participants defined contracts for each following week related to newly acquired information and skills for exercise, diet, stress management, or joint protection. Progress on the previous week's contract is reported back to the group, where members are rewarded with praise for success or are given group support and problem solving to address barriers for unattained goals. The feedback, problem solving and goal adjustment is important for skills mastery and self-efficacy. Contracting has been used for other wellness courses for people with chronic illnesses including the self-help management Community Wellness Class for people with multiple sclerosis, designed by faculty at The Washington University Program in Occupational Therapy (Neufeld, 1994).

Reinterpretation of symptoms or physiological cues can facilitate performance of new healthy behaviors and increased self-efficacy. At a cognitive level, a therapist can try to debunk myths about the likelihood of certain symptoms and their implications, based on research findings. Positive self talk can also shape one's reactions to symptoms and improve coping. In group programs or individually, a person could practice at positive interpretation of symptoms during guided role play. Relaxation training and guided imagery can also help counteract problematic internal states that interfere with performance of desired skills. Being aware of activity contraindications is important, as is instructing people on proper techniques and pacing. However, talking oneself through a task has long been a strategy to support new learning following a neurological deficit.

While working with individuals, groups, or in training peer trainers to lead programs, occupational therapists can address factors that facilitate observational learning. They can also design programs that support increased perceived self-efficacy for behavior that maximizes health. Contracting and reinterpretation of symptoms can also improve the acquisition of health-promoting behaviors and preventive skills.

Health Belief Model

The Health Belief Model was constructed to understand and predict preventive health behaviors or health promotion actions, especially related to specific health risks (Janz and Becker, 1984). It emphasizes four components (Figure 22-8). *Perceived severity* and *perceived susceptibility* are the individuals' assessments of the magnitude of the health threat and the likelihood of their personal vulnerability to the risk. *Barriers* and *benefits* of taking action are weighed in subjective ways. Examples of barriers include financial costs, efforts, stigma. Benefits could be long term, as with improved well being from exercise, or short term, as in the case of financial savings or decreased social ostracism from quitting smoking. A fifth component, *cues to action,* serves as a reminder of plans to pursue the health behavior. Placing exercise clothes beside the bed at night is a cue to action for morning exercise. Signs on the refrigerator about healthy snacks is a cue to improve eating habits. Someone who is trying to do stretching and repositioning at the computer terminal to decrease muscle strain and tension could set a buzzer or computer signal for designated intervals as a reminder or cue to take a stretch. Although it is intuitively appealing, the model does not adequately address social or environmental factors. Decisions and actual actions are not necessarily consistent. The Health Belief Model can play a role in development of materials or programs, but should not be used by itself. More recent users of the Health Belief Model have also addressed self-efficacy in their interventions (Rosenstock, Strecher & Becker, 1988).

Community Empowerment

Community empowerment provides a framework to examine the health education needs of groups or communities, particularly for disenfranchised or disadvantaged groups. It involves social action to enable people to gain mastery over their lives and health by changing their social and political environment (Kari & Michels, 1991; Labonte, 1989,

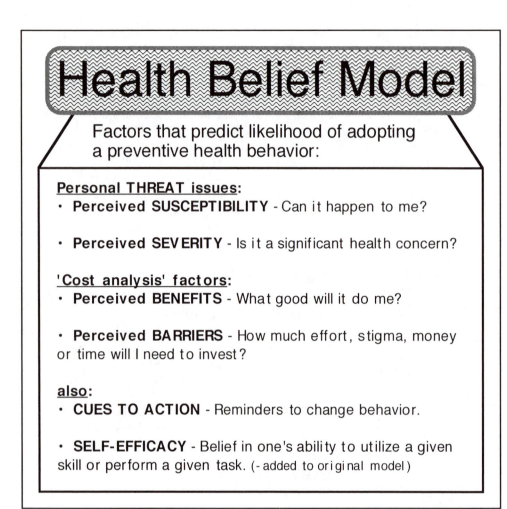

Figure 22-8. Health Belief Model.

1990; Minkler, 1989; Rousseau, 1993; Wallerstein & Bernstein, 1988). Community empowerment has foundations in community and social psychology as well as community organization, critical theory, and especially Paolo Freire's approach to literacy education. Freire (1985) developed innovative literacy programs for Brazilian peasants after finding only children's-type materials available that were foreign to the needs of adults. He chastised traditional education as a banking model with the expert teacher depositing selected chunks of information into passive students whose background was irrelevant to the process. Freire designed a system that actively involves students and teachers in collaboration. In his system, students are active agents, building knowledge and skills that integrate with past experiences that help them address future needs (Freire, 1985; McMurray, 1991; Shor, 1993; Shor & Freire, 1987).

Key components of community empowerment are listening, dialogue, and implementation of change (Figure 22-9). *Listening* to community members facilitates the educator/ health worker's understanding of the community's needs. Listening, rather than telling or directing, is essential to empowerment education. *Dialogue* with community members addresses concerns and problems identified. Tangible "codes" can be used to facilitate the dialogue, especially with low literacy groups or where language may be difficult. Codes could take many forms: role plays, stories, photos, or songs (Wallerstein & Bernstein, 1994). These codes stimulate dialogue with critical thinking about problems and action plans. Dialogue is followed by collective *implementation of change*.

Empowerment can address community organization, group development, political action, or personal behavior each of which can influence the health of individuals and the entire community. A prime example of community empowerment is the Independent Living movement, which has "enabled persons with disabilities to reframe as social pathology what previously had been framed as individual pathology. That is, disability was reconceptualized as resulting from a social environment that disregarded the existence of people with disabilities by making it difficult, if not impossible for them to participate in public life" (Robertson & Minkler, 1994, pp. 297-298). The model can be used in

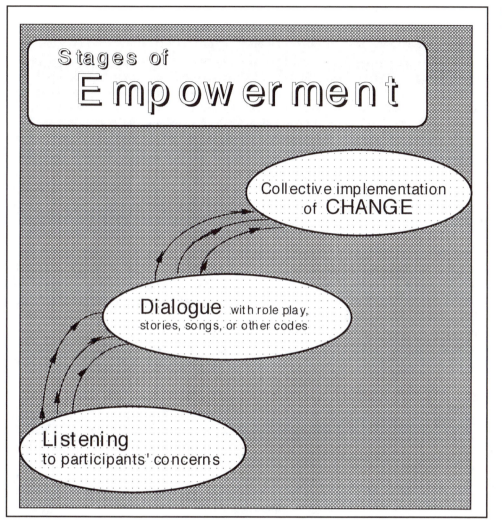

Figure 22-9. Stages of empowerment.

many settings. Healthy Cities/Healthy Communities, as described earlier in the chapter, utilizes the empowerment approach. Occupational therapists also used it to design a nursing home model of governance that helped residents increase their sense of control (Kari & Michels, 1991).

OCCUPATIONAL THERAPY ROLES

Prevention and health promotion are not new for occupational therapy. The founders of the profession supported a holistic approach that embraced wellness and health promotion, with services provided for groups as well as individuals (Reitz, 1992). Some of the new trends in health care enact the writings of Adolph Meyer and others who laid the foundation of occupational therapy in the 1920s. Occupational therapists in all institutional settings, even in acute care, can utilize principles and strategies of prevention and health promotion to foster self health management and empowerment. Client-

centered service delivery (Law, Baptiste & Mills, 1995) is a prime example. Bringing together individuals with similar conditions or goals for group sessions that involve shared leadership can also initiate self-help and empowerment.

Community settings offer special opportunities and challenges for health care. Over three decades ago, West identified several roles that occupational therapists needed to assume to address prevention including evaluator, consultant, supervisor, and researcher (West, 1967). In the Canadian Seniors' Health Promotion Project (Letts, Fraser, Finlayson, & Walls, 1993), occupational therapists add networking, collaborating, and planning to the list of occupational therapy roles. Today, with managed care and the growing emphasis on community health, occupational therapists must develop more opportunities for indirect service roles. Occupational therapists can act as consultants, program planners, staff trainers/educators, researchers, community health advisors, primary care providers, policy makers, case managers, and advocates—for individuals, groups, and communities. They need to collaborate with clients' families, employers, neighbors, and teachers with an active role in the community (Baum & Law, 1997).

The 1990 Member Data Survey from AOTA showed that the largest percentages of occupational therapists were in school systems and hospital or clinic settings. Health promotion and prevention initiated in these settings can lay the foundation for personal empowerment, self-efficacy, and therefore increased performance in daily living. Many other settings could provide even more important opportunities for occupational therapists to address prevention and health promotion in ways that could improve quality of life and the health of society. Businesses or factories could benefit from occupational therapists who provide ergonomic consultation. Facility managers, supervisors, and housing managers could be educated about how environment affects health and performance. Occupational therapists have training in compliance and accommodation strategies for the Americans with Disabilities Act (ADA). They need to be politically active with input to policy makers that ensures social policy and its enactment to guarantee access to resources that can enable maximal function by removing community barriers for all citizens.

PROGRAM EXAMPLES

Occupational therapy can make significant contributions to individuals' health throughout the life span using health promotion and prevention strategies. They can also promote healthier communities and a society that facilitates maximal performance and wellness of all citizens. Some examples of occupational therapy practice that illustrate the strategies and theories described in this chapter follow (Table 22-3).

Parent and Child Health

Most experts agree that play is essential for child development; it is the occupation of childhood (Reilly, 1974). Children with disabilities are often deprived of play opportunities, particularly free play, because of their functional limitations and their dependence on caregivers. Missiuna and Pollock propose that play deprivation could constitute a secondary disability by hindering occupational development (Missiuna & Pollock, 1991). They identified several barriers to free play for children with disabilities: limitations imposed by caregivers, physical and personal limitations of the child, environmental barriers, and social barriers. These barriers are risk factors which could be addressed by occupational therapy consultation with parents, teachers, and caregivers. Information can be provided about the child's capabilities and needs, ways to structure the environment, and selection of appropriate activities to facilitate active free play.

Parenting presents a variety of challenges and has been described as a neglected human occupation that could benefit from occupational therapy attention to the parents' perspectives (Llewellyn, 1994). Esdaile (1996) developed a community-based, play-focused intervention for mothers of preschoolers to address parent-child play interactions, reduce stress, and educate mothers on child development. Mothers attended ten weekly sessions to develop knowledge and skills in the following areas: learning through play; preschool behavior and imaginative activity; stress management and relaxation techniques for mothers and children; and use of structured activity for skill development and problem solving. Participants reported that the program was useful and enjoyable; several of them helped develop community play groups. The program had unanticipated secondary prevention effects: 23% of the participants subsequently linked into services for child or marital difficulties. Olson, Heany and Soppas-Hoffman (1989) implemented a community outreach activity group for at-risk mothers and children, demonstrating important potential contributions of occupational therapy for preventive psychiatry. Social learning theory principles and techniques were used with play activities to promote the development of adaptive behavior in mother-child interactions.

Occupational therapists, with knowledge of the developmental process, activity, and environment, can intervene to prevent disabilities in schools, home, and childcare settings. Schaaf and Davis (1992) describe multiple roles that occupational therapists can serve to promote health in children who are at risk or those who have disabilities. They propose a collaborative teaching approach involving child, parents, other caregivers, and the entire team. The authors cite the following goals for OT to promote health and wellness for children and families in any setting:

1. *Preventing or reducing the primary problems resulting directly from risk conditions*
2. *Preventing secondary problems by aiding the child in the development of appropriate adaptive skills or mechanisms*
3. *Encouraging parenting that reinforces positive developmental patterns*
4. *Strengthening family development ... and enhancing parent-child interactions and bonding*
5. *Facilitating the child's own adjustment to outside environments (school and community groups) through environmental adaptations, teacher training, and community advocacy. (Schaaf & Davis, 1992, p. 274)*

Occupational therapists can also address social problems that challenge individual and community health. Examples include youth enrichment and violence prevention (Kniepmann & Flanagan, 1995), as well as prevention, early identification, and intervention for childhood lead poisoning (Hotz, Kniepmann & Kohn, in press).

TABLE 22-3
Program Examples Across the Lifespan

Program	Demonstrates or applies
Parent and child health programs	Prevention-all three levels, health promotion, social learning, theory, community empowerment
Adolescence	All of the above
Independent Living Movement	Community empowerment, tertiary prevention with focus on social policy and environmental changes
Cross cultural community programming (Native American community)	Needs assessment techniques, empowerment
Worksite programs	Primary and secondary prevention, health promotion, Social Learning Theory
Self help with chronic illness	Social Learning Theory, especially self-efficacy Health promotion and prevention
Older adults - fall prevention	Primary and secondary prevention, Health Belief Model
Older adult information and information services	Health promotion

Adolescence

Youth with disabilities need to ensure that they will maximize their options for work and community living. Brollier, Shepherd, and Markley (1994) outline a team approach that starts in early school years to focus on real life activities through functional skills training. The occupational therapist helps support performance through modification of tasks or of the environment with suggestions for accessibility, work simplification, positioning, assessment, recommendations, and training for use of assistive technology.

Chandler, O'Brien, & Weinstein (1996) outlined occupational therapy contributions to transition planning, with attention to performance skills both at home and in school. Task-oriented and social skills relevant to work settings that interest the individual youth can simulate real work situations. A mock grocery store, a simulated assembly line, actual cafeteria jobs, and vocational training in carpentry, gardening, mechanical jobs, and child care can be provided in the school settings. Training programs such as these provide opportunities to use social learning from role models.

Independent Living

The Independent Living Movement demonstrates community empowerment for health promotion and prevention. Frieden and Cole (1985) identified three barriers to independence for people with spinal cord injury: Environmental, personal, and economic. They suggest that independence is a "mind process": the ability to make independent decisions that influence one's life. A program for selecting, training,

and directing a personal attendant to assist with self care tasks rather than spending enormous time and effort to do it for oneself would be an example. Independent living emphasizes adapting and changing the environment more than restoring client's abilities. Individuals with disabilities want to identify their needs, interests, and goals, rather than depending on direction and help from experts. Health care professionals can serve as consultants or employees for independent living centers to assist them in the accomplishment of their goals. In Australia, Price and Lightbody (1994) involved peer facilitators and community members for instruction in community living skills for people with spinal cord injuries. Their program included lectures, discussion, role play, problem solving, and decision making to ease the transition from hospital to community living. By involving peer facilitators and experiential learning, the concepts of social learning for health promotion and skill development for prevention are used. Many other examples exist which demonstrate these concepts. Please refer to the Recommended Reading list at the end of this chapter to find such examples.

Cross-cultural Community Programming

Community health promotion and psychosocial primary prevention programs were developed by DeMars (1992) for a Native American tribe in British Columbia, Canada. Distressed by school problems and a high rate of dropouts, tribal leaders obtained government funding to develop new educational programs. An occupational therapist was contacted to develop a life skills program for the community.

Following a literature review, a needs assessment of the community was conducted. Readings and discussion with members of the community enabled the therapist to learn much more about the values, interests, and habits of the tribe, as well as their health and educational concerns. In this way, DeMars could develop a culture specific program. She changed the title from "Life Skills and Vocational" to "Leisure Skills/Career Development." The entire community was involved. She facilitated workshops to enable children to learn from elders, who were respected role models in the tribe. Vocational training, as well as academic preparation, were provided. Long term follow-up and outcome measures showed that attendance at school increased by over 50%, tardiness decreased, and most of the recommendations were implemented and endorsed by the community. This program demonstrates several components of social learning theory in a culturally sensitive way for health promotion and prevention. Active involvement of the community members in defining needs and designing programs increased community empowerment.

Worksite Programs

Employee Management Advisory Teams (EMATs) are being established in a large urban medical center to address ergonomic issues for health care workers. The project is a joint effort of the Washington University Medical School and the CDC. The purpose of this project is to evaluate the effectiveness of participatory teams in decreasing the incidence of musculoskeletal disorders. Participatory teams have been shown to provide effective practical ways to identify occupational safety and health problems in industrial settings and to implement intervention strategies. A critical part of a participatory approach is the cohesiveness of the "team" and its ability to determine intervention strategies. Addressing this critical issue early in the ergonomics process is crucial (Bohr, personal communication, 1996). Because of the need for skills in group process, communication, and problem solving skills, occupational therapy is critical to sustaining the groups over time. The occupational therapy role has focused on facilitating group interaction. Three groups of employees are involved:

1. Transporters and orderlies, who are at risk for back and lower extremity injury;
2. lab workers, who typically have high rates of upper extremity fatigue and stress
3. ICU nurses, who have multiple job stressors including long work shifts, psychological stress, heavy lifting, prolonged standing, and awkward posture.

Baseline evaluations have documented individual worker's discomfort levels as well as concerns about work stress-

es. Employees were asked to rate their pain at the end of the day and try to relate that to job tasks or environmental factors. Based on their analysis and guidance for the project advisors, EMAT decides on a strategy for intervention and oversees its implementation. Strategies may include different techniques, using different equipment, or performing stretching exercises. This program uses primary prevention with populations at risk. It addresses an important opportunity for the future of the profession. According to an earlier article, "As industry tries to control its health care costs, prevention strategies can be directed toward the identification of risk factors within industrial sites to prevent such injuries. OTs assess factors that threaten or impair performance" (Baum, 1991, p. 488). A number of publications demonstrate ways that occupational therapists can address prevention or health promotion in work settings. Allen described two programs that addressed office environments (Allen, 1986). Carayon and Smith (1992) provide extensive background and practical guidelines to prevent or minimize physical and mental strain in computerized workplaces. Child care programs present a variety of health risks that can be addressed by occupational therapists who are familiar with ergonomics (King, Gratz, Scheuer & Claffey, 1996).

Self-Help with Chronic Illness

The Arthritis Self-Management Program (ASMP) uses social learning theory to enable people to feel more control over their symptoms (Lorig & Holman, 1993). A 6-week program is taught to about 15 participants and their significant others in community settings. Participants tailor their own exercise and cognitive pain management routines. Additionally, the program covers nutrition, communication, and problem solving. The program promotes and reinforces self-efficacy through the group sessions. Results indicate that improvements in health are strongly associated with improved self-efficacy. Change in health behavior (such as increased exercise) had a weaker association with improved health status. Follow-up study 4 years later showed that self-efficacy not only persisted but increased, and the number of physician visits decreased by 43%. This program demonstrates how self-efficacy and other components of social learning theory can be used to enhance a sense of control and maximize performance of people with chronic diseases.

Older Adults—Fall Prevention

Prevention of falls among the elderly, which often lead to death or disability, is a national priority (U.S. Department of Health and Human Services, 1991). Over 1500 older adult members of Group Health Cooperative, a health maintenance organization, participated in a randomized study to test a multicomponent educational intervention (Wagner, LaCroix,

Grothaus, Leveille, Mecht, Artz, Odle & Buchner, 1994). The experimental group spent 60 to 90 minutes with a nurse educator to identify risk factors, establish a health status baseline, and design appropriate interventions for risk reduction. Exercise and social activity were recommended for all. Follow-up behavioral intervention addressed other risk factors according to individual needs: Sedentary lifestyle, alcohol use, home safety problems, medication, and hearing or vision problems. The control group received usual care and a third group received a single, general session with a nurse about chronic disease prevention. After 1 year, the intervention group had a lower incidence of functional decline and falls. After a second year, these group differences were smaller however the cost savings from 1 additional year of independence is an important finding.

This program involved only nurses, but its lessons could be expanded by occupational therapists. Risk identification can utilize the health belief model, addressing severity, susceptibility, benefits, and barriers that need to be addressed in order to increase preventive practices. Group educational sessions for skill building could be guided by social learning theory—with peer educators, role modeling, and self-efficacy enhancing techniques. Occupational and physical therapists published a model to address person/individual, environmental, and societal areas for primary, secondary, and tertiary prevention of falls (Holliday, Cott, & Torresin, 1992). They propose comprehensive multidisciplinary services, recommending research on environment and technology transfer to address this problem.

Older Adult Services and Information System

As life expectancy is increasing, health promotion efforts should address post-retirement needs. Older Adult Services and Information System (OASIS) is a partnership of health care personnel and senior volunteers working together to enhance the quality of life for older adults (Mann, Edwards & Baum, 1986). OASIS is designed to offer retired adults opportunities to study and engage in arts and humanities programs; it provides courses, lectures, socialization, community service opportunities, and special projects. Programs are designed to promote intellectual, social, and psychological health. Through its diverse programs, it provides access to secondary prevention and provides a new health promotion model for people who are at risk for disabilities, or may develop risks in the future. Older adults play central roles in operating OASIS centers, planning programs, and training new volunteers. Occupational therapists have been involved in initial design, grant writing, consultation, screening, and classes. Occupational therapy students participate as volunteers on selected projects.

CONCLUSION

Occupational therapy can make dramatic contributions to the health of society by shifting its attention from institutional care to community settings and by addressing health promotion and prevention in all phases of its programming. Knowledge and skills from public health and health education can facilitate maximal occupational performance to improve quality of life for people of all ages. Collaboration with others is essential to this endeavor. The scientific framework of the profession enables occupational therapists to carefully investigate the effects of well-designed interventions. Building knowledge about occupation and its contributions to health promotion and prevention will be a major determinant of the health of a society that is aging and living with chronic disease and disability. We need to disseminate our results in ways that promote replication of new models for health services. We have the knowledge and skills to take the lead and shape expanded horizons of health and healthy policies for a better world.

STUDY QUESTIONS

1. Explain the three levels of prevention and give examples of how occupational therapy can address each level in various settings (schools, hospitals, communities).

2. Describe at least three key national or international resources that can guide your involvement in health promotion and prevention activities. If you are not in the United States, find out about health initiatives in your own country or international resources such as the World Health Organization that could provide a foundation for your practice.

3. What are the similarities between tertiary prevention and rehabilitation? Describe rehabilitation from a prevention standpoint.

4. Outline ways that occupational therapists could implement primary prevention programs for people with disability, including ideas for how to adapt existing primary prevention programs to include people with special needs.

5. Identify a topic and target audience for a prevention or health promotion program. Select at least two needs assessment techniques and formulate strategies or questions to gather information about the target audience.

6. What is self-efficacy and why is it important for health behavior change? Explain ways that you could help others build their self-efficacy.

7. Search peer-reviewed literature to find articles about

prevention programs that involve behavior change or change of the environment. Identify ways that occupational therapists could enrich the programs.

8. Analyze the health problems of a disadvantaged or minority community. Identify ways that the community empowerment approach could be combined with efforts to change social health policy in ways that address the problems.

9. Formulate examples of health promotion topics that occupational therapists could address for people with disabilities along each stage of the lifespan. You could use the Healthy People 2000 priority areas as a basis for identifying topics.

RECOMMENDED READINGS

Barney, K. F. (1991). From Ellis Island to assisted living: Meeting the needs of older adults from diverse cultures. *American Journal of Occupational Therapy, 45,* 586-593.

Baum, C. M. (1980). Eleanor Clarke Slagle Lecture: Occupational therapists put care in the health system. *American Journal of Occupational Therapy, 34,* 505-516.

Bazyk, S. (1989). Changes in attitudes and beliefs regarding parent participation and home programs: An update. *American Journal of Occupational Therapy, 43,* 723-728.

Becker, M. H., & Maiman, L. A. (1980). Strategies for enhancing patient compliance. *Journal of Community Health, 6,* 113-135.

Bell, B., Gaventa, J., & Peters, J. (Eds.). (1990). *We make the road by walking: Conversations on education and social change.* Philadelphia: Temple University Press.

Bruce, M. L., Seeman, T. E., Merrill, S. S., & Blazer, D. G. (1994). The impact of depressive symptomatology on physical disability: MacArthur studies of successful aging. *American Journal of Public Health, 84,* 1796-1799.

Canadian Association of Occupational Therapists. (1991). *Occupational therapy guidelines for client-centred practice.* Toronto: Canadian Association of Occupational Therapists Publications ACE.

Chin, R., & Benne, K. (1969). General strategies for effecting changes in human systems. In K. Benne & R. Chin (Eds.), *The planning of change.* New York: Holt, Rinehart & Wilson.

Dyck, I. (1993). Health promotion, occupational therapy and multiculturalism: Lessons from research. *Canadian Journal of Occupational Therapy, 60,* 120-129.

Edwards, D. F. (1994). Prevention of performance deficits. In B. R. Bonder & M. B. Wagner (Eds.), *Functional performance in older adults.* Philadelphia: F. A. Davis Company.

Esdaile, S. A. (1996). A play-focused intervention involving mothers of preschoolers. *American Journal of Occupational Therapy, 50,* 113-123.

Epp, J. (1986). *Achieving health for all: A framework for health promotion.* Ottawa: Health and Welfare Canada.

Finlayson, M., & Edwards, J. (1995). Integrating the concepts of health promotion and community into occupational therapy practice. *Canadian Journal of Occupational Therapy, 62,* 70-75.

Grady, A. P. (1995). Building inclusive community: A challenge for occupational therapy: 1994 Eleanor Clarke Slagle Lecture. *American Journal of Occupational Therapy, 49,* 300-310.

Hahn, H. (1984). Reconceptualizating disability: A political science perspective. *Rehabilitation Literature, 45,* 362-365.

Hoffman, K., & Dupont, J. (1992). *Community health centres and community development.* Ottawa: Health & Welfare Canada: Cat.# H3N-261.1992E.

Humphry, R. (1989). Early intervention and the influence of the occupational therapist on the parent-child relationship. *American Journal of Occupational Therapy, 43,* 738-742.

Jaffe, E. G. (1985). Nationally speaking—Transition in Health care: Critical planning for the 1990's part two. *American Journal of Occupational Therapy, 39,* 499-503.

Jaffe, E. G. (1986). Nationally Speaking—The role of occupational therapy in disease prevention and health promotion. *American Journal of Occupational Therapy, 40,* 749-752.

Kerr, N., & Meyerson, L. (1987). Independence as a goal and a value of people with physical disabilities. Some caveats. *Rehabilitation/Psychology, 32,* 173-180.

Lange, B. K. (1988). Ethnographic interview: An occupational therapy needs assessment tool for American Indian and Alaska Native alcoholics. *Occupational Therapy in Mental Health, 8,* 61-80.

Law, M. (1991). Muriel Driver Memorial lecture. The environment: A focus for occupational therapy. *Canadian Journal of Occupational Therapy, 58,* 171-179.

Law, M., & Dunn, W. (1993). Perspectives on understanding and changing the environments of children with disabilities. *Physical and Occupational Therapy in Pediatrics, 13,* 1-17.

Llewellyn, G. (1994). Parenting: A neglected human occupation—Parents' voices not yet heard. *Australian Occupational Therapy Journal, 41,* 173-176.

Madill H., Townsend E., & Schultz, P. (1989). Implementing a health promotion strategy in occupational therapy education and practice. *Canadian Journal of Occupational Therapy—Revue Canadienne d' Ergotherapie, 56:* 6772.

Maurer, K. E., & Teske, Y. R. (1989). Barriers to occupational therapy in wellness. *Occupational Therapy in Health Care, 5,* 57-67.

McComas, J., & Carswell, A. (1994). A model for action in health promotion: A community experience. *Canadian Journal of Rehabilitation, 7,* 257-265.

McLeroy, K. R., & Clark N. M. (1995) Creating capacity through health education: What we know and what we don't. *Health Education Quarterly, 22,* 273-89.

McLeroy, K. R., Clark, N. M., Simons-Morton, B. G., Forster, J., Connell, C. M., Altman, D., & Zimmerman, M. A. (1995). Creating capacity: Establishing a health education research agenda for special populations. *Health Education Quarterly, 22,* 390-405.

Minkler, M. (1985). Building supportive ties and sense of community among the inner city elderly: The Tenderloin senior outreach project. *Health Education Quarterly, 12,* 303-314.

Mirotznik, J., Feldman, L., & Stein, R. (1995). The health belief model and adherence with a community center-based, supervised coronary heart disease exercise program. *Journal of Community Health, 20,* 233-245.

Miyake, S., & Kraml-Angle D. (1989). From hospital to community—the health care challenge of the 1980's. *Occupational Therapy in Health Care, 5,* 115-1989.

Olson L., Heany, C., & Soppas-Hoffman, B. (1989). Parent-child activity group treatment in preventive psychiatry. *Occupational Therapy in Health Care, 6,* 29-43.

Patterson, M., & Geber, G. (1991). Preventing mental health problems in children with chronic illness or disability. Parent-to-Parent Conference (1990, Tampa, Florida), *Children's Health Care, 20,* 150-161.

Pope, A. M. (1992). Preventing secondary conditions. *Mental Retardation, 30,* 347-354.

Quinn, P. (1995). Social work and disability management policy; yesterday, today and tomorrow (review). *Social Work in Health Care, 20,* 67-82.

Rothman, J. (1992). Problem-solving approach to health and wellness: An educational model. In J. Rothman & R. Levine (Eds.), *Prevention practice: Strategies for physical therapy and occupational therapy.* Philadelphia: W. B. Saunders Company.

Spencer, E. A. (1989). Toward a balance of work and play: Promotion of health and wellness. *Occupational Therapy in Health Care, 5,* 87-99.

Twible, R. L., & Henley, E. C. (1993). A curriculum model for a community development approach to community-based rehabilitation. *Disability, Handicap & Society, 8,* 43-57.

VanDeusen, J. (1995). What is the role of the occupational therapist in managed care? *American Journal of Occupational Therapy, 49,* 833-834.

Vanier, C., & Hebert, M. (1995). An occupational therapy course on community practice. *Canadian Journal of Occupational Therapy*—Revue Canadienne d'Ergotherapie, 62: 76-81.

Waller, J. (1994). Reflections on a half century of injury control. *American Journal of Public Health, 84*(4), 664-670.

Wallerstein, N., & Bernstein, E. (1988). Empowerment education: Freire's ideas adapted to health education. *Health Education Quarterly, 15,* 379-394.

Werner, D., & Bower, B. (1982). *Helping health workers learn.* Palo Alto, CA: Hesperian Foundation.

Williams, K. A. (1992). Consultative work programs for cumulative trauma disorders. In J. Rothman & R. Levine (Eds.), *Prevention practice: Strategies for physical therapy and occupational therapy.* Philadelphia: W. B. Saunders Company.

Yang, E. M., Fink, A., Mirsch, S. M., Robbins, A. S., & Rubenstein L. V. (1995). Helping practices reach primary care goals—Lessons from the literature. *Archives of Internal Medicine, 155,* 1146-1156.

Yerxa, E. J. (1994). Dreams, dilemmas, and decisions for occupational therapy practice in a new millennium: An American perspective. *American Journal of Occupational Therapy, 48,* 586-589.

REFERENCES

Allen, V. (1986). Health promotion in the office. *American Journal of Occupational Therapy, 40,* 764-770.

American Occupational Therapy Association. (1979). Role of the occupational therapist in the promotion of health and prevention of disabilities (position paper). *American Journal of Occupational Therapy, 33,* 50-51.

American Occupational Therapy Association. (1989). Role of the occupational therapist in the promotion of health and prevention of disabilities (position paper). *American Journal of Occupational Therapy, 43,* 806.

American Occupational Therapy Association. (1990). *Member data survey.* Rockville, MD: Author.

Bandura, A. (1977). *Social learning theory.* Englewood Cliffs, NJ: Prentice-Hall.

Bandura, A. (1986). *Social foundations of thought and action: A social cognitive theory.* Englewood Cliffs, NJ: Prentice Hall.

Baum, C. M. (1991). The environment: Providing opportunities for the future. *American Journal of Occupational Therapy, 45,* 487-490.

Baum, C. M. (1995). Personal communication.

Baum, C. M., & Law, M. (1997). Occupational therapy practice: Focusing on occupational performance. *American Journal of Occupational Therapy.*

Bohr, P. (1996). Personal communication.

Brollier, C., Shepherd, J., & Markley, K. F. (1994). Transition from school to community living. *American Journal of Occupational Therapy, 48,* 346-353.

Carayon, P., & Smith, R. A. (1992). Physical and mental strain in computerized workplaces: Causes and remedies. In J. Rothman & R. Levine (Eds.), *Prevention practice—Strategies for physical therapy and occupational therapy.* Philadelphia: W.B. Saunders Co.

Caserta, M. S. (1995). Health promotion and the older population: Expanding our theoretical horizons. *Journal of Community Health, 20,* 283-292.

Chandler, J., O'Brien, P., & Weinstein, L. (1996). The role of occupational therapy in the transition from school to work for adolescents with disabilities. *Work, 6,* 53-59.

Clark, N. M., & McLeroy, K. R. (1995). Creating capacity through health education: What we know and what we don't. *Health Education Quarterly, 22,* 273-289.

Community Practice Team. (1996). *Creating partnerships for healthier communities.* St. Louis: Program in Occupational Therapy, Washington University School of Medicine.

Daltroy, L. M., & Liang, M. H. (1993). Arthritis education: Opportunities and state of the art. *Health Education Quarterly, 20,* 3-16.

DeJong, G. (1995). *Preventing and managing secondary conditions in an era of managed care.* Syracuse, NY: Conference on Secondary Conditions and Aging with a Disability.

DeMars, P. A. (1992). An occupational therapy life skills curriculum model for a native American tribe: A health promotion program based on ethnographic field research. *American Journal of Occupational Therapy, 46,* 727-36.

Finn, G. (1972). The occupational therapist in prevention programs.

American Journal of Occupational Therapy, 26, 59-66.

Freire, P. (1985). *The politics of education: Culture, power, and liberation.* Translated by P. Macedo. South Hadley, MA: Bergin & Garvey Publishers, Inc.

Frieden, L., & Cole, J. A. (1985). Independence: The ultimate goal of rehabilitation for spinal cord injured persons. *American Journal of Occupational Therapy, 39,* 734-739.

Gage, M., & Polatajko, M. (1993). Enhancing occupational performance through an understanding of perceived self-efficacy. *American Journal of Occupational Therapy, 48,* 452-461.

Green, L. W., & Johnson, K. W. (1983). Health education and health promotion. In E. Mechanic (Ed.), *Handbook of health, health care, and the health professions.* New York: Macmillan.

Grossman, J. (1991). A prevention model for occupational therapy. *American Journal of Occupational Therapy, 45,* 33-41.

Hancock, T. (1988). The future of public health in Canada. *Canadian Journal of Public Health, 79,* 416-419.

Hancock, T. (1993a). Health, human development and the community ecosystem: Three ecological models. *Health Promotion International, 8,* 41-47.

Hancock, T. (1993b). The evolution, impact and significance of the healthy cities/healthy communities movement. *Journal of Public Health Policy, 14,* 5-18.

Hancock, T. (1993c). Creating healthier communities. Seeing the vision, defining your role. *Healthcare Forum Journal, 36,* 30-36.

Hennekens, C. H., & Buring, J. E. (1987). *Epidemiology in medicine.* Boston: Little, Brown and Company.

Holliday, P., Cott, C., & Torresin, W. (1992). Preventing accidents/falls by the elderly. In J. Rothman & R. Levine (Eds.), *Prevention practice: Strategies for physical therapy and occupational therapy.* Philadelphia: W. B. Saunders Company.

Hotz, M., Kniepmann, K., & Kohn, L. (accepted, 1996). Occupational therapy in pediatric lead exposure prevention. *American Journal of Occupational Therapy.*

Institute for Alternative Futures. (1992). *Healthy people in a healthy world: The Belmont vision for health vare in America.* Alexandria, VA: Author.

Jaffe, E. G., & Epstein, C. F. (1992). *Occupational therapy consultation: Theory, principles and practice.* St. Louis: Mosby Year Book.

Janz, N. K., & Becker, M. H. (1984). The health belief model: A decade later. *Health Education Quarterly, 11,* 1-48.

Johnson, J. A. (1986). Wellness and occupational therapy. *American Journal of Occupational Therapy, 40,* 753-758.

Joint Committee on Health Education Terminology. (1991). Report of the Joint Committee on Health Education Terminology. *Journal of Health Education, 22,* 97-108.

Kari, N., & Michels, P. (1991). The Lazarus project: The politics of empowerment...nursing home models of governance. *American Journal of Occupational Therapy, 45,* 719-725.

Kimmey, J. R. (1993). *A new paradigm for health reform.* Unpublished manuscript.

King, P. M., Gratz, R., Scheuer, G., & Claffey, A. (1996). The ergonomics of child care: Conducting worksite analyses. *Work, 6,* 25-32.

Kniepmann, K., & Flanagan, J. (1995). Violence prevention for

children and families. American Occupational Therapy Association conference. Denver, CO.

Labonte, R. (1989). Community empowerment: Reflections on the Australian situation. *Community Health Studies, 13,* 347-349.

Labonte, R. (1990). Empowerment: Notes on professional and community dimensions. *Canadian Review of Social Policy, 26,* 1-12.

Law, M., Baptiste, S., & Mills, J. (1995). Client-centred practice: What does it mean and does it make a difference? *Canadian Journal of Occupational Therapy, 62,* 250-257.

Learnard, L. T., & Devereaux, E. (1992). Occupational therapy update: A model for community practice. *Hospital and Community Psychiatry, 43,* 869-871.

Leavell, H. R., & Clark, E. G. (1965). *Preventive medicine for the doctor in his community: An epidemiological approach* (2nd ed.). New York: McGraw-Hill.

Letts, L., Fraser, B., Finlayson, M., & Walls, J. (1993). *For the health of it! Occupational therapy within a health promotion framework.* Toronto: Canadian Association of Occupational Therapists Publications ACE.

Lorig, K., & Holman, M. (1993) Arthritis self-management studies: A twelve year review. *Health Education Quarterly, 20*(1), 17-28.

Mahowald, M. L., Steveken, M. E., Young, M., & Ytterberg, S. (1988). The Minnesota arthritis training program: Emphasis on self-management, not compliance. *Patient Education and Counseling, 11,* 235-241.

Mann, M., Edwards, D. F., & Baum, C. M. (1986). OASIS: A new concept for promoting the quality of life for older adults. *American Journal of Occupational Therapy, 40,* 784.

Marge, M. (1988). Health promotion for people with disabilities: Moving beyond rehabilitation. *American Journal of Health Promotion, 2*(4), 29-44.

Maynard, M. (1986). Health promotion through employee assistance programs: A role for occupational therapists. *American Journal of Occupational Therapy, 40,* 771-776.

McKillip, J. (1987). *Needs analysis: Tools for the human services and education.* Newbury Park, California: Sage Publication.

McLeroy, K. R., Bibeau, D., Steckler, A., & Glanz, K. (1988). An ecological perspective on health promotion programs. *Health Education Quarterly, 15,* 351-378.

McMurray, A. (1991). Advocacy for community self-empowerment. *International Nursing Review, 38,* 19-21.

Minkler, M. (1989). Health education, health promotion and the open society: An historical perspective. *Health Education Quarterly, 16,* 17-30.

Missiuna, C., & Pollock, N. (1991). Play deprivation in children with physical disabilities: The role of the occupational therapist in preventing secondary disability. *American Journal of Occupational Therapy, 45,* 882-888.

Moore, C. (1987). *Group techniques for idea building.* Newbury Park, CA: Sage Publication.

Mullen, P. D., Evans, D., Forster, J., Gottlieb, N. H., Kreuter, M., Moon, R., O'Rourke, T., & Strecher, V. (1995). Settings as an important dimension in health education/promotion policy, programs & research. *Health Education Quarterly, 22*(3), 329-345.

National Center for Health Statistics. (1981). Health characteristics of persons with chronic activity limitation: U.S., 1979. Vital and Health Statistics, Series 10, No. 137. DHHS Pub #(PHS) 82-1565. Hyattsville, MD: U.S. Departments of Health and Human Services.

Neufeld, P. (1994). Community programming for Parkinson's disease and Multiple Sclerosis. American Occupational Therapy Association Annual Conference. Boston, MA.

Patrick, D. L. (1994). Toward an epidemiology of disablement. *American Journal of Public Health, 84,* 1723-1725.

Price, G., & Lightbody, S. (1994). A community living skills education programme within spinal cord injury rehabilitation. *Australian Occupational Therapy Journal, 41,* 37-40.

Reilly, M. (1974). *Play as exploratory learning.* Beverly Hills, CA: Sage.

Reitz, S. M. (1992). A historical review of occupational therapy's role in preventive health and wellness. *American Journal of Occupational Therapy, 46,* 50-55.

Robertson, D., & Keller, C. (1992). Relationships among health beliefs, self efficacy, and exercise adherence in patients with coronary artery disease. *Heart and Lung, 21,* 56-63.

Robertson, A., & Minkler, M. (1994). New health promotion movement: A critical examination. *Health Education Quarterly, 21,* 295-312.

Rosenstock, I. M., Strecher, V. J., & Becker, M. H. (1988). Social learning theory and the health belief model. *Health Education Quarterly, 15,* 175-183.

Rothman, J., & Levine, R. (Eds.). (1992). *Prevention practice: Strategies for physical therapy and occupational therapy.* Philadelphia: W. B. Saunders Company.

Rousseau, C. (1993). Community empowerment: The alternative resources movement in Quebec. *Community Mental Health Journal, 29,* 535-546.

Schaaf, R. C., & Davis, W. S. (1992). Promoting health and wellness in the pediatric disabled and "at risk" population. In J. Rothman & R. Levine (Eds.), *Prevention practice: Strategies for physical therapy and occupational therapy.* Philadelphia: W. B. Saunders Co.

Shor, I., & Freire, P. (1987). *A pedagogy for liberation: Dialogues for transforming education.* South Hadley, MA: Begin & Garvey.

Shor, I. (1993). Education in politics—Paolo Freire's critical pedagogy. In P. McLaren & P. Leonard (Eds.), *Paolo Freire: A critical encounter.* London: Routledge.

Shugars, D. A., O'Neil, E. H., & Bader, J. D. (Eds.). (1991). *Healthy America, practitioners for 2005, An agenda for action for U.S. health professional schools.* Durham, NC: The Pew Health Professions Commission.

Simmons, J. J., Nelson, E. C., Roberts, E., Salisbury, Z. T., Kane-Williams, E., & Benson, L. (1989). A health promotion program: Staying healthy after 50. *Health Education Quarterly, 16,* 461-472.

Simons-Morton, B. D., Greene, W., & Gottlieb, N. (1995). *Introduction to health education and health promotion.* Prospect Heights, Illinois: Waveland Press.

Snell, R. (1993). Medical rehabilitation and public policy.

Steckler, A., Allegrante, J. P., Altman, D., Brown, R., Burdine, J. N., Goodman, R. M., & Jorgensen, C. (1995). Health education strategies: Recommendations for future research. *Health Education Quarterly, 22*(3), 307-328.

Stuifbergen, A. K., & Becker, M. A. (1994). Predictors of health-promoting lifestyles in persons with disabilities. *Research in Nursing & Health, 17,* 3-13.

Tarlov, A., & Pope, A. (1991). *Disability in America: Toward a national agenda for prevention.* Institute of Medicine. National Academy Press: Washington, D.C.

Thier, S. (1990). The future of disease prevention. *Journal of General Internal Medicine, 5,* S136-137.

Townsend, B. (1991). Beyond our clinics: A vision for the future. *American Journal of Occupational Therapy, 45,* 871-873.

Twible, R. L. (1992). Consumer participation in planning health promotion programmes: A case study using the nominal group technique. *Australian Occupational Therapy Journal, 39,* 13-18.

U. S. Department of Health and Human Services, Public Health Services. (1990). *Healthy people 2000—National health promotion and disease prevention objectives.* DHHS Publication No. (PHS) 91-50212. Washington, DC: U.S. Government Printing Office.

U. S. Department of Health and Human Services. (1991). National Conference on The Prevention of Primary and Secondary disabilities: Building partnerships towards health—Reducing the risks for disability. Atlanta: Centers for Disease Control and Prevention.

Wagner, E. M., LaCroix, A. Z., Grothaus, L., Leveille, S. G., Mecht, J. A., Artz, K., Odle, K., & Buchner, D. M. (1994). Preventing disability and falls in older adults: A population-based randomized trial. *American Journal of Public Health, 84,* 1800-1806.

Wallerstein, N., & Bernstein, E. (1994). Introduction to community empowerment, participatory education, and health. *Health Education Quarterly, 21,* 141-149.

Warheit, G., Bell, R., & Schwab, J. (1977). *Needs assessment approaches: Concepts and methods.* Rockville, MD: National Institute of Mental Health.

West, W. (1967). The occupational therapist's changing responsibility to the community. *American Journal of Occupational Therapy, 21,* 312-316.

Wiemer, R. (1972). Some concepts of prevention as an aspect of community health. *American Journal of Occupational Therapy, 26,* 1-9.

Wilcock, A. A. (1993). Keynote paper: Biological and sociocultural aspects of occupation, health and health promotion. *British Journal of Occupational Therapy, 56,* 200-203.

World Health Organization. (1986a). A discussion document on the concept and principles of health promotion. *Health Promotion, 1,* 73-78.

World Health Organization. (1986b). Ottawa charter for health promotion. Reprinted in Health Promotion, 1987, 1: iii-v.

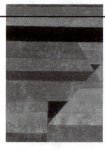

CHAPTER CONTENT OUTLINE

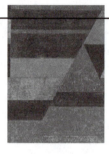

ABSTRACT

This chapter provides an introduction to outcomes research in rehabilitation. The NCMRR model is used as a framework for discussing the need for outcomes research in occupational therapy. The chapter also discusses the differences between program evaluation and quality assurance activities and scientifically designed outcome studies. The medical outcomes movement represents a shift away from morbidity and mortality data to patient- or client-centered measures of the impact of care. These client-centered assessments are thought to evaluate quality of life. Several conceptual models of quality of life used in medical treatment studies, or clinical trials, are described. Methodological issues in outcome research are reviewed, with particular emphasis on different approaches to measurement.

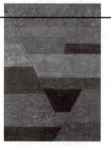

KEY TERMS

CARF

Quality Improvement (QI) Systems

Program Evaluation (PE) Systems

Morbidity

Mortality

Functional Outcomes

Quality of Life

Utility

Cost Effectiveness

Cost Utility Analysis

Behavioral Competence

Calman's Gap

Clinimetric measurement

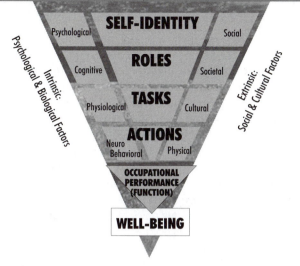

CHAPTER 23

The Effect of Occupational Therapy on Function and Well-Being

Dorothy Farrar Edwards, PhD

OBJECTIVES

The information in this chapter is intended to help the reader:

1. understand the linkage between occupational performance and health, productivity and well-being

2. describe the theoretical and practical contributions of outcomes research to the delivery of occupational therapy services

3. differentiate between quality improvement (QI) and program evaluation (PE) activities and scientifically designed outcome studies

4. identify three theoretical models which support the shift from medical measures of outcome (such as mortality) to measures of functional limitation, disability and quality of life in rehabilitation outcome studies

5. explain the different conceptual approaches to measuring quality of life including: Utility, Economic, Psychosocial and Community Centered Models

6. compare and contrast psychometric and clinometric measurement methods

7. discuss the role of occupational therapy in the evolving science of rehabilitation outcomes research.

"Is occupational therapy a sufficiently vital and unique service for medicine to support and society to reward?"

Mary Riley, 1962

Introduction

Occupational therapists have always focused, both in theory and in practice, on the person's need for occupation. Occupations, are the chunks of daily activity which define our lives. Through occupation we express who we are, what is of value, and who we wish to be. Occupations are embedded in the daily lives of people. When illness or loss occurs we restore our sense of self through a return to the occupations that were meaningful in the past, and the acquisition of new activities that will provide meaning and a sense of purpose in the future (Zemke & Clark, 1996). This concept is so fundamental to occupational therapy practice that it is often assumed that the types of methods used to measure the outcomes of occupational therapy interventions will reflect occupational performance. However, many of the scales used to document outcomes fall short of this goal. The growing emphasis on rehabilitation outcomes has opened up exciting opportunities for occupational therapists to demonstrate the value of occupation as treatment outcomes are documented.

This chapter will address the theoretical and practical contributions of outcomes research to the delivery of occupational therapy services. According to the Institute of Medicine, disability is not solely a medical issue: "In cases where the initial disabling condition cannot be prevented, much can be done to prevent or reduce the consequences and the progression toward disability and secondary conditions" (Disability in America, 1991, p. 9). Consumers, family members, insurers, professional organizations and regulatory agencies are all asking occupational therapists to be more accountable to those who consume or pay for their services (Wilkerson, 1995). Occupational therapists have a significant role to play in the development and implementation of outcome studies that focus attention on the interventions that avoid, retard, or reverse the effects of disabling conditions. Occupational therapists must become active players in the outcomes movement by demonstrating the contributions of occupational performance to health, productivity, and well-being. Failure to do this will put occupational therapy at risk in this rapidly changing health care environment.

Managed care organizations use outcome evaluation to address issues across the full spectrum of health care delivery. From the manager's perspective this approach ensures a process of ongoing and end stage quality evaluation (Ellenberg, 1996). Health care systems use critical pathways and program evaluation to monitor the effectiveness of care. Critical pathways, also known as care paths, are standard treatment plans created for specific diagnoses. In a critical pathways approach multidisciplinary teams work together to define the most efficient and effective treatment protocols by examining utilization and outcome data as indicators of program quality. Under the right circumstances this process not only produces continuous improvement in the quality of care, it has the added benefit of increasing collaboration among health care professionals (Hurley, 1994). Three essential elements of this process are client satisfaction, quality of care and financial stability (Meier, 1994). It is easy to understand why health care systems place value on this approach, as a satisfied consumer is more likely to return to the system when they need more care. Consumer satisfaction also brings in more revenues to the system.

The implementation of outcomes research within rehabilitation settings is challenging occupational therapists to develop creative approaches to assessment, treatment and program evaluation without increasing the cost of care. To achieve this goal it is important to understand the different perspectives which have influenced the evolution of outcomes research in rehabilitation. Outcomes research is a broad and complex topic. Outcome data can be used in two related, but distinctly different ways. Outcomes data has been used to study the impact of medical treatments and public health interventions on large populations of individuals with health problems or persons at risk for disease or disability. Program evaluation, another form of outcome assessment, uses standardized measures of outcome. In this case the goal is to document the degree to which a given program produces sustained, practical improvement in patient function (Johnson, Wilkerson & Maney, 1993).

Quality Improvement and Program Evaluation in Medical Rehabilitation

Medical rehabilitation facilities implement program evaluation for many reasons. These include, but are not limited to: accreditation, internal quality improvement, documentation of effectiveness of care for third party payors, and measuring consumer satisfaction.

In the United States, medical rehabilitation facilities rely on two independent accrediting organizations: the Joint Commission on Accreditation of Health Organizations (JCAHO) and the Commission on Accreditation of Rehabilitation Facilities (CARF). JCAHO accreditation is required for hospital licensure and reimbursement. As a part of the accreditation process, JCAHO requires facilities to develop and maintain quality improvement (QI) systems. CARF accreditation is voluntary, and is sought by rehabilitation programs to attest to their commitment to maximizing the benefits of rehabilitation to disabled persons. CARF requires an outcome-oriented program evaluation (PE) system in order to document functional gains achieved by patients treated by the facility. The UDS (Uniform Data System) which is based on the FIM (Functional

Independence Measure) is an example of a national data system used for multidisciplinary program evaluation (Hamilton, Granger, Sherwin, Zielezny & Tashman, 1987).

The growing emphasis on management tools for program evaluation has stimulated the development of new products designed to help occupational therapists measure outcomes. For example, occupational and physical therapists working together with other members of the American Society of Hand Therapists (ASHT) have joined with surgeons from the American Society of Surgery of the Hand to create a national outcomes database called UE-NET. The database is managed by the ASHT. They were motivated to create UE-NET to avoid being forced to use outcomes measures and management tools imposed by systems with less knowledge and experience with hand injuries (ASHT, 1996).

Two proprietary applications which interface with UE-NET have also been developed with input from occupational therapists to evaluate hand and upper extremity rehabilitation programs. The information obtained through these systems are said to enable therapists to "simplify treatment practices, provide cost effective application, increase practice income and take advantage of important national outcome studies (Ellenberg, 1996). These systems will become more common as all types of patient populations and treatment settings are included in managed care systems.

Patient/client satisfaction measures are a standard part of QI/PE systems. Patient satisfaction questionnaires ask patients to rate their satisfaction with care. Questions generally focus on issues such as timeliness of service, cleanliness and attractiveness of the facilities, and the friendliness or helpfulness of the staff. This information is important, for marketing and facilities management uses but should not be confused with quality of life and life satisfaction scales used by outcomes researchers.

It is important to understand the distinctions between QI and PE programs and scientifically designed outcome studies. Johnson and his colleagues state that "Although PE and QI data systems are often useful research tools, by themselves these systems are not designed to discover new causal knowledge: only well-controlled research can accomplish this" (Johnson, Wilkerson & Maney, 1993, p. 242).

THEORETICAL MODELS FOR REHABILITATION OUTCOME RESEARCH

Earlier chapters describe different models for the field of occupational therapy. These models guide terminology, measurement, and hypotheses for practice as well as define questions for scientific research. The two major models of disability are the International Classification of Impairments, Disabilities and Handicaps (ICIDH), and the "functional lim-

itation" or Nagi framework. These frameworks address the pathway from pathology to various types of functional outcomes (Verbrugge & Jette, 1994) and provide the foundation for shifting attention from the medical consequences of a disabling event (measured by mortality or morbidity data), to the impact of functional limitation and disability on quality of life. The Institute of Medicine Model presented in *Disability in America* illustrates the impact of risk factors and the disabling process on quality of life.

Disability in America was part of a large and diverse movement raising awareness of the impact of disabilities on American society. These efforts led to the drafting of the Americans with Disabilities Act (ADA). The passage of the ADA in 1990 fostered many changes in the way that people in the United States respond to persons with disabilities. In addition to the emphasis on accessibility, employment and civil rights, the ADA has also had an impact on health care system delivery and research on the effectiveness of rehabilitation interventions. As part of the implementation of the ADA, subsequent legislation (PL 101-613) established the National Center for Medical Rehabilitation Research (NCMRR) to enhance the quality of life for persons with disabilities through support of research on restoration, replacement, enhancement or prevention of the deterioration of function (NIH, 1993).

The NCMRR plan presents a conceptual model with five overlapping domains relevance to the study of disability. The five domains are: pathophysiology, impairment, functional limitation, disability and societal limitation. This model is similar to both the World Health Organization and the Nagi Disability in America schema. Table 23-1 presents a comparison of these models and the operational definitions for each domain. The NCMRR model challenges rehabilitation professionals to categorize assessments and interventions into the relevant domains so that outcome studies can be designed to answer questions at each level of the model. The model also helps to organize multidisciplinary studies: Each discipline can point to areas of shared interest as well as areas of specific relevance. The full impact of a disease or disabling event can only be fully understood if there are reliable and valid data available along the entire continuum from pathophysiology to societal limitation.

RESEARCH PRIORITIES IN TREATMENT EFFECTIVENESS

The NCMRR plan defined critical needs in the field of rehabilitation. Two are of relevance for this chapter. They are: 1) the lack of measurement tools and systems that can be used to 2) assess the effectiveness of treatment interventions.

A measurement system is needed to integrate findings of many different outcomes in the whole context of a person

TABLE 23-1

Terminology in Disability Classification

Classification Schema Proposed by	Impact on the Person with Disability				Impact On Others	
WHO	Disease	Impairment	Disability	Handicap disadvantage in life roles		
NAGI DISABILITY IN AMERICA MODEL	Pathophysiology	Impairment	Functional Limitations	Disability		
PHS TASK FORCE	Underlying cause	Organ level	Person level	Interaction of environment on person	Family	Community
NCMRR	Pathophysiology	Impairment	Functional limitation	Disability	Societal limitation	

Pathophysiology: Interruption of or interference with normal physiological and developmental processes or structures. Impairment: Loss or abnormality of cognitive, emotional, physiological, or anatomical structure or function, including all losses or abnormalities, not just those attributable to the initial pathophysiology. Functional limitation: Restriction or lack of ability to perform an action in the manner or within the range consistent with the purpose of an organ or organ system. Disability: Inability or limitation in performing tasks, activities, and roles to levels expected within physical and social contexts.	Societal limitation restriction, attributable to social policy or barriers (structural or attitudinal), which limits fulfillment of roles or denies access to services and opportunities that are associated with full participation in society.

with disability, without these, investigations in the field of rehabilitation will remain isolated snapshots of a few variables. They will not help us to understand how each affects the life of a person with a disability. Government, private insurance, and individuals are becoming increasingly skeptical of claims that devices and therapies are effective and efficient in restoring, increasing or preventing further loss of function (NIH, 1993).

Occupational therapists must be able to provide scientific evidence for the interventions that impact the persons they serve. There are many interesting and important questions for occupational therapists to address. For example:

- How does engagement in meaningful activities contribute to a person's improved brain function and suc-

cessful long term integration into productive pursuits, families and communities?
- What factors enable persons with disabilities to perform self care and/or create and manage support networks to provide assistance in activities of daily life?
- What are the intervention strategies that contribute to optimal function, including self-sufficiency, social integration, improved health status, and employment in persons with chronic disease and disabilities?

These questions about the impact of occupational therapy are not new. Similar questions were raised by Mary Reilly (1962) and Wilma West (1968) in the 1960s. It is critical for occupational therapists to contribute information to answer these questions.

DETERMINING EFFECTIVENESS: SHIFTING FROM MORTALITY AND MORBIDITY TO FUNCTIONAL OUTCOMES

The rapid growth of managed care in response to the need for cost containment in the United States has drawn our attention to the payor's perspective of quality and effectiveness. Health care providers must be able to document the benefits of treatment. Payment will increasingly be denied for treatments that are not supported by objectively quantified outcomes (Thomas, 1993). The pressure to produce evidence of both efficacy and efficiency in order to remain competitive in a cost-driven market may lead OTs to measure immediate gains in functional performance rather than long-term maintenance of function and reintegration of individuals into the family and community activities (Wilkerson, 1995). The types of variables selected by a profession as the best indicators of outcome will ultimately determine the types of treatments promoted by the profession. Understanding the evolution of medical outcomes from mortality (death) and morbidity (disease and symptom) variables to measures of well-being and quality of life may help occupational therapists define the measures which capture their unique contributions to rehabilitation.

In the 1800s and early 1900s, the health care system focused almost exclusively on the control of infectious disease. In 1900, the leading causes of death and disability were diseases such as diphtheria, smallpox, measles, typhoid fever and tuberculosis. Prevention efforts were directed toward controlling or eradicating infectious diseases through public health activities, such as sanitation, clean water, regulation of food processing, and immunizations (Reuter, Klebe, & Cislowski, 1986). Mortality rates were the primary index of the effectiveness of treatment or prevention programs. Decreased mortality was seen as the most positive outcome of treatment, and was also favored because it was "hard" data and the meaning of this outcome was not difficult to describe or understand. According to Kaplan and Anderson (1990), the major problem with mortality as an outcome is that mortality rates consider only the dead and ignore the living. Also, many common disabling conditions such as arthritis have little impact on mortality. Thus, there was a need to define and measure nonfatal outcomes.

Public health activities such as sanitation, clean water, regulation of food, and creation of hospitals to treat persons with contagious diseases like tuberculosis, and immunization programs, drastically reduced the number of deaths due to infectious diseases. As life expectancy increased, the methods of evaluating the efficacy of public health and medical treatment programs shifted from mortality statistics to mor-

bidity data. Morbidity is defined as the prevalence, or rate of disease in a particular area or population. Morbidity data are used by epidemiologists to track the health status of the population. Morbidity estimates may also include the number of days of reduced activity, such as time away from work, days in the hospital, or number of hospital admissions.

Morbidity studies are often used to examine the "cost" of health problems in terms of lost productivity, health care utilization, or social service needs. These studies also introduced measures of function and role performance as essential components of multidimensional health status assessment. Attention shifted away from the extent and severity of the pathology of a disease to the impact of the disease on the patient's ability to perform activities of daily living. Thus, the door was opened to include the person's evaluation of his or her health status in general, and their personal judgment of the impact of the disease or disabling condition on their social and emotional well-being.

FUNCTIONAL ASSESSMENT OF MEDICAL OUTCOMES

Interest in functional outcomes is not new. According to John Ware (1993), a leading scientist in the field of medical outcomes research, papers appeared as early as 1914 in the medical literature stressing the importance of a patient's perspective in determining the effectiveness of care. Ware (1993, p. 3) cites the work of Lembcke, who wrote in 1952: " The best measure of quality is not how well or frequently a medical service is given, but how closely the result approaches the fundamental objectives of prolonging life, relieving distress, restoring function and preventing disability."

Functional assessment began with the measurement of the impact of physical disability on activities of daily living (Spector, 1992). Physical functioning refers to the performance of, or the capacity to perform a variety of physical activities normal for people in good health (Stewart & Kamberg, 1993). The measurement of physical function has been plagued by conceptual and methodological problems. One problem is associated with defining the appropriate content of the scale. Stewart and Kamberg (1993) note that since all activities of daily living are physical, theoretically all activities could be included. A second issue raised by these authors involves the level of exertion or effort required. Scales that are designed for special populations, such as the elderly, may not be appropriate for the evaluation of health status in more varied groups. If the activities are not strenuous enough there is a problem with ceiling effects, or too many people receiving perfect scores. In this case high scores represent the absence of significant physical limitations rather than a positive state of physical functioning.

Perhaps the most important issue for rehabilitation professionals relates to whether the extent of difficulty or the need for help in the form of another person or adaptive equipment should be scored in functional tests. Should a person who can walk with a cane receive the same score as a person who covers the same distance without one? Several scales assign the same score to performance with or without assistive devices, however most scales assign lower scores to activities performed with adaptive equipment. Does this mean that persons who use attendants to dress in order to go to work are less independent than those who dress themselves but do not work?

The Katz ADL scale and the Barthel Index, both developed in the 1960s, represent two different approaches to the measurement of basic activities of daily living. The original version of the Katz ADL scale was created as a performance-based measure of six functions: bathing, dressing, toileting, transfers from bed to chair, continence and feeding (Katz, Ford, Moscowitz, Jackson & Jaffe, 1963). The scale was used to document recovery from stroke, hip fracture and rheumatoid arthritis. Later versions of the scale were modified for use in personal interviews when direct observation of performance was not possible or practical. The interview form of the scale has been widely used for studies of community resident elderly (Branch, Katz, Kniepmann, & Paspidero, 1984).

The Barthel Index (Mahoney & Barthel, 1965) was developed in a chronic hospital setting and has been used to monitor progress for severely disabled persons in comprehensive medical rehabilitation. The Functional Independence Measure (FIM) (Keith, Granger & Hamilton, 1987) has recently replaced the Barthel Index as the standard functional measure in medical rehabilitation, however, the Barthel Index is still widely used in neurological research, especially in stroke studies. A three-level ordinal scoring scheme is used for each Barthel item: can do by oneself, can do with the help of someone else, and cannot do at all. Weights ranging from 0 to 15 are used to create an aggregate score. The Barthel Index is not a hierarchically ordered scale, the score is the sum of the items. According to Spector (1992), interpretation of the Barthel scores is difficult because it is not certain that a lower score implies more disability. For example, the same total score may result from a number of different profiles. A person who is unable to walk or climb stairs but whom is independent in dressing, and grooming and other self-care items, may have the same score as a person who needs assistance with self-care but is independent in mobility. Persons tested in environments that support performance of basic activities of daily living through the presence of adaptive equipment or barrier-free designs will have higher scores than persons of the same ability tested under less supportive conditions.

The FIM was created to address a wider range of functions than either the Katz or the Barthel. It has become the primary tool for documenting the outcome of rehabilitation services (Granger, Ottenbacher, Baker & Sehgal, 1995). Standardized functional status measures were developed in response to a Congressional mandate to create a system for Medicare patients in need of rehabilitation (Velozzo, Megahles, Pan & Leiter, 1995). The use of measures like the FIM was seen as a better approach to documenting treatment effectiveness than conventional quality assurance studies which examined the process of rehabilitation programs (i.e., the presence of goals, hours of operation, the inclusion of the patient in goal-setting). There are many reasons for the growing acceptance of the FIM as a rehabilitation outcome measure. First, the 18 activities included are thought to be essential for survival, they do not require unusual skill, and they are not culturally or socially stereotyped. Second, subscribers to the Uniform Data System (UDS) for medical rehabilitation receive a variety of standard reports that allow a facility to evaluate efficacy in comparison to national norms for similar facilities or patient populations. There are many advantages to standardized functional measures like the FIM. However, the FIM does not adequately address the cognitive skills needed for independence. The heavy emphasis on musculoskeletal function as an index of the impact or benefit of rehabilitation may disenfranchise many consumers that continue to need rehabilitation to return to full independence. Persons with cognitive impairment can be very successful when the environment is designed to support their occupation. If reimbursement is tied to the FIM the very services which support the core values of occupational therapy may no longer be possible.

The adoption of physical function scales as outcome indicators represented an important shift away from physiologic and symptom-based measures of health status, but this shift was an intermediate step toward the goal of measuring health status rather than disease states. While the ability to perform simple and complex activities of daily living is an important component of health status it does not represent the totality of health and well-being. Health is defined by the WHO as "not merely the absence of disease, but complete physical, social, and psychosocial well-being" (World Health Organization, 1958). Occupational therapists, through their interventions enable people to regain health as well as function.

QUALITY OF LIFE AS AN OUTCOME

In response to concerns about selecting variables that were too narrow the scientific research in health outcomes moved to a more global construct called "health related quality of life." While there is no single, standard definition of quality of life, there is general agreement that quality of life as a scientific outcome is defined by patients' perceptions of performance in four areas: physical and occupational function, psychological

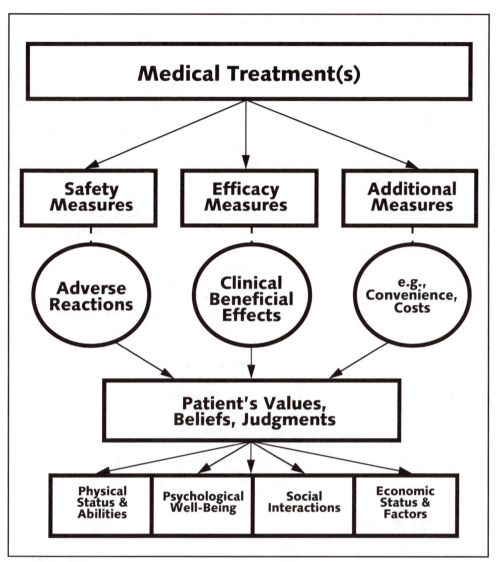

Figure 23-1. A Model For Evaluating the Impact of Medical Treatment on Quality of Life.

state, social interaction and somatic, or bodily, state (Schipper, Clinch, & Powell, 1990). This construct emphasizes the "functional effect" of an injury or illness and subsequent therapy on the day-to-day comings and goings of a free, living individual. The patient (person) serves as his or her own control, the comparisons are made against his or her own expectation or experience of function. It is the ultimate client-centered measure since no one can truly define the meaning of the four areas for someone else (Guyatt et al., 1991).

Spilker (1990) suggests that the major domains of quality of life can be represented by four categories: 1) physical status and functional abilities, 2) psychological status and well-being, 3) social interactions, and 4) economic status and factors. Spilker presents a model which illustrates how a medical treatment can be examined within the context of the different levels and types of responses. The patient's values, beliefs and judgments act as a filter and place the clinical benefits of the

treatment within the framework of his or her life experience. Studies have shown that physicians cannot accurately predict the impact of a treatment on the patient's quality of life (QOL) (Slevin, Plant, Lynch, Drinkwater, & Gregory, 1988). While there is no empirical data on the success of other health professionals in predicting a person's response to treatment, it is possible that occupational therapists would also have difficulty predicting the impact of treatment on the individual's perceived QOL. Spilker's model is presented in Figure 23-1.

Spilker (1990) noted that some authors who report on QOL include may only include of one these broad domains in a study. While it is not essential for an investigator to study all areas in a clinical trial, trials that evaluate only one domain should be distinguished from trials that are more inclusive.

It is important to interpret QOL data within the larger circumstances of the person. For example, factors outside of the treatment situation can have a major impact on the outcome.

A person who loses a job or is hurt in an accident may not have enough money to pay for all of the prescribed or recommended treatment. It is essential to identify barriers to full compliance or participation in a treatment program before drawing conclusions about effectiveness. Spilker suggests that in population-based models of health care considerations of resource availability, allocation, and consumption would have to be included, as well as the impact of a patient's QOL on the community.

Occupational therapists can make a significant contribution to the understanding of QOL. Occupational performance, or the means to engage in meaningful occupations, is the essence of QOL. Occupational therapists must systematically translate this core value into practice by using assessments that capture the importance of occupation to health and well-being because it is important to interpret QOL data within the larger circumstances of the person. Factors outside of the treatment situation can have a major impact on the outcome. It is essential to identify barriers to full compliance or participation in a treatment program before drawing conclusions about effectiveness (Rogers & Holm, 1994).

CONCEPTUAL MODELS OF QUALITY OF LIFE

While there is consensus about the four domains which define the construct of QOL, the scales that have been developed do not conform to a single conceptual model. Schipper, Clinch and Powell (1990) identified five different conceptual models of QOL measurement within the two main areas of economic and psychosocial impact. These conceptual models include: utility; psychological; community reintegration; Calman's Gap principle and community-centered approaches, and will be briefly described.

Utility Approaches

The utility approach to QOL is also known as the time trade-off concept. Some people prefer survival at any cost, while other individuals would not want to live under certain circumstances. For example, when a group of healthy individuals was presented with two alternative treatments for laryngeal cancer which differed in length of survival and preservation of voice, the majority of the respondents indicated that they would trade off 14% of their full life expectancy in order to avoid loss of the ability to speak (MacNeil, Weischselbaum, & Pauker, 1981). The original utility/time trade-off studies were conducted with healthy subjects in order to gauge the feelings about treatment options in general. Today, the same techniques are used to help patients work their way through complicated decisions about treatment alternatives. This research attempts to

operationalize the day-to-day decisions we make to maximize our QOL. The utility approaches have been used to study the economic impact of health care services. The standard utility measures try to capture the satisfaction or enjoyment the consumer experiences. Most health economists do not measure utility directly. Instead, they conduct studies designed to pose questions about treatment conditions to samples of people who do *not* have the health problem. The most common methods are known as the standard gamble and time trade-off techniques (Torrance, 1986). The time trade-off approach offers a subject a choice between living for *t* years in perfect health or *t* years in an alternative less desirable health state (the one for which the analyst wants the utility score). The utility value is the ratio of the shorter period of good health to the longer period of the less desirable state (t) or x/t.

Some individuals may prefer survival at any cost, while others may believe that life is not worth living under some circumstances. In a study of a large group of people (N=209) at high risk for stroke severe motor impairment was rated as an outcome significantly worse than death (Solomon, Glick, Russo, Lee, & Shulman, 1994). In other words, for this group of individuals increased life expectancy was not worth the resultant loss of autonomy associated with severe motor impairment. Thus, if a new treatment for stroke was associated with the possibility of motor impairment, the utility of the treatment would be low in persons who relied heavily on mobility to preserve their autonomy.

The approach is difficult for many occupational therapists to understand and accept because they do not often equate disability and disadvantage. They also know that people who would never choose to be disabled find that living with a disability usually brings with it enhanced meaning and valuable contributions.

The standard gamble procedure offers a subject a choice between two alternatives: living in the health state in "Choice A" with certainty, or taking a gamble with treatment (Feeny, Labelle & Torrance, 1990). This approach has been used extensively to study treatment alternatives in cancer where the alternative treatments may offer the possibility of greater life expectancy but at the risk of significant side effects. One of the most frequently cited studies involved the treatment of laryngeal cancer. MacNeil et al. (1981) presented groups of normal individuals with two treatment alternatives for laryngeal cancer. The first treatment offered was laryngectomy (removal of the voicebox and vocal cords) which offers the possibility of longer survival but total loss of the ability to speak. The second treatment option was radiation therapy with a risk of shorter survival, but preservation of the ability to speak. The study suggests that the majority of respondents would be willing to "trade-off" life expectancy in order to retain the ability to speak.

Economic Approaches

Economists are interested in linking costs to the consequences of health care. The cost of care includes direct costs such as professional fees, drugs, diagnostic tests, and hospital charges as well as indirect costs such as lost earnings, and the burden or responsibilities of care assumed by families or friends (Feeny & Torrance, 1989). There are three major approaches to the study of economics and QOL, cost-effectiveness, cost benefit, and cost utility. These terms should be understood by practitioners as they frequently enter into conversations and are often used incorrectly.

Cost-effectiveness studies compare the dollar value of the resources used to clinical effects produced by treatment. For example, a study of community education programs to reduce the risk of strokes may report the findings in terms of average reductions in the blood pressure of program participants. The reductions in blood pressure can then be used to project a decrease in the incidence of stroke within the same population. The most important feature of this design is that the investigator does not need to assign a dollar value to the outcome (Drummond, Stoddard & Torrance, 1987).

Cost-utility analyses examine the dollar value of the health care resources expended to the QOL outcomes produced by the clinical effects of the intervention. Traditionally the QOL measure is expressed in terms of quality adjusted life years (QUALYS). QUALYS are used to integrate measures of well-being with survival measures. Coronary artery bypass surgery has been studied extensively using this method. In these studies, symptom reports and activity limitations were used to generate the QUALYS scores. The Veterans' Administration found that the estimated net cost per quality adjusted life year gained from the surgery was $3,800 for left main artery disease to $30,000 for one vessel disease. The cost analysis included the direct cost of the surgery, as well as the savings attributed to prevention of subsequent events (CASS, 1983). Cost-utility analyses differ from cost-effectiveness studies in that they incorporate QOL measures into the results.

Cost-benefit analyses focus on the dollar value of resources saved or created as a result of a given treatment. This research strategy has been widely used to demonstrate the cost savings associated with prevention and public health programs. The application of cost-benefit analyses to direct treatment programs has been challenged from an ethical perspective. The assignment of dollar figures to peoples' lives and functions makes many investigators uncomfortable, particularly given the wide array of religious, cultural and personal values in our society. There are concerns that this type of analysis might be used to withhold or decrease the availability of treatments based on some external standard of value.

Psychosocial Approaches

The psychological view of QOL reflects the patient's per-

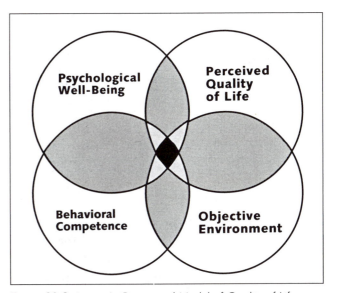

Figure 23-2. Lawton's Conceptual Model of Quality of Life: Inteaction Among Four Critical Domains.

ception of the impact of the disease or disability. This perception is the product of the person's experience of the symptoms, how he labels and communicates the distress they cause, the experience of being unable to function normally, and the coping strategies used by the person and his family to gain some control over the disorder (Kleinman, 1986). This approach to the measurement of psychological states grew out of the recognition that coping strategies and personality type have an influence on the function of the immune system. The importance of perception has also been observed in the wide range of responses to similar medical states, such that simply knowing a diagnosis and the clinically defined severity will not lead to accurate predictions of function.

There is some confusion about the term "quality of life." Several authors (Spilker, 1990; Gill & Feinstein, 1994) suggest that most of the studies of QOL presented in the medical literature use the terminology without definition. This means that "quality of life" is substituted for other terms related to health such as health status, functional status, or emotional well-being. Lawton (1991) reviewed all of the published medical QOL studies and concluded that: 1) all of the studies used measures that were plausible indicators of QOL, and 2) the components represented a jumble of content and levels of generality. Lawton defines QOL as the multidimensional evaluation, by both intrapersonal and social-normative criteria, of the person-environment system of the individual in time past, current and anticipated. This definition is consistent with the WHO definition of health. According to Lawton, QOL is based on the interaction of four key concepts. These concepts are psychological well-being, perceived QOL, behavioral competence, and the objective environment. This model is illustrated in Figure 23-2.

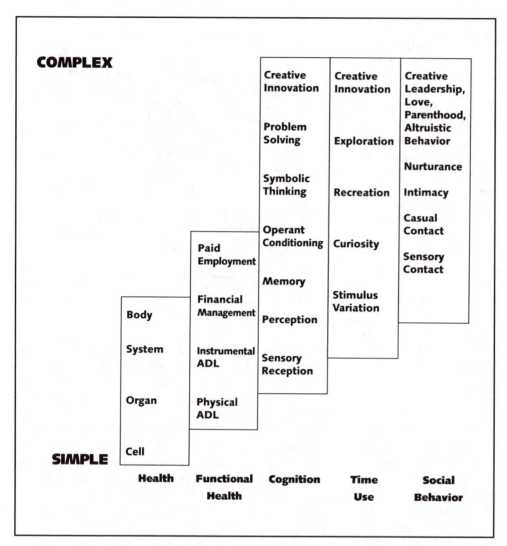

COMPLEX

Creative Innovation

Creative Innovation

Creative Leadership, Love, Parenthood, Altruistic Behavior

Problem Solving

Exploration

Nurturance

Symbolic Thinking

Recreation

Intimacy

Casual Contact

Operant Conditioning

Paid Employment

Curiosity

Sensory Contact

Memory

Financial Management

Stimulus Variation

Body

Perception

System

Instrumental ADL

Sensory Reception

Organ

Physical ADL

Cell

SIMPLE

Health   **Functional Health**   **Cognition**   **Time Use**   **Social Behavior**

Figure 23-3. The Hierarchical Progression of Behavioral Competence: An Illustration of the Link Between Occupational Performance and Quality of Life.

Of particular importance to occupational therapists is the contribution of behavioral competence, as defined by Lawton (1991), to QOL. Behavioral competence encompasses the continuum from physical health through social interaction. Behavioral competence is expressed through active engagement in life tasks, or occupation. This construct incorporates the elements of occupational performance addressed by occupational therapists. The link between occupational performance and QOL emerges very clearly in this model. Lawton's schema of behavioral competence is presented in Figure 23-3.

As interest in using QOL measures to document rehabilitation outcomes grows, it is very important for occupational therapists to use scales that measure all domains (physical, social, psychological and environmental) since many of the measures used to evaluate QOL very heavily on assessment of physical well-being and minimize the social and emotional aspects of health.

Wood and Williams (1987) proposed the term "reintegration to normal living" as a proxy for QOL. Wood includes the person's satisfaction with mobility, self care abilities, daily activities, recreational activities, social activities, family roles, personal relationships, presentation of self and general coping skills as the types of roles and responsibilities necessary for everyday life. In this context QOL is associated with the factors which enable a person to do what one has or wants to do, but does not necessarily mean that the person is free of disease or symptoms. This approach is far more appropriate for the evaluation of the impact of chronic disease than symptom-based profiles. This concept is particularly appropriate for persons with disabilities where a cure is unlikely, because it de-emphasizes the physical and physiological domains in favor of satisfaction with participation in meaningful roles and activities. It is also of great interest to occupational therapists as these issues are consistent with the concept of occupation. There are several scales which were designed to assess this domain. Perhaps the best known is the Reintegration to Normal Living Index (Wood-Dauphinee, Opzoomer, Williams, Marchand, & Spitzer, 1988). The goal

---

TABLE 23-2

Reintegration to Normal Living Index Items

1. I move around in my living quarters as I feel necessary (wheelchairs, other equipment, or other resources may be used).

2. I move about my community as I feel necessary (wheelchairs, other equipment, or other resources may be used).

3. I am able to take trips out of town as I feel necessary (wheelchairs, other equipment, or other resources may be used).

4. I am comfortable with how my self-care needs (dressing, feeding, bathing, toileting) are met (adaptive equipment, supervision, or assistance may be used).

5. I spend my days in a work activity that is necessary or important to me (work activity could be paid employment, housework, volunteer work, school, etc.) (adaptive equipment, supervision, or assistance may be used).

6. I am able to participate in recreational activities (hobbies, crafts, sports, reading, television, games, computers, etc.) as I want to (adaptive equipment, supervision, or assistance may be used).

7. I am able to participate in social activities with family, friends, or business acquaintances as is necessary or desirable to me (adaptive equipment, supervision, or assistance may be used).

8. I assume a role in my family which meets my needs and those of other family members. Family means people with whom you live or relatives with whom you do not live but see on a regular basis (adaptive equipment, supervision, or assistance may be used).

9. In general, I am comfortable with my personal relationships.

10. In general, I am comfortable with myself when I am in the company of others.

11. I feel that I can deal with life events as they happen.

---

of this scale is to help document how a person is able to resume "living" his or her life after incapacitating illness or trauma. Reintegration is defined as the ability to do what one wants or feels one has to do, not that one is free of symptoms or even disability. This scale focuses on the interaction of the person with his or her environment by examining both objective indicators and the person's perspective of physical, social and psychosocial dimensions. The scoring does not penalize the person for the use of adaptive equipment or social or emotional support. For example, the ADL question states "I am happy with how my self-care needs are met" (adaptive equipment, supervision or assistance may be used). The items are rated on either a 10-point Likert scale with descriptive phrases "does not describe my situation" and "fully describes my situation" at opposite ends of the rating scale, or using a yes/no dichotomous rating. This QOL scale seems to be a better measure of occupational performance and person-environment fit than systematic functional assessments like the FIM or handicap measures like the CHART (Whiteneck, Charlifue, Gerhart, Overholser & Richardson, 1992). The CHART uses 27 objective questions to measure deviation from roles generally fulfilled by persons without disability or handicap. The scale does not include subjective evaluations of role performance. The Reintegration to Normal Living Scale items are presented in Table 23-2.

Another approach to measuring community participation and reintegration is to measure participation in meaningful activity. Oakly, Sunderland, Hill, Phillips, Makahon, and Ebner (1991), an occupational therapist at the National Institutes of Health (NIH) is using an activity index as part of a series of chronic disease outcome studies. Similarly, Baum (1995) uses an activity card sort to assess the impact of a disabling event or disease on activity patterns. Both of these measures are client-centered, in that only activities of value to the person are scored. These indexes are designed to determine the number of activities given up, as well as the number of new activities adopted. Preliminary results with both measures across a variety of populations suggest that activity measures are sensitive indicators of QOL.

Calman (1984) defined QOL as the gap between a person's expectations and achievements. The smaller the gap, the higher the QOL. If the person is unable to achieve his goals the gap increases and QOL declines. Expectations and achievements change over time, so the gap will vary with the changing circumstances. Calman suggested that QOL reflects the impact of illness on the individual. Professionals have an important role to play in helping the person to set realistic expectations in light of his or her capacities. If the goals are unrealistic the patient may become frustrated, increasing the gap and decreasing QOL. Another gap may exist between the person's actual achievements and his potential achievements. This type of gap is indicative of lack of fit between the person and his or her environment. When the resources necessary to support performance are not available the gap increases and QOL declines. This conceptualization should challenge the occupational therapist to plan client-centered services to overcome deficits in occupational performance. Calman does not recommend a specific scale to identify the gap between the person and his environment. However, the Canadian Occupational Performance Measure (COPM), a client-centered assessment which provides a quantitative rating of the person's ability and satisfaction associated with the performance of life tasks is a good measure of this construct.

Community-Centered Concept

The community-centered concept was proposed by Ware (1984) to provide a sense of the impact that illness has on the broader community. This model is defined by a group of concentric circles starting with the physiologic parameters of disease in the center, surrounded in turn by personal functioning, psychological stress and well-being, general health perceptions and social/role functioning as the exterior circle. The impact on the community is seen in terms of the content of the exterior circle which refers to the an individual's capacity to perform activities associated with his or her usual role including employment, schoolwork or homemaking and parental responsibilities. Ware and his colleagues have developed a series of outcome measures which operationalize this concept of well-being.

Ware (1995) notes that the emphasis needs to be on the factors that people value most. The Medical Outcomes Study (MOS) adopted a three-part model that included traditional clinical measurement of symptoms and problems, generic or global ratings of health, and the social and emotional status of the person (Tarlov, Ware, Greenfield, & Hays, 1989; Ware, 1991). The SF-36 MOS Short-Form 36 has become the most widely used scale for evaluating medical treatments in large populations. Ware suggests that the methodology developed for the MOS supports the triangulation of a comprehensive health measurement model. According to Ware, "generic measures focus on health concepts valued by everyone, regardless of age, disease, or treatment group. They represent basic human values, for example, how a person feels and how well he or she can function." These categories permit the comparisons of the burden of one disease relative to another and the relative benefits of different treatments. The MOS framework of physical and mental health indicators is presented in Chapter 5.

Methodological Issues in Outcomes Research

The importance of outcomes research cannot be overstat-

ed. Occupational therapists must understand that the outcomes movement is well underway and must decide what contributions they will make. There are many efforts underway to build systems of outcomes. An alternative approach follows which will lead us into a discussion of how these measures are scored.

Clinimetric versus Psychometric Measurement

The new QOL measurement tools are challenging measures that have been used previously by occupational therapists. The following discussion is presented to facilitate an understanding of the controversy surrounding clinical versus statistical or research implications of measurement.

Rating scales or indices that are constructed to measure the severity of clinical symptoms, co-morbidity, or functional status often use terms like "none," "mild," "moderate," or "severe" to create ordinal or ranked response categories. These terms are used as a means of capturing information from the individual about the experience of a disease or the effects of a disability (Feinstein, 1987). Unlike laboratory data which relies on the measurement of physical or physiological effects of an illness, these types of ratings have not been accepted as "hard" information that can be trusted scientifically. Only variables of proven scientific merit have been included in computerized data banks or examined in statistical studies of medical interventions. The reliance on "hard" data meant that the subjective experience of the person was absent from outcome studies, and limited the applicability of the findings to the very people that the studies were designed to aid. These omissions produced major flaws in the art and science of patient care (Feinstein, 1987, p. 3).

Over the past 20 years, the use of psychometric clinical indexes has grown dramatically. At the same time, Feinstein and colleagues have fostered the parallel growth of a new approach to measurement called clinimetrics. Clinimetric and psychometric measurement strategies share common goals including accurate measurement of attributes (reliability) and prediction of different states or status (validity) (Wright & Feinstein, 1992). The differences lie in the mathematical and statistical techniques used to determine reliability and validity and in the rules which guide the creation of an index or scale. Psychologists and educators have used psychometric approaches to measure psychological phenomena and educational achievement. Psychometric approaches require the creation of large numbers of items in order to fully survey the attributes, while clinimetric measures try to capture the attributes in the fewest number of items possible. Psychometric measures also require homogeneity, that is that the items in the scale represent only one domain at a time. Clinimetric measures include items that represent many domains in order to document the impact of disease or disability on a global phenomenon like function or QOL. A comparison of these two approaches is presented in Table 23-3.

The rehabilitation literature reflects the growing dissatisfaction with the use of psychometric methods to create and evaluate functional scales. Rehabilitation professionals traditionally have used ordinal scales which limits how these scales can be used to study outcomes (Merbitz, Morris, & Grip, 1989; Fisher, Harvey, Taylor, Kilgore & Kelly, 1994). A new technique called Rasch analysis is used to determine the reliability and validity of clinical measures. Rasch analysis makes it possible to scale the items scores and place them in a hierarchical order. This item hierarchy is similar to a Guttmann scale. This means that if a person passes a difficult item, he or she, will also be able to successfully pass a simple item. The analysis also mathematically transforms the item scores to allow an investigator to sum items and generate total scores which can be used to study effectiveness and QOL. Structural equation modeling is another statistical technique that can be used to evaluate the reliability and validity of clinical measures (Edwards, Chen & Diringer, 1995). It too, will be used in analyses of treatment effectiveness.

Issues in Outcome Research

Ottenbacher (1995) has written extensively about methodological problems that limit the success of rehabilitation outcomes research. He suggests that investigators often confuse clinical and statistical significance. They often confound this problem by failing to report details of the statistical analyses and results, including problems of low statistical power. Statistical power is the ability of a study to detect a significant difference that really does exist. Many investigators report that there were no significant differences between treated and untreated groups of patients. Unfortunately, if the sample sizes are small, or if the performance of the subjects was highly variable, the results may lead the investigator to *erroneously* conclude that there are no differences between the groups. This is known as a Type II error. Ottenbacher also notes the absence of replication studies designed to confirm the previous findings of treatment efficacy (or lack of efficacy). The failure to establish consensus leads to statistical confusion, calls to abandon quantitative methods in favor of alternative research strategies, and to delays in developing a useful body of knowledge on rehabilitation interventions.

The growing interest in documenting the outcome of rehabilitation is due in part, to health care reform and the implementation of cost-containment programs. Occupational therapists are being challenged to "demonstrate the value of occupational therapy interventions by providing objective and persuasive evidence of the effectiveness of occupational therapy interventions for the various patient populations served" (Rogers & Holm, 1994, p. 871). While health care

---

TABLE 23-3
Comparison of Psychometric and Clinimetric Approaches to Measurement

Psychometric Measurement
Reliability examined
Validity examined
Large numbers of items used to measure domains
Focus on homogeneity of measures (single construct in each scale)
Redundant/similar items used to test consistency of response
Items summed to create interval measures

Clinimetric Measurement
Reliability examined
Validity examined
Scales have as few items as possible
Focus on heterogeneity of measures (multiple constructs in each scale)
No repetition of items
Generally ordinal level of measurement

---

reform has been the primary impetus for outcome studies, occupational therapy researchers have also recognized the scientific merit of studies of treatment effectiveness. The growth of the body of knowledge about occupation is one of the benefits of outcomes research. The design and implementation of new treatment strategies is fueled by the findings of scientific studies which explain the complex interactions among the intrinsic and extrinsic factors which support occupational performance. Thus, even if third-party payment for occupational therapy services were not an issue, the profession would still need to commit time and resources to studying the outcomes of treatment to build a body of knowledge to support best practices.

What outcomes should occupational therapists measure? According to Rogers and Holm (1994), the outcome of occupational therapy is the functional consequence for the patient, of the therapeutic actions implemented by the occupational therapist. Their examples of potential outcomes of therapy included: stronger muscles, increased independence in dressing, or return to work. Each of these outcomes is indicative of "function." The term *function* has many meanings. If you look up function in the dictionary you will find it defined as role, use, activity, capacity, job, position, pursuit or place (Baum et al., 1994). In addition to the many meanings of the term, many disciplines believe that they promote or facilitate functional independence. In light of these factors what unique contributions do occupational therapists make to the understanding of function, and correspondingly to support therapeutic interventions designed to facilitate or enhance function?

The answer lies in the core values and scientific foundations of occupational therapy. Occupational therapists address the occupational performance needs of persons through the therapeutic use of meaningful activities. Standardized functional performance scales like the FIM do not really measure occupational performance. While it is very important to document the effects of treatment on standardized functional measures, the scores on these scales do not represent the true or long-term outcome of occupational therapy services. QOL measures, particularly scales like the Reintegration to Normal Living Index or the COPM are better tools for demonstrating occupational therapy outcomes.

Lang and Marek (1992) have written about the role of outcomes research in supporting clinical practice in nursing. Their careful examination of the interface between outcome assessment and nursing practice provides guidance to occupational therapists committed to the same process. These authors suggest that health care is a multidimensional phenomenon. It is provided in multiple sites, by multiple providers, with multiple environmental and organizational variables influencing the outcome. The optimal approach would be to expand the concept of care beyond one episode (or location) so that the longitudinal outcomes can be examined.

The NCMRR model operationalized this approach. An example of a comprehensive outcome study based on the NCMRR model is presented. Figure 23-4 illustrates a measurement model designed to study the outcomes of stroke. This model was developed by a multidisciplinary team of rehabilitation professionals working together to develop more reliable and valid measures for determining the effectiveness of stroke treatments. The professions/disciplines involved in this study include: neurology, occupational therapy, nursing, rehabilitation medicine, psychology, social work and health care economics. Each member of the research team can test hypotheses about outcomes at each level of the model. For example, the neurologist is interested in treatments designed to reduce brain swelling that may result from brain ischemia soon after the stroke occurs. The outcome variable of interest in the intensive care unit (ICU) is the Glasgow Coma Scale which measures consciousness and reactivity to simple stimuli. In this case the outcome is a pathophysiology measure which is obtained immediately. The health economist wants to know if aggressive treatment of brain swelling will result in reduced costs due to fewer days in the hospital. If so, an expensive treatment delivered in the ICU may result in cost savings when the total cost of the stroke is examined. However, the treatment may not produce any significant differences on upper extremity tests such as the Williams' Latch Board which is considered to be assessment of functional limitation, or changes in the Functional Independence Measure (FIM). The measures at the

disability level which examine executive function, activity patterns and functional ability rather than functional limitations will begin to capture the impact of the stroke on the occupational performance of the person. The measures of societal limitation such as community integration, well-being and career burden allow us to evaluate the fit between persons and their environments. Thus, there is no single measure of treatment outcome. The particular research questions will lead to the selection of appropriate dependent (or outcome) variables. The most important step in the development of any outcome study is framing the question. Occupational therapists need to decide which domain or domains along the continuum from pathophysiology to societal limitation best reflect(s) the impact of occupational therapy interventions. However, disability measures such as the FIM do not fully depict person-environment fit or occupational performance.

There are important functional outcomes to be documented at each stage of the treatment process. Occupational therapists can and should be involved in measurement in many different settings with different types of functional outcomes and methodologies depending the type of intervention. This model requires the use of standardized measurement tools that are reliable and valid. The American Occupational Therapy Association (AOTA) and the American Occupational Therapy Foundation (AOTF) have defined an agenda for occupational therapy outcomes research. This agenda includes:

- Devising an occupational therapy minimum data set to facilitate research across sites and settings.
- Developing function outcomes measures that are sensitive to occupational therapy interventions.
- Devising strategies to incorporate research examining the effectiveness of occupational therapy interventions into existing programs examining the effectiveness and outcomes of medical treatments.
- Developing practice-based research networks to investigate occupational therapy effectiveness in targeted populations.
- Fostering the development of occupational therapy scientists in research methods and designs appropriate for studying the effectiveness of occupational therapy interventions.
- Advocating for the inclusion of essential occupational therapy variables in national health databases.

AOTA and AOTF support this agenda by providing research consultation for investigators, mentoring for future grant recipients, and funding for effectiveness studies.

The proposed research agenda supports the development of sensitive and reliable measures of function. Multidimensional functional status measures like the FIM are being used to document the effectiveness of rehabilitation treatments and to create a prospective payment system for rehabilitation

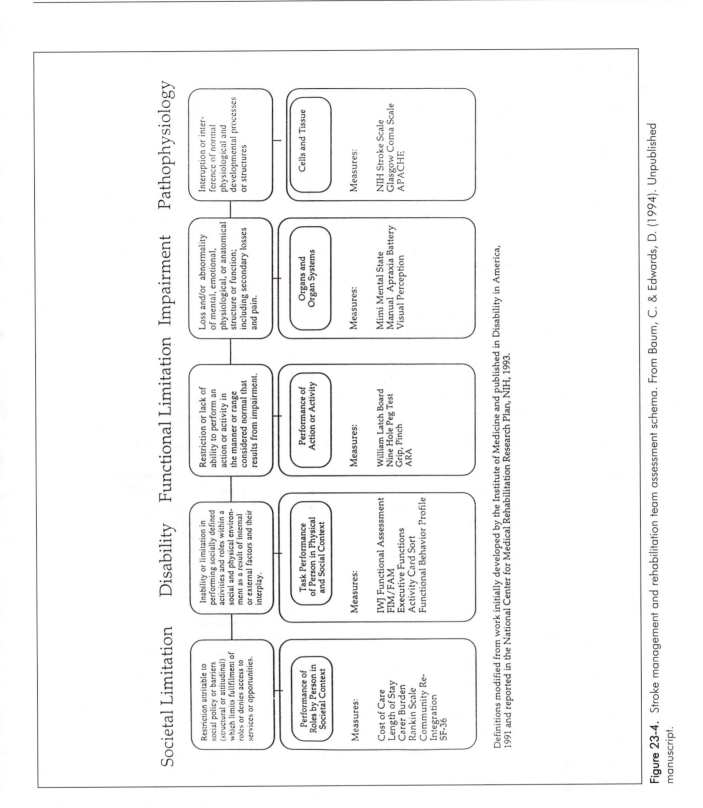

Figure 23-4. Stroke management and rehabilitation team assessment schema. From Baum, C. & Edwards, D. (1994). Unpublished manuscript.

services. Some have proposed the adoption of a single outcome measure that all therapists would use. The goal of mandating one measure is to promote the collection of standardized functional outcomes by the majority of occupational therapists. This would enable occupational therapists to conduct large-scale studies of the outcomes of occupational therapy (Velozo, 1994). As yet, that one instrument has not been chosen.

The use of standardized measures is essential for large-scale outcomes studies. It is important to identify the measure or measures which best describes the impact of occupational therapy. However, the full impact or outcome of occupational therapy is much greater than the performance of daily living tasks as measured by the FIM or other standardized functional measures.

QOL has become a primary outcome for all care. It is also becoming the predominant measure of clinical research. (Spilker, 1990). The emphasis on QOL is very important for occupational therapists. Occupational therapy is based on the assumption that QOL is achieved through occupational performance or function. According to Law and Baum, "Occupational performance reflects the individual's dynamic experience of engaging in daily occupations within the environment" (1994, p. 12).

Occupational therapists should not just be interested in measuring QOL, they should be interested in *improving* QOL through interventions that help the client engage in purposeful daily occupations that address the goals that he or she has set.

The reason that occupational therapy is moving into a major role in health care is because of our focus. By helping individuals achieve their goals, the overall outcome, QOL, should be improved. Actually, Mary Reilly was right in 1962 when she said that individuals influence their health through occupation. Now we are challenged to prove it.

STUDY QUESTIONS

1. Describe the contributions that occupational therapists can make to the evolving science of rehabilitation outcomes research.

2. Identify the types of progam evaluation used by managed care organizations. Distinguish between consumer satisfaction and quality improvement (QI)/program evaluation (PE) methods.

3. Differentiate between outcome data used to study the impact of medical treatments or public health interventions and program evaluations used to document patient function.

4. Review the historical evolution of functional indices as outcome measures. Compare and contrast the measures which emphasized physical functioning to those that assess quality of life.

5. Describe the different conceptual models of quality of life (utility, economic, psychosocial and community-centered). How do each of these models reflect the core beliefs of occupational therapy?

6. Consider Lawton's model of quality of life. How does the fit between the person and his or her environment influence each of the four components of this model?

7. What are the advantages and disadvantages of using a functional measure such as the FIM as the standard indicator of the effectiveness of occupational therapy interventions?

8. Review the similarities and differences in clinimetric and psychometric measurement strategies. Describe the strengths and limitations of each approach.

REFERENCES

American Society of Hand Therapists. (1996). *UE-NET Informational Brochure*. Chicago, IL: Author.

Baum, C. M. (1995). The contribution of occupation to function in person's with Alzheimer's disease. *Journal of Occupational Science, 2*, 55-67.

Baum, C., & Edwards, D. (1994). Stroke management and rehabilitation team assessment schema. Unpublished manuscript.

Baum, C. M., & Law, M. (1994). Occupational therapy practice. Paper presented at the Can-Am Conference, Boston, MA.

Branch, L. G., Katz, S., Kniepmann, K., & Paspidero, J. A. (1984). A prospective study of functional status among community elders. *American Journal of Public Health, 74*, 266-268.

Calman, K. C. (1984). Quality of life in cancer patients—An hypothesis. *Journal of Medical Ethics, 10*, 124-127.

CASS Principal Investigators and Their Associates. (1983). Coronary artery surgery study (CASS): A randomized trial of of coronary artery bypass surgery: Quality of life in patients randomly assigned to treatment groups. *Circulation, 68*, 951-960.

Drummond, M. F., Stoddard, G. L., & Torrance, G. W. (1987). *Methods for the economic evaluation of health care programmes*. Oxford: Oxford University Press.

Edwards, D. F., Chen, Y. W., & Diringer, M. N. (1995). The Unified Stroke Scale is reliable and valid in ischemic and hemorrhagic stroke. *Stroke, 26*, 1852-1858.

Ellenberg, D. B. (1996). Outcomes research: The history, debate and implications for the field of occupational therapy. *American Journal of Occupational Therapy, 50*, 435-441.

Feeny, D., Labelle, R., & Torrance, G. W. (1990). Integrating economic evaluations and quality of life assessments. In B. Spilker (Ed.), *Quality of life assessments in clinical trials*. New York: Raven Press.

Feeny, D., & Torrance, G. W. (1989). Incorporating utility based qualify of life assessment measures in clinical trials. *Medical*

Care, 27, S190-S204.

Feinstein, A. R. (1987). *Clinimetrics.* New Haven/London: Yale University Press.

Fisher, W. P., Harvey, R. F., Taylor, P., Kilgore, K. M., & Kelly, C. K. (1994). Rehabits: A common language for rehabilitation. *Archives of Physical Medicine and Rehabilitation, 76,* 113-122.

Gill, T. M., & Feinstein, A. R. (1994). A critical appraisal of quality of quality of life measurements. *Journal of the American Medical Association, 272,* 619-626.

Granger, C. V., Ottenbacher, K. J., Baker, J. G., & Sehgal, A. (1995). Reliability of a brief outpatient functional assessment measure. *Archives of Physical Medicine and Rehabilitation, 74,* 469-475.

Guyatt, G., Feeny, D., & Patrick, D. (1991). Issues in quality of life measurement in clinical trials. *Controlled Clinical Trials, 12,* 81S-90S.

Hamilton, B. B., Granger, C. V., Sherwin, F. S., Zielezny, M., & Tashman, J. S. (1987). A uniform national data system for medical rehabilitation. In M. J. Fuhrer (Ed.), *Rehabilitation outcomes: Analysis and measurement* (pp. 137-147). Baltimore, MD: Paul H. Brookes,.

Hurley, M. (1994). Focusing on outcomes. *RN,* 57-60.

Johnson, M. V., Wilkerson, D. L., & Maney, M. (1993). Evaluation of the quality and outcomes of medical rehabilitation programs. In DeLisa J. A. (Ed.), *Rehabilitation medicine: Principles and practice.* Philadelphia: J.B. Lippincott.

Kaplan, R. M., & Anderson, J. P. (1990). *The general health policy model: An integrated approach.* New York: Raven Press.

Katz, S., Ford, A. B., Moskowitz, R. W., Jackson, B. A., & Jaffe, M. W. (1963). Studies in illness in the aged. The index of ADL: A standardized measure of biological and psychosocial function. *Journal of the American Medical Association, 185,* 914-919.

Keith, R. A., Granger, C. V., & Hamilton, B. B. (1987). The functional independence measure: A new tool for rehabilitation. In M. G. Eisenberg & R. C. Grzesiak (Eds.), *Advances in clinical rehabilitation,* 1, New York: Springer-Verlag.

Kleinman, A. (1986). Culture, quality of life and cancer pain. In V. Ventrafriedda (Ed.), *Assessment of quality of life and cancer treatment,* Exerpta Medica International Congress Series, 702, 43-50.

Lang, N. M., & Marek, K. D. (1992). Outcomes that reflect clinical practice. In *Patient outcomes research: Examining the effectiveness of nursing practice.* Proceedings of the State of the Science Conference sponsored by the National Center for Nursing Research, September 11-13, 1991. U.S. Department of Health and Human Services, Public Health Service, National Institutes of Health, NIH publication number 93-3411, 27-38.

Lawton, M. P. (1991). A multidimensional view of quality of life in frail elders. In J. Birren (Ed.), *The concept and measurement of quality of life in frail elders* (pp. 4-23). San Diego: Academic Press.

MacNeil, B., Weischselbaum, R., & Pauker, S. (1981). Tradeoffs between quality and quality of life in laryngeal cancer. *New England Journal of Medicine, 305,* 983-987.

Mahoney, F. I., & Barthel, D. W. (1965). Functional evaluation: The Barthel Index. *Maryland State Medical Journal, 14,* 914-919.

Meier, B. (1994, Oct. 6). Rx for a system in crisis. *New York Times Sunday Magazine.*

Merbitz, C., Morris, J., & Grip, J. C. (1989) Ordinal scales and the foundation of misinference. *Archives of Physical Medicine and Rehabilitation, 70,* 308-312.

National Institutes of Health. (1993). Research Plan For the National Center For Medical Rehabilitation Research. U.S. Public Health Service Publication No. 93-3509.

Oakly, F., Sunderland, T., Hill, J. L., Phillips, S. L., Makahon, R., & Ebner, J. D. (1991). The daily activities questionnaire: A functional assessment for people with Alzheimer's disease. *Physical and Occupational Therapy in Geriatrics, 10,* 67-81.

Ottenbacher, K. J. (1995). Why rehabilitation research does not work (as well as we think it should). *Archives of Physical Medicine and Rehabilitation, 76,* 123-129.

Pope, A. M., & Tarlov, A. R. (1991). *Disability in America: Toward a national agenda for prevention.* Washington DC: National Academy Press.

Reilly, M. (1962). Occupational therapy can be one of the great ideas of 20th century medicine. *American Journal of Occupational Therapy, 16,* 87-105.

Reuter J., Klebe, E., & Cislowski, J. (1986). Health promotion and disease prevention for the elderly. Congressional Research Service Report, 36-40 EPW. Library of Congress.

Rogers, J. R., & Holm, M. (1994). Nationally speaking: Accepting the challenge of outcome research: Examining the effectiveness of occupational therapy practice. *American Journal of Occupational Therapy, 48,* 871-876.

Schipper, H., Clinch, J., & Powell, V. (1990). Definitions and conceptual issues. In B. Spilker (Ed.), *Quality of life assessments in clinical trials.* New York: Raven Press.

Slevin, M. R., Plant, H., Lynch, D., Drinkwater, J., & Gregory, W. M. (1988). Who should measure quality of life, the doctor or the patient? *British Journal of Cancer, 57,* 109-112.

Solomon, N. A., Glick, H., Russo, C. J., Lee, J., & Shulman, K. A. (1994). Patient preferences for stroke outcomes. *Stroke, 25,* 1721-1725.

Spector, W. D. (1992). Functional disability scales. In B. Spilker (Ed.), *Quality of life assessments in clinical trials.* New York: Raven Press.

Spilker, B. (1990). Introduction. In B. Spilker (Ed.), *Quality of life assessments in clinical trials.* New York: Raven Press.

Stewart, A. L., & Kamberg, C. J. (1993). Physical functioning measures. In A. L. Stewart & J. Ware (Eds.), *Measuring function and well-being: The medical outcomes study approach.* Durham, NC: Duke University Press.

Tarlov, A. R., Ware, J. E., Greenfield, S., & Hays, R. D. (1989). The medical outcomes study: An application of methods for monitoring the results of health care. *Journal of the American Medical Association, 262,* 925-930.

Thomas, R. L. (1993). The national pain data bank. *Rehabilitation Management, 6,* 117-119.

Torrance, G. W. (1986). Measurement of health state utilities for economic appraisal. *Journal of Health Economy,* 1-30.

Velozzo, C. A. (1994). Should occupational therapy choose a single functional outcome measure? *American Journal of Occupational Therapy, 48,* 946-947.

Velozzo, C. A., Megalhes, L. C., Pan, A. W., & Leiter, P. (1995). Functional scale discrimination at admission and discharge: Rasch analysis of the Levels of Rehabilitation Scale-III. *Archives of Physical Medicine and Rehabilitation, 76,* 705-712.

Verbrugge, L. M., & Jette, A. M. (1994). The disablement process. *Social Science and Medicine, 38,* 1-14.

Ware, J. E. (1995). The status of health assessment. *Annual Review of Public Health, 16,* 327-354.

Ware, J. E. (1993). Measures for a new era of health assessment. In A. L. Stewart & J. Ware (Eds.), *Measuring function and well-being: The medical outcomes study approach.* Durham, NC: Duke University Press.

Ware, J. E. (1991). Conceptualizing and measuring generic health outcomes. *Cancer, 67,* (Suppl 3), 774-779.

Ware, J. E. (1984). Conceptualizing disease impact and treatment outcomes. *Cancer, 53,* 2316-2323.

West, W. L. (1968). Professional responsibility in times of change. *American Journal of Occupational Therapy, 22,* 9-15.

Wilkerson, D. (1995). Developing outcomes management tools. *Rehabilitation Management, 8,* 114-118.

Whiteneck, C. G., Charlifue, S. W., Gerhart, K. A., Overholser, J. D., & Richardson, G. N. (1992). Quantifying handicap: A new measure for long-term rehabilitation outcomes. *Archives of Physical Medicine and Rehabilitation, 73,* 519-526.

Wood, S., & Williams, J. I. (1987). Reintegration to normal living as a proxy for quality of life. *Journal of Chronic Disease, 40,* 491-499.

Wood-Dauphinee, S. L., Opzoomer, M. A., Williams, J., Marchand, B., & Spitzer, W. O. (1988). Assessment of global function: The reintegration to normal living index. *Archives of Physical Medicine and Rehabilitation, 69,* 583-590.

World Health Organization. (1958). *The first ten years of the World Health Organization.* Geneva: Author.

Wright J. G., & Feinstein A. R. (1992) A comparative contrast of clinimetric and psychometric methods for constructing indexes and scales. *Journal of Clinical Epidemiology, 45,* 1201-1218.

Zemke, R., & Clark, F. (1996). Preface. In R. Zemke & F. Clark (Eds.), *Occupational science: The evolving discipline.* Philadelphia: F.A. Davis.

Appendix A

Uniform Terminology for Reporting Occupational Therapy Services, Third Edition

Used by permission of The American Occupational Therapy Association, Inc., Rockville, Maryland.

This is an official document of The American Occupational Therapy Association. This document is intended to provide a generic outline of the domain of concern of occupational therapy and is designed to create common terminology for the profession and to capture the essence of occupational therapy succinctly for others.It is recognized that the phenomena that constitute the profession's domain of concern can be categorized, and labeled, in a number of different ways. This document is not meant to limit those in the field, formulating theories or frames of reference, who may wish to combine or refine particular constructs. It is also not meant to limit those who would like to conceptualize the profession's domain of concern in a different manner.

INTRODUCTION

The first edition of Uniform Terminology was approved and published in 1979 (AOTA, 1979). In 1989, the Uniform Terminology for Occupational Therapy, Second Edition (AOTA, 1989) was approved and published. The second document presented an organized structure for understanding the areas of practice for the profession of occupational therapy. The document outlined two domains. PERFORMANCE AREAS (activities of daily living [ADL], work and produc-tive activities, and play or leisure) include activities that the occupational therapy practitioner (1) emphasizes when determining functional abilities. PERFORMANCE COMPONENTS (sensorimotor, cognitive, psychosocial, and psychological aspects) are the elements of performance that occupational therapists assess and, when needed, in which they intervene for improved performance.This third edition has been further expanded to reflect current practice and to incorporate contextual aspects of performance. Performance Areas, Performance Components, and Performance Contexts are the parameters of occupational therapy's domain of concern. Performance areas are broad categories of human activity that are typically part of daily life. They are activities of daily living, work and productive activities, and play or leisure activities. They are activities of daily living, work and productive activities, and play or leisure activities. Performance components are fundamental human abilities that to varying degrees and in differing combinations are required for successful engagement in performance areas.These components are sensorimotor, cognitive, psychosocial, and psychological. Performance contexts are situations or factors that influence an individual's engagement in desired and/or required performance areas. Performance contexts consist of temporal aspects (chronological age, developmental age, place in life cycle, and health status) and environmental aspects (physical, social, and cultural considerations). There is an interactive relationship among performance areas, performance components, and performance contexts. Function in performance areas is the ultimate concern of occupational therapy, with performance components considered as they relate to participation in performance areas. Performance areas and performance components are always viewed within performance contexts. Performance contexts are taken into consideration when determining function and dysfunction relative to performance areas and performance components, and in planning intervention. For example, the occupational therapist does not evaluate strength (a performance component) in isolation. Strength is considered as it affects necessary or desired tasks (performance areas). If the individual is interested in homemaking, the occupational therapy practitioner would consider the interaction of strength with homemaking tasks. Strengthening could be addressed through kitchen activities, such as cooking and putting groceries away. In some cases, the practitioner would employ an adaptive approach and recommend that the family switch from heavy stoneware to lighter weight dishes, or use lighter weight pots on the stove to enable the individual to make dinner safely without becoming fatigued or compromising safety.Occupational therapy assessment involves examining performance areas, performance components, and performance contexts. Intervention may be directed toward elements of performance areas (e.g. dressing, vocational exploration), performance components (e.g., endurance, problem solving), or the environmental aspects of performance contexts. In the last case, the physical and/or social environment may be altered or augmented to improve and/or maintain function. After identifying the performance areas the individual wishes or needs to address, the occupational therapist assesses the features of the environments in which the talks will be performed. If an individual's job requires cooking in a restaurant as opposed to leisure cooking at home, the occupational therapy practitioner faces several challenges to enable the individual's success in different environments. Therefore, the third critical aspect of performance is the performance context, the features of the environment that affect the person's ability to engage in functional activities.This document categorizes specific activities in each of the performance areas (ADL, work and productive activities, play or leisure). This categorization is based on what is considered "typical", and is not meant to imply that a particular individual characterizes personal activities in the same manner as someone else. Occupational therapy practitioners embrace individual differences, and so would document the unique pattern of the individual being served, rather than forcing the "typical" pattern on him or her and family. For example, because of experience or culture, a particular individual might think of home management as an ADL task rather than "work and produc-

tive activities" (current listing). Socialization might be considered part of play or leisure activity instead of its current listing as part of "activities of daily living", because of life experience or cultural heritage.

EXAMPLES OF USE IN PRACTICE

Uniform Terminology, Third Edition defines occupational therapy's domain of concern, which includes performance areas, performance components, and performance contexts. While this document may be used by occupational therapy practitioners in a number of different areas (e.g., practice, documentation, charge systems, education, program development, marketing, research, disability classifications, and regulations), it focuses on the use of uniform terminology in practice. This document is not intended to define specific occupational therapy interventions. Examples of how performance areas, performance components, and performance contexts translate into practice are provided below.

• An individual who is injured on the job may have the potential to return to work and productive activities, which is a performance area. In order to achieve the outcome of returning to work and productive activities, the individual may need to address specific performance components such as strength, endurance, soft tissue integrity, time management, and the physical features of performance contexts, like structures and objects in his or her environment. The occupational therapy practitioner, in collaboration with the individual and other members of the vocational team, uses planned interventions to achieve the desired outcome. These interventions may include activities such as an exercise program, body mechanics instruction, and job site modifications, all of which may be provided in a work hardening program.

• An elderly individual recovering from a cerebral vascular accident may wish to live in a community setting, which combines the performance areas of ADL with work and productive activities. In order to achieve the outcome of community living, the individual may need to address specific performance components, such as muscle tone, gross motor coordination, postural control, and self-management. It is also necessary to consider the sociocultural and physical features of performance contexts, such as support available from other persons, and adaptations of structures and objects within the environment. The occupational therapy practitioner, in cooperation with the team, utilizes planned interventions to achieve the desired outcome. Interventions may include neuromuscular facilitation, practice of object manipulation, and instruction in the use of adaptive equipment and home safety equipment. The practitioner and individual also pursue the selection and training of a personal assistant to ensure the completion of ADL tasks. These interventions may be provided in a comprehensive inpatient rehabilitation unit.

• A child with learning disabilities is required to perform educational activities within a public school setting. Engaging in educational activities is considered the performance area of work and productive activities for this child. To achieve the educational outcome of efficient and effective completion of written classroom work, the child may need to address specific performance components. These include sensory processing, perceptual skills, postural control, motor skills, and the physical features of performance contexts, such as objects (e.g., desk, chair) in the environment. In cooperation with the team, occupational therapy interventions may include activities like adapting the student's seating in the classroom to improve postural control and stability, and practicing motor control and coordination. This program could be developed by an occupational therapist and supported by school district personnel.

• The parents of an infant with cerebral palsy may ask to facilitate the child's involvement in the performance areas of activities of daily living and play. Subsequent to assessment, the therapist identifies specific performance components, such as sensory awareness and neuromuscular control. The practitioner also addresses the physical and cultural features of performance contexts. In collaboration with the parents, occupational therapy interventions may include activities such as seating and positioning for play, neuromuscular facilitation techniques to enable eating, facilitating parent skills in caring for and playing with their infant, and modifying the play space for accessibility. These interventions may be provided in a home-based occupational therapy program.

• An adult with schizophrenia may need and want to live independently in the community, which represents the performance areas of activities of daily living, work and productive activities, and leisure activities. The specific performance categories may be medication routine, functional mobility, home management, vocational exploration, play or leisure performance, and social interaction. In order to achieve the outcome of living independently, the individual may need to address specific performance components such as topographical orientation, memory, categorization, problem solving, interests, social conduct, time management, and sociocultural features of performance contexts, such as social factors (e.g., influence of family and friends) and roles. The occupational therapy practitioner, in cooperation with the team, utilizes planned interventions to achieve the desired outcome. Interventions may include activities such as training in the use of public transportation, instruction in budgeting skills, selection of and participation in social activities, and instruction in social conduct. These interventions may be provided in a community-based mental health program.

• An individual with a history of substance abuse may

need to reestablish family roles and responsibilities, which represent the performance areas of activities of daily living, work and productive activities, and leisure activities. In order to achieve the outcome of family participation, the individual may need to address the performance components of roles, values, social conduct, self-expression, coping skills, self-control, and the sociocultural features of performance contexts, such as custom, behavior, rules, and rituals. The occupational therapy practitioner, in cooperation with the team, utilizes planned intervention in achieve the desired outcomes. Interventions may include roles and values exercises, instruction in stress management techniques, identification of family roles and activities, and support to develop family leisure routines. These interventions may be provided in an inpatient acute care unit.

PERSON-ACTIVITY-ENVIRONMENT FIT

Person-activity-environment fit refers to the match among skills and abilities of the individual; the demands of the activity; and the characteristics of the physical, social, and cultural environments. It is the interaction among the performance areas, performance components, and performance contexts that is important and determines the success of the performance. When occupational therapy practitioners provide services, they attend to all of these aspects of performance and the interaction among them. They also attend to each individual's unique personal history. The personal history includes one's skills and abilities (performance components), the past performance of specific life tasks (performance areas), and experience within particular environments (performance contexts). In addition to personal history, anticipated life tasks and role demands influence performance.

When considering the person-activity-environment fit, variables such as novelty, importance, motivation, activity tolerance, and quality are salient. Situations range from those that are completely familiar, to those that are novel and have never been experienced. Both the novelty and familiarity within a situation contribute to the overall task performance. In each situation, there is an optimal level of novelty that engages the individual sufficiently and provides enough information to perform the task. When too little novelty is present, the individual may miss cues and opportunities to perform. When too much novelty is present, the individual may become confused and distracted, inhibiting effective task performance.

Humans determine that some stimuli and situations are more meaningful than others. Individuals perform tasks they deem important. It is critical to identify what the individual wants or needs to do when planning interventions. The level of motivation an individual demonstrates to perform a particular task is determined by both internal and external factors. An individual's biobehavioral state (e.g., amount of rest, arousal, tension) contributes to the potential to be responsive. The features of the social and physical environments (e.g., persons in the room, noise level) provide information that is either adequate or inadequate to produce a motivated state.

Activity tolerance is the individual's ability to sustain a purposeful activity over time. Individuals must not only select, initiate, and terminate activities, but they must also attend to a task for the needed length of time to complete the task and accomplish their goals.

The quality of performance is measured by standards generated by both the individual and others in the social and cultural environments in which the performance occurs. Quality is a continuum of expectations set within particular activities and contexts.

UNIFORM TERMINOLOGY FOR OCCUPATIONAL THERAPY—THIRD EDITION OUTLINE

I. Performance Areas

A. Activities of Daily Living
  1. Grooming
  2. Oral Hygiene
  3. Bathing/Showering
  4. Toilet Hygiene
  5. Personal Device Care
  6. Dressing
  7. Feeding and Eating
  8. Medication Routine
  9. Health Maintenance
  10. Socialization
  11. Functional Communication
  12. Functional Mobility
  13. Community Mobility
  14. Emergency Response
  15. Sexual Expression

B. Work and Productive Activities
  1. Home Management
    a. Clothing Care
    b. Cleaning
    c. Meal Preparation/Cleanup
    d. Shopping
    e. Money Management
    f. Household Maintenance
    g. Safety Procedures
  2. Care of Others
  3. Educational Activities

  4. Vocational Activities
    a. Vocational Exploration
    b. Job Acquisition
    c. Work or Job Performance
    d. Retirement Planning
    e. Volunteer Participation

C. Play or Leisure Activities
  1. Play or Leisure Exploration
  2. Play or Leisure Performance

II. Performance Components

A. Sensorimotor Component
  1. Sensory
    a. Sensory Awareness
    b. Sensory Processing
      (1) Tactile
      (2) Proprioceptive
      (3) Vestibular
      (4) Visual
      (5) Auditory
      (6) Gustatory
      (7) Olfactory
    c. Perceptual Processing
      (1) Stereognosis
      (2) Kinesthesia
      (3) Pain Response
      (4) Body Scheme
      (5) Right-Left Discrimination
      (6) Form Constancy
      (7) Position in Space
      (8) Visual-Closure
      (9) Figure Ground
      (10) Depth Perception
      (11) Spatial Relations
      (12) Topographical Orientation
  2. Neuromusculoskeletal
    a. Reflex
    b. Range of Motion
    c. Muscle Tone
    d. Strength
    e. Endurance
    f. Postural Control
    g. Postural Alignment
    h. Soft Tissue Integrity
  3. Motor
    a. Gross Coordination
    b. Crossing the Midline
    c. Laterality
    d. Bilateral Integration
    e. Motor Control
    f. Praxis

g. Fine Motor Coordination/Dexterity
h. Visual-Motor Integration
i. Oral-Motor Control

B. Cognitive Integration and Cognitive Components
1. Level of Arousal
2. Orientation
3. Recognition
4. Attention Span
5. Initiation of Activity
6. Termination of Activity
7. Memory
8. Sequencing
9. Categorization
10. Concept Formation
11. Spatial Operations
12. Problem Solving
13. Learning
14. Generalization

C. Psychosocial Skills and Psychological Components
1. Psychological
a. Values
b. Interests
c. Self-Concept

2. Social
a. Role Performance
b. Social Conduct
c. Interpersonal skills
d. Self-Expression
3. Self-Management
a. Coping Skills
b. Time Management
c. Self-Control

III. Performance Contexts

A. Temporal Aspects
1. Chronological
2. Developmental
3. Life Cycle
4. Disability Status

B. Environmental Aspects
1. Physical
2. Social
3. Cultural

Appendix B

Resources

Obtaining additional information in many areas is essential. Turning to educational institutions, libraries, and professional associations has always been a logical step. Now with the advent of the Internet and the World Wide Web, vast amounts of information have been opened up to the general public, as well as the health care professional. Listed below are some ideas of how to seek out information on:

- Resource Organizations
- Manufacturers of Technological Resources
- Adaptive Equipment and Devices

I. Educational Institutions

Colleges and universities, particularly those with multiple programs in rehabilitation, have a wealth of resources on which to draw. Whether in the department, in the library, or associations or organizations on campus, this should be the first place to turn.

II. Libraries

Whether public or academically affiliated, libraries can also provide a vast array of material, either on-site, available through inter-library loan, or on-line. Most larger libraries have numerous print or electronic indices that provide the next step for a search for answers or contacts.

III. Professional Associations

The American Occupational Therapy Association is an important resource for information. They can be reached at:

The American Occupational Therapy Association
4720 Montgomery Lane
PO Box 31220
Bethesda, MD 20824-1220
301-652-2682
Fax: 301-652-7711
www.aota.org

Other associations such as The American Physical Therapy Association and The American Speech-Language-Hearing Association, can be reached via traditional methods as well as through the World Wide Web. These associations, and many others, provide valuable information on the profession, as well as resources for the professional. If you are interested in specific manufacturers or devices, many times these association conventions provide a centralized location to meet with manufacturers and view various products.

IV. On-line Resources

The explosive growth of information on the World Wide Web is expected to continue. There are many sites that serve as search engines, or indices to the World Wide Web.

Two of many general ones are:

Yahoo
www.yahoo.com

Lycos
www.lycos.com

Two medical-related resources of value are:
Achoo: On-line Healthcare Services
www.achoo.com

Medical Matrix
www.slackinc.com/matrix/

The professional organizations listed on the previous page can be located at:

AOTA Home Page
www.aota.org

APTA Home Page
www.apta.org

American Speech-Language-Hearing Association
www2.asha.org/asha/

Finally, many sites have been created which have active links to areas of value. A selected listing includes:

Occupational Therapy Internet World
www.mother.com/~ktherapy/ot/

Occupational Therapy Talk Back
www.seagull.net/whitson/ot/talkback.htm/

Occupational Therapy Internet Links
www.iop.bpmf.ac.uk/home/trust/ot/otlinks.htm

Slack Incorporated Publishers
Occupational Therapy & Physical Therapy Internet Directory
www.slackinc.com/otpt/otpt.htm

The Hosford Muscle Tables: Skeletal Muscles of the Human Body
www.ptcentral.com/muscles/

OTPT Pages: Occupational Therapy & Physical Therapy at Puget Sound
otpt.ups.edu/

Occupational Outlook Handbook
stats.bls.gov./oco/ocos078.htm

The Occupational Therapy Journal of Research
www.slackinc.com/allied/otjr/otjrhome.htm

Community Information & Referral
www.cirs.org/

One reminder, a troubling part of on-line services is the frequency of changes of their addresses, or URLs. If the sites listed cannot be found, as a last resort enter their name in one of the search engines listed above.

Appendix C

General Guidelines for Stages of Practice

(Canadian Association of Occupational Therapists)

The following general guidelines were taken from GUIDELINES FOR THE CLIENT-CENTRED PRACTICE OF OCCUPATIONAL THERAPY.

a. Referral Guidelines

i. The therapist should receive a referral from an authorized source in accordance with the policy of the service.

ii. The therapist should determine the appropriateness of the referral and the eligibility of the individual for an occupational therapy program. This may be done in an interview or by review of records.

iii. When the referral is received the therapist should document:
   - the date of receipt;
   - referral source; and
   - the kind of services requested.

iv. If the referral is appropriate, the therapist should undertake a general assessment of the individual.

v. If the referral is inappropriate, the therapist should recommend alternatives to the referral source.

vi. The documentation should be done within a time frame that is in accordance with the policy of the service.

b. Assessment Guidelines

i. The therapist should gather data and outline the purposes of the assessment.

ii. The therapist should obtain additional relevant information regarding history, education, work records and family from the individual and family/significant others.

iii. This global assessment should include an evaluation and documentation of the individual's abilities and deficits in the following areas:
   occupational performance areas
   - self-care
   - productivity
   - leisure

   performance components
   - mental
   - physical
   - sociocultural
   - spiritual

environment
- physical
- social
- cultural

The therapist should document occupational performance and determine if more detailed and specific evaluation is required.

The therapist should ensure complete assessment either within the service or by referral to other professionals.

iv. The therapist should analyze the assessment data, formulate impressions of the presenting problem(s) and make recommendation.

v. This assessment should be documented within a defined time interval following receipt of the referral.

c. Program Planning Guidelines

i. The therapist should determine and document a program plan consistent with the assessment data and the recommendations obtained in the assessment.

ii. The program plan should be developed to include a:
- statement of measurable goals both short-term and long-term;
- selection of a theoretical approach/frame of reference appropriate to the individual's needs;
- selection of methods of intervention;
- schedule for the implementation of the plan;
- tentative discharge plan; and
- evaluation schedule

iii. The program plan goals and methods must be developed in conjunction with:
- goals of the individual and/or family;
- program plans of other professionals; and
- available resources (institutional and community).

iv. The program plan should be developed within a defined interval following completion of the assessment.

d. Intervention Guidelines

i. The therapist should implement the program according to the program plan.

ii. The therapist should document the occupational therapy services provided and the individual's progress toward the goals at a frequency recommended by the service.

iii. The therapist should regularly (or as determined by the service) reevaluate and document changes in the individual's occupational performance and the performance components of those skills.

iv. The program plan should be modified in accordance with these changes.

v. The therapist should communicate at regular intervals (or as determined by the service) with other involved professionals and family/significant others.

vi. The therapist should review and refine the discharge plan.

e. Discharge Guidelines

i. The therapist should terminate services when the individual has achieved the goals or when maximum benefit has been derived from occupational therapy services.

ii. A discharge plan should be finalized and documented.

iii. The plan should be consistent with:
- the individual's functional abilities and deficits, goals, prognosis and community resources; and
- the discharge plan of other involved professionals.

iv. Time should be allocated for the coordination and effective implementation of the plan.

v. The therapist should document a discharge summary in accordance with the policies of the service. This could include the individual's functional status, goal attainment, unmet goals, plans for ongoing services and further recommendation.

vi. The client - therapist relationship should be terminated.

f. Follow-up Guidelines

i. The therapist should reevaluate the individual at an appropriate time interval following discharge.

ii. The reevaluation results should be documented.

iii. If the individual requires further service, the therapist should refer to the service needed.

g. Program Evaluation Guidelines

i. The therapist should evaluate the effectiveness and efficiency of the program with respect to:
• adherence to the process guidelines as described above; and
• outcome - i.e., results of intervention.

From: *Occupational Therapy Guidelines for Client-centred Practice* (1991). Published by the Canadian Association of Occupational Therapists. Reprinted with permission of CAOT Publications and Health Canada.

Appendix D

Code of Ethics

(Canadian Association of Occupational Therapists)

This code of ethics has been published and distributed by the Canadian Association of Occupational Therapists to guide and assist the members in meeting and maintaining proper standards of professional conduct. The Code of Ethics shall be construed as a general guide and not a denial of the existence of other duties equally imperative and other rights not specifically mentioned.

Certain terms used in the Code require definition as follows:

"Member" means an Individual or Life Member of the Association and any person eligible for Individual Membership in the Association. "Client" means a person to whom a member renders professional services.

ARTICLE ONE

The member shall possess the qualities of integrity, loyalty, reliability and shall maintain a standard of professional competency as required by the profession, and shall at all times demonstrate behaviour which reflects the member's professional interest and attitude.

ARTICLE TWO

The welfare of the client shall be the primary concern of the member. Without limiting the generality of the foregoing, in furtherance of this goal the member shall:

a. provide service at the highest possible level of professional skill;
b. demonstrate respect for the client and appreciation of the particular need of the client;
c. respect confidentiality of all client information;
d. report to the appropriate authority any alleged unethical conduct or inappropriate practice of occupational therapy of another member.

ARTICLE THREE

A member shall recognize and accept responsibility to the relevant employing agency, to other health care colleagues, and to the community at large, and furthermore thereof shall:

a. maintain comprehensive, accurate and up-to-date records of professional activities which include the nature, extent, duration and outcome of occupational therapy intervention;
b. co-operate and maintain appropriate communication with other health care colleagues or services dealing with the client in order that the combined desired results are achieved in the treatment of that client;

c. be professionally responsible for all treatment and services rendered by the member, or by other personnel including students, who are under the direct supervision of the member;

d. respect and uphold the dignity of each individual with whom the member is associated within the profession of occupational therapy;

e. provide no misrepresentation regarding information relating to the practice of the profession of occupational therapy or regarding the provision of occupational therapy services to individual clients;

f. maintain an appropriate relationship with members of the public in order to facilitate the promotion of the goals and functions of the profession of occupational therapy;

g refrain from endorsing any goods or services related to the practice of occupational therapy without having made an objective assessment of those goods and services.

ARTICLE FOUR

The members shall endeavour to maintain and improve their professional knowledge and skill, and in this regard shall maintain a progressive attitude.

ARTICLE FIVE

The members shall recognize and accept their responsibilities to the profession and to professional organizations, and shall do everything within their means to provide for the growth and development of occupational therapy.

ARTICLE SIX

A member shall be responsible for the prompt identification and proposed resolution of conflicts of interest. If a real or potential conflict of interest arises, the member will take all reasonable steps to resolve conflict of interest by informing all parties of the need to resolve the situation in a manner that is consistent with the code of ethics.

A member shall not exploit any relationship established as a therapist to further their own physical, emotional, financial, political, or business interests at the expense of the best interest of clients. This includes, but is not limited to: soliciting clients of the member's employer for private practice; using coercion or taking advantage of trust or dependency to engage in sexual activities or to initiate/continue treatment of a client where it is ineffective, unnecessary or no longer indicated; breaching an agreement with a client or employer regarding the use of resources for provision of services; securing or accepting significant financial or material benefit for activities which are already awarded by salary or other compensation; and prejudicing others against a colleague for reasons of personal gain.

Adopted from the British Columbia Society of Occupational Therapists' Code of Ethics June 1983. Revised by the Canadian Association of Occupational Therapists, 1996. *Reprinted with permission of the Canadian Association of Occupational Therapists.*

Glossary

Abbreviation Expansion Program—software that allows a person to rapidly enter a few defined characters (abbreviation) to print out an expanded long string of characters (expansion) on a computer or communication aid. This system saves the user typing time and effort.

Absolute endurance—muscular endurance when force of contraction tested does not consider individual differences in strength.

Accessibility—the degree to which an exterior or interior environment is available for use, in relation to an individual's physical and/or psychological abilities.

Accommodation—the process whereby the organization of information within a schema must be revised or altered due to the inability to fit new information into any existing mental category.

ACSM—American College of Sports Medicine.

Active stretch—stretch produced by internal muscular force.

Activity pattern analysis—any method for determining the type, amount, and organization of activities which occupy the lives of individuals on a recurring basis.

Activity—productive action required for development, maturation, and use of sensory, motor, social psychological, and cognitive functions. Activity may be productive without yielding an object. It is also a valuable vehicle to acquire, maintain or redevelop skills necessary to fulfill occupational roles and provide satisfaction.

Activity configuration—an evaluation tool which identifies the patient's use of time, the value of one's daily activities and the changes one would like to make in time management and routines.

Acuity—the ability of the sensory organ to receive information.

Adaptation—a change a person makes in his or her response approach when that person encounters an occupational challenge. This change is implemented when the individual's customary response approaches are found inadequate for producing some degree of mastery over the challenge.

ADL—activities of daily living; the typical life tasks required for self-care and self-maintenance, such as grooming, bathing, eating, cleaning the house and doing laundry.

Aerobic metabolism—energy production utilizing oxygen.

Aerobic power—maximal oxygen consumption; the maximal volume of oxygen consumed per unit time.

Affect—the emotion conveyed in a person's face or body; the subjective experiencing of a feeling or emotion.

Affective state—the emotional or mental state of an individual, which can range from unconscious to very agitated; sometimes referred to as behavioral state.

Affordance—anything which the environment can offer the individual which is pertinent to the role challenge and can facilitate role competence. Aspects of the environment perceived by the person which combine with the person's effectancies to produce competence. Affordances are objective aspects of the environment which must be known and valued by the person. Thus, affordances have a psychological basis.

Agency—psychological term expressing the action orientation of humans.

Agonist—a muscle that resists the action of a prime mover.

Agreement, Index of—a numerical value that indicates the amount of agreement between scores assigned by two or more raters. Values usually range from 0.00 (no agreement) to 1.00 (perfect agreement).

Alarm reaction—the body's immediate response to imposed stress.

American National Standards Institute—a clearinghouse and coordinating body for voluntary standards activity on the national level.

Analog—a continuous information system; for example, a clock with dials that move continuously on a continuum (as opposed to a digital clock).

Analogical reasoning—the process of reasoning based on prior experiences.

Analogue—a contrived situation created in order to elicit specific patient behaviors and allow for their observation.

Anaphylactic shock—a condition in which the flow of blood throughout the body becomes suddenly inadequate due to dilation of the blood vessels as a result of allergic reaction.

Anosognosia—awareness; insight.

ANOVA—a statistical test for comparing groups (analysis of variance).

Anteriolateral system—this is located in the anterior (front) and side portions of the spinal cord and appears to be responsible for processing pain and temperature information.

Aphasia—the absence of cognitive language processing ability which results in deficits in speech, writing, or sign communication. Aphasia occurs most often in people suffering left hemisphere stroke.

Apraxia—inability to motor plan or execute purposeful movement.

Archetypal places—settings in the physical environment that support fundamental human functions, including taking shelter, sleeping, mating, grooming, feeding, excreting, storing, establishing territory, playing, routing, meeting, competing, and working (Spivack, 1973).

Architectural barrier—structural impediment to the approach, mobility, and functional use of an interior or exterior environment.

Arousal—an internal state of the individual characterized by increased responsiveness to environmental stimuli.

Arteriosclerosis—thickening and hardening of the arteries.

ASCII—a standardized coding scheme that uses numeric values to represent letters, numbers, symbols, etc. ASCII is an acronym for American Standard Code for Information Interchange and is widely used in coding information for computers. For example, the letter "A" is "65" in ASCII.

Assessment—a process by which data are gathered, hypotheses formulated, and decisions made for further action.

Assimilation—the expansion of data within a given category or subcategory of a schema by incorporation of new information within the existing representational structure without requiring any reorganization or modification of prior knowledge.

Assistive technology—equipment or device designed to help persons with disabilities increase functional capacities or meet the requirements of everyday living.

Atherosclerosis—deposits of fat and cholesterol in arteries.

ATP—assistive technology practitioner.

Auditory cues—sound prompts or signals which guide or facilitate behavior.

Augmentative Alternative Communication—a method or device which increases a person's ability to communicate. Examples include non-electronic devices such as communication boards, or electronic devices such as portable communication systems which allow the user to speak and print text.

Autistic—a mental disorder characterized by non-communicative, non-interactive behaviors and exclusion from reality.

Autogenic facilitation—the ability to stimulate one's own muscle to contract (muscle spindle).

Autogenic inhibition—the ability to inhibit action in one's own muscle (GTO).

Automatic processes—processes that occur without much attentional effort.

Autonomic nervous system—that part of the nervous system concerned with the control of involuntary bodily functions.

Autonomy—reflected in the ability to make choices and have control over the environment.

Avoidance—A psychological coping strategy whereby the source of stress is ignored or avoided.

Balance—the ability to maintain a functional posture through motor actions which distribute weight evenly around the body's center of gravity.

Balance of occupations—a belief, not substantiated by research, that a general configuration of daily occupations can contribute to health and well-being.

Balance of power—complementary functions of brain regions which result in well modulated behavioral responses to environmental stimuli.

Balanced muscle tone—muscle tone that is satisfactory for normal movement.

Ballistic stretch—repeated rhythmic movements at the outer limits of range of motion.

Basal ganglia—an intricate internal motor circuitry of the CNS, its primary structures are the caudate nucleus, the putamen, and the globus pallidus. The basal ganglia network is primarily responsible for initiating movement and for regulating stereotypic movements.

Basic ADL—those ADL tasks which pertain to self-care, mobility and communication.

Battery—an assessment approach or instrument with several parts.

Behavior setting, physical—location in which a standing pattern of behavior occurs irrespective of the particular inhabitants of the setting.

Behavioral assessment—a systematic and quantitative method for observing and assessing behaviors.

Behavioral setting—a milieu in which the specific environment dictates the kinds of behaviors that occur there, independent of the particular individuals who inhabit the setting at the moment.

Bilateral integration—the ability to perform purposeful movement that requires interaction between both sides of the body in a smooth and refined manner.

Biofeedback—a training program designed to enhance control of the autonomic (involuntary) nervous system by monitoring biological signals or responses and feeding them back to the individual in expanded signals.

Biomedical reasoning—the process of reasoning from a biomedical perspective. It is typically directed at identifying malfunctioning body parts and is characterized by hypothetical-deductive thinking.

Biomedical rehabilitation—a goal-oriented and time-limited process aimed at enabling an impaired person to reach an optimum mental, physical and/or social functional level (United Nations, 1983).

Biopsychological assessment—an evaluation used to determine how the central nervous system influences behavior and understand the relationship between physical state and thoughts, emotions and behavior.

Blocked practice—one task is practiced repeatedly before practicing another task.

Body image—the subjective picture people have of their physical appearance.

Body scheme—the perception of one's physical self through proprioceptive and interoceptive sensations.

Bottom-up performance component approach—approach to assessment which emphasizes a microlevel subcomponent level of analysis.

Bottom-up processing—when processing starts with the sensory signal and works up from the bottom or is "data driven."

Bradykinesia—slowed or depressed movements.

Broca's area—located in the frontal lobe, and through connections with Wernicke's area, it integrates information for expressive language.

Calman's Gap—the gap between a person's expectations and achievements.

Capacity—the immediate potential of the individual to perform tasks which support occupational performance.

Card sort—an approach to gathering information that requires the person being evaluated to consider information contained on separate index cards and to separate or sort the cards according to a specific set of instructions.

Cardiac output—the volume of blood pumped from the heart per unit of time. Cardiac output is the product of heart rate and stroke volume.

Caregiver—one who provides care and support to a person.

CARF (Commission on the Accreditation of Rehabilitation Facilities)—U.S. organization which sets standards and recognizes compliance through voluntary accreditation.

Cause and effect—when something occurs as a result of a motion or activity.

Center of gravity—the point at which the downward force created by mass and gravity is equivalent or balanced on either side of a fulcrum.

Centrifugal control—the brain's ability to regulate its own input.

Cerebellum—located just behind the brain stem and just under the occipital lobe of the cortex, it is able to orchestrate motor activity by monitoring the ongoing sensory input that contributes to the need to move, and by comparing that input with the early drafts of one's plan about moving.

Characteristic behavior—behavior typical of one's performance under everyday conditions.

Checklist—a type of assessment approach whereby a list of abilities, tasks, or interests is presented and those items meeting a designated criterion are checked. An interest checklist, for example, might list a number of activities in varied categories and ask the respondent to check those which are viewed as most interesting.

Chronobiology—the study of biological and environmental timing processes which influence daily life.

Classical conditioning—a method of eliciting specific responses through the use of stimuli that occur within a period of time that permits an association to be made between them. Also called *Pavlovian conditioning*, after the Russian scientist who made the technique famous.

Client-centered—a collaborative relationship with individuals in the client's environment (family, teachers, independent living specialists, employers, neighbors, friends) to assist the client to obtain the skills and make the modifications to remove barriers that would create a social disadvantage.

Client-centered rehabilitation—a therapeutic orientation whereby clients engage the assistance and support of a therapist to facilitate the achievement of their goals, in an environment of understanding, trust and acceptance.

Clinical reasoning—the process of ongoing, interactive reasoning related to your clinical role and interaction with clients at an individual, group, or population level.

Clinimetric measurement—an approach to measurement which attempts to document the impact of disease or disability in a global fashion with few items and multiple constructs.

Closed question—a question which asks for a specific response, e.g., one that may be answered with a "yes" or a "no."

Cocontraction—simultaneous contraction of antagonistic muscle groups which act to stabilize joints.

Cognition—mental processes which include thinking, perceiving, feeling, recognizing, remembering, problem solving, knowing, sensing, learning, judging and metacognition.

Cognitive complexity—features of an environment that affect its information-processing demands, such as variety, familiarity, pace, complexity, and responsiveness potential of stimuli.

Colles Wrist Fracture—the transverse fracture of the distal end of the radius (just above the wrist).

Commitment—the degree of importance attached to an event by an individual, based on his or her beliefs and values. The degree of commitment is an important element in motivation.

Community-based rehabilitation—a strategy with community development for the rehabilitation, equalization of opportunities and social integration of all people with disabilities. CBR is implemented through the combined efforts of people with disabilities themselves, their families and communities, and the appropriate health, education, vocational and social services (ILO/UNESCO/WHO, 1994).

Community forum—a needs assessment technique that invites residents/members of the target population to discuss their concerns at open "town hall" type meetings.

Community mental health movement—during the 1960s, government, medical and community organizations supported treatment approaches which would keep patients living in the community rather than confined in long-term hospitals.

Compensatory action of the nervous system—the action that occurs when the central nervous system attempts to respond to stimuli without the usual full complement of information.

Competence—the ability to interact effectively with the environment while maintaining individuality and growth (White, 1960). Achievement of skill equal to the demands of the environment.

Competition—rivalry for objects, for resources, facilities or position in an organization.

Comprehensive battery—a battery of tests which measure different components of cognitive functioning and perceptual and motor functioning.

Computerized assessment—an assessment which includes the administration, scoring, and interpretation of test results done by a sophisticated computer program.

Concentric contraction—a muscular contraction during which the muscle fibers shorten in an attempt to overcome resistance.

Construct—a conceptual structure used in science for thinking about the factors underlying observed phenomena.

Construct validity—in research, the extent to which a test measures the construct (mental representation) variables that it was designed to identify.

Contact oriented approach to reasoning—where a clinical problem is examined in terms of the problem, definition, and content.

Contextual modifications—cues from the therapist, task environment, and/or individual which affect task performance.

Control parameter—a critical factor or variable that will cause a change or shift in motor behavior.

Convergence—the ability of the brain to respond only after receiving input from multiple sources.

Coordination—a property of movement characterized by the smooth and harmonious action of groups of muscles working together to produce a desired motion.

Coping—the process through which individuals adjust to the stressful demands of their daily environment.

Corporal potentiality—the ability to screen out vestibular and postural information at conscious levels in order to engage the cortex in higher order cognitive tasks.

Cortically programmed movements—movements that are based on input from structure in the cortex (motor strip or basal ganglia).

Corticorubrospinal pathway—this descending pathway serves limb control, from the motor cortex through the red nucleus in the brain stem and onto the spinal cord.

Corticospinal pathway—oversees the finely tuned movements of the body by controlling finely tuned movements of the hands; this pathway travels from the motor cortex to the spinal neurons that serve the hand muscles.

Cost benefit analysis—a process used to evaluate the economic efficiency of new policies and programs by comparing an outcome and the costs required to achieve it.

Cost containment—an approach to health care which emphasizes reduced costs.

Crisis interview—an interview used to identify crisis problems and immediate interventions following an emergency.

Criterion—particular standard or level of performance of expected outcome.

Criterion validity—in measurement, a test which predicts the specific behaviors required to function in, meet the standards of, and be successful in daily life.

Cue—subjective or objective clinical data about a client.

Cultural style—collections of furnishings, objects, and decor with generally accepted cultural connotations of certain lifestyles or behavior patterns.

Culture—things that human beings learn as members of a social group.

Database—a collection of data organized in information fields in electronic format.

Decision making—the process of making decisions, i.e., the choice of certain preferred courses of action over others.

Declarative memory—memory for factual information; "knowing that."

Deductive reasoning—a serial strategy where conclusions are drawn on the basis of premises which are assumed to be true.

Defense mechanisms—unconscious processes which keep anxiety producing information out of conscious awareness. Some common examples include compensation, denial, rationalization, sublimation and projection.

Degrees of freedom—the options or directions available for movement from a given point.

Dependence—the need to be influenced, nurtured or controlled.

Dermatome—the area on the surface of the skin that is served by one spinal segment.

Deviance—a sociological term for behavior which deviates from the expected norm.

Dexterity—skill in using the hands, usually requiring both fine and gross motor coordination.

Diagnosis—the decision in which the clinician selects a particular description of the underlying cause of the client's clinical problem(s) over other alternatives.

Diagnostic hypothesis—a tentative explanation of the nature of a clinical problem or situation.

Diagnostic interview—an interview used by a professional to classify the nature of dysfunction in a person under care.

Disability—the inability or limitation in performing socially defined activities and roles expected of individuals within a social and physical environment as a result of internal or external factors and their interplay.

Disability behavior—the ways in which people respond to bodily indications and conditions that they come to view as abnormal. It includes how people monitor themselves, define and interpret symptoms, take remedial action, and use sources of help.

Disease—a deviation from the norm of measurable biological variables as defined by the biomedical system. It refers to abnormalities of structure and function in body organs and systems.

Disinhibition—the inability to suppress a lower brain center or motor behavior like a reflex, indicative of damage to higher structures of the brain.

Distractibility—the level at which competing sensory input are able to draw attention away from tasks at hand.

Distribution—refers to manner through which a drug is transported by the circulating body fluids to the sites of action.

Disuse atrophy—the wasting or degeneration of muscled tissue which occurs as a result of inactivity or immobility.

Divergence—the brain's ability to send information from one source to many parts of the central nervous system simultaneously.

Domain—specific occupational performance area; occupational performance domains are work (including education), self-care and self-maintenance, and play/leisure.

Dorsal columns—touch-pressure and proprioceptive pathways housed in the back portion of the spinal cord.

Dorsolateral fasciculus—touch-pressure and proprioceptive pathways for the lower extremities; located in the back and side portion of the spinal cord.

DRG—diagnosis related group.

Dualism—a Cartesian concept that describes two linked parts, i.e., mind and body.

Dyadic activity—an activity involving another person.

Dynamic flexibility—amount of resistance of joint(s) to motion.

Dynamic strength—the force of muscular contraction in which joint angle changes.

Dynamometer—device used to measure force produced from muscular contraction.

Dysdiadochokinesia—the inability to perform rapid alternating movements.

Dysfunctional hierarchy—the levels of dysfunction including impairment, disability and handicap.

Dysmetria—the inability to stop a movement at a desired position.

Dyssynergia—a lack of smoothness of movement due to the lack of reciprocal action in opposing muscle groups.

Eccentric contraction—a muscular contraction during which the length of muscle fibers is increased.

Ecology of Human Performance—a framework for considering the transaction among persons, tasks, and the contexts (i.e., temporal, cultural, social, and physical environments) for daily life.

Economy of effort—the idea of identifying task performance strategies which yield satisfactory results without unnecessary expenditures of time, energy or equipment.

Effectance—the sub-set of the individual's abilities pertinent to the task challenges posed by role demands.

Efficacy—having the desired influence or outcome.

Effortful processes—processes which require much attentional effort.

Ego—in psychoanalytic theory, one of three personality structures. It controls and directs one's actions after evaluating reality, monitoring one's impulses and taking into consideration one's values and moral and ethical code. The executive structure of the personality.

Electronic communication system—see Augmentative communication.

Emotion-focused coping—coping strategies that focus on managing the emotions associated with a stressful episode.

Empathy—while maintaining one's sense of self, the ability to recognize and understand the emotions and state of mind of another person.

Empirical base—knowledge based upon the observations and experience of master clinicians.

Emulator—a device which imitates the action of another; for example, a terminal emulator is a system which is not a terminal *per se*, but is designed to operate like one.

Encoding (cognitive)—those processes or strategies used to initially store information in memory.

Encoding (electronic)—technique for increasing the number of selections possible from a limited number of input options. Morse code is an example where a full alphabet is encoded to dashes and dots.

Endurance—the ability to sustain effort. A distinction should be made between cardiovascular endurance and muscular endurance.

Environment—the external social and physical conditions or factors which have the potential to influence an individual.

Environmental assessment—the process of identifying, describing and measuring factors external to the individual which can influence performance or the outcome of treatment. These can include space and associated objects, cultural influences, social relationships and systems and available resources.

Environmental contingencies—those factors in the environment that influence the patient's performance during an evaluation.

Environmental Control Unit (ECU)—a device that allows those with limited physical ability to operate other electronic devices by remote control.

Environmental (extrinsic) factors—include the cultural, economic, institutional, political, and social context from the perspective of the person.

Environmental fit—the process of matching the individual's capacities with opportunities for action in the physical, social, and cultural environments.

Environmental press—the tendency of environments to encourage or require certain types of behavior.

Epicritic sensation—the ability to localize and discern fine differences in touch, pain, and temperature.

Epigenesis—the notion that elements of each developmental stage are represented in all developmental stages.

Episodic memory—memory for personal episodes or events that have some temporal reference.

Equipment—a device which usually cannot be held in the hand and is electrical or mechanical (e.g., table or electrical saw or stove); devices can be specifically designed to assist function or compensate for absent function, or they can be labor-saving and convenience gadgets.

Ergometer—a device which can measure work done, i.e., bicycle ergometer, arm crank ergometer.

Ergometry—measurement of work.

Ergonomics—the field of study which examines and optimizes the interaction between the human worker and the non-human work environment.

Essential fat—stored body fat that is necessary for normal physiologic function and found in bone marrow, nervous system, and all body organs (also sex characteristic fat deposits in women).

Establish/restore interventions—address person variables; the therapist identifies what the person's skills and abilities are, and designs interventions to improve the person's skills.

Ethnicity—a component of culture that is derived from membership in a racial, religious, national, or linguistic group or subgroup, usually through birth.

Ethology—the systematic study of the formation of the core characteristics of being human.

Evaluation—the process of obtaining and interpreting data necessary for treatment.

Excess disability—a disability that occurs above and beyond that which should occur given the person's actual limitations. Excess disability results when the individual is not allowed to do things to retain the skills necessary to perform the tasks.

Exchange relationship—a social concept which views interaction as exchanges of value. For example, the grandfather who teaches his grandson how to fish is exchanging knowledge and experience for the company and affection that the grandson may bring to the interaction.

Exercise prescription—a scientifically based regimen of exercise provided with a particular functional goal in mind.

Exertional angina—paroxysmal thoracic pain due most often to anoxia of the myocardium precipitated by physical exertion (also called angina).

Exhaustion—depletion of energy with consequent inability to respond to stimuli.

Expertise—the possession of a large body of knowledge and procedural skill that allows the solution of most domain problems effectively and efficiently.

Explanatory model—unique mental model held by an individual about an illness episode, containing knowledge, thoughts, and feelings about etiology, timing and mode of onset of an illness, the pathophysiological process, the natural history and the severity of the illness, ethnoanatomy and ethnophysiology, and appropriate treatments and their rationale.

Explicit memory—memory which involves the conscious retrieval of information.

Explorative framework—a structure or framework developed and used to guide exploration and understanding of the problem and its boundaries.

External stimulation—factors in the area where the activity is being performed which may enhance or impede performance.

Extrinsic motivation—stimulation to achieve or perform that initiates from the environment.

Face validity—the dimension of a test by which it appears to test what it purports to test.

Factor analysis—a statistical test which examines relationships of many variables and their contribution to the total set of variables.

Fatigue—decreased ability to maintain a contraction at a given force.

Figure-ground perception—the person's ability to distinguish shapes and objects from the background in which they exist.

Flexibility—the range of motion at a joint or in a sequence of joints.

Flow—term describing the subjective quality of an experience.

Frames of reference—conceptual systems which organize applied knowledge in occupational therapy (mechanisms for linking theory to practice).

Frequency counts—the process of counting specific behaviors which occur during an identified time period.

FRG—functional related group.

Function—as used by an occupational therapist, function describes a behavior related to the performance of a task.

Functional electrical stimulation (FES)—the stimulation of nerves from surface electrodes in order to activate specific muscle groups for facilitating function.

Functional independence—ability to successfully perform the day-to-day activities expected of the person (depending on culture, age, and gender).

Functional limitations—restrictions or lack of ability to perform an action or activity in the manner or within the range considered normal that results from impairment or failure of an individual to return to the preexisting level or function. This is synonymous with occupational therapists' description of performance components.

General adaptation syndrome (GAS)—the term used by Hans Selye to describe the body's generalized response to noxious stimuli in the environment. This syndrome consists of an alarm reaction, a resistance stage, and an exhaustion stage.

Generalization—skill and performance in applying specific concepts to a variety of related solutions.

Geniculostriate system—visual system pathways that transmit information for identifying the nature of the objects in the environment.

Goal state—a predetermined situation in which problem solution is directed towards the goal.

Golgi tendon organ (GTO)—sensory receptors in the tendons of muscles which monitor tension of muscles.

Goniometer—instrument for measuring movement at a joint.

Graded activity—an activity which has been modified in one or more of a variety of ways in order to provide the appropriate therapeutic demand or challenge for a patient. The characteristics of activities useful for therapy can be graduated, or incrementally changed, so that a desired level of performance can be attained.

Graded Exercise Test—physical performance of measured, incremental workloads with measurement of physiologic response. Used to assess physiologic response to exercise stress for determination of cardiac and respiratory status.

Graphesthesia—ability to identify letters or designs on the basis of tactile input to the skin.

Gratification—the ability to receive pleasure, either immediate (immediately upon engaging in activity) or delayed (after completion of the activity).

Group—a plurality of individuals (three or more) who are in contact with one another, who take each other into account, and who are aware of some common goal.

Group roles—patterns of behavior shared by group members and necessary for the group to function and meet its goals. They are often categorized as expressive instrumental.

Gustatory—sense of taste.

Guttman scale—a specific type of behavioral measurement scale which, when scored, results in an inclusive hierarchy of performance. Items on such a scale are ordered in such a way as to ensure that if one performs a given item satisfactorily, then one must also have the ability to perform all previous items at a designated criterion level of performance.

Habits—behaviors performed at an automatic or preconscious level.

Habituate—process of accommodating to a stimulus through diminished response.

Habituation subsystem—a conceptual subsystem in the Model of Human Occupation that houses the ability to organize skills into roles and routines.

Hallucinations—to sense (e.g., see, hear, smell or touch) something that does not exist externally.

Handicap—defined by the World Health Organization as a disadvantage for a given individual, resulting from an impairment or disability, that limits or prevents the fulfillment of a role that is normal (depending on age, sex, and cultural factors) for that individual.

Handicapping situation—a barrier to the performance of an activity (a non-accessible building, an attitude discrimination, a policy that denies access).

Health—the physical, mental and social well-being of the person. Includes a focus on the individual's ability to function optimally in his or her environment.

Health education—a combination of educational, organizational, economic, and environmental supports for behavior conducive to health.

Health policy—the set of initiatives taken by government to direct resources toward promoting and maintaining the health of its citizens.

Helplessness—psychological state characterized by a sense of powerlessness or the belief that one is not capable of meeting an environmental demand competently.

HETI Model (Human-Environment-Technology model)—a conceptual framework designed to convey the relationship between human performance deficits and the use of technologies to address these deficits.

Heuristic—clinical reasoning strategies, or shortcuts, that simplify complex cognitive tasks.

History—a type of interview, either structured or unstructured, during which information about specific areas of functional performance is elicited. Historical information can be gathered directly from the patient or client or indirectly through reports of others who are familiar with one's past performance.

History-taking interview—an interview used to elicit information about the patient's medical, family, marriage, sexual and occupational histories.

Holistic—a concept in which understanding is gained by examination of all parts working as a whole.

Homonymous hemianopia—the visual field is limited to one side; usually due to optic tract damage.

Human—an organism that maintains and balances itself in the world of reality and actuality by being in active life and active use.

Human factors engineering—the engineering field which investigates and optimizes function of interactions between humans and machines.

Hydrostatic weighing—underwater weighing to determine body volume; body volume is used to determine body density, from which body composition can be calculated.

Hypermobility—a condition of excessive motion in joints.

Hyperplasia—increased number of cells.

Hypertonus—a muscular state wherein muscle tension is greater than desired, spasticity; hypertonus increases, resistance to passive stretch.

Hypertrophy—increased cell size leading to increased tissue size.

Hypothesis—a hypothesis is used as a basis for further investigation in which it may be proved or disproved. Experienced clinicians usually entertain a number of hypotheses when making clinical decisions.

Hypothetical-deductive thinking—a reasoning process that uses first principles to logically derive solutions.

Hypotonicity—a decrease in the muscle tone and stretch reflex of a muscle resulting in decreased resistance to passive stretch and hyporesponsiveness to sensory stimulation.

Hypotonus—a muscular state wherein muscle tension is lower than desired, flaccidity; hypotonus decreases resistance to passive stretch.

Hypoxia—deficiency of oxygen.

ICIDH—International Classification of Impairments, Disability, and Handicap developed by the World Health Organization.

Id—in psychoanalysis, the unconscious part of the psyche which is the source of primitive, instinctual drives and strives for self preservation and pleasure. The primary process element of personality.

Ideation—an internal process in which the nervous system gathers information from stimuli in the environment or recruits information from memory stores to formulate an idea about what to do.

Illness—the experience of devalued changes in being and in social function. It primarily encompasses personal, interpersonal, and cultural reactions to sickness.

Impairment—the loss and/or abnormality of mental, emotional, physiological, or anatomical structure or function; this term includes all losses or abnormalities, not just those attributable to the initial pathophysiology, and also includes pain as a limiting experience.

Incidence—the number of newly developed cases or events of a given illness or injury in a population during a designated time period, expressed as the number of new "cases" divided by the total number at risk (Hennekens & Buring, 1987).

Independence—having adequate resources to accomplish everyday tasks.

Independent living movement—a political movement to promote a view of disability as a socially constructed phenomenon. Independent living represents a new attitude, a new set of organizing principles, and a new approach to service delivery, aimed to ensure people with disabilities access to housing, health care, transportation, employment, education, and mobility. These aims are achieved through self-help and peer support, research and service development, and referral and advocacy.

Index individual—a person of interest in any social group; in studies of social support, the person who receives the support.

Individual Education Plan (IEP)—a legislated interdisciplinary plan required for special education students in the U.S.

Inductive reasoning—generation and testing of a hypothesis on the basis of evidence to indicate its validity.

Inference—a possible result or conclusion that could be deduced from evaluation data.

Informant interview—an interview in which the therapist gathers information about the patient or environment from significant others.

Informational support—a type of social support which informs, thereby reducing anxiety over uncertainty.

Institutionalization—the effects of dehumanizing and depersonalizing characteristics of the environment that result in apathy, a significant decrease in motivation and activity and increased passivity of an individual.

Instrumental ADL—instrumental activities of daily living; originated by Lawton to refer to those essential self-maintenance activities which are necessary for independent living that are not considered basic ADL or self-care tasks.

Insurance denial—when a third party has denied payment for a service; organizations may appeal denials if they believe the criteria have not been equitably applied.

Intake interview—an interview in which the therapist identifies the patient's needs and his or her suitability for treatment.

Integrative functional approach—approach to assessment which combines the microlevel and macrolevel of analysis.

Intelligence—the intelligence quotient is the relationship of mental age to chronological age. As commonly used, the potential or ability to acquire, retain and use experience and knowledge to reason and problem solve.

Interdependence—a concept which recognizes the mutual dependencies of individuals within social groups.

Interface—the program or device that links the way two or more pieces of equipment, or person/machine units work together. There is an interface between the computer and printer, keyboard and computer, persons and wheelchair control, etc.

Internal postural control—the ability of the body to support and control its own movement without reliance on supporting structures in the environment.

Internality—general term given for the extent to which people feel that their actions can influence their environment.

International Classification of Diseases—disease classification system developed by the World Health Organization.

Interval scales—measurement scales that include scores where there is an equal distance between each adjacent value, but there is no set zero point.

Intrinsic motivation—stimulation to achieve or perform that initiates from within oneself.

Inventory—an assessment comprised of a list of items to which the patient gives responses.

Isokinetic strength—force generated by a muscle contracting through a range of motion at a constant speed.

Isometric contraction—contraction of a muscle during which shortening or lengthening is prevented.

Isometric strength—force generated by a contraction in which there is no joint movement and minimal change in muscle length.

Isotonic contraction—contraction of a muscle during which the force of resistance remains constant throughout the range of motion.

Isotonic strength—force of contraction in which a muscle moves a constant load through a range of motion.

Judgment—the ability to use data or information to make a decision.

Key informant approach—a needs assessment technique that asks information of individuals ("key informants") who are selected for their assumed familiarity with the needs of the community as a whole or with the target population for a potential program.

Kinesthesia—a person's sense of position, weight and movement in space. The receptors for kinesthesia are located in the muscles, tendons and joints.

Labeling theory—a sociological theory which questions the medical model of psychiatric diagnosis and treatment. The theory suggests that symptoms and illness are deviations from the norm of social behavior and should not be labeled as illness.

Lateral trunk flexion—the ability to move the trunk from side to side without moving the legs, which is essential for maintaining balance.

Learning—the enduring ability of an individual to comprehend and/or competently respond to changes in information from the environment and/or from within the self. As one learns about the environment, alterations occur in the definition of the self and possible behaviors; as one learns about the self, alterations occur in the definition of the environment and possible behaviors.

Leisure—that category of occupations for which freedom of choice and enjoyment seem to be the primary motives.

Levels of processing—the durability of the memory trace is a function of the level to which the information was encoded.

Life roles—daily life experiences that occupy one's time, including roles of student, homemaker, worker (active or retired), sibling, parent, mate, son, daughter, and peer.

Lifestyle—a pattern of daily occupations over time that are stable and predictable, through which an individual expresses his or her self-identity.

Likert scale—a point system which is used to rank a particular level of skill, function or attitude.

Limbic system—a primitive system that serves arousal, emotional tone, and memory functions.

Locus of control—a psychological term referring to one's orientation to the world of events. Persons with an internal locus of control believe they can influence the outcome of events. Those with an external locus of control, conversely, believe that the outcome of events is largely a matter of fate or chance, i.e., that they cannot have influence over the outcome of events.

Long-term memory—permanent memory store for long-term information.

Long-term support system—ensuring that individuals have access to the services that are needed to support independent living.

LOS—length of stay; the duration of hospitalization, usually expressed in days.

Lower motor neuron—sensory neuron found in the anterior horn cell, nerve root or peripheral nervous system.

Managed care—in the United States, a general term which refers to any of a number of changes in the delivery of health care with the primary objective being to manage or contain costs.

Master care plan—the treatment plan, which includes the list of patient problems and identifies the treatment team's intervention strategies and responsibilities.

Mastery—the achievement of skill to a criterion level of success.

Maximal Oxygen Consumption (max VO₂, maximal oxygen uptake, aerobic capacity)—the greatest volume of oxygen used by the cells of the body per unit time.

Mean—the arithmetic average.

Meaning—the personal significance of an event as interpreted by an individual.

Meaninglessness—lack of belief in the value, usefulness or importance of daily occupations or lives.

Mechanical efficiency—the amount of external work performed in relation to the amount of energy required to perform the work.

Mechanistic view (reductionism)—supports that the mind and body should be viewed as separate and that the human being, like a machine, can be taken apart and reassembled if its structure and function are sufficiently well understood.

Medial longitudinal fasciculus (MLF)—pathway in the brain stem that connects the vestibular system with the cranial nerves that serve eye muscles (III, IV, VI).

Median—the value or score that most closely represents the middle of a range of scores.

Medicare—In the U.S., a federally funded health insurance program for the elderly, certain disabled people, and most individuals with end-stage renal disease.

Medicare Part A—In the U.S., the Hospital Insurance Program (HI) of Medicare, which covers hospital inpatient care, care in skilled nursing facilities, and home health care.

Medicare Part B—In the U.S., the Supplemental Medical Insurance Program (SMI) of Medicare, which covers hospital outpatient care, physicians' fees, home health care, comprehensive outpatient rehabilitation facility fees, and other professional services.

Memory processes—the strategies for dealing with information which are under the individual's control.

Memory structure—the unvarying physical or structural components of memory.

Mental status exam—a standardized diagnostic procedure used to evaluate intellectual, emotional, psychological and personality function.

Metabolism—the process by which the body inactivates drugs (also called biotransformation).

Metacognition—the process of thinking about one's thoughts; this allows reflection and behavioral change.

Mobility sphere—a territory within which individuals regularly travel in their daily activity patterns. Its dimensions depend on distances that the person can travel by ambulation or available modes of transportation, as well as on the accessibility features of the environment.

Mode—the value or score in a set of scores that occurs most frequently.

Monitoring—determining a patient's status on a periodic or ongoing basis.

Motivation—the inclination to act.

Motor control—the ability to move.

Motor planning—ability to organize and execute movement patterns to accomplish a task.

Motor unit—one alpha motor neuron, its axon, and all muscle fibers attached to that axon.

Multiaxial evaluation—the five axes of DSM IV which are used to establish a psychiatric diagnosis that can aid in treatment planning and predicting intervention outcome.

Multidimensional maps—the pictures of self and environment that are created within the central nervous system after receipt and analysis of multisensory input.

Muscle endurance—sustained muscular contraction, measured as repetitions of submaximal contractions (isotonic) or submaximal holding time (isometric).

Muscle spindles—sensory receptors in the tendons of muscles which monitor tension of muscles.

Muscle strength—a non-specific term relating to muscle contraction, often referring to the force generated by a single maximal isometric contraction.

Muscle tone—the amount of tension or contractibility among the motor units of a muscle; often defined as the resistance of a muscle to stretch or elongation.

MVC—maximum voluntary contraction.

Narrative—the interpretation of events through stories.

Narrative documentation—system of documentation which uses summary paragraphs to describe evaluation data and treatment progress.

Narrative reasoning—an aspect of clinical reasoning requiring understanding the "life stories" of clients.

National health insurance—a form of insurance sponsored by a national government intended to pay for health services used by its citizens.

Naturalistic observation—during an evaluation, the assessor's observation of the patient performing in his or her natural environment.

Needs assessment—systematic gathering of information about strengths, problems, resources, and barriers in a given population or community. Results of needs assessment are the basis of program planning.

Networking—a process that links people and information in order to accomplish objectives.

Neuromuscular re-education—specific treatment regimens carried out by occupational and physical therapists to improve motor strength and coordination in persons with brain or spinal cord injuries.

Neuropsychological—a specialty area of cognitive research that explores the neurological basis of behavior.

Neurosis—an emotional disorder in which reality testing is not seriously disturbed; a diagnostic category used prior to DSM III.

Nominal scales—measurement scales that contain information that is categorical and mutually exclusive, that is, it can only be contained in one category.

Normality—the range of behavior considered acceptable by a social group or culture.

Norm-referenced test—any instrument which uses the typical scores of members of a comparison group as a standard for determining individual performance.

Norms—standards of comparison derived from measuring an attribute across many individuals to determine typical score ranges.

Noticing—the act of knowing; awareness of critical issues.

Novitiate—the beginning stages or apprenticeship within a professional career.

Object relations—in psychoanalytic theory, the investment of psychic energy in objects and events in the world; sometimes seen exclusively as the bond(s) between two persons.

Objective measure—a method of assessment which is not influenced by the emotions or personal opinion of the assessor.

Obligatory reflexive response—a reflex which is consciously present in a motor pattern; this reflex may dominate all other movement components.

Observer bias—when the previous experiences of the therapist influence his or her observations and interpretation of behaviors being assessed.

Obtrusive observation—when the patient is aware of being observed by the therapist for the purpose of evaluation of cognitive, physical and/or psychosocial performance.

Occupation—engagement in activities, tasks, and roles for the purpose of productive pursuit, maintaining oneself in the environment, and for purposes of relaxation, entertainment, creativity, and celebration; activities in which people are engaged to support their roles.

Occupational adaptation (the process)—a series of actions, internal to the individual, which unfold as the individual is faced with occupational challenge. The individual engages in this process with the intention to produce a response that will result in an experience of relative mastery over the challenge.

Occupational adaptation (the state)—a state of competency toward which human beings aspire. The existence and strength of this state in an individual is a function of the extent to which occupational responses have been effective in producing relative mastery over occupational challenges and the extent to which such responses have successfully generalized to a variety of occupational challenges.

Occupational behavior—the set of responses which allow the individual to maintain role competence.

Occupational development—the systematic progression of change which occurs across the life span in response to an individual's role-based challenges.

Occupational factors—include the self-maintenance, work, home, leisure and family roles and activities of the person.

Occupational performance—accomplishment of tasks related to self-care/self-maintenance, work/education, play/leisure, and rest/relaxation; the unique term used by occupational therapy to express function as it reflects the individual's dynamic experience of engaging in daily occupations within the environment.

Occupational performance component—any subsystem that contributes to the performance of self-care/self-maintenance, work/education, play/leisure, and rest/relaxation.

Occupational science—the study of occupation.

Occupational status—a collective term encompassing occupational performance components, occupational performance, and occupational role performance.

Occupational therapy—a health discipline concerned with enabling function and well-being.

Occupational therapy diagnosis—a descriptive problem statement that succinctly describes actual or potential occupational status dysfunctions that are amenable to intervention with occupational therapy procedures and modalities.

Occupational therapy treatment process—the generalization of the steps or stages that typically occur in professional interactions with clients.

Occupations—the ordinary and familiar things that people do every day.

Olfactory—sense of smell.

On-line—a monitor linked to an off-site computer.

Open-ended question—a question which may have multiple responses rather than a definite answer.

Open system—a system of structures that functions as a whole and maintains itself by means of input from the environment and organismic change occurring as needed.

Operant—a form of conditioning in which reinforcement is contingent upon the occurrence of the desired response.

Operant conditioning—a form of conditioning in which reinforcement is contingent upon the occurrence of the desired response

Order—the desired state of affairs, which is an absence of disease in medicine and competence in the performance of work, play or self-care. Disorder is defined as disease in medicine and performance dysfunction in occupational therapy.

Ordinal scales—measurement scales that contain information that can be rank ordered.

Orthostatic hypotension—lowered blood pressure when a person changes from a horizontal to an erect position.

Osteoporosis—reduction in bone mass associated with loss of bone mineral and matrix occurring when bone resorption is greater than formation.

Outcome measure—an instrument designed to gather information on the efficacy of service programs; a means for determining if goals or objectives have been met.

Overflow—clinical term for unwanted movement in a part of the body inappropriate to the action being performed.

Oxygen consumption—the oxygen used by the mitochondria.

Parallel interventions—method of applying technology while at the same time providing therapy to maximize abilities for an individual for more powerful technology.

Parasthesia—an abnormal sensation, such as burning or prickling.

Participant-observer—a descriptor which can be applied when a therapist observes and evaluates a patient's performance while engaged in an activity with the patient.

Passive stretch—stretch applied with external force.

Pathophysiology—an interruption or interference of normal physiological and developmental processes or structures.

Patient management interview—an interview used by multiple professionals to identify the type of intervention or treatment needed.

Patient-related consultation—when the occupational therapist shares information with other professionals regarding patients who are not presently receiving occupational therapy services (AOTA, 1979, p. 6).

Patterns of help-seeking—culturally distinct ways in which people go about finding help at particular times in an illness. It refers to both the range of options (often categorized as the biomedical, popular, and traditional health sectors) and the decision-making process.

Percent body fat—percent of body weight that is fat, includes storage fat (expendable), essential fat, and sex specific fat reserve.

Perception—ability to interpret incoming sensory information.

Perceptual motor skill—the ability to integrate perceptual (sensory) input with motor output in order to accomplish purposeful activities.

Perceptual trace—memory for past movement; the internal reference of correctness.

Performance subsystem—a subsystem in the model of human occupation that includes neuromuscular skills, process skills, and communication/interaction skills.

Perseveration—continued, meaningless repetition of a specific behavior.

Person(s)—individuals who possess unique characteristics including those that are physical, emotional, and spiritual. Each individual can assume a variety of roles (such as parent, worker, and friend) simultaneously.

Person (intrinsic) factors—the neurobehavioral, cognitive, physical, and psychosocial strengths and deficits presented by the person.

Personality—the unique characteristics and traits which typify a person's behavior.

Personality trait—a distinguishing feature that reflects one's characteristic way of thinking, feeling and/or adapting.

Person-environment fit—the degree to which individuals have adapted to their unique environments.

Person-Environment-Occupational Performance Model—a model of occupational therapy practice which considers the individual, the situations or environments in which they find themselves, and their engagement in daily occupations with the objective of providing multiple options for client-centered intervention.

Physical environment—that part of the environment which can be perceived directly through the senses. The physical environment includes observable space, objects and their arrangement, light, noise, and other ambient characteristics which can be objectively determined.

Piagentian—a set of concepts and constructs ascribed to Jean Piaget, a Swiss psychologist who studied child development.

Plasticity—the ability of the central nervous system to adapt structurally or functionally in response to environmental demands.

Play—category of occupations characterized by choice, expression and development.

Policy—laws or decisions that guide one's actions, including the distribution of funds and sources.

Poor registration—when persons have difficulty registering stimuli due to high thresholds and act in accordance with those thresholds, they tend to have a dull or uninterested appearance. Their nervous systems fail to provide them with adequate activation to sustain focus on tasks or contextual cues.

Position in space—the person's awareness of the place of his or her body in space.

Post formal thought—a theoretical construct used to describe the changes noted in adolescence and adulthood that flow on from more regular cognitive development models described by people such as Piaget.

Postrotary nystagmus—reflexive movement of the eyes that occurs after quick rotational movements have ceased; used as indicator of level of processing of vestibular information.

Praxis—cognitive process by which the individual creates, organizes, and plans motor acts.

Press—the behavioral influences exerted by an environment.

Prevalence—the proportion of people who currently have a given condition, calculated as the number of existing cases of a disease divided by the total population at a given point in time.

Prevention—efforts that limit the progression of disease at any point along its course. It can be differentiated into three levels: primary, secondary, and tertiary.

Prevent intervention—occurs when therapists use their expertise to anticipate problems in the future, and design interventions to keep negative outcomes from occurring.

Primary appraisal—that part of the appraisal process in coping whereby the individual determines whether a stressful episode poses a situation of potential harm, threat, or challenge.

Primary prevention—efforts that support or protect the health and well-being of the general population.

Primatology—the study of primates.

Prime mover—that muscle with the principal responsibility for a given action. For example, the biceps brachii is the prime mover for flexing the arm at the elbow.

Principle of overload—the concept that repeated imposition of a stress above that normally experienced will produce physiologic adaptation.

Problem-focused coping—coping strategies that are directed at the source of stress itself, rather than at feelings or emotions associated with the stress.

Problem-oriented documentation—a structured system of documentation originated by Weed which has four basic components: subjective data, objective data, a problem list and a plan for treatment.

Problem-oriented process model—a conceptual model in which emphasis is on the process surrounding the problem definition.

Problem space—the boundaries or limitations that define the problem definition and guide the area of concepts that need to be considered.

Problem solving—the process which determines an appropriate course of action.

Procedural knowledge—the ability to demonstrate understanding by applying it.

Procedural memory—knowledge for the necessary procedures to perform some activity; the so-called "knowing how."

Process-oriented approach to reasoning—where a clinical problem is examined in terms of the problem solving process or talk stages.

Prognosis—a forecast or advanced indication of the course and outcome of a diagnosis.

Program evaluation—measuring the effectiveness or goal-attainment of programs.

Projective activities—ambiguous stimuli onto which an individual can project inner needs, thoughts, feelings and concerns.

Projective assessment—an evaluation approach which uses unstructured stimuli to elicit patient responses that suggest personality type, characteristics and unconscious material.

Prophylactic—preventive.

Proprioception—the ability to identify the position of the body and its parts in space, and in relation to each other.

Prospective memory—remembering to carry out some action in the future.

Protective extension response—a reflexive act consisting of extending one's arms in front of the head to protect the face and head during forward falling.

Protopathic sensation—gross sensory abilities in the extremities, allowing one to detect light moving touch, pain and temperature, but without the ability to make fine discrimination of extent.

Proxemics—study of humans' use of space.

Psychological constructs—psychological concepts; terms (without universal definitions) commonly used to describe mental states.

Psychometric interview—an interview in which a psychologist does formal psychological testing.

Psychometric techniques (tests)—methods for measuring personality, interest and attitude (frequently used in psychology).

Psychosis—a severe mental disorder causing extreme personality disorganization, loss of reality orientation and poor function in society.

Public good—general welfare or benefit to the majority or large contingent of citizens.

Purposeful activity—actions which are goal directed.

Qualitative research—methods for knowing which consider the unique properties of a natural setting without a reliance on quantitative data.

Quality improvement—evaluative processes aimed at increasing identified and desired service outcomes.

Quality of life—concept defined by an individual's perceptions of overall satisfaction with his or her living circumstances, including physical status and abilities, psychological well-being, social interactions, and economic conditions.

Random practice—tasks practiced in a mixed order.

Rates under treatment—needs assessment technique that examines data from service delivery sites such as clinics, hospitals, schools, and mental health centers to ascertain who (socio-demographically) is using what kinds of services.

Ratio scales—measurement scales that contain values that are equally distant from each other and are characterized by the presence of an absolute zero value.

Raw score—an unadjusted score derived from observations of performance; frequently, the arithmetic sum of a subject's responses.

Re-entry programs—rehabilitation programs designed to maximize independence. These programs are usually the final rehabilitation program after hospitalization and rehabilitation programs are completed. Re-entry programs are usually outpatient or community programs.

Reactivity—a characteristic of assessment instruments whereby the act of administering the assessment changes the behavior of the person being evaluated, thus distorting the representativeness of the findings.

Reality testing—the ability to know what is real and what is fantasy, usually accomplished through structured activity.

Reasoning—the use of one's ability to think and draw conclusions, motives, causes, or justifications which will form the basis of actions.

Receptive field—the receptor area served by one neuron.

Receptor—the specific site at which a drug acts through forming a chemical bond.

Reductionistic—an approach to understanding where the problem is broken into parts and the parts are viewed and managed separately.

Reflex—a subconscious, involuntary reaction to an external stimulus.

Relative endurance—muscular endurance when force of contraction tested is based on percentage of measured strength.

Relative mastery—the extent to which the person experiences the occupational response as efficient (use of time and energy), effective (production of the desired result), and satisfying to self and society.

Release phenomenon—the ongoing action of one part of the central nervous system without modulation from a complementary functional component.

Reliability—confidence that scores reflect true performance; an index of the amount of measurement error in a test.

REM (Rapid eye movement)—REM sleep is a stage of sleep thought to be important for adequate rest and health.

Repetitions maximum (RM)—maximum weight that can be lifted in isotonic contraction; one RM = maximum weight that can be lifted one time, two RM = maximum weight that can be lifted twice, etc.

Representative assembly—the policy-making body of the American Occupational Therapy Association.

Re-privatize—to return responsibility to the private sector as opposed to public responsibility.

Resistance development—adaptation which decreases physiologic response to a chronic stressor.

Resource environment—facilities available to an individual within his or her life space that may meet his or her instrumental (survival) or symbolic needs.

Responsivity—the level that the sensory input facilitates reaction or noticing.

Rest/relaxation—performance during time not devoted to other activity and during time devoted to sleep.

Reticulospinal tract—pathways that support action of the flexors and extensors of the neck for postural control.

Retrospective memory—remembering information that occurred in the past.

Retrospective recording—waiting until the evaluation is completed to record observations of patient function.

Rituals—patterns of behavior that have strong elements of symbolism attached to them.

RM (Repetition Maximum)—maximum weight that can be lifted in isotonic contraction. One RM = maximum that can be lifted one time; two RM = maximum weight that can be lifted twice, etc.

Role—a set of behaviors that have some socially agreed upon functions and for which there is an accepted code of norms.

Role competence—achievement of the behaviors which have some socially agreed-upon function and for which there is an accepted code of behavioral norms or expectations.

Routines—occupations with established sequences, such as the related sequence of tasks that characterizes personal care (bathing, dressing, grooming) at the start of the day.

RPE (Rating of Perceived Exertion)—psychophysical scale for subjective rating of exertion during work.

RTS—rehabilitation technology supplier.

Saccule—organ in the inner ear that transmits information about linear movement in relation to gravity.

Sample of behavior—selected test items chosen because they constitute a subset of the behaviors that need to be assessed.

Scanning—a technique for making selections on a device such as a communication aid, computer, or environmental control system. Scanning involves moving sequentially through a given set of choices, and making a selection when the desired position is reached. Types of scanning include automatic, manual, row-and-column, and directed.

Schema theory—the notion that standard routine performances occur in given situations in a typical sequence and with typical kinds of participants; within the general framework or structure the details of a given performance may vary but the basic structure remains consistent.

Schemata—the basic units of all knowledge. Each simple organization of experience and knowledge by the mind make up the original "schema" or framework which represents our everyday experiences. Each experience, thought and idea is a structural element in an organizational matrix which integrates each person's experiences and history into a meaningful set of categories, each filled with data from one's memory of prior events.

Schemes—structural elements of cognition.

Screening—review of a patient case to determine if occupational therapy services are necessary.

Screening instrument—an assessment device used for purposes of identifying potential problem areas for further in-depth evaluation.

Secondary conditions (also called secondary disabilities)—pathology, impairments, or functional limitations derived from the primary condition.

Secondary prevention—efforts directed at populations who are considered "at risk" by early detection of potential health problems, followed by the interventions to halt, reverse, or at least slow the progression of that condition.

Self-actualization—the process of striving to achieve one's ultimate purpose in life with accompanying feelings of accomplishment and personal growth.

Self-care activities—personal activities an individual performs to prepare for and maintain a daily routine.

Self concept—a person's view of self in relation to others and the environment.

Self-efficacy—a belief in one's ability to perform a given task successfully. It predicts the likelihood that someone will attempt a given behavior and continue working at it, despite possible difficulties, in new situations.

Self-identity—the composite, unique view of self that a person works at shaping to establish acceptance in the social community.

Self-maintenance—occupations pursued to enable participation in the social world, related to personal care and existence in the community.

Self monitoring—a process whereby the patient records specific behaviors or thoughts as they occur.

Self-report—a type of assessment approach where the patient reports on his or her level of function or performance.

Semantic compaction—a technique for reducing the number of selections a user must make to generate a phrase on a voice-output communication aid. Symbols for semantic units are used rather than number or letter codes (see Encoding).

Semantic differential—a structured approach to measuring the perceived value of objects or events, developed by Osgood.

Semantic memory—memory for general knowledge.

Semicircular canals—organ in the inner ear that transmits information about head position.

Sensation avoiding—when persons have low thresholds and develop responses to counteract their thresholds, they might appear to be resistant and unwilling to participate.

Sensation seeking—when persons have high thresholds, but develop responses to counteract their thresholds, they engage in behaviors to increase their own sensory experiences. They add movement, touch, sound, and visual stimuli to every experience.

Sensitivity—the extent to which an assessment instrument detects a disorder when it is truly present.

Sensitivity to stimuli—due to low thresholds, persons who act in accordance with those thresholds tend to seem hyperactive or distractible. They have a hard time staying on tasks to complete them or to learn from their experiences because their low neurological thresholds keep directing their attention from one stimulus to the next, whether it is part of the ongoing task or not.

Sensitization—the process of a receptor becoming more susceptible to a given stimulus.

Sensory registration—the brain's ability to receive input and select that which will receive attention and that which will be inhibited from consciousness.

Sensory integration—the ability to organize sensory information to make an adaptive response to the environment.

Sensory or body disregard—a condition characterized by lack of awareness of one side of the body.

Sensory memory—memory store which holds sensory input in its uninterpreted sensory form for a very brief period of time.

Sex identification—the assigning of a masculine or feminine connotation to a given activity.

Short-term memory—a limited capacity memory store which holds information for a brief period of time; the so-called "working memory."

Sign of behavior—patient responses which are viewed as "indirect manifestations" (or signs) of one's underlying personality.

Situation-specific—in psychosocial assessment, those behaviors and tasks which must be mastered to function every day in a particular environment.

Skin fold measurement—a method for estimating percent of body fat by measuring subcutaneous fat with skin fold calipers.

Social climate—the combined variables in the social environment that directly or indirectly influence individual behavior, and that are influenced by individual behavior.

Social disadvantage or handicap—results when an individual is not able to fulfill a role that he or she expects or is required to fill.

Social environment—those social systems or networks within which a given person operates; the collective human relationships of an individual, whether familial, community, or organizational in nature, constitute the social environment of that individual.

Social indicators—an approach to needs assessment that examines data from public records—census, county health department, police records, housing offices.

Social support—the social relatedness and interactions with others that are perceived by the individual as supplying emotional, physical, and social resources.

Social support—the experience of being cared for and loved, valued and esteemed, and able to count on others should the need arise.

Social systems—organized interactions among individuals, as within marriages, families, communities, and organizations, both formal and informal.

Socialization—the development of the individual as a social being and a participant in society that results from a continuing, changing interaction between a person and those who attempt to influence him or her.

Societal limitations—when societal policy, attitudes and actions (or lack of actions) create a physical, social or financial barrier to access health care, housing or vocational/avocational opportunities.

Software—programs that run on computers.

Somatic motor system—serves the voluntary muscles. These pathways cannot operate without sensory input and processing.

Somatotopic—the organization of cells in the somatosensory system which enables one to identify the exact skin surface touched.

Spasticity—an increase in the muscle tone and stretch reflex of a muscle resulting in increased resistance to passive stretch of the muscle, and hyper-responsivity of the muscle to sensory stimulation.

Special interest groups—collectives of individuals and organizations who are bound by beliefs about specific issues and/or populations, and who seek to influence decisions about the allocation of resources.

Specialized battery—a battery of tests which measure a more specific component of cognitive functioning, such as attention or language.

Specificity—an instrument's ability to accurately identify subjects possessing a specific trait.

Spinocerebellar tracts—pathways in the side portion of the spinal cord that transmit body position proprioceptive information to the cerebellum.

Spiritual meaning—meaning, usually symbolic, related to one's concerns with matters that transcend physical life.

Spirituality—concern with the non-material aspects of existence.

Stabilizer—any muscle that acts to fix one attachment of a prime mover or hold a bone steady to provide a foundation for movement.

Standard deviation—mathematically determined value used to derive standards scores and compare raw scores to a unit normal distribution.

Standard scores—raw scores mathematically converted to a scale that facilitates comparison.

Standardization—a method by which test scores of a typical population are derived, thus allowing subsequent test scores to be analyzed in light of that broad population; standardization requires a rigorous process of data collection and comparison.

Standardized assessment—tests and evaluation approaches with specific norms, standards and protocol.

Standardized battery—a battery of tests in which the testing and scoring procedures are well-defined and fixed and the interpretation involves the use of standardized norms.

Static flexibility—range of motion in degrees that joint(s) will allow.

Static strength—the force of muscular contraction in which there is no change in angle of involved joints.

Static stretch—holding the lengthened position without movement.

Step test—graded exercise test in which subject is required to rhythmically move up and down steps of gradually increasing height.

Stereognosis—the ability to identify common objects by touch with vision occluded.

Stereotypic behavior—repeated, persistent postures or movements, including vocalizations.

Stigma—an undesirable difference that becomes a basis for separating an individual bearing such traits from the rest of society.

Stimulus-arousal properties—the alerting potential of various sensory stimuli, generally thought to be related to their intensity, their pace, and their novelty.

Storage fat—adipose tissue found primarily subcutaneously and surround the major organs.

Strength—a nonspecific term relating to muscle contraction, often referring to the force generated by a single maximal isometric contraction.

Stress—the individual's general reaction to external demands, or stressors. Stress results in psychological as well as physiological reactions.

Stressors—external events that place demands on an individual above the ordinary.

Stroke volume—the amount of blood pumped out of the heart on each beat.

Structured activities—activities which have rules and can be broken down into manageable steps and which are preplanned and preorganized.

Sub-ASIS Bar—an orthotic bar included in seating and positioning systems placed snugly below the Anterior Superior Iliac Spine of the pelvis to maintain a forward tilt of the pelvis and better postural alignment.

Subjective measure—an assessment designed to identify the patient's own view of problems, performance, etc.

Superego—in psychoanalytic theory, one of three personality components. It houses one's values, ethics, standards and conscience.

Suppression—the ability of the central nervous system to screen out certain stimuli so that others may be attended to more carefully.

Symbolic associations—an object's broader, cultural connotations and its narrower, idiosyncratic associations for individuals or families.

Symbols—abstract representations of perceived reality.

Sympathetic nervous system—that part of the autonomic nervous system that mobilizes the body's resources during stressful situations.

Synergist—any muscle that functions to inhibit extraneous action from a muscle that would interfere with the action of prime mover.

Tacit—implied understanding that isn't verbalized.

Taxonomy—a system of naming and differentiating objects or phenomena.

Technology transfer—the process by which knowledge is applied.

Temporal environment—the manner in which social and cultural expectations influence behavior by organizing the time during which activities occur and the amount of time devoted to them.

Tenodesis splint—orthosis fabricated to allow pinch and grasp movements through use of wrist extensors in substitution for finger flexors.

Tensiometer—device use to measure force produced from an isometric contraction.

Tertiary prevention—efforts that attempt to maximize function and minimize the detrimental effects of illness or injury.

Test protocol—the specific procedures that must be followed when assessing a patient; formal testing procedures.

Test sensitivity—an instrument's ability to detect change in a variable being measured.

Theories—the products of the scientific disciplines, whose task it is to explain natural phenomena.

Third party payment—payment for health (or other) services by someone other than the person receiving them.

Thought disorder—disturbance in thinking, including distorted content (ideas, beliefs and sensory interpretation) and distorted written and spoken language (e.g., word salad, loose associations, echolalia).

Threat minimization—a psychological coping strategy whereby emotions are managed through "playing down" the importance or significance of a stressor.

Threshold—the point at which a stimulus characteristic is identified.

Time-related measures—an assessment in which the patient records the thoughts, feelings and/or behaviors which occur during a specific time period; time sampling and duration are included.

Tolerance—the psychological and physiological accommodation or adaptation to a chemical agent over time.

Tone—state of muscle contraction determined by resistance to stretch.

Tone (tonus)—the status or condition of muscle as characterized by resistance to stretch.

Tonotopic—the organization of cells within the auditory system which enables one to identify the exact sound heard.

Top-down functional approach—approach to assessment which emphasizes a macrolevel functional level of analysis.

Top-down processing—when processing starts with higher order stored knowledge and depends upon contextual information or is "conceptually driven."

Topographic—the organization of cells in the visual system which enables one to identify the exact location and features of the stimulus.

Transaction—implies a dynamic situation in which individuals alter their performance based on their perceptions of changing conditions in the environment.

Transfer appropriate processing—the concept that the cognitive processes used while learning determine the type of criterial task on which one will best perform when evaluated for what has been learned.

Transparent access—complete emulation usable with all or an entire major class of software. For example, a successful keyboard emulating interface provides transparent access to standard software using alternate keyboards.

Tunnel vision—the visual field is limited to one side; the peripheral fields are lost, usually due to damage to the optic chiasm.

Type A behavior—a cluster of personality traits that includes high achievement motivation, drive, and a fast paced lifestyle.

Unconscious proprioceptive pathways—pathways in the side portion of the spinal cord that transmit body position information to the cerebellum.

Universal access design—concept of designing the built environment to permit access regardless of physical or sensory capability.

Unobtrusive observation—observation for assessment which minimizes reactivity.

Unstructured activities—activities which are not preplanned or broken down into steps.

Upper motor neuron—neurons of the cerebral cortex that conduct stimuli from the motor cortex of the brain to motor nuclei of cerebral nerves of the ventral gray columns of the spinal cord.

Utricle—organ in the inner ear that transmits information about linear movement in relation to gravity.

Validity—the degree to which a test measures what it is intended to measure.

Values—beliefs and interpretive statements that influence choice, conduct and meaning.

Vestibular—sense of one's orientation in space.

Vestibulo-ocular—pathways that support coordination of head and eye movements.

Vestibulospinal tracts—pathways that support action of the flexors and extensors of the neck for postural control.

Visual cues—visual signs or indicators which guide or facilitate behavior.

Visual neglect—inattention to visual stimuli occurring in the space on the involved side of the body.

Visual orientation—awareness and location of objects in the environment and their relationship to each other and to oneself.

Visual perception—the brain's ability to understand sensory input to determine size, shape, distance and form of objects.

Volitional subsystem—a subsystem in the model of human occupation that includes one's values, interests, and feelings of personal causation.

Weight shift—bearing the body's weight from one leg to another; shifting the center of gravity.

Well-being—a subjective sense of overall contentment, thought to be defined by affective state and life satisfaction.

Well-defined problem—a situation in which most parameters are known and there is consensus about an optimum solution.

Wernicke's area—located at the intersection of the parietal, occipital, and temporal lobes, and processes information to enable the brain to interpret language. In the left hemisphere, Wernicke's area processes speech communication, while in the right hemisphere, the area processes information to interpret nonverbal communication.

WHO—World Health Organization.

Word prediction—technique used in software to guess the current word or next word when beginning letters or the previous word, respectively, is typed.

Work—a category of occupation in which an individual engages for the primary purpose of subsistence.

Work/education—skill and performance in purposeful and productive activities in the home, in employment, in school, and in the community.

Work setting—any environment in which an individual performs productive activity.

Work space—the physical area in which one performs work.

Index of Assessments

Index